D1243220

Management
of Head and Neck
Cancer

Edited by

Rodney R. Million

M.D.

American Cancer Society Ashbel C. Williams,
    M.D., Memorial Professor of Clinical
    Oncology, and
Chief, Division of Radiation Therapy
University of Florida College of Medicine
Gainesville, Florida

Nicholas J. Cassisi

D.D.S., M.D.

Professor and Chief
Division of Otolaryngology
University of Florida College of Medicine
Gainesville, Florida

19 CONTRIBUTORS

Management of Head and Neck Cancer A Multidisciplinary Approach

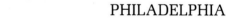
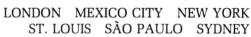

J. B. Lippincott Company

PHILADELPHIA

LONDON   MEXICO CITY   NEW YORK
ST. LOUIS   SÃO PAULO   SYDNEY

The authors and publisher have exerted every effort to ensure that drug selection and dosage set forth in this text are in accord with current recommendations and practice at the time of publication. However, in view of ongoing research, changes in government regulations, and the constant flow of information relating to drug therapy and drug reactions, the reader is urged to check the package insert for each drug for any change in indications and dosage and for added warnings and precautions. This is particularly important when the recommended agent is a new or infrequently employed drug.

Sponsoring Editor: Richard Winters
Manuscript Editor: Lee Henderson
Indexer: Sandra King
Art Director: Maria S. Karkucinski
Designer: Patrick Turner

Production Supervisor: N. Carol Kerr
Production Assistant: S. M. Gassaway
Compositor: TAPSCO, Inc.
Printer/Binder: The Murray Printing Company

3 5 6 4 2

Library of Congress Cataloging in Publication Data
Main entry under title:

Management of head and neck cancer.

  Bibliography: p.
  Includes index.
  1. Head—Cancer—Treatment. 2. Neck—Cancer—Treatment. I. Million, Rodney R. II. Cassisi, Nicholas J. [DNLM: 1. Head and neck neoplasms—Therapy. WE 707 M2665]
  RC280.H4M26 1984   616.99'49106   83-7975
  ISBN 0-397-50619-8

This text is dedicated to our mentors, Gilbert H. Fletcher, M.D., and Joseph H. Ogura, M.D., who have contributed so much to the understanding and management of head and neck cancer, as well as giving us an excellent start.

R.R.M.
N.J.C.

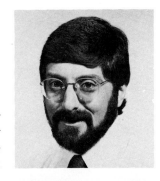

Assistant Professor
Division of Radiation Therapy
University of Florida College of Medicine
Gainesville, Florida   **Francis J. Bova, Ph.D.**

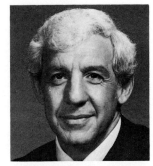

Professor and Chief
Division of Otolaryngology
University of Florida College of Medicine
Gainesville, Florida   **Nicholas J. Cassisi, D.D.S., M.D.**

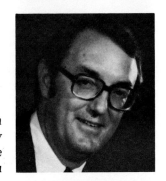

Professor and Chairman
Department of Surgery
University of Florida College of Medicine
Gainesville, Florida   **Edward M. Copeland III, M.D.**

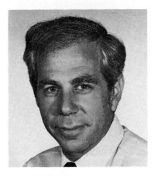

Speech Pathologist
Department of Audiology and Speech
Pathology
Gainesville Veterans Administration
Hospital
Gainesville, Florida   **Lewis P. Goldstein, Ph.D.**

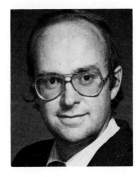

Associate Professor
Department of Radiology
University of Florida College of Medicine
Gainesville, Florida   **Derek J. Hamlin, M.D.**

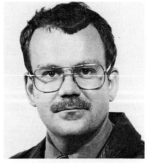

*Associate Professor of Radiology
University of Toronto, and
Staff Radiation Oncologist
Princess Margaret Hospital
Toronto, Ontario*

**Andrew R. Harwood, M.B., Ch.B.,
F.R.C.P.(C)**

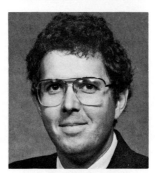

*Assistant Professor
Division of Otolaryngology
University of Florida College of Medicine
Gainesville, Florida*

John H. Isaacs, Jr., M.D.

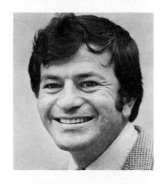

*Assistant Professor
Department of Removable Prosthodontics
University of Florida College of Dentistry
Gainesville, Florida*

Alan C. Levin, D.D.S.

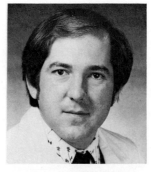

*Assistant Professor
Division of Radiation Therapy
University of Florida College of Medicine
Gainesville, Florida*

Robert B. Marcus, Jr., M.D.

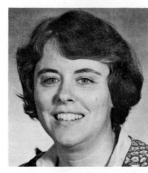

*Editorial Assistant
Division of Radiation Therapy
University of Florida College of Medicine
Gainesville, Florida*

Patricia J. McCarty

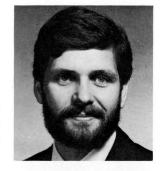

Assistant Professor
Division of Radiation Therapy
University of Florida College of Medicine
Gainesville, Florida   **William M. Mendenhall, M.D.**

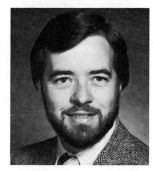

Associate Professor
Division of Otolaryngology
University of Florida College of Medicine
Gainesville, Florida   **Gerald E. Merwin, M.D.**

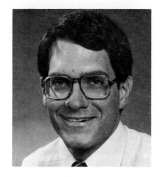

American Cancer Society
Ashbel C. Williams, M.D., Memorial
Professor of Clinical Oncology, and
Chief, Division of Radiation Therapy
University of Florida College of Medicine
Gainesville, Florida   **Rodney R. Million, M.D.**

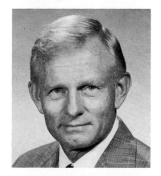

Assistant Professor
Division of Radiation Therapy
University of Florida College of Medicine
Gainesville, Florida   **James T. Parsons, M.D.**

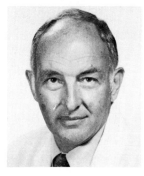

Professor
Department of Surgery
University of Florida College of Medicine
Gainesville, Florida   **William W. Pfaff, M.D.**

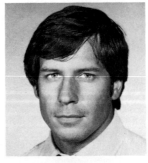

Associate Professor
Division of Medical Oncology
University of Florida College of Medicine
Gainesville, Florida   **Warren E. Ross, M.D.**

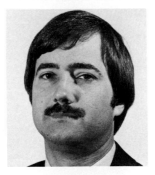

Assistant Professor
Department of Surgery
University of Florida College of Medicine
Gainesville, Florida   **Thomas O. Rumley, M.D.**

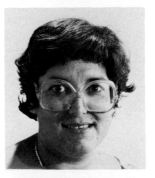

Collections Manager
Division of Radiation Therapy
University of Florida College of Medicine
Gainesville, Florida   **Marguerite C. Sigal, M.Ed.**

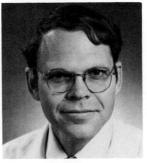

Associate Professor
Division of Radiation Therapy
University of Florida College of Medicine
Gainesville, Florida   **Timothy L. Thar, M.D.**

Management of Head and Neck Cancer: A Multidisciplinary Approach is a result of 10 years of close cooperation between the authors in the management of head and neck neoplasms at the University of Florida. Lip service is often given to cooperative multidisciplinary cancer management, but for us it is a reality.

This text represents our current philosophy in the management of head and neck tumors. We recognize that there are many successful treatment alternatives in the management of head and neck cancer and do not argue that our approach is the only one or the best. Treatment results are reviewed yearly to determine areas that need change or refinement. To base treatment recommendations on the last "success" or "failure" is irrational. We have outlined our usual treatment recommendations in the various chapters, but we never hesitate to individualize recommendations based on the specific problem. After all, there are approximately 35 different anatomical sites in the head and neck. Each site may present with a myriad of clinical situations and each patient with different personal requirements. It is clearly impossible to cover every clinical situation in the text, and therefore the physician must remain flexible and innovative to individualize where needed.

Our general approach to the management of the neck is presented once, in Chapter 4, General Principles for Treatment of Cancers in the Head and Neck: Selection of Treatment for the Primary Site and for the Neck ("Management of the Neck"); special situations are considered in the individual chapters.

Space is allocated preferentially to radiation therapy over surgery, since there are other texts emphasizing the surgeon's viewpoint and surgical technique. This should not be construed to mean that we fail to recognize the importance of operation, but rather to highlight the possible uses and advantages of radiation therapy.

Rodney R. Million, M.D.
Nicholas J. Cassisi, D.D.S., M.D.

Acknowledgments

It was decided from the outset to obtain independent reviews of each chapter to detect errors of commission or omission. Robert D. Lindberg, M.D., was the primary editorial consultant and completed the reviews in his usual meticulous and knowledgeable fashion.

Additional thanks for editorial review go to Gilbert H. Fletcher, M.D., and H. Rodney Withers, M.D., Ph.D., for review of Chapter 13, Time–Dose–Volume Relationships in Radiation Therapy, and Chapter 14, The Effect of Radiation on Normal Tissues of the Head and Neck; Helmuth Goepfert, M.D., and Oscar M. Guillamondegui, M.D., F.A.C.S., for review of Chapter 28, Major Salivary Gland Tumors; Helmuth Goepfert, M.D., for review of Chapter 19, Larynx, and Chapter 32, Carcinoma of the Thyroid; K. Kendall Pierson, M.D., for review of Chapter 26, Carcinoma of the Skin, and Chapter 27, Melanoma of the Head and Neck; Dempsey S. Springfield, M.D., and William F. Enneking, M.D., for review of Chapter 34, Adult Mesenchymal Tumors Presenting in the Head and Neck; William F. Hanafee, M.D., for assistance on the radiology sections; Glenn E. Sheline, Ph.D., M.D., for review of Chapter 32, Carcinoma of the Thyroid; and Thomas Ervin, M.D., for review of Chapter 8, General Principles for Treatment of Cancers in the Head and Neck: Chemotherapy.

Carla J. Lenkey served as medical illustrator for most of the figures and anatomical displays.

A. W. Peter van Nostrand, M.D., F.R.C.P.(C), permitted us to use his excellent whole-organ sections of the larynx, pyriform sinus, and nasopharynx.

Professor Ugo Fisch generously allowed us to reproduce the cervical lymphangiograms from his book *Lymphography of the Cervical Lymphatics.*

William R. Panje, M.D., F.A.C.S., supplied the original photographs of five midface skin cancers.

Karl Storz GmbH and Co., Tuttlingen, West Germany, generously supported the publication of the color photographs in Chapter 3, Examination With Fiberoptic Equipment, and Chapter 19, Larynx.

William C. Calton and the entire staff of the Learning Resources Center, University of Florida, spent endless hours producing photographs and figures suitable for publication.

Denise Hair, Carlton Thompson, and Jane Rogers spent many hours performing the endless administrative tasks associated with a first edition.

Patricia J. McCarty and Diane E. Dreves, editorial assistants, did yeoman work in preparing the manuscript; the text would have been impossible without them.

Contents

Management
of Head and Neck
Cancer

History of Diagnosis and Treatment of Cancer in the Head and Neck

PATRICIA J. McCARTY
RODNEY R. MILLION

HEAD AND NECK CANCER IN EARLY PEOPLES

Treatment of Head and Neck Cancer by Primitive Peoples

The history of the earliest treatment of cancer is obscure. To make conclusions about early primitive populations based on observations of later primitive populations is risky. The findings described below can only suggest possibilities about ancient practices.

In a review of surgery practiced by primitive peoples, Ackerknecht theorized that their failure to develop surgical therapy was due mostly to the widespread magical beliefs about the causation of disease. Primitive peoples would use sophisticated techniques for ritual mutilation or punishment without applying these same techniques in situations in which they might have saved lives.

Ackerknecht called the Masai of East Africa the "primitive master surgeons."[6] They and some of their East African neighbors performed many kinds of operations with iron knives, using thorns for sutures and tendons to suture vessels to stop bleeding. Surgeons formed a separate occupational class and operated on people and animals. Some of the head and neck procedures carried out in primitive Africa included scarification of inflamed tonsils, enucleation of eyes, excision of neck glands in cases of trypanosomiasis, cauterization of neck tumors, and removal of the uvula.

The natives of one Polynesian island were reported to operate successfully on lipomas, tuberculous neck glands, and old ulcers, using only shark teeth as scalpels.[6]

In America, the pottery of the ancient Peruvians shows numerous instances of mutilated noses and lips, but these may have resulted from disease processes rather than surgical operations. If the mutilations were deliberately inflicted, the purpose was more likely punitive or religious rather than medical, although surgical treatment of nose or lip cancer could have produced this appearance.[6]

Paleopathologic Evidence for Head and Neck Cancers

The "Kanam mandible," a fossilized mandibular fragment found in East Africa by Leakey, was deformed by an irregular lesion that was "fairly extensive, extending onto the lingual and labial surfaces of the jaw in the region of the symphysis."[19,86] This fossil probably dates back to the Middle Pleistocene (more than 500,000 years ago), making this the oldest known instance of a tumor in a human species. It was interpreted as an osteogenic sarcoma by Lawrence, but others interpreted it as a reaction to trauma.[85,128]

Benign neoplasms, both primary osteoma and bony reactions to meningioma, hemangioma, fibroma, or nasal polyps, have been described in ancient skulls. One benign neoplasm destroyed most of the nasal bones, the left inner orbit, and the left maxilla and much of the palate in a young adult male in neolithic Denmark; it may have been a juvenile angiofibroma.[19] Some disseminated lesions—either widespread metastases or multiple myelomas—have also been reported.[19,162]

1

TABLE 1-1. Paleopathologic Evidence for Primary Carcinoma and Ameloblastoma in the Head and Neck in Ancient and Medieval Peoples

Geographic Location	Era	Age/Sex	Probable Primary Site	Description of Bone Destruction
1. Tepe Hissar, Iran	3500–3000 B.C.	Adult man	?	Extensive destruction of the left facial bones (maxilla, palatine, and zygoma) and the floor of the left orbit; obliteration of the left maxillary sinus; penetration of the floor of the left nasal fossa, extending to the right of the midline; all of the left upper teeth and right central incisor missing
2. Egypt	Old Kingdom, III–V Dynasty, 2686–2345 B.C.	30–35-yr-old man	Maxillary sinus and palate	Destruction of the left maxillo-alveolar regions, part of the palate, the medial and lateral pterygoid plates, and part of the inferior concha; 26 secondary lesions scattered over the skull
3. Northwest of Naga-ed-Dêr, Upper Egypt	VI–XII Dynasty, 2345–1786 B.C.	35–45-yr-old woman	Nasopharynx most likely; possibly nasal cavity, oral cavity, or pharynx	Greater part of the facial skeleton and the sphenoid region of the skull base destroyed; center of the tumor (if growth was symmetrical) in the epipharynx to the right of midline; also a small separate honeycomb area on the squamous part of the right temporal bone
4. Southern part of Egyptian Nubia	New Kingdom, 1567–1085 B.C.	Elderly woman	?	Erosion of the base of the skull affected the left half of the sphenoid bone; also, there were other lesions on top of the vault, including a frontal perforation
5. Nubia	A.D. 300–600	Man	Nasopharynx or sphenoid sinus	Massive destruction from the cribriform plate back nearly to the foramen magnum, and destruction of almost all of the sphenoid bone, the nasal turbinates and vomer, and the posterior part of the palate
6. El-Barsha, Menya province, Upper Egypt	A.D. 500 ± 100	30–35-yr-old man	Nasopharynx or maxillary sinus	Erosion from the pterygoid fossa into the maxillary sinus (piece of linen cloth in ear)
7. Baselland, Switzerland	"Frühmittelalter" period (early Middle Ages)		Ethmoid sinus or skin	Destruction of part of the frontal region: the right upper orbital margin and the nasal bones to the left of the upper orbital margin
8. Caen, France	A.D. 1100–1200	Man <40 yr old	Maxillary antrum	60-mm × 40-mm tumor of the right maxilla, extending up to the orbit and down to the nasal orifice; a rectangular hole in the zygomatic bone; all maxillary teeth missing
9. Czersk, Poland	A.D. 1000–1300	40–50-yr-old man	Mandible	Expansile lesion of the middle segment of the right side of the mandible; ameloblastoma by gross appearance and x-ray

Very few ancient skulls have been reported to show evidence of primary head and neck carcinoma. Table 1-1 includes nine such cases, two of which may show evidence of therapeutic efforts. In case 6, from upper Egypt in the Early Christian era, a tumor (possibly nasopharyngeal) had eroded through the pterygoid fossa into the maxillary sinus. A piece of linen cloth was found in the right external auditory meatus, indicating, possibly, that therapy had been performed for severe pain or discharge.[50] In case 8, a skull found in the ossuary of a 12th-century French castle revealed that a huge maxillary tumor had invaded the orbit and nose. A rectangular hole had been cut in the man's zygomatic bone an appreciable time before his death, judging by the healing that had taken place in the bone, which may represent an effort to relieve excruciating pain.[41]

The evidence for tumors in ancient skulls is frequently debatable, for trauma, infection, and postmortem damage can result in similar bony changes. There is also argument about the incidence of head and neck cancer in the ancient past. Since few people lived beyond 50 years of age, there was not a large population in the most cancer-prone age-group. There may actually have been a relatively high incidence of nasal, nasopharyngeal, or paranasal sinus cancers in some ancient populations. Wells, for instance, discussed the possible relationship of inhalation of wood smoke or peat smoke to the occurrence of sinusitis and sinus cancer in people who lived in poorly ventilated huts.[164] He found a 6.8% incidence of changes resulting from severe sinusitis in a series of Anglo-Saxon skulls.

Head and Neck Cancer in Ancient Civilizations

The oldest medical documents, on Egyptian papyri, describe tumor treatment. The Edwin Smith papyrus, a surgical treatise written about 1600 B.C. or earlier, mentions what is probably breast cancer, but no head and neck tumors. The Ebers papyrus, written about 1500 B.C. or earlier, describes medical rather than surgical treatment; it is essentially a collection of drug recipes with a fragmentary description of the diseases they are intended to treat.[26] Among the diseases mentioned are an "eating ulcer of the gums" and an "illness of the tongue," descriptions too vague to allow us to decide whether the lesions were neoplastic.[31]

The ancient Greek physicians definitely recognized cancer, especially breast cancer. Around 400 B.C., Hippocrates referred to what was probably tongue cancer in his *Prorheticon* when he described chronic ulcers of the edge of the tongue, which he said were common and related to the presence of sharp teeth rubbing against the tongue.[105] Hippocrates also reported that "a man who had a carcinoma in his pharynx and was cauterized by us got well."[99]

The Greco-Roman physician Asklepiades is credited with the use of tracheotomy, probably for diphtheria, around 50 B.C.[103] He rejected the Hippocratic doctrine of the four humors and was the founder of the Methodist school of medicine in Rome.

About A.D. 30, Celsus compiled an encyclopedia of the Roman medical knowledge of his time. He described cancer treatment in this way: "Some physicians used caustic remedies. Some cauterized, and others operated with the knife. The remedies, however, never did any good to anybody."[137] Nevertheless, he described an operation for cancer of the lip and, probably, plastic repair of the lip after removal of the tumor.[68] He also wrote about necrotic ulcers that caused foul breath, which were treated with cauterization. He advised splitting the nostril if necessary to treat ulcers in the nose and then suturing the nostril. Such ulcers, he said, would heal slowly.[110] These ulcers must have had a variety of causes; if they were malignant, it is unlikely that they would have healed. Celsus also mentioned many other head and neck procedures, such as uvulotomy, nasal polypectomy, and an operation for removal of goiter. He wrote that hardened tonsils might be scratched out with a fingernail or hooked up and dissected out.[110] He also described the wiring of loose teeth and the use of a dental mirror.[138]

Local drug therapy during Celsus's time included the use of metallic salts (copper and lead), sulfur, and arsenic pastes. Such remedies were commonly used on ulcers of any type and were therefore applied to malignant ulcers as well.[137] The arsenic paste, which was used into the 20th century, might actually have had some true antineoplastic effect.

By the time of Galen (A.D. 129–199), the humoralists were ascendant, and Galen's great synthesis and forceful

---

◄ *Note: Case 1:* Skull no. 33-23-36 from Hissar II. Reported (with photograph) by Krogman, who thought destruction was due to "inflammatory condition," perhaps secondary to "sinus infection brought about by dental disease."[83] Wells called it "a naso-pharyngeal lesion."[163] Brothwell said destruction "could well be the result of carcinoma."[19] According to Ho, "There was no description of destruction of bone in the immediate vicinity of the nasopharynx. There are, therefore, no grounds to interpret from these findings that the primary condition could be nasopharyngeal carcinoma."[71]

Case 2: Skull no. 236, Duckworth Laboratory, Cambridge, England. Reported by Wells, who examined the skull by x-ray and transillumination.[161] Also pictured in Brothwell, Ho, and Wells.[19,71,164] Ho examined the skull and thought that the primary site was probably the maxillary alveolus or the floor of the maxillary sinus, rather than the nasopharynx, and that the most likely diagnosis, especially in view of the secondary lesions in the cranial vault, should be multiple myeloma.

Case 3: Skull no. 12-5046, tomb 217, cemetery 100, Lowie Museum of Anthropology, Berkeley, California. Reported with photographs by Strouhal.[145]

Case 4: From Grave no. 204/15. Batrawi called the lesion an "unexplained erosion of the base of the skull."[13] Judging by pictures in Batrawi's report, Brothwell thought it should be reexamined as a possible neoplasm.[19]

Case 5: X-group skeleton no. 188B. Derry described destruction in detail.[44] Elliott Smith and Dawson said the lesion was suggestive of "epithelioma of the naso-pharynx."[48] The lesion was pictured by Brothwell.[19] Ho said that the "site and appearance of the destruction are consistent with a diagnosis of either carcinoma of the sphenoid sinus or nasopharyngeal carcinoma."[71]

Case 6: Skull no. 58. Reported by El-Rakhawy and co-workers and described by Strouhal.[50,145]

Case 7: Skull D. 10, Kantonsmuseum, Liestal. Described as postmortem erosion by Hug.[74] Brothwell studied the skull and believed the destruction was caused by a destructive tumor in the region of the frontal sinuses.[19]

Case 8: Ossuary under Chapelle Saint-Georges inside Château de Caen. Reported with photographs by Dastugue.[41]

Case 9: From a medieval burial ground; only the mandible was preserved. Reported with photographs by Gladykowska–Rzeczycka.[62]

development of the humoral theory made it the basis for medical practice for some 1500 years. In this theory, cancer was supposed to be the result of overproduction of "black bile" and its local thickening or concentration, which was particularly likely to occur on the face, lips, or breast.[97] Because the local lesion was thought to be a manifestation of systemic disease, local treatment such as surgery was discouraged. Unsuccessful surgical treatment would have supported the theory.

Galen, an accomplished surgeon, gave the following instructions for cancer operations: "If you attempt to cure cancer by surgery, begin by cleaning out the melancholic tumor by cathartics" (i.e., first treat the systemic disease). "Make accurate incisions surrounding the whole tumor so as not to leave a single root. Let the blood flow and do not check it at once, but make pressure on the surrounding veins, so as to squeeze out the thick blood. Then treat as other wounds."[99] He advocated the use of cautery, both to achieve hemostasis and to destroy any remnants of cancer.[118] He also described the surgical removal of a goiter and of nasal polyps, and uvulectomy was apparently a very common operation, performed for a variety of conditions.[159] In passing, Galen mentioned a hard tumor of the tongue, which he said he would discuss in a later book; unfortunately, the later book has been lost.[105]

Galen was also an experimental physiologist and anatomist. He demonstrated the function of the recurrent laryngeal nerve, proving the connection of the vocal cords to the brain. He cut the nerve in a pig (in an attempt to determine whether the nerve had any effect on respiration) and was surprised to find that, although it continued breathing, the pig could no longer squeal. He repeated the experiment in dogs, goats, and monkeys with similar results, and he described accidental severance of the nerve in patients during goiter operations, which rendered them mute also.[159]

Galen also described accurately the anatomy of the throat: the thyroid, cricoid, and arytenoid cartilages and the epiglottis; their ligaments; the muscles of the larynx and nearby structures; and the tensing and stretching of the vocal cords.[159]

The only other ancient medical writings having any pertinence to the modern Western treatment of cancer are the works of the ancient Indian physicians, especially the legendary Sushruta. In his work he combined the system of hygiene, preventive medicine, and a healthful regimen of living taught by the high-caste Brahmin physicians with the practical techniques of the surgeons, who had previously been illiterate and of low caste. Sushruta described the removal of tumors. He sutured wounds with flax, sinews, or hair, using a variety of needles. In his writings he listed 101 blunt and 20 sharp surgical instruments. Cauterization and methods of hemostasis were described, and anesthesia was produced by alcoholic drinks.[157]

The early Indian surgeons developed great skill in plastic surgery, partly because the ears and nose were frequently amputated as a punishment, even for minor infractions, and partly because defects often occurred as a result of the constant warfare. Sushruta described in detail his method of reconstructing a missing nose:

> First the leaf of a creeper, long and broad enough to cover fully the whole of the severed or clipped off part, should be gathered; and a patch of living flesh, equal in dimension to the preceding leaf, should be sliced off (from down upward) from the region of the cheek and, after scarifying it with a

knife, swiftly adhered to the severed nose. Then the cool-headed physician should steadily tie it up with a bandage decent to look at and perfectly suited to the end for which it has been employed. The physician should make sure that the adhesion of the severed parts has been fully effected and then insert two small pipes into the nostrils to facilitate respiration, and to prevent the adhesioned flesh from hanging down.[146]

The wound was then treated with powders, bandaged in cotton, and sprinkled with sesame oil. The patient was given clarified butter to drink, was anointed with oil, and was treated with purgatives after his meals were digested. When the donor site was healed, the nose could also be considered healed. If adhesion was incomplete, the area could again be scarified and bandaged together. Also, the surgeon could attempt to elongate or shorten the new nose if its length was not quite right. Sushrata also described reconstruction of severed lips and earlobes.[168]

MEDIEVAL AND RENAISSANCE CANCER TREATMENT

The very early medical writings, although fragmentary and often obscure in meaning, were the basis of Western medicine until sometime after 1600. As the Roman empire disintegrated, Byzantine and later Arab physicians inherited the Egyptian, Greek, and Roman medical treatises and preserved them, with occasional personal additions, through the centuries. These medieval writers mentioned cancer only occasionally, and they mentioned cancer of the head and neck area, usually of the tongue or lips, even less often.

Probably the greatest Byzantine medical writer was Paul of Aegina (7th century). His work is primarily a compilation of earlier writings, but he was himself a practicing surgeon, and he occasionally inserted information from his own experience. His works were translated into Arabic, and with other similar Byzantine works they formed the basis of Arabic medicine. He advocated bleeding, cauterization, and open treatment of surgical wounds. In his discussion of tracheotomy, he quoted Antyllus, a great Roman surgeon (circa A.D. 150) whose works are otherwise lost:

> Wherefore, bending the patient's head backwards, so as to bring the windpipe better into view, we are to make a transverse incision between two of the rings, so as that it may not be the cartilage which is divided, but the membrane connecting the cartilages. If one be more timid in operating, one may first stretch the skin with a hook and divide it, and then, removing the vessels aside, if they come in the way, make the incision.

He then continued:

> We judge that the windpipe has been opened from the air rushing through it with a whizzing noise, and from the voice being lost. After the urgency of the suffocation has passed over, we pare the lips of the incision so as to make them raw surfaces again, and then have recourse to sutures, but sew the skin only, without the cartilage.

Paul also discussed neck dissection for scrofulous (but not for carcinomatous) neck nodes.[119]

The 10th-century Spanish Muslim physician Albucasis, (Abu'l-Quasim) of Córdoba, wrote the only medieval Arabic textbook of surgery. Most of his book was taken from Paul of Aegina, but he inserted some case histories from his own practice. He depended heavily on Galen. Albucasis said that cancer "should not be attacked with a sharp instrument, at least not when it is so fixed in an organ that it cannot be radically excised," and he advocated cauterization for cancer excision and hemostasis.[20,168]

Avenzoer (Ibn Zuhr), of 11th-century Córdoba, was the only Muslim physician actually to advance the knowledge of cancer through his descriptions of cancer of the stomach and esophagus. He diagnosed and treated cancer of the esophagus with sounds or dilators made of silver or tin.[68]

This garbled collection of translations of ancient texts and later additions was then translated again—this time from Arabic into Latin. Other medical texts were preserved by the Byzantines. Both Arabic and Byzantine medical texts were available to physicians at Salerno (in southern Italy), which by the late 11th century had become a center of medical knowledge, particularly of practical surgical knowledge.[104] In his *Surgery*, compiled in 1170, Master Roger of Salerno taught that cancer should be completely excised by knife or cautery, if possible, or that it should be otherwise treated with caustic ointments. If located close to major nerves or arteries, it was best left alone. Scrofulous neck nodes were excised if they were very enlarged, but apparently cancerous nodes were not.* Goiter was treated first with a drug that contained ashes of sponge and seaweed (both containing iodine), but if this treatment failed, the goiter was removed surgically.[36] Roger gave an illustration of the special forceps he used for uvulotomy, which apparently was still a common operation, and in an early effort at producing surgical anesthesia, the Salernitan surgeons described the use of the "soporific sponge," which was soaked in the juice of hyoscyamus and poppy.[36,125]

In the 1500s the work of the first of the modern anatomists began, with Italy as the center of activity. It was at this time, for example, that the anatomy of the ear—the eustachian tube, tympanic membrane, and semicircular canals—was elucidated. The cerebral vessels and cranial nerves were described, as were the larynx and the musculature of the pharynx and palate. The great anatomists were practicing surgeons as well. Fallopius (Gabriele Fallopio), for instance, devised a polyp snare, "a steel wire looped inside a tube through which it could be drawn, thus cutting off the polyp."[110] Perhaps the most renowned Italian surgeon–anatomist was Fabricius of Acquapendente (Gerolamo Fabrizio). Among his surgical achievements were the attempt to improve the technique for tracheotomy, the development of a silver cannula for feeding through the nose, and the invention of an angulated scissors for the extraction of polyps. His surgical works, one section of which was entitled "Tumors," were reprinted every few years until 1729.[22,94]

Plastic surgery was badly needed during the 1500s to replace missing or mutilated lips, ears, palates, and, particularly, noses. There was a virulent epidemic of syphilis, warfare resulted in blade and arrow wounds, and punitive mutilation was widely practiced—Pope Sextus V (1521–1590), for example, ordered the amputation of the nose as a punishment for theft. The most famous 16th-century plastic surgeon was Gaspare Tagliacozzi of Bologna, although he probably derived his techniques from other Italian surgeons, such as the contemporary Vianeo family of Calabria, Aranzio of Bologna, the Sicilian Brancas (father and son) from the previous century, and others. The elder Branca used flaps of skin from a patient's face to form a nose (the Indian method). His son used the skin of the patient's arm and extended the method to repair lips and ears as well. Most of these early practitioners guarded their methods as family secrets, but Tagliacozzi of Bologna, whatever the origin of his techniques, publicized his work and found his services in great demand. He published a book detailing his methods in 1597, complete with illustrations (Fig. 1-1). For restoration of the nose or lip, he cut a flap from the anterior surface of the arm and applied it to the appropriate area. The arm was then held in place by a sort of sling until the flap adhered to the face. To replace a missing ear, he used sliding flaps, taking a section from the parieto-occipital region to form the upper part of the ear and a section from the upper triangle of the neck to form the lobe.[21] Tagliacozzi's success was not approved of by the religious authorities of the day, who thought it derived from the Devil. After his death, nuns were said to have heard a voice at night saying that Tagliacozzi was damned, and his remains were removed from consecrated ground. Restorative surgery was not practiced again for some 200 years.[21,94,104,138]

Another approach used at this time was to construct a prosthesis to replace missing parts. The Danish astronomer Tycho Brahe lost most of the bridge of his nose in a duel in 1566 and replaced it with a prosthesis made of a copper–silver alloy, painted to match his skin and glued in place. He was a nobleman, wealthy and vain of appearance, and he would undoubtedly have sought surgical repair of the defect had such been available.[8,89]

In the mid–16th century Amatus Lusitanus published an account of his method of replacing a part of the palate that had been destroyed by syphilis:

> I ordered a goldsmith to prepare a golden-headed nail; the head of the nail was round and broad enough to close the total circumference of the foramen, whereas the tip of the nail was narrow and round; in its center an ear, lentil-shaped, was prominent. To the said tip, or spike, of the nail a small sponge was fitted, and this the patient had to introduce at the same time into the foramen where it expanded with moisture and so remained fixed in position. Thereby he was able to speak correctly as if nothing ailed him.[90]

Ambroise Paré, a 16th-century French surgeon, was ingenious in devising prostheses for the soldiers who were mutilated by war, which by his time included the use of gunpowder. He published illustrations of artificial eyes, noses, and ears that he had devised (Fig. 1-2), and he even made an artificial tongue, which was attached by a string to the patient's neck.[117,127] He apparently applied these methods to cancer patients also. He wrote of the "erosion or eating of a pestulent carbuncle or ulcerated cancer so that the teeth may be seen to lie bare with great deformity," and he said that "If the loss or consumption of lip be not very great it may be repaired by that way I have described

---

* Hayes Martin noted that "Up until the latter part of the 19th century, most cervical lymphadenopathies were grouped under the general term 'scrofula,' especially if they were associated with 'eruptions' of the skin or oral mucous membranes. Under such conditions, it is obvious that errors in diagnosis would be likely to occur in the cases of oral cancer in which cervical lymphadenopathy appeared as the first or as one of the early symptoms."[105]

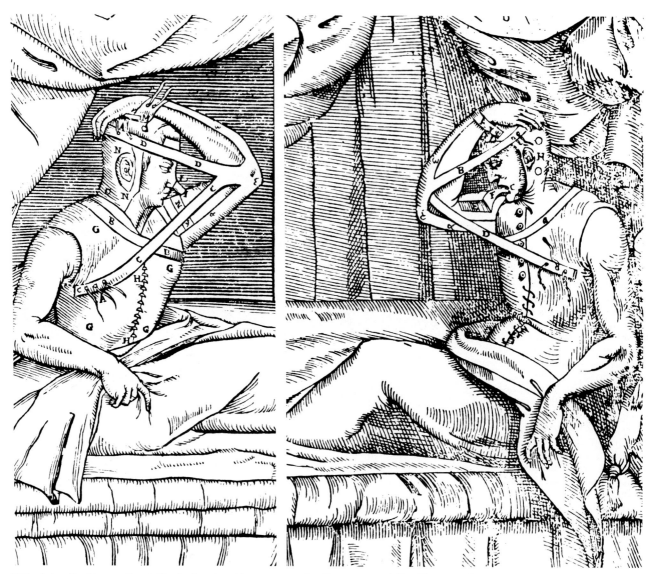

FIG. 1-1.   Tagliacozzi's method of restorative surgery for the nose and lip, illustrated in his *De Curtorum Chirurgia per Insitionem* (1597). (*Left*) Rhinoplasty. (*Right*) Lower lip restoration. (*Left* from Margotta R: The Story of Medicine, p. 180. Verona, Arnoldo Mondadori, Editore, 1968. *Right* from Singer C, Underwood EA: A Short History of Medicine, 2nd ed, p 99. New York, Oxford University Press, 1962)

in the cure of hare lips or ulcerated cancer, but if it be great, then there must be a tip of gold made for it."[127]

One of Paré's case reports describes his operation for lip cancer in a 50-year-old man:

> Pass a threaded needle through the cancer so the thread held in the left hand can lift and control the cancer without any of it escaping. One can then cut to good flesh with scissors in the right hand; and cut so that a layer of good flesh of the lip remains to serve as a base and foundation for regeneration of flesh in place of the portion amputated, supposing the cancer has not taken root and spread from top to bottom. This done, having let enough blood flow from within and without, at the right and left of the amputation, make deep enough incisions with the razor so that later, when one would draw together and unite the edges of the wound, as in the case of harelip, the flesh would be more obedient to the thread and needle.[69]

The greatest of the German surgeons of the time was Fabricius Hildanus (Wilhelm Fabry of Hilden, near Düsseldorf, who practiced in Germany and in Berne). In his *Century of Surgical Cases* he described a number of cases of cancer in which he carried out extensive operations.[68] His cases of head and neck cancer (or tumor) included the removal in 1605 of a "fleshy excrescence" from the external ear canal of a 19-year-old girl who had a 10-year history of otorrhea and deafness but no pain. He placed ligatures, which he tightened daily with special forceps of his own design, around the pedicle of the tumor. On the seventh day of treatment the tumor came away, and the root was cauterized twice daily for 2 days. Eight years later, the patient was still well.[80]

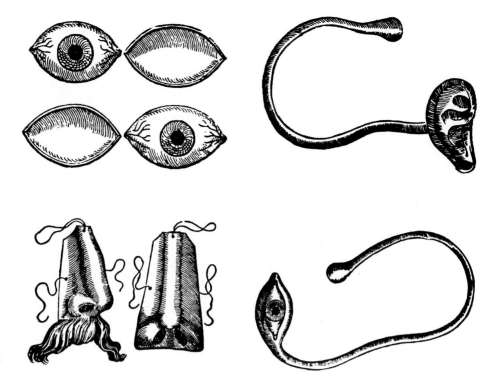

FIG. 1-2. Examples of prostheses devised by Paré, from *Of the Means and Manner to Repair or Supply the Natural or Accidental Defects or Wants in Man's Bodie.* (Roberts AC: Facial reconstruction by prosthetic means. Br J Oral Surg 4:157–182, 1966)

Like Paré, Fabricius invented surgical instruments and devised prostheses. For example, he invented an instrument for blowing styptic powder onto an enlarged uvula: a tube, bent at one end, with a small copper spoon attached at that end for holding the powder and a leather bag attached at the other end for an insufflator. He invented a complicated instrument for removal of nasal polyps, and he improved a tube used to remove foreign bodies from the pharynx. He also described a successful palatal obturator.[80]

Paré and Fabricius Hildanus were practical men rather than scholars—barber–surgeons rather than university physicians. They both realized the importance of the study of anatomy, the area of great medical breakthroughs in their time. Galen's humoral theory still held sway in more scholarly circles and offered little basis for any kind of realistic cancer treatment.

THE DEVELOPMENT OF PRESENT-DAY CANCER OPERATIONS

In the late 18th century Paris became the center of the medical world. The Parisian physicians discarded much of the humoralist system in favor of "localism," the idea that disease, including cancer, might have a local rather than systemic origin and could therefore be treated in its early stages. This provided a theoretical basis for the development of cancer surgery. The Parisian physicians were strong believers in postmortem dissections and developed the study of gross pathology. In keeping with the 18th-century penchant for classifying, they began to sort out cancer from other kinds of growths and ulcers and even to recognize different kinds of cancer. Parisian medicine was almost totally clinical in its orientation, however, and resisted the new areas of microscopy, experimental physiology, and medicinal chemistry. The Germans were not so conservative, though, and they were able in their uni-versities to combine the best of the Parisian emphasis on physical examination, statistics, and macroscopic pathologic anatomy with the new equipment (such as the achromatic microscope) and experimental methods. Germany thus became the new center of the medical world, particularly for surgery, in the 19th century.[5]

In the mid-19th century anesthesia and antisepsis were developed, both of which were crucial for the development of modern surgery. First was anesthesia, the use of which began in the 1850s. It made patients more willing to undergo operations and enabled them to lie quietly while the surgeon did careful, methodical work. The great advances in operative technique began with this innovation, and the beginnings of all the modern, complex operations for head and neck cancer can be traced to this era.[110] Then, beginning in the 1870s, antibacterial methods began to be adopted—first antisepsis for a brief time, then asepsis. As a result, a patient who survived an operation was less likely to die of infection.

Along with the development of anesthesia and antisepsis, a third necessity for effective cancer therapy was the development of microscopic pathology. The 19th-century technical revolution in this field was described by Long:

> In the first decades of the 19th century, men were cutting slices of fresh tissue by hand and examining them under the microscope. At the close of the century, they were hardening tissues in appropriate fluids, embedding them in rigid materials to facilitate cutting, slicing them with machinery into incredibly thin sections, and coloring them with combination stains which sharply contrasted the varying cellular elements.[97]

John Hughes Bennett, a surgeon, lectured on histology at Edinburgh University beginning in 1841 and included microscopic demonstrations of morbid histology. Hughes Bennett published a book about cancer in 1849 that included for the first time both clinical case histories and microscopic descriptions of tumors.[68] His description of the relationship of clinical medicine and microscopic pathology has a very modern ring: "It is not the recognition, by means of the microscope, of certain cells and fibers, which will enable us to assert with certainty the existence of Cancer; but that their detection in particular places, and accompanying peculiar forms of growth, permits us to do so."[75]

The great systematizer of microscopic pathology was Rudolf Virchow. In his greatest work, *Cellular Pathology* (1858), Virchow asserted that all cells arose from preexisting cells but that sometimes normal cells could transform into malignant ones.[97] He believed that the malignant cells were localized to one area in the beginning. As Ackerknecht has said, "The whole emphasis with Virchow was on local causes, local beginnings of tumors."[4] This concept encouraged the use of surgery at the earliest stage of the disease. Virchow thought that metastases were caused by a chemical produced by tumors rather than by transported tumor cells, and he thought that carcinoma arose from connective rather than epithelial tissue (although he was less sure of this later in his life, after Thiersch, Waldeyer, and others had demonstrated otherwise).[4]

The great surgeons of the late 19th century operated with increasing confidence and ingenuity. In the time of Paré and Fabricius Hildanus, surgery was a distasteful profession on the borderline of reputable medical practice, but by the late 19th century, surgery had become the main focus of advancing medical science. This was the start of the current age of cancer therapy.

Oral Cancer

In the Middle Ages, the oral tongue was often cut, torn, or burned off as a punishment for heresy or *lese majesty* or to prevent the telling of secrets. According to Hayes Martin, the tongue was drawn from the mouth, usually by a sharp hook, and the protruding portion was cut off from below.[105] Many of the victims survived, especially after it was found that the use of a red-hot knife resulted in less bleeding. Some of the victims had enough tongue musculature remaining to enable them to speak. These reports must have encouraged surgeons in their first efforts to treat tongue cancer and the other serious afflictions of the tongue that were probably even more common in those days, such as gangrene, syphilis, or congenital macroglossia. Some of the patients recovered, but even those who survived the operation itself frequently died later of infection. Several early operations for tumors of the tongue were reported. In 1664, Pietro de Marchetti of Padua, who was also known for the resection of ulcers or cancers of the lip and gingiva, cut and burned away a hard tumor "the size of a hazel nut" from the underside of the tongue. In 1676, the English surgeon Richard Wiseman described two cases of fungating oral cancer in his *Chirurgical Treatise*. He cauterized the tumors, but both patients had neck node metastases and died of their disease shortly thereafter.[3,25,107]

In the 18th century, there were scattered reports of operations for tongue tumors by German, English, Italian, and French surgeons. Their techniques varied: some used a knife, some used scissors. Sometimes the affected portion of the tongue was tied off with ligatures. Some surgeons had an assistant hold the patient's tongue with a piece of linen, others used forceps. They controlled bleeding through cautery or the application of ice or a caustic.[25]

The major proponent of glossectomy at this time was the French surgeon Antoine Louis, who in 1759 improved operative hemostasis by ligating the vessels that supplied the involved portion of the tongue prior to the operation.[3]

In the late 1700s Benjamin Bell described operations for tongue, lip, and buccal cancers in his book, *A System of Surgery*. This Edinburgh surgeon wrote that "cancers, in very few instances, perhaps none, ever arise from a general affection of the system; but, on the contrary, are, at their first appearance, almost always local."[15] He reported that while "cancers occasionally occur in every part of the body," the "under lip is more frequently attacked with cancer than any other part of the body." He blamed most treatment failures on delay in performing an operation. Some of Bell's precepts for treating cancer have held up amazingly well for 200 years. He advised using a scalpel rather than caustics or pastes, saying that the surgeon should "extirpate every part that is diseased," including any part adherent to the tumor, if possible: "Even every indurated gland in the neighborhood of a cancerous sore, should just as certainly be taken away as the ulcer itself; for if allowed to remain, a return of the disease may with certainty be looked for." If it was not possible to extirpate all the disease, he thought the operation should not be performed at all—for instance, when the cancer had spread to other parts of the body, or when it was adherent to the trachea or a large artery. He concluded, "Whatever the risk may be, however, if the diseased parts can be all removed, the operation should certainly be advised. For as we know of no other remedy upon which any dependence can be placed for the cure of cancer it is surely better to submit to some risk than to be left to certain misery and death."[15]

Bell found that lip cancer and cheek cancer could be treated effectively by excision, but that when excision was done in the usual way, "by removing the diseased parts only, and allowing them to heal without drawing them together," the cosmetic and functional result was very poor. For cancers extending over the entire lip, no repair was possible after the cancer was removed, but he advocated that, whenever possible, the lip should be repaired by the method he used for harelip (Fig. 1-3). Bell found that by using this method he could remove up to half of the lower lip and still achieve a good functional result and minimal deformity. The same method of repair was advised for buccal cancer, for which his excision began and ended at the angle of the mouth, circling around the lesion. The surgeon was then to bring the sides of the cut "neatly together" and pin, which according to Bell produced very good results.[15]

Bell allowed that excision of much of the tongue was "a very formidable operation" during which the "symptom of hazard" was the "very sudden discharge of blood." He advised the use of ligatures, which he said could be used more often and at greater depth in the mouth than was commonly thought. Cautery was a last resort. Bell advised that not every surgeon should attempt operations on the tongue, because they required "that steady, deliberate coolness, which a natural firmness of nerves, conjoined with much experience, alone can give."[15]

Well into the 19th century, the method of strangulating the affected area with ligatures was used in cases of tongue cancer (Fig. 1-4). Patients may have been less afraid of this method than of being cut by a knife, but the method was painful and the danger of hemorrhage and infection was very great while the tied-off portion was sloughing. Another treatment method involved the use of caustics. As Butlin and Spencer described in 1900, "The tongue was drawn out, stabs made round the growth, and into the punctures arrowhead-like pieces of chloride of zinc were inserted."[25]

In 1819 Conrad J. M. Langenbeck applied wedge resection, an operation already in use for cancers of the lower lip, to the tongue. He used sutures to achieve hemostasis. This is considered to have been the first modern, systematic, scalpel excision of tongue cancer.[25,105]

In 1831 Michael Jaeger was the first to divide the cheek in order to remove a tongue cancer. The patient survived the operation, and the wound healed.[25]

In 1838 Giorgio Regnoli of Pisa removed a patient's tongue through a T-shaped submental incision (a "pull-through" operation; Fig. 1-5). The patient was a 14-year-old girl who had some sort of tumor the size of a hen's egg occupying most of her tongue. He drew the tongue down through the incision, encircled the tongue entirely with ligatures proximal to the tumor, and cut off all parts of the tongue beyond the ligatures with scissors, using cautery as needed. The stump was returned to the mouth; the external wound was left partly open for drainage. The wound was completely healed in 6 weeks, and the patient was able to swallow and to speak with the hypertrophied stump.[25,34]

Philibert Roux reported the case of a 35-year-old man who had had a tumor of the tongue for 5 months. It began as an ulcer and was attributed to smoking. By the time of the operation in 1839 it occupied the entire left half of the patient's tongue. Roux commenced the operation by tying the left lingual artery. He freed the tongue from the floor of mouth, the lower jaw, and the anterior tonsillar pillar and then used a bistoury (a long, narrow knife) from underneath to remove the entire left half of the tongue (*i.e.*, he performed a hemiglossectomy). There was no hemor-

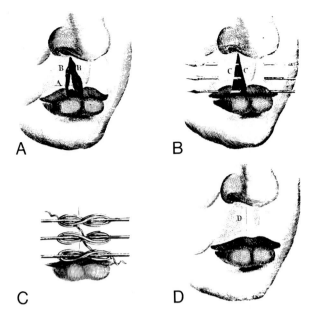

FIG. 1-3. Benjamin Bell's method for repair of harelip, which he also recommended for use after excision of lip and cheek cancers. (*A*) Appearance of the defect prior to repair. (*B*) After cut and insertion of pins. Bell wrote "Edges of cut ought to be smooth, equal, and exactly of the same length on each side, so that when drawn together, no inequality may be perceptible." The pins were made of gold with removable steel points that were taken off after the ligatures were applied. (*C*) Appearance immediately after the completion of the operation. (*D*) Final result. (Bell B: A System of Surgery, 6th ed, vol 5, plate XLIV. Edinburgh, Bell and Bradfute, 1796)

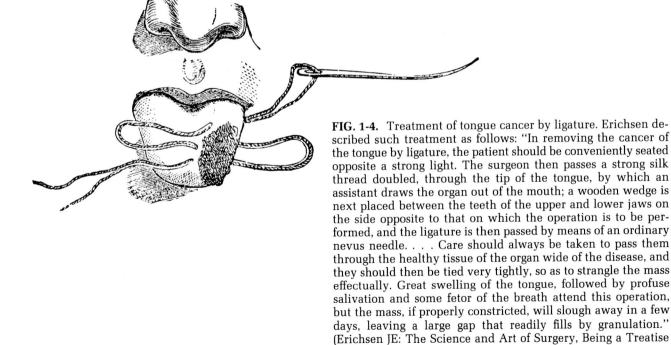

FIG. 1-4. Treatment of tongue cancer by ligature. Erichsen described such treatment as follows: "In removing the cancer of the tongue by ligature, the patient should be conveniently seated opposite a strong light. The surgeon then passes a strong silk thread doubled, through the tip of the tongue, by which an assistant draws the organ out of the mouth; a wooden wedge is next placed between the teeth of the upper and lower jaws on the side opposite to that on which the operation is to be performed, and the ligature is then passed by means of an ordinary nevus needle. . . . Care should always be taken to pass them through the healthy tissue of the organ wide of the disease, and they should then be tied very tightly, so as to strangle the mass effectually. Great swelling of the tongue, followed by profuse salivation and some fetor of the breath attend this operation, but the mass, if properly constricted, will slough away in a few days, leaving a large gap that readily fills by granulation." (Erichsen JE: The Science and Art of Surgery, Being a Treatise on Surgical Injuries, Diseases, and Operations, p 655. Brinton JH [ed]. Philadelphia, Blanchard and Lea, 1854)

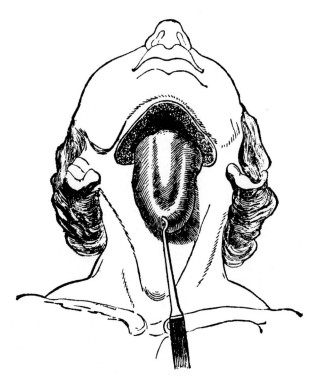

FIG. 1-5. The American surgeon Samuel D. Gross noted that the "remarkable feat of excising the whole tongue has recently been performed several times in Europe." He illustrated Regnoli's method, calling it the "operation affording the most easy access to the affected organ." (Gross SD: A System of Surgery: Pathological, Diagnostic, Therapeutic, and Operative, 3rd ed, vol II, p 472. Philadelphia, Blanchard and Lea, 1864)

rhage. The patient reportedly "spoke immediately afterward without difficulty," and the wound healed well. In 1900 Butlin and Spencer called this the first "major operation for the removal of a carcinomatous tumour such as might be carried out at the present time."[25]

Roux, one of the greatest surgeons of his era, is also said to have divided the lower jaw vertically for an operation on the tongue, the predecessor of later mandible-splitting techniques. Charles Sédillot in 1844 also divided the lower jaw, using an angular cut. "The jaw was fixed [i.e., reunited] by a gold plate and by silk threads between the teeth."[25]

During the last half of the 19th century, écraseurs were briefly in vogue for operations on the tongue. An écraseur included a loop of wire or chain that was tightened around the affected part of the patient's body. The procedure was completed more rapidly than a ligature procedure, in hours or even minutes rather than days, and, unlike scalpel excision, produced a sort of tourniquet effect that prevented primary hemorrhage. Severe bruising and frequent infections resulted, however, and the location of the cut was difficult to control precisely; curved needles were sometimes inserted through the tongue to prevent the loop from slipping forward. More than one écraseur could be used in different directions, and the loop could be introduced in various ways, such as through the mouth or from below or after division of the jaw (Fig. 1-6).[25,66]

A "galvano-écraseur" was described in the medical literature as early as 1851. It provided a hot, cauterizing

cutting surface by means of an electric current that ran through the cutting loop. Although it was at that time a difficult and uncertain instrument, it was used and improved throughout the second half of the century.[25]

All these operations were improved and enlarged upon after the advent of anesthesia. In 1862 Theodor Billroth modified the submental operation by raising a musculocutaneous flap by means of a U-shaped submental incision to gain access to the oral cavity. In the same year he also divided the ramus of a patient's mandible in two places, turned down the resulting flap of skin and bone to remove the tongue, and then restored the bone in place with wire sutures. In 1875 Bernhard von Langenbeck reported the removal of enlarged regional lymph nodes as well as of the tongue cancer, and Billroth also emphasized the importance of removing involved regional nodes. As early as 1881, Billroth's results (reported by his student Anton Wölfler) indicated that the prognosis in patients with involved nodes that were treated by radical excision was similar to that of patients without clinically involved nodes—that is, the cancer could be cured even after it spread to the regional lymph nodes.[3,25,105]

FIG. 1-6. Gross illustrated a glossectomy technique using two écraseurs and wrote, "In order to avoid the hemorrhage attendant upon this operation, Chassaignac has proposed the substitution of the écraseur for the knife, and it may readily be perceived that if there are any cases in which such an instrument is applicable, this is one of them. The patient, being under the influence of chloroform, would experience no pain, and the ablation being performed slowly would be almost bloodless." Gross wrote, however, that, in general, little could be achieved by glossectomy, and he did not recommend the operation, writing instead that, "So cruel a procedure could hardly have any other than a fatal termination." (Gross SD: A System of Surgery: Pathological, Diagnostic, Therapeutic, and Operative, 3rd ed, vol II, p 472. Philadelphia, Blanchard and Lea, 1864)

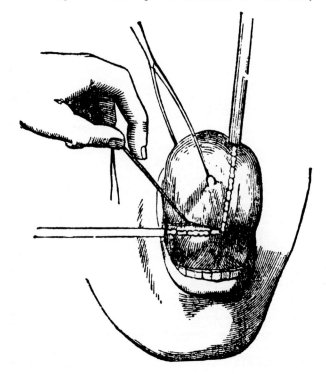

Theodor Kocher, best remembered for his operations on the thyroid, probably achieved the lowest operative mortality of his day for glossectomy through careful dissection, meticulous hemostasis, and rigorous antisepsis. He used an incision that ran downward along the sternocleidomastoid muscle and then up diagonally to form a triangular submental flap. In this way he had access to the submandibular lymph nodes, the lingual artery, and the oral cavity for removal of any part of the tongue, including the base. His results from 1880 onward brought about the eventual end of the écraseur, ligature, and caustic methods described above.[3] The English surgeon Walter W. Whitehead standardized the techniques for operations through the mouth during the late 1800s, achieving a 3% mortality rate in generally less-advanced cases.[25]

By 1900 Butlin and Spencer reported a 12% overall mortality rate in 333 patients who were operated on for tongue cancer in four clinics (two German clinics, Kocher's and Krönlein's; two English clinics, Whitehead's and Butlin's). Mortality for simple removal of some or all of the tongue was 7%; mortality increased to 20% to 25% for operations performed through the submental area and those that involved removing the "glands" beneath the jaw or splitting the jaw. In these same 333 cases, 199 patients were considered to be evaluable for cure; 40 (20%) were free of disease for at least 3 years.[25]

It was during this era that Ulysses S. Grant suffered throat cancer. He is the only American president known to have died of cancer. Grant was a very heavy cigar smoker, smoking as many as 12 cigars a day for 20 years or more. He had been a heavy drinker also, although probably not after he achieved positions of responsibility. In June 1884, when he was 63 years old, Grant noticed soreness in his right tonsillar area. His family doctor was in Europe until October, so Grant waited for him to return before seeking treatment. He was immediately referred to a New York throat specialist, John H. Douglas, who kept a diary throughout the months of his devoted attendance on Grant. The diary has not been published, but it is now in the Library of Congress. At the time of Douglas's first examination, Grant's tongue was "swollen, and hard at the base, and to the right side," and the soft palate was inflamed. An enlarged lymph node was noted under the angle of the mandible on the right. In keeping with the custom of that time, Grant was informed that the disease was "serious," but the word "cancer" was not used. Grant was told to stop smoking, which he did. Because his teeth were in bad repair, he was sent to a dentist, Frank Abbott, who pulled three rotten teeth, filled several others, and cleaned the remainder. George F. Shrady, a noted New York surgeon and the editor of the *Medical Record*, was called in for consultation. Apparently, an operation was discussed among his physicians but was never recommended to Grant owing to the extent of the required surgery (removal of the entire tongue and the "glandular structures under the right angle of the lower jaw"), the uncertainty of cure, and the high risk of immediate mortality associated with the operation. Only local treatment was prescribed, including various antiseptic gargles and topical pain relievers. In February 1885, a biopsy was taken after cocaine had been used as a local anesthetic and a squamous cell carcinoma was revealed.[49] The public clamored for news, and weekly bulletins were issued in the *Medical Record*. As his disease pursued its inexorable course, Grant was writing his memoirs. Victimized by a large-scale swindle, he had been left virtually penniless several months before his illness was discovered. In great distress at the thought of leaving his family destitute, he was persuaded by Samuel Clemens (Mark Twain), a personal friend, to write his memoirs as a means of providing for his family after his death. With cocaine and morphine prescribed for control of pain, Grant worked on the manuscript throughout his illness, despite the constant threat of suffocation and at least one severe hemorrhage. He finally completed his memoirs less than a week before his death on July 23, 1885. The memoirs were published by Clemens and were a great success, eventually providing over $450,000 in royalties for Grant's family.[17,113,142,167]

A more successfully treated case was that of Grover Cleveland, who was President at the time his cancer was discovered. The manner in which his case was handled raises questions about the right of the public to know if the President is seriously ill. In June 1893, the President's physician, Major Robert M. O'Reilly (who was later to become Surgeon General), was asked to examine a "rough place" on the president's hard palate. He discovered "an ulcerative surface nearly as large as a quarter with cauliflower granulations."[112,135] O'Reilly called in a surgeon, Joseph D. Bryant, of New York, who found an oval lesion "extending from the inner surface of the molar teeth to within a quarter of an inch of the median line of the roof of the mouth and encroaching somewhat upon the anterior part of the soft palate" (Fig. 1-7).[112] A biopsy specimen was submitted to William H. Welch of Johns Hopkins, who apparently diagnosed an epithelial cancer.[112]

The President agreed to have an operation. Because the country was in the midst of the "Financial Panic of 1893," he insisted on strict secrecy regarding the nature of his illness. He and his associates believed that any publicity would jeopardize his management of the crisis.[111,135]

Bryant was a good choice for surgeon. He had previously read a paper entitled "A History of Two Hundred and Fifty Cases of Excision of the Superior Maxilla" to the New York State Medical Society. Only two of the cases were from his own experience, but he was certainly familiar with the indications and risks of the operation. He reported a 14% mortality rate for the series.[23,112]

On June 30 the President left Washington and boarded a friend's yacht at New York City, purportedly for a vacation. In fact, Cleveland's physicians had made preparations to do the operation on board the yacht. In addition to O'Reilly and Bryant, the surgical team included John F. Erdmann, Bryant's surgical assistant; William W. Keen, a distinguished Philadelphia surgeon; Edward G. Janeway, a prominent New York City internist; and Ferdinand Hasbrouck, a New York City dentist who was skilled in the use of nitrous oxide as an anesthetic.[112] The yacht's "saloon" had been fitted out as an operating room. The necessary drugs and gases had been brought aboard, as well as the surgical instruments and two storage batteries for an electric cautery and electric light. The crew was told that the President was having dental work done.

On July 1, the President's mouth and the surgeon's hands and instruments were thoroughly disinfected. The surgeons donned aprons over their street clothing. There was considerable worry about Cleveland's general medical condition. He drank socially and smoked cigars heavily, was very fat, and had mild chronic nephritis, but after a careful examination Janeway pronounced him fit for the operation. Just after noon, as the yacht steamed toward Long Island Sound, the operation commenced. Bryant operated, with Erdmann and Keen assisting, while Janeway kept watch over the President's general condition. Anesthetics used in the course of the operation included cocaine, nitrous

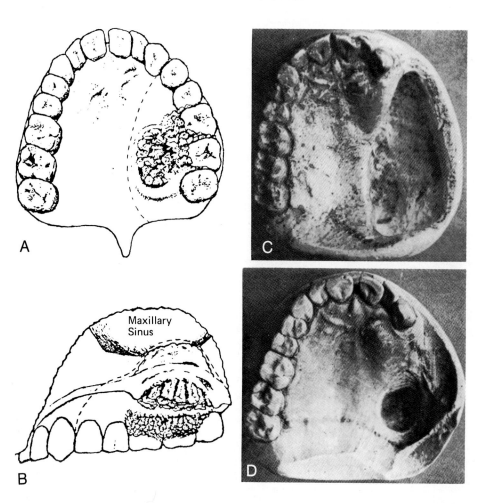

FIG. 1-7. President Cleveland's tumor. (*A* and *B*) Sketches reconstructing Cleveland's tumor, based on descriptions by physicians who examined him. The dotted lines represent the extent of the surgery. (*C*) Cast of Cleveland's upper jaw made in July 1893 by prosthodontist Kasson C. Gibson; the defect measured $2\frac{1}{2} \times {}^{13}\!/_{16}$ inches. (*D*) Cast made 4 years later, in 1897, shows defect measuring only ${}^{11}\!/_{16}$ inch $\times$ ${}^{7}\!/_{16}$ inch. (*A* and *B* from Brooks JJ, Enterline HT, Aponte GE: The final diagnosis of President Cleveland's lesion. Trans Stud Coll Physicians Phila 10:1–25, 1980; *C* and *D* from Morreels CL Jr: New historical information on the Cleveland operations. Surgery 62:542–551, 1967)

oxide, and ether, with the aim being to use ether as little as possible because of the President's potential medical problems. According to Keen, the first incisions were made in the gum and hard palate. The cheek was then dissected loose, and the front of the jaw was chiseled loose from the first bicuspid to the posterior extremity of the bone. The palatal process was divided, and the bone was removed. Because the growth was found to extend as "a gelatinous mass" into the maxillary sinus, "it was determined to remove all of the jaw except the floor of the orbit and the intermaxillary portion."[112] The operation, though extensive, was entirely intraoral. Bleeding was controlled by the electric cautery, pressure, hot water, and one ligature. The electric light was reported to have been very useful. The operation was completed before two o'clock, and the President's condition was very good.[112]

Cleveland was out of bed the second day after the operation and on July 5 was able to walk from the yacht when it arrived at his summer home, where he went into seclusion. His recovery was interrupted, however, when Bryant, who remained in attendance, decided that "a suspicious looking growth" on the inner margin of the wound should be removed."[112] Janeway, Keen, and Erdmann again boarded the yacht, where Bryant operated again on July 17, removing the suspicious tissue and recauterizing the entire surface of the wound.

Thereafter, recovery was apparently smooth, although when the packing was removed from the wound, the President's speech was said to resemble "cleft palate speech."[112]

Kasson C. Gibson, a New York City prosthodontist, set up a dental laboratory in the President's summer home and fabricated a prosthesis of vulcanized rubber that was attached to a dental plate. On his original cast of Cleveland's upper jaw, now in the possession of the New York Academy of Medicine, it can be seen that the original surgical defect measured about $2\frac{1}{2}$ inches by ${}^{13}\!/_{16}$ inch (see Fig. 1-7C).[112]

Suspicion had been aroused by the circumstances of the President's precipitate departure from Washington, and rumors soon spread that he was ill. His family and Cabinet members specifically denied that the President had cancer.[112] Cleveland returned to Washington, and on August 7 he addressed a special session of Congress. He was found to look and sound better than he had before leaving Washington, an improvement attributed to rest and sea air. The secret seemed safe.[112]

On August 29, however, a detailed and mostly factual account of the operation was published in the Philadelphia *Press*. Hasbrouck was the weak link in the conspiracy. His story was relayed to Elisha J. Edwards, a correspondent for the *Press*, and Hasbrouck confirmed it. The story was specifically and vigorously denied by everyone else involved in the case, even to the point of outright lies. The President's public appearance on August 7 with no scar on his face and no speech defect did much to discredit Edwards's story. The reporter's reputation suffered and was not restored until long after he and Cleveland both were dead.[70,111,112]

Cleveland's oral defect closed through the years. A cast taken by Gibson in 1897 shows it to be less than an inch in diameter (see Fig. 1-7D).[112] Cleveland died in 1908, apparently the result of cardiovascular and renal disease and an intestinal blockage of uncertain origin.[18]

The story of Cleveland's illness was finally made public in 1917. Keen, then 80 years old and retired from practice, had kept a scrapbook of clippings, notes, and letters about the operation. He published the full story in a book entitled *The Surgical Operation on President Cleveland in 1893* and in the *Saturday Evening Post*.[112]

Cleveland's physicians disagreed over the histology of the tumor, and all of the original pathology reports have apparently been lost. More than 80 years after the operation, in an effort to settle the question, samples of the tissue (preserved in the Mütter Museum of the College of Physicians of Philadelphia) were examined by modern pathologists. Their opinion was that the tumor was a verrucous carcinoma, accounting for the initial cauliflowerlike appearance described by O'Reilly, the differences of opinion regarding histology, and the lack of recurrence of the tumor in the 15 years that Cleveland lived after the operation.[18]

Cancer of the Larynx and Pharynx

The treatment of laryngeal and hypopharyngeal cancer was complicated by the fact that, although ancient physicians knew such tumors occurred, a technique for examining the larynx was not developed until the mid–19th century. Credit for the invention of mirror laryngoscopy is generally given to Manuel Garcia, whose description of his self-examination of his larynx expresses the spirit of scientific endeavor in the 19th century (or, indeed, in any century):

> I placed against the uvula the little mirror (which I had heated in warm water and carefully dried); then, flashing upon its surface with the hand mirror a ray of sunlight, I saw at once, to my great joy, the glottis wide open before me, and so fully exposed, that I could perceive a portion of the trachea. When my excitement had somewhat subsided, I began to examine what was passing before my eyes. The manner in which the glottis silently opened and shut, and moved in the act of phonation, filled me with wonder.[60]

Garcia was not really the first to use a mirror to visualize the larynx. For instance, in 1829 Benjamin Babington demonstrated a "glottiscope" with a single mirror upon which sunlight was concentrated by means of a hand lens. The clumsy device included a built-in tongue depressor. Babington himself reportedly used his glottiscope for many years to examine patients, but no one else adopted his apparatus.[32,64,149]

Garcia was able to examine himself as he did because he was a trained singer and could consciously control his tongue and throat muscles. He was born into a family of professional musicians; his parents and his two sisters were famous opera singers. They were Spanish by nationality, but they toured all over Europe and America. His father established a voice training school in Paris, and in about 1830 Manuel decided (since his voice was not good enough for an operatic career) to join his father in teaching. In the 19th-century manner, he was very serious and scientific in pursuing his chosen profession. He studied in the Mil-

itary Hospital of Paris for a year or two in an effort to learn all that medicine could teach him about the human voice. He also became thoroughly familiar with the anatomy of the larynx by dissecting many human and animal specimens at home. He published a paper in 1840 on the human voice, and later he published others on his methods of teaching singing. Perhaps his most famous pupil was Jenny Lind, the "Swedish Nightingale." He was not satisfied with these activities, however, as is clear from what he later said, "During all the years of study and investigation of the problems of voice production, one wish was ever uppermost in my mind—if only I could see the glottis."[136] In 1850 he was appointed Professor at the Royal Academy of Music in London. Thereafter, England became his home, and it was to the Royal Society of England that he presented his discovery of mirror examination. It is typical, however, that his 1855 paper was not about laryngoscopy *per se*; it was instead a highly technical discussion on the production of voice—different from those that preceded it because he no longer had to theorize about the movements of the larynx that corresponded to various tones, since he could actually watch them being made.[32,59,82,136]

Garcia's report was met with apathy in England, but Ludwig Van Türck of Vienna worked on a similar device that made use of sunlight and a hand mirror during the summer of 1857, giving up in disgust when the cloudy days of autumn arrived. He gave one of his instruments to Johann Czermak of Budapest, who thought of having the examiner wear a perforated concave ophthalmoscopic mirror over his eye to gather and reflect a beam of artificial light. Czermak's idea really made routine laryngoscopy possible. He and Türck both took up laryngology with enthusiasm, later writing books disputing each other's claim of priority in the use of the laryngoscope. Morell Mackenzie, the first English laryngologist, learned the technique in Czermak's Budapest clinic in 1859. The first laryngoscopic mirror was introduced in New York in 1858, and by 1861 a paper about laryngoscopy was read to the New York Academy of Medicine. Within a decade of Garcia's report, the technique of laryngoscopy was accepted, and laryngology was on its way to becoming an established specialty.[32]

Garcia continued his distinguished career as a teacher and voice specialist until he retired at the age of 96. In 1905, on the occasion of his 100th birthday, he was honored as the "Father of Laryngology" at a celebration in London arranged by Felix Semon, the dean of English laryngologists at the time. Whether or not Garcia may be said to have invented the technique of mirror laryngoscopy, he was the first to report his systematic observations of the larynx.[76,82,136]

The early laryngologists, particularly Mackenzie in England, the German surgeon Viktor von Bruns, and Jacob D. Solis-Cohen, of Philadelphia, became skilled in performing laryngeal treatment through the mouth.[33,149] A specialized set of surgical instruments was developed for such operations. Very few malignant tumors could be treated successfully through the mouth, however. Thyrotomy, the exposure of the larynx by splitting the thyroid cartilage, had been described for the treatment of laryngeal polyps by the 18th-century Parisian surgeon Pierre J. Desault, and 100 years later it was still sometimes called "Desault's operation."[47,129] After the introduction of anesthetics, thyrotomy, or laryngofissure, was performed more frequently for piecemeal removal of tumors followed by cauterization, often in cases much too advanced to be cured by this procedure. By 1868 there was disillusionment with thyrotomy because it was recognized that this procedure was inadequate in most cases of malignancy.[150]

At his clinic in Vienna, Billroth was at this time preparing to carry out total laryngectomy. Vincenz Czerny, then one of Billroth's surgical assistants, performed a series of successful laryngectomies on dogs and published the results of 1870. It became a question of waiting for the right patient, and he appeared in November, 1873, a 36-year-old teacher of religion who had a biopsy-proven cancer beneath the true vocal cords. He had been treated through the mouth with cauterization and partial excision, but the tumor recurred, and it was decided that an "external operation" was the only hope for cure. Billroth first performed laryngofissure and removed the tumor with scissors and a curet. The patient was soon found to have extensive recurrence. Billroth at this time planned curettage of the entire larynx,

but during surgery on December 31st the tumor was found to be too extensive for this procedure to offer any hope of cure. The man was allowed to awaken, and his consent to total laryngectomy was obtained. Billroth then performed the operation along the lines that Czerny's experiments had established. He had considerable difficulty controlling bleeding, but he managed to perform an extensive dissection that included the base of the epiglottis and the first two tracheal rings; he sutured the tracheal and pharyngeal openings to the skin and brought the edges of the esophagus together (Fig. 1-8). Four hours later he had to reoperate to place ligatures to control bleeding from the left superior laryngeal artery. Amazingly, the patient did not develop any infection. The sutures and ligatures were removed after 3 days, leaving a midline wound, with the tracheal stoma below and the pharyngeal fistula above. The patient was fed by tube at first, but the pharyngeal fistula began

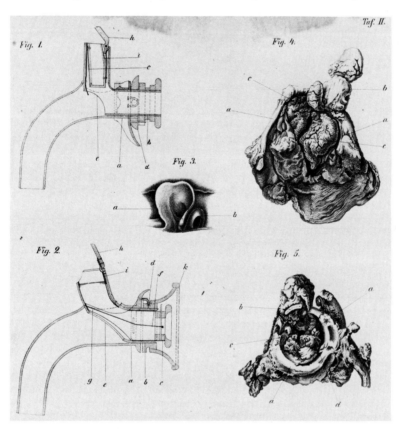

FIG. 1-8.   Plate illustrating Gussenbauer's report of Billroth's original laryngectomy. *Fig. 1* is the first artificial larynx Gussenbauer constructed. (*a*) Tracheal limb of tube. (*b*) Pharyngeal limb of tube. (*c*) This part shifts upward on phonation. The rotating ring (*d*) serves to fixate the tubes. The opening (*e*) communicates with the trachea. Plate (*h*) is kept open by a spring (*i*). The vibratory device quickly filled with mucus. *Fig. 2* is the improved version, which was quite successful. Letter designations are the same as in *Fig. 1*; in addition, *f* is the frame in which the metal vibrating tongue is fastened, and *k* is the respirator affixed to the pharyngeal tube. *Fig. 3* is the laryngoscopic view at the time of the patient's discharge. (*a*) Epiglottis. (*b*) Catheter introduced from below into the pharyngeal opening. *Fig. 4* is the excised larynx, from above. (*a*) Boundaries of laryngeal entrance. (*b*) Portion of epiglottis that was excised. (*c*) Supraglottic extension of cancer. *Fig. 5* is the excised larynx, from below. (*a*) Cricoid cartilage. (*b*) Part of trachea. (*c*) Subglottic extension of cancer. (*d*) Mucous membrane not yet involved by cancer. (Gussenbauer C: Über die erste durch Th. Billroth am Menschen ausgeführte Kehlkopf-Exstirpation und die Anwendung eines künstlichen Kehlkopfes. Arch Klin Chir 17:343–356, 1874)

to close, and he was able to swallow liquids on the 8th day after surgery and solids by the 18th day. Czerny and Karl Gussenbauer, another of Billroth's surgical assistants, had already done some work with dogs toward devising an artificial larynx, and Gussenbauer was now assigned the task of helping the patient speak again. He was able to provide an artifical larynx that enabled the patient to speak loudly and clearly, but with a monotonous tone (see Fig. 1-8). The patient was discharged in March 1874, but he suffered local recurrence of the tumor and died later in the year.[2,46,67,143,160] The artificial larynx, which shunted air from the trachea to the pharynx, was based on the same principle as the modern-day Singer-Blom and Panje devices. (See Chapter 20, Speech Rehabilitation After Total Laryngectomy.)

This was probably the first laryngectomy, and certainly it was the first performed for cancer. Despite the dangers of the operation, others followed in quick succession in Czechoslovakia, Poland, Germany, and Italy. The first total laryngectomy in the United States was performed in 1879. The patient survived the operation but committed suicide a week later. In 1883, Solis-Cohen published a collection of 65 laryngectomy case reports in which over one third of the patients mentioned had died within a month of the operation.[140]

Treatment of laryngeal cancer became the subject of international controversy, in both medical and lay publications, when Prince Frederick, the middle-aged Crown Prince of Germany, developed a laryngeal lesion in March 1887. It was first treated with cauterization through the mouth, but it quickly regrew. By May the tumor was distinctly larger than ever and the mobility of the vocal cords was lessened. A laryngotomy was recommended for direct visualization of the tumor and, if possible, removal. It was decided, however, to request one more expert consultation, and (at the behest of the Crown Princess, eldest daughter of Queen Victoria of England) the English laryngologist Morell Mackenzie was summoned. Mackenzie disagreed with the conclusion of the German physicians, contending that there should be proof that the condition was malignant before a major operation was undertaken. He recommended biopsy, which was done three times during May and June. The specimens were submitted to Virchow himself, who was a friend and admirer of the Crown Prince and who reported that they showed no evidence of malignancy. To the despair of the German physicians, only minimal transoral treatment was carried out, despite the malignant behavior of the lesion, until November, by which time the tumor had grown to such an extent that only a total laryngectomy with its high risk of operative mortality held any possibility of success (Fig. 1-9). Prince Frederick decided against it. In February 1888, he underwent a tracheotomy to relieve stridor. Carcinoma was diagnosed in March by Wilhelm Waldeyer based on sputum specimens. Frederick lived long enough to succeed to the throne on March 9, but he died on June 15. At the autopsy, the last he ever performed, Virchow found laryngeal carcinoma with metastases in cervical lymph nodes. The crown then passed to Frederick's militant son, the Emperor William II, who led Germany into World War I. Whether his peace-loving father could have prevented this conflict can only be a subject for speculation. The medical repercussions were also felt for some years, particularly the question of whether biopsy should or should not be carried out prior to treatment in cases of laryngeal disease. An acrimonious and undignified dispute was carried out in print between the German physicians and Mackenzie on this and the other disputed points in the case, beginning even before their royal patient's death. Mackenzie died with his reputation marred by this episode, although later writers have been more balanced in their judgment of his career.[30,61,98,102,115,116,151]

The results of laryngectomy were greatly improved by the technique developed by Glück in Germany in 1881 and by Solis-Cohen in the United States whereby the trachea and larynx were elevated above the level of the wound, preventing the entry of blood into the lungs during the procedure, and the hypopharyngeal defect was closed, lessening the risk of postoperative aspiration.[33,150] In 1913, Glück and Soerensen reported that only 22 of 244 patients had died intraoperatively and that 24 patients had survived 4 to 15 years following total laryngectomy for carcinoma of the larynx. It should be noted that these were more advanced cases; they performed thyrotomy or hemilaryngectomy in less advanced cases, with excellent results. The value of laryngectomy was still widely disputed.[42,129]

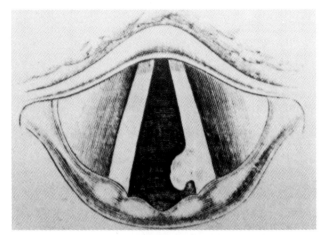

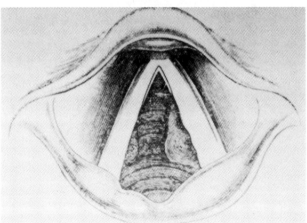

FIG. 1-9. Drawings by Morell Mackenzie of the laryngoscopic appearance of Crown Prince Frederick's laryngeal tumor, published in his 1888 book, *The Fatal Illness of Frederick the Noble.* (*Top*) Representation of the initial examination in May 1887. (*Bottom*) Drawing of the Prince's condition in November 1887, when Mackenzie had to admit that the tumor was probably malignant. (Gerlings PG: Laryngeal carcinoma—Some considerations with reference to the illness of Emperor Frederick III. Eye Ear Nose Throat Monthly 47:566–571, 1968)

Later Surgical Developments

Technical improvements in the surgical techniques for head and neck cancer operations came rapidly and included improved methods of producing anesthesia, the development of specialized instruments, and refinements of the operative method. However, dramatic lowering of operative mortality rates depended mostly on meticulous preoperative and postoperative care of the patient, techniques for which were developed by Chevalier Jackson of Philadelphia, George W. Crile of Cleveland, and John E. MacKenty of New York, among many others. In this preantibiotic era, precautions taken before, during, and after surgery to lessen the infection rate were of crucial importance. Postoperative care now included nasogastric tube feeding and elaborate care to prevent or treat aspiration. Statistics were also improved by more knowledgeable selection of patients for the operations.[78,95] In the mid–20th century the list of supportive measures grew with the discovery of antibiotics, the use of blood transfusions, a better understanding of blood chemistry, and still further improvements in anesthetics and in operative and rehabilitative techniques.[129]

Surgeons could focus on their actual goal—control of the cancer—once patients began routinely to survive the operative procedures. It had long been recognized that control of the primary tumor was not enough, in many cases, to cure the patient of cancer. Early attempts to cope surgically with neck lymph node metastases reached a culmination in 1906 when Crile, after the model of Halsted's treatment of breast cancer, advocated en bloc resection of the "entire lymphatic-bearing tissue" in the neck, on one or both sides, for patients with a wide variety of head and neck tumors when the neck nodes were enlarged. A less radical block excision of the pertinent lymphatic drainage area was advised when there was no palpable neck disease present.[39]

The English surgeon Wilfred Trotter established the modern system for naming, diagnosing, and treating pharyngeal cancers on the basis of the natural history of the tumors.[165] Writing in 1913, he described the manifestations of and the best therapy for tumors of each of five anatomical areas: nasopharynx, oropharynx, epilarynx, pyriform sinus, and hypopharynx.[154] He said that neck nodes were characteristic for nasopharyngeal tumors, and the presentation of hearing loss, trigeminal pain, and partial paralysis of the palate (which he described in 1911) is still known as "Trotter's triad."[153,165] He said that these tumors were frequently "endotheliomata of a peculiar and characteristic type," which were found also at times in the tonsil and occurred mostly in young males (probably this category included lymphoepithelioma, not described until 1921).[154] For nasopharynx tumors, curative treatment was generally not possible. Tumors of the oropharynx, including the tonsil, the anterior tonsillar pillar, and the base of the tongue, showed a "marked tendency to longitudinal spread [which] renders free longitudinal exposure an essential necessity in the operative technique."[154] Cancer of the base of the tongue was particularly serious because of "the remarkable tendency it has to grow into the substance of the tongue without in the early stages ulceration or projection at the surface" and because it produced few early symptoms and resulted in presentation at an advanced stage.[154] The epilaryngeal tumors were those referred to by others as "extrinsic tumors of the larynx," which arose on the epiglottis or aryepiglottic fold. Unlike others, Trotter found that these lesions were "the most hopeful of all malignant pharyngeal tumors" because of their tendency to produce symptoms at an early stage; he thought that total laryngectomy was often unnecessary in treating them.[154] In the case of tumors of the pyriform sinus, however, he could only be pessimistic. Its depths were, according to him, "quite inaccessible to laryngoscopic examination."[154] The tumors produced no early symptoms and often presented as "obviously malignant glands in the neck without ostensible primary tumour."[154] Indeed, typically there was invasion of the thyroid cartilage by the primary tumor, which was "sometimes mistaken for a gland."[154] This was the only pharyngeal tumor, in his experience, for which "that terrible operation," a total laryngectomy, was always required, because it was always advanced at the time of the operation.[154] He found that early diagnosis was possible for hypopharyngeal carcinomas, but that treatment was frequently delayed owing to the mistaken belief that the tumors were inoperable. He also noted that although most other pharyngeal tumors occurred mostly in men, hypopharyngeal cancers occurred frequently in women. As to treatment, Trotter recommended "lateral pharyngotomy by the transthyroid route," as he termed it in a later (1920) paper, to provide the necessary "free and untroubled access to the part."[155] He advised excising a ½-inch margin for early tumors and a ¾-inch to 1-inch margin for moderately advanced cases, with a larger margin in the direction in which the tumor was known to have a propensity to spread. Margins were to be determined by pathologic examination rather than by anatomy. As for treatment of the neck, he attributed to the otolaryngologist Henry Butlin the rule that "the gland operation should be as much a part of the treatment as the removal of the primary growth."[154] If there were few or no palpable neck metastases, the operation was limited to removal of "all lymphoid tissue" above the thyroid cartilage, but it was extended horizontally "to comprise about four fifths of the circumference of the neck."[154] If there was extensive lymph node involvement, the operation was unilateral, but its course extended downward and included the sacrifice of the spinal accessory nerve, the sternocleidomastoid muscle, and the jugular vein.[154]

The increasingly radical efforts of the early 20th-century surgeons to cure patients of head and neck cancers sometimes produced the unhappy result of a patient without recurrence of cancer who was so maimed by the treatment that his extended life span was miserable in quality. The cartoon character "Andy Gump" was probably based on a real man, a patient treated by radical surgery for lip cancer at Johns Hopkins in 1915, who lived in upstate New York in the same small town where cartoonist Sidney Smith lived as a boy. Andy Gump was depicted as having no lower jaw, a defect that caused him no apparent disability and produced only a comic disfigurement; the reality, of course, was grim. An unsuccessful lawsuit filed by the cured patient in 1928 charged that the cartoonist had disgraced and humiliated him, but it would be fairer to say that the lifesaving surgery itself had caused his problems.[141]

Plastic surgeons and prosthedontists developed new techniques and materials in their efforts to repair the mutilations of war. The early work on skin grafting by Reverdin, Ollier, and Thiersch was done around the time of the Franco-Prussian War (1870–1871), but prior to World War I there was really no specialty of plastic surgery. This war offered ample work to those interested in reconstructive operations.[101] As the Dutch oral surgeon Johannes Esser put it in his 1917 paper, "As I made in Austria over 700 plastic operations on war-cripples I enlarged my practical experience, especially in repairing defects of the face in an important manner."[52] He described the neck and cheek flap, centered on the external maxillary artery, for reconstruction of upper lip and cheek defects; the nasolabial flap for lower lip defects; and the use of a mold of Stent's dental compound, wrapped in a "Thiersch graft" raw side out, to hold the graft in place in a cavity. He noted that plastic operations should leave neither uncovered tissue nor excess skin folds, for "a beautiful plastic is always a mathematically correct and maximally economical one."[52] Harold D. Gillies did his first plastic surgery on British troops in World War I and later went on to establish the specialty of plastic surgery in England. He described the many uses he had found for the tubed pedicle flap in his textbook, *Plastic Surgery of the Face*, published in 1920. Vilray P. Blair, already known as a reconstructive surgeon before the war, led the American section on oral and plastic surgery. He later developed the method of raising large flaps, describing in his "The Delayed Transfer of Long Pedicle Flaps" in 1921, and he described the use of the larger, thicker split-thickness skin graft in 1929. In 1938 the invention of the dermatome by Earl C. Padgett made it easier to obtain skin grafts, just in time for use in World War II.[35] These new techniques could often be applied to the rehabilitation of cancer patients after radical surgery. In the 1950s Vahram Bakamjian, of Roswell Park, raised a tube flap from the cervical area to repair the defect left by radical cancer surgery and used the pectoral flap to cover the wound in the neck.[11,12]

Sigmund Freud suffered and eventually died from a carcinoma of the hard palate, diagnosed in 1923 when Freud was 67 years old. He underwent a total of 33 operations and numerous x-ray and radium treatments for his disease. Freud's biographer, Ernest Jones, published the case notes of Hans Pichler, the distinguished Viennese oral surgeon who cared for Freud from the first radical operation for recurrence in 1923 until Freud left Vienna in 1938 for England as a refugee from Nazism. In October 1923, Pichler described "a crater-shaped typical ulcer at the posterior part of the [maxillary tuberosity] with slight infiltration into the palatoglossal fold continuing into the buccal mucous membrane and over the margin of the mandible."[79] Pichler first performed "typical clearance of the submaxillary glands" and ligature of the external carotid artery on October 4. Some of the lymph nodes appeared "suspicious," but no malignancy was found microscopically. On October 11, Pichler resected the maxilla and part of the ascending mandibular ramus on the right side. The soft palate was mostly preserved, and the wound was covered by a "Thiersch-graft" taken from the left upper arm. A preliminary prosthesis was put in place at the time of the operation. After receiving the pathologist's report, Pichler immediately reoperated, cutting an additional 1½-cm margin in the soft palate and removing the pterygoid process, until the margins again appeared clear.[79]

For the remaining 16 years of his life Freud struggled with his prosthesis, which he dubbed "the monster." He had great difficulty inserting and removing it, owing in part to its large size and in part to trismus dating from his initial operation. He was in pain much of the time, and his speech was always more or less defective; he never again gave lectures. Despite frequent construction of new prostheses and adjustments of old ones, his prosthesis almost never fit properly, not too surprising in view of the

constant threat of recurrence, with repeated operations and radiation treatments* and the subsequent postsurgical, postirradiation changes in his tissues. In addition, he had always had sinusitis off and on, and this problem continued. Despite all this, Pichler paradoxically concluded, on July 5, 1925, that the psychiatrist's problems with his prosthesis were "mainly nervous." Freud continued to work during these years, teaching, seeing patients, and writing, as much as his illness allowed. Definite tumor recurrence was diagnosed in 1936, and finally, in May 1939, in London, a tumor was found "high above in antrum," and it was noted that "Operation not indicated any more." Some additional radiation treatments were given, and Freud survived until September.[40,79]

RADIATION THERAPY IN HEAD AND NECK CANCER

Early X-ray Therapy

In January 1896, Röntgen's discovery of x-rays was publicized throughout the world. The medical usefulness of the new rays was immediately obvious, and the March 1896 issue of *Index Medicus* listed more than 40 published papers dealing with the subject. As soon as the effects of the rays on tissues were observed, x-ray treatment of cancer was tried, and head and neck cancers were among the first to be treated. In fact, on February 3, 1896, Voight reported to the Medical Society of Hamburg that he had irradiated a case of pharyngeal cancer and that the patient's pain had been relieved. For this effect to have occurred by February 3, the treatments were probably administered sometime in January.[29,158]

Emil Grubbé, of Chicago, administered x-ray therapy to a patient with breast cancer on January 29, 1896, making him the first in the United States to administer radiotherapy. He and his partner, Albert Schmidt, a German glassblower, had been producing vacuum tubes, mostly electric light bulbs but also Geissler tubes and a small mica-vane radiometer tube. Grubbé was a freshman medical student (and teacher of physics and chemistry) at Hahnemann Medical College of Homeopathy in 1896 when Röntgen's discovery was reported. He claimed that he experimented with cathode-ray tubes and that he tested them by watching the image of his hand on a fluoroscopic screen.[72] As Hodges recounted in his biography,

> Toward the end of January, 1896, Emil noticed severe itching on the back of the left hand followed shortly by swelling, inflammation, pain, blistering, loss of hair (epilation), and eventually breaking down of the skin (desquamation). That was the state of affairs, he says, when on January 27, 1896, he attended a faculty meeting of the medical college where he was both student and teacher. Several of his physician

---

* Freud's radiation therapist early in the course of his disease was Guido Holzknecht, of whom Jones writes: "Holzknecht, who had been a former patient of Freud's, was the leading radiologist in Vienna and one of the pioneers of that science. Like so many of those pioneers he was also a victim and was now [in 1931] in hospital dying of cancer, which an amputation of his right arm had failed to arrest; he died a few months later. Freud and Schur [Dr. Max Schur, Freud's internist] visited him, none of them being under any illusion, and when they parted Freud said, 'You are to be admired for the way you bear your fate.' Holzknecht replied, 'You know I have only you to thank for that.' "[79]

colleagues and teachers, noticing that his hand was bandaged, inquired about it and when the bandage had been removed offered therapeutic suggestions. One of the group, Dr. J. E. Gilman, instead of advising as to treatment expressed the belief that if x-rays could be so damaging to normal tissues they might be effective against disease tissues such as neoplasm. This idea impressed the other physicians who were present and two of them offered to send Emil cancer patients if he cared to make a therapeutic trial. In this manner, the ground was laid for the birth of radiation therapy.

At 10:00 A.M., on Wednesday, January 29, 1896, Mrs. Rose Lee, a patient of Dr. R. Ludlam, came to Emil's little place at 12 Pacific Avenue and he administered the first of eighteen treatments to a carcinoma of her left breast which had recurred after a first and then a second operation. The treatment reduced her pain, but she died about a month after the first visit.[72]

Grubbé was kept busy treating patients for cancer and other diseases while he completed his medical education, and he had a long career in radiology. Like many of the pioneers in the field, he developed radiation-induced skin cancers that caused him great suffering, although he survived to be 85 years old. He was very concerned late in his life with the question of priority in the use of radiation therapy, and he willed his fortune to the University of Chicago on the condition that a biography be written, which he hoped would document his claims. This task was carried out with sympathy, skill, and a strict regard for the truth by Paul C. Hodges,* and the resulting biography, *The Life and Times of Emil H. Grubbé,* makes fascinating reading for anyone interested in the early days of radiology.[72]

As the effects of radiation on skin were recognized, many dermatologists experimented with the new treatment medium (Fig. 1-10). At the 1902 meeting of the American Medical Association Section on Cutaneous Medicine and Surgery, the use of x-rays was reported for a variety of skin conditions, ranging from acne and eczema to lupus and cutaneous tuberculosis, as well as for cancers.[152] The fact that radiation would cause hair to fall out was discovered in 1896 and led to its widespread use for epilation in cases of ringworm of the scalp.

Skin cancers were an obvious target for radiation therapy, and two Swedish physicians, general practitioners in Stockholm, successfully treated facial skin cancers in 1899. Tage Sjögren treated a patient with basal cell carcinoma of the left lower eyelid and cheek with a total of 100 10-minute exposures over several months, producing total regression of the tumor but also producing a late dermatitis on the eyelid that resulted in ectropion of the lower lid.[57] Tor Stenbeck treated a woman with basal cell carcinoma of the nose with 99 treatments beginning July 4, 1899, and extending over several months. The patient was presented to the Swedish Society of Medicine in December 1899 and was presented to the Second International Congress of Radiologists in Stockholm in 1928, having survived nearly

---

* Before the cumulative long-term effects of radiation were widely known, the early radiologists often calibrated their machines on themselves. Dr. Hodges, who was a radiologist in Peking, China, from 1919 to 1927, calibrated his machines on his own legs, which many years later showed numerous round, depressed scars (the size and appearance of cigarette burns) resulting from this technique. Many early radiologists died as a result of radiation-induced cancers of the skin or soft tissues, leukemia, or aplastic anemia.[73] (Hodges PC: Personal communication, 1982)

30 years after treatment.[16] By 1904, the author of one early textbook of radiology commented that "the treatment of external forms of carcinoma, including those of breast, tongue, and cervix uteri, by the Röntgen rays has become a recognized method."[14]

In September 1902, William Scheppegrell, a New Orleans otolaryngologist, reported his experience with the use of x-ray treatment for larynx cancer to the American Electrotherapeutic Association. The patient was a 57-year-old lawyer from western Louisiana who had suffered hoarseness for 6 months prior to consulting Scheppegrell in April 1902. He was found to have a tumor of the left side of the larynx with paresis of the left vocal cord. The patient had just been injured in a street accident while on his way to see Scheppegrell and had to recuperate before his cancer could be treated. In June he returned, and the tumor had grown to the point that respiration was impeded, the vocal cord was paralyzed, ulceration had set in, and his voice was reduced to a husky whisper. To Scheppegrell's experienced eye, the lesion appeared to be a typical carcinoma of the intrinsic larynx. There was as yet no evident lymph node involvement. The patient was offered "laryngotomy" as treatment but declined the operation. Scheppegrell had used x-rays to treat laryngeal tuberculosis with good results and proposed that this treatment be tried, warning the patient that x-rays had been proven effective only in very superficial carcinomas. The patient agreed to a trial of treatment. Scheppegrell used a high-tension Tesla coil to generate the current, and he decided to use a tube with medium vacuum, providing more penetration than was needed to treat superficial disease but less than that required for chest examination. In what was certainly one of the first references to elective node irradiation, he said "The face and chest of the patient were protected with specially prepared paraffin paper, no effort being made to limit the rays to the diseased area by means of lead foil. The object was to utilize the effects of the treatment on the neighboring tissues and on the lymphatic glands, in case these had been involved in the malignant process."[130] The patient was seated with his head bent back to expose the neck as thoroughly as possible to the x-rays. He had a 10-minute exposure every day for 20 days, with little apparent result except decrease in pain. He was sent home to await results before deciding whether to continue the treatment. Six days later Scheppegrell was discouraged when he received a letter from the patient's wife, reporting that he was feverish, in pain, and expectorating blood clots. However, when the patient returned on July 24, Scheppegrell found the result to be almost incredible. Most of the tumor had disappeared, taking with it a large part of the left vocal cord. The patient's acute illness had apparently resulted from the sloughing process. X-ray treatment was recommended and was continued for an additional 10 days, at which time the ulceration in the larynx had completely healed and the patient was sent home. Scheppegrell published the case in the New York Medical Journal (as well as in the British and French literature) with follow-up as of October 25, 1902, at which time the patient was in excellent condition with no evidence of recurrence. His voice had improved, and he had resumed his law practice.[130–132] Unfortunately, when Charles Allen (a New York dermatologist) cited the case in his 1904 radiotherapy textbook, he added, "This patient, I am informed, subsequently died from the disease."[7]

Leonard Dobson, of London, reported a case of advanced larynx cancer treated by radiation during 1901 and 1902.

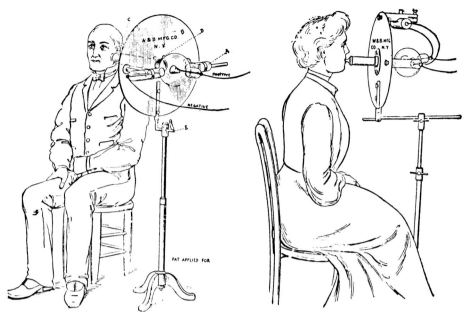

FIG. 1-10. Treatment of facial skin and intraoral cancer with an x-ray tube mounted behind an "Allen shield," illustrated by dermatologist Charles W. Allen of New York in his 1904 radiation therapy textbook. He reported that he had used this apparatus "constantly for about two years with much satisfaction. It is a great saving of time, as the patient has only to sit before the opening in the disk, and is also saved the discomfort of a mask or metallic covering to the body. . . . Treatment can be applied to any area in any position of patient." While cautioning that "we cannot to-day rely fully upon the ray alone," he was nevertheless enthusiastic about the results of x-ray treatment: "Let not the man arise who will cry, 'Away with x-ray for inoperable cancer!' until he can proclaim a nearer approach to a cure." (Allen CW: Radiotherapy and Phototherapy Including Radium and High-Frequency Currents, Their Medical and Surgical Applications in Diagnosis and Treatment, p 103. New York, Lea Brothers, 1904)

The tumor initially involved the neck lymph nodes and was considered to be too advanced for an operation. By October 1901, the patient, a 64-year-old man, could not speak above a whisper and required tracheostomy for dyspnea. He was weak and cachectic. As a desperation measure, x-ray treatments were begun. The report is vague as to the details of the treatment, but apparently the patient received daily 5-minute exposures over the course of several months. The neck nodes all but disappeared, and the primary tumor decreased greatly in size. The patient could talk again and take long walks. In June 1902, treatments were temporarily discontinued because he suddenly developed a severe skin reaction; they were resumed after the skin healed, and the tumor continued to shrink. Although treatments were reduced to 3-minute sessions three times a week, very soon "the skin again gave way."[45] At this time it was decided to switch to "electrotherapy" using high-frequency current. X-rays were tried again from time to time, but "one short exposure even was sufficient to create an angry blush of the skin."[45] The patient remained well until the autumn of 1902, when "a small abscess formed and burst at the side of the tracheotomy wound, leaving a fistulous track which never afterwards completely healed."[45] About November 1902, the tumor began to grow again, and by March 1903 it was noted to have regained its original size. The patient went slowly downhill. Finally, "the whole right side of the neck necrosed," and he died of hemorrhage in August 1903.[45] Dobson noted that although ultimately the patient had died, his life was much longer and better in quality than seemed possible when the x-ray treatments were started.[45]

The radiation sources available at this time produced large amounts of "soft" radiation, automatically producing a proportionately greater effect on the skin and superficial tissues. Some early therapists attempted to avoid severe radiation reactions by giving extremely cautious doses over a prolonged period of time, as in the Swedish skin cases. Other early therapists assumed that the immediate effects of radiation, those that are now considered acute side-effects, were the important ones—they thought the tumor would burn up as if cauterized or would necrotize and slough as if resected.[24] In order to maximize such a result, these therapists emphasized applying the largest possible dose in the shortest possible time.

There was initially no way at all to measure the radiation being applied or to predict its effect on the patient. In 1902, Guido Holzknecht of Vienna developed a "pastille radiometer," based on the observation that certain chemicals would change color upon exposure to roentgen rays. His initial "chromoradiometer" was not very successful, but by 1910 he had developed a system that consisted of a 4½-inch-long celluloid band that was colorless at one end and shaded through orange to deep brown at the other, which was compared to an exposed pastille to determine the radiation dosage (the darker the color of the exposed pastille, the higher the dose). The deepest color indicated an "epilation dose" when the pastille was placed halfway between the skin and the source of radiation. If the pastille was placed directly on the skin, the measured dose was only about one fourth as great, so higher doses could be measured. The reading had to be taken less than 1 minute after the radiation exposure because the color faded rapidly.[123] The system was inexact and subjective, but, according to Quimby, it was the best available at the time. The only alternative was still more subjective: direct observation of the effects of radiation on the skin. This was expressed in terms of the "erythema dose," the amount of radiation required to produce reddening of the skin when given in a single dose. The amount of radiation required to produce this effect would vary, of course, from patient to patient and from one radiation source to another, but the concept of the erythema dose was widely used nevertheless.

Considering the indeterminate amount and quality of radiation produced by the early tubes and the general ignorance of the biologic effects of radiation, it is little wonder that massive, sometimes fatal necrosis of soft tissue, bone, and cartilage often occurred in the first patients treated for head and neck cancer. At the same time, since only the superficial tissues were receiving tumoricidal doses of radiation, cancer cures were few. Probably only skin cancers or other very superficial malignancies were actually cured in the earliest period of therapy development, although radiation was tried on almost everything, malignant or otherwise.

The more extensive tumors, especially those extending into deeper tissues, would show a good apparent response but would then come back. As James Ewing later commented, "This fact proved most disconcerting, and I well remember my own feeling of amazement and incredulity upon finding that a tumor process once caused to regress and apparently disappear could start to grow again from the remnants of damaged cells."[53] By 1910, there was disillusionment with the new modality, and it was feared that its uses as a curative agent were strictly limited.

Early Radium Therapy

One way around the limitations of superficial treatment was to try to place the radiation source directly onto the tumor, either by inserting it into a body cavity or by surgically exposing the tumor. X-ray tubes were awkward to use in this way, and "curie therapy" using natural radiation sources was begun soon after radium was discovered in 1898 by the Curies. The biologic effects of radium exposure were discovered inadvertently by Becquerel in 1901, when he left a tube of radium in his vest pocket for several hours. Fourteen days later, a reaction occurred on the underlying skin. Pierre Curie realized the possible medical value of radium and gave some to a Paris physician for experimentation. Only very minute amounts of radium were then available, but radium therapy was reported in Paris in 1901, in the United States in 1903, and in Germany, England, and Russia in 1904. For head and neck cancer, applicators consisting of tubes containing radium salts (perhaps 25 mg of radium in one or two tubes) were inserted into the mouth or (as suggested by Alexander Graham Bell in 1903—see Chapter 13, Time–Dose–Volume Relationships in Radiation Therapy) buried in tumors. Perhaps the best of these early applicators was reported in 1908 by Henri Dominici, of the Radium Institute of Paris. The "Dominici tube" enclosed the radium in platinum, which filtered out much of the less energetic radiation and thus decreased the side-effects of treatment. Walter C. Stevenson, of Dublin, devised the method of sealing "radium emanation," radon gas, in tiny capillary tubes that could then be loaded into hollow needles and inserted into a tumor, distributing the dose of radiation much more evenly than was possible by any other method. Stevenson reported good results in cases of parotid cancer, cancer of the floor of the mouth, and "malignant glands of the neck," among others (Fig. 1-11). This method, first used in 1914, was the forerunner of modern interstitial therapy.[88,144]

Many of the early experimenters with curie therapy were surgeons. In the United States, Robert Abbe, better known as a pioneer plastic surgeon (creator of the Abbe flap), began the use of radium in the treatment of head and neck cancer at St. Luke's Hospital in New York in 1903.[1] In 1912 Henry H. Janeway was appointed chief of cancer surgery and radiation therapy at Memorial Hospital in New York. Janeway was motivated in his radical experimentation partially by the fact that he himself suffered from ameloblastoma of the mandible, which was first diagnosed in 1905, was operated on many times, and was treated with various types of radiation therapy before finally causing his death in 1921.[53] Among other techniques, Janeway treated his patients with glass capillary seeds containing radon, which he distributed into the tumors. The radiation was essentially unfiltered and caused severe reactions, although as Ewing stated, "If the patient could stand the ordeal, he was often rewarded by an unexpected cure of extensive disease."[53] Janeway was able to report cures of lip, tongue, and tonsil cancers using this method.

> All cases of carcinoma of lip, tongue, tonsil, skin, in his service were immediately assigned to radiation therapy. . . . The radical nature of this step may be revealed by the fact that the first cases of lip cancer treated by interstitial irradiation were done surreptitiously and the cases were exhibited only after all traces of the disease had disappeared, and all protests were throttled.[53]

Gioacchino Failla, Janeway's radiation research chief at Memorial after 1915, developed gold casing for the radon seeds in 1924 (only one of Failla's many contributions to clinical radiation physics through the years). Because the gold covering filtered out most of the beta radiation, these seeds produced fewer side-effects and were used in the treatment of head and neck tumors for many years.[54]

The Beginnings of Modern Radiation Therapy

The development of x-ray therapy was left primarily to the radiologists. As Ewing expressed it,

> The atmosphere of roentgen therapy was quite obnoxious to conservative minds. The noisy racket of the transformer, the noxious gases exhaled from the tubes in ill-ventilated rooms, and the retching of nauseated patients, created a repulsive contrast to the solemn ceremonies of the surgical amphitheater. . . . All one could really do was to place the patient under the machine and hope for the best.[53]

Physicists attempted very early to develop objective means for measuring radiation output. After the more reliable Coolidge tube was introduced in 1913, it was feasible to express radiation output in terms of the known milliamperage and kilovoltage of the tube, and by adding the factors of exposure time and source-to-skin distance to the equation, a dose could be calculated (e.g., skin dose) for any given beam. This formula was developed sufficiently enough by 1927 that MacKee could publish a set of dose tables, and his technique of dose prescription was used, particularly by dermatologists, for many years.[123]

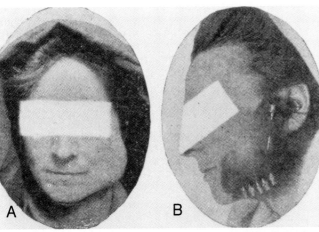
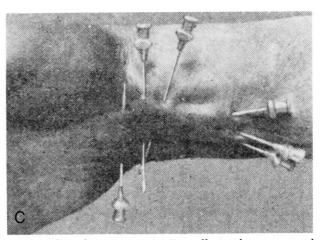

FIG. 1-11. One of the first interstitial "radium emanation" needle implants reported by Walter C. Stevenson, of Dublin, was in a case of unresectable "mixed parotid sarcoma." (*A*) Prior to treatment, the tumor was fixed and the patient had severe trismus. (*B*) Placement of the needles for the third implantation. Needles, containing varying amounts of radon, were left in place for 1 to 2½ days. According to Lederman, patients went home after the needles were inserted and returned for their removal.[88] After four implants, 7 weeks from the start of treatment, the tumor was much smaller and no longer fixed, and the patient could open her mouth. (*C*) The needles can be seen in more detail in a photograph of the implant of a painful "fibrous scar" of the wrist. (Stevenson WC: Preliminary clinical report on a new and economical method of radium therapy by means of emanation needles. Br Med J 2:9–10, 1914)

The ionization effect of radiation was recognized by Röntgen only a few weeks after he discovered x-rays, and this effect was used along with the other methods mentioned above to measure radiation. In 1914 Szilard detailed the requirements for a practical, objective radiation meter and described an ionization chamber that was the forerunner of modern instruments. An internationally recognized radiation unit, the roentgen, was defined and adopted in 1928.[123]

Claudius Regaud, head of the radiobiologic laboratory of the Radium Institute in Paris, began after World War I to study the effects of x-rays in animals. He found that it was impossible to sterilize the testicles of a ram or rabbit with a single dose of radiation without causing extensive tissue destruction, but if the dose was divided into several fractions, sterilization could be achieved without serious tissue damage. Regaud theorized that the rapidly dividing testicular cells might be analogous to cancer cells, and on this basis Henri Coutard began treating head and neck cancers at the Institute with fractionated doses of x-rays in 1919. This work was the foundation of modern external-beam radiation therapy.[81] After careful experimentation with varying dosage schedules, Coutard concluded that the best results were obtained by repeating small doses of radiation daily for several weeks. The x-ray machines he used were so low in output that each patient was treated for at least 50 minutes a day, ranging up to periods of 3 to 4 hours a day that were divided into a morning and an afternoon session. Treatments were administered 7 days a week, with occasional days of rest if the treatment continued for more than 25 days. The best results were obtained when he treated patients with cancer of the tonsillar region for 30 to 40 days; patients with cancer of the lower pharynx for 24 to 31 days; and patients with cancer of the larynx for 15 to 21 days. In general, smaller tumors could be given lower total doses over shorter periods, whereas

larger treatment fields required higher doses over lengthier periods. Coutard used some of the early dosimeters—in 1932 he mentioned both "ionometric apparatus" and the "colorimetric scale of Holzknecht, with disks of platinocyanide of barium"—but his main guide to correct dosage was the reaction produced in the patient's tissues.[37] Coutard developed this subjective evaluation into almost an art. He made careful drawings of the tumor response and the radiation reaction as they occurred in each patient. He found that all the patients who were cured by irradiation from 1920 to 1926 had a definite pattern in their radiation response, and he concluded that this pattern was a necessary prerequisite to cure. About 13 to 14 days after the start of treatment, "radioepithelitis of the mucosa" appeared, evolving to denudation and false membrane formation and then healing totally by 26 to 28 days into the treatment. At this time the skin reaction, "radioepidermitis," would begin, healing in turn by the 42nd day. If these reactions did not occur in just this pattern, recurrence was bound to happen.[28,37,92] Late effects were often severe; for example, of eight patients treated by Coutard for hypopharyngeal cancer during 1932 and 1933, four were alive and free of recurrence after 5 years. Three had severe skin changes and sclerosis of the treated areas, and one required permanent tracheostomy. All four survivors later died of second cancers appearing in the irradiated area between the sixth and tenth year after treatment.[9]

In 1926 François Baclesse joined Coutard, and in 1936 he became chief of the radiation therapy department at the Radium Institute. He gradually extended the treatment courses in order to reduce the severe acute and late reactions in normal tissues. He used somewhat higher total doses, but smaller daily doses, which he administered over 60 to 74 days, and he reduced the size of the treatment portal partway through the treatment when possible.[9,38,55,84,92]

During the late 1920s and 1930s, therapists in Europe and the United States gradually adopted the "Coutard technique." Maurice Lenz, of New York City, who trained in Paris, commented in 1934 that "Coutard's method of roentgen therapy of cancer of the upper respiratory tract is being used more widely each year."[93] He noted that the use of machines of higher milliamperage resulted in shorter treatment times, making the method practical for treating large numbers of patients in a clinical setting.[92]

Coutard himself ended his career in the United States in Colorado Springs. According to Juan A. del Regato, Coutard treated and cured a Colorado mining tycoon named Spencer Penrose who had carcinoma of the larynx in Paris in the early 1930s when del Regato was in training there.* Seven years later, Penrose developed a second primary cancer in his esophagus. Coutard was by this time practicing in Chicago, and Penrose went there to be treated again by radiation but did not like the summer weather in Chicago. He bought an up-to-date General Electric 400-kV radiation therapy unit and had it installed in his home, a large estate located behind the Broadmore Hotel in Colorado Springs, so that he could complete his therapy at home in comfort. The treatment this time was unavailing, and Penrose died in 1939 of the esophageal cancer. Penrose had donated his radiation treatment machine to the Sisters of Charity at the Gluckner Hospital in Colorado Springs, and when they told him they had no place to put the equipment, he built a new wing on the hospital to house it. After her husband's death, Mrs. Penrose, childless and wealthy, wished to establish a cancer treatment center in Colorado Springs as a memorial to her husband. Coutard, then over 60 years old, was offered every inducement to move to Colorado Springs, and he became Director of Research of the Penrose Tumor Clinic in 1941. He spent the last years of his life in Colorado Springs, where he enjoyed frequent hikes in the Rockies, before returning to France in 1949 at the age of 73. Dr. William Moss, en route to Manchester for a 1-year fellowship in radiation therapy, sailed on the same ship; he relates that Coutard unfortunately became quite eccentric in his last years.† Coutard died in France in 1950.[10,43] Dr. del Regato became head of the brand new Penrose Cancer Hospital in 1949 and was its director for 25 years.

Treatment of Nasopharynx Cancer

Nasopharynx tumors were scarcely ever recognized before the 20th century. In 1901 Jackson found only 13 cases in the world medical literature.[77] Godtfredsen attributed to Michaux the first (1845) report of a histologically verified nasopharyngeal tumor; the patient, a 45-year-old man who had suffered increasing difficulty in swallowing for a year, died immediately following Michaux's attempt to extirpate the tumor.[63]

---

* Another famous patient treated at the Radium Institute while Dr. del Regato was in training there was the French writer François Mauriac (1885–1970). Dr. del Regato relates that Mauriac had had a hemilaryngectomy for larynx cancer in 1932 but had developed a recurrence about a year later. The recurrent tumor was cured by radiation therapy. Mauriac was thus able to continue his career as a distinguished novelist (1952 Nobel laureate) and political and religious writer (del Regato JA: Personal communication, 1982). His voice for the rest of his life was "a hoarse whisper."[139]

† Moss W: Personal communication, 1982.

Martin theorized that the failure to recognize nasopharynx tumors was due to the lack of early symptomatology referable to the nasopharynx and the propensity for early metastatic spread; in many cases the patient would die of metastatic disease before the primary site was apparent.[108] With the resources of 20th-century medicine, nasopharynx tumors began to be diagnosed more frequently. In 1911 Trotter was able to elucidate the clinical syndrome. He hoped that this might lead to earlier diagnosis and might permit successful surgical treatment. He said that all eight patients on whom he had attempted radical excision had had advanced disease at diagnosis and that all had suffered recurrence by 15 months.[153]

Because the results of surgery were so poor, radiation therapy was attempted very early, but the early x-ray tubes could not deliver an adequate dose to the tumor. Applicators were devised to hold radium in the nasopharynx, directly against the tumor, but long-term results were poor.

Lymphoepithelioma was described in 1921 as a pharyngeal tumor with distinctive histologic and clinical features.[126,133] It was found to be more sensitive to radiation than the typical squamous cell carcinoma. Although the nature and even the existence of lymphoepithelioma as a pathologic entity were later disputed, most reported series of nasopharyngeal cancers since the 1930s have included separate statistics for lymphoepithelioma and in general have shown it to have a better cure rate than squamous cell carcinomas.

As early as 1920 radiation therapy was the treatment of choice for the primary lesion, although there was still some controversy regarding treatment of the neck metastases that were so prominent a feature of this disease. Irradiation of a nasopharynx tumor was (and still is) a test of the expertise of the therapist. Delivering an adequate dose to the tumor in the middle of the head while avoiding overdosage of the normal tissues (skin, brain, eyes, ears, and so on) was a serious technical problem, especially when all that was available were 200-kV x-rays and radium or radon seeds. In addition, therapists only gradually came to understand the patterns of spread of the tumor—especially into the base of skull—well enough to be able to define the tumor volume. Recurrence often resulted from underestimation of the tumor spread rather than from the lack of means to deliver an adequate dose.

The two radiation techniques most often used during the 1930s and 1940s were the Coutard technique, in which 200-kV x-rays or teleradium were used to deliver a 6- to 8-week course by way of several lateral or anterior fields, and the Radiumhemmet technique, which involved two 2-week courses of external therapy with an intracavitary radium application in between. By the late 1930s, reported cure rates ranged from 0 to about 25% at 5 years. Furstenberg, of Ann Arbor, Michigan, reported 1 of 40 patients alive at 2 years and concluded that "the prognosis remains hopelessly futile."[58] His patients were treated by "radical excision, electrocoagulation, x-ray and radium therapy in various combinations."[58] In 1931, the Radiumhemmet, using their combination of external and intracavitary treatment, had achieved a 5-year survival rate of 11.4% in 70 cases.[63] From the Mayo Clinic, an overall 5-year survival rate of 8.9% was reported, 15.6% (5/32) for patients without neck metastases on admission. The patients were treated with intracavitary radium plus external x-ray or teleradium therapy.[114] Lederman wrote, "The results of radiotherapy are universally poor and ours are no exception."[87] Averaging the results of several series from this era, he found a 15% overall cure rate. This was in line with his own results for patients treated from 1933 to 1955 with 200 kV: about 13% survival at 5 years.[87]

A few therapists achieved better results. Lenz wrote that about 25% of patients could be expected to survive for at least 5 years.[91] Using 200-kV x-rays, he reported a 5-year survival rate in 2 of 14 patients with carcinoma and in 6 of 17 with lymphoepithelioma. Martin, of Memorial Hospital, used a combination of intracavitary radium or radon seeds plus a 200-kV external beam administered by way of angled anterior fields. He listed the many "gloomy reports" in the literature, but his results were more hopeful: 20 of 80 patients (25%) were free of disease after 5 years or more. If there were no neck node metastases at the time of admission, the 5-year survival rate was 39%. He also analyzed survival by histology: 11 patients of 51 (22%) for carcinoma, 6 out of 14 (43%) for lymphoepithelioma.[108]. At M. D. Anderson Hospital, the 5-year absolute survival rate for patients treated with orthovoltage radiation was approximately 30%. In order to achieve these results with orthovoltage, very complex techniques had to be used if severe side-effects and complications were to remain within tolerable limits (Fig. 1-12).

The use of supervoltage radiation equipment began in the early 1950s. The supervoltage radiation was important because, with its skin-sparing qualities, therapists could deliver higher doses to larger fields more easily. The technique of irradiation was still the key factor. By the early 1960s, improved cure rates were reported from major centers. In 1963 a series from Massachusetts General Hospital revealed a 48% 5-year survival rate for patients treated with supervoltage radiation (2 MeV Van de Graaff). The analysis took into account not just survival rate and histology, but also the stage of the disease and the site of failure. One subgroup of patients, comprising those with involvement of the cranial nerves, the paranasal sinuses, or the base of the skull, was found to have a very poor prognosis.[96] Similar results were reported for M. D. Anderson Hospital, where it was found that involvement of the base of the skull or of the cranial nerves resulted in virtually no cures.[56] The treatment technique was modified at M. D. Anderson Hospital in 1962 by increasing the dose to the base of the skull for T3 and T4 lesions; as a result, the local control for the T4 lesions increased from essentially 0 to approximately 50%, and there was an improvement in the overall cure rate. As a result of sophisticated analysis of radiation dosage, treatment volume, and sites of failure, doses were subsequently increased for the T1 and T2 lesions beginning in 1972. The incidence of local control of these less advanced lesions increased from 76% (42 of 55 patients) for patients treated from 1954 to 1971 to 94% (16 of 17 patients) for those treated from 1972 to 1977. Thanks to the meticulous treatment technique, no central nervous system (CNS) complications resulted from the increased dose. Overall, for the 251 nasopharynx cases treated at M. D. Anderson Hospital from the first use of supervoltage radiation in 1954 until 1977, the 5-year survival rate was 52%.[109]

Elective Neck Irradiation

It was gradually recognized that radiation treatment could also be used for neck disease and that it could be used electively for possible subclinical neck disease. Douglas Quick, of Memorial Hospital, was one of the first to advocate

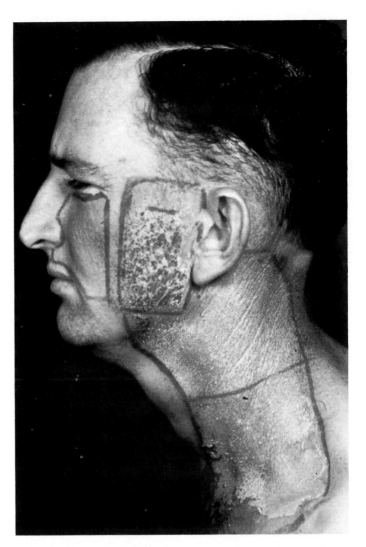

FIG. 1-12. The orthovoltage technique for carcinoma of the nasopharynx adopted at M. D. Anderson Hospital consisted of eight portals. The nasopharynx was treated through two lateral portals tilted 10° posteriorly and two anterior portals tilted 20° to 30° medially. The four upper and lower neck portals were treated separately with the patient supine and the head rotated away from the side being treated. The superior margin of the lateral portal was approximately 2 cm above the zygoma. With the differential absorption in bone plus the dose reduction at the periphery of an orthovoltage portal, the dose in the base of skull would be too low to cure many advanced cases. The figure shows the skin reaction at the completion of the radiation therapy course. It was necessary to treat all eight portals each day in order to avoid moist desquamation. The skin of the lower neck was less tolerant of radiation than the skin of the upper neck, and the upper neck was less tolerant than the facial skin. It required 8 to 9 weeks to deliver 4500 rad to the lower neck. Treatment of the primary lesion could sometimes be completed in 7 to 8 weeks, but 9 to 10 weeks was often necessary because of the severe mucositis. The local control with orthovoltage was 67% (24 of 36 patients), and the neck control was 71%. For comparison, the initial supervoltage results (1954–1960) showed a local control of 76% (45 of 59 patients) and regional control of 81%.

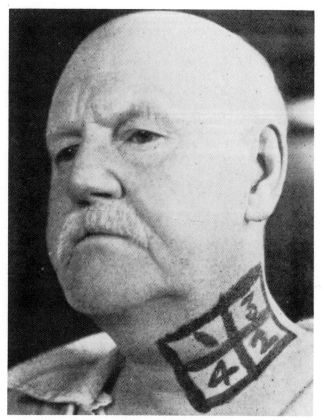

FIG. 1-13. Neck treatment portals for Sir Stanford Cade's teleradium technique, which he considered "the best method of external irradiation of the cervical lymphatic field." The teleradium unit at Westminster Hospital, London, could treat a field 3.5 cm in diameter, so four to six ports of entry were required. As Cade described it, "The treatment of the neck . . . requires on an average 60 exposures or 12 hours per port. The dose delivered at a depth of 4 cm from the skin varies from 4000 to 6000 r. The maximum skin dose is 7000 to 9000 r. Moist peeling of the skin occurs at the end of the fourth week. Healing is rapid, and is complete in 2 or 3 weeks." (Cade S: Malignant Disease and Its Treatment by Radium, pp 181–182. Bristol, John Wright and Sons, 1949)

elective neck irradiation in the 1920s. Describing the procedure there, he said "Patients presenting with no palpably enlarged metastatic nodes on admission for treatment, are subjected to heavy external irradiation and kept under routine observation."[122] In 1928 he reported that of 289 patients with tongue cancer without clinically involved neck nodes at the time of admission, 103 (36%) later developed neck node metastases. This perhaps represented a slight improvement over what would have been expected without any neck treatment at all. Quick used a combination of a 4-g radium pack and x-ray therapy from both sides of the neck.[121,122] In 1933, Bernard Widmann, of Philadelphia General Hospital, reported the results of elective neck irradiation in patients with carcinoma of the lip. Of 52 patients who had elective neck irradiation, 17% developed neck node metastases; of 72 patients whose necks showed no clinical signs of cancer and were not irradiated, 51% developed neck node metastases. Widmann used "high-voltage roentgen rays" (which in that era meant probably 200 kV) or radium packs.[166]

With the equipment then available, it was difficult to deliver an adequate, well-distributed dose to the neck. For example, the crusty surgeon Stanford Cade, of Westminster Hospital, London, was puzzled, frustrated, and disillusioned by his failure with elective neck irradiation. He had observed some modest success with irradiation of grossly enlarged cervical lymph nodes and properly reasoned that occult disease could be managed by "prophylactic" irradiation. However, his results, as reported in his classic book *Malignant Disease and Its Treatment by Radium*, were disappointing: "In my own series of 100 cases that were [electively] treated, the incidence of metastasis was only slightly smaller than in the group of 50 patients where no treatment was given and the patient kept under observation."[27] This led Cade to recommend ipsilateral radical neck dissection in cancers of the tongue or the floor of the mouth after irradiation of the primary site. Why did Cade have such poor results? For one thing, he was using a teleradium device that could irradiate only a tiny (3.5-cm square) portal. The numbered squares shown in Figure 1-13 were tiny separate treatment fields, almost sure to give an erratic dose pattern. (As Cade himself noted, "the actual distribution of radiation so provided leaves much to be desired.")[27] But more importantly, only the midneck was irradiated; the subdigastric and submandibular lymph nodes were completely ignored. In light of these factors, it is little wonder that his elective irradiation was unsuccessful.

Development of Supervoltage Radiation Therapy

Enthusiasm for radiation therapy once again waned in the 1940s as the delayed effects of radiation became apparent. For example, Hayes Martin, an enthusiastic proponent of radiation therapy in the 1930s, wrote the following in a 1948 review article:

> Fractionated radiation therapy for cancer of the larynx brought about some promising initial results. . . . Such early hopes have not been sustained by the experience of the past twenty years. Radiation therapy will cure a small percentage of cases of laryngeal cancer, both extrinsic and intrinsic. This method of treatment, however, is uncertain and fraught with serious complications that may arise at any time, even years following completion of therapy.[106]

Martin turned instead to radical surgery.[100]

It was thought that better results could be obtained if higher doses could be delivered at the proper depth without producing disastrous side-effects; this led to the development of megavoltage radiation sources. Low-megavoltage (1 MeV–2 MeV) Van de Graaff generators came into clinical use in the 1940s, but it was after World War II that supervoltage treatment became practical on a large scale. Cobalt-60 could be produced in a nuclear reactor in large enough quantities to make a high-dose-rate, economical teletherapy unit feasible, and the first such units were developed in the United States and Canada in 1951.[134] In a 1958 review, E. Dale Trout reported that about 200 cobalt-60 units were in use throughout the world. By 1973 the number was over 1100.[156]

One of the authors (Million) began his training at M. D. Anderson Hospital on the first cobalt-60 unit in the United States, a ceiling-mounted unit that was developed through a joint effort by the Oak Ridge Institute of Nuclear Studies and the M. D. Anderson Hospital and was manufactured by General Electric.[65] Collimation was accomplished with a set of removable lead cones; the maximum field size was 15 cm × 15 cm. The unit was awkward beyond belief and required considerable dexterity and a suitable vocabulary of four-letter words to accomplish certain techniques.

Accelerators for the production of x-rays were first developed in the 1940s. By 1958, Trout reported that a dozen betatrons were in use for cancer therapy, and several linear accelerators were then in use in England and at Stanford in the United States.[156] Accelerators could also be used to administer electron-beam therapy, and the first experimental use of this modality began in the 1950s. Betatrons and linear accelerators of increasingly high energy were put in use during the 1960s, and electron-beam treatment units became standard equipment during the 1970s.

Development of the Current Concept of Radiation Oncology

Gilbert Fletcher (and his associate, Fernando Bloedorn) must receive a great deal of the credit for modernizing the radiation treatment of head and neck cancers. Doses were pushed to previously unheard-of levels, and cure rates went up, often accompanied by an increase in complications. Repeated analyses of the specific cause of failure (e.g., local recurrence, regional metastases, distant metastases) and complications led to numerous refinements in the techniques of head and neck irradiation.

It is easy to see the development of radiation therapy as a succession of machines, each more powerful than the one before, but in his review entitled "The Evolution of the Basic Concepts Underlying the Practice of Radiotherapy from 1949 to 1977" Fletcher wrote about the developments in radiobiology and treatment planning that he considered far more important than the changing capabilities of the machines used to deliver the radiation.[55] He noted that the prevailing concepts in 1949, when he entered the field, were (1) an "all or none cancerocidal dose," linked with the histology of the disease; (2) a homogeneous dose of irradiation to the entire target volume; (3) the use of a single treatment modality, either irradiation or surgery; (4) postoperative irradiation, used only for recurrence, rather than electively; and (5) the acceptance of only radical surgical procedures for use in cancer cases. He then went on to describe the changes that had taken place. Fundamental discoveries in radiation biology were made in the 1950s, such as the discovery that the effect of radiation on cells was dependent on the presence of molecular oxygen, which was followed by the discovery of areas of hypoxic cells in human tumors.[124,148] In 1956 the survival curve for irradiated cells was found to be exponential.[120] The concept of the steep sigmoid-shaped dose–response curve was developed, demonstrating that small differences in radiation dose could produce wide differences in the result of treatment. The curve was found to be applicable both to tumor control and to damage to normal tissues. Finally, Fletcher listed the ways in which these new concepts were applied to radiation therapy during the 1970s. First, the volume of cancer was more important than the histology in determining the dose of radiation required for cure. Larger tumors, containing higher proportions of hypoxic cells, would require higher doses of radiation for control than small tumors. Second, the dose did not have to be homogeneous through the entire area of interest but could reflect the varying concentrations of tumor that were present. The "shrinking field" technique, originated by Baclesse, was used to deliver lower doses to large areas surrounding a tumor mass for control of "subclinical disease" (disease statistically assumed to be present, but not clinically evident) and to deliver higher doses to a smaller field centered over the bulk of the tumor. Third, irradiation could be used as a supplement to surgery in situations in which it was most likely to be successful (e.g., the treatment of microscopic or small-volume cancer), just the opposite of the early days when radiation treatment was reserved for the hopelessly large, unresectable tumors. Fourth, as a corollary, large tumors should be resected, if possible. Fifth, since the dose–response curve was very steep, an optimum dose, which varied with the clinical situation, had to be determined and maintained. Sixth, conservative surgical resection might be combined with modest doses of radiation to yield a better quality of life for the patient than either modality alone.[55]

The fractionation schedules in radiation therapy are still being investigated and revised. The dissociation of acute and late effects on normal tissues as reported recently by Thames and co-workers supports the current interest in multiple daily fractions.[147]

During these years, the specialty of radiation oncology was coming of age. Fletcher estimated that there were 25 full-time radiation therapists in the United States in 1949, compared with more than 1500 in 1980.[55] Many of the early American radiation therapy specialists, such as Maurice Lenz, Traian Leucutia, Isadore Lampe, Franz Buschke, Juan A. del Regato, Gilbert H. Fletcher, Fernando Bloedorn, and many others, were foreign born and trained in Europe. However, in the early years, most radiation therapy in this country was administered by general radiologists with only 6 to 12 months of training in radiation therapy. Dermatologists were also briefly trained in the technical aspects of radiation therapy, and they administered superficial therapy for skin conditions. (Some, such as Jesshill Love, went on to become full-time radiation therapists). Despite the best efforts of the pioneers, radiation therapy was long considered a technical skill (and the therapists as "button pushers") rather than a respectable oncologic specialty. Three-year radiation therapy training programs emerged in the 1960s, but it was not until 1978 that the "general radiology" option (combining diagnostic and therapeutic training) was totally discontinued in the United States in favor of separate training programs. At the University of Florida the training period in radiation therapy was extended as of September 1983 from 4 years to 5 in order to further improve the quality of training by allowing for 8 months of additional time in radiation therapy and 4 months of additional elective time in surgery, medicine, radiology, pathology, and clinical research.

Sophisticated treatment planning dates from the early 1960s, when computers were first used for external-beam and interstitial isodose distributions. In the 1980s the next phase of treatment planning is just beginning, with the use of the computed tomography (CT) scan added to correct for tissue inhomogeneities. The need for radiation physicists, dosimetrists, and therapeutic technicians is only just beginning to be met on a broad scale as the 1980s begin, and the training of these specialized support personnel is currently a top priority in the field of radiation therapy.

REFERENCES

1. Abbe R: Radium in surgery. JAMA 47:183–185, 1906
2. Absolon KB, Keshishian J: First laryngectomy for cancer as

performed by Theodor Billroth on December 31, 1873: A hundred anniversary. Rev Surg 31(2):65–70, 1974

3. Absolon KB, Rogers W, Aust JB: Some historical developments of the surgical therapy of tongue cancer from the seventeenth to the nineteenth century. Am J Surg 104:686–691, 1962

4. Ackerknecht EH: Rudolf Virchow, Doctor, Statesman, Anthropologist, pp 98–105. Madison, University of Wisconsin Press, 1953

5. Ackerknecht EH: Medicine at the Paris Hospital 1794–1848, pp 122–124. Baltimore, Johns Hopkins Press, 1967

6. Ackerknecht EH: Primitive surgery. In Brothwell D, Sandison AT: Diseases in Antiquity: A Survey of the Diseases, Injuries and Surgery of Early Populations, pp 635–650. Springfield, IL, Charles C Thomas, 1967

7. Allen CW: Radiotherapy and Phototherapy Including Radium and High-Frequency Currents, Their Medical and Surgical Applications in Diagnosis and Treatment, pp 103, 190. New York, Lea Brothers, 1904

8. Ashbrook J: Tycho Brahe's nose. Sky and Telescope 6:353, 358, 1965

9. Baclesse F: Roentgentherapy in cancer of the hypopharynx. JAMA 140:525–529, 1949

10. Baclesse F: Coutard (1876–1949). J Radiol Electrol 31:475, 1950

11. Bakamjian V: A technique for primary reconstruction of the palate after radical maxillectomy for cancer. Plast Reconstr Surg 31:103–117, 1963

12. Bakamjian V, Littlewood M: Cervical skin flaps for intraoral and pharyngeal repair following cancer surgery. Br J Plast Surg 17:191–210, 1964

13. Batrawi AM: Report on the human remains. Mission Archéologique de Nubie 1929–1934, p 186 and Plate XV. Cairo, Government Press, 1935 (cited in Brothwell [19])

14. Beck C: Röntgen Ray Diagnosis and Therapy, p 390. New York, D. Appleton, 1904

15. Bell B: A System of Surgery, 6th ed, vol 2, p 387; vol 4, pp 482–486; vol 5, pp 93–97 and Plate 44. Edinburgh, Bell and Bradfute, 1796

16. Berven E: The development and organization of therapeutic radiology in Sweden. Radiology 79:829–841, 1962

17. Bickmore JT: Grant's cancer. Trans Am Acad Ophthalmol Otolaryngol 80:366–374, 1975

18. Brooks JJ, Enterline HT, Aponte GE: The final diagnosis of President Cleveland's lesion. Trans Stud Coll Physicians Phila 2:1–25, 1980

19. Brothwell D: The evidence for neoplasms. In Brothwell D, Sandison AT: Diseases in Antiquity: A Survey of the Diseases, Injuries and Surgery of Early Populations, pp 320–340. Springfield, IL Charles C Thomas, 1967

20. Brown AJ: Old masterpieces in surgery: The surgery of Albucasis. Surg Gynecol Obstet 38:428–429, 1924

21. Brown AJ: Old masterpieces in surgery: The plastic surgery of Tagliacozzi. Surg Gynecol Obstet 39:518–519, 1925

22. Brown AJ: Old masterpieces in surgery: The Pentateuch and Operations of Surgery by Hieronymus Fabricius of Acquapendente. Surg Gynecol Obstet 39:842–843, 1925

23. Bryant JD: A history of two hundred and fifty cases of excision of the superior maxilla. Trans Med Soc State NY, 1893, p 63 (cited in Morreels [112])

24. Buschke F: Radiation therapy: Historical perspectives. Radiol Clin Biol 40:217–220, 1971

25. Butlin HT, Spencer WG: Diseases of the Tongue, pp 346–366; 393–397. London, Cassell & Co, 1900

26. Butterfield WC: Tumor treatment, 3000 B.C. Surgery 60:476–479, 1966

27. Cade S: Malignant Disease and Its Treatment by Radium, 2nd ed, Vol II, pp 153–183. Baltimore, Williams & Wilkins, 1949

28. Cantril ST: Radiation therapy in cancer of the larynx. A review. Am J Roentgenol Radium Ther Nucl Med 81:456–474, 1959

29. Case JT: History of radiation therapy. In Buschke F: Progress in Radiation Therapy, Vol 1, pp 13–41. New York, Grune & Stratton, 1958

30. The case of the late Emperor Frederick. Br Med J 2:836–841, 1888

31. Christ JE: A historical perspective of the floor of the mouth. Surg Gynecol Obstet 149:745–750, 1979

32. Clerf LH: Manuel Garcia's contribution to laryngology. Bull NY Acad Med 32:603–611, 1956

33. Clerf LH: Jacob DaSilva Solis–Cohen, M.D.: Pioneer laryngologist. Ann Otol Rhinol Laryngol 81:599–602, 1972

34. Conley JJ, Vonfraenkel PH: Historical aspect of head and neck surgery. Ann Otol Rhinol Laryngol 65:643–655, 1956

35. Converse JM: Plastic surgery: The twentieth century: The period of growth (1914–1939). Surg Clin North Am 47:261–278, 1967

36. Corner GW: Salernitan surgery in the twelfth century. Br J Surg 25:84–99, 1937

37. Coutard H: Roentgen therapy of epitheliomas of the tonsillar region, hypopharynx, and larynx from 1920 to 1926. Am J Roentgenol Radium Ther 28:313–331, 1932

38. Coutard H: Principles of x-ray therapy of malignant diseases. Lancet 2:1–8, 1934

39. Crile GW: Excision of cancer of the head and neck with special reference to the plan of dissection, based on one hundred and thirty-two operations. JAMA 47:1780–1786, 1906

40. Curtis TA, Cantor R: The maxillofacial rehabilitation of President Grover Cleveland and Dr. Sigmund Freud. J Am Dent Assoc 76:359–361, 1968

41. Dastugue J: Tumeur maxillaire sur un crâne du moyen-âge. Bull Cancer 52:69–72, 1965

42. Delavan DB: A history of thyrotomy and laryngectomy. Laryngoscope 43:81–96, 1933

43. del Regato JA: Henri Coutard, M.D., 1879–1950. Radiology 54:758, 1950

44. Derry DE: Anatomical report. Archeological Survey of Nubia, Bulletin 3:29, 1909 (cited in Brothwell [19])

45. Dobson LC: A case of carcinoma of the larynx treated by x-ray and high frequency currents. West London Med J 9:46–49, 1904

46. Donegan WL: An early history of total laryngectomy. Surgery 57:902–905, 1965

47. Durham AE: On the operation of opening the larynx by section of the cartilages, etc., for the removal of morbid growths. Medico-Chir Trans 55:17–90, 1872

48. Elliot Smith G, Dawson WR: Egyptian Mummies, p 157. London, George Allen & Unwin, 1924

49. Elliott GR: The microscopical examination of specimens removed from General Grant's throat. Medical Record 27:289–290, 1885

50. El-Rakhawy MT, El-Eishi HI, El-Nofely A, Gaballah MF: A contribution to the pathology of ancient Egyptian skulls. Anthropologie (Bruenn) 9:71–78, 1971

51. Erichsen JE: The Science and Art of Surgery, Being a Treatise on Surgical Injuries, Diseases, and Operations, p 655. Brinton JH (ed). Philadelphia, Blanchard and Lea, 1854

52. Esser JF: Studies in plastic surgery of the face. Ann Surg 65:297–315, 1917

53. Ewing J: Early experiences in radiation therapy. Am J Roentgenol Radium Ther 31:153–163, 1934

54. Failla G: The development of filtered radon implants. Am J Roentgenol Radium Ther 16:507–525, 1926

55. Fletcher GH: The evolution of the basic concepts underlying the practice of radiotherapy from 1949 to 1977. Radiology 127:3–19, 1978

56. Fletcher GH, Million RR: Malignant tumors of the nasopharynx. Am J Roentgenol Radium Ther Nucl Med 93:44–55, 1965

57. Freund L: Elements of General Radio-Therapy for Practitioners, p 291. Lancashire GH (trans). New York, Rebman Company, 1904

58. Furstenberg AC: Malignant neoplasms of the nasopharynx. Surg Gynecol Obstet 66:400–404, 1938

59. Garcia M: Observations on the human voice. Proc R Soc Lond 1855, pp 399–410

60. Garcia M: Physiological observations on the human voice. Transactions of the Seventeenth International Medical Congress, Vol 3, p 197. London, 1881 (quoted in Thomson [149])

61. Gerlings PG: Laryngeal carcinoma—Some considerations with reference to the illness of Emperor Frederick III. Eye Ear Nose Throat Monthly 47: 566–571, 1968

62. Gladykowska-Rzeczycka J: Mandibular tumor in a male skeleton from a medieval burial ground in Czersk. Folia Morphol (Warsz) 37:191–196, 1978

63. Godtfredsen E: Ophthalmologic and neurologic symptoms at malignant nasopharyngeal tumours: A clinical study comprising 454 cases with special reference to histopathology and the possibility of earlier recognition. Acta Psychiat Neurol, Suppl 34, 1944

64. Goldman JL, Roffman JD: Indirect laryngoscopy. Laryngoscope 85:530–533, 1975

65. Grimmett LG, Kerman HD, Brucer M, Fletcher GH, Richardson JE: Design and construction of a multicurie cobalt teletherapy unit. A preliminary report. Radiology 59:19–31, 1952

66. Gross SD: A System of Surgery: Pathological, Diagnostic, Therapeutic, and Operative, 3rd ed, Vol II, p 472. Philadelphia, Blanchard and Lea, 1864

67. Gussenbauer C: Ueber die erste durch Th. Billroth am Menschen ausgeführte Kehlkopf-Exstirpation und die Anwendung eines künstlichen Kehlkopfes. Arch Klin Chir 17:343–356, 1874

68. Haagensen CD: An exhibit of important books, papers, and memorabilia illustrating the evolution of the knowledge of cancer. Am J Cancer 18:42–126, 1933

69. Hamby WB: The case reports and autopsy records of Ambroise Paré, p 69. Springfield, IL, Charles C Thomas, 1960 (Translated from Malgaigne JP: Oeuvres Completes d'Ambroise Paré, Paris, 1840)

70. Harding WG II: Oral surgery and the presidents—A century of contrast. J Oral Surg 32:490–493, 1974

71. Ho JHC: Nasopharyngeal carcinoma. Adv Cancer Res 15:57–92, 1972

72. Hodges PC: The Life and Times of Emil H. Grubbe, pp 21–24. Chicago, University of Chicago Press, 1964

73. Hodges PC: An autobiographical sketch. Perspectives in Biology and Medicine 17:17–66, 1973

74. Hug E: Die Anthropologische Sammlung im Kantonsmuseum Baselland. Liestal, Kantonsmuseum Baselland, 1959 (cited in Brothwell [19])

75. Hughes Bennett J: On Cancerous and Cancroid Growths. London, Simpkin, Marshall and Co and Samuel Highley, 1849

76. Huizinga E: Sir Felix Semon. Arch Otolaryngol 84:473–478, 1966

77. Jackson C: Primary carcinoma of the nasopharynx: A table of cases. JAMA 37:371, 1901

78. Jackson C, Babcock WW: Laryngectomy for carcinoma of the larynx. Surg Clin North Am 11:1207–1227, 1931

79. Jones E: The Life and Work of Sigmund Freud, Vol 3, The Last Phase, 1919–1939, pp 89–99, 101–103, 126, 157, 240–246, 468–495. New York, Basic Books, 1957

80. Jones EWP: The life and works of Guilhelmus Fabricius Hildanus (1560–1634), Part II. Med Hist 4:196–209, 1960

81. Kaplan HS: Historic milestones in radiobiology and radiation therapy. Semin Oncol 6:479–489, 1979

82. Kernan JD: Manuel Garcia: The artist and scientist. Bull NY Acad Med 32:612–619, 1956

83. Krogman WM: The skeletal and dental pathology of an early Iranian site. Bull Hist Med 8:28–48, 1940

84. Lacassagne A: François Baclesse (1896–1967). J Radiol Electrol 49:185–186, 1968

85. Lawrence JWP: A note on the pathology of the Kanam mandible. In Leakey LSB: The Stone Age Races of Kenya, 2nd ed, Appendix A, p 139. Oosterhout NB, The Netherlands, Anthropological Publications, 1970

86. Leakey LSB: The Stone Age Races of Kenya, 2nd ed, pp 19–20, plates II–V. Oosterhout NB, The Netherlands, Anthropological Publications, 1970

87. Lederman M: Cancer of the Nasopharynx: Its Natural History and Treatment, pp 102–110. Springfield, IL, Charles C Thomas, 1961

88. Lederman M: The early history of radiotherapy: 1895–1939. Int J Radiat Oncol Biol Phys 7:639–648, 1981

89. Lee DC: Tycho Brahe and his sixteenth century nasal prosthesis. Plast Reconstr Surg 50:332–337, 1972

90. Leibowitz JO: Amatus Lusitanus and the obturator in cleft palates. J Hist Med 13:492–494, 1958

91. Lenz M: Roentgen therapy of primary cancer of the nasopharynx. Am J Roentgenol Radium Ther 48:816–832, 1942

92. Lenz M: The early workers in clinical radiotherapy of cancer at the Radium Institute of the Curie Foundation, Paris, France. Cancer 32:519–523, 1973

93. Lenz M, Coakley CG, Stout AP: Roentgen therapy of epitheliomas of the pharynx and larynx. Am J Roentgenol Radium Ther 32:500–507, 1934

94. Leonardo RA: History of Surgery, pp 141–144. New York, Froben Press, 1943

95. Lewis FO: Outstanding points in laryngectomy as developed by Mackenty and some of the other ideas relating to this operation. Laryngoscope 43:97–102, 1933

96. Little JB, Schulz MD, Wang CC: Radiation therapy for cancer of the nasopharynx. Long-term follow-up on 113 adequately treated patients. Arch Otolaryngol 77:621–624, 1963

97. Long E: A History of Pathology, pp 23, 124, 128–129. New York, Dover Publications, 1965

98. Lucente FE: The impact of otolaryngology on world history. Trans Am Acad Ophthalmol Otolaryngol 77:424–428, 1973

99. Lund FB: Hippocratic surgery. Ann Surg 102:531–547, 1935

100. MacComb WS: A biographical treatise of Dr. Hayes E. Martin. Am J Surg 136:414, 1978

101. McDowell F: Wars and skin grafting: From Bismarck to Hitler. Plast Reconstr Surg 42:76–77, 1968

102. McInnis WD, Egan W, Aust JB: The management of carcinoma of the larynx in a prominent patient, or did Morell Mackenzie really cause World War I? Am J Surg 132:515–522, 1976

103. Major RH: A History of Medicine, Vol 1, p 165. Springfield, IL, Charles C Thomas, 1954

104. Margotta R: The Story of Medicine, pp 122, 180, 184. Lewis P (ed). New York, Golden Press, 1968

105. Martin HE: The history of lingual cancer. Am J Surg 48:703–716, 1940

106. Martin HE: Cancer of the head and neck. III. Cancer of the larynx. JAMA 137:1366–1376, 1948

107. Martin HE: Richard Wiseman on cancer. Cancer 4:906–912, 1951

108. Martin HE, Blady JV: Cancer of the nasopharynx. Arch Otolaryngol 32:692–727, 1940

109. Mesic JB, Fletcher GH, Goepfert H: Megavoltage irradiation of epithelial tumors of the nasopharynx. Int J Radiat Oncol Biol Phys 7:447–453, 1981

110. Mettler CC: History of Medicine, pp 890–898, 1060, 1066–1067. Philadelphia, P Blakiston Co, 1947

111. Miller JM: Stephen Grover Cleveland. Surg Gynecol Obstet 113:524–529, 1961

112. Morreels CL Jr: New historical information on the Cleveland operations. Surgery 62:542–551, 1967

113. Nelson RB III: The final victory of General U. S. Grant. Cancer 47:433–436, 1981

114. New GB, Stevenson W: End results of malignant lesions of the nasopharynx. AMA Arch Otolaryngol 38:205–209, 1943

115. Ober WB: The case of the Kaiser's cancer. Pathol Annu 5:207–216, 1970

116. Pack GT, Campbell R: Historical case records of cancer: The

laryngeal cancer of Frederick III of Germany. Ann Med Hist 2:151–170, 1940

117. Paré A: Ten Books of Surgery with the Magazine of the Instruments Necessary for It, pp 261–262. Linker RW, Womack N (trans): Athens, Georgia, University of Georgia Press, 1969

118. Park R: An epitome of the history of carcinoma. Bulletin of the Johns Hopkins Hospital 14:289–294, 1903

119. Paul of Aegina: The Seven Books of Paulus Aegineta. Adams F (trans), 1844 (quoted in Zimmerman and Veith [168])

120. Puck TT, Marcus PI: Action of x-rays on mammalian cells. J Exp Med 103:653–666, 1956

121. Quick D: Surgery and radiation in the treatment of cancer of the buccal cavity. Report of the International Conference on Cancer (British Empire Cancer Campaign), pp 146–152. Bristol, John Wright & Sons, 1928

122. Quick D: Treatment of cancer of the lip and mouth. Am J Roentgenol Radium Ther 21:322–327, 1929

123. Quimby EH: The history of dosimetry in roentgen therapy. Am J Roentgenol Radium Ther 54:688–703, 1945

124. Read J: The effect of ionizing radiations on the broad bean root. Part X. The dependence of the x-ray sensitivity on dissolved oxygen. Br J Radiol 25:89–99, 1952

125. Reichborn-Kjennerud I: The School of Salerno and surgery in the North during the saga era. Tjomsland A (trans): Ann Med Hist 9:321–337, 1937

126. Reverchon L, Coutard H: Lympho-epithelioma de l'hypopharynx. Comptes Rendus Soc Franc d'Otol Laryngol Rhinol 34:209–214, 1921 [cited in Godtfredsen [63]]

127. Roberts AC: Facial reconstruction by prosthetic means. Br J Oral Surg 4:157–182, 1966

128. Sandison AT: Letter: Kanam mandible's tumor. Lancet 1:279, 1975

129. Schechter DC, Morfit HM: The evolution of surgical treatment of tumors of the larynx. Surgery 57:457–479, 1965

130. Scheppegrell W: A case of cancer of the larynx cured by the X rays. NY Med J 76:984–986, 1902

131. Scheppegrell W: A case of cancer of the larynx cured by the X rays. J Laryngol Rhinol Otol 18:70–76, 1903

132. Scheppegrell W: Un cas de cancer du larynx gueri par les rayons X. Rev Hebd Laryngol Otol Rhinol 1:305–311, 1903

133. Schmincke A: Über lymphoepitheliale Geschwülste. Beitr Path Anat Allg Path 68:161–170, 1921

134. Schulz MD: The supervoltage story. Am J Roentgenol Radium Ther Nucl Med 124:541–559, 1975

135. Seelig MG: Cancer and politics: The operation on Grover Cleveland. Surg Gynecol Obstet 85:373–376, 1947

136. Shaw H: Manuel Garcia—A centenary tribute. J Laryngol Otol 69:343–346, 1955

137. Sigerist HE: The historical development of the pathology and therapy of cancer. Bull NY Acad Med 8:642–653, 1932

138. Singer C, Underwood EA: A Short History of Medicine, 2nd ed, pp 53–55, 98–99. New York, Oxford University Press, 1962

139. Smith MA: François Mauriac, pp 43–44. New York, Twayne, 1970

140. Solis Cohen J: Does excision of the larynx tend to the prolongation of life? Transactions of the College of Physicians of Philadelphia, pp 353–369, April 4, 1883

141. Steckler RM, Edgerton MT, Gogel W: "Andy Gump." Ann Surg 128:545–547, 1974

142. Steckler RM, Shedd DP: General Grant: His physicians and his cancer. Am J Surg 132:508–514, 1976

143. Stell PM: The first laryngectomy. J Laryngol Otol 89:353–358, 1975

144. Stevenson WC: Preliminary clinical report on a new and economical method of radium therapy by means of emanation needles. Br Med J 2:9–10, 1914

145. Strouhal E: Ancient Egyptian case of carcinoma. Bull NY Acad Med 54:290–302, 1978

146. Sushruta: An English Translation of The Sushruta Samhita. Based on the original Sanskrit text, edited and published by KKL Bhishagratna, Vol 1, pp 152–154. Calcutta, Wilkins Press, 1907 (quoted in Zimmerman and Veith [168])

147. Thames HD Jr, Withers HR, Peters LJ, Fletcher GH: Changes in early and late radiation responses with altered dose fractionation: Implications for dose–survival relationships. Int J Radiat Oncol Biol Phys 8:219–226, 1982

148. Thomlinson RH, Gray LH: The histological structure of some human lung cancers and the possible implications for radiotherapy. Br J Cancer 9:539–549, 1955

149. Thomson St.C: The history of the laryngoscope. Laryngoscope 15:181–184, 1905

150. Thomson St.C, Colledge L: Cancer of the Larynx, pp 75–88, 136–146. London, Kegan Paul, Trench, Trubner and Co, 1930

151. Thorwald J: The Triumph of Surgery, pp 195–206. New York, Pantheon Books, 1960

152. Transactions of the Section on Cutaneous Medicine and Surgery of the American Medical Association, 1902, pp 90–146. Chicago, American Medical Association, 1903

153. Trotter W: On certain clinically obscure malignant tumours of the nasopharyngeal wall. Br Med J 2:1057–1059, 1911

154. Trotter W: Principles and technique of the operative treatment of malignant disease of the mouth and pharynx. Lancet 1:1075–1081, 1913

155. Trotter W: A method of lateral pharyngotomy for the exposure of large growths in the epilaryngeal region. J Laryngol Rhinol Otol 35:289–295, 1920

156. Trout ED: History of radiation sources for cancer therapy. In Buschke F (ed): Progress in Radiation Therapy, Vol 1, pp 42–61. New York, Grune & Stratton, 1958

157. Veith I: The surgical achievements of ancient India: Sushruta. Surgery 49:564–568, 1961

158. Voight A: Behandlung eines inoperablen Pharynxkarzinoms mit Röntgenstrahlen. Ärztlichen Verein in Hamburg, November 3, 1896 (cited in Case [29])

159. Walsh J: Galen's writings and influences inspiring them. Part IV. Ann Med Hist 9:34–61, 1937

160. Weir NF: Theodore Billroth: The first laryngectomy for cancer. J Laryngol Otol 87:1161–1169, 1973

161. Wells C: Ancient Egyptian pathology. J Laryngol Otol 77:261–265, 1963 (cited in Wells [164])

162. Wells C: Two mediaeval cases of malignant disease. Br Med J 1:1611–1612, 1964

163. Wells C: Bones, Bodies, and Disease: Evidence of Disease and Abnormality in Early Man, pp 70–75. New York, Frederick A Praeger, 1964

164. Wells C: Disease of the maxillary sinus in antiquity. Medical and Biological Illustration 27:173–178, 1977

165. Whicker JH, Devine KD: Wilfred Batten Lewis Trotter, 1872 to 1939: His legacy to pharyngeal surgeons. Arch Otolaryngol 97:423–425, 1973

166. Widmann BP: Carcinoma of the lip: Results of roentgen and radium treatment. Am J Roentgenol Radium Ther 32:211–217, 1934

167. Wold KC: Ulysses S. Grant—His last battle. Tic 34(7):10–12, 1975

168. Zimmerman LM, Veith I: Great Ideas in the History of Surgery, pp 56–67, 81–89. Baltimore, Williams & Wilkins, 1961

The Natural History of Squamous Cell Carcinoma

RODNEY R. MILLION

EPIDEMIOLOGY

The estimated number of new head and neck cancer cases (excluding skin cancer) for 1982 in the United States was approximately 37,700; this represented about 5% of the total new cancer cases for that year.[38] The ratio of occurrence for males versus females was approximately 3:1 to 4:1. Head and neck cancers are usually diagnosed when the patient is past the age of 40, except for salivary gland and nasopharyngeal tumors, which may occur in younger age groups. There has been no major change in the incidence of head and neck cancer over the past 3 decades in either the male or female population, which is a bit surprising, since a common etiologic factor, cigarette smoking, has resulted in a large increase in lung cancer. Cigarette smokers have an increased risk for multiple head and neck primary lesions and also lung cancer. Alcohol has also been implicated as a causative factor for certain head and neck cancers, and the effects of alcohol and tobacco seem to be additive.[43]

PRIMARY LESION

Most squamous cell (epidermoid) carcinomas and their variants begin as surface lesions, but occasionally they may arise from ducts of minor salivary glands, in which case they originate below the surface of the visible mucosa. This latter phenomenon is more likely to occur in the floor of the mouth, the base of the tongue, and the nasopharynx. The very early surface lesions may show only erythema and a slightly elevated, smooth or minimally roughened mucosa. These are the so-called red lesions, which always deserve consideration for biopsy.

The early asymptomatic red lesions may be either carcinoma *in situ* or invasive carcinoma. About one third will have a component of leukoplakia. Pure white lesions turn out to be carcinoma *in situ* or invasive carcinoma in approximately 10% of cases biopsied. The most common sites for detection of asymptomatic red lesions are the floor of the mouth, the oral tongue, the soft palate, the anterior tonsillar pillar, and the retromolar trigone—areas that may be easily examined by dentists and physicians. Asymptomatic red lesions of the pharyngeal walls, supraglottic larynx, and hypopharynx have occasionally been detected during routine follow-up of head and neck cancer patients.

Each anatomical site has its own peculiar spread patterns, and these will be described separately in the following chapters. Muscle invasion is a common feature, and a tumor may spread along muscle or fascial planes for a surprising distance from the palpable or visible lesion. A tumor may attach to periosteum or perichondrium quite early, but actual bone or cartilage invasion is usually a late event. Bone and cartilage act as a barrier to spread, and these structures are generally spared until the neoplasm has explored easier avenues of growth. A tumor that encounters cartilage or bone in its path will usually be diverted and spread along a path of less resistance. Slow-growing neoplasms of the gingiva may produce a pressure defect or saucerization of the underlying bone with minimal or no bone invasion detected by microscopic examination of the specimen.

Entrance of a tumor into the parapharyngeal space allows superior or inferior spread from the base of the skull to the root of the neck, but most parapharyngeal space involvement is confined above the hyoid.

Spread inside the lumen of a duct, such as those of the sublingual, submaxillary, and parotid glands, is not a prevalent pattern. The nasolacrimal duct is frequently invaded in ethmoid sinus carcinoma and nasal carcinoma.

Perineural spread is an important pathway for tumor spread; no site or histology is immune to this growth pattern. Squamous cell carcinoma and its variants and minor salivary gland tumors, especially adenoid cystic carcinoma, may show this pattern. Local recurrence increases the likelihood of perineural involvement, and tumors may track along a nerve to the base of the skull. Peripheral perineural spread (*i.e.*, growth away from the central nervous system) has been seen. Patients with perineural invasion will often develop minor neurologic symptoms. Some nerve palsies are secondary to compression or entrapment rather than to actual nerve invasion.

LYMPHATIC SPREAD

The risk of lymph node metastasis may be predicted by the differentiation of the tumor (the more poorly differentiated, the greater the risk), by the size and depth of penetration of the primary lesion, and by the availability of capillary lymphatics. The risk of lymphatic spread increases with recurrent lesions.

No histology is excluded from lymphatic spread; mere access to the capillary lymphatics determines the opportunity for it. Minor salivary gland tumors and sarcomas, for example, assume a risk of lymphatic metastasis similar to squamous cell carcinoma for each anatomical site. For instance, a minor salivary gland tumor or sarcoma arising in the nasopharynx would have a relatively high risk for lymphatic metastasis, while the same tumors would have

a relatively low risk should they arise from the maxillary antrum.

It is common for a patient to present with a metastatic lymph node and, despite an extensive workup, have the site of origin remain undetermined. If only the neck is treated, a primary lesion may appear at a later date, but for many of these patients one never appears. This strongly suggests spontaneous healing of the initial lesion.

The risk of subclinical disease in the lymph nodes in a patient with a neck that shows no clinical evidence of cancer may be determined either by studying the incidence of positive nodes found in elective neck dissection specimens or by counting the number of necks initially normal that become positive when the neck is not treated.

The relative risk for cervical metastatic disease for squamous cell carcinomas developing at various sites is outlined in Table 2-1.[29]

The relative incidence of clinically positive lymph nodes by anatomical site and T stage is shown in Table 2-2. The risk for clinically positive nodes and more advanced neck disease increases with the T stage, except for the nasopharynx and hypopharynx.

There is usually an orderly progression of lymph node involvement, but skips and random involvement may occur.

Well-lateralized lesions spread to ipsilateral neck lymph nodes. Lesions on or near the midline and lateralized tongue and nasopharyngeal lesions may spread to both sides, but they tend to spread to the side occupied by the bulk of the lesion. Patients with clinically positive lymph nodes in the ipsilateral side of the neck are at risk for contralateral disease, especially if the nodes are large or if multiple lymph nodes are involved. Obstruction of the lymphatic pathways caused by surgery or radiation therapy will also shunt the lymphatic flow to the opposite side of the neck. This shunting occurs mainly through anastomotic channels by way of the submaxillary and submental shuttle.[11]

TABLE 2-1. Incidence of Lymph Node Metastasis by Site of Primary in Head and Neck Squamous Cell Carcinomas

Site	N+ at Presentation	N0 Clinically, N+ Pathologically	N0 → N+ With No Neck Treatment
Floor of mouth	30%–59%[15,17,21]	40%–50%[18,40]	20%–35%[1,6,31]
Gingiva	18%–52%[5,9,15,28]	19%[5]	17%[1,5]
Hard palate	13%–24%[8,10,28]		22%[1]
Buccal mucosa	9%–31%[15,21]		16%[1]
Oral tongue	34%–65%[15,17,20,21]	25%–54%[3,9,16,23,40]	38%–52%[16,20,31,41]
Nasopharynx	86%–90%[4,26,32]		19%–50%*[19,33]
Anterior tonsillar pillar/retromolar trigone	39%–56%[2,22,25]		10%–15%[39]
Soft palate/uvula	37%–56%[2,22,25]		16%–25%[25]
Tonsillar fossa	58%–76%[4,17,22,26,32]		22%†[37]
Base of the tongue	50%–83%[22,32,35,39]	22%[35]	
Pharyngeal walls	50%–71%[22,32,35,39]	66%[35]	
Supraglottic larynx	31%–54%[17,39]	16%–26%[35,36]	33%[12,36]
Hypopharynx	52%–72%[9,35,39]	38%[35]	

* T1N0 patients only.

† Patients received preoperative irradiation.

(Mendenhall WM, Million RR, Cassisi NJ: Elective neck irradiation in squamous cell carcinoma of the head and neck. Head Neck Surg 3:15–20, 1980)

TABLE 2-2. Percentage of Clinically Detected Nodal Metastasis on Admission, by T Stage—2044 Patients (M. D. Anderson Hospital, 1948–1965)

Primary Site	Stage	Percentage N0	N1	N2–N3
Oral tongue*	T1	86	10	4
	T2	70	19	11
	T3	52	16	31
	T4	24	10	66
Floor of the mouth*	T1	89	9	2
	T2	71	18	10
	T3	56	20	24
	T4	46	10	43
Retromolar trigone/ anterior tonsillar pillar†	T1	88	2	9
	T2	62	18	20
	T3	46	21	33
	T4	32	18	50
Soft palate†	T1	92	0	8
	T2	64	12	24
	T3	35	26	39
	T4	33	11	56
Tonsillar fossa†	T1	30	41	30
	T2	32	14	54
	T3	30	18	52
	T4	10	13	76
Base of the tongue†	T1	30	15	55
	T2	29	14	56
	T3	26	23	52
	T4	16	8	76
Oropharyngeal walls†	T1	75	0	25
	T2	70	10	20
	T3	33	22	44
	T4	24	24	52
Supraglottic larynx‡	T1	61	10	29
	T2	58	16	26
	T3	36	25	40
	T4	41	18	41
Hypopharynx§	T1	37	21	42
	T2	30	20	49
	T3	21	26	54
	T4	26	15	58
Nasopharynx‖	T1	8	11	82
	T2	16	12	72
	T3	12	9	80
	T4	17	6	78

* T stage defined by Lindberg.[24]
† T stage defined by Fletcher and co-workers.[13]
‡ T stage defined by Fletcher and co-workers.[14]
§ T stage defined by MacComb and co-workers.[27]
‖ T stage defined by Chen and Fletcher.[7]

(Lindberg R: Distribution of cervical lymph node metastases from squamous cell carcinoma of the upper respiratory and digestive tracts. Cancer 29:1446–1449, 1972)

When well-lateralized lesions metastasize contralaterally, the subdigastric node is the one most commonly involved. Occasionally the subdigastric may be bypassed, in which case the midjugular or low jugular is most often affected. When lymph node metastases appear in an unexpected distribution, a careful search must be made for a second primary. The lymphatic collecting trunks empty into the venous system at the root of the neck, but very rarely, retrograde lymph node metastases in the ipsilateral axilla may be associated with involvement of the lower neck nodes.

DISTANT SPREAD

The incidence of distant metastases for 5019 cases reviewed by Merino and co-workers was about 11% for squamous cell carcinoma of all head and neck sites.[30] The incidence by site and stage is shown in Tables 2-3 and 2-4. The risk of distant metastases was similar for patients treated by radiation therapy or surgery when compared by stage. As expected, the risk of distant metastasis increases with T stage, N stage, and total stage, but it is most dependent on

TABLE 2-3. Incidence of Distant Metastasis by Site—Head and Neck Squamous Cell Carcinoma (5019 Cases*)

Primary Site	Incidence of Distant Metastasis
Oral cavity	7.5%
Faucial arch	6.7%
Oropharynx	15.3%
Nasopharynx	28.1%
Paranasal sinuses and nasal cavity	9.1%
Supraglottic larynx	15.0%
Vocal cord	3.1%
Hypopharynx	23.6%
Total	10.9%†

* Minimum 2-year follow-up.
† Excludes 41 patients in whom distant metastasis was found only at autopsy.
(Adapted from Merino OR, Lindberg RD, Fletcher GH: An analysis of distant metastases from squamous cell carcinoma of the upper respiratory and digestive tracts. Cancer 40:145–151, 1977)

TABLE 2-4. Risk of Distant Metastasis by Stage

Stage	Risk	T Stage	Risk	N Stage	Risk
I	2%	T1	5.2%	N0	4.9%
II	5.7%	T2	9.6%	N1	11.8%
III	8.5%	T3	12.7%	N2	21.8%
IV	19.5%	T4	16.1%	N3	27.1%

(Adapted from Merino OR, Lindberg RD, Fletcher GH: An analysis of distant metastases from squamous cell carcinoma of the upper respiratory and digestive tracts. Cancer 40:145–151, 1977)

TABLE 2-5. Risk of Distant Metastasis Related to Initial Neck Control—Primary Sites in Oral Cavity, Clinically Negative Neck, No Elective Neck Treatment, Primary Lesion Controlled

No. Patients	Neck Control	Percentage With Distant Metastases
387	Neck remained negative	3%
94	Neck became positive	11%

(Data from Jesse RH, Barkley HT, Lindberg RD, Fletcher GH: Cancer of the oral cavity: Is elective neck dissection beneficial? Am J Surg 120:505–508, 1970)

TABLE 2-6. Risk of Distant Metastasis Related to Initial Neck Control—Primary Sites in Oral Tongue, Floor of Mouth, and Faucial Arch; N1, N2A, N2B Neck Disease; Primary Lesion Controlled

No. Patients	Neck Control	Percentage With Distant Metastases
134	Neck controlled by initial treatment	12%
46	Neck not controlled by initial treatment	24%

(Data from Northrop MF, Fletcher GH, Jesse RH, Lindberg RD: Evolution of neck disease in patients with primary squamous cell carcinoma of the oral tongue, floor of mouth, and palatine arch, and clinically positive neck nodes neither fixed nor bilateral. Cancer 29:23–30, 1972)

TABLE 2-7. Risk of Distant Metastasis Related to Initial Neck Control—Primary Sites in Oral Cavity and Faucial Arch; N3A, N3B Neck Disease

No. Patients	Neck Control	Percentage With Distant Metastases
20	Primary and neck controlled by initial treatment	5%
45	Primary or neck not controlled by initial treatment	31%

(Data from Votava C Jr, Jesse RH Jr, Lindberg RD, Fletcher GH: Management of cervical nodes, either fixed or bilateral, from squamous cell carcinoma of the oral cavity and faucial arch. Radiology 105:417–420, 1972)

neck stage. The lung is the most common site of distant metastasis, accounting for 52% of the first-recognized sites. Mediastinal metastases are uncommon, representing only 3%. Almost half of the metastases are recognized by 9 months, 80% are recognized by 2 years, and 90% are recognized by 3 years. The risk of distant metastasis doubles in patients who develop a recurrence above the clavicle: the risk is 16.7% for those who have a recurrence, even if they are salvaged, and 7.9% for those who never develop a recurrence.

The incidence of distant metastasis is strongly related to initial control, particularly control of the neck (Tables 2-5 through 2-7). Although squamous cell carcinoma can spread from the primary site to a distant site without involvement of the intervening lymphatics, the lymphatic system is probably the common pathway to the venous system. The available data strongly suggest that a significant percentage of distant metastasis occurs as a result of failure to achieve initial neck control. In other words, *untreated occult neck disease may shed tumor into the lymphaticovenous system and produce distant metastases while the lymph node is slowly growing to a size that can be detected.* Although some patients with neck recurrences can be regionally salvaged, many of these patients eventually die owing to distant metastasis.

REFERENCES

1. Ash CL: Oral cancer: A twenty-five year study. Am J Roentgenol Radium Ther Nucl Med 87:417–430, 1962
2. Barker JL, Fletcher GH: Time, dose, and tumor volume relationships in megavoltage irradiation of squamous cell carcinomas of the retromolar trigone and anterior tonsillar pillar. Int J Radiat Oncol Biol Phys 2:407–414, 1977
3. Beahrs OH, Devine KD, Henson SW: Treatment of carcinoma of the tongue: End-results in one hundred sixty-eight cases. Arch Surg 79:399–403, 1959
4. Berger DS, Fletcher GH, Lindberg RD, Jesse RH: Elective irradiation of the neck lymphatics for squamous cell carcinomas of the nasopharynx and oropharynx. Am J Roentgenol Radium Ther Nucl Med 111:66–72, 1971
5. Cady B, Catlin D: Epidermoid carcinoma of the gum: A 20-year survey. Cancer 23:551–569, 1969
6. Campos JL, Lampe I, Fayos JV: Radiotherapy of carcinoma of the floor of the mouth. Radiology 99:677–682, 1971
7. Chen KY, Fletcher GH: Malignant tumors of the nasopharynx. Radiology 99:165–171, 1971
8. Chung CK, Rahman SM, Lim ML, Constable WC: Squamous cell carcinoma of the hard palate. Int J Radiat Oncol Biol Phys 5:191–196, 1979
9. del Regato JA, Spjut JH: Ackerman and del Regato's Cancer: Diagnosis, Treatment, and Prognosis, 5th ed, pp 264, 281, 341–342, 345. St. Louis, CV Mosby, 1977
10. Eneroth CM, Hjertman L, Moberger G: Squamous cell carcinomas of the palate. Acta Otolaryngol (Stockh) 73:418–427, 1972
11. Fisch U: Lymphography of the Cervical Lymphatic System. Philadelphia, WB Saunders, 1968
12. Fletcher GH: Elective irradiation of subclinical disease in cancers of the head and neck. Cancer 29:1450–1454, 1972
13. Fletcher GH, Jesse RH, Healey JE Jr, Thoma GW Jr: Oropharynx. In MacComb WS, Fletcher GH: Cancer of the Head and Neck, pp 179–212. Baltimore, Williams & Wilkins, 1967
14. Fletcher GH, Jesse RH, Lindberg RD, Koons CR: The place of

radiotherapy in the management of the squamous cell carcinoma of the supralottic larynx. Am J Roentgenol Radium Ther Nucl Med 108:19–26, 1970

15. Fletcher GH, MacComb WS, Braun EJ: Analysis of sites and causes of treatment failures in squamous cell carcinomas of the oral cavity. Am J Roentgenol Radium Ther Nucl Med 83:405–411, 1960

16. Frazell EL, Lucas JC: Cancer of the tongue: Report of the management of 1554 patients. Cancer 15:1085–1099, 1962

17. Goffinet DR, Gilbert EH, Weller SA, Bagshaw MA: Irradiation of clinically uninvolved cervical lymph nodes. Can J Otolaryngol 4:927–933, 1975

18. Hardingham M, Dalley VM, Shaw HJ: Cancer of the floor of the mouth: Clinical features and results of treatment. Clin Oncol 3:227–246, 1977

19. Ho JHC: An epidemiologic and clinical study of nasopharyngeal carcinoma. Int J Radiat Oncol Biol Phys 4:183–198, 1978

20. Horiuchi J, Adachi T: Some considerations on radiation therapy of tongue cancer. Cancer 28:335–339, 1971

21. Jesse RH, Barkley HT, Lindberg RD, Fletcher GH: Cancer of the oral cavity: Is elective neck dissection beneficial? Am J Surg 120:505–508, 1970

22. Jesse RH, Fletcher GH: Metastases in cervical lymph nodes from oropharyngeal carcinoma: Treatment and results. Am J Roentgenol Radium Ther Nucl Med 90:990–996, 1963

23. Kremen AJ: Results of surgical treatment of cancer of the tongue. Surgery 39:49–53, 1956

24. Lindberg R: Distribution of cervical lymph node metastases from squamous cell carcinoma of the upper respiratory and digestive tracts. Cancer 29:1446–1449, 1972

25. Lindberg RD, Barkley HT, Jesse RH, Fletcher GH: Evolution of the clinically negative neck in patients with squamous cell carcinoma of the faucial arch. Am J Roentgenol Radium Ther Nucl Med 111:60–65, 1971

26. Lindberg RD, Jesse RH: Treatment of cervical lymph node metastasis from primary lesions of the oropharynx, supraglottic larynx, and hypopharynx. Am J Roentgenol Radium Ther Nucl Med 102:132–137, 1968

27. MacComb WS, Healey JE Jr, McGraw JP, Fletcher GH, Gallager HS, Paulus DD: Hypopharynx and cervical esophagus. In MacComb WS, Fletcher GH: Cancer of the Head and Neck, pp 213–240. Baltimore, Williams & Wilkins, 1967

28. Martin CL, Craffey EJ: Cancer of the gums. Am J Roentgenol Radium Ther Nucl Med 67:420–427, 1952

29. Mendenhall WM, Million RR, Cassisi NJ: Elective neck irradiation in squamous-cell carcinoma of the head and neck. Head Neck Surg 3:15–20, 1980

30. Merino OR, Lindberg RD, Fletcher GH: An analysis of distant metastases from squamous cell carcinoma of the upper respiratory and digestive tracts. Cancer 40:145–151, 1977

31. Million RR: Elective neck irradiation for TXNO squamous carcinoma of the oral tongue and floor of mouth. Cancer 34:149–155, 1974

32. Million RR, Fletcher GH, Jesse RH: Evaluation of elective irradiation of the neck for squamous cell carcinoma of the nasopharynx, tonsillar fossa, and base of tongue. Radiology 80:973–988, 1963

33. Moench HC, Phillips TL: Carcinoma of the nasopharynx: Review of 146 patients with emphasis on radiation dose and time factors. Am J Surg 124:515–518, 1972

34. Northrop MF, Fletcher GH, Jesse RH, Lindberg RD. Evolution of neck disease in patients with primary squamous cell carcinoma of the oral tongue, floor of mouth, and palatine arch, and clinically positive neck nodes neither fixed nor bilateral. Cancer 29:23–30, 1972

35. Ogura JH, Biller HF, Wette R: Elective neck dissection for pharyngeal and laryngeal cancers: An evaluation. Ann Otol Rhinol Laryngol 80:646–651, 1971

36. Putney FJ: Elective versus delayed neck dissection in cancer of the larynx. Surg Gynecol Obstet 112:736–742, 1961

37. Rolander TL, Everts EC, Shumrick DA: Carcinoma of the tonsil: A planned combined therapy approach. Laryngoscope 81:1199–1207, 1971

38. Silverberg E: Cancer statistics, 1982. CA 32:15–31, 1982

39. Southwick HW: Elective neck dissection for intraoral cancer. JAMA 217:454–455, 1971

40. Southwick HW, Slaughter DP, Trevino ET: Elective neck dissection for intraoral cancer. Arch Surg 80:905–909, 1960

41. Spiro RH, Strong EW: Discontinuous partial glossectomy and radical neck dissection in selected patients with epidermoid carcinoma of the mobile tongue. Am J Surg 126:544–546, 1973

42. Votava C Jr, Jesse RH, Lindberg RD, Fletcher GH: Management of cervical nodes, either fixed or bilateral, from squamous cell carcinoma of the oral cavity and faucial arch. Radiology 105:417–420, 1972

43. Wynder EL: The epidemiology of cancers of the upper alimentary and upper respiratory tracts. Laryngoscope (Suppl 8) 88:50–51, 1978

Examination With Fiberoptic Equipment

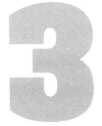

RODNEY R. MILLION
NICHOLAS J. CASSISI

The fiberoptic telescopes (FOT), both rigid and flexible, are an important addition to outpatient examination and photography (Figs. 3-1 through 3-5). The advantage of the FOT over conventional tools is that it enables the examiner to obtain a better view of the laryngeal surface of the epiglottis, the anterior commissure, the nasal cavity, and the nasopharynx. It also makes it easier to examine a patient with an abnormal epiglottis (e.g., a horseshoe or edematous epiglottis) or a large, active tongue.

Indirect mirror laryngoscopy affords a better panorama of the larynx and hypopharynx and should not be discarded.

Almost every patient can be adequately examined with the rigid FOT. The flexible FOT is useful in situations in which the epiglottis occludes the view of the larynx and in patients with a hyperactive gag reflex that cannot be controlled with a local anesthetic. The field of vision is smaller with the flexible FOT than with the rigid FOT.

The fiberoptic laryngoscope can be inverted to view the nasopharynx, and this technique is preferred over mirror examination. A small-diameter (3-mm) fiberoptic nasoscope may be used to examine the entire nasal cavity and for an anterior examination of the nasopharynx. In a small percentage of patients, especially children, satisfactory examination of the nasopharynx, nose, and larynx may require a general anesthetic.

PHOTOGRAPHY

Photographs of the larynx, pharynx, nasopharynx, and nasal cavity are made on a routine basis in the outpatient clinic (Plates l through 9 in this chapter). The Karl Storz endoscopic camera is attached to a rigid fiberoptic laryngoscope equipped with a photographic sheath.* The xenon light source produces light for both examination and photography and has the advantage over flash-generated light, which must be recycled before subsequent photographs can be made. We currently use Kodak Ektachrome ASA 400 film, which is push-processed to ASA 1200. Several photographs should be made in order to ensure obtaining a few good ones. An entire roll is exposed for new lesions if there may not be another opportunity to take photographs. A local anesthetic is suggested for even the most cooperative patient, since the added bulk and weight of the camera and the shooting process often cause slight jiggling of the scope.

Photographs taken with the small-diameter nasoscope are clear and sharp, but difficult to interpret because of the small field of vision. We have no experience with photography with the flexible FOT.

The rigid FOT may be connected to a movie camera or video camera for motion studies.

* Special thanks to Karl Storz GmbH, Tuttlingen, West Germany. Distributed in the U.S. by Karl Storz Endoscopy-America, Inc., 10111 W. Jefferson Blvd., Culver City, CA 90230.

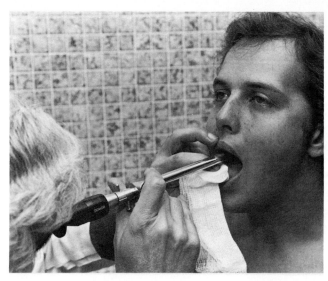

FIG. 3-1. Karl Storz rigid fiberoptic laryngoscope with photographic sheath. The distal viewing window is warmed in a bead (dental) sterilizer to prevent fogging. The tongue is held as for indirect mirror examination. The scope is rotated 90° as it is inserted over the tongue to avoid gathering saliva on the distal viewing window. The distal scope often rests against the posterior pharyngeal wall. The posterior pharyngeal wall may be difficult to visualize with a 90° telescope.

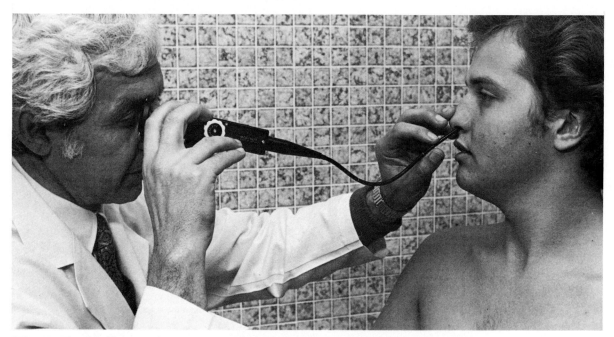

FIG. 3-2. Flexible fiberoptic laryngoscope. A local anesthetic is applied to the oropharynx and larynx. A 4% cocaine solution may be used to shrink and anesthetize the nasal mucosa. The flexible scope is sometimes required for anxious patients with a hyperactive gag reflex; a few may require intramuscular sedation. The distal viewing window is warmed and inserted under direct vision. If the viewing window becomes covered with secretions, it may be cleared by wiping it gently across the epiglottis. The tip of the scope may be curved up to 90° during examination.

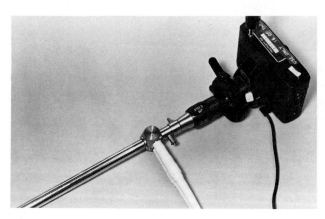

FIG. 3-3. Karl Storz endoscopic camera attached to a 90° fiberoptic laryngoscope with a photographic sheath. The motor drive for advancing film is built into the camera. Only 16 of the possible 20 frames are exposed to avoid placing an excessive work load on the small winding motor. Shrink sheaths (white) have been added where the fiberoptic cables join with the laryngoscope to avoid inadvertent loosening of the connections. Regular 35-mm camera bodies may be adapted so that they may be attached to the fiberoptic laryngoscope, but they have the disadvantage of added weight and bulk, which can render them awkward to handle.

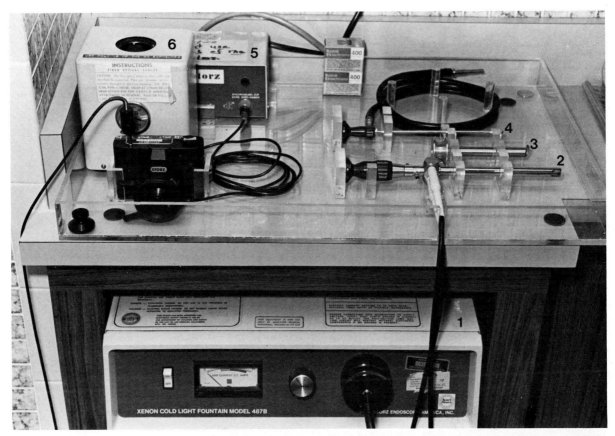

FIG. 3-4. (1) Karl Storz xenon light source. (2) Karl Storz fiberoptic laryngoscope (90°) with photographic sheath. (3) Soft palate retractor. (4) Karl Storz fiberoptic nasoscope (30°). (5) AC adapter for camera winding motor. (6) Bead sterilizer.

FIG. 3-5. Bulb release for activating camera shutter. This arrangement frees both hands for holding the scope and the patient's tongue. (Shoe courtesy of G. H. Bass & Co.)

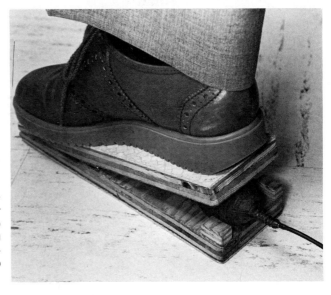

ADDENDUM (August 1984): The photographic system was modified in 1984, and the quality of the photographs has improved as a result. An Olympus OM-2N camera body was substituted for the Karl Storz camera shown in Figure 3-3. A Karl Storz adapter was needed to make the proper connection. The weight added by the Olympus camera body requires two people to steady the apparatus during photography rather than one person. One person holds the patient's tongue, while the other manages the camera and endoscope. The foot pedal with bulb release (Fig. 3-5) is still used. Use of the bead sterilizer (heater) was discontinued because the beads tended to scratch the surface of the distal viewing window; hot water is now used to prevent fogging.

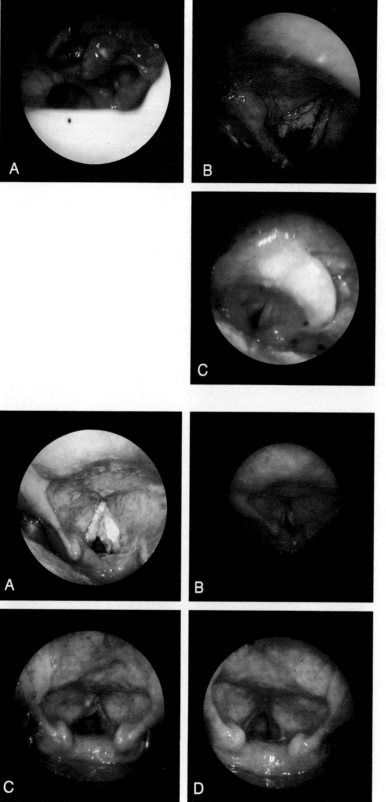

PLATE 1. (A) Early squamous cell carcinoma of the vocal cord in a 60-year-old woman. The larynx was very small, and the tip of the epiglottis rested against the posterior pharyngeal wall and prohibited outpatient examination of the larynx. The right half of the tip was amputated with a biopsy forceps. Photograph was taken 1 year after radiation therapy. Patient was free of disease at 5 years. (B) Squamous cell carcinoma of the left vocal cord with subglottic extension and involvement of the posterior left false cord and the face of the arytenoid in a patient with a 3-year history of hoarseness and left-sided sore throat. The cord was fixed (T3N0). Treatment was 7440 rad (120 rad twice a day) over 6 weeks, cobalt-60. The inferior treatment border was 2.5 cm below the cricoid cartilage. (C) Three years after treatment. Mobility has returned to normal.

PLATE 2. (A) Squamous cell carcinoma of both vocal cords with subglottic extension, 1 cm to 1.5 cm, and early involvement of the right false cord. Both cords were mobile (T2N0). Treatment was 6300 rad/28 fractions/5 weeks, cobalt-60. (B) No evidence of disease at 3½ years. (C) Squamous cell carcinoma of both vocal cords with involvement of the anterior commissure, left anterior false cord, and petiole of the epiglottis. The mobility of the left vocal cord was reduced (T2N0). Treatment was 6750 rad/30 fractions/6 weeks, cobalt-60. (D) One month after completion of therapy. Patient was free of disease at 5 years.

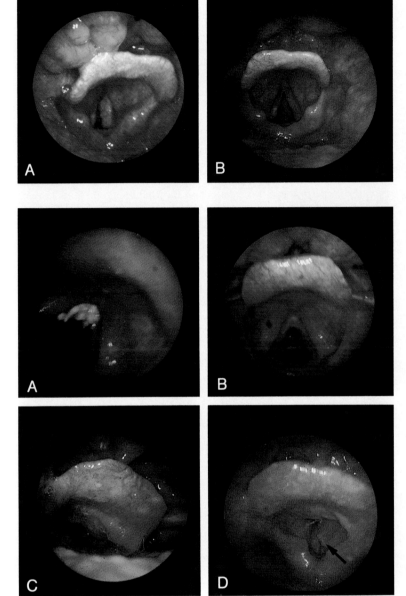

PLATE 3. (A) Squamous cell carcinoma of the right vocal cord (T1N0). There was about 2 mm of normal-appearing right vocal cord anteriorly. Treatment was 6300 rad/28 fractions/5½ weeks, cobalt-60. (B) Photograph taken 2 years after treatment. NED at 5 years.

PLATE 4. (A) Squamous cell carcinoma of the vocal cord (T2N0). Horseshoe-shaped lesion involving both vocal cords and the anterior commissure, with a 5-mm subglottic extension anteriorly and minimal involvement of the left false cord. Treatment was 6300 rad/5½ weeks (225 rad/fraction), cobalt-60 (3-field technique). (B) Photograph taken 4 months after treatment. NED 4 years. (C) Direct and indirect laryngoscopy revealed a large lesion of the right infrahyoid epiglottis in a 70-year-old man with a 3-month history of a sore throat and a 1-month history of hoarseness. The larynx was rotated clockwise. There was involvement of the right aryepiglottic fold, the medial wall of the pyriform sinus, and the right posterior false cord (not shown on this photograph). Mobility of the right arytenoid was sluggish. The vocal cords were normal. (D) Photograph at 2 months after treatment. The patient was treated with radiation therapy. There was a suspicion of persistence in the right false cord (*arrow*). Biopsies on three occasions were negative. The patient was free of disease at 2½ years; he had moderate supraglottic edema and hoarseness but no pain or airway obstruction. There was considerable fibrosis in the neck and persistent submental edema.

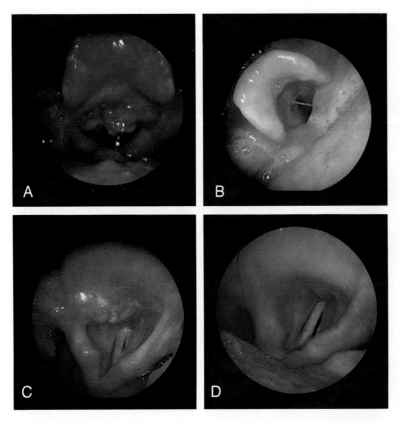

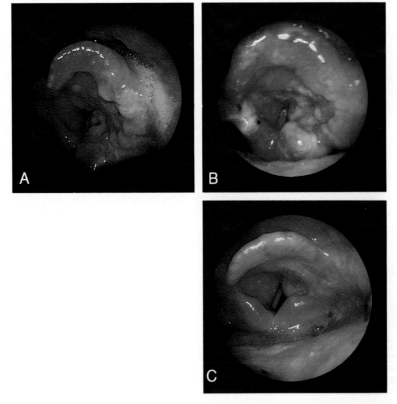

PLATE 5. (A) A 64-year-old man presented with a 6-month history of dysphagia, hoarseness, and a cough that produced mucus, sometimes mixed with blood. Past history included coronary artery disease, hypertension, pulmonary emphysema, and adenocarcinoma of the prostate. He had an exophytic, bulky squamous cell carcinoma of the infrahyoid epiglottis with minimal involvement of the false cords and aryepiglottic folds (T2N0). The anterior commissure and true vocal cords were free of disease. Irradiation was recommended because the patient was medically unsuitable for supraglottic laryngectomy and a borderline risk for total laryngectomy. He received 7000 rad/ 7 weeks, cobalt-60. (B) Photograph taken 3 years after treatment. NED at 5 years. (C) A 68-year-old man who was admitted for lens implant was noted to have a mass in the left upper neck. Examination revealed a squamous cell carcinoma of the infrahyoid epiglottis with multiple bilateral neck nodes (T2N3B). The largest lymph node on the left was 5 cm × 3 cm, and the largest lymph node on the right was 3 cm × 2 cm. All of the lymph nodes were mobile. The photograph shows a lesion of the infrahyoid epiglottis with minimal extension to the aryepiglottic fold and pharyngoepiglottic fold. Radiation therapy was elected for treatment of the primary lesion because of the desirability of combining radiation therapy and neck dissection for management of the neck. High-energy x-rays (17 MV) were selected in view of the planned bilateral neck dissection. The radiation treatment plan included 7000 rad/7 weeks, 17 MV, to the primary and upper neck. The lower neck received 5000 rad/5 weeks, 8 MV x-ray. The posterior upper neck received 1000 rad, 10 MeV electrons. Staged neck dissection followed at 1 month and 2 months after radiation therapy. (D) Photograph taken at 20 months; there was essentially no edema. NED at 30 months.

PLATE 6. (A) Squamous cell carcinoma of the right aryepiglottic fold with extension to the false cord, the pharyngoepiglottic fold, and the vallecula and across the midline of the epiglottis (T3N0) in a 52-year-old woman. The surgical alternative was total laryngectomy. The treatment plan was the administration of 4500 rad and reevaluation. (B) There was an estimated 65% regression at 4500 rad, and it was recommended that full-dose radiation therapy be completed. (C) Patient was free of disease at 3½ years.

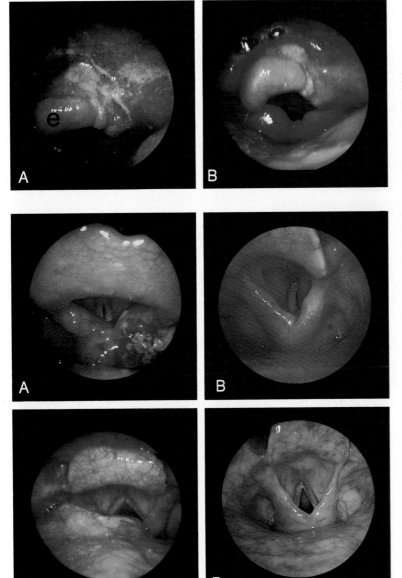

PLATE 7. (*A*) Squamous cell carcinoma of the tip of the epiglottis with extension to the right vallecula and pharyngoepiglottic fold. The epiglottis (e) was partially destroyed by tumor (T3N0). (*B*) At 3 months, there was persistent cartilage exposure, but the patient was essentially asymptomatic. There was complete healing at 1 year, and the patient was free of disease at 6 years.

PLATE 8. (*A*) There was an exophytic lesion on the medial wall of the right pyriform sinus, extending to the aryepiglottic fold and just onto the laryngeal surface of the epiglottis. The left postcricoid area was invaded submucosally. The right vocal cord was immobile, probably owing to invasion of the cricoarytenoid muscle or joint (T3N3B—Stage IV). (*B*) The final dose to the pyriform sinus and the lymph nodes was 7400 rad/6 weeks (120 rad twice a day). The enlarged lymph nodes disappeared after 4000 rad, and it was decided that the neck should be observed. The vocal cord regained full mobility 2 months after treatment. The patient's voice and swallowing were normal at 4 years. (*C*) Squamous cell carcinoma of the posterior pharyngeal wall (T2N0). The treatment plan called for 6000 rad/6 weeks, cobalt-60, and gold grain implant, 2000 rad to 2500 rad. (*D*) Three years NED.

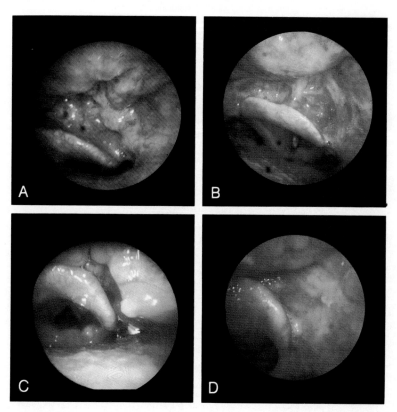

PLATE 9. (*A*) Squamous cell carcinoma of the base of the tongue (T2N3B [N2B–N2B]) in an 82-year-old man. The base of the tongue received 7500 rad/40 fractions/9 weeks (6500 rad, cobalt-60; 1000 rad, 8 MV x-ray). There was no neck dissection. (*B*) Photograph taken 22 months after treatment. NED at 3 years. (*C*) A 71-year-old woman presented with a 4-month history of a lump in the right side of her throat. There was a 4 × 5-cm submucosal lesion in the right base of the tongue, extending to the vallecula. The neck was negative. Biopsy showed low-grade mucoepidermoid carcinoma. The treatment plan was 7500 rad tumor dose/8½ weeks, cobalt-60. There was 70% regression at completion of the treatment. (*D*) There was complete disappearance of the tumor at 5 months (patient was free of disease at 30 months).

General Principles for Treatment of Cancers in the Head and Neck: Selection of Treatment for the Primary Site and for the Neck

RODNEY R. MILLION
NICHOLAS J. CASSISI

Surgery and radiation therapy are the only curative treatments for carcinoma arising in the head and neck. Chemotherapy, used alone, is not curative, and its role as an adjunct to surgery, radiation therapy, or both is being investigated.

Most early-stage head and neck squamous cell carcinomas can be cured by an operation or by irradiation, and each modality generally produces similar cure rates for lesions that are similar in size. The decision as to which form of treatment to use then rests on such factors as the functional and cosmetic result, the general stage of the patient's health, and the preference of the patient and his family. Some patients prefer to join in the selection of treatment, but most prefer to be presented with the options and told which is the best treatment for them. The prior experience of a close friend or relative involving an operation or radiation therapy is occasionally a major factor.

ADVANTAGES OF AN OPERATION

The advantages of an operation over radiation therapy, assuming comparable cure rates, *may* include the following:

1. A limited amount of tissue is exposed to treatment.
2. Treatment time is shorter.
3. The risk of immediate and late radiation sequelae is avoided.
4. Irradiation is reserved for a subsequent head and neck primary tumor that may not be as suitable for an operation. For example, a patient might have an early lesion that would usually be treated by radiation therapy, but because the remainder of the mucosa has premalignant changes suggesting a higher than usual probability of a second tumor, an operation might be selected instead.
5. Pathologic examination of tissues permits patients with more extensive disease than originally determined to be identified; for these patients, immediate postoperative irradiation can be added to the treatment.

ADVANTAGES OF RADIATION THERAPY

The advantages of irradiation *may* include the following:

The threat of a major operation is avoided. An operative mortality rate of only 1% to 2% may seem high to the patient, since there is no immediate threat from radiation therapy.

No tissues are removed. Resection of even a relatively small lesion may produce a functional or cosmetic defect. This risk must be weighed against the risk of a radiation necrosis.

Elective irradiation of the lymph nodes can be included with little added morbidity, whereas the surgeon must either adopt an attitude of "wait and see" or proceed with elective neck dissection. This is important for lesions with a high rate of spread to the lymph nodes, especially where there is a high opportunity for bilateral spread (e.g., the midline floor of the mouth, the base of the tongue, the soft palate, the hypopharynx, the supraglottic larynx, and the nasopharynx) and when large clinically positive lymph nodes are present in the ipsilateral side of the neck.

The surgical salvage of irradiation failures is more likely to succeed than the salvage of a surgical failure by operation, irradiation, or both. When irradiation is unsuccessful in treating a primary lesion, the disease almost always recurs in the center of the original lesion; disease recurring at the margins of the primary lesion is uncommon. A rescue operation can often be done that would be similar in scope to the initial operation, albeit with a greater risk for a serious complication. In some cases the rescue operation may entail a much more severe functional or cosmetic loss than if the operation had been performed initially. For example, if an epiglottic lesion suitable for supraglottic laryngectomy is treated by radiation therapy and the treatment fails, then the rescue procedure is often a total laryngectomy.

Rescue of a surgical failure may be attempted by operation, radiation therapy, or both. Surgical recurrences usually develop at the margins of the resection, in or near the suture line. It is difficult to distinguish the normal surgical scar from recurrent disease, and diagnosis of recurrence is often delayed. The response of the tumor to radiation therapy under these circumstances is poor. Surgical failures that present as small mucosal recurrences, however, can often be salvaged by either an operation or radiation therapy or by both.

Multiple simultaneous primary lesions can be treated. It is not unusual for a patient to present for treatment with more than one squamous cell carcinoma occurring simultaneously in the head and neck area, and it usually is advantageous to use radiation therapy initially. From June 1964 to October 1978, 28 patients were identified at the University of Florida as having simultaneous head and neck carcinomas. The soft palate and the floor of the mouth is the most frequent combination of areas in which carcinomas occur. The number of patients who were free of disease after 18 months is shown in Table 4-1 by T and N stage. Radiation therapy alone was administered for the primary lesions in 24 patients, with immediate neck dissection added in 4 patients. Four patients had irradiation followed by immediate resection of one primary lesion. The overall results are reasonably good because many of the patients presented with relatively small primary lesions. However, when one of the lesions is a T3 or T4, the cure rate is poor. A summary of the treatment results by stage is given in Table 4-2.

Frequently, the radiation therapist finds a second primary lesion when the patient is referred for consultation for one lesion. It is incumbent on the consulting physician to look carefully at all mucosal areas because of the possibility of a second lesion and the obvious change in treatment planning its presence would require. An odd distribution of lymph node metastases is often a clue to a second primary lesion.

INFLUENCE OF HISTOLOGY (SQUAMOUS CELL CARCINOMA AND ITS VARIANTS)

The vast majority of malignant head and neck neoplasms arise from the surface epithelium and are therefore squamous cell carcinoma or one of its many variants, including lymphoepithelioma, spindle cell carcinoma, verrucous carcinoma, and undifferentiated carcinoma.

TABLE 4-1. Simultaneous Multiple Primary Lesions:* Absolute Survival Free of Disease at 18 months (28 Patients)

Highest T stage	N0	N1	N2B	N3B
T1	3/3	0/0	1/1	0/1
T2	5/7	4/5	1/2	1/2
T3	0/2	0/1	1/1	0/2
T4	0/1	0/0	0/0	0/0

* Two or more squamous cell carcinomas separated by at least 1 cm.
Note: University of Florida data; patients treated 6/64–10/78; analysis 4/80 by S. Westgate, MD.

TABLE 4-2. Simultaneous Multiple Primary Lesions: Summary of Treatment Results

Stage	Total No. Patients	Control With Initial Treatment	Surgical Salvage Primary	Surgical Salvage Neck	Absolute Survival—NED at 18 Mo	Failure at >18 Mo	Absolute Survival—NED at 4 Yr
I	3	2/3	1/1	0/0	3/3	0	1/2
II	7	4/7	1/3	0/0	5/7	0	4/6
III	8	3/8	1/1	0/0	4/8	1 DM	2/5
IV	10	3/10	1/2	0/1	4/10	1 P	1/6
Total	28	12/28 (43%)	4/7	0/1	16/28 (57%)		8/19 (42%)

(NED, no evidence of cancer; DM, distant metastases; P, primary failure)

Note: University of Florida data; patients treated 6/64–10/78 (through 4/76 for 4-year survival); analysis 4/80 by S. Westgate, MD.

As a general rule, the less-differentiated tumors usually have a higher incidence of positive lymph nodes and a higher risk for distant metastasis than low-grade lesions of comparable size and from similar anatomical sites. This factor is taken into consideration during treatment planning. The local and regional control of squamous cell carcinoma by radiation therapy is not much affected by grade, although the survival rate is lower for a high-grade tumor, owing to the increased rate of distant metastasis. The presence of a lymphoid stroma (lymphoepithelioma) predicts a better local and regional control rate and survival when treated by irradiation compared to garden-variety squamous cell carcinoma.

During a course of radiation therapy, the response rate or disappearance rate of high-grade carcinomas is usually more rapid than that of low-grade lesions. The physician is prone to label these rapidly responding tumors "radiosensitive," but the rate of disappearance does not correlate in a linear fashion with radiocurability. (See Chapter 13, Time–Dose–Volume Relationships in Radiation Therapy.)

The gross and microscopic morphology or growth pattern plays a role in treatment results. Some squamous cell carcinomas tend to grow in an exophytic pattern with pushing borders; these lesions usually have a lower rate of lymph node metastasis and are more readily encompassed by an operation or by interstitial irradiation because the borders are well defined and the chance of missing the margins during surgery or irradiation is low. These discrete lesions tend to respond better to treatment, whether they are managed by surgery, radiation therapy, or both.

Some squamous cell carcinomas (usually the poorly differentiated ones) tend to be markedly infiltrative, with fingers of tumor cells far beyond the visible or palpable lesion. This growth pattern is associated with a higher rate of regional lymph node metastases and is generally more difficult to encompass by an operation. Since irradiation portals usually have a generous margin around the obvious lesion, it is less likely that the margins will be missed with radiation therapy, but control by radiation therapy alone is also less likely to be achieved for this growth pattern than for the more discrete lesions.

Undifferentiated lymphomas and undifferentiated carcinomas may appear similar under the microscope. Unless the clinical picture and histologic reading are definitely those of lymphoma, it is better to treat the lesion as if it were carcinoma.

Differentiating between tumor recurrence and radiation necrosis following irradiation is not always easy. Since recurrence usually implies major ablation, the clinical picture must fit the diagnosis. Several examples of misdiagnosis of recurrent cancer have been seen in which the patient had a major cancer operation for recurrence, only to find that in fact he had a radiation necrosis that might have healed with conservative therapy. The opinion of a highly qualified pathologist is invaluable in avoiding such a situation.

Lymphoepithelioma

Lymphoepithelioma is a carcinoma with a lymphoid stroma. The lymphoid stroma may or may not be present in regional lymph nodes or distant metastases. Lymphoepithelioma occurs at anatomical sites that have lymphoid aggregates in the submucosa, namely, the nasopharynx, tonsil, and base of the tongue. It has a higher rate of cure by radiation therapy than squamous cell carcinoma.

Verrucous Carcinoma

Verrucous carcinoma is a "grade one-half" squamous cell carcinoma that is most often found in the oral cavity, particularly on the gingiva and the buccal mucosa. It usually has an indolent growth pattern and is often associated with the chronic use of snuff or chewing tobacco. Verrucous tumors resemble warts: they are white or pink and exophytic, with distinct margins and multiple filiform processes that produce a roughened, cobblestone surface. The lesion may be soft or firm to palpation, depending on the degree of keratinization and associated inflammation. Often in cases of verrucous carcinoma the patient has multiple biopsies that indicate an obvious lesion, but the pathologist returns a diagnosis of hyperkeratosis or pseudoepitheliomatous hyperplasia. Eventually cancer therapy may be recommended only on the appearance of the lesion and observation of its continued growth. If the pathologist can readily make a diagnosis of carcinoma from histologic examination, the diagnosis of verrucous carcinoma is unlikely.

There is a great deal of controversy about the response of verrucous carcinoma to radiation therapy. Perez and co-workers reported eight patients with verrucous carcinoma who were treated by irradiation; all eight tumors recurred.[23] In three cases the histologic picture evolved to a markedly undifferentiated picture.

Kraus and Perez-Mesa reviewed 105 cases of verrucous carcinoma.[13] Seventeen of the lesions were treated by radiation therapy, and all recurred. Four of the recurrences showed an anaplastic transformation, and all four patients died of metastatic disease. None of the patients treated surgically developed metastases.

Fonts and co-workers reported ten patients with verrucous carcinoma, but five patients actually had well-differentiated squamous cell carcinoma.[11] Three patients developed anaplastic transformation; five patients were free of disease 1 to 3½ years after radiation therapy.

We have seen typical verrucous carcinomas disappear with radiation therapy and not recur during long periods of follow-up. It is our policy to select surgery for verrucous carcinoma whenever possible, but we do not hesitate to try radiation therapy first if the morbidity (e.g., from total laryngectomy or glossectomy) is unacceptable. Pathologists vary widely in the criteria they use to diagnose verrucous carcinoma, which probably explains some of the conflicting data, and many of the radiation therapy failures were treated with low-dose schemes. Nevertheless, prudence dictates the use of an operation when reasonable.

Spindle Cell Carcinoma

A component of spindle cells resembling sarcoma is intermixed with squamous cell carcinoma in an estimated 2% to 5% of malignant specimens taken from the upper aerodigestive tract. This picture is variously described in the literature as pleomorphic carcinoma, sarcomatoid squamous cell carcinoma, squamous cell carcinoma with spindle cell variant, pseudosarcoma, and spindle cell squamous cell carcinoma, among others. For the most part, these lesions cannot be distinguished grossly from the usual squamous cell carcinoma. In some, the spindle cell component is relatively minor; in others, it dominates the picture and the squamous cell component is difficult to find. The sarcomatoid component may have features that are consistent with malignant fibrous histiocytoma. The lymph node metastases may show only the spindle cell component, only the carcinomatous element, or a mixture of both. This pattern may be seen anywhere that squamous cell carcinoma is found in the head and neck area. Leventon and Evans reported 20 cases of spindle cell carcinoma.[14] All of the patients with superficially invasive tumors were cured, whereas only one of the ten patients with deep invasion was cured. The tumors responded both to surgery and radiation therapy, with six of the survivors being treated by operation, three by irradiation only, and two by combined treatment. Six of the tumors were said to have occurred in previously irradiated areas, and five of these patients eventually died of deeply invasive tumors. There are no data to compare the effectiveness of surgery and radiation therapy. It is our policy to disregard the spindle cell element in treatment decisions.

MANAGEMENT OF THE PRIMARY SITE

Patients with early-stage lesions (T1 N0-1, T2 N0-1) usually have a favorable prognosis when managed by either surgery or radiation therapy, and combined treatment should be avoided because it only increases the morbidity and provides little or no benefit (Fig. 4-1).[19] In the few instances of failure salvage is often achieved by a second procedure.

FIG. 4-1. American Joint Committee stage grouping.[2] T represents the primary lesion and N represents the neck. Stage IV represents a wide spectrum of disease. One patient may have a T1 or T2 lesion with treatable N2 or N3 neck disease and represent a reasonable candidate for curative therapy, while another may have either a far-advanced primary lesion or far-advanced neck disease that is virtually a hopeless situation. *Do not adopt the habit of recommending a plan of management based on T, N, or total stage. Within each stage is a variety of situations for which the treatment plan must be individually tailored to the patient.* (Million RR, Cassisi NJ, Wittes RE: Cancer in the head and neck. In DeVita VT Jr, Hellman S, Rosenberg SA [eds]: Cancer: Principles and Practice of Oncology, pp 301–395. Philadelphia, JB Lippincott, 1982)

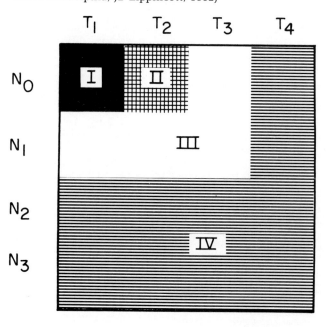

Patients with moderately advanced lesions may benefit from combined therapy in some instances, but if either radiation therapy or surgery is reasonably successful by itself, then one modality may be held in reserve if treatment fails. When combined therapy is selected, it should be aggressive, since there is rarely a chance for salvage after combined approaches.

The most difficult decision is whether to offer a curative attempt to patients with very advanced lesions. There are always anecdotal cases of patients whose advanced disease was cured. However, at best the cure rate for some very advanced lesions may be estimated at 1% to 2%. The question then becomes, is it rational to put 100 patients through major therapy with a treatment-related mortality rate of 5% to 10% and a high morbidity rate in order to cure 1 or 2 patients? Many of these patients with advanced lesions are in very poor general medical condition, and treatment with radical surgery, radiation therapy, or both is simply unrealistic. However, if the patient is in relatively good condition, and especially if he is young, then a curative approach may be considered. The patient and family must be presented the facts and assist in the decision. Frequently, when faced with a low-yield major ablative procedure the patient will select a palliative course, usually radiation therapy. Palliative surgery is used in selected cases (usually when radiation therapy has already been tried) to relieve major symptoms or reduce nursing care (e.g., in the case of tumor fungating into the skin). There are patients with very advanced disease for whom even a short course of palliative radiation therapy is considered inadvisable if symptoms can be controlled by other means. Experimental chemotherapy may be advised for advanced lesions, and often there is spectacular, if temporary, tumor regression. The best treatment may be only observation; 2% to 3% of patients seen in our clinic receive no cancer therapy, and 5% to 10% receive only palliative measures, usually radiation therapy.

MANAGEMENT OF THE NECK

Management of carcinoma that involves the neck lymph nodes is closely tied to management of the primary lesion, but certain general principles can be outlined. Death due only to failure to control metastatic tumor in the neck if the primary tumor is controlled should be an uncommon event if surgery and radiation therapy are used to maximum advantage. Variations in the management of the neck will be discussed under specific anatomical areas in later chapters.

Anatomy of the Lymphatic System of the Head and Neck

The lymphatic system arises embryonically by a budding from the venous system, which explains the close anatomical association of the two drainage systems. One of the normal functions of the lymphatic system is to reabsorb the large protein molecules and lymphocytes from the interstitial space and to return them to the bloodstream. The blood capillaries have narrow endothelial junctions and do not normally reabsorb large molecules and lymphocytes. The capillary lymphatics, on the other hand, have relatively open endothelial junctions that permit the larger molecules to be absorbed, and this probably explains why tumor cells enter the lymphatic system more readily than the vascular system.

CAPILLARY LYMPHATICS

Capillary lymphatics originate in the form of a closed cul-de-sac; the efferent vessels anastomose to form a network of lymph vessels. There are no capillary lymphatics in the epithelium, central nervous system, cartilage, bone, bone marrow, eyeball, membranous labyrinth, or placenta.[25,27] Muscle and fat contain few capillary lymphatics. There are a few capillary lymphatics in the periosteum or perichondrium but none within the bone and cartilage. The fact that there are no capillary lymphatics in the eyeball and very few within the orbit explains the low rate of lymphatic metastases for tumors arising in orbital tissues.[25]

Since there are no capillary lymphatics in the epithelium, a tumor must penetrate the lamina propria before lymphatic invasion can occur. In the mucosa and skin, the blood capillaries are generally closer to the surface than the lymphatic capillaries. In the superficial layer, the lymphatic capillaries are usually finer in diameter than in the deeper layers. The richness of the capillary network in any given head and neck site may be predicted by the relative incidence of lymph node metastases. The density of the capillary lymphatic network does not necessarily correspond to the density of the vascular capillary system. The nasopharynx and pyriform sinus have the most profuse networks of capillary lymphatics. The paranasal sinuses, middle ear, and vocal cord have few or no capillary lymphatics, which is in agreement with their low rate of lymph node metastasis when tumor is confined to these sites. The capillary lymphatic system, particularly in the larynx and trachea, tends to atrophy with age.

LYMPHATIC TRUNKS

The capillary lymphatics converge to form lymphatic trunks that have semilunar valves that direct flow to a lymph node. However, the dermal lymphatic vessels are without valves, and once cancer invades this system, flow is unpredictable and erratic, with skin nodules surfacing at remote distances from the original area of skin invasion. The lymphatic trunks eventually empty into a large vein, usually near the junction of the internal jugular vein and the axillary vein, the so-called venous angle. However, the lymphatic vessels, particularly the lymphatic vessels of the thyroid, may on occasion empty directly into the internal jugular vein or subclavian vein well above the venous angle. Lymphaticovenous connections exist between lymphatic trunks and veins or within the lymph node. The lymphaticovenous connections between vessels are probably of little importance until a lymphatic trunk is obstructed. Lymphaticovenous connections are occasionally observed in otherwise normal lymphangiograms. The lymphatic trunks do not have an absorbing function, only a transporting function. The direction of lymphatic flow for each anatomical site is predictable and will be outlined as each site is discussed in later chapters. Aberrant pathways may occur. Tiny intercalated nodes may occur anywhere along a lymph channel. Obstruction of a lymph channel has the effect of rerouting the lymphatic flow. Complete obstruction by surgical transection will cause major changes in the expected pathway of lymph node metastasis. Radiation therapy causes partial obstruction, and the degree of obstruction is dose dependent. Lymph nodes that are replaced by tumor may cause partial or complete obstruction, especially when the mass becomes large enough to compress or invade the afferent lymphatic trunks.

LYMPH NODES

There are an estimated 150 to 350 lymph nodes above the clavicles, nearly one third of the total lymph nodes in the body. The arrangement of the lymph nodes in the head and neck region is shown in Figure 4-2. The nomenclature

FIG. 4-2. Arrangement of lymph nodes in the head and neck. (Redrawn from Rouvière H: Anatomy of the Human Lymphatic System, p 27. Tobias MJ [trans]. Ann Arbor, MI, Edwards Brothers, 1938)

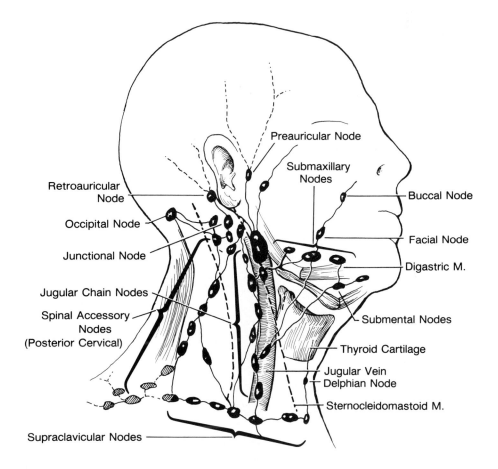

Preauricular Node

Submaxillary Nodes

Buccal Node

Retroauricular Node

Facial Node

Occipital Node

Digastric M.

Junctional Node

Jugular Chain Nodes

Spinal Accessory Nodes (Posterior Cervical)

Submental Nodes

Thyroid Cartilage

Jugular Vein
Delphian Node

Sternocleidomastoid M.

Supraclavicular Nodes

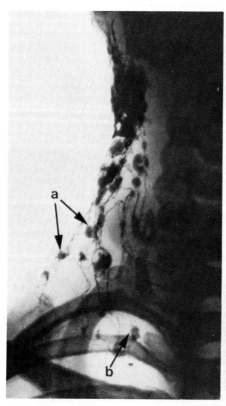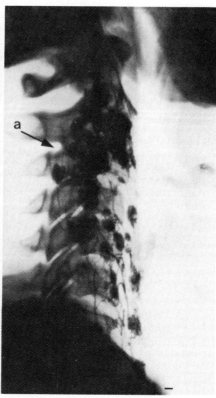

FIG. 4-3. Normal cervical lymphatics as shown by lymphangiography. Early filling image shows contrast still in lymphatic trunks. The beaded appearance of the lymphatic trunks is due to the semilunar valves. *a,* Spinal accessory lymph nodes; *b,* Supraclavicular lymph nodes. (Fisch U: Lymphographische Untersuchungen über das zervikale Lymphsystem [Fortschritte der Hals-Nasen-Ohrenheilkunde, vol 14], pp 53–162. Basel, Karger, 1966)

associated with the cervical lymph nodes is burdened by a variety of synonyms, some of which are listed in Table 4-3. The normal cervical lymphatics as shown by lymphangiography are depicted in Figures 4-3 through 4-5.[8] The normal internal jugular vein (IJV) is evident in Figure 4-6 on anteroposterior and lateral views of the neck.[8]

TABLE 4-3.	Synonyms for Names of Cervical Lymph Node Chains
Name Used in This Text	**Synonym**
Internal jugular chain (8–32 nodes)	Deep cervical chain
Spinal accessory chain (6–10 nodes)	Posterior cervical nodes
Supraclavicular nodes	Transverse cervical chain
Junctional nodes	Parapharyngeal nodes
	Superior or high internal jugular vein nodes
	Nasopharyngeal node
	Base of skull nodes
	Nodes of Krause
Submaxillary	Submandibular
Subdigastric nodes (1–5 nodes in adults)	Tonsillar node
	Principal node (of Küttner)
	Infradigastric nodes
Middle jugular chain	Omohyoid nodes
Lower jugular chain	
Lateral retropharyngeal node	Node of Rouvière
Retroauricular nodes	Mastoid nodes

The intercalated lymph nodules are inconstant, minute (1-mm to 2-mm) lymph nodes that occur along the course of a lymph vessel between its origin and its entrance to a larger lymph node. These nodules could become involved and replaced by tumor and appear as satellite nodules. This is probably an uncommon event, but it may account for the odd recurrence.

The IJV lymph nodes are located in relation to the IJV from the jugular fossa at the base of the skull to the termination of its lymphatic trunks at the base of the neck. They are subdivided into an anterior group and a lateral group according to their relationship to the IJV. The highest IJV nodes lie near the base of the skull in the poststyloid portion of the lateral pharyngeal space and are referred to as the junctional lymph nodes. They lie deep to the sternocleidomastoid muscle, the posterior belly of the digastric muscle, and the tail of the parotid and thus are difficult to detect, even when enlarged. These lymph nodes form a rather extensive lymphoid aggregate. They are often referred to as the parapharyngeal lymph nodes, since they occupy the parapharyngeal space. Until recently we were under the impression that the so-called parapharyngeal lymph nodes were a group of lymph nodes lying in the parapharyngeal space and distinct from the highest IJV lymph nodes. In fact, they are the same. The term *junctional lymph nodes* derives from the junction of the spinal accessory and IJV lymphatic chains.

The remainder of the IJV lymph nodes are customarily divided for practical purposes into upper, middle, and lower. The upper group begins at the lower border of the posterior belly of the digastric muscle and is referred to as the subdigastric lymph nodes. Virtually all head and neck malignancies spread to the subdigastric area, either primarily or secondarily. The nodes lie anterior or lateral to the IJV and may be palpated in front of the sternoclei-

ered only by the skin and thin platysma muscle and thus are quite superficial.

The supraclavicular lymph nodes lie in the lower neck along the upper margin of the clavicle and communicate with the spinal accessory chain. They are actually a continuation of part of the axillary chain and join other efferent trunks from the axilla before ending in the venous angle. They receive lymph from the head and neck, the ipsilateral upper extremity, the breast, the thorax, and the abdomen.

The submaxillary lymph nodes (three to six in number) are related to the submaxillary gland, the undersurface of the mandible, and the anterior facial vein (see Fig. 4-2). These lymph nodes drain the lips, floor of the mouth, buccal mucosa, upper and lower gums, nasal vestibule, skin of

FIG. 4-5. Normal cervical lymphangiogram. Note the relationship of the spinal accessory lymph nodes (*arrows*) to the spinous processes. (Fisch U: Lymphographische Untersuchungen über das zervikale Lymphsystem [Fortschritte der Hals-Nasen-Ohrenheilkunde, vol 14], pp 53–162. Basel, Karger, 1966)

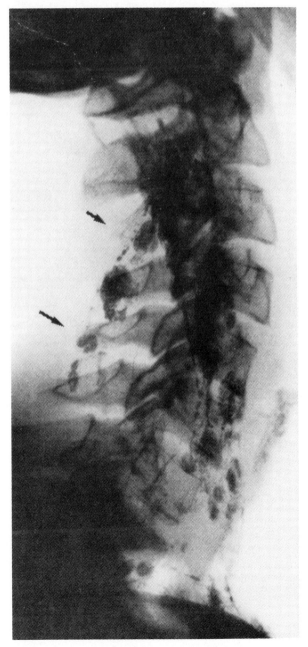

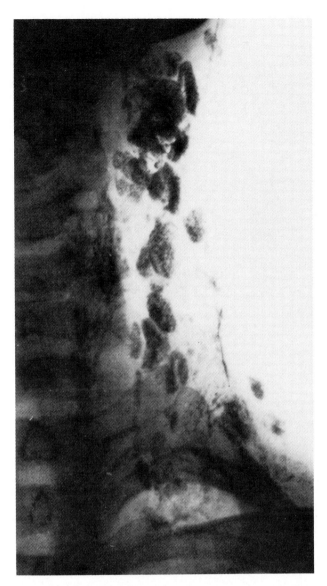

FIG. 4-4. Normal cervical lymphangiogram, late image. Twenty-three lymph nodes were counted between the mastoid tip and the hyoid bone. (Fisch U: Lymphographische Untersuchungen über das zervikale Lymphsystem [Fortschritte der Hals-Nasen-Ohrenheilkunde, vol 14], pp 53–162. Basel, Karger, 1966)

domastoid muscle, deep to it, or, less commonly, behind it. One of the subdigastric lymph nodes, the principal node, is normally large and elliptic and can be detected in most people even when normal. The midjugular lymph nodes lie deep to the sternocleidomastoid at a level between the thyroid notch and the cricoid cartilage. The low jugular nodes assume a more anterior and medial relationship to the IJV and lie quite close to the trachea; these nodes are less constant than the upper and middle IJV lymph nodes.

The lymph nodes of the spinal accessory chain (usually six to ten nodes) are distributed along the general course of the spinal accessory nerve (see Fig. 4-5). The superior nodes of the spinal accessory chain blend with the upper IJV lymph nodes (see Fig. 4-3). The middle and lower spinal accessory chain nodes diverge posteriorly and become continuous with the supraclavicular chain. They are cov-

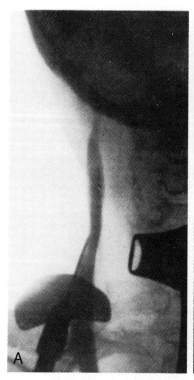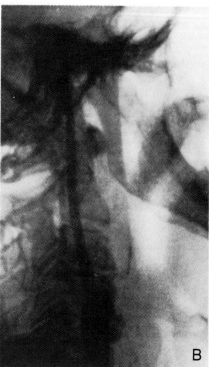

FIG. 4-6. Anteroposterior (*A*) and lateral (*B*) roentgenograms of the internal jugular vein. Compare relationship of the internal jugular vein with the cervical lymph nodes in Figures 4-3 through 4-5. (Fisch U: Lymphographische Untersuchungen über das zervikale Lymphsystem [Fortschritte der Hals-Nasen-Ohrenheilkunde, vol 14], pp 53–162. Basel, Karger, 1966)

the anterior face including the medial eyelids, tongue, palate, and submaxillary and sublingual salivary glands.

The submental lymph nodes lie in the midline between the anterior bellies of the digastric muscle and between the hyoid bone and symphysis menti; they are external to the mylohyoid muscle. They receive lymph from the lip, chin, and cheeks and to a lesser extent from the floor of the mouth, anterior lower gingiva, and tip of the tongue. The efferent vessels drain to the submaxillary or subdigastric lymph nodes.

The occipital lymph nodes (one to six in number) receive lymph from the occipital scalp and the skin of the upper nape of the neck. The nodes lie in the posterior midline and laterally in the angle formed by the sternocleidomastoid muscle and trapezius muscle insertions.

The retroauricular nodes (one or two in number when present) are located behind the pinna in relationship to the mastoid bone. They receive lymph vessels from the parietal scalp and skin of the ear.

A discussion of the parotid lymph nodes is presented in Chapter 28, Major Salivary Gland Tumors.

The preauricular lymph nodes (one to four in number when present) lie superficial to the fascia in immediate relationship to the tragus and the superficial temporal vessels. They are important in the spread of skin cancer and in lymphomas. They receive lymph from the skin of the frontal scalp, temple area, and nose, eyelids, pinna, external auditory canal, upper eyelid, and malar area. There is a pathway for drainage of the eustachian tube to this set of nodes.[25]

The facial and buccal nodes are inconstant intercalated lymph nodules located in the subcutaneous tissues along the anterior facial vein. They may be found just posterior to the nasolabial fold, 2 cm to 3 cm behind the commissure of the lip (buccal node) or overlying the external surface of the mandible near the mental foramen.

The lateral retropharyngeal lymph nodes lie beneath the pharyngeal constrictor muscle and lateral to the anterior rectus capitis muscle and fascia and anterior to the lateral masses of C1 and occasionally C2 (Fig. 4-7). The internal carotid artery and the upper pole of the superior cervical ganglion of the sympathetic chain are just lateral to these nodes and separated only by a layer of fascia. These nodes atrophy with age, but at least one node can usually be found and they are rarely totally absent. They receive lymph from the nasal cavity, nasopharynx, pharyngeal walls, hard and soft palate, middle ear, and eustachian tube. (See Chapter 24, Nasopharynx, for a detailed review of the lateral retropharyngeal lymph nodes.)

The medial retropharyngeal lymph nodes are tiny, inconstant, intercalated nodes that lie near the midline of the posterior pharyngeal wall in contact with the pharyngeal wall and range from the base of skull to the level of the hyoid.

There is a group of small midline prelaryngeal and paratracheal nodes that are sometimes important in the spread of cancers of the larynx, hypopharynx, and thyroid gland. The prelaryngeal nodes are usually located in relation to the cricothyroid membrane but may be above or below this site. They are seen on whole organ sections and are quite small when normal or even when replaced by tumor.[22] The largest one seen clinically was no more than 1.5 cm in diameter, and they are frequently 2 mm to 3 mm in diameter even when enlarged by tumor. The midline prelaryngeal node is often referred to as the Delphian node,* because when involved by tumor it is said to herald

---

* The first nodes to be exposed at the time of surgery for thyroid carcinoma are the midline lymph nodes anterior to the larynx and trachea. There is always one node in the midline in relationship to the thyrocricoid area, commonly two or three, occasionally four. This node or group of nodes has been termed *the*

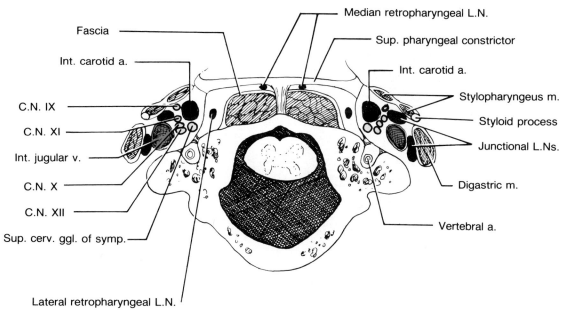

FIG. 4-7. Anatomical relationships of medial and lateral retropharyngeal lymph nodes at level of C1.

bad news (oracle of Delphi).[6] The Delphian node receives lymph from the upper anterior portion of the body of both thyroid lobes, from the upper poles, and from the isthmus. It also receives lymph from the larynx.

The paratracheal nodes and their lymphatic vessels provide a potential route of spread to the superior mediastinal lymph nodes, but in actual practice this is an uncommon event, partly because these lymph nodes are uncommonly invaded by cancer in the first place.

OBSERVATIONS ON THE PATHOPHYSIOLOGY OF THE CERVICAL LYMPHATICS

There are several observations regarding the normal and diseased cervical lymphatic system that should be stressed.

The risk of lymphatic spread is most dependent on the availability and relative denseness of the capillary lymphatics and is largely independent of histology. Tumors with "pushing borders" are less likely to develop lymphatic metastases, and true verrucous carcinoma, the ultimate in "pushing borders," almost never invades the lymphatic system. The majority of sarcomas originate in tissues such as muscle, bone, or cartilage and therefore have little opportunity for lymph node involvement. However, they will metastasize by way of the lymphatic system once they spread to involve areas with capillary lymphatics. Even basal cell carcinoma of the skin, which has a very low rate of lymphatic spread, will eventually invade the lymphatic system, but usually only after multiple recurrences.

Neoplasms mostly show a radial growth pattern. It is unlikely that the lymphatic trunks, which have a transporting function, play a role in local growth and spread of a neoplasm. If the tumor cells that enter the lymphatic system were to sprout random tumor colonies along the course of the transporting vessels, then one would expect to see numerous noncontiguous satellite nodules, an uncommon feature in head and neck carcinoma. Likewise, operations that do not remove the intervening lymphatic vessels would not succeed. For example, a discontinuous excision of the tongue and radical neck dissection does not remove the intervening lymphatic vessels, but it is a successful procedure. However, when the lymphatic vessels become obstructed, tumor cells pile up in the lymphatics and may colonize the vessel.

Injection of the lymphatics of the human larynx prior to laryngectomy shows two patterns of lymph flow. Injection of the deeper lymphatics reveals a unilateral flow without crossover. Injection of the superficial submucosal lymphatics shows a nondirectional pattern of flow to both sides.[24] It is doubtful, however, that the lymphatics have much to do with local spread of tumor, either in the larynx or elsewhere.

Normal cervical lymphangiograms following a retroauricular injection show a strictly ipsilateral flow without contralateral cervical filling.* A surgical incision that interrupts the IJV trunks (e.g., for biopsy of a lymph node) causes nearly complete ipsilateral obstruction, as do some enlarged metastatic lymph nodes (Figs. 4-8 and 4-9). Radiation therapy causes partial obstruction secondary to a diminution in the number and size of the lymphatic trunks and lymph nodes, and the degree of obstruction is dose related. Hyperplastic nodes without cancer can also produce a lymphatic blockage.

Roentgenograms of the neck following cervical lymphangiography and radical neck dissection often show remaining lymph nodes, particularly in the junctional area.

Delphian node by Dr. Oliver Cope because it is exposed first and, if diseased, will foretell the nature of the disease process to be found in the thyroid gland. The name Delphian was suggested to Dr. Cope by Dr. Raymond V. Randall, then a fourth-year medical student at Harvard Medical School attending the Thyroid Clinic at Massachusetts General Hospital.[6]

* We are indebted to Dr. U. Fisch, a head and neck surgeon at the University of Zurich, who has studied the cervical lymphatics by lymphangiography and reported his data in an excellent monograph, *Lymphography of the Cervical Lymphatic System.*[8]

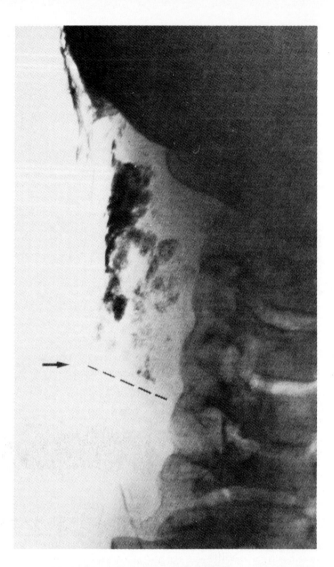

The junctional area is the weak spot in the standard radical neck dissection and is an occasional site of recurrence (Fig. 4-10).

When cervical lymphangiography is done after radical neck dissection, a persistent ipsilateral obstruction is observed; there is a subcutaneous diversion of the lymph flow toward the submaxillary area with submental shunting to the contralateral lymph nodes. Lymph is thus diverted to the opposite side after unilateral neck dissection (Figs. 4-11 and 4-12). When a bilateral neck dissection is done, the lymph is shunted to the dermal lymphatics, which will reconstitute across a surgical scar and eventually provide an escape pathway (Fig. 4-13).

Further obstruction of the lymphatic pathways occurs with the addition of irradiation to a neck dissection or to a bilateral neck dissection. It is of clinical importance to irradiate as little of the skin as possible in patients undergoing neck dissection plus radiation therapy in order to preserve some element of the dermal lymphatic system to help reduce lymphedema. This same tactic has been found necessary in the irradiation of the extremities in patients with sarcomas. Preservation of a strip of normal "skin" reduces the risk of lymphedema. In the head and neck cancer patient, the strip of skin to be preserved when possible is in the submental area and the anterior midline neck. It may require considerable technical effort to shield small strips of skin, but this sparing is often the difference between lymphedema and little or no lymphedema, particularly of the larynx.

FIG. 4-8. Cervical lymphangiogram following incisional biopsy. Note the almost complete lymphatic obstruction. (Fisch U: Lymphographische Untersuchungen über das zervikale Lymphsystem [Fortschritte der Hals-Nasen-Ohrenheilkunde, vol 14], pp 53–162. Basel, Karger, 1966)

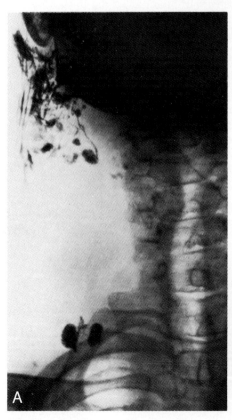
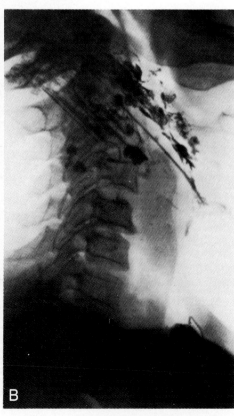

FIG. 4-9. Cervical lymphangiogram in patient with carcinoma of the hypopharynx and large right cervical lymph node metastases (late image). Note persistence of contrast medium in lymphatic vessels due to obstruction by tumor in lymph nodes. Two supraclavicular lymph nodes are filled. (A) Anteroposterior. (B) Lateral. (Fisch U: Lymphographische Untersuchungen über das zervikale Lymphsystem [Fortschritte der Hals-Nasen-Ohrenheilkunde, vol 14], pp 53–162. Basel, Karger, 1966)

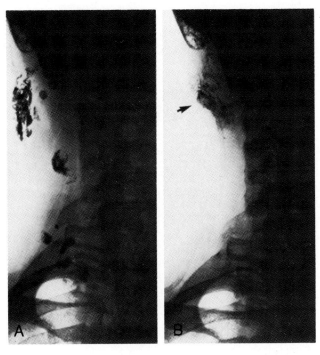

FIG. 4-10. (*A*) Preoperative cervical lymphangiogram. (*B*) Postoperative film 2 days after radical neck dissection. Arrow indicates a lymph node suspicious for metastatic carcinoma. Residual metastatic carcinoma was later confirmed by histologic examination. (The silhouette of the suction catheter is seen.) (Fisch U: Lymphographische Untersuchungen über das zervikale Lymphsystem [Fortschritte der Hals-Nasen-Ohrenheilkunde, vol 14], pp 53–162. Basel, Karger, 1966)

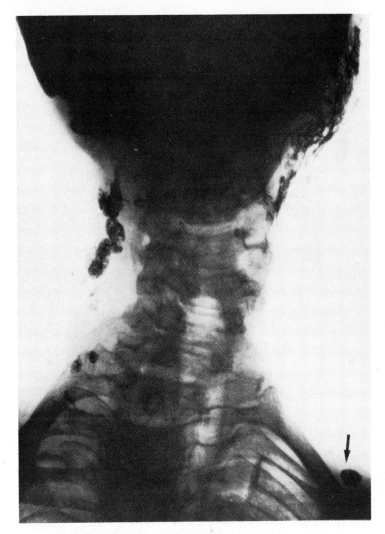

FIG. 4-11. Left cervical lymphangiogram 5 years after radical neck dissection. There is diversion of lymph across the submental space to the contralateral internal jugular chain. Note the low left supraclavicular node lying in the lateral supraclavicular space (*arrow*). (Fisch U: Lymphographische Untersuchungen über das zervikale Lymphsystem [Fortschritte der Hals-Nasen-Ohrenheilkunde, vol 14], pp 53–162. Basel, Karger, 1966)

FIG. 4-12. (*A*) Cervical lymphangiogram 13 months after radical neck dissection. There is filling of fine lymphatic channels along the mandible, and numerous small lymph nodes can be seen. The arrow points to the submental diversion of the lymph to the contralateral side. (*B*) Left cervical lymphangiogram 5 years after radical neck dissection (same patient as in Fig. 4-11). Arrows point to the submental diversion to the opposite side. (Fisch U: Lymphographische Untersuchungen über das zervikale Lymphsystem [Fortschritte der Hals-Nasen-Ohrenheilkunde, vol 14], pp 53–162. Basel, Karger, 1966)

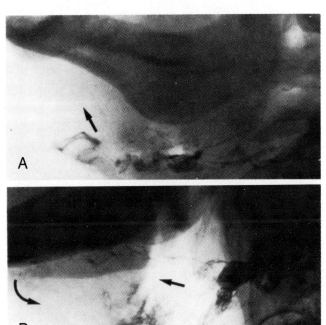

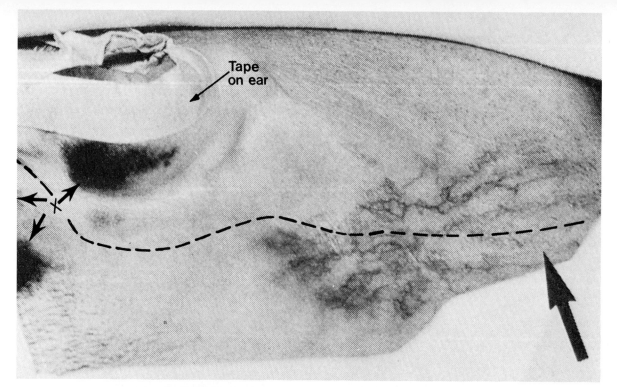

FIG. 4-13. Retroauricular injection (x) of patent blue dye 3 years after bilateral radical neck dissection. The dye is picked up by the dermal lymphatics and carried toward the submaxillary area. The large arrow points to the incision (*dashed line*). The dermal lymphatic vessels have regrown across the scar, allowing lymph flow to the submental area. (Fisch U: Lymphographische Untersuchungen über das zervikale Lymphsystem [Fortschritte der Hals-Nasen-Ohrenheilkunde, vol 14], pp 53–162. Basel, Karger, 1966)

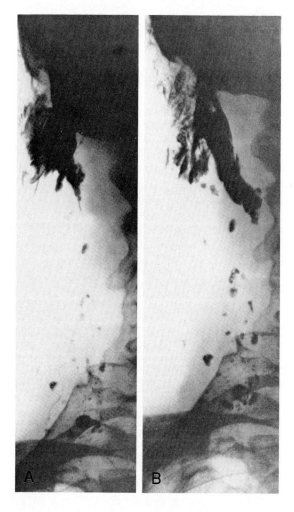

FIG. 4-14. Cervical lymphangiogram 7 months after 7000 rad. (*A*) Filling phase. Note fine caliber and decreased number of lymphatic vessels. (*B*) Late phase. Lymph nodes are small and irregularly but densely filled by the contrast medium. The reduced diameter of the vessels causes an increase in intralymphatic pressure, which results in extensive extravasation of contrast medium in the junctional area. (Fisch U: Lymphographische Untersuchungen über das zervikale Lymphsystem [Fortschritte der Hals-Nasen-Ohrenheilkunde, vol 14], pp 53–162. Basel, Karger, 1966)

Radiation therapy without radical neck dissection causes a decrease in the number and caliber of the lymph vessels, and the nodes decrease in size (Fig. 4-14). Complete lymphatic obstruction such as that seen with neck dissection does not occur within the range of clinically used doses. Radiation therapy does not "seal off" the lymphatics, but it certainly produces a partial obstruction. The degree of lymphatic change is dose and volume related. Following high-dose radiation therapy to both sides of the neck, lymph flow is diverted anteriorly to the submental space (just as with surgical obstruction) and an accumulation of lymph occurs in the submental space, creating an unsightly, but painless bag of water, which is referred to as a "wattle" because it resembles a turkey wattle. This lymphedema gradually disappears in 6 months to 1 year.

RELATIONSHIP OF LYMPHATICS AND
THE CEREBROSPINAL FLUID

Although the majority of the cerebrospinal fluid is absorbed by the arachnoid villi and passes mainly into the dural sinuses, there are avenues for cerebrospinal fluid to escape directly into the lymphatic system. One of the major avenues is by way of the arachnoid sheaths of the olfactory nerves, which penetrate the cribriform plate and then connect with capillary lymphatics in the submucosa of the olfactory nasal submucosa. This route of absorption of cerebrospinal fluid is probably relatively unimportant, but it can be demonstrated in both humans and animals that blood and other proteins and particles may escape from the anterior cranial fossa through this route. Similar connections have been observed in the spinal cord and brain stem. There also may be a similar connection in the region of the jugular bulb. Földi has shown that complete surgical obstruction of the cervical lymphatics leads to a neurologic syndrome that he called lymphogenic encephalopathy, which is characterized by increased cerebrospinal fluid pressure, cerebral edema, papilledema, lymphedema of the soft tissues of the head and neck, and lethargy.[10] It seems reasonable that part of the central nervous system syndrome associated with ligation of the internal jugular veins, especially bilateral ligation, is due not only to venous obstruction but also to the simultaneous lymphatic obstruction.

Physical Examination of the Neck

Staging of carcinoma of the neck is almost totally dependent on physical examination, although computed tomographic (CT) scanning will probably play a role in the future. The technique of physical examination will be described in detail, since it is not generally taught in medical schools or in standard physical diagnosis texts.

At least 3 to 5 minutes are needed to perform a thorough neck examination. It is important to repeat the examination at every opportunity and even more important to compare findings among several examiners. Detailed drawings complement the written report and are an essential part of the medical record.

The preferred position is with the patient sitting and the examiner standing behind. Since many examination chairs have a head rest or cannot be lowered sufficiently, it is often necessary to move the patient to a regular chair or stool so that the patient's neck is opposite the examiner's waistline. It is common to observe neck examinations being done by patting the neck with the fingers; this method is not acceptable for examination of the jugular chain lymph nodes (Fig. 4-15).

We prefer to start at the sternal notch and work upward. The suprasternal notch, the space that extends into the upper mediastinum, and the space behind the insertion of the sternocleidomastoid muscle to the clavicle are explored with the index finger (Fig. 4-16). Normally nothing should be felt except the anterior wall of the trachea. Clinically positive lymph nodes are frequently found in this area, but only the top or side of the lymph node may be felt. The nodes are usually located 1 cm to 2 cm from the midline. Metastatic lymph nodes from lung and breast cancers as well as metastatic nodes from cancers arising below the diaphragm are frequently felt in this area. *This is one of the most commonly missed physical findings.* Since the discovery of a metastatic node in this position is so meaningful, it should be carefully sought before major operative or radiation procedures are enlisted. The differential diagnosis of a hard, discrete mass in this area includes thyroid mass, aneurysm of a major vessel, and mediastinal mass.

When the examination of the internal jugular chain is begun and the neck is grasped, the patient instinctively extends the neck, thereby tensing the sternocleidomastoid muscle (Fig. 4-17). Since the internal jugular chain lymph nodes lie deep to the sternocleidomastoid, it is essential

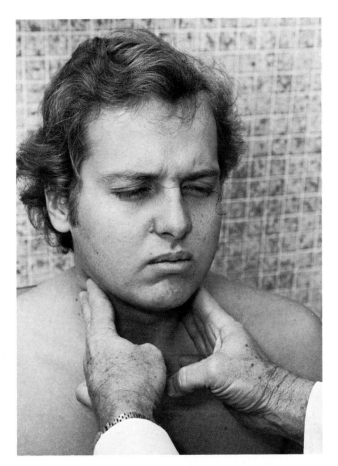

FIG. 4-15. Neck examination: improper technique.

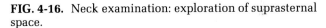

FIG. 4-16. Neck examination: exploration of suprasternal space.

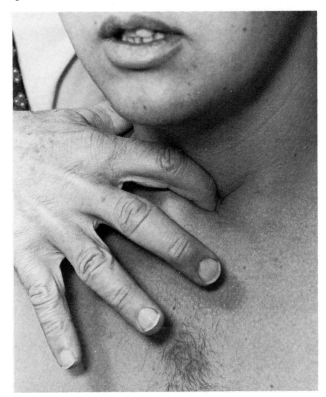

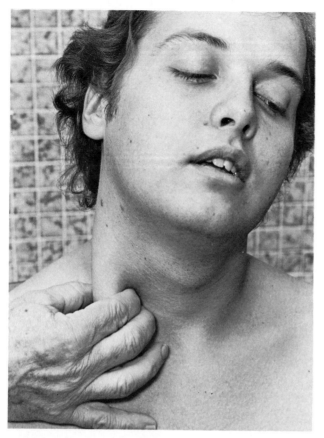

FIG. 4-17. Neck examination: neck extended to contra-lateral side; sternocleidomastoid muscle is tensed.

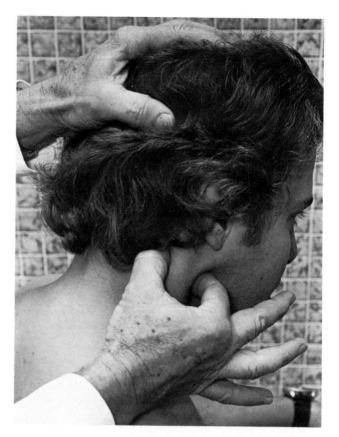

FIG. 4-18. Neck examination: hand on occiput is used to control the head. The neck is flexed forward and to the side that is being examined.

FIG. 4-19. Neck examination: the thumb and index finger form a C to palpate beneath the sternocleidomastoid muscle.

FIG. 4-20. Diagram of technique shown in Figure 4-19.

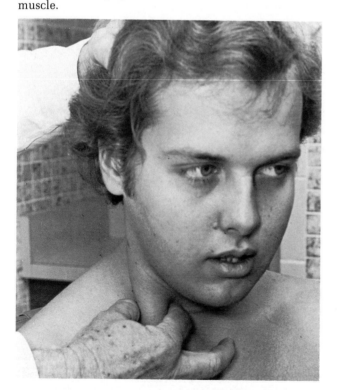

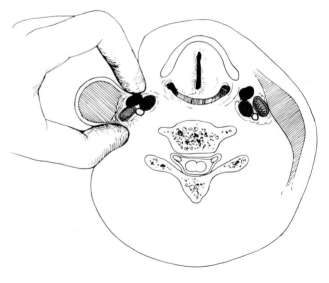

to have the neck muscles relaxed. Therefore, one hand is placed on the patient's occiput in order to flex the head forward and slightly to the side being examined (Figs. 4-18 and 4-19). If the patient is tense, gentle rocking of the head along with gentle massage of the neck will often obtain the relaxation necessary. The right neck is examined with the right hand and the left neck, with the left hand.

The internal jugular chain lymph nodes lie deep to the sternocleidomastoid muscle in the lower neck; in the upper neck some of the nodes lie at the anterior border of the sternocleidomastoid. The thumb and index finger form a C around the sternocleidomastoid muscle (Fig. 4-20). The tips of the examining thumb and fingers nearly meet on most patients. As one proceeds up the jugular chain, the thumb and index finger are in constant motion, using a wiggle-waggle maneuver. Positive lymph nodes in the lower jugular area are often small, mobile, and deep, and only slow, careful, gentle, repeated examinations will find them. Most clinically positive lymph nodes will be found in the upper jugular chain. The carotid artery and carotid bulb are identified by the pulsation in the vessel. The pressoreceptors in the carotid bulb respond to external pressure as well as internal vascular pressure. Stimulation will produce a drop in blood pressure and slowing of the pulse. The response is more sensitive in older patients. Patients may develop slight faintness or sudden syncope and collapse. Palpation of the bulb must be gentle and *must not be done simultaneously on both sides.* Palpation of the carotid artery may rarely cause an atheromatous plaque to be splintered from the artery. In one such instance, the patient noted a sudden change in vision in the ipsilateral eye during neck examination. Eye examination confirmed that a branch of a retinal vessel had been occluded, presumably from a small thrombotic plaque entering the ophthalmic artery.

The subdigastric lymph node(s) (tonsillar node) is the largest normal node in the neck and can be identified in many people. A metastatic lymph node mass may be deep in the neck in the subdigastric area, and only the external surface of the mass may be felt. The junctional lymph nodes are difficult to palpate, particularly in men, because the well-developed sternocleidomastoid muscle and the posterior belly of the digastric muscle intervene, and the attachment of the muscles to the mastoid tip restricts the examining fingers.

There are a number of normal structures that may be confused with a jugular chain lymph node. The lateral tip of the transverse process of C1 or C2 may feel like a 1-cm to 2-cm lymph node. The transverse process is especially conspicuous in patients with long, thin necks. The tail of the parotid gland becomes firm, discrete, and globular in older, obese patients, especially men, and resembles a lymph node. This mass lies just below the ear lobe, between the horizontal ramus of the mandible and the tip of the mastoid. The palpable parotid tails are usually symmetrical, which gives a clue to their identity; clinically positive nodes in the tail of the parotid are unusual except in parotid malignancies, skin cancers, or occasionally lymphomas or leukemias. The carotid bifurcation (carotid bulb) may be quite prominent in older people and feel like a subdigastric lymph node. Gentle palpation to determine pulsation of the vessel helps to distinguish the vessel from the node. The differential diagnosis is especially difficult when a 1.5-cm to 2-cm node is closely approximated to the carotid bifurcation. Localized atheromatous plaques along the carotid produce a localized fusiform enlargement that may be confused with a small lymph node.

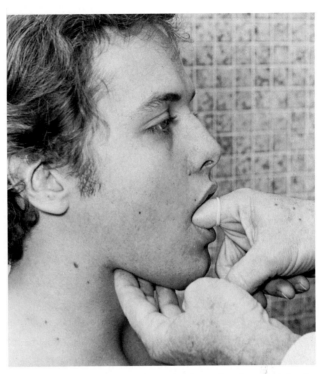

FIG. 4-21. Neck examination: bimanual palpation of submandibular and submental lymph nodes and submandibular gland.

Both the submaxillary and submental nodes are examined bimanually with one index finger in the floor of the mouth (Fig. 4-21). The submaxillary lymph nodes lie along the horizontal ramus of the mandible. The submaxillary gland may be small and firm and tucked up underneath the mandible, especially in younger patients. More frequently the gland lies in the neck just below the mandible, especially in older people. If the submaxillary duct is obstructed by tumor, the gland may be enlarged, firm, tender, and immobile. Several lymph nodes lie in juxtaposition to the submaxillary gland (see Fig. 4-2), and small lymph nodes are located inside the capsule of the gland. It is impossible to distinguish between an enlarged submaxillary gland and an enlarged lymph node and whether an enlarged, firm submaxillary gland is enlarged due to obstruction or radiation effect as opposed to cancer. If the mass is tender or painful, it suggests inflammation rather than cancer, but the finding is not reliable. Needle biopsy is helpful, but removal of the submaxillary gland is the only reliable means of making a diagnosis. The most common errors in evaluating the neck have been made in underestimating the findings in the submaxillary gland until the diagnosis of metastatic cancer was all too obvious and the disease was unmanageable. An enlarged submaxillary mass is better managed by action than by observation.

The submental lymph nodes lie in the midline between the anterior bellies of the digastric muscles. The most commonly involved submental lymph node lies just anterior to the hyoid; rarely, a node is found to be positive just behind the symphysis of the mandible.

Examination of the spinal accessory and supraclavicular lymph nodes requires only light, gentle palpation of the neck. Preauricular lymph node examination is often overlooked. These nodes lie just anterior to the tragus and may be very small when first involved by tumor. Examination of the superficial mastoid, occipital, mental, facial, and Delphian lymph nodes completes the examination.

RELIABILITY OF NECK EXAMINATION

The reliability of the neck examination depends on the experience and ability of the examiner, the gross anatomy of the individual neck, and whether the neck has been surgically violated.

Personal observations over many years have made it vividly obvious that there is a wide range of abilities among physicians in the skills of physical diagnosis, and this is particularly true in the neck examination. The neck examination is not difficult, it is just not properly taught in medical schools nor in most residencies. This difference in diagnostic ability surely explains many of the differences in the incidence of clinically positive or clinically negative neck examinations.

A fat, thick, or muscular neck may be difficult to evaluate, and one should allow for this fact in treatment planning.

A recent surgical procedure such as incisional biopsy, major operation, or tracheostomy usually prevents satisfactory examination of the neck.

Neck Lymph Node Staging

The American Joint Committee on Cancer (AJCC) classification system is adopted for this book:[2]

NX   Minimum requirements to assess the regional nodes cannot be met.

N0   No clinically positive node

N1   Single clinically positive homolateral node 3 cm or less in diameter

N2   Single clinically positive homolateral node more than 3 cm but not more than 6 cm in diameter or multiple clinically positive homolateral nodes, none more than 6 cm in diameter

N2A   Single clinically positive homolateral node more than 3 cm but not more than 6 cm in diameter

N2B   Multiple clinically positive homolateral nodes, none more than 6 cm in diameter

N3   Massive homolateral node(s), bilateral nodes, or contralateral node(s)

N3A   Clinically positive homolateral node(s), one more than 6 cm in diameter

N3B   Bilateral clinically positive nodes (in this situation, each side of the neck should be staged separately; that is, N3B: right, N2A; left, N1)

N3C   Contralateral clinically positive node(s) only

The current AJCC neck staging is acceptable and easy to apply. The concept of whether or not a node is fixed has been discarded, since there is too much disagreement among clinicians regarding what is fixed and what is not fixed.

The N3B stage is a wastebasket with relatively favorable, treatable situations (e.g., N1–N1 or N2–N1) mixed with advanced, untreatable situations. The N3C stage is rarely seen on presentation and should alert the clinician to look for a second primary lesion.

Management of the Clinically Negative Neck

The incidence of subclinical disease in the regional lymphatics when the neck is clinically negative is shown in Table 2-1 in Chapter 2. The risk for subclinical disease for any single primary lesion may be estimated by the size or T stage of the primary lesion (see Table 2-2 in Chapter 2) and the differentiation of the neoplasm. The nasopharynx and the pyriform sinus are the exceptions to gauging the risk of subclinical disease by T stage, since both show little correlation between T stage and neck disease. The explanation lies in the very dense capillary lymphatic networks of these two areas and the propensity to lymphatic spread with early lesions. A policy of "wait and see" may be adopted for the N0 neck in order to avoid unnecessary treatment, and the neck may often be successfully treated if clinically positive nodes appear. However, even though the delayed neck treatment may be judged successful, these patients are at an increased risk to develop distant metastasis and have a poorer prognosis (see Tables 2-5 through 2-7 in Chapter 2).[16,21] Elective neck treatment is indicated, therefore, when the associated morbidity is low and has the added advantage of giving complete treatment initially and simplifying the follow-up neck examinations because of its high success rate.

ELECTIVE NECK IRRADIATION

There is a large volume of data supporting the success of irradiation in eradicating subclinical disease in regional lymphatics.[3,4,9,15,16–18,20,21]

The results for elective neck irradiation when the primary lesion is controlled are shown in Tables 4-4 through 4-7. Assuming a conservative 25% overall risk for subclinical disease in the regional lymph nodes, the calculated efficiency is at least 90% for doses in the range of 4500 rad to 6000 rad/4½ to 6 weeks. If the primary lesion recurs, however, there is a renewed chance for lymphatic spread and the neck is at considerable risk even if elective neck irradiation has been given. If the primary lesion is to be treated with external-beam irradiation, then elective neck irradiation incurs little or no added cost and, if properly done, little added morbidity. Elective neck irradiation is not recommended for small, superficial, T1 lesions of the anterior floor of the mouth and anterior two thirds of the oral tongue (see Table 4-4) in which the risk of subclinical disease in the lymph nodes is small (less than 10%), since the external-beam portals required to irradiate the submaxillary and subdigastric nodes must include a large amount of normal mucosa and the majority of both parotid glands.[17] The acute and late side-effects of the elective neck irradiation do not justify its use in these low-risk cases.

For the patient with a lesion of the floor of the mouth or oral tongue who has no clinically evident neck disease, elective neck irradiation when indicated is usually confined to the first-echelon nodes in the upper neck; the lower neck is included for the larger lesions, for poorly differentiated histology, or when the neck is difficult to examine.

Elective neck irradiation usually includes the entire neck, frequently on both sides, for lesions of the nasopharynx, oropharynx, hypopharynx, and supraglottic larynx.

When there are clinically positive neck nodes present, elective neck irradiation may be given to those portions of the neck that are clinically negative, such as the contralateral neck, or the lower neck when the upper neck only has positive lymph nodes.

The results of partial neck irradiation as compared with whole neck irradiation for lesions originating in the nasopharynx, tonsillar fossa, base of the tongue, and faucial arch are shown in Table 4-5.[4] Partial neck irradiation was usually prescribed for patients with earlier stages of neck disease (only 6.5% had N3A or N3B), in which case the neck was not completely irradiated. Twelve percent (22 patients) developed new lymph node disease in areas initially negative when both the primary lesion and the clinically positive nodes (if present) were controlled. Three patients had recurrences in electively irradiated areas, and the other 19 developed recurrences either at the edge of the treatment portal or well outside the irradiated field.

In the group of 284 patients with whole neck irradiation, of whom 35% had N3 neck disease, only 7 patients had recurrences in areas initially clinically negative; five recurrences were within electively irradiated areas, and two were outside irradiation portals in the submental area.

TABLE 4-4. Efficacy of Elective Neck Irradiation (ENI) With Primary Tumor Controlled (125 Patients)

Primary Stage	No. of Patients With Neck Controlled/ No. of Patients With Primary Lesion Controlled		
	No ENI	Partial ENI	Whole ENI
T1	11/12	17/18	9/10
T2	6/8	17/17	22/22
T3	0/1	10/10	18/18
T4	1/1	5/5	3/3
Total	18/22 (82%)*	49/50 (98%)*	52/53 (98%)*

* Significance level = 0.01, using exact test procedures.[1]
Note: University of Florida data; patients treated 10/64–6/76; minimum 2-year follow-up.
(Mendenhall WM, Million RR, Cassisi NJ: Elective neck irradiation in squamous cell carcinoma of the head and neck. Head Neck Surg 3:15–20, 1980)

TABLE 4-5. Comparison of Partial and Whole Neck Irradiation* in Squamous Cell Carcinomas of the Nasopharynx, Tonsillar Fossa, Base of Tongue, and Faucial Arch

	No. Patients	Percentage N3	Neck Failures in Areas Initially Clinically Negative†
Partial neck irradiation	185	6.5%	12%
Whole neck irradiation	284	35%	2.5%

* Radical neck dissection was added after radiation therapy in 24 patients with partial neck irradiation and in 58 patients with whole neck irradiation.
† Primary lesions and initial clinically positive neck disease were controlled.
(Data from Berger DS, Fletcher GH, Lindberg RD, Jesse RH Jr: Elective irradiation of the neck lymphatics for squamous cell carcinomas of the nasopharynx and oropharynx. Am J Roentgenol Radium Ther Nucl Med 111:66–72, 1971)

TABLE 4-6. Failure of Initial Ipsilateral Neck Treatment—596 Patients With Carcinoma of the Tonsillar Fossa, Base of Tongue, Supraglottic Larynx, or Hypopharynx

Treatment	Stage							
	N0			N1	N2A	N2B	N3A	N3B
	No Treatment	Partial	Complete					
Irradiation		15%	2%	15%	27%	27%	38%	34%
Surgery	55% (16/29)	35%	7%	11%	8%	23%	42%	41%
Combined		1/5	0/6	0	0	0	23%	25%

Note: M. D. Anderson Hospital data; patients treated 1948–1967.
(Adapted from Barkley HT Jr, Fletcher GH, Jesse RH, Lindberg RD: Management of cervical lymph node metastases in squamous cell carcinoma of the tonsillar fossa, base of tongue, supraglottic larynx, and hypopharynx. Am J Surg 124:462–467, 1972)

TABLE 4-7. Cervical Metastasis Appearing in the Contralateral N0 Neck—596 Patients With Carcinoma of the Tonsillar Fossa, Base of Tongue, Supraglottic Larynx, or Hypopharynx

Treatment	N0	N1	N2A	N2B	N3A
Radiation	4%	2%	9%	7%	0
Surgery	25%	17%	23%	43%	33%
Combined	0/6	0	0	11%	0

Note: M. D. Anderson Hospital data; patients treated 1948–1967.
(Adapted from Barkley HT Jr, Fletcher GH, Jesse RH, Lindberg RD: Management of cervical lymph node metastases in squamous cell carcinoma of the tonsillar fossa, base of tongue, supraglottic larynx, and hypopharynx. Am J Surg 124:462–467, 1972)

ELECTIVE NECK DISSECTION

Surgeons have argued for many years over the relative merits of elective neck dissection as compared with observation.[12] It is a difficult decision to recommend a full radical neck dissection with the resulting cosmetic and functional losses, unless the potential benefit is considerable. However, recent operative modifications reduce this morbidity. The so-called functional neck dissection popularized by Bocca* preserves the spinal accessory nerve, the jugular vein, and the sternocleidomastoid muscle and works as well as radical neck dissection for subclinical (N0) disease.[5] This concept can be extended to the supraomohyoid neck dissection, which differs from the Bocca neck dissection in that the lower internal jugular chain nodes below the omohyoid muscle are not removed because of their insignificant risk for metastases in certain oral cavity lesions. This concept is similar to elective neck irradiation for early oral cavity lesions in which only the first-echelon nodes are irradiated.

For lesions of the oral cavity, an elective supraomohyoid neck dissection on one or both sides may be better classified as a staging procedure. If the nodes are negative, no further treatment is given. If the nodes are positive, the neck dissection is completed or postoperative radiation therapy is

* Dr. George Crile described a functional neck dissection in 1906. He indicated that only the regional lymphatics were removed if there were "no palpable glands," and in the discussion following his presentation to the American Medical Association he stated that the sternomastoid muscle and internal jugular vein were removed only when neck metastases had already occurred.[7] Bocca credits O. Suarez of Argentina (1963) for describing the technique of conservative neck dissection.[26]

used. These two forms of neck dissection are at least 90% to 95% effective and create relatively few side-effects. Functional supraomohyoid neck dissection is not sufficient treatment, however, for lesions of the oropharynx, larynx, or hypopharynx (see Table 4-6). There is significant risk that a supraomohyoid neck dissection will miss tumor in the lower neck. The functional neck dissection is a more difficult and longer procedure than the standard radical neck dissection.

Management of the Clinically Positive Neck

The rate of treatment failure of neck disease by N stage and therapeutic category reported from M. D. Anderson Hospital is shown in Table 4-6.[3] The irradiation preceded the operation if the primary site was to be treated by radiation therapy or if a node was fixed or borderline resectable. The operation preceded the irradiation if the primary site was to be treated surgically.

Radical neck dissection is sufficient treatment for the ipsilateral neck for patients with N1 or N2A disease. Radiation therapy is added for other N stages and/or for control of contralateral subclinical disease (see Table 4-7).[3] Invasion through the capsule of the node or the finding of multiple positive nodes in the specimen is an indication to add postoperative radiation therapy regardless of the clinical stage.

Radiation therapy alone is sufficient for patients with small N1 (0 to 2 cm) disease, but it should usually be combined with a neck dissection for large N1 (3 cm), N2A, or N3A disease. The decision to add neck dissection for N2B and N3B disease is individualized, based on the diameter of the largest node or the multiplicity of palpable nodes. For example, a patient's disease may be staged N2B on the basis of a 2-cm subdigastric node and two 1-cm nodes in the middle and lower jugular chain; this neck might be treated with radiation therapy alone. However, another patient with N2B disease may have a 3-cm to 4-cm neck node and several other small nodes, and neck dissection should be added if possible. If the enlarged nodes disappear completely and early during the course of the radiation therapy, the likelihood of control by radiation therapy alone is improved and neck dissection may be withheld. However, it is always safer to add the neck dissection immediately after radiation therapy, since the detection of neck node recurrence after high-dose radiation therapy is difficult because of fibrosis and salvage is generally unsatisfactory. Large, fixed nodes (over 5 cm to 6 cm) may receive 6000 rad to 8000 rad prior to neck dissection; some of the specimens will show "no viable tumor," and quite a few patients will have the disease controlled in the neck (Fig. 4-22).

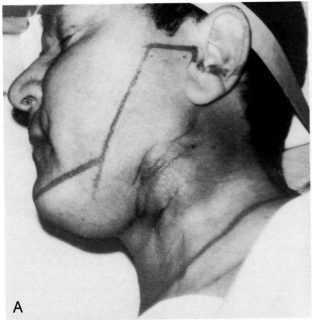

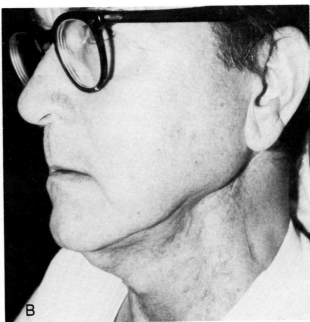

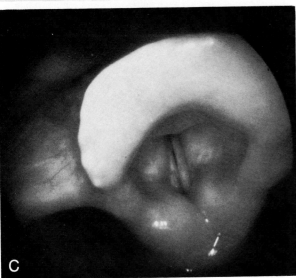

FIG. 4-22. T1N3A squamous cell carcinoma of the pyriform sinus treated with 6000 rad to the primary lesion and 8000 rad to the left neck mass. The final 2000 rad to the neck mass was delivered through a reduced portal. A radical neck dissection was done 1 month later; the specimen showed no viable tumor cells. The patient is alive, free of disease, as of January 1982 (4 years from start of treatment). (A) Left neck with treatment portals. The 8 × 7-cm neck mass had infiltrated the skin and was stuck to the mandible and base of skull and surrounded the neurovascular sheath. (B) Appearance of neck 3 years following radiation therapy and neck dissection. (C) Appearance of larynx and hypopharynx 3 years after radiation therapy and neck dissection. There is mild (+1) bilateral arytenoid and aryepiglottic fold edema. No evidence of disease at 4 years.

REFERENCES

1. Agresti A, Wackerly D: Some exact conditional tests of independence for R × C cross-classification tables. Psychometrika 42:111–125, 1977

2. American Joint Committee on Cancer: Manual for Staging of Cancer, 2nd ed, p 27. Philadelphia, JB Lippincott, 1983

3. Barkley HT Jr, Fletcher GH, Jesse RH, Lindberg RD: Management of cervical lymph node metastases in squamous cell carcinomas of the tonsillar fossa, base of tongue, supraglottic larynx, and hypopharynx. Am J Surg 124:462–467, 1972

4. Berger DS, Fletcher GH, Lindberg RD, Jesse RH Jr: Elective irradiation of the neck lymphatics for squamous cell carcinomas of the nasopharynx and oropharynx. Am J Roentgenol Radium Ther Nucl Med 111:66–72, 1971

5. Bocca E, Pignataro O: A conservation technique in radical neck dissection. Ann Otol Rhinol Laryngol 76:975–987, 1967

6. Cope O: Surgery of the thyroid. In Means JH, DeGroot LJ, Stanbury JB (eds): The Thyroid and Its Diseases, 3rd ed, pp 561–598. New York, McGraw-Hill, 1963

7. Crile G: Excision of cancer of the head and neck: With special reference to the plan of dissection based on one hundred and thirty-two operations. JAMA 47:1780–1786, 1906

8. Fisch U: Lymphographische Untersuchungen über das zervikale Lymphsystem (Fortschritte der Hals-Nasen-Ohrenheilkunde, vol 14), pp 53–162. Basel, Karger, 1966. [English edition: Fisch U: Cervical lymphography following irradiation of the neck. In: Lymphography of the Cervical Lymphatic System, pp 47–146. Philadelphia, WB Saunders, 1968]

9. Fletcher GH: Elective irradiation of subclinical disease in cancers of the head and neck. Cancer 29:1450–1454, 1972

10. Földi M: Lymphogenous encephalopathy. In Mayerson HS (ed): Lymph and the Lymphatic System, pp 169–198. Springfield, IL, Charles C Thomas, 1968

11. Fonts EA, Greenlaw RH, Rush BF, Rovin S: Verrucous squamous cell carcinoma of the oral cavity. Cancer 23:152–160, 1969

12. Jesse RH, Barkley HT, Lindberg RD, Fletcher GH: Cancer of the oral cavity: Is elective neck dissection beneficial? Am J Surg 120:505–508, 1970

13. Kraus FT, Perez-Mesa C: Verrucous carcinoma: Clinical and pathologic study of 105 cases involving oral cavity, larynx and genitalia. Cancer 19:26–38, 1966

14. Leventon GS, Evans HL: Sarcomatoid squamous cell carcinoma of the mucous membranes of the head and neck: A clinicopathologic study of 20 cases. Cancer 48:994–1003, 1981

15. Lindberg RD, Barkley HT Jr, Jesse RH, Fletcher GH: Evolution of the clinically negative neck in patients with squamous cell carcinoma of the faucial arch. Am J Roentgenol Radium Ther Nucl Med 111:60–65, 1971

16. Mendenhall WM, Million RR, Cassisi NJ: Elective neck irradiation in squamous cell carcinoma of the head and neck. Head Neck Surg 3:15–20, 1980

17. Mendenhall WM, Van Cise WS, Bova FJ, Million RR: Analysis of time–dose factors in squamous cell carcinoma of the oral tongue and floor of mouth treated with radiation therapy alone. Int J Radiat Oncol Biol Phys 7:1005–1011, 1981

18. Million RR: Elective neck irradiation for TXN0 squamous carcinoma of the oral tongue and floor of mouth. Cancer 34:149–155, 1974

19. Million RR, Cassisi NJ, Wittes RE: Cancer in the head and neck. In DeVita VT Jr, Hellman S, Rosenberg SA (eds): Cancer: Principles and Practice of Oncology, pp 301–395. Philadelphia, JB Lippincott, 1982

20. Million RR, Fletcher GH, Jesse RH Jr: Evaluation of elective irradiation of the neck for squamous cell carcinoma of the nasopharynx, tonsillar fossa, and base of tongue. Radiology 80:973–988, 1963

21. Northrop MF, Fletcher GH, Jesse RH, Lindberg RD: Evolution of neck disease in patients with primary squamous cell carcinoma of the oral tongue, floor of mouth, and palatine arch, and clinically positive neck nodes neither fixed nor bilateral. Cancer 29:23–30, 1972

22. Olofsson J, Van Nostrand AWP: Growth and spread of laryngeal and hypopharyngeal carcinoma with reflections on the effect of preoperative irradiation. Acta Otolaryngol Suppl. 308, 1973

23. Perez CA, Kraus FT, Evans JC, Powers WE: Anaplastic transformation in verrucous carcinoma of the oral cavity after radiation therapy. Radiology 86:108–115, 1966

24. Pressman JJ, Simon MB, Monell C: Anatomical studies related to the dissemination of cancer of the larynx. Trans Am Acad Ophthalmol Otolaryngol 64:628–638, 1960

25. Rouviere H: Anatomy of the Human Lymphatic System, pp 1–28, 77–78. Tobias MJ (trans). Ann Arbor, MI, Edwards Brothers, 1938

26. Suarez O: El problema de las metastasis linfáticas y alejadas del cáncer de laringe e hipofaringe. Rev Otorrinolaringol (Santiago, Chile) 23:83–99, 1963

27. Yoffey JM, Courtice FC: Lymphatics, Lymph and the Lymphomyeloid Complex, p 15. London, Academic Press, 1970

General Principles for Treatment of Cancers in the Head and Neck: Surgery

5

RODNEY R. MILLION

NICHOLAS J. CASSISI

Make accurate incisions surrounding the whole tumor so as not to leave a single root.

—GALEN (A.D. 129–199)

Many patients who present with head and neck malignancies are older, undernourished individuals who use alcohol and tobacco to excess. Medical problems such as diabetes, pulmonary disease, and cardiovascular disease are often present. All such factors must be considered and corrected prior to offering the choice of surgery to these patients. There are relatively few absolute contraindications to surgery, but if the medical problems are so severe that the risk with anesthesia is high, then surgery is contraindicated unless there is no feasible alternative and the patient strongly urges that the operation be done. A myocardial infarction within the previous 3 months is a contraindication to surgery. A relative contraindication to surgery is the presence of simultaneous double primary lesions that cannot be encompassed in a single operative procedure; individualization is required for these cases.

MANAGEMENT OF THE PRIMARY LESION

The surgical goal in management of a primary lesion is complete excision with immediate reconstruction to a socially acceptable level of function and cosmesis.

Surgery must be considered the therapeutic modality of choice if the cure rate is at least as great as with radiation therapy, if the functional and cosmetic deformities are acceptable to the patient, or if the anticipated complications from irradiation are severe enough to ultimately require surgery. The skills of the surgeon are a consideration; for instance, it would be better to treat an early lesion of the infrahyoid epiglottis with radiation therapy than with a total laryngectomy if the supraglottic laryngectomy is not in the surgeon's armamentarium, since a total laryngectomy is always an option for salvage.

Lesions in certain anatomical sites lend themselves well to surgery (e.g., small lesions of the lip, the retromolar trigone, the tip of the tongue, the gingiva, the epiglottis, and the skin).

The surgeon must exercise prudent judgment in advising excision of advanced lesions. A few patients may be cured, but others may become functional or cosmetic cripples and wish they were dead. Some physicians justify their decision to perform excision with the attitude that "if we don't do something, the patient will die." These decisions vary with the experience and aggressiveness of the surgeon; the patient and his family must be totally informed of the probable chance of cure and the functional and cosmetic problems so that they may select the proper option. It is unwise to talk a patient into undergoing a major operative procedure only to have a bitter patient and family as a reward for the effort.

MANAGEMENT OF THE NECK*

Arterial Supply to the Skin of the Neck and Its Influence on Neck Dissection Incisions

The incision that is selected for neck dissection is based, first of all, on whether or not the primary site is to be resected, since the exposure of the primary lesion governs the choice of incision. A large variety of incisions are available to the surgeon, and each has advantages and disadvantages. Knowledge of the vascular supply to the cervical skin is an important factor in selecting the incision most likely to heal without necrosis, especially when prior radiation therapy has been administered. A simplified schematic of the arterial supply to the skin of the neck is provided in Figure 5-1, *center*. The arterial supply tends to run in a superior–inferior direction. The facial, occipital, and transverse cervical arteries are often ligated during the operation. Numerous arterial loops are shown on cadaver injection studies. The venous drainage is from above and is interrupted by any horizontal incision.[8]

The popular Hayes Martin incision (Fig. 5-1, *upper left*) affords excellent anatomical exposure, but it places the trifurcate junction over the carotid and risks exposure and rupture of that vessel.[17] The MacFee incision (Fig. 5-1, *upper right*) avoids a trifurcate junction, but it may not provide adequate exposure for a surgeon who is not experienced with the technique.[15] The cosmetic result is excellent. A neck incision commonly used by Cassisi and similar to that proposed by Ogura, Freund, Schobinger, Conley, and others (Fig. 5-1, *lower left*) provides good exposure, minimal interruption of the blood supply, and satisfactory cosmetic result.[1,9,19] The vertical limb is placed far posterior so that there is virtually no need to dissect and elevate the posterior flap. The posterior flap is supplied with blood by the descending branch of the occipital artery from above and by the ascending branch of the transverse artery from below. In the event that radiation therapy has been used prior to surgery, this posterior flap will receive little or no irradiation. Therefore, one has an essentially normal segment of skin to suture to the front flaps, and the trifurcation is posterior to the common carotid. The horizontal limb of the incision allows satisfactory exposure of the submaxillary and submental area. The vertical limb tends to drift anteriorly as it heals; as a result, its final position is somewhat farther forward than might be imagined, based on its initial position (Fig. 5-2). This modification in the neck incision is one of the changes that has enabled neck dissection to be performed without catastrophic complications after the delivery of high doses of radiation therapy (6000 rad to 8000 rad) to large, fixed neck nodes.

For tumors in some anatomical sites, the risk of metastatic disease in the submental or submaxillary nodes is essentially nonexistent (e.g., supraglottic carcinoma with no palpable neck nodes), and the area need not be resected. A single-limb incision (Fig. 5-3) is useful in these cases, since it avoids the trifurcate junction and provides satisfactory anatomical exposure except in the submental area. It is therefore useful for those lesions with no risk for

---

* For "Anatomy of the Head and Neck Lymphatics," see Chapter 4, General Principles for Treatment of Cancers in the Head and Neck: Selection of Treatment for the Primary Site and for the Neck.

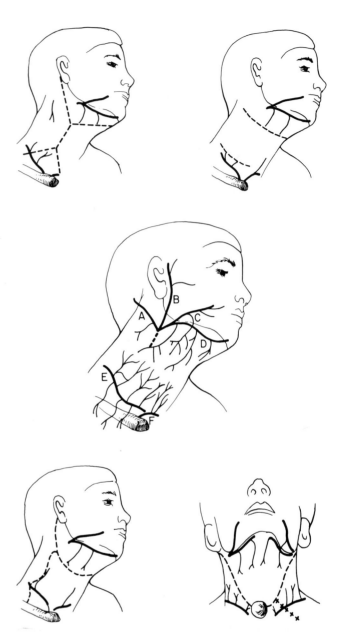

FIG. 5-1. Simplified schematic of the normal arterial supply to the skin of the neck and the effect of four commonly used incisions. (*Center*) Normal arterial supply to the skin of the neck: *A,* Occipital artery and the descending branch; *B,* Superficial temporal artery; *C,* Facial artery, *D,* Submental branch of facial artery; *E,* Transverse cervical artery; *F,* Subscapular artery. (*Upper left*) Incision recommended by Martin (1951).[17] (*Upper right*) Incision recommended by MacFee (1960).[15] (*Lower left*) Incision recommended by Cassisi. This is a modification of the incisions recommended by Ogura (1969), Freund (1967), Conley (1966), and Schobinger.[1,10,19] (*Lower right*) Apron flap described by Durante (1905), often employed for laryngectomy and neck dissection.[7] Two trifurcate junctions occur at the tracheostome in an area with a depleted blood supply; as a result, wound infection and necrosis may occur. (Redrawn from Freeland AP, Rogers JH: The vascular supply of the cervical skin with reference to incision planning. Laryngoscope 85:714–725, 1975)

submental or submandibular metastases. It is especially useful for irradiated patients.

If the patient is to receive postoperative radiation therapy, the radiation therapist must decide whether to cover the entire area of the surgical dissection. It is customary to include the entire surgical field, but incisions that extend far beyond the conventional radiation field require an increased volume of irradiation and minor changes in treatment planning. Although this can be done, especially when electron-beam therapy is available, it unnecessarily complicates the radiation therapy and should be avoided when possible.

Normal Venous Drainage of the Head and Neck

The intracranial and extracranial arrangement of the veins of the head and neck area is shown in Figure 5-4.

Except for a few small veins around the larynx, the veins of the head and neck are *without valves,* and therefore venous blood may be readily shunted to an alternate route when a vein is ligated or obstructed.

Venous blood leaves the cranium through the internal jugular veins, the emissary veins, the diploic veins, and the vertebral veins. The internal jugular vein and even the external jugular vein may be preserved in conservative neck dissections, but in the usual radical neck dissection, the internal jugular vein and the external jugular vein are ligated, thereby removing two major escape routes for blood leaving the brain (see Fig. 5-4). The normal vertebral veins are estimated to be adequate to carry the overload created by ligation of both internal jugular veins.[2,12] The vertebral veins and posterior emissary veins communicate with the occipital plexus and represent a major escape route after radical neck dissection.[12] The nape of the neck should be suspended in the postoperative period to prevent occlusion of this venous system by pillows or dressings. The head rests on a pillow or "doughnut," and there should be room to place a hand between the neck and the bed.*

Anomalies of the venous system are frequent, however, so the capacity to shunt venous blood from right to left or *vice versa* may be poor. The confluence of the venous sinuses is particularly important in the rerouting of blood flow. Venous blood from the superior sagittal sinus flows into the right transverse sinus, which is often larger than the left transverse sinus. Blood from the straight sinus flows into the left transverse sinus. The junction of these veins (confluence) may at times be nearly or completely separate and may thus eliminate the major pathway for the shunting of blood from side to side. Rohrbach reported the autopsy findings for a patient who died after a left neck dissection; the patient's right transverse sinus and internal jugular vein were underdeveloped—"the size of a knitting needle," according to Rohrbach.[21] These anomalies may account for the rare reports of acute difficulties that arise after ligation of one internal and one external jugular vein.[25] Carotid angiograms taken with and without compression of the internal jugular vein may be used in special cases to establish the patency of the anastomoses between the right and left venous system.

Ligation of one or both internal and external jugular veins is regularly accompanied by an immediate rise in

* Levine H: Personal communication, 1982.

the cerebrospinal fluid pressure. The rise in pressure is due to the accumulation of intracranial venous blood, which displaces the cerebrospinal fluid into the spinal canal. The cerebrospinal fluid pressure regularly returns to normal a short time after the ligation of one internal jugular vein; however, after a second jugular vein has been ligated, the pressure may remain elevated unless cerebrospinal fluid is removed.

Failure of the venous-lymphatic system to compensate produces a clinical picture of lymphedema of the facial structures, especially of the eyelids; cyanosis; and other signs and symptoms consistent with a sudden increase in intracranial pressure. Patients prefer to sleep with the head elevated, which assists venous drainage. Pressure on the posterior neck should be avoided postoperatively to prevent further obstruction of the suboccipital venous plexus and perhaps of the dermal lymphatics.

The ligation of the internal and external jugular veins in conjunction with radical neck dissection is further complicated by the surgical obstruction of the lymphatic trunks. A small proportion of the cerebrospinal fluid is absorbed through lymphatic capillary connections with the central nervous system, which are located in the cribriform plate and possibly in the jugular bulb (see Chapter 4).

Fascial Compartments of the Neck

The lymph nodes are separated from the muscles, vessels, and nerves by their respective aponeuroses (Fig. 5-5). Bocca and Pignataro provide a detailed discussion of the fascial compartments of the neck.[3]

CERVICAL LYMPHADENECTOMY

The concept of en *bloc* removal of the regional neck nodes has undergone major modification in the 80 years since it was first described, around the turn of the century. In early years, the indications for radical neck dissection were tightly restricted to favorable situations. In 1940, Duffy indicated that the primary lesion must be controlled, limited to one side of the oral cavity, and well differentiated; that the enlarged cervical metastases must be limited to one or two contiguous groups, with no perforation of the lymph node capsule and no contralateral metastases; that there must be no distant metastases; and that the patient must be in good general condition.[6] By 1951, Martin had reduced the number of contraindications and indicated that neck dissection should be done when (1) there was clinical evidence of cancer in the cervical lymphatics, (2) the primary disease was either controlled or was going to be resected in connection with the neck dissection, (3) there was a reasonable chance of resection of the cervical metastatic tumor, (4) there was no evidence of distant metastases, and (5) surgery was more likely to be successful than radiation therapy.[17]

Contraindications to Neck Dissection

There remain few absolute contraindications to neck dissection. Contraindications include the presence of multiple intradermal nodules, solid adherence of the tumor to the base of the skull or the cervical spine, and medical contraindications.

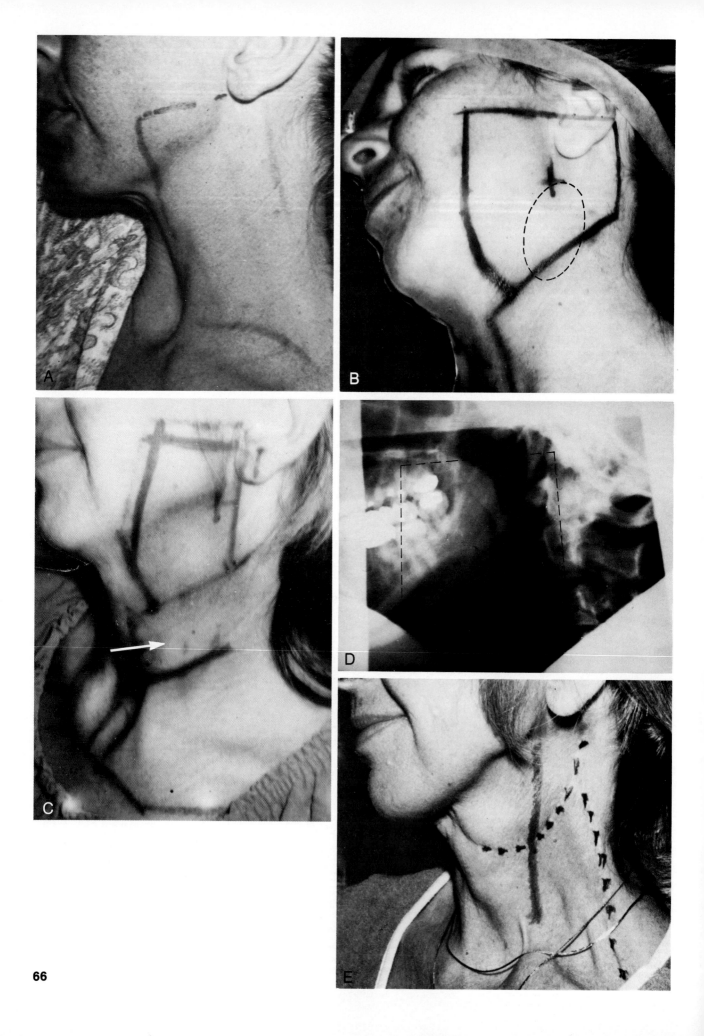

◄ **FIG. 5-2.** A 43-year-old woman presented with a left neck mass that had enlarged over the previous year. A primary lesion of the left base of the tongue was discovered; biopsy revealed anaplastic squamous cell carcinoma. The lesion extended from the midline of the tongue to the glossotonsillar sulcus and onto the lower pole of the tonsillar fossa. There was a fairly discrete mobile mass, 6 cm × 3 cm, in the left jugulodigastric area (T3N3A—stage IV). (A) The patient had received 1800 rad through parallel opposed rectangular portals prior to consultation. Note borderline coverage of the base of the tongue and the upper jugular chain, junctional, and spinal accessory lymph nodes. The lower jugular chain was not included. The entire larynx was in the treatment portal. (B) Revised cobalt-60 portals. Note difference in portal borders compared with A. The superior margin is 2 cm higher to ensure adequate coverage of the base of the tongue and the junctional lymph nodes. The lower neck received 5000 rad through a separate anterior portal in order to avoid unnecessary irradiation of the larynx, hypopharynx, and spinal cord; the junction between the upper and lower portals falls across the 6-cm lymph node (*dashed line*). (C) Portal reduction at 5000 rad. The spinal cord was excluded from the upper portal, and the superior and anterior margins were reduced 1 cm. Through a reduced anterior portal (*arrow*), 1000 rad was added to the lower portion of the metastatic lymph node. (D) Roentgenogram of treatment portal shown in B. *Dashed lines* represent reduced portal adopted at 5000 rad. Treatment was completed through parallel opposed fields, cobalt-60, 6500 rad tumor dose/7 weeks; 1000 rad was added to the base of tongue through a submental boost. The final tongue dose was estimated at 7500 rad. The maximum dose to the left neck node was 7000 rad to 7500 rad; the minimum dose was 6000 rad. The patient had a left radical neck dissection 4 weeks following radiation therapy. The specimen was negative for tumor. Her postoperative course was uneventful, and she was discharged from the hospital in 1 week. (E) Appearance of neck 7½ years after treatment. The *solid line* represents the carotid artery. The *dashed line* represents the scar of the radical neck dissection. Note the relationship of the posterior limb of the incision and the trifurcate junction to the artery. The upper portion of the posterior flap lies on the posterior edge of the irradiation portal and received little or no irradiation. The lower portion of the posterior flap received approximately 4000 rad.

FIG. 5-3. Single-limb incision.

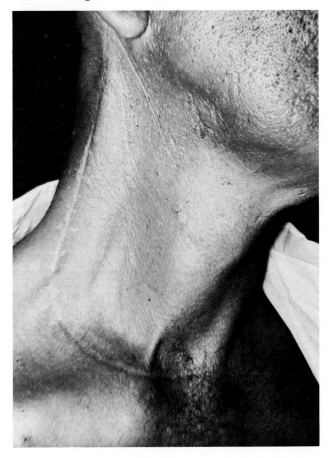

RELATIVE CONTRAINDICATIONS

SKIN INVASION

The extension of a tumor through the platysma into the skin is a relative contraindication to lymphadenectomy (see Fig. 4-22). As soon as a tumor enters the dermal lymphatics, spread is erratic, and because the tumor has often extended a considerable distance beyond the obvious skin involvement, it generally cannot be removed by surgery alone. Attempts to treat this type of patient with surgery alone would be no more successful than attempts to treat patients with inflammatory breast cancer by surgery alone. We have treated some patients with limited skin involvement in whom radiation therapy was used first to control the tumor in the dermal lymphatics and then the involved skin was removed at the time of radical neck dissection. The radiation therapy is administered in full therapeutic doses in this situation.

BONE OR PERIOSTEAL INVASION

Large neck masses may become attached to the transverse processes of the cervical spine, the base of the skull, or the mandible. Bone films are usually normal. Neck dissection is still possible in some instances after high-dose radiation therapy. A portion of the mandible, the mastoid tip, or rarely a portion of a transverse process may be removed. The high-dose irradiation reduces the size of the mass, and a pseudocapsule forms, which aids in the dissection. These are not cases for the beginning surgeon, because the potential for a surgical disaster is high.

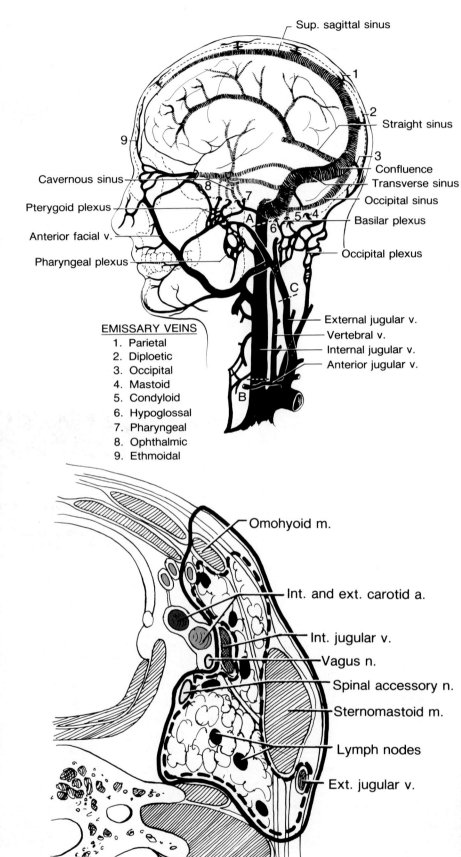

Sup. sagittal sinus

Straight sinus

Confluence
Transverse sinus
Occipital sinus
Basilar plexus

Occipital plexus

Cavernous sinus
Pterygoid plexus
Anterior facial v.
Pharyngeal plexus

External jugular v.
Vertebral v.
Internal jugular v.
Anterior jugular v.

EMISSARY VEINS
1. Parietal
2. Diploetic
3. Occipital
4. Mastoid
5. Condyloid
6. Hypoglossal
7. Pharyngeal
8. Ophthalmic
9. Ethmoidal

FIG. 5-4. Head and neck venous system. *A* and *B* represent the usual sites for ligation of the internal jugular vein during a neck dissection. *C* represents the location for ligation of the external jugular vein. (Redrawn from Eycleshymer AC, Jones T [eds]: Hand-Atlas of Clinical Anatomy, p 53. Philadelphia, Lea & Febiger, 1925)

Omohyoid m.

Int. and ext. carotid a.

Int. jugular v.

Vagus n.

Spinal accessory n.

Sternomastoid m.

Lymph nodes

Ext. jugular v.

FIG. 5-5. Comparison of radical neck dissection and conservative neck dissection. The solid line indicates the structures usually removed with a radical neck dissection, and the dashed line indicates the limits of the conservative neck dissection. (Redrawn from Bocca E, Pignataro O: A conservative technique in radical neck dissection. Ann Otol Rhinol Laryngol 76:975–987, 1967)

INVASION OF THE CAROTID VESSELS

Large neck masses attach to the carotid vessels, but they rarely invade the wall to any significant depth. This diagnosis may be suspected preoperatively by the size and location of the mass and by the relative immobility of the mass, particularly in the up and down directions. A computed tomographic (CT) scan with contrast medium may be of help in assessing resectability preoperatively. The external carotid may be sacrificed, but ligation of the common carotid and the internal carotid produces a substantial risk of stroke. If high-dose irradiation (6000 rad to 8000 rad) is administered prior to neck dissection, a fibrous capsule develops around the tumor, and it frequently can be dissected free of the carotid. A segment of the common carotid or the internal carotid may be resected and the vessel reunited with a graft, but the risk of stroke is still present.

CLINICALLY POSITIVE LOW NECK DISEASE

There is a belief among some surgeons and radiation therapists that clinically positive nodes in the lower neck are related to such a high rate of distant metastasis or regional treatment failure that a curative approach is not warranted. However, we have observed several patients with pathologically positive lower neck nodes who have been cured. Patients with extensive lower neck disease are seldom suitable for curative therapy.

Surgical Options for Neck Dissection

As recently as 10 to 20 years ago, it was considered bad practice to do anything but a full radical neck dissection, but this concept is gradually changing, and the surgeon has a number of modified neck dissections to choose from that may be used in various circumstances. Surgeons have begun to depart from the traditional standard radical neck dissection in which the sternocleidomastoid muscle, the internal and external jugular veins, and the spinal accessory nerve along with the submaxillary gland are removed as a single unit. The supraomohyoid neck dissection as described by Crile has been resurrected, and the functional neck dissection as described by Suarez in Argentina and Bocca in Italy proved that the sternocleidomastoid muscle, internal jugular vein, and spinal accessory nerve could be preserved without any loss in regional control when the procedure was used in patients with a clinically negative neck or small mobile nodes.[3,5,24]

The concept of combining surgery and radiation therapy, especially elective neck irradiation, has also helped change the surgeon's options in neck dissection.

The M. D. Anderson Hospital group led by Jesse indicated that a regional or partial neck dissection was sufficient surgery following whole neck irradiation in instances where only one or two contiguous neck nodes were clinically involved. The radiation therapy was expected to sterilize subclinical disease in the unresected nodes, and the surgical excision was expected to remove any residual cancer not sterilized by the radiation.* The risk of neck recurrence for 310 neck dissections managed at the M. D. Anderson Hospital between 1970 and 1975 is analyzed in Table 5-1. The operating surgeon was free to select the neck dissection, based on the distribution of neck disease.[13] The highest recurrence rate occurred in the oral cavity cases: 26 of the 39 regional failures (66%) occurred in the patients with oral cavity lesions. Partial neck dissection coupled with radiation therapy was associated with a low regional failure rate (11%) when used in selected cases. The failure rate in oral cavity cases was higher, partly because the irradiation portals were smaller and the doses were lower than with oropharynx, hypopharynx, and larynx cases.

Simple excision of a positive lymph node followed by high-dose radiation therapy is a surprisingly effective

* There was considerable hue and cry and general misunderstanding about this concept when it was introduced by Jesse. Many surgeons considered (and still do) that anything less than a radical neck dissection was doomed to failure. The radiation therapists mistakenly thought that the operation was a simple "lumpectomy" after radiation therapy, rather than a regional node dissection.

TABLE 5-1. Risk of Neck Recurrence After Neck Dissection

	Therapeutic (N+)*		Elective (N0)*	
	Surgery Alone	Surgery + Radiation Therapy	Surgery Alone	Surgery + Radiation Therapy
Partial neck dissection	4/13 (27%)	8/72 (11%)	4/54 (7%)	2/32 (6%)
Spinal accessory nerve spared	1/12	2/8	0/3	0/1
Radical neck dissection	9/37 (25%)	8/57 (15%)	1/12	0/9
Total	32/199 (16%)		7/111 (6%)	
Total recurrence rate for oral cavity lesions	20/79 (25%)		6/61 (10%)	
Total recurrence rate excluding patients with oral cavity lesions	12/120 (10%)		1/50 (2%)	

* Number of patients with recurrence/number treated.
Note: M. D. Anderson Hospital data; patients treated 1970–1975.

(Adapted from Jesse RH, Ballantyne AJ, Larson D: Radical or modified neck dissection: A therapeutic dilemma. Am J Surg 136:516–519, 1978)

treatment, although the treatment is not usually planned in this fashion. For example, suppose that a neck mass is excised for diagnosis, and squamous cell carcinoma is diagnosed. The primary lesion may or may not be discovered, and the patient is subsequently treated only by radiation therapy. The success for this combination is quite high in spite of theoretical considerations to the contrary (see Chapter 16, The Unknown Primary).

RADICAL NECK DISSECTION

In a standard radical neck dissection, the superficial and deep cervical fascia, with its enclosed ipsilateral lymph nodes, is removed with the sternocleidomastoid muscle, the omohyoid muscle, the internal and external jugular veins, the spinal accessory nerve, and the submaxillary gland. The incisions used by the surgeon are to a large extent governed by the primary lesion if it is also to be resected.

The main advantages of the full radical neck dissection are the improved anatomical exposure, especially near the base of the skull, and the wider margins of excision. Nodes larger than 2 cm to 3 cm have often penetrated the nodal capsule, and the sternocleidomastoid and omohyoid muscles may be invaded by the tumor. Removal of the sternocleidomastoid provides better exposure near the base of the skull and allows a high ligation of the internal jugular vein and more complete removal of junctional lymph nodes.

RADICAL NECK DISSECTION WITH SPARING OF THE SPINAL ACCESSORY NERVE

The degree of functional loss resulting from severance of the spinal accessory nerve varies, since innervation of the trapezius may be partly supplied by branches of the anterior rami of the third and fourth cervical nerves. Atrophy of the trapezius is followed by a shoulder drop and a reduced ability to pick up and carry heavy objects. Shoulder pain is a frequent side effect. The functional deformity that occurs with the sacrifice of the spinal accessory nerve appears justified when the disease is extensive. The functional loss and discomfort may be somewhat minimized with physical therapy.

Preservation of the spinal accessory nerve is especially important for individuals who, for occupational reasons, require use of the trapezius muscle. In general, it is specified for patients with no clinically enlarged nodes or with small, clinically positive, mobile nodes located away from the base of skull and for patients with clinically positive necks that become clinically negative after radiation therapy. Sparing of the spinal accessory nerve is contraindicated if there are clinically palpable nodes high in the jugular chain, because it interferes with adequate dissection. The decision to save or sacrifice the nerve is often made at the time of neck dissection, and the patient must not be promised that the nerve can be preserved. Preservation of the nerve does not guarantee return of function, because it is often stretched and sometimes fails to recover full activity. The incidence of neck recurrence reported for series in which the spinal accessory nerve was saved is given in Table 5-2.[4,13,14,22]

FUNCTIONAL NECK DISSECTION

The functional neck dissection as popularized by Bocca removes only the superficial and deep cervical fascia along

TABLE 5-2.   Neck Recurrence Reported for Series in Which the Spinal Accessory Nerve Was Saved

Institution	Percentage of Patients With Nerve Saved	Neck Recurrence*
Indianapolis[14]	22%	7/98 (7%)
Mayo Clinic[22]	36%	7/89 (8%)
Karolinska[4]	64%	7/80 (9%)
M. D. Anderson[13]	66%	21/205 (10%)

* Number of patients with recurrence/number treated.

with its enclosed nodes, leaving intact the sternocleidomastoid and omohyoid muscles, the internal jugular vein, and the spinal accessory nerve (see Fig. 5-5). Bocca and Pignataro report no higher incidence of neck failure with their procedure even in clinically positive necks, than with a standard radical neck dissection.[3]

The elective functional neck dissection is used if there are no clinically positive nodes in the neck or if there are only small, clinically positive, mobile nodes. Bilateral functional neck dissection may be done for midline lesions.

One of the major advantages of the functional neck dissection is the preservation of the sternocleidomastoid, which provides excellent coverage of the carotid vessels in the event of a wound necrosis. Approximately one half to one third of the sternocleidomastoid muscle mass is lost owing to reduced blood supply, but the muscle continues to function if the spinal accessory nerve is preserved. Sparing the nerve preserves the function of the trapezius and sternocleidomastoid. Although the internal jugular vein may be spared, it may be sacrificed on one side with almost no risk; in fact, sacrificing it makes the operation a bit easier. If bilateral simultaneous functional neck dissection is planned, the first internal jugular vein should be spared, if possible, in case it must be ligated on the second side.

The disadvantage to the functional neck dissection is that the access to the junctional lymph nodes is poorer and the operating time longer compared with the radical neck dissection.

SUPRAOMOHYOID NECK DISSECTION

The supraomohyoid neck dissection is a functional regional neck dissection in which the internal jugular chain lymph nodes above the omohyoid muscle, the junctional lymph nodes, the upper spinal accessory lymph nodes, the submaxillary gland with its prevascular and postvascular nodes, and the submental lymph nodes are removed.

The supraomohyoid neck dissection may be used when a small primary lesion of the oral cavity is to be excised and the neck is clinically negative; in such a case, the first echelon of nodes is removed. If the nodes are found to be positive at the time of the operation, the dissection is extended to a full neck dissection. Another indication for the supraomohyoid neck dissection occurs in cases in which the primary lesion is to be treated with radiation therapy and the patient has one or two large upper neck nodes. Irradiation is administered to the primary lesion and the entire neck on one or both sides. After irradiation, there is a residual, ill-defined mass in the upper neck. If a supraomohyoid neck dissection is used in this situation, the sternocleidomastoid muscle and perhaps the spinal accessory nerve may be preserved.

Bilateral supraomohyoid neck dissection may be performed in patients with bilateral upper neck disease (Fig. 5-6). Both dissections may be done simultaneously if one internal jugular vein can be preserved. Fewer complications occur, however, if the second neck dissection is carried out 4 to 6 weeks after the initial neck dissection.

BILATERAL RADICAL NECK DISSECTION

Bilateral radical neck dissection is usually prescribed for patients with bilateral clinically positive nodes. The indications for and timing of bilateral radical neck dissection

vary according to the initial management of the primary lesion. We generally do not recommend simultaneous bilateral radical neck dissection, especially in conjunction with resection of the primary lesion, because the risk for serious complications is often greater than the chance for cure. Staged bilateral neck dissection is safer, even though it requires two separate operations. Prolonged facial and central nervous system edema may occur after bilateral ligation of the lymphatic and venous systems. The venous and lymphatic systems eventually compensate over a period of 1 to 2 years in those fortunate enough to survive (Fig. 5-7). If the primary lesion is to be treated by radiation therapy alone, both sides of the neck are irradiated, followed by staged neck dissections.

If and when bilateral internal jugular vein ligation is

FIG. 5-6. A 54-year-old man with poorly differentiated squamous cell carcinoma of the base of the tongue and the vallecula with extension to the epiglottis and left pharyngoepiglottic fold. There was a 3-cm jugulodigastric node on the right and a 4-cm jugulodigastric node on the left (T3N3B). He received a tumor dose of 6000 rad/7 weeks, through parallel opposed fields, cobalt-60, followed by a 1000-rad submental boost to the primary lesion. The lower neck received 5000 rad. There was complete disappearance of the primary lesion after 2000 rad; the nodes were 50% smaller at the completion of treatment. Six weeks later, the patient underwent bilateral supraomohyoid neck dissection. There was no tumor in the nine left neck nodes and seven right neck nodes. There were suspicious nodes located on the left spinal accessory nerve, and the nerve was sacrificed. A large lymph node was found in the right midjugular area, and approximately 1 cm of the sternocleidomastoid muscle was resected; the right spinal accessory nerve was spared. The patient had an uneventful postoperative course and was discharged 7 days later. He had no significant edema and was free of disease 4½ years after the start of treatment. (A) Prior to treatment. (P, posterior pharyngeal wall; E, epiglottis; V, right vallecula) (B) Treatment portals. (C) Primary site 3 years after the start of treatment. (D and E) Appearance of the neck 3 years after treatment. Note the preservation of sternocleidomastoid muscles and freedom from significant edema or fibrosis. Approximately one third to one half of the sternocleidomastoid muscle mass is lost; the motor nerve to the sternocleidomastoid muscle is the spinal accessory nerve, which was preserved on the right but sacrificed on the left.

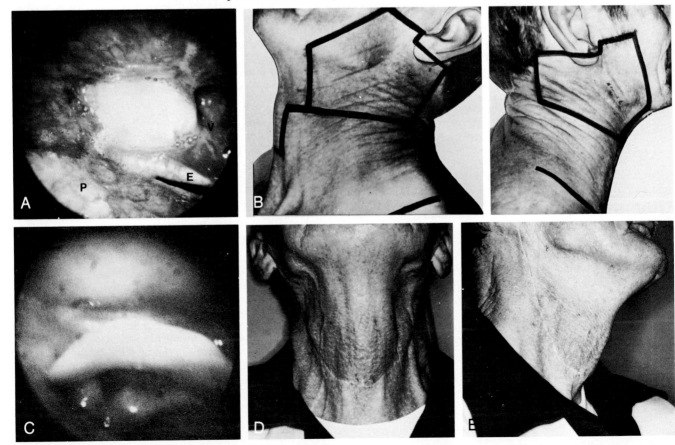

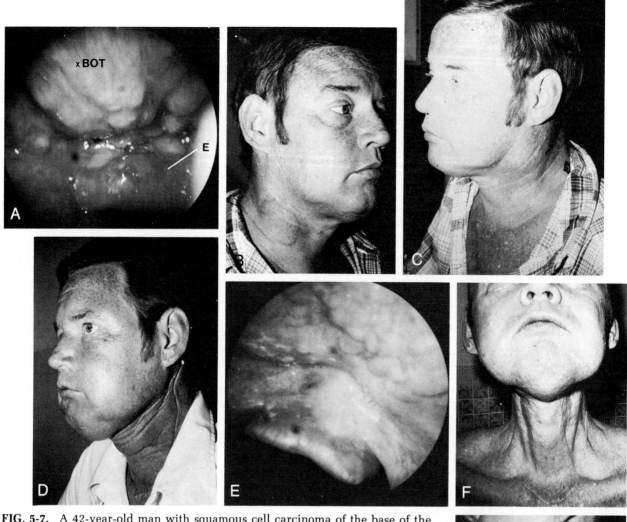

FIG. 5-7. A 42-year-old man with squamous cell carcinoma of the base of the tongue and bilateral cervical lymphadenopathy (T3N3B [N2A, N2A]—stage IV). (*A*) Large lesion in the vallecula, extending laterally to both pharyngoepiglottic folds and the lingual surface of the epiglottis and extending anteriorly to the circumvallate papillae. (*BOT*, base of tongue; *E*, epiglottis) (*B*) Matted nodes measuring 3 cm × 4 cm in the right midjugular region. (*C*) Subdigastric mass measuring 4 cm × 5 cm in the left neck. The primary and upper neck received a tumor dose of 7400 rad/6 weeks, delivered at 120 rad twice a day. Bilateral electron strips added 1260 rad to the spinal accessory lymph nodes. Both sides of the lower neck received 6000 rad/6 weeks. There was persistent disease in both sides of the neck 1 month after radiation therapy was completed. Simultaneous bilateral modified neck dissections were done by Ogura; both internal jugular veins were spared. The pathology report showed necrotic tumor in large neck nodes. (*D*) Lymphedema 1 month after neck dissection. Edema slowly disappeared over a 2-year period. There were minimal problems with wound healing. (*E*) Two years after the start of treatment, the patient was without evidence of disease at the primary site. (*F* and *G*) Appearance of the neck at 22 months. There was mild lymphedema, which was accentuated by loss of muscle. The patient described a "tight, constricting sensation" in the neck.

likely, it is preferable to perform a two-stage procedure, which allows time for the vascular and lymphatic systems to compensate. Radiation therapy is used to hold disease in the unoperated side of the neck in check during this interval. It is important that the radiation therapist shield as much normal skin as possible to reduce the radiation effect on the dermal lymphatics.

The long-term survivors of radiation therapy and bilateral neck dissection complain of difficulty in swallowing, a tight, restrictive sensation in the neck, discomfort in the shoulders, and facial swelling. Although their quality of life is acceptable, most of these patients have nagging complaints for the rest of their lives.

POSTEROLATERAL NECK DISSECTION

The posterolateral neck dissection is used to resect lymph nodes associated with skin malignancies (melanomas and squamous cell carcinomas) that arise from the posterior scalp, occiput, and nape of the neck.[11] The regional lymph nodes at risk would include the retroauricular, suboccipital, and spinal accessory nodes. The retroauricular nodes lie in the soft tissues, either on or just behind the mastoid. The suboccipital nodes are divided into three subgroups: (1) the superficial occipital nodes, which are closely related to the cutaneous branch of the occipital artery and the greater occipital nerve at the insertion of the trapezius to the inferior nuchal line; (2) the deep occipital nodes, which lie underneath the superficial layer of the deep cervical fascia next to the splenius capitis; and (3) one lymph node, which is usually located along the splenius portion of the occipital artery. The occipital and retroauricular nodes drain to the spinal accessory chain and sometimes to the internal jugular chain.

If the primary lesion is located on the scalp close to the ear, the lymph nodes in the parotid area may also be at risk. A complete regional node dissection for such lesions would include not only a posterolateral neck dissection but also the removal of the lymph nodes of the parotid area and a conventional neck dissection to remove the lymph nodes of the internal jugular chain.

TECHNIQUE

If the primary lesion is present and lies close to the neck dissection limits, it may be incorporated into the neck dissection specimen. Skin flaps are elevated from the posterior edge of the sternocleidomastoid to the posterior midline. The trapezius is separated from the nuchal line and resected down to the level of C3 to C4. The lymph nodes are removed along with the occipital artery. The spinal accessory nerve may or may not be preserved, depending on whether the lymph nodes are clinically negative or positive. The spinal accessory nerve forms the inferior limits of the dissection if the lymph nodes are negative. The nodes of the upper internal jugular vein are dissected by retracting the sternocleidomastoid muscle anteriorly. Whether or not the sternocleidomastoid should be removed depends on the clinical situation. No major cosmetic or functional deformity is noted other than that commonly associated with spinal accessory nerve loss, even for those patients who undergo bilateral dissection. A high rate of regional control is reported for this procedure, which is used mainly for malignant melanoma of the scalp.[11]

Complications of Neck Dissection

FACTORS AFFECTING COMPLICATION RISKS

The risk of operative mortality and morbidity is affected primarily by four factors:

1. Prior irradiation. The total dose of radiation given, the volume of tissues irradiated, the radiation energy (i.e., the degree of skin-sparing), and the time elapsed between the irradiation and the operation affect the risk of a complication.
2. Resection of the primary lesion. Neck dissection without resection of the primary site, with or without prior radiotherapy, carries far less risk of a complication than dissection combined with resection of the primary lesion, particularly when the oral cavity or pharynx must be entered.
3. Tumor extent in the neck. Patients with minimal tumor involvement have fewer complications than those with large masses that require more extensive resection.
4. The general medical and nutritional status of the patient.

INTRAOPERATIVE COMPLICATIONS

LIGATION OF NERVES

A number of cranial and cervical nerves are at risk to be ligated during the neck dissection. Any or all of these have been reported to have been ligated at one time or another. The risk is proportionately greater when a large mass involves the nerve or lies near it, in which case the ability to dissect out the mass and preserve the nerve is reduced. The facial, vagus, spinal accessory, and hypoglossal nerves; the lingual nerve; the brachial plexus; the phrenic nerve; and the cervical nerves are all at some risk. The marginal mandibularis of the facial nerve and the anterior cervical nerves are commonly severed as part of the neck dissection. The incidence of unintentional ligation of nerves is less than 5%.

VASCULAR COMPLICATIONS

Air emboli may enter the venous system secondary to a hole in the internal jugular vein. Also, a tumor may involve the carotid sheath, and, during an attempt to literally scrape the tumor off the carotid artery, the vessel wall may be injured. Both of these complications are quite uncommon. Bilateral ligation of the internal jugular veins may produce increased intracranial pressure, manifested by sudden death, convulsions, eye complications, or nasal hemorrhage. Cerebrovascular complications may occur from (1) an embolism resulting from an ulcerated carotid plaque, (2) intravascular thrombosis, (3) unintentional ligation of the internal carotid artery, (4) ligation of an external carotid artery with prior internal carotid occlusion, and (5) a transient decrease in cerebrovascular perfusion.[23]

LYMPHATIC COMPLICATIONS

A chylous fistula occurs in about 2% of patients who undergo neck dissection, owing to the severing of the thoracic duct or a tributary. If the chylous drainage persists, it may be necessary to attempt to suture the leak. Chylothorax may occur in some cases.

PULMONARY COMPLICATIONS

Pneumothorax may occur, particularly in operations involving the thyroid, since the neck dissection also involves the removal of paratracheal nodes, which often extend into the upper mediastinum. The pleura at the apex of the mediastinum may inadvertently be torn.

POSTOPERATIVE COMPLICATIONS

IMMEDIATE COMPLICATIONS

Pneumothorax may not be recognized during the operation, since the lung does not collapse until the cuff of the endotracheal tube is deflated. Failure to recognize this complication may result in serious consequences.

Development of a hematoma, a seroma, or an infection with resultant necrosis of the wound or flap is the most common immediate postoperative complication. This may be prevented by catheter drainage when the patient is at an increased risk for this problem. Facial lymphedema is commonly seen in the immediate postoperative period, but it begins to regress within a few days if neck dissection is done on only one side. In cases in which a bilateral neck dissection is performed or in which there has been prior radiation therapy, the edema is slower to disappear.

DELAYED COMPLICATIONS

Delayed complications include the breakdown of flaps, the exposure of the carotid artery, and the potential development of carotid rupture. Although this latter complication is relatively uncommon, it is the most common cause of operative mortality. There may be times when the carotid must be ligated if coverage cannot be obtained and rupture is imminent, even though ligation of the carotid puts the patient at risk for paraplegia or even sudden death. The risk of stroke is considerably less when the vessel is ligated electively rather than at the time of rupture.

Laryngeal lymphedema may develop, and if it is sufficiently severe a tracheotomy may be required. Lymphedema of the face usually persists to some degree, especially after bilateral neck dissection. This side-effect gradually disappears over time. Prior radiation therapy increases the severity and duration of the lymphedema.

One of the most common side-effects of radical neck dissection results from the loss of the spinal accessory nerve and the subsequent atrophy of the trapezius muscle. There is considerable variation in the innervation of the trapezius muscle; sometimes a portion of the innervation comes from the anterior cervical nerves. However, when there is complete atrophy of the trapezius, there is a subsequent shoulder drop, and the patient will often complain of shoulder pain. Shoulder drop puts some stress on the brachial plexus, and this is aggravated by cold weather or unusual activity.

Even if the spinal accessory nerve is spared, it may not recover function for several months owing to the considerable stretching that occurs during the operative procedure. Physical therapy may reduce the side-effects of this complication. Younger patients seem to adapt more easily than older patients. When possible, a nerve graft, using a portion of the greater auricular nerve, may be used to span the resected portion of the spinal accessory nerve.

Some patients complain of difficulty in swallowing after neck dissection has been performed, even though they have had no radiation therapy or surgical treatment involving the swallowing muscles. The cause is not entirely clear.

Gustatory sweating has been reported after radical neck dissection in six patients; the onset was from 1 month to 5 years after surgery.[18]

Patients who have a functional neck dissection or supraomohyoid neck dissection have fewer problems overall than those who have a radical neck dissection.

COMPLICATIONS OF BILATERAL RADICAL NECK DISSECTION

After bilateral radical neck dissection, the patient's face may appear purple and swollen owing to venous congestion and the associated lymphedema. The purplish discoloration subsides within a day or two, but the lymphedema persists.

A tall, thin, lanky person usually has fewer complications and side-effects from the bilateral operation than a short, obese, "no-neck" patient.

Razack and co-workers reported on 61 patients who underwent simultaneous bilateral radical neck dissection; 75% of the patients had bilateral clinically positive disease, and 75% had T3 or T4 primary lesions.[20] The operative mortality rate at 30 days was 10% (6 of 61 patients). Seven patients had intraoperative hypotensive episodes, and three died without regaining consciousness. There was an 11% rate of postoperative life-threatening carotid artery hemorrhage. The complications of surgery, many of which were associated with resection of the primary lesion, are listed in Table 5-3. The 3-year and 5-year survival rates were 20% and 12.5%. The same authors also reported on 63 patients who had nonsimultaneous bilateral radical neck dissection; 58% were operated on 6 to 12 months after the first radical neck dissection. The operative mortality rate was 3.2% The survival rates at 3 years and 5 years for this group of more favorably staged cases were 60% and 38%, respectively. There were no postoperative deaths when one or both internal jugular veins were preserved.

McGuirt and McCabe compared the complications of a second neck dissection (91 patients) with the complications resulting from a first neck dissection (606 patients).[16] Eleven of the bilateral neck dissections were simultaneous, and 80 were nonsimultaneous (17 were performed within 1 month of the first dissection, and the remainder were done

---

TABLE 5-3. Postoperative Complications for Simultaneous and Nonsimultaneous Bilateral Radical Neck Dissection

Complication	Simultaneous No. Patients (%)	Nonsimultaneous No. Patients (%)
Total number of patients	61 (100%)	63 (100%)
Facial edema and swelling	39 (63%)	19 (30%)
Wound infection	39 (63%)	9 (14%)
Orocutaneous fistula	22 (36%)	4 (6%)
Carotid artery blowout	7 (11%)	0 (0%)
Pulmonary infection	10 (16%)	0 (0%)
Cyanosis	5 (8%)	0 (0%)
Major flap loss	3 (4.9%)	0 (0%)
Unconsciousness	3 (4.9%)	0 (0%)
Mortality	6 (10%)	2 (3.2%)

(Adapted from Razack MS, Baffi R, Sako K: Bilateral radical neck dissection. Cancer 47:197–199, 1981)

TABLE 5-4.   Complications of Bilateral Versus Unilateral Neck Dissection

Complications	First Dissection (606 Patients) Percentage	Second Dissection (91 Patients) Percentage
Major surgical		
Death	2.8	0
Carotid rupture	1.3	1.1
Fistula	19.2*	19.0*
Minor surgical (*e.g.,* wound necrosis, infection, separation)	25.0	18.7
Flap elevation	5.8	7.7
Other		3.3

* Includes only patients having communications of neck and aerodigestive tract.

(McGuirt WF, McCabe BF: Bilateral radical neck dissections. Arch Otolaryngol 106:427–429, 1980. Copyright © American Medical Association, 1980)

after a longer interval, usually for delayed contralateral metastases). The surgical complications in the two groups are compared in Table 5-4.

OPERATIVE MORTALITY

The mortality rate after ipsilateral neck dissection without resection of the primary lesion and without prior radiation therapy is less than 1%. When the neck dissection is combined with resection of the primary lesion, it takes on the operative mortality for the primary lesion. For bilateral, nonsimultaneous, staged neck dissections, the operative mortality is low, 0 to 3.2%.[16,20] Simultaneous bilateral radical neck dissection was associated with a 10% operative mortality rate in Razack's series.[20]

REFERENCES

1. Babcock W, Conley J: Neck incisions in block dissection. Arch Otolaryngol 84:554–557, 1966
2. Batson OV: Anatomical problems concerned in the study of cerebral blood flow. Fed Proc 3:139–144, 1944
3. Bocca E, Pignataro O: A conservation technique in radical neck dissection. Ann Otol Rhinol Laryngol 76:975–987, 1967
4. Carenfelt C, Eliasson K: Cervical metastases following radical neck dissection that preserved the spinal accessory nerve. Head Neck Surg 2:181–184, 1980
5. Crile G: Excision of cancer of the head and neck. With special reference to the plan of dissection based on one hundred and thirty-two operations. JAMA 47:1780–1786, 1906
6. Duffy JJ: Treatment of cervical nodes in intraoral cancer. Surg Gynecol Obstet 71:664–671, 1940
7. Durante F: A new operative method for the total extirpation of the larynx. Int Clin 1:122–124, 1905
8. Eycleshymer AC, Jones T: Hand-Atlas of Clinical Anatomy, p 53. Philadelphia, Lea & Febiger, 1925
9. Freeland AP, Rogers JH: The vascular supply of the cervical skin with reference to incision planning. Laryngoscope 85:714–725, 1975
10. Freund HR: Technique of radical neck dissection. In Principles of Head and Neck Surgery, pp 96–101. New York, Appleton-Century-Crofts, 1967
11. Goepfert H, Jesse RH, Ballantyne AJ: Posterolateral neck dissection. Arch Otolaryngol 106:618–620, 1980
12. Guis JA, Grier DH: Venous adaptation following bilateral radical neck dissection with excision of jugular veins. Surgery 28:305–328, 1950
13. Jesse RH, Ballantyne AJ, Larson D: Radical or modified neck dissection: A therapeutic dilemma. Am J Surg 136:516–519, 1978
14. Lingeman RE, Stephens R, Helmus C, Ulm J: Neck dissection: Radical or conservative. Ann Otol Rhinol Laryngol 86:737–744, 1977
15. MacFee WF: Transverse incisions for neck dissection. Ann Surg 151:279–284, 1960
16. McGuirt WF, McCabe BF: Bilateral radical neck dissection. Arch Otolaryngol 106:427–429, 1980
17. Martin H, DelValle B, Ehrlich H, Cahan WG: Neck dissection. Cancer 4:441–499, 1951
18. Myers EN, Conley J: Gustatory sweating after radical neck dissection. Arch Otolaryngol 91:534–542, 1970
19. Ogura JH, Biller HF: Conservation surgery in cancer of the head and neck. Otolaryngol Clin North Am 2:641–665, 1969
20. Razack MS, Baffi R, Sako K: Bilateral radical neck dissection. Cancer 47:197–199, 1981
21. Rohrbach R: Über Gehirnerweichung nach isolierter Unterbindung ver Vena jugularis interna. Beitr Z Klin Chir 17:811–827, 1896–1897
22. Roy PH, Beahrs OH: Spinal accessory nerve in radical neck dissections. Am J Surg 118:800–804, 1969
23. Sobel SM, Freeman R, Thawley S, Little J, Beven E: Management of inadvertent injury to the carotid artery during head and neck surgery. Head Neck Surg 4:475–482, 1982
24. Suarez O: El problema de las metastasis linfáticas y alejadas del cáncer de laringe e hipofaringe. Rev Otorrinolaringol (Santiago, Chile) 23:83–99, 1963
25. Sugarbaker ED, Wiley HM: Intracranial pressure studies incident to resection of the internal jugular vein. Cancer 4:242–250, 1951

General Principles for Treatment of Cancers in the Head and Neck: Radiation Therapy

RODNEY R. MILLION
NICHOLAS J. CASSISI

6

SELECTION OF PATIENTS

Prior high-dose irradiation to the head and neck area, even if given years previously, is a contraindication to radiation therapy, unless the new cancer is clearly out of the prior radiation portals. There are a few exceptions to this rule, such as recurrent lymphoepithelioma of the nasopharynx, but curative reirradiation is rarely successful and the risk of major necrosis is high. An operation should be the treatment of choice, with reirradiation used only in desperate or special circumstances.

A history of low-dose irradiation (e.g., for acne) is a relative contraindication. The history of prior irradiation may be missed, since the irradiation was often given years ago. Irradiated skin has a characteristic appearance, and persistent questioning will frequently confirm the suspicion. Radiation therapy records are usually not available, and one must depend on the appearance of the skin and mucosa to guess the possible radiation dose.

The majority of patients with squamous cell carcinoma of the oral cavity, oropharynx, hypopharynx, and larynx either are or were confirmed tobacco or alcohol users. These patients are at a slightly greater risk to develop a radiation necrosis or edema if they continue their unsavory habits with zeal. However, if they moderate or stop smoking, drinking, or both, the risk of a complication is similar to that for other patients. The history of tobacco or alcohol use is not usually a decisive factor in treatment selection. The alcoholic is likely to refuse a major operation but is also rather intolerant of the acute side-effects of irradiation once treatment is started. About 50% of the patients who smoke will stop immediately when advised to do so, about 25% will decrease their tobacco use, and the remaining 25% do not alter their habit.

A common reason for selecting radiation therapy instead of an operation is a concomitant medical condition. Radiation therapy has essentially a zero acute mortality rate, and it makes no sense to offer the patient an operation if the risk of an operative death is significant.

Young patients are best treated by an operation, all other factors being equal, since the risk of a late-appearing radiation complication is ever present, especially for lesions of the oral cavity and pharynx (Table 6-1).[4] Elderly or frail patients are frequently referred for radiation therapy even though they have a lesion preferably treated by an operation. A long, drawn-out, 7- to 8-week course of irradiation may be more wearing than an operation, which may entail only 7 to 14 days of hospitalization.

Adult patients with squamous cell carcinoma of the head and neck treated by high-dose radiation therapy alone have no greater chance of a second head and neck cancer than those treated by an operation.[4]

The risk for developing a second primary cancer for 1163 patients with squamous cell carcinoma who were clinically free of disease for at least 5 years after initial treatment is outlined in Table 6-2.[4] There is essentially no difference in the risk of a second cancer either in the initial site, in a

TABLE 6-1.   Complications of Treatment Occurring After 5 Years in 720 Irradiated Patients With No Evidence of Disease at 5 Years

Site	No. Patients	No. Compli- cations (%)	Type of Complication				
			Soft Tissue Ulcers	Bone Necrosis	Excessive Fibrosis	Peripheral Neuropathy	Miscella- neous
Oral cavity and faucial arch	319	24 (7.5)	10*	12*	1	1	0
Pharynx (naso-, oro-, hypo-)	132	21 (15.9)	1	3	5	8†	4
Larynx	252	2 (0.8)	0	0	1	0	1
Nasal cavity and paranasal sinuses	17	0 (0)	0	0	0	0	0

* One patient with additional fistula.
† One patient with bilateral neuropathy.
Note: M. D. Anderson Hospital data; patients treated 1/48–12/65; analysis 8/73.

(Kogelnik HD, Fletcher GH, Jesse RH: Clinical course of patients with squamous cell carcinoma of the upper respiratory and digestive tracts with no evidence of disease 5 years after initial treatment. Radiology 115:423–427, 1975)

TABLE 6-2.   Relative Risk of a New Primary Cancer Occurring After 5 Years by Modality of Treatment of Squamous Cell Carcinoma: 1163 Patients, All Anatomical Sites

Site	Modality of Treatment		
	Surgery	Irradiation	Preoperative or Postoperative Irradiation
Same location	1.8% (6/337)	2.8% (20/720)	1.9% (2/106)
Vicinity	4.2%* (14/337)	2.6%* (19/720)	6.6%* (7/106)
Remote sites in the oral cavity and pharynx	4.7% (16/337)	5.4% (39/720)	7.5% (8/106)
Lung and esophagus	3.3% (11†/337)	5.4% (39‡/720)	5.7% (6§/106)

* Average incidence is 3.1% for the surgery and irradiation groups. This figure is statistically different from 6.6% (*p* = 0.07).
 † 10 lung, 1 esophagus.
 ‡ 27 lung, 11 esophagus, 1 trachea.
 § 4 lung, 2 esophagus.
Note: M. D. Anderson Hospital data; patients treated 1/48–12/65; analysis 8/73.

(Kogelnik HD, Fletcher GH, Jesse RH: Clinical course of patients with squamous cell carcinoma of the upper respiratory and digestive tracts with no evidence of disease 5 years after initial treatment. Radiology 115:423–427, 1975)

TABLE 6-3.   Incidence of Neck Disease Appearing More Than 5 Years After Treatment in Patients With the Initial Primary Lesion and Neck Disease Controlled and No Squamous Cell Carcinoma Found Below the Clavicles: 1163 Patients, All Anatomical Sites

Modality of Treatment to the Primary Lesion	Incidence
Surgery	1.2% (4/337)
Irradiation	1.4% (10/720)
Combination surgery and irradiation	0 (0/106)

Note: M. D. Anderson Hospital data; patients treated 1/48–12/65; analysis 8/73.
(Kogelnik HD, Fletcher GH, Jesse RH: Clinical course of patients with squamous cell carcinoma of the upper respiratory and digestive tracts with no evidence of disease 5 years after initial treatment. Radiology 115:423–427, 1975)

marginal site, or in remote head and neck sites for the categories of surgery alone, radiation therapy alone, and combined treatment. The follow-up was 8 to 25 years. The soft palate group had the highest incidence (33%) of new head and neck squamous cell carcinomas 5 years following successful treatment.

The risk of late-appearing neck disease (more than 5 years) is shown in Table 6-3, and the incidence of late-appearing distant metastasis is indicated in Table 6-4.[4]

The rate of radiation therapy complications after 5 years is shown in Table 6-1. The majority occur in T2–T3 lesions. Late-appearing surgical complications are quite uncommon.

Radiation-induced sarcomas are almost never seen when high-dose radiation is given to adults; the estimated risk is less than 1% for patients treated in the second decade and 3% to 5% for those treated in the first decade. One of the common radiation-induced neoplasms in the head and neck area is papillary carcinoma of the thyroid, which is highly curable; the others (e.g., osteosarcoma, fibrosarcoma) are frequently incurable.

A few patients have a fear of radiation therapy. If this fear is not easily reconciled, one should not force the issue.

PRIMARY SITE IRRADIATION

The head and neck represents one of the few areas where both the primary lesion and the regional nodes can be readily evaluated and observed during a course of radiation therapy. Even the invisible sinus lesions can be mapped with some assurance by tomography and computed tomographic (CT) scans. Careful plotting of the primary lesion should be accomplished by precise diagrams and clinical photographs. Multiple examiners and multiple examinations help refine minute details. One has only to know the usual patterns of spread to include the possible microscopic extensions that are not visible or palpable. Study of the patterns of spread of moderately advanced and advanced lesions gives valuable clues to possible routes of subclinical extension for early lesions. One of the major advantages of irradiation compared with surgery is the ability to cover potential avenues of spread with less morbidity; a marginal failure after radiation therapy is an uncommon finding. There is no simple rule as to the margin in centimeters around a tumor. One must gauge the initial margins by the known patterns of spread, the history of the growth rate, the histology, and the gross appearance (e.g., discrete, well defined, exophytic vs. vague, ill defined, infiltrative).

Shrinking Fields

The principle of shrinking fields is used to minimize the effects of a large treatment volume. The outer 1-cm to 3-cm perimeter of the treatment volume usually includes only tissues having the possibility of containing subclinical disease.* If these tissues have not been surgically disturbed, 4500 rad to 5000 rad should be sufficient to sterilize minimal amounts of squamous cell carcinoma, and the first reduction may occur at this dose level. Additional reductions are usually made at 6000 rad and 7000 rad. An interstitial implant to residual disease is considered a shrinking field technique. The final treatment portals are often quite small and are referred to as "boosts," "booster treatments," or "coned down" to the center of the resolving mass. The final small fields are often used, however, to raise the dose in an undertreated zone to the same level as the remainder of the treatment volume. This situation occurs when there is a low dose owing to lack of homogeneity within a treatment field and the actual dose is less than the specified tumor dose. This may occur because the tumor may be near the edge or corner of the field or due to partial shielding of the beam by bone. This maneuver is simply referred to as "make-up treatment." With the use of computers, CT scan, *in vivo* dosimetry, irregular field computations, and special water phantom measurements, low-dose areas can be estimated and the dose adjusted.

Tailored Fields

Radiation beams exit from the machines as squares or rectangles and require tailoring of the beam by secondary

* *Subclinical disease* refers to disease statistically known to be present but that cannot be seen or palpated in areas accessible to physical examination nor seen on highly efficient roentgenographic studies.

TABLE 6-4.	Incidence of Distant Metastases Appearing After 5 Years in Patients With the Initial Primary Lesion and Neck Disease Controlled and No Squamous Cell Carcinoma Found Below the Clavicles: 1163 Patients, All Anatomical Sites

Modality of Treatment to the Primary Lesion	Incidence
Surgery	1.2% (4/337)
Irradiation	0.6% (4/720)
Combination surgery and irradiation	2.8% (3/106)

Note: M. D. Anderson Hospital data; patients treated 1/48–12/65; analysis 8/73.

(Kogelnik HD, Fletcher GH, Jesse RH: Clinical course of patients with squamous cell carcinoma of the upper respiratory and digestive tracts with no evidence of disease 5 years after initial treatment. Radiology 115:423–427, 1975)

collimation to fit the individual situation and, in the case of cobalt-60, to reduce the penumbra. Very few clinical situations call for a square or rectangular portal.

Lead alloy blocks are placed on a tray between the patient and the machine to produce the irregular fields required for head and neck therapy.

There is a disparity between radiation therapy centers in the tailoring of portals and the volume of tissues included, which explains some of the discrepancies reported for radiation side-effects as well as for local and regional control.

REGIONAL NODE IRRADIATION

The regional nodes are included in the treatment planning for the primary lesion.

For almost all primary lesions of the head and neck, the subdigastric node area (i.e., sentinal node, tonsillar node) is the major drainage site. For oral cavity lesions, the submaxillary nodes are also at high risk. For lesions of the nasopharynx, soft palate, and posterior tonsillar pillar, the junctional and spinal accessory lymph nodes are also commonly involved. There is usually an orderly progression of lymphatic spread along the jugular chain. Patients with clinically positive neck nodes are at some risk for contralateral neck disease, even if the primary lesion is small and well lateralized. When lymphatic obstruction develops from tumor or lymph node biopsy, the lymph flow is diverted. One common shunt is the submental pathway to the contralateral subdigastric and midjugular nodes.[3]

Clinically Negative Neck

When the nodes are clinically negative and the risk of subclinical disease is 15% to 20% or greater, the lymph nodes are included and receive a minimum dose of 4500 rad to 5000 rad. In the treatment portals used for cancers of the oropharynx, supraglottic larynx, and hypopharynx, most of the high-risk upper neck nodes are automatically included with the primary lesion. For oral cavity, nasopharynx, large glottic, nasal cavity, and paranasal sinus lesions, the portals must be extended to include the nodes. Innovative treatment techniques must be devised to include the lymph nodes but to keep mucosal irradiation to a minimum. The criteria for elective lymph node irradiation depend on several features:

1. Primary site and overall risk of subclinical disease
2. Risk for bilateral subclinical disease
3. Histologic grade
4. Size of the primary lesion (T stage)
5. Difficulty of neck examination
6. Relative morbidity for extending the lymph node coverage related to the risk of subclinical disease
7. Likelihood that the patient will return for frequent follow-up examinations
8. Suitability of the patient for a radical neck dissection should tumor appear in the neck

Elective neck irradiation for primary lesions of the oral cavity usually includes the submaxillary and subdigastric lymph nodes and, occasionally, the midjugular nodes. For primary lesions of the oropharynx, nasopharynx, supraglottic larynx, and hypopharynx the entire jugular chain, spinal accessory, junctional, and lower neck nodes are usually included; the risk for subclinical disease in the lower neck and spinal accessory groups in some cases is admittedly quite small when findings in the upper neck are negative. Using the well-tailored en *face* lower neck field adds little morbidity and ensures control of neck disease.

The justification for elective irradiation of the lower jugular and supraclavicular nodes is emphasized by Sagerman and co-workers, who reviewed 72 patients given 5000 rad/5 weeks preoperative irradiation for stage III and IV glottic, supraglottic, and pyriform sinus cancers.[11] Thirty-one patients were treated with only lateral opposing portals that did not include the lower neck, and 41 had similar portals but also an added 5000 rad through a separate lower neck portal. Ten of the 31 (32%) treated with the two-field technique died with a recurrence, while only 4 of the 41 (10%) developed a recurrence when the lower neck field was added. The complication rate was no different in the two groups.

Clinically Positive Nodes

The treatment plan for the patient with clinically positive lymph nodes depends on the management of the primary lesion; on the size, number, and location of the palpable lymph nodes; and whether the patient will accept a neck dissection.

If the primary lesion is to be treated by radiation therapy alone, then the clinically positive lymph nodes plus the contiguous clinically negative lymph nodes are included. If the contralateral neck is clinically negative, it may also be electively treated; an estimation of the risk must be made for each anatomical site and the extent of gross disease.

The relative control with radiation therapy alone versus radiation therapy followed by neck dissection is shown in Table 6-5. (See Tables 4-8 and 4-9 in Chapter 4 for similar information.) At first glance, one might conclude that neck dissection does not add anything to regional control for neck disease staged N1 and N2. Since the cases are heavily selected by node size, fixation, multiplicity of nodes, and response to radiation therapy, the less favorable cases within each N stage are referred for neck dissection.

The 2-year neck disease control related to size of the largest node and the preoperative dose is given in Table 6-6. The primary lesion was managed by radiation therapy, and a planned neck dissection was added within 3 months. When the specimen was negative, the neck disease control was 87%, compared with 59% (p = 0.06) when the specimen was positive. Failure at the primary site was associated with a 62% neck recurrence rate (8 of 13) compared with 10% neck recurrence (3 of 33) with the primary lesion controlled a minimum of 2 years. The total complication rates, which increased with doses above 6000 rad, are shown in Table 6-7. Soft tissue and bone disorders are radiation therapy complications and are not thought to be increased by the neck dissection. Almost all of the severe (3+) or fatal complications (3) occurred at the high dose levels.

If neck dissection is to follow radiation therapy, the dose to the nodes varies with size, location, mobility, and response to irradiation. A preoperative dose of 5000 rad to 6000 rad is usually sufficient for 3-cm to 6-cm nodes, but the dose is increased if there are adverse clinical findings.

TABLE 6-5. Control of Neck Disease With Radiation Therapy Alone Versus Radiation Therapy Plus Neck Dissection (Primary Lesion* Treated and Controlled by Radiation Therapy)

Neck Treatment	Neck Disease Stage (No. of Heminecks Controlled/No. of Heminecks Treated)		
	N1	N2	N3
Radiation therapy	34/34 (100%)	18/25 (72%)	16/39 (41%)
Radiation therapy plus neck dissection	12/14 (85%)	13/17† (76%)	23/27 (85%)

* Primary sites included oral tongue, floor of the mouth, soft palate, base of the tongue, tonsillar fossa, supraglottic larynx, and pyriform sinus.

† Excluding two operative deaths.

Note: University of Florida data.

TABLE 6-6. Control of Neck Disease With Radiation Therapy Followed by Neck Dissection: Primary Lesion Managed Initially by Radiation Therapy—46 Patients; 47 Evaluable Heminecks (No. Controlled/No. Treated)

Maximum Node Diameter	Minimum Node Dose (rad)			
	3000–4000	4000–5000	5000–6000	6000–7000
3–4 cm	1/2	7/11	8/9	0/0
5–6 cm	0/3	5/6	3/3	2/3
7–8 cm	0/0	1/1	3/4	4/5

Note: University of Florida data; patients treated 10/64–2/79; analysis 4/81 by B. D. Greenberg, MD.

TABLE 6-7. Complications Relative to Subcutaneous Dose: Primary Lesion Managed Initially by Radiation Therapy Alone, Preoperative Radiation Therapy Plus Surgery to Neck (63 Patients*)

Complication	Maximum Subcutaneous Dose (rad)		
	3000–5000	5000–6000	6000–7000
Fistula			
2+	0	0	1
3+	0	1	0
Soft tissue			
1+	1	1	5
2+	0	2	2
3+	0	1	1
Bone			
1+	0	0	2
2+	0	3	2
3+	0	0	1
Edema (2+)	0	1	0
Flap separation/delayed healing			
1+	2	1	2
2+	0	0	3
3+	0	1	5
Fibrosis			
1+	1	1	0
2+	0	1	1
Trismus (1+)	0	1	0
Hypoglossal nerve palsy	0	1	1
Nonfatal carotid rupture	0	0	1
Laryngeal necrosis	0	0	1 (fatal)†
Postoperative pulmonary embolus	0	0	1 (fatal)
Postoperative cardiac arrhythmia	0	0	1 (fatal)
Total No. of complications	4	15	30
Fraction of patients with complications	2/6	10/16	19/41

* Includes 17 patients not eligible for neck control analysis in Table 6-6.

† Total laryngectomy led to fatal flap separation with carotid rupture.

Note: University of Florida data; patients treated 10/64–2/79; analysis 4/81 by B. D. Greenberg, MD.

A 6-cm node may be freely mobile, located in the upper neck, but judged to be free of the carotid, with a good tumor-free space between the mass and the base of skull, spine, and mandible; large doses are not required in this situation. A 6-cm mass located higher in the neck and seemingly fixed or tethered to the base of skull, skin, or neurovascular bundle gives the surgeon more technical difficulty. Therefore, the prescribed dose is usually 6000 rad to 7000 rad or even higher in special cases. The same reasoning follows for masses larger than 7 cm, and the regional control can be surprisingly good with acceptable complications. It must be stressed that these large doses are not delivered to the entire neck but just to the mass.

If the node mass lies behind the plane of the spinal cord,

TABLE 6-8. **Results of Treatment of Positive Neck Lymph Nodes With Irradiation Alone: Lymph Node Control Versus Treatment Technique (No. Controlled/No. Treated)***

Size (cm)	Continuous Course	Split Course
<1.0	5/5	2/2
1.0	29/35 (83%)	19/23 (83%)
1.5–2.0	42/49 (88%)	20/24 (83%)
2.5–3.0	14/19 (74%)	10/18 (56%)
3.5–6.0	14/20 (70%)	10/17 (59%)
≧7.0	0/2	0/5

* Excluded: <5000 rad for nodes ≦1.0 cm and <5500 rad for nodes ≧1.5 cm.

Note: University of Florida data; patients treated 10/64–4/80; analysis 3/83.

(Mendenhall WM, Million RR, Bova FJ: Analysis of time-dose factors in clinically positive neck nodes treated with irradiation alone in squamous cell carcinoma of the head and neck. Int J Radiat Oncol Biol Phys, in press. Copyright 1984, Pergamon Press, Ltd)

TABLE 6-9. **Dose Guidelines for Squamous Cell Carcinoma Metastatic to the Cervical Lymph Nodes**

Node Size (cm)	Dose (rad)	
	1000 rad/week	900 rad/week
≦1.0	6000	6500
1.5–2.0	6500	7000
2.5–3.0	7000	7500
3.5–6.0	7500	8000

Note: Based on University of Florida data; patients treated 10/64–4/80; analysis 3/83 by W. M. Mendenhall, MD.

electrons or parallel opposed AP and PA portals with wedges may be necessary to obtain the required dose. Large lymph nodes may not show much regression during the course of the radiation treatments, but they will often show major change by the time the patient returns in 4 to 6 weeks for neck dissection. The node mass frequently has a thick capsule at this time that facilitates removal.

If neck dissection is undesirable from a medical standpoint, radiation therapy alone will cure a significant number of patients with positive neck nodes (Table 6-8).[5] The control of the involved lymph nodes seems to parallel the response and control of the primary lesion. The final dose to the lymph nodes is gauged by their original size (Table 6-9). An interstitial implant may be used in selected cases for a boost dose. The dose for lymphoepitheliomatous nodes may be 500 rad to 1000 rad less if they show rapid, early regression.

Patients with bilateral neck disease require individualized planning with the surgeon. If the neck disease is minimal on one side, then irradiation may be used for control on that side and neck dissection is used on the side that has the major disease (N2A, N2B, N3A).

If there is major bilateral neck disease, then bilateral

neck dissection follows the radiation therapy. The neck dissections are preferably done in two stages. Major lymphedema may be anticipated but will gradually subside in 1 to 2 years.

Metastatic disease to the lower neck nodes is often curable. There is some indirect evidence that when comparing N stages (N2B, N3A, N3B) with or without metastatic cancer in the lower neck nodes, the risk of distant metastasis is similar.

GENERAL PRINCIPLES OF IRRADIATION TECHNIQUES FOR THE CERVICAL LYMPHATICS

Except for the nasal cavity and the paranasal sinuses, the first-echelon lymph nodes are included in the treatment portals along with the primary lesions. Some of the common configurations used are shown in Figures 6-1 through 6-5. A typical portal for a lesion of the anterior floor of the mouth or anterior one third of the oral tongue and clinically negative neck is demonstrated in Figure 6-1A. The submaxillary and subdigastric nodes are included to the level of the thyroid notch. The posterior border includes the sternocleidomastoid muscle, but the junctional lymph nodes and spinal accessory chain are not included. The superior border is modified (primary lesion permitting) to exclude a portion of the parotid gland. A strip of skin and subcutaneous tissue should be spared in the submentum, if possible, to reduce edema and fibrosis. If the lesion is advanced or poorly differentiated, a midjugular or lower neck portal may be added (see Fig. 6-1B). A single ipsilateral portal may be used for a well-lateralized lesion of the oral tongue with a clinically negative neck; parallel opposed portals would be used for anterior lesions of the floor of the mouth.

A portal arrangement for a clinically negative neck for carcinomas of the oropharynx is shown in Figure 6-2A. The posterior border includes the spinal accessory chain. The posterior limb of the superior border is 2 cm to 3 cm above the mastoid tip to encompass the junctional lymph nodes. This border would usually pass just below or through the external auditory canal in order to include adequately the jugular fossa. The inferior border is the thyroid notch, unless there is extension of the primary lesion below the hyoid level. The lower neck portals to be used when there is no disease in the upper neck or it is minimally involved are shown in Figure 6-2B and C. The lateral borders in the lower neck are set just around the root of the neck when the risk of disease is small. The lower neck portal is modified when there are enlarged lymph nodes in the neck (see Fig. 6-2D). The lateral borders are placed laterally at the junction of the clavicle with the trapezius only in situations in which there is a major risk for supraclavicular disease, such as with major disease in the upper neck or in very poorly differentiated tumors or carcinomas of the nasopharynx.

Separation of the upper and lower neck portals at or near the thyroid notch is a very important technical point, since it eliminates or reduces unnecessary irradiation to the larynx, hypopharynx, and spinal cord. Failure to adopt this technique adds greatly to the acute and chronic sequelae.

The separation between the upper and lower neck portals is a common line. It is our practice to include the line in the treatment of the upper neck portal and to exclude it in the treatment of the lower neck portal. Radiation ther-

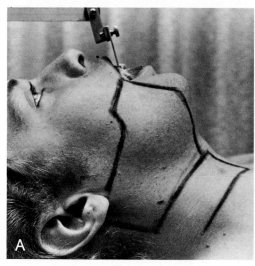

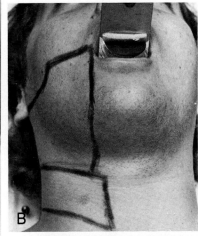

FIG. 6-1. Portal used to irradiate a primary tumor of the anterior oral cavity along with first-echelon clinically negative lymph nodes. A separate, optional midjugular portal is used when a clinically negative neck is associated with an advanced or poorly differentiated primary tumor of the oral cavity. (*A*) Lateral view. (*B*) Anterior view.

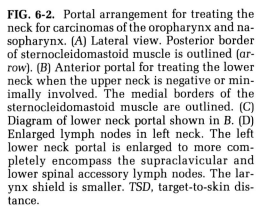

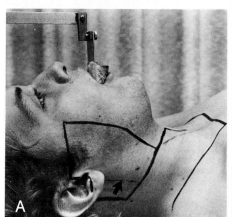

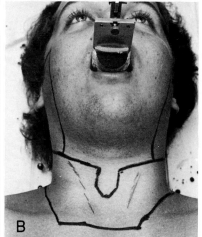

FIG. 6-2. Portal arrangement for treating the neck for carcinomas of the oropharynx and nasopharynx. (*A*) Lateral view. Posterior border of sternocleidomastoid muscle is outlined (*arrow*). (*B*) Anterior portal for treating the lower neck when the upper neck is negative or minimally involved. The medial borders of the sternocleidomastoid muscle are outlined. (*C*) Diagram of lower neck portal shown in *B*. (*D*) Enlarged lymph nodes in left neck. The left lower neck portal is enlarged to more completely encompass the supraclavicular and lower spinal accessory lymph nodes. The larynx shield is smaller. *TSD*, target-to-skin distance.

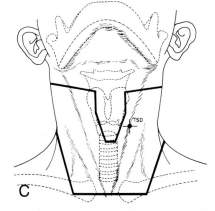

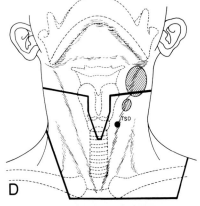

FIG. 6-3. Portal configuration for primary lesions of the supraglottic larynx, large glottic tumors, and hypopharyngeal tumors. (*A*) Lateral view. The posterior border of the sternocleidomastoid muscle is outlined. (*B*) Anterior view of lower neck portal that encompasses lower jugular chain lymph nodes for a patient with a clinically negative neck. A small shield is inserted over the trachea. The borders of the right sternocleidomastoid muscle are marked with a dashed line. The portal would be enlarged in the presence of clinically involved lymph nodes.

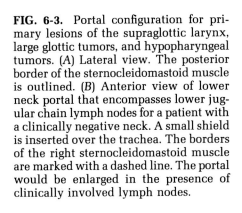

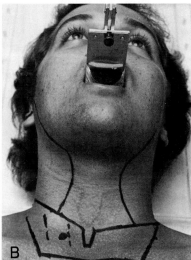

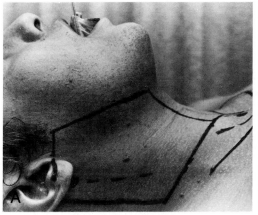

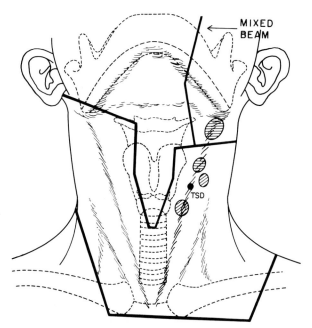

FIG. 6-4. Portal arrangement to irradiate the opposite upper neck and both sides of the lower neck in conjunction with mixed photon and electron beam therapy to the primary lesion. *TSD,* target-to-skin distance.

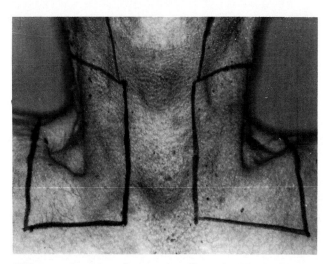

FIG. 6-5. *Incorrect* design of midline shielding of an anteroposterior low neck portal. The lower jugular lymph nodes are shielded or at best in a marginal-dose area.

apists not trained in this technique voice opposition to the practice of separating the upper and lower neck portals, fearing overtreatment or undertreatment and subsequent complications or recurrences. Recurrences have not been identified at the site of the junction because, if anything, there is almost always a slight overtreatment rather than an undertreatment. It is uncommon to see a strip of moist desquamation at the junction, but it may occur. Thousands of patients have been treated using this technique, and its advantages in excluding normal tissue far outweigh the minor disadvantage of an occasional strip of subcutaneous fibrosis or moist desquamation. It makes no sense to unnecessarily irradiate the larynx, hypopharynx, cervical

esophagus, and a long length of cervical spinal cord to save a possible minor change in the skin and subcutaneous tissue. It has been our customary plan to slant the junction line between the upper and lower neck portals upward (see Fig. 6-2A) in order to further exclude small portions of the larynx (arytenoids), pharynx, and spinal cord.

Some therapists have advocated mathematical formulas for calculating the separation between the upper and lower neck portals; we have no experience with this method.

A typical portal configuration for primary lesions of the supraglottic larynx, large glottic tumors, and tumors of the pharyngeal walls and pyriform sinus is shown in Figure 6-3A. The submaxillary lymph nodes are not included unless there is major disease in the upper neck. The junctional, lateral retropharyngeal, and spinal accessory lymph nodes are included for pharyngeal wall and pyriform sinus cancers. Lesions confined to the larynx in a patient with a clinically negative neck require only the internal jugular vein lymph node chain to be treated. In these situations, incidental irradiation of most of the normal larynx as well as the cervical spinal cord is unavoidable. However, it is difficult to include the entire lower neck through lateral portals, because of the shoulders. The lower neck portal used for this situation is shown in Figure 6-3B. In this case, the lower border of the upper neck fields has already encompassed most or all of the larynx. Therefore, only a very small, short midline shield may be used to protect a bit of the subglottic area, trachea, and spinal cord. The most important reason to put a small midline shield in this location is because both lateral portals and the lower neck portal are aimed at a common point on the spinal cord, and the shield helps to reduce potential overdosage.

When the primary lesion is treated with a unilateral mixed photon and electron beam, a special neck portal is designed to include both sides of the low neck and the contralateral upper neck (Fig. 6-4) when the opposite neck is at risk for subclinical disease. The photon contribution to the contralateral subdigastric region must be considered in the calculations.

The shield that is placed over the larynx must be carefully designed. The internal jugular vein lymph nodes lie adjacent to the most posterolateral margin of the thyroid cartilage, so that the shield cannot cover the entire cartilage without producing a low-dose area in those nodes. Likewise, the shield can extend inferiorly, usually to the level of the cricoid or the first two tracheal rings, but the shield must be tapered since the nodes tend to lie closer to the midline as the lower neck is approached. It is not at all unusual to observe a lower neck portal that extends out to the shoulders, encompassing supraclavicular nodes that have very little risk, and a larynx block that partially shields the high-risk middle jugular nodes and completely misses the lower jugular lymph nodes (Fig. 6-5). The major risk is usually in the midjugular nodes when the upper neck is clinically negative, and it is essential that they be adequately treated. Failure to taper the "larynx" shield will result in shielding of the lower internal jugular vein lymph nodes.

When clinically positive lymph nodes are present, for any of the primary sites, then the neck portals increase proportionally not only to cover the obvious gross disease but also to include contiguous areas that are then at risk. If neck dissection cannot be added, the dose must be raised by photon boost (Fig. 6-6), appositional electron portal, or interstitial implant.

Frequently, there is a large upper neck node, and a decision must be made as to placement of the line that sep-

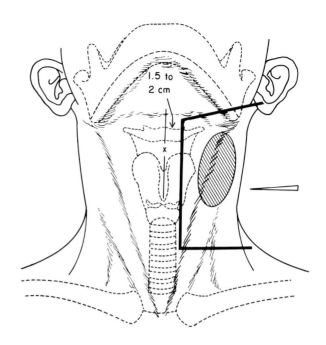

FIG. 6-6. Photon portal to boost neck node. Parallel opposed anterior and posterior neck portals with wedges are used. The medial border is usually 1.5 cm to 2.0 cm from the midline.

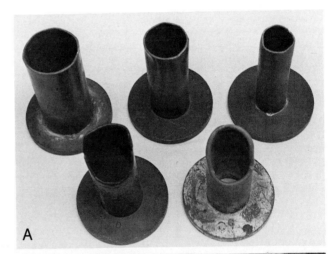

FIG. 6-7. Lead cones for orthovoltage intraoral therapy. (*A*) Cones fabricated in the hospital shop. Note that the two cones in the lower half of the photograph have been trimmed to fit the anatomy and coated with wax for comfort and cleanliness. (*B*) The positioning of the cone is checked each day by the physician. A good localizer, such as the one shown, is essential to final positioning. The patient holds a panic button, which will release the brake in case of difficulty.

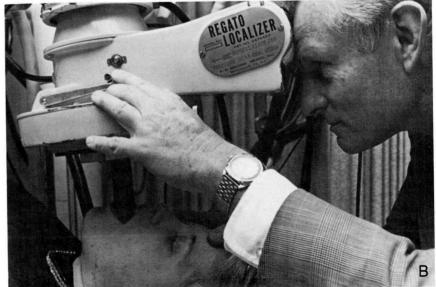

arates the upper and lower neck portals. It is our practice to draw the line across the positive lymph node if necessary in order to put the separation near the thyroid notch. Since these patients frequently have a neck dissection in any case, it is not felt to be critical that the separation be placed away from the lymph node. The major advantage in this situation is still thought to be in the avoidance of unnecessary irradiation of the larynx, hypopharynx, and cervical spinal cord as opposed to a possible problem created by the junction line. No treatment failures have been identified that could be related to placement of the junction of the upper and lower neck portals through a large node.

RADIATION THERAPY TOOLS

The radiation therapist has a wide range of tools available that help deliver the high doses required with as few side-effects as possible. (See Chapter 15, Treatment Planning for Irradiation of Head and Neck Cancer.)

External-Beam Therapy

A range of photon energies from cobalt-60 to 22 MeV or higher allows physical distribution of the beam to be tailored to the treatment volume. The great majority of external-beam plans consist of opposed lateral portals; these arrangements may be weighted to the side of the lesion. Single lateral portals may be used when part of the treatment is by interstitial therapy.

Intraoral Cone Therapy

An intraoral cone may be used to deliver part or all of a treatment. This form of therapy has the advantage of using a small portal (2 cm to 5 cm in diameter) directly applied to the lesion, thereby excluding normal tissues. The depth doses from 250 kV intraoral cone therapy diminish rapidly due to the short target-to-skin distance. The effective treatment area with a small-diameter orthovoltage field is constricted by the reduction of depth dose at the edges. Patient cooperation and experience on the part of the physician are essential to avoid missing the tumor (Fig. 6-7). Intraoral cone therapy may also be done with electrons.

Electron-Beam Therapy

Electron-beam therapy is generally available and has its major application in the management of head and neck cancer. Electrons may be used alone or mixed with photon beams to tailor the treatment volume to the target area. The higher-energy electrons have the disadvantage of increasing skin reactions and bone absorption compared with photon beams. Mixed beams of photons and electrons are useful in well-lateralized lesions of the parotid, tonsillar area, buccal mucosa, ear, and nasal vestibule; in neck masses; and in selected skin cancers.

Electrons are also used to add radiation to the posterior neck after the dose limits to the spinal cord have been reached.

There is constriction of the effective treatment area with electrons compared with photons, and when the beams are mixed, the electron beam portal is larger by 1 cm.

Interstitial Therapy

Numerous studies attest to the enhanced control of floor of mouth and oral tongue cancers when all or part of the therapy is given by interstitial treatment.[6] Interstitial treatment is also used for lip, nasal vestibule, parotid, soft palate, buccal mucosa, and posterior pharyngeal wall tumors; neck masses; and other special situations.

The advantages are that a smaller volume is treated and the dose is given in a shorter period of time. The disadvantage is that the skills required for interstitial implant are not generally available.

TIME/DOSE/FRACTIONATION

A more complete discussion of this topic is given in Chapter 13, Time–Dose–Volume Relationships in Radiation Therapy.

Conventional external-beam treatments of the head and neck employ a single daily treatment, 5 days a week, with a daily tumor dose that usually varies from 180 rad to 225 rad. The larger daily tumor doses (200 rad to 225 rad) shorten the overall treatment time and decrease the total dose, but they also increase the acute sequelae and possibly the late complications. Smaller daily doses to the tumor (170 rad to 190 rad) require more treatment days and a slightly increased total dose to accomplish the same control rate but produce fewer acute and late radiation effects on normal tissue. *Small differences in total dose (300 rad to 500 rad) may significantly affect the chance of local and regional control.* The specified tumor dose is based on the *volume of tumor* (size, diameter, T stage) and to a lesser degree on the *site of origin.* The regression rate during treatment reflects the mitotic rate of the tumor but does not accurately predict the control rate, and it is not used to select the dose. If there is persistent abnormality on physical examination at the completion of treatment, a higher rate of recurrence can be predicted.

Tumor doses have been derived empirically from retrospective analysis. The dose-response data are summarized by anatomical site and T stage from reports of the University of Florida and M. D. Anderson Hospital in Table 6-10.[7,8,10,12–15] Because of vagaries in specification of tumor dose, staging of lesions, and portal design, these time–dose schemes will not necessarily produce the same results in other departments, but they do serve as a guideline. Formulas (e.g., nominal standard dose) are not recommended for use in adjusting dose schemes, since extrapolation beyond known empirical treatment schemes cannot be accurately predicted.

Other fractionation schemes have been tried, but they generally fail to improve local control or reduce the complication rate. Split-course schemes, which insert a rest period halfway through the treatment course, have been in vogue during the past decade, but no one has produced convincing evidence that local control is as good as with conventional treatment plans. The advantage of a split course is touted as allowing the severe mucosal reactions to heal part way through treatment, thereby reducing the suffering of the patient. A comparison of continuous-course and split-course schemes for each T stage, reported by Parsons and co-workers, is presented in Table 6-11.[10] The local control and survival rates were poorer with the split-course scheme, and the complication rates were not re-

TABLE 6-10. Guidelines to Time–Dose Schedules (Rad/Week) for Various Head and Neck Squamous Cell Carcinomas (5 Fractions/Week)

Stage	Percent Local Control	Oropharynx* (UF)[10]	Tonsil (MDAH)[13]	Anterior Tonsillar Pillar/Retromolar Trigone (MDAH)[1]	Glosso-tonsillar Sulcus (MDAH)[14]	Base of Tongue (MDAH)[15]	Pharyngeal Wall (MDAH)[7]	Pyriform Sinus (UF)[8]	Supraglottic Larynx (UF)†	Supraglottic Larynx (MDAH)[12]
T1	99		6300/6–6700/7	7000/7		6600/6–7000/7		6000/7–6500/8	6000/6–6250/7	6000/6
	95	6000/6–6500/7				6300/6				
	85						7000/6			
T2	99		6600/6–7000/7	7200/7						
	95	6000/6–6500/7								
	90					6750/6–7250/7				
T3	99		6800/6–7200/7	7500/7–7½		6900/6–7300/7				
	80									
	65	6400/7–6800/8								
T2 + T3	99			7000/6–7500/7						
	90				6750/6–7000/7	6750/6–7250/7		6500/7–7000/8	6700/7½–7000/8	6500/6–7000/7½
	85						6600/6–7250/7			
	80									
T4	50			7500/7½						
T3 + T4	99		6800/6–7200/7				7000/6			
	≅50						6000/6			
	≅25									

* Includes tonsillar region, base of the tongue, and soft palate: 221 cases.
† Unpublished University of Florida data; patients treated 10/64–11/77; analysis 11/79 by S. L. Golder, MD.
(UF, University of Florida data; MDAH, M. D. Anderson Hospital data)

(Million RR, Cassisi NJ, Wittes RE: Cancer in the head and neck. In DeVita VT Jr, Hellman S, Rosenberg SA [eds]: Cancer: Principles and Practice of Oncology, pp. 301–395. Philadelphia, JB Lippincott, 1982)

TABLE 6-11. Comparison by Tumor Site of Continuous-Course Versus Split-Course External-Beam Irradiation (No. Patients With Local Control/No. Treated)

Disease Site	Stage T1–T2*		Stage T3		Stage T4	
	Split Course (6200 rad)†	Continuous Course (6100 rad)†	Split Course (6600 rad)†	Continuous Course (6600 rad)†	Split Course (6600 rad)†	Continuous Course (6600 rad)†
Oral cavity‡	4/8	2/5	2/5	1/3	No data	No data
Oropharynx‡	17/24	39/45	9/22	8/15	1/18	2/7
Nasopharynx	4/4	3/3	5/6	3/3	2/6	6/10
Hypopharynx	2/4	10/17	2/11	5/7	1/8	0/6
Supraglottic larynx	4/6	11/12	4/4	4/7	1/2	0/2
Total	31/46 (67%)	65/82 (79%)	22/48 (46%)	21/35 (60%)	5/34 (15%)	8/25 (32%)

* 40% of the split-course patients had T1 lesions versus 35% of the continuous-course patients.

† Median dose of external irradiation.

‡ Patients with oral cavity and oropharynx primary lesions who received interstitial irradiation were excluded.

Note: University of Florida data; patients treated 9/64–8/76; analysis 8/78.

(Adapted with permission from Parsons JT, Bova FJ, Million RR: A reevaluation of split-course technique for squamous cell carcinoma of the head and neck. Int J Radiat Oncol Biol Phys 6:1645–1652, 1980. Copyright © 1980 by Pergamon Press, Ltd.)

TABLE 6-12. Local Control of Primary Lesion With Twice-a-Day Fractionation ± Neck Dissection* (Minimum 2-Year Follow-up)

Stage	Local Control
T2	2/5† (40%)
T3	11/14‡ (79%)
T4	4/19 (21%)

* 14 patients excluded from local control analysis; died of intercurrent disease <2 years after treatment with the primary lesion controlled.

† 2 local failures received low doses of 6960 rad each.

‡ 1 local failure received only 6000 rad.

Note: University of Florida data; patients treated 3/78–7/81; analysis 7/83 by J. T. Parsons, MD.

duced. (See Tables 13-12 through 13-16 and Figures 13-22 through 13-24 in Chapter 13.)

A number of fractionation schemes have been tried in which treatments are given only one, two, three, or four times per week instead of five times per week. In these schemes the daily dose is higher. When these schemes are compared with five fractions per week, the local control is better with five treatments per week and the complication rates are less.[2,16]

Multiple daily fractionation schemes, mainly twice-a-day fractionation, have been used in recent years for advanced squamous cell carcinomas of the head and neck. The hope was that local and regional control would be improved and the complication rate would be reduced. Twice-a-day fractionation, 5 days per week, has been in use at the University of Florida since 1977. A dose of 120 rad is given twice daily with at least a 4-hour interval between treatments. A total dose of 7400 rad or 7680 rad is delivered in 43 to 44 days. The acute mucosal reactions are similar to those seen with 190 rad to 200 rad/day for large-volume treatment portals; the skin reactions are either similar or slightly greater than with once-a-day fractionation schemes.

Thirty-seven patients were treated by radiation therapy alone; 13 by radiation therapy followed by a neck dissection; and seven by radiation therapy followed by resection of the primary lesion and a neck dissection. The rate of local control for the primary lesion is shown in Table 6-12. Data on control of neck disease when the primary lesion was controlled are given in Table 6-13.

The absolute survival free of disease with a minimum 2-year follow-up is shown in Table 6-14. The complications were judged to be no worse and perhaps slightly less compared with one fraction per day. One of the advantages is that the overall treatment time is shortened from the 7 to 8 weeks required for once-a-day treatment to 6 to 6½ weeks for twice-a-day fractionation. However, the actual number of treatments given each patient is significantly increased (64 vs. 40), which is somewhat of a burden on a busy radiation therapy department. It is not clear at this time whether there is a worthwhile clinical advantage to this fractionation scheme.

RADIATION THERAPY FOR PALLIATION

If the goal is palliation, radiation therapy is the modality most often selected. Excellent, durable palliation may sometimes be obtained by a 1000-rad tumor dose given twice with a 1-week interval or 3000 rad/10 fractions/2 weeks. A full course of radical irradiation may be prescribed in selected situations. The relief of moderate to severe pain may require radical doses. The typical tumor regression after two doses of 1000 rad for a massive epidermoid carcinoma of the tongue is shown in Figure 6-8. This method of palliation is simple to apply, has few acute side-effects, and often produces amazing tumor regression and a few cases of long-term control.

TABLE 6-13. Neck Control With Control of Primary Disease With Twice-a-Day Fractionation (No. Heminecks Controlled/No. Treated)

Hemineck Stage	Radiation Therapy Alone	Radiation Therapy Plus Neck Dissection	Total
N0	16/17*		16/17
N1	9/10	5/5	14/15
N2A	2/2	2/2	4/4
N2B	3/5	5/5	8/10
N3A	0/2†	3/3	3/5
Total			45/51‡ (88%)

* Failure occurred after 3600 rad.
† Incomplete treatment (distant metastases prior to radical neck dissection) in 2 patients.
‡ 2/6 salvaged by radical neck dissection.
Note: University of Florida data; patients treated 3/78–7/81; analysis 7/83 by J. T. Parsons, MD.

TABLE 6-14. Absolute Disease-Free Survival at 2 Years With Twice-a-Day Fractionation

Treatment	Stage II	Stage III	Stage IVA	Stage IVB
Radiation therapy ± radical neck dissection	0/1	4/6	10/20	4/23
Preoperative radiation therapy plus surgery		2/2	2/2	1/3
Total	0/1 (0)	6/8 (75%)	12/22 (55%)	5/26 (19%)

Note: University of Florida data; patients treated 3/78–7/81; analysis 7/83 by J. T. Parsons, MD.

FIG. 6-8. A 55-year-old man presented with a sore throat that he had had 6 months. (*A*) Examination prior to treatment revealed a massive lesion of the oral tongue with extension to the base of the tongue, floor of the mouth, and left lower gingiva with invasion of the mandible. There were bilateral clinically involved lymph nodes. Biopsy showed squamous cell carcinoma (T4N3B). Palliative radiation therapy was recommended, and 2000 rad was delivered in two fractions, 1 week apart. There was a 35% decrease in tumor 1 week after the first 1000-rad treatment; there were no acute side-effects at that point. (*B*) Examination 6 weeks after completion of treatment revealed 80% regression and relief of symptoms. There was palpable induration in the tongue. The pros and cons of surgical excision consisting of total glossectomy, laryngectomy, hemimandibulectomy, and bilateral neck dissection were discussed with the patient; he elected no further therapy.

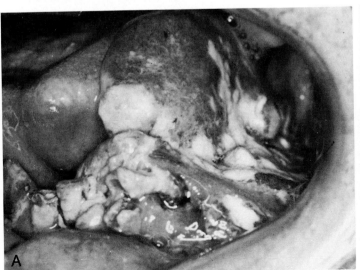
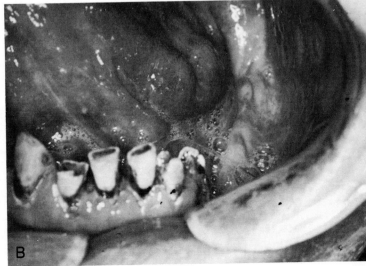

REFERENCES

1. Barker JL, Fletcher GH: Time, dose and tumor volume relationships in the megavoltage irradiation of squamous cell carcinomas of the retromolar trigone and anterior tonsillar pillar. Int J Radiat Oncol Biol Phys 2:407–414, 1977

2. Cox JD, Byhardt RW, Komaki R, Greenberg M: Reduced fractionation and the potential of hypoxic cell sensitizers in irradiation of malignant epithelial tumors. Int J Radiat Oncol Biol Phys 6:37–40, 1980

3. Fisch U: Cervical lymphography following irradiation of the neck. In Lymphography of the Cervical Lymphatic System, pp 142–163. Philadelphia, WB Saunders, 1968

4. Kogelnik HD, Fletcher GH, Jesse RH: Clinical course of patients with squamous cell carcinoma of the upper respiratory and digestive tracts with no evidence of disease 5 years after initial treatment. Radiology 115:423–427, 1975

5. Mendenhall WM, Million RR, Bova FJ: Analysis of time-dose factors in clinically positive neck nodes treated with irradiation alone in squamous cell carcinoma of the head and neck. Int J Radiat Oncol Biol Phys, in press

6. Mendenhall WM, Van Cise WS, Bova FJ, Million RR: Analysis of time–dose factors in squamous cell carcinoma of the oral tongue and floor of mouth treated with radiation therapy alone. Int J Radiat Oncol Biol Phys 7:1005–1011, 1981

7. Meoz-Mendez RT, Fletcher GH, Guillamondegui OM, Peters LJ: Analysis of the results of irradiation in the treatment of squamous cell carcinomas of the pharyngeal walls. Int J Radiat Oncol Biol Phys 4:579–585, 1978

8. Million RR, Cassisi NJ: Radical irradiation for carcinoma of the pyriform sinus. Laryngoscope 91:439–450, 1981

9. Million RR, Cassisi NJ, Wittes RE: Cancer in the head and neck. In DeVita VT Jr, Hellman S, Rosenberg SA (eds): Cancer: Principles and Practices of Oncology, pp 301–395. Philadelphia, JB Lippincott, 1982

10. Parsons JT, Bova FJ, Million RR: A re-evaluation of split-course technique for squamous cell carcinoma of the head and neck. Int J Radiat Oncol Biol Phys 6:1645–1652, 1980

11. Sagerman RH, Chung CT, King GA, Dala P, Yu WS: High-dose preoperative irradiation of the lower neck and supraclavicular fossae. AJR 132:357–359, 1979

12. Shukovsky LJ: Dose, time, volume relationships in squamous cell carcinoma of the supraglottic larynx. Am J Roentgenol Radium Ther Nucl Med 108:27–29, 1970

13. Shukovsky LJ, Fletcher GH: Time-dose and tumor volume relationships in the irradiation of the squamous cell carcinoma of the tonsillar fossa. Radiology 107:621–626, 1973

14. Shukovsky LJ, Fletcher GH, Baeza MR: Results of irradiation in squamous cell carcinomas of the glossopalatine sulcus. Radiology 120:405–408, 1976

15. Spanos WJ Jr, Shukovsky LJ, Fletcher GH: Time, dose, and tumor volume relationships in irradiation of squamous cell carcinomas of the base of tongue. Cancer 37:2591–2599, 1976

16. Wiernik G, Bleehen NM, Brindle J, Bullimore J, Churchill-Davidson IFJ, Davidson J et al: Sixth Interim Progress Report of the British Institute of Radiology fractionation study of 3F/week versus 5F/week in radiotherapy of the laryngopharynx. Br J Radiol 51:241–250, 1978

General Principles for Treatment of Cancers in the Head and Neck: Combining Surgery and Radiation Therapy

RODNEY R. MILLION
NICHOLAS J. CASSISI

The head and neck region is one of the most common areas treated by a combination of surgery and radiation therapy. Either preoperative or postoperative radiation therapy may be used, and there are advocates for each. Analysis of available data suggests that there is little or no difference in local-regional control or survival comparing the two sequences; the major difference is the increased operative morbidity associated with operations performed after radiation therapy.

Within our own institutional experience with postoperative irradiation, an improved local and regional control rate was reflected in a higher 5-year survival rate (Fig. 7-1).[1,3,7] El-Badawi and co-workers have reported an improved 5-year survival rate for pyriform sinus cancer treated by combined treatment compared with surgery alone (see section on pyriform sinus in Chapter 21, Hypopharynx: Pharyngeal Walls, Pyriform Sinus, and Postcricoid Pharynx).[2]

Combined modality therapy should be avoided when a high cure rate (70% or greater) is predicted by either surgery or radiation therapy alone. In many patients who develop local or regional failure, salvage can be achieved by secondary procedures. Fifteen to 20% will die of other causes within 5 years, and approximately 5% will develop another head and neck cancer.

The advantages of postoperative compared with preoperative radiation therapy include less operative morbidity, more meaningful margin checks at the time of the operation, a knowledge of tumor spread for radiation treatment planning, safe use of a higher radiation dose, and no chance that the patient will refuse surgery.

The disadvantages of postoperative radiation therapy include the larger treatment volume necessary to cover surgical dissections and scars, a delay to the start of radiation therapy with possible growth of tumor (especially contralateral neck nodes), and the higher dose required to accomplish the same rate of local-regional control.

PREOPERATIVE RADIATION THERAPY

Preoperative radiation therapy instead of postoperative radiation therapy is recommended for the following situations:

A trial of radiation therapy (5000 rad) is given to judge the response of the primary lesion. The patient is reevaluated with the surgeon, and a decision is made to continue for cure by radiation therapy or to stop the irradiation and proceed in 4 to 6 weeks to an operation. This philosophy is selected for moderately advanced lesions that have a reasonable chance to respond favorably to radiation therapy, thereby avoiding a major ablative procedure. The pyriform sinus and larynx are common primary sites for use of this strategy. There is no proof that one can select patients on this basis, but the concept is used by many groups and seems to work. In our practice, about four of five patients selected for a trial will complete a full course of radiation therapy. On the other hand, a few patients initially selected for a full course of radiation therapy are reevaluated after 5000 rad of treatment because the response is so poor, and irradiation is stopped and an operation is recommended.

A neck node that is on the borderline of resectability or inoperable is a reason to give radiation therapy before surgery. The dose to the primary lesion depends on whether it is to be treated for cure by radiation therapy or to be resected at the time of neck dissection. If the primary lesion is to be treated for cure by radiation therapy, then the treatment of the major neck mass is continued to a dose of 6000 rad to 8000 rad through a reduced portal. Most large nodes will become resectable, and approximately 50% of the specimens contain no residual carcinoma. The control of the neck disease in this situation is quite respectable, and the complications are acceptable (see Tables 6-6 and 6-7 in Chapter 6).

However, when the primary lesion is to be resected in addition to the neck nodes, the preoperative doses prescribed are tempered by the increased complications expected.

The results for control of neck disease when both the primary lesion and the neck disease are managed by preoperative radiation therapy and surgery are shown in Table 7-1. The disease was not controlled in necks with masses 5 cm to more than 8 cm in size and with doses less than 5000 rad; four neck masses were unresectable at the time of surgery because of fixation to the base of skull or neurovascular bundle. The incidence of pathologically negative neck specimens was only 15%. When the primary lesion was controlled, the neck disease was controlled in 84% (16/19) compared with 25% (3/12) with primary failure. The major (3+) complication rate increases once the aerodigestive tract is breached by operation (Table 7-2). It is quite obvious that large lymph nodes should receive more than 4500 rad to 5000 rad; a reduced portal could be used for the lymph node boost to try to avoid increasing the surgical morbidity associated with resection of the primary lesion.

If reconstruction and rehabilitation will delay the start of postoperative radiation therapy by more than 6 weeks, then preference may be given to the use of preoperative radiation therapy.

If simultaneous primary lesions are present, then preoperative irradiation may be used (see Chapter 4).

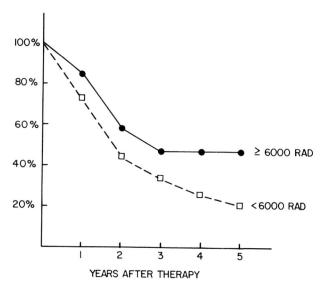

FIG. 7-1. Actuarial survival of the 65 patients evaluable for local disease control after radical surgery followed by postoperative irradiation for advanced squamous cell carcinomas of the oral cavity, oropharynx, pyriform sinus, supraglottic larynx, and glottic larynx.[1] The p value of the difference between the two curves was 0.10 by the Gehan method.[3] (University of Florida data; patients treated 10/64–9/76; minimum 2-year follow-up) (Reprinted with permission from Marcus RB Jr, Million RR, Cassisi NJ: Postoperative irradiation for squamous cell carcinomas of the head and neck: Analysis of time–dose factors related to control above the clavicles. Int J Radiat Oncol Biol Phys 5:1943–1949, 1979. Copyright © 1979, Pergamon Press, Ltd.)

Dermal invasion necessitates the preoperative use of radiation therapy.

There are only a few clinical situations in which an unresectable primary lesion can be converted to a resectable lesion with preoperative radiation therapy. The full therapeutic dose is delivered in these cases prior to operation.

An ususual lesion in which radiation therapy was used to cure part of the primary lesion and surgery was used to resect only a portion of the lesion, thus necessitating

TABLE 7-1. Control of Neck Disease With Preoperative Radiation Therapy Followed by Resection of the Primary and Neck Dissection: 32 Patients; 35 Evaluable* Heminecks (No. of Heminecks Controlled/No. of Heminecks Treated)

Maximum Node Diameter	Minimum Node Dose (rad)			
	3000–4000	>4000–5000	>5000–6000	>6000–7000+
3–4 cm	4/5	12/16	1/2	1/1
5–6 cm	0/1	0/5	1/2	0/0
7–8+ cm	0/0	0/3	0/0	0/0

* Includes four patients with unresectable neck masses at the time of surgery after 3300 rad (5 cm), 4400 rad (4 cm), 4700 rad (8 cm), and 5000 rad (7 cm).

Note: University of Florida data; patients treated 10/64–2/79; analysis 4/81 by B. D. Greenberg, MD.

TABLE 7-2. Complications—Preoperative Radiation Therapy Followed by Resection of the Primary Lesion and Neck Dissection (38 Patients*)

	Maximum Subcutaneous Dose (rad)		
Complication	3000–5000	5000–6000	6000–7000
Fistula			
1+	0	1	0
2+	0	0	1
3+	4	2	1
Bone exposure			
1+	0	2	0
2+	0	0	1
Edema			
2+	1	0	0
Flap separation/delayed healing			
1+	2	0	1
2+	5	1	1
3+	5	3	1
Carotid rupture	2	1	0
Pharyngeal stricture	2	0	0
Laryngeal necrosis	0	1	0
Aspiration pneumonia	0	1 (fatal)	1
Postoperative hemorrhage (7 units)	1	0	0
Total No. of complications	22	12	7
Fraction of patients with complications	17/23	9/10	4/5

* Includes 6 patients not evaluable for analysis of control of neck disease (see Table 7-1).
Note: University of Florida data; patients treated 10/64–2/79; analysis 4/81 by B. D. Greenberg, MD.

"cutting across" an area that had been involved by cancer prior to irradiation, is shown in Figure 7-2.

The dose for preoperative radiation therapy is usually 5000 rad/5 to 6 weeks to the primary lesion; neck masses over 5 cm in diameter should receive a higher dose. Short treatment schemes using a few large fractions followed immediately by surgery have shown little or no advantage in comparison with surgery alone.[4,5,8] Moderate-dose schemes, 3000 rad to 4000 rad, have not shown any great increase in control rates. A dose of 5000 rad will control a large percentage of subclinical disease in lymph nodes and also reduce the recurrence rates for the primary site. A few venturesome groups have tried higher doses, 6000 rad to 6500 rad to the primary site and neck, but the morbidity may exceed the gain in cures.

POSTOPERATIVE RADIATION THERAPY

Postoperative radiation therapy is considered when the risk of recurrence above the clavicles exceeds 20%.

The operative procedure should require only one stage and should be of such magnitude that irradiation is started no later than 6 weeks after surgery and preferably no later than 4 weeks. The operation should be undertaken only if it is believed to be highly likely that all gross disease will be removed and that margins will be negative. It is fashionable to talk about *debulking* or *cytoreductive* operations prior to radiation therapy. These terms have no precise meaning and should be avoided because they may imply partial removal of gross disease (cut-through), a maneuver that probably reduces the chance of control by radiation therapy rather than enhancing it.

The radiation therapist is frequently called on to decide the type of further treatment based on the pathologist's report following surgery. Positive margins or close margins are definitely an indication for radiation therapy, but the failure rate with negative margins is substantial. Looser and co-workers compared the clinical significance of negative and positive margins for 1775 previously untreated squamous cell carcinomas of the head and neck (excluding glottic and skin).[6] Only 3.5% were scored as having positive margins. The incidence of recurrence at the primary site was 31.7% for patients with negative margins and 71% for those with positive margins. There was no difference whether the positive margin was due to carcinoma *in situ*, invasive tumor, or close margin (within 5 mm). Other indications for postoperative irradiation may be cartilage or bone invasion, perineural spread, and high-grade histology.

The findings in the neck dissection are frequently the indication for postoperative radiation therapy. If there are multiple positive nodes, invasion through the capsule, or high-grade histology, then a high risk of recurrence in both the dissected neck and the contralateral neck can be predicted.

The referring surgeon is sometimes insistent that the patient receive postoperative radiation therapy, even though there is no good indication for it; it is usually best to follow the surgeon's intuition. (See Chapter 13, Time–Dose–Volume Relationships in Radiation Therapy, for full discussion of the results of postoperative radiation therapy.)

Greenberg analyzed the regional control rate for postoperative radiation therapy in 30 patients (34 necks) with N2 and N3 neck disease. There were no N3A patients, since they received preoperative radiation therapy. The control of the neck disease related to N stage and dose is

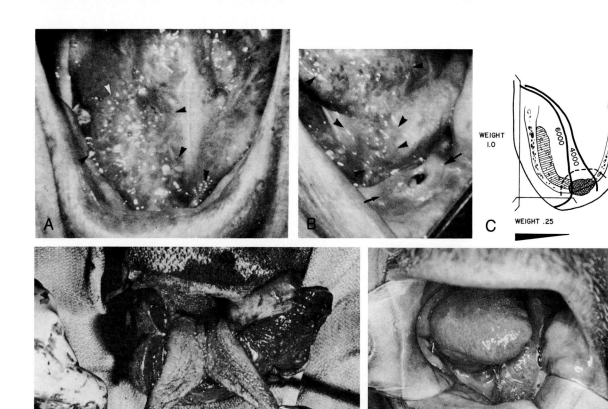

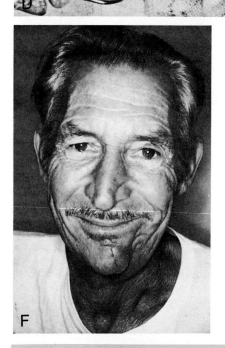

FIG. 7-2. A 58-year-old man presented with squamous cell carcinoma of the right floor of the mouth with extension to the left lower gingiva (T4N1). (*A*) Superficial involvement of the entire right floor of mouth, extending to the third molar region (*arrows*). (*B*) The tumor extended across the midline floor of mouth (*arrowheads*) to involve the left gingiva. The underlying mandible was invaded by tumor (*arrows*). (*C*) Radiation treatment plan: 6000 rad/9 weeks, split course, cobalt-60, was delivered to the superficial lesion of the floor of the mouth. The gingival lesion received 4000 rad to 5000 rad. The lesion of the floor of the mouth had completely healed prior to surgery. The dashed line indicates the margins of excision. (*D*) A partial mandibulectomy with tongue flap reconstruction was done 6 weeks following radiation therapy. (*E*) Postoperative appearance of oral cavity. (*F*) Patient was free of disease at 7 years.

TABLE 7-3. Analysis of Neck Disease Control—Postoperative Radiation Therapy: 30 Patients, 34 Evaluable Heminecks (No. Controlled/No. Treated)

Clinical Neck Stage	No. Patients	Minimum Node Dose (rad)			
		3000–4000	4000–5000	5000–6000	6000–7000+
N2A	4	0/0	2/2	1/1	1/1
N2B	13	1/1	6/6	3/5	1/1
N3B	13*	0/0	9/12	2/2	2/3

* Seventeen heminecks evaluable in 13 N3B patients.

Note: University of Florida data; patients treated 10/64–2/79; analysis 4/81 by B. D. Greenberg, MD.

TABLE 7-4.   Complications—Postoperative Radiation Therapy (35 Patients*)

Complication	Maximum Subcutaneous Dose (rad)		
	3000–5000	5000–6000	6000–7000
Fistula			
1+	0	0	3
2+	0	0	1
3+	0	1	0
Edema			
1+	0	1	1
2+	0	1	0
Flap separation/delayed healing			
1+	0	2	1
2+	1	1	3
Fibrosis			
1+	0	0	1
2+	0	0	1
Aspiration (3+)	0	1	0
Postoperative pneumonia	0	0	1
Total No. of complications	1	7	12
Fraction of patients with complications	1/7	6/11	10/22

* Includes 5 patients not evaluable for analysis.

(1+, healed in 6 months or less with conservative treatment only; 2+, healed with conservative treatment only in >6 months; 3+, required a surgical procedure for treatment of complication)

Note: University of Florida data; patients treated 10/64–2/79; analysis 4/81 by B. D. Greenberg, MD.

given in Table 7-3. The control rate is exceptionally high compared with preoperative radiation therapy (see Table 7-1), which reflects selection of patients with mobile, resectable nodes and use of higher doses of radiation for this sequence of therapy. When the primary lesion was controlled, the neck disease was controlled in every patient (28/28); when treatment of the primary lesion failed, the neck disease was not controlled (0/3). Total complications, which are considerably less frequent and less severe compared with preoperative radiation therapy to the neck, are presented in Table 7-4.

REFERENCES

1. Cutler SJ, Ederer F: Maximum utilization of the life table method in analyzing survival. J Chronic Dis 8:699–712, 1965
2. El-Badawi SA, Goepfert H, Fletcher GH, Herson J, Oswald MJ: Squamous cell carcinoma of the pyriform sinus. Laryngoscope 92:357–364, 1982
3. Gehan EA: A generalized Wilcoxon test for comparing arbitrarily singly-censored samples. Biometrika 52:203–223, 1965
4. Ketcham AS, Hoye RC, Chretien PB, Brace KC: Irradiation twenty-four hours preoperatively. Am J Surg 118:691–697, 1969
5. Lawrence W Jr, Terz JJ, Rogers C, King RE, Wolf JS, King ER: Preoperative irradiation for head and neck cancer: A prospective study. Cancer 33:318–323, 1974
6. Looser KG, Shah JP, Strong EW: The significance of "positive" margins in surgically resected epidermoid carcinomas. Head Neck Surg 1:107–111, 1978
7. Marcus RB Jr, Million RR, Cassisi NJ: Postoperative irradiation for squamous cell carcinomas of the head and neck: Analysis of time-dose factors related to control above the clavicles. Int J Radiat Oncol Biol Phys 5:1943–1949, 1979
8. Strong EW: Preoperative radiation and radical neck dissection. Surg Clin North Am 42:271–276, 1979

General Principles for Treatment of Cancers in the Head and Neck: Chemotherapy

WARREN E. ROSS

Carcinoma of the upper aerodigestive system represents a source of continuing challenge and frustration to the medical oncologist. Twenty years after methotrexate was found to have single-agent activity in this group of tumors, the precise role of chemotherapy remains to be defined. Indeed, it is fair to say that, at present, chemotherapy exerts no significant impact on long-term survival and only occasionally provides brief palliation. However, a new wave of enthusiasm has been generated by the introduction of cisplatin into the armamentarium and by the recognition that a major response can be achieved in most patients with advanced squamous cell cancer of the head and neck if chemotherapy is administered prior to surgery or irradiation. Responses even in this setting are generally not durable, but they may render some patients candidates for curative procedures who might otherwise have received only palliative measures.

The difficulties encountered in the pharmacologic management of this group of patients result both from the nature of the tumor and from a series of problems posed by this particular patient population. As a group, squamous cell malignancies are only moderately responsive to chemotherapy, and squamous cell cancers of the head and neck area are no exception. In addition, the setting in which they occur often limits the extent to which chemotherapy may be used. Nutritional deficiencies frequently coexist with continuing alcohol abuse. Indeed, a high frequency of subclinical folate deficiency has been documented in a study by Hellman and co-workers.[19] Such deficiencies are certain to reduce the patient's tolerance to drugs with an already unfavorable therapeutic index. It is not uncommon for patients to present with draining fistulas, areas of severe ulceration, or continuing aspiration. Mucositis subsequent to previously administered radiation therapy may be exacerbated or "recalled" by several of the commonly used drugs. Finally, since these malignancies frequently occur in older patients who have long histories of various forms of self-abuse, it is not uncommon for there to be compromised function of heart, lungs, kidneys, or liver, thereby altering drug disposition and increasing the risk of organ toxicity.

Despite the obstacles encountered in drug therapy of head and neck cancer, there is little question that an effective chemotherapy program would rapidly assume a major therapeutic role. There exists a need to find ways of improving local and regional control, avoiding deforming surgical procedures, reducing the incidence of distant metastases, treating recurrences when surgery and radiation therapy are no longer an option, and reducing the dose of radiation and thus the complication risk.

The location of head and neck cancers presents several opportunities to increase the response rates to chemotherapy. Intra-arterial drug administration has been used with equivocal results by a number of investigators over the years. In 1975, Goldsmith and Carter surveyed the literature on this approach and concluded that the response rate was not substantially different from that achieved with intravenous administration and thus that this approach could not be justified in light of the increased risks, inconvenience, and expense involved.[17] Improvements in technique appear to have improved the safety and efficacy of this approach, and randomized trials are being done to reassess its role as an adjunct to surgery and radiation therapy.

The accessibility of head and neck cancers would seem to make them ideal candidates for hyperthermia, either as an independent treatment modality or as a means of increasing responses to chemotherapy and radiation therapy. Early data are encouraging; a pilot study of hyperthermia combined with either doxorubicin (Adriamycin) or bleomycin was reported by Arcangeli and co-workers.[3] Eight patients received doxorubicin and six patients received bleomycin for nodal metastases from squamous cell cancer. In addition to chemotherapy, half the nodes received high-frequency hyperthermia (43°C) every other day. All nodal areas treated with both modalities responded, while only 5 of 14 areas responded to chemotherapy alone. These preliminary findings merit further investigation.

Tumor accessibility should also facilitate tumor sampling for studies of drug sensitivity by the human tumor stem cell assay. Mattox and Von Hoff have reported successful application of this technique to head and neck cancer.[28] They were able to grow tumor cell colonies in soft agar from 23 of 36 tumors and demonstrated limited sensitivity to either bleomycin, methotrexate, or cisplatin in the small number of patients studied. These investigators observed that cloning efficiency was inversely related to the degree of differentiation of the sample and to survival at 3 months from the time of biopsy. One application suggested for the assay would be to detect residual viable tumor in sites that appear to be histologically free of disease following radiation therapy or surgery.

The inability to make an accurate prediction of the clinical response to chemotherapy in patients with head and neck cancer has prompted several investigators to attempt to identify those factors that influence the response rate. The heterogeneity of head and neck tumors and the diversity of regimens employed, as well as the relatively low overall response rates, make interpretation of existing data difficult, but several factors have emerged consistently enough to warrant consideration. A history of previous therapy, either surgery or irradiation, usually reduces the response rate to all subsequently administered drugs, singly or in combination. The reasons for this are not well understood, but they may relate to changes in vascular supply or tumor growth characteristics. Overlapping toxicities, expecially exacerbation of radiation mucositis by a variety of drugs, not infrequently compromise drug dose. There are few data regarding the effect prior chemotherapy exerts on second-line chemotherapy treatment, but experience in other tumor systems suggests that this, too, will be an important prognostic factor.

A second major determinant of response to chemotherapy appears to be patient performance status. Amer and co-workers found that patients with a 70% performance status or better by the Karnofsky scale responded more frequently (32% vs. 13%) and lived longer (median survival 29 weeks vs. 9 weeks) following chemotherapy than those with a lower score.[2]

Patients with less advanced tumors also respond to chemotherapy more frequently. Although smaller tumors are more responsive, this generally does not translate into a survival advantage, again emphasizing the ineffectiveness of chemotherapy in altering the natural course of these diseases. The presence of distant metastases has been found by some groups to reduce response rates drastically, while others have not confirmed this observation. It may well be that drug selection accounts in part for these discrepancies. Other suggested prognostic factors, which are currently shrouded in some dispute, are the site of disease and the degree of tumor differentiation.

SINGLE-AGENT THERAPY

Systematic evaluation of single-agent activity in head and neck cancer has been infrequent, and, as a consequence, reliable data are available for only a few drugs. The published literature on the subject is further complicated by response rates inflated by the inclusion of patients experiencing less than 50% tumor regression and of "complete responses" that are unconfirmed histologically and by the failure to provide information on the important prognostic factors noted previously. For these reasons, tabulated data, such as published by Goldsmith and Carter (Table 8-1), must be viewed with some caution and comparison of one agent to another is clearly not reasonable.[17]

TABLE 8-1. Single-Agent Activity in Head and Neck Cancer

		Response	
Drug	Patients	>50% Tumor Regression	Overall Rate
5-Fluorouracil	118	18	15%
6-Mercaptopurine	45	6	12%
Hydroxyurea	18	7	39%
Mechlorethamine HCl	66	5	7.5%
Cyclophosphamide	77	28	36%
Chlorambucil	34	5	14.7%
Vinblastine	35	10	29%
Procarbazine	31	3	10%

(Modified with permission from Goldsmith MA, Carter SK: The integration of chemotherapy into a combined modality approach to cancer therapy: V. Squamous cell cancer of the head and neck. Cancer Treat Rev 2:137–158, 1975. Copyright © Academic Press Inc [London] Ltd.)

Methotrexate

The most extensively studied agent in the management of head and neck cancer is methotrexate. The original observations of its activity have been followed by an extensive literature regarding the optimal dose, route, and schedule of administration. While not all issues in this debate have been resolved, several points of practical importance have emerged that are agreed on by most investigators. When methotrexate is given in "standard" doses, better activity is observed when the drug is given intermittently rather than daily. Treatment on a weekly or biweekly schedule is preferable to a monthly schedule. Indeed, no schedule of administration has proved superior to that employed by Leone and associates in one of the earliest clinical trials reported.[25] Thirty-five patients with advanced head and neck cancer, most of whom had previously undergone surgery or irradiation, received methotrexate, 60 mg/m², on a weekly schedule. There were 9 complete and 11 partial responses, for a total response rate of 67%. The median duration of response was 128 days. The chief toxicity encountered was oral mucositis, which occurred in 69% of the patients. The response rate (and the incidence of toxicity) reported in this series is somewhat higher than the 30% to 50% response rate obtained by most investigators using methotrexate, but it points out that, as a general rule, response rates are variable and comparison of other regimens with that of methotrexate must be done in a direct, randomized fashion to be meaningful. The short duration of response observed is characteristic of all trials of single agents in the treatment of head and neck cancer and undoubtedly results from the presence of a large population of resistant cells from the onset of therapy. The dose-limiting toxicity in the trial of Leone and associates was oral mucositis, but other series report myelosuppression as the dose-limiting factor with these types of regimens. The frequency and severity of mucositis depend to some extent on the extent of previous irradiation and on the nutritional status of the patient.

Intra-arterial administration of methotrexate has also been employed in an effort to enhance efficacy and to avoid systemic toxicity. Goldsmith and Carter reviewed 340 cases treated in this manner and found a cumulative response rate that did not differ from that observed with intravenous administration of methotrexate.[17] The failure of intra-arterial therapy to increase tumor cell kill significantly, despite the higher local drug concentrations achieved at the tumor site, is of considerable interest and may, in fact, have presaged the failure of so-called high-dose methotrexate regimens given intravenously. In any event, it confirms the profound resistance of a large subpopulation of tumor cells to this particular drug.

Perhaps no aspect of the chemotherapy of head and neck cancer has been as controversial as the use of high doses of methotrexate followed by folinic acid rescue. This method has been used with apparent success in other solid tumors and was rapidly applied to head and neck cancer in the early 1970s. It is based on experimental studies of mouse L1210 leukemia in which the therapeutic index of methotrexate was improved by rescuing normal cells from the cytotoxicity of methotrexate with folinic acid. The latter represents the end product of the metabolic pathway normally inhibited by intracellular methotrexate. Such rescue allows very high doses of methotrexate to be employed, thus presumably overcoming mechanisms of resistance based on reduced cellular uptake of drug. Initial efforts to apply this technique to human cancer were complicated by the fact that the high concentrations of methotrexate excreted by the kidneys resulted in intratubular drug precipitation and consequent renal failure. This problem was subsequently overcome through the use of rigorous hydration and forced alkaline diuresis.

Analysis of results obtained with high-dose methotrexate is clouded by the lack of uniformity of dose and scheduling of both the methotrexate and the folinic acid rescue. Experimental tumor models indicate that there is considerable difference in the results obtained when the timing of the rescue and the dose of the rescue agent are varied. Thus, it is difficult at present to make a categorical statement regarding the efficacy of the method. An early trial reported by Levitt and co-workers compared methotrexate given in doses of 120 mg to 1000 mg/m² with folinic acid rescue to standard doses of methotrexate.[26] They found a similar response rate, but less myelosuppression and fewer treatment-related deaths in the group treated with the higher doses. This stimulated much interest in the technique for head and neck cancer, but unfortunately a number of trials directly comparing various methotrexate dose levels have been reported, and the weight of evidence suggests that high-dose regimens, as currently designed, offer no significant advantage with regard to response rate or duration (Table 8-2). Indeed, in the study of Deconti and Schoenfeld, methotrexate given weekly at conventional doses produced better response durations and survival.[10] Furthermore, toxicity in several of these trials was more severe in the groups treated with the higher doses. In summary, it appears that the optimal use of methotrexate includes weekly or biweekly administration at a dose of 40 mg to 60 mg/m². Whether intravenous administration offers any advantage over oral administration is not clear.

Cisplatin

A second major therapeutic agent in head and neck cancer is cisplatin. While experience with this drug is more limited than that for methotrexate, there is little question that it has achieved an important place in the therapeutic armamentarium. Cisplatin is a heavy metal coordination complex that exerts its antitumor effect by binding to deoxyribonucleic acid (DNA), thereby inhibiting template activity. Initial studies of cisplatin suggested that the dose-limiting toxicity would be renal tubular damage, but subsequent employment of aggressive hydration and forced diuresis with furosemide and/or mannitol has allowed dose escalation to the point that bone marrow suppression and nausea and vomiting have become the dose-limiting toxicities.

The response rate in head and neck cancer to cisplatin when used as a single agent is reported to be 25% to 40%. In comparing series that used various doses, the frequency of response does not appear to increase beyond a dose of approximately 50 mg/m² given every 3 weeks. The duration of response to cisplatin is similar to that of methotrexate (i.e., 2 to 4 months). The failure to improve either the response rate or the duration by escalating doses of cisplatin again suggests the presence of a large population of tumor cells that are either markedly resistant to the drug or are so poorly vascularized that adequate drug levels are not achieved.

Patient tolerance to cisplatin has been severely limited by vomiting, which is resistant to most antiemetic mea-

TABLE 8-2. **Randomized Trials of Methotrexate Dose–Response Relationship**

Study	Regimens	No. Patients	Response Rate	Response Duration	Survival
DeConti and Schoenfeld[10]	MTX 40–60 mg/m² IV weekly	81	26%	4.4 months	5.1 months
	MTX 240 mg/m² IV plus LV 25 mg po q6h × 8 doses beginning 42 hr after MTX	80	24%	1.4 months	4.4 months
	MTX/LV as above plus CTX 500 mg/m² IV plus Ara-C 300 mg/m² IV	76	18%	1.6 months	3.3 months
Vogler and co-workers[39]	MTX 125 mg/m² po q6h × 4 doses plus LV	49	27%	6.3 months	N/A
	MTX 15 mg/m² po q6h × 4 doses	44	27%	5.8 months	N/A
	MTX 60 mg/m²/wk IV	61	34%	5.4 months	N/A
Woods and co-workers[40]	MTX 50 mg/m² IV	11	45%	N/A	N/A
	MTX 500 mg/m² IV plus LV	16	31%	N/A	N/A
	MTX 5000 mg/m² IV plus LV	12	50%	N/A	N/A

(MTX, methotrexate; LV, leukovorin; CTX, cyclophosphamide; Ara-C, cytosine arabinoside; N/A, not available)

sures. This is a particularly difficult problem in patients with head and neck cancer, who tend to be older and more debilitated than the general population. Fortunately, it now appears that this problem may be overcome in many patients by administering high doses of metoclopramide.[18]

Bleomycin

A complex glycopeptide, bleomycin is a bacterial product that is cytotoxic by virtue of its ability to produce strand scission in DNA. The initial trials of bleomycin reported from Japan, where the drug was developed, suggested a response rate of approximately 60%. However, in a review of 298 patients treated with bleomycin in US trials, only 64 patients (21%) experienced objective response.[6] This response rate is apparently not improved by administration by continuous infusion. Despite the fact that the drug is thought to exhibit cell-cycle phase specificity in experimental animal tumor systems, Krakoff and associates observed only two responses in 11 patients who received 0.25 mg/kg/day of bleomycin by continuous infusion for 7 to 10 days.[24] The duration of infusion was determined by mucocutaneous toxicity. By whatever schedule, the low response rate, the occasionally severe mucositis, the skin reactions, and the risk of lung fibrosis have limited its usefulness as a single agent in the treatment of head and neck cancer. In fact, the principal features of bleomycin that render it useful are its lack of bone marrow toxicity, which allows its use in combination with other agents, and the possibility that it enhances the effect of radiation therapy.

Other Single-Drug Studies

In addition to methotrexate, cisplatin, and bleomycin there are scattered small series in the literature that suggest that other agents may have a modicum of activity in the treatment of head and neck cancer. Interpretation of response rates in these studies of second-line agents is especially difficult because many of these patients have received pre-vious chemotherapy in addition to surgery and radiation therapy. Thus, response rates may be lower than might be achieved if the drugs were used initially. The lack of good data on single-agent activity in head and neck cancer is a potent argument for studying previously untreated patients in the phase II trials of these single agents. Caveats notwithstanding, it would appear that single agents that have some effect on head and neck cancer, but that have not been adequately studied, include hydroxyurea, 5-fluorouracil, cyclophosphamide, vinblastine, dibromodulcitol, and mitomycin C. Finally, there are a few agents that have been studied in a sufficient number of patients to conclude that they are not effective in the treatment of head and neck cancer. These include 6-mercaptopurine, nitrogen mustard, procarbazine, dianhydrogalactitol, the epipodophyllotoxins VP16 and VM26, and peptichemio. Further studies of these agents do not appear warranted.

COMBINATION CHEMOTHERAPY

Administration of chemotherapeutic agents in combination has significantly improved the response rate and duration in a number of solid tumors. Thus, it was natural that investigators would apply this principle to advanced head and neck cancer. This area of investigation is still in an early phase and it is impossible to assess its ultimate role, but there are indications that response rates, if not durations, may be improved when active agents are used in combination. Unfortunately, the toxicities encountered with combination chemotherapy are correspondingly greater as well and drug-related deaths have been reported in several series. Most of the agents that have been employed either have overlapping toxicities or have the potential to interact with one another in such a way as to enhance toxicity. Oral mucositis is commonly observed following treatment with cisplatin, methotrexate, 5-fluorouracil, vinblastine, vincristine, and bleomycin, while bone marrow suppression is a problem when all but the last two agents are used. Renal tubular damage resulting in renal failure may occur as a result of treatment with cisplatin or high-dose methotrexate. Since both of these

TABLE 8-3. Combination Regimens Containing Cisplatin

Study	Drugs	No. Patients	No. Previously Treated	Response Rate	Response Duration
Hong and Shapshay[21]	CP, Bleo	55	7	73%	N/A
Elias and co-workers[11]	CP, Bleo, MTX	33	11	67%	N/A
Glick and co-workers[16]	CP, Bleo	29	0	48%	N/A
Spaulding and co-workers[37]	VCR, Bleo, CP	28	0	97%	N/A
Al-Sarraf and co-workers[1]	Bleo, CP, MTX	22	0	86%	N/A
Creagan and co-workers[8]	CTX, CP, Ad	27	27	64%	7 months
Vogl and Kaplan[38]	CP, Bleo, MTX	37	32	51%	3 months
Ervin and co-workers[13]	Bleo, CP, MTX	29	14	100%	N/A
Caradonna and co-workers[5]	Bleo, CP, MTX	19	17	74%	4 months

(CP, cisplatin; Bleo, bleomycin; MTX, methotrexate; VCR, vincristine; CTX, cyclophosphamide; Ad, Adriamycin; N/A, not available)

TABLE 8-4. Selected Combination Regimens Not Containing Cisplatin

Study	Drugs	No. Patients	No. Previously Treated	Response Rate	Response Duration
Price and co-workers[33]	VCR, Bleo, MTX, HU, 5-FU, LV ± Ad	117	27	67%	N/A
Miyamoto[29]	Bleo, MTX	33	N/A	66%	N/A
Holoye and co-workers[20]	Bleo, CTX, MTX, 5-FU, ± VCR	49	N/A	55%	N/A
Cortes and co-workers[7]	Bleo, CTX, MTX, 5-FU	39	33	54%	11 months (CR) 7 months (PR)
Molinari and co-workers[30]	VCR, Bleo, MTX	84	"Most"	62%	6.9 months (CR) 3.9 months (PR)

(VCR, vincristine; Bleo, bleomycin; MTX, methotrexate; HU, hydroxyurea; 5-FU, 5-fluorouracil; LV, leukovorin; Ad, Adriamycin; CTX, cyclophosphamide; CR, complete response; PR, partial response; N/A, not available)

drugs, as well as bleomycin, are primarily eliminated by renal excretion, nephrotoxicity can increase the risk of organ failure in other sites as well. Cognizance of these potential hazards, however, has resulted in regimens that exhibit encouraging activity and tolerable levels of toxicity.

Evaluating the relative efficacy of drug combinations in head and neck cancer is complicated by the fact that as interest in this form of therapy increases, patients are being treated at earlier phases of their disease. In patients with disease previously treated by radiation therapy and/or surgery, it has yet to be conclusively demonstrated that response rates to the combination chemotherapy regimens are superior to those for single-agent therapy. Indeed, despite the encouraging results obtained by some investigators in heavily pretreated patients (Table 8-3), a study by David and Kessler indicated that cisplatin alone was not less active than a combination of cisplatin, methotrexate, and vincristine.[9] On the other hand, in previously untreated patients, response rates to combination therapy ranging from 70% to 100% are commonly reported, and it seems unlikely that any single agent currently available could consistently achieve this level of activity.

Of the regimens that have produced objective (complete and partial) responses in greater than 50% of patients, only a few have not contained cisplatin (Table 8-4). One of these, the Price–Hill regimen, resulted in a response rate

of 75% in previously untreated patients.[33] This is a combination of seven different agents administered in a complex schedule based on tumor cell kinetic theory. Unfortunately, 27% of patients (32 of 117) entered into the trial were considered inevaluable. Similarly, in the study of Molinari and co-workers, there were 29% (24 of 84 patients) considered inevaluable.[30] One encouraging note, however, is that while the response rate to bleomycin, cyclophosphamide, methotrexate, and 5-fluorouracil (B-CMF) reported by Cortes and associates was only 54%, the median duration of complete response was 11 months and that for partial response was 7 months.[7] These are considerably longer than what is generally reported and merit verification. Also of note was the fact that pulmonary metastases responded in seven of eight patients.

Based on available evidence, it would appear that the most active drug combinations include cisplatin. Selected series of the most active cisplatin-containing regimens are listed in Table 8-3. Of those shown, several merit individual consideration. Al-Sarraf and co-workers treated 22 patients with stage III–IV head and neck cancers with cisplatin, vincristine, and bleomycin prior to surgery or radiation therapy.[1] There were 27% clinical complete remissions and 59% partial remissions. Interestingly, of the 6 patients in whom complete remissions were reported, 4 were found to have microscopic disease at surgery. Using only cisplatin and bleomycin, Hong and Shapshay reported results virtually identical to those of Al-Sarraf, while Glick, using a nearly identical regimen, obtained only a 48% partial response rate with no complete responses.[16,21] The reason for the discrepancy in the two series is unclear, but it may relate to seemingly minor differences in schedules of drug administration and to the small numbers of patients. Durations of response to chemotherapy are generally not available for these studies because most patients received subsequent therapy (i.e., irradiation or surgery) prior to relapse.

The studies of Creagan and co-workers, Vogl and Kaplan, Caradonna and co-workers, and Ervin and co-workers are of note because of the high response rates reported in previously treated patients.[5,8,13,38] As noted, this is contrary to the results of most investigators but suggests the possibility that certain subgroups of previously treated patients may demonstrate an increased response rate. If this is confirmed in large trials, it would constitute a major advance in the treatment of head and neck cancer.

In summary, the state of the art of combination chemotherapy is in flux. It would appear that the response rates to combination regimens are superior to those of single agents, especially in previously untreated patients. It is unclear, however, what impact these improved response rates will have on survival.

COMBINED MODALITY THERAPY

Many investigators have tried to take advantage of the distinct, but limited, activity of chemotherapy for head and neck cancer by combining it with the more traditional modalities of irradiation and surgery. There are several theoretical considerations that suggest that such a multidisciplinary approach might be fruitful.

Control of the primary site could be improved by at least two mechanisms. First, significant reduction of tumor would effectively result in a down-staging of advanced primary lesions, thus increasing the likelihood of permanent control by irradiation or surgery. Ervin and co-workers suggest that this may be an attainable objective at present in at least some patients.[12] Of 21 patients with "inoperable" stage III–IV squamous cell carcinoma of the head and neck treated with weekly high-dose methotrexate, 11 demonstrated objective tumor regression. Nine of the 11 were then rendered disease free following irradiation and/or surgery, while only 3 of the 10 nonresponders achieved complete remission. Long-term control of the primary site and nodal metastases was better in the responders. These differences in response appear to have translated into increased survival, since 6 of 11 responders are free of disease at a minimum of 38 months' follow-up.

The second mechanism for improving local control by chemotherapy is by sensitizing the tumor to the lethal effects of radiation. Such radiosensitization has been demonstrated in experimental animal tumor models, but there has yet to be convincing evidence for such a phenomenon in humans.

Another potential benefit of chemotherapy-induced reduction of the primary lesion is that less extensive and disfiguring surgical procedures might be feasible in some patients. Unfortunately, there is no evidence that this objective is within sight. Attempts to reduce the magnitude of the operation after preoperative radiation therapy are associated with a high failure rate. The surgeon depends on seeing and palpating the extent of disease to determine surgical margins. When these parameters are lost, either from radiation therapy or chemotherapy, there is a tendency to reduce the scope of the procedure, and this translates into an increased risk of recurrence. The preoperative treatment (i.e., radiation therapy or chemotherapy) nearly eliminates the use of frozen section examination of the margins by the pathologist. These two problems are particularly problematic when an entire organ is not removed; the tongue is a particularly difficult area in which to determine adequate margins at the time of resection, and preoperative treatment makes it even worse.

Finally, by analogy with other solid tumors such as Ewing's sarcoma and testicular carcinomas, it is reasonable to expect that effective chemotherapy may reduce the risk of distant metastasis by eliminating microscopic foci of tumor that have formed prior to control of the primary site.

In designing a combined modality approach it is obvious that the timing of chemotherapy with respect to irradiation or surgery depends on the therapeutic objective. Primary site down-staging and reduction of intraoperative dissemination require that the chemotherapy begin at least several weeks prior to the onset of definitive local therapy. Radiosensitization, if it occurs, would likely be optimal if chemotherapy were given concomitantly with irradiation. On the other hand, elimination of preexisting distant metastases will require an extended course of chemotherapy following local control. Most studies have employed only a brief course of chemotherapy just prior to, and occasionally during, radiation treatments. Such an approach appears to be well justified, since the infirmities of the patient population limit tolerance to aggressive chemotherapy, and responses to chemotherapy are generally only of a few months' duration in any case. Also, since control of the primary site, and not distant metastases, poses the major obstacle to cure in most of these patients, it seems reasonable to focus the therapy on this problem.

Over the past 20 years, a number of trials have suggested a major benefit from the use of chemotherapy as part of the primary treatment plan. Unfortunately, many of these trials are uncontrolled pilot studies in which results are compared with previously published historical controls with little attention to prognostic stratification or other variables. One of the better studies employing historical controls was that of O'Connor and co-workers.[32] They reported that a kinetically based combination of vincristine, bleomycin, and methotrexate improved initial disease control as well as disease-free survival when given to 92 patients with advanced head and neck cancer immediately prior to, during, and just after radiation therapy. The control group was composed of 92 patients treated at the same institution during the 4 years immediately prior to the study. However, confidence in these results is mitigated by the fact that 26 patients were not allowed to participate in the combination treatment because of medical "unfitness," thus raising a question about comparability between the control and treatment groups.

Even some of the randomized trials are difficult to interpret because of problems in design. A study reported by Nervi and associates presents a useful example.[31] These workers administered methotrexate intra-arterially to 72 patients with cancer of the oral cavity, oropharynx, and maxillary antrum prior to definitive irradiation and compared the outcome to 68 patients treated only with irradiation. A survival advantage resulting from combined modality treatment was observed only in the patients with intraoral cancers with T1 or T2 lesions at the time of irradiation. However, the patients with the smaller lesions were given additional radiation therapy in the form of interstitial radium implants. While it is true that the downstaging effected by chemotherapy resulted in more patients becoming eligible for the interstitial implants, it is not clear whether the improved outcome derived from a therapeutic effect of methotrexate or simply from the fact that the combined modality group became weighted with respect to the additional irradiation.

Those well-designed randomized trials of combined modality therapy for advanced head and neck cancer that have been published suggest that the use of such an approach is sharply limited. As expected, methotrexate has been the most frequently used agent in combined modality studies. There are several randomized studies employing this drug prior to radiation therapy, and, despite differences in dose and schedule, all have concluded that no improvement in survival was observed.[15,23,36]

Bleomycin has also been investigated. Shanta and Krishnamurthi performed a randomized study in which patients with cancer of the oral cavity in India received either radiation therapy and concomitant intra-arterial bleomycin (10 mg to 15 mg, administered intra-arterially three times a week) or radiation therapy alone.[35] Severe mucositis resulted in the bleomycin group, which received only 5500 rad to 6000 rad total dose, while the control group received 6500 rad. However, 58% of the combined modality patients were disease free at 2 years' follow-up, versus 17% of the control group. Interestingly, these workers found that the effects of intravenously administered bleomycin were equivalent to those from intra-arterial administration. A more recent randomized trial from a different group in India failed to demonstrate any benefit from bleomycin when it was used in a schedule similar to that of Shanta and Krishnamurthi.[34]

The EORTC also studied concomitantly administered bleomycin in a randomized trial.[4] Ninety-nine patients with epidermoid carcinoma of the oropharynx who received bleomycin, 15 mg, administered intramuscularly or intravenously twice a week, for the first 5 weeks of radiation therapy were compared with a control group of 87 patients who received irradiation alone. The total dose of radiation delivered was the same in both groups, but weight loss, profound weakness, mucositis, and epidermatitis were significantly more common in the combined modality group. There was no significant difference in tumor response or survival when compared with irradiation alone, with a median follow-up of 15 months. Two other randomized studies of the use of bleomycin as an adjunct to irradiation have also failed to demonstrate a survival advantage.[14,22] The dramatic difference in results obtained by Shanta and others remains unexplained.

One randomized trial comparing 5-fluorouracil administered concomitantly with radiation versus radiation alone for cancer of the oral cavity and oropharynx has demonstrated a significant survival benefit in the combined modality group.[27] Although this benefit was limited to patients with oral cavity primary tumors, it is significant because of the long-term follow-up (2 to 13 years). Also of note is the fact that while local control was improved by the brief course of chemotherapy during the irradiation, the frequency of distant metastasis was unchanged.

In summary, the available data suggest that combining chemotherapy with radiation therapy may increase the initial response rate in some patients but will likely not affect survival except in a limited number of circumstances. These disappointing results are not surprising. In general, the drugs employed were of limited efficacy and the tumors treated were quite advanced. Newer trials using the more potent regimens containing cisplatin are underway. It is hoped that the dramatically increased response rates observed with these regimens will at last make an impact on long-term survival.

CONCLUSION

Having reviewed the available data on the efficacy of chemotherapy for head and neck cancers, it is appropriate to attempt to provide some perspective on the state of the art and to suggest some guidelines for the practitioner faced with treating these difficult tumors. These comments are particularly directed at the treatment of patients outside the study setting.

It is an unfortunate fact that the medical oncologist most frequently encounters patients whose head and neck cancer is far advanced. Frequently, patients have received surgery, radiation therapy, or both. They are elderly, cachectic, depressed, and desperate. If potentially curative chemotherapy were available for these patients, it might be reasonable (although still difficult) to muster up the courage to approach them aggressively. Such therapy is not available. Thus, the goal in these patients is always palliation, and because of the limitations and risks of chemotherapy, palliation does not always result from its use. For the patient with far-advanced disease, who is nonambulatory and has draining fistulas and problems with deglutition, chemotherapy clearly poses greater risks than potential benefits. These patients are best managed with aggressive nursing care and other supportive measures. However, many patients with previously treated advanced head and neck cancer are, after careful evaluation, reasonable candidates for chemotherapy, and the physician must then decide which of the many available regimens to choose. Since combination chemotherapy, with or without cisplatin, has not proved superior to the use of methotrexate alone in this setting, it is difficult to justify the enhanced morbidity and cost that attends its use. A weekly intravenous bolus of methotrexate, 40 mg to 60 mg/m^2 (or even oral methotrexate), will significantly reduce tumor size in 25% to 40% of patients, and many of these patients will report symptomatic improvement as well. The principal toxicities (i.e., myelosuppression and mucositis) are predictable, dose dependent, and manageable. Because responses are generally seen within the first 4 weeks if they are to occur, patients not responding appropriately can have their management altered before serious toxicity occurs. As previously noted, higher doses of methotrexate combined with folinic acid rescue are neither more effective nor less toxic. Failure to respond to methotrexate, or tumor regrowth after an initial regression, usually portends inexorable progression, and the likelihood of response to subsequent agents is very low.

With increasing frequency the medical oncologist is being referred patients who have advanced (unfavorable stage III or IV) cancer on initial presentation to a physician. These are the patients for whom the traditional therapeutic approach with surgery or irradiation holds little promise for cure and significant risk for disfigurement or other morbidity. Assuming the patient is ambulatory and has reasonable cardiac, renal, and hepatic function, this is a circumstance in which combination chemotherapy may be more effective than single-agent therapy. A regimen containing cisplatin and either bleomycin or methotrexate in one of the schedules noted in Table 8-3 will provide a 50% to 80% probability of achieving a partial regression, with a few patients undergoing a complete remission. There is no basis for using cisplatin doses greater than 50 mg/m², nor is there any reason to believe that three-drug combinations are superior to two-drug combinations. Whether high-dose, weekly administered methotrexate with folinic acid rescue will provide equivalent responses in this setting or not, it is not available to most physicians and it does not appear to offer any major advantage. It is important to note, however, that even in the previously untreated patient, the response duration is likely to be 3 to 6 months, and thus, if possible, the response should be consolidated with surgery or radiation therapy at the earliest possible opportunity. Should a complete remission result, adjuvant chemotherapy may be considered, but there are no data to support its employment. Is the probability of cure enhanced by such an aggressive approach in this setting? Unfortunately, no data exist from prospective randomized trials that would support such a hope. The radiation therapist should continue to specify treatment plans and dose based on the initial extent of the lesion, not on the down-staged lesion. Likewise, the surgeon should plan an operation based on the original lesion. Preliminary data already show residual tumor in surgical specimens after complete response, and the residual tumor is not necessarily confined to the center of the lesion.* *It is absolutely essential that the surgeon and/or radiation therapist see the patient for examination prior to initiation of chemotherapy because their treatment plans are totally dependent on physical findings.*

Finally, in summarizing the status of chemotherapy for head and neck cancer, it is apparent that much progress must be made before this modality can assume a routine role in management.

* Ervin T: Personal communication, 1982.

REFERENCES

1. Al-Sarraf M, Amer MH, Vaishampayan G, Loh J, Weaver A: A multidisciplinary therapeutic approach for advanced previously untreated epidermoid cancer of the head and neck: Preliminary report. Int J Radiat Oncol Biol Phys 5:1421–1423, 1979
2. Amer MH, Al-Sarraf M, Vaitkevicius VK: Factors that affect response to chemotherapy and survival of patients with advanced head and neck cancer. Cancer 43:2202–2206, 1979
3. Arcangeli G, Cividalli A, Mauro F, Nervi C, Pavin G: Enhanced effectiveness of Adriamycin and bleomycin combined with local hyperthermia in neck node metastases from head and neck cancers. Tumori 65:481–486, 1979
4. Cachin Y, Jortay A, Sancho H, Eschwege F, Madelain M, Desaulty A, Gerard P: Preliminary results of a randomized E.O.R.T.C. study comparing radiotherapy and concomitant bleomycin to radiotherapy alone in epidermoid carcinomas of the oropharynx. Eur J Cancer 13:1389–1395, 1977
5. Caradonna R, Paladine W, Ruckdeschel JC, Goldstein JC, Osone JE, Jaski JW, et al: Methotrexate, bleomycin, and high-dose cis-dichlorodiammineplatinum (II) in the treatment of advanced epidermoid carcinoma of the head and neck. Cancer Treat Rep 63:489–491, 1979
6. Carter SK: The chemotherapy of head and neck cancer. Semin Oncol 4:413–424, 1977
7. Cortes EP, Kalra J, Amin VC, Attie J, Eisenbud L, Khafif R et al: Chemotherapy for head and neck cancer relapsing after radiotherapy. Cancer 47:1966–1970, 1981
8. Creagan ET, Fleming TR, Edmonson JH, Ingle JN, Hoods JE: Cyclophosphamide, adriamycin, and cis-diamminedichloroplatinum II in the treatment of patients with advanced head and neck cancer. Cancer 47:240–244, 1981
9. Davis S, Kessler W: Randomized comparison of cis-diamminedichloroplatinum versus cis-diammeninedichloroplatinum, methotrexate, and bleomycin in recurrent squamous cell carcinoma of the head and neck. Cancer Chemother Pharmacol 3:57–59, 1979
10. DeConti RC, Schoenfeld D: A randomized prospective comparison of intermittent methotrexate, methotrexate with leucovorin, and a methotrexate combination in head and neck cancer. Cancer 48:1061–1072, 1981
11. Elias EG, Chretien PB, Monnard E, Kahan T, Brouchelle WH, Wiernik PH et al: Chemotherapy prior to local therapy in advanced squamous cell carcinoma of the head and neck: Preliminary assessment of an intensive drug regimen. Cancer 43:1025–1031, 1979
12. Ervin TJ, Kirkwood J, Weichselbaum RR, Miller D, Pitman SW, Frei E: Improved survival for patients with advanced carcinoma of the head and neck treated with methotrexate-leucovorin prior to definitive radiotherapy or surgery. Laryngoscope 91:1181–1190, 1981
13. Ervin TJ, Weichselbaum R, Miller D, Meshad M, Posner M, Fabian R: Treatment of advanced squamous cell carcinoma of the head and neck with cisplatin, bleomycin, and methotrexate (PBM). Cancer Treat Rep 65:787–791, 1981
14. Eschwege F, Richard JM, Sancho-Garnier H: Résultats préliminaires d'un essai thérapeutique de l'O.E.R.T.C. sur le rôle de l'association bléomycine-radiothérapie dans le traitement des cancers de l'oropharynx. J Radiol Electrol 59:634–635, 1978
15. Fazekas JT, Sommer C, Kramer S: Adjuvant intravenous methotrexate or definitive radiotherapy alone for advanced squamous cancers of the oral cavity, oropharynx, supraglottic larynx or hypopharynx: Concluding report of an RTOG randomized trial on 638 patients. Int J Radiat Oncol Biol Phys 6:533–541, 1980
16. Glick JH, Marcial V, Richter M, Velez-Garcia E: The adjuvant treatment of inoperable stage III and IV epidermoid carcinoma of the head and neck with platinum and bleomycin infusions prior to definitive radiotherapy: An RTOG pilot study. Cancer 46:1919–1924, 1980
17. Goldsmith MA, Carter SK: The integration of chemotherapy into a combined modality approach to cancer therapy: V. Squamous cell cancer of the head and neck. Cancer Treat Rev 2:137–158, 1975
18. Gralla RJ, Itri LM, Pisko SE, Squillante AE, Kelsen DP, Braun DW et al: Anti-emetic efficacy of high-dose metoclopramide: Randomized trials with placebo and prochlorperazine in patients with chemotherapy-induced nausea and vomiting. N Engl J Med 305:905–909, 1981
19. Hellman S, Ianotti AT, Bertino JR: Determination of levels of serum folate in patients with carcinoma of the head and neck treated with methotrexate. Cancer Res 24:105–113, 1964
20. Holoye PY, Byers RM, Gard DA, Goepfert H, Guillamondegui OM, Jesse RH: Combination chemotherapy of head and neck cancer. Cancer 42:1661–1669, 1978
21. Hong WK, Shapshay SM: Treatment of previously untreated stage III and IV squamous cell carcinoma of the head and neck. Otolaryngol Clin North Am 13:521–528, 1980
22. Kapstad B, Bang G, Rennaes S, Dahler A: Combined preoperative treatment with cobalt and bleomycin in patients with head and neck carcinoma: A controlled clinical study. Int J Radiat Oncol Biol Phys 4:85–89, 1978
23. Knowlton AH, Percarpio B, Bobrow S, Fischer JJ: Methotrexate and radiation therapy in the treatment of advanced head and neck tumors. Radiology 116:709–712, 1975

24. Krakoff IH, Cvitkovic E, Currie V, Yeh S, Lamonte C: Clinical pharmacologic and therapeutic studies of bleomycin given by continuous infusion. Cancer 40:2027–2037, 1977

25. Leone LA, Albala MM, Rege VB: Treatment of carcinoma of the head and neck with intravenous methotrexate. Cancer 21:828–837, 1968

26. Levitt M, Mosher MB, DeConti RC, Farber LR, Skeel RT, Marsh JC et al: Improved therapeutic index of methotrexate with "leukovorin rescue." Cancer Res 33:1729–1734, 1973

27. Lo Theodore CM, Wiley AL Jr, Ansfield FJ, Brandenburg JH, Davis HL Jr, Gollin FF et al: Combined radiation therapy and 5-fluorouracil for advanced squamous cell carcinoma of the oral cavity and oropharynx: A randomized study. Am J Roentgenol 126:229–235, 1976

28. Mattox DE, Von Hoff DD: In vitro stem cell assay in head and neck squamous carcinoma. Am J Surg 140:527–530, 1980

29. Miyamoto T: A sequential combination of bleomycin and mitomycin C in the treatment of advanced squamous cancers. Recent Results Cancer Res 63:179–190, 1978

30. Molinari R, Mattavelli F, Cantù G, Chiesa F, Costa L, Tancini G: Results of a low-dose combination chemotherapy with vincristine, bleomycin and methotrexate (V-B-M) based on cell kinetics in the palliative treatment of head and neck squamous cell carcinoma. Eur J Cancer 16:469–472, 1979

31. Nervi C, Arcangeli G, Badaracco G, Cortese M, Morelli M, Starace G: The relevance of tumor size and cell kinetics as predictors of radiation response in head and neck cancer: A randomized study on the effect of intraarterial chemotherapy followed by radiotherapy. Cancer 41:900–906, 1978

32. O'Connor AD, Clifford P, Dalley VM, Durden-Smith DJ, Edwards WG, Hollis BA: Advanced head and neck cancer treated by combined radiotherapy and VBM cytotoxic regimen: Four-year results. Clin Otolaryngol 4:329–337, 1979

33. Price LA, Hill BT, Calvert AH, Dalley M, Levene A, Busby ER et al: Improved results in combination chemotherapy of head and neck cancer using a kinetically-based approach: A randomized study with and without Adriamycin. Oncology 35:26–28, 1978

34. Shah PM, Shukla SN, Patel KM, Patel NL, Buboo HA, Patel DD: Effect of bleomycin-radiotherapy combination in management of head and neck squamous cell carcinoma. Cancer 48:1106–1109, 1981

35. Shanta V, Krishnamurthi S: Combined therapy of oral cancer bleomycin and radiation: A clinical trial. Clin Radiol 28:427–429, 1977

36. Shanta V, Sundaram K: The combined therapy of oral cancer. Gann Monogr Cancer Res 19:159–170, 1976

37. Spaulding MB, Klotch D, Grillo J, Sanani S, Lore JM: Adjuvant chemotherapy in the treatment of advanced tumors of the head and neck. Am J Surg 140:538–542, 1980

38. Vogl SE, Kaplan BH: Chemotherapy of advanced head and neck cancer with methotrexate, bleomycin, and cis-diamminedichloroplatinum (II) in an effective outpatient schedule. Cancer 44:26–31, 1979

39. Vogler WR, Jacobs J, Moffitt S, Valex-Garcia E, Goldsmith A, Johnson L, Mackay S: Methotrexate therapy with or without citrovorum factor in carcinoma of the head and neck, breast and colon. Cancer Clin Trials 2:227–236, 1979

40. Woods RL, Tattersall MHN, Sullivan J: A randomized study of three doses of methotrexate in patients with advanced squamous cell cancer of the head and neck (abstr). Proc Am Assoc Cancer Res 20:262, 1979

Flaps and Grafts for Reconstruction

JOHN H. ISAACS, Jr.
NICHOLAS J. CASSISI

A major factor limiting surgical management of cancers of the head and neck has been the reconstructive techniques for providing coverage, contour, and restoration of function. Although prosthetic appliances, flaps, and grafts have been used for many years, the surgeon has been able to extend the boundaries of his surgery only through the modifications that occur with constant application. Prosthetic devices and implantable materials will be discussed in Chapter 10, Maxillofacial Prosthetics.

GRAFTS

Among the types of grafts available to the surgeon are autografts, which will be discussed first and in greater detail, and xenografts and allografts, which will be discussed briefly.

Autografts

An autograft removes biologic material from its normal location and from its blood supply in the body and transfers it to another part of the body. It must establish a new blood supply to remain viable. Several types of autografts are used in head and neck surgery, including skin, mucous membrane, dermal, bone, cartilage, fat, and nerve grafts.

The major disadvantages of autografts are the limited amount of material that can be obtained, the prolonged surgery required, and the additional scarring. However, the advantages of being readily available and having immune compatibility make these the most frequently used grafts.[6,11]

SKIN AND MUCOUS MEMBRANE GRAFTS

Skin grafts are the most commonly used of all grafts. They are classified as either full thickness or split thickness. If the entire epidermis and dermis are used, the graft is called a full-thickness skin graft. These grafts must obtain a blood supply from the periphery as well as from the base of the new site, and therefore are limited in size if they are to remain viable. The donor site must be closed primarily or covered with another graft. If the entire epidermis and only part of the dermis are used, the graft is referred to as a split-thickness skin graft. Split-thickness skin grafts can be thick or thin, depending on the amount of dermis used. Thick grafts contract less than thin grafts, but it is more difficult for a thick graft to take because the new blood vessels must support more tissue. The donor site for split-thickness skin grafts will reepithelialize, so closure is not required.[1]

The surgeon must bear in mind that tissue transferred to a new site will retain its original characteristics; for example, a hair-bearing skin graft transferred to the mouth will continue to grow hair. Mucous membrane grafts are very similar to skin grafts, but their use is limited because of the small amount of tissue available.

ANATOMY

The skin is composed of two principal layers: (1) the epidermis, or superficial layer, and (2) the dermis, or deep layer. The thickness of the epidermis varies from 0.3 mm to 1.5 mm in different areas of the body; the eyelids, penis, and inner surfaces of the upper arm have the thinnest epidermis. The dermal layer of skin is extremely variable in thickness and contains the skin appendages (Fig 9-1).[12]

SOURCES AND USES

Skin can be obtained from anywhere on the body surface, but the usual donor sites for split-thickness skin grafts are the thighs, buttocks, and lower abdomen. Full-thickness skin grafts are often obtained from the postauricular area.

Skin and mucous membrane grafts are used whenever coverage is needed for viable tissue that has it own blood supply but lacks epithelial coverage and is too large to be closed primarily.[17]

Full-thickness skin grafts from behind the ear can be used to cover the defect after a basal cell carcinoma is removed from the tip or dorsum of the nose (Fig. 9-2). The color match is excellent, and the donor site can be closed primarily. Various types of flaps can also be used to fill such a defect, with excellent cosmetic results; however, recurrences are more readily diagnosed when skin grafts are used.

Split-thickness skin grafts may be used to line the cheek after a partial maxillectomy. This provides coverage and allows for the use of a prosthetic device.[6,11,18]

DIFFICULTIES IN USING SKIN GRAFTS

When skin grafts are used sometimes there is less than a 100% take. It may also be difficult to obtain a good color match.

DERMAL GRAFTS

Dermal grafts are similar to skin grafts except that the epithelium is not used. After the dermis has been removed, the epithelium is returned to the donor site. Dermal grafts are usually placed deep in tissues, but they may be used superficially in the oral cavity. As with skin grafts, dermal grafts must become vascularized at their new site.[1,6,13]

ANATOMY

See the section on anatomy under Skin Grafts.

SOURCES AND USES

Dermal grafts are obtained from any skin surface, especially the abdomen, buttocks, or thighs. They are commonly used to provide additional protection to the carotid artery after radical neck dissection, since they have the capacity for epithelializing when exposed to air. Dermal grafts can also be used to provide facial contouring and to line the oral cavity.[1,19]

DIFFICULTIES IN USING DERMAL GRAFTS

Fibrosis and shrinking may occur when dermal grafts are used.

BONE GRAFTS

Bone grafts are used primarily when structural rigidity is needed and occasionally when bulk is required. Because of its rigidity, cortical bone is often used in combination with medullary bone and periosteum, which have a greater number of osteoblasts (bone-forming cells), allowing for development of new bone.[1,4,6,11]

ANATOMY

Cortical bone provides rigidity or bulk but contains very few osteoblasts. Cancellous bone is found inside the cortical bone and contains more osteoblasts than does cortical bone. Periosteum, a tough outer covering of bone, also contains osteoblasts.

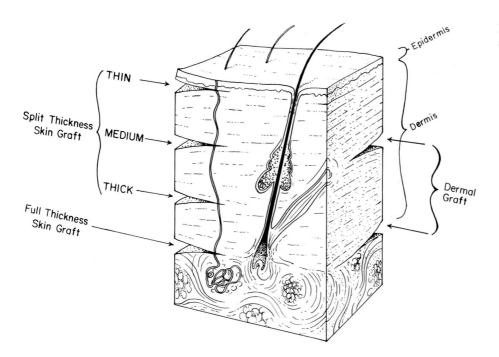

FIG. 9-1. Anatomy of skin for skin and dermal grafts.

SOURCES AND USES

The iliac crest and rib are the most commonly used sources of bone grafts. Bone grafts are most often used for mandibular reconstruction, although they may also be used for nasal reconstruction and facial recontouring. When used for mandibular reconstruction, cancellous bone is sometimes held in place in the body by setting the bone inside a cobalt–chromium alloy mesh tray.

DIFFICULTIES IN USING BONE GRAFTS

Harvesting the bone graft may be difficult. The donor site is often very painful. Pneumothorax can occur after taking a rib graft. There may be a tendency for the bone to reabsorb and fibrose over a period of time. Occasionally, the bone graft does not take.

CARTILAGE GRAFTS

Cartilage is used wherever semirigidity is required. Disadvantages include the limited availability of suitable material, absorption, migration, and movement. An advantage is that cartilage can be taken as a composite graft (i.e., skin and cartilage).[1,5,6,11]

ANATOMY

Cartilage is an avascular matrix of ground substance and fibers with scattered chondrocytes. It tends to maintain its original shape.

SOURCES AND USES

Cartilage for grafts, either alone or as part of a composite graft, is readily obtained from the concha of the ear or the septum of the nose. Cartilage may also be obtained from the cartilaginous portion of the ribs. Cartilage grafts are most often used in laryngeal and tracheal reconstruction. Costochondral cartilage grafts are used to reconstruct the external ear. Composite grafts of skin and ear cartilage may be used for reconstruction of the nasal ala (Fig. 9-3).

FAT GRAFTS

Fat is used for contour or to provide bulk. In most patients in this country, it is easily obtained. It is seldom used because it is too readily absorbed; however, this problem can be avoided to some extent by using a composite dermal-fat graft.[1,6,11,13]

ANATOMY

Fat is poorly vascularized and therefore seldom revascularizes. If a dermal fat graft is taken, the dermis picks up a good blood supply and there is less absorption.

SOURCES AND USES

Fat is generally obtained from the abdomen; the left lower quadrant is used to avoid confusion with an appendectomy scar. It is used to obliterate frontal sinus cavities and, occasionally, for facial contouring.

DIFFICULTIES IN USING FAT GRAFTS

The major difficulty found in the use of fat grafts is absorption.

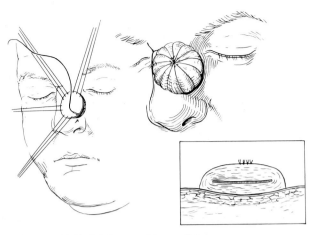

FIG. 9-2. Full-thickness skin graft to nose.

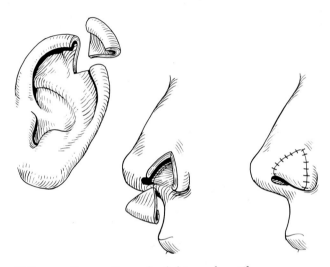

FIG. 9-3. Composite graft of skin and cartilage.

NERVE GRAFTS

Nerve grafts are generally used to provide a pathway for regrowth of axons from severed nerves. There must be no tension, and approximation should be as exact as possible. A limited number of very fine (8-0 or 10-0) sutures are used to minimize trauma. A small portion of nerve ending must be excised in order to remove scar tissue before grafting. The epineurium is removed, and the perineurium is sewn together. It is important that the diameter of the graft be as equal as possible to the removed nerve, even if this requires multiple lengths of grafts. The purpose of nerve grafting is to provide a pathway for regrowth of axons from the viable nerve cell bodies. The nerve axon segment in the graft does not remain viable; the remaining supporting cell, however, provides a guide for the regenerating axon fibers, directing them to the distal nerve segment.[9,11]

ANATOMY

A nerve consists of a cell body, usually centrally located, and an axon, a long extension of that body. Axons are often covered with a myelin sheath produced by Schwann cells, especially outside the central nervous system. The nerve is protected by layers of epineurium, perineurium, and endoneurium.

SOURCES AND USES

The two most frequent donor sites are the greater auricular nerve and the sural nerve. Nerve grafts are most frequently used for facial nerve reconstruction after resection of parotid or temporal bone tumors.

DIFFICULTIES IN USING NERVE GRAFTS

The two major problems when using nerve grafts are scarring at the anastomosis and inability to control the direction of nerve regrowth, which results in synkinesis.

FASCIAL, MUSCLE, AND TENDON GRAFTS

Fascial, muscle, and tendon grafts are used in head and neck surgery in rare and specific instances, such as the use of fascial slings in patients with facial nerve paralysis.[6,11]

Allografts and Xenografts

Allografts (grafts from the same species) and xenografts (grafts from another species) are not used extensively in head and neck surgery, but they are often used as temporary coverage on burn patients since the major problem with allografts and xenografts is rejection by the host. Material that has been cleaned and freeze dried to make it antigen free has found some use and may prove more useful in the future.[11]

FLAPS

The major difference between grafts and flaps is that flaps carry their own blood supply. The blood supply to most cervical cutaneous flaps is by way of capillary vessels that travel through the skin's pedicle; cutaneous flaps have no anatomically recognized arteriovenous system. A flap with this vascular arrangement is called a random pattern flap. If the flap includes an anatomically recognized arteriovenous system, it is called an axial pattern flap. A special subdivision of axial pattern flaps is myocutaneous flaps. These flaps depend on the blood supply that serves the muscle. The skin then gets its blood supply from the underlying muscle. This type of flap has found increasing use in reconstructing defects caused by head and neck cancer surgery.[1,6]

Random Pattern Flaps

Random pattern flaps can be positioned almost anywhere. However, for many of these flaps the blood supply must be developed in stages before moving the flap. This procedure is time consuming, usually requiring 2 weeks, and is defined as "delaying" the flap.

The bilobed flap is a combination of two random pattern flaps, one slightly smaller than the other (Fig. 9-4).

Axial Pattern Flaps

Axial pattern flaps have been extremely useful in all types of reconstruction. The development of myocutaneous flaps has expanded their use.

DELTOPECTORAL FLAPS

One of the best known and most useful of all axial pattern flaps is the deltopectoral, or Bakanjian, flap, which is based on the second, third, and fourth anterior perforating branches of the internal mammary arteries. Blood supply comes from arteries in subcutaneous tissues above the muscle. Thus, the deltopectoral flap need not contain any muscle. The advantages of deltopectoral flaps include their longer lengths, which result from multiple arteries running through the flaps, and less need for delaying the flaps (Fig. 9-5).[6,7,17]

MYOCUTANEOUS FLAPS

Use of the myocutaneous axial pattern flap has become increasingly popular because of its versatility. It is very durable, seldom fails, and, except for the sternocleidomastoid flap, is found outside the head and neck irradiation portals. The major myocutaneous flaps used by the head and neck surgeon are the pectoralis major, the trapezius, the sternocleidomastoid, and the latissimus dorsi.

PECTORALIS MAJOR

Use of the pectoralis major flap has become very popular in head and neck surgery because of its many clinical applications and advantages. The pectoralis major is a fan-shaped muscle whose fibers run horizontally in the cephalad portion and obliquely in the lower portion from the sternum to the shoulder. The major vascular pedicle is

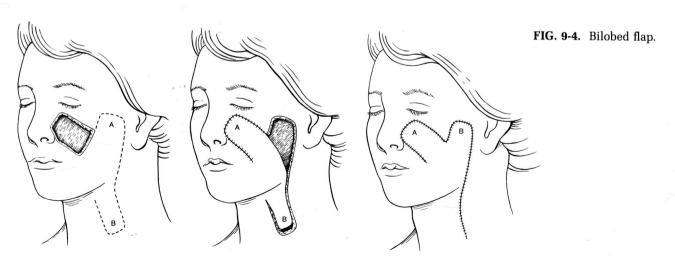

FIG. 9-4. Bilobed flap.

the thoracoacromial artery, a branch of the subclavian artery. The nerve supply is the lateral pectoral nerve from the brachial plexus. The vascular pedicle descends at a right angle from the middle of the clavicle until it meets the xiphoid acromial line, at which point it turns and proceeds medially along this line. The skin paddle can be outlined over the vascular pedicle to conform to the surgical defect (Fig. 9-6).[2]

The lateral portion of the flap is incised first. The underlying muscle fibers are then split by sharp and blunt dissection until a plane between the vascular pedicle above and the level of the ribs below is reached. The pectoral muscle can then be elevated by blunt finger dissection. With the use of a large breast retractor to lift the pectoralis major, the axial neurovascular bundle can be seen. The skin is incised to be included with the full thickness of underlying muscle, except for the proximal portion of the skin paddle, which is incised only down to the muscle. The remainder of the axial base is dissected to the clavicle. The flap may then be placed where it is needed. It is often brought into position by tunneling it subcutaneously. If there is a raw surface after positioning the flap, it can be covered with a split-thickness skin graft. This would be necessary if the flap were used to reconstruct a cheek, since epithelium is needed on both the inner and outer surfaces.

The following areas can be covered by pectoralis major flaps: oropharynx, hypopharynx, cheek defects, orbital defects, and temporal bone dissections.

The advantages of the pectoralis major flap are its versatility and the large amounts of skin and muscle available. Disadvantages include the occasional need for a split-thickness skin graft to close the donor site and the difficulty of use in women because of breast tissue.[2] The flap's bulk can be cumbersome at times.

TRAPEZIUS

The trapezius myocutaneous flap is based on three principal vascular territories that overlay the trapezius muscle;

the occipital artery, the suprascapular artery, and the transverse cervical artery provide the major blood supply to the trapezius myocutaneous flap. The anterior incision works well as the vertical limb in a neck dissection if it follows the border of the trapezius. The posterior incision parallels the anterior incision, extending up the midline of the posterior neck. The skin and muscle flap is then elevated. If a thin distal flap is needed, the distal part of the flap with the deep fascia is elevated, leaving bare trapezius muscle. The suprascapular and transverse scapular arteries are sacrificed at this point. The spinal accessory nerve may or may not be sacrificed. At the neck–shoulder angle the vascular pedicle of the transverse cervical artery is identified and preserved by using blunt finger dissection between the trapezius and supraspinatus muscles. Anterior mobility is gained by posteriorly dividing the nuchal fascia in the midline. If both the transverse cervical artery and occipital artery are preserved, then a 12-cm × 42-cm flap

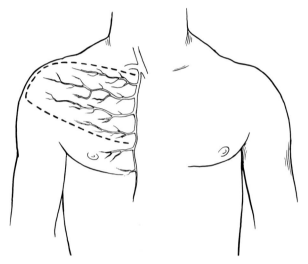

FIG. 9-5. Deltopectoral flap.

FIG. 9-6. Pectoralis major flap.

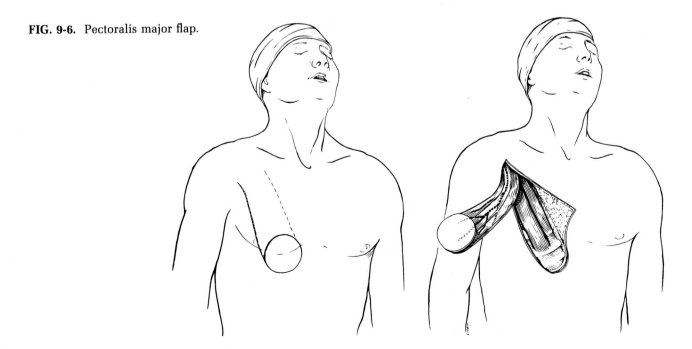

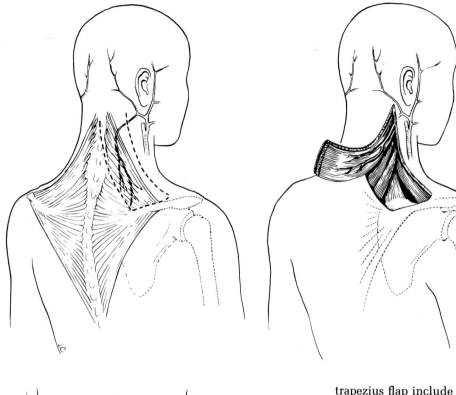

FIG. 9-7. Trapezius flap.

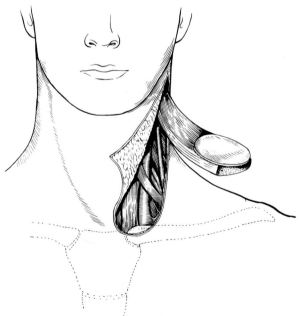

FIG. 9-8. Sternocleidomastoid flap.

can be obtained. If the transverse cervical artery is sacrificed and a delay is not possible, then the flap should be only 8 cm × 25 cm (Fig. 9-7).[3,8,14,16,17]

The clinical uses of a trapezius flap include defects of the lower two thirds of the face, neck, temporal fossa, oropharynx, hypopharynx, and cervical esophagus. A composite flap with the spine of the scapula may be used in mandible reconstruction.

The advantages of the trapezius flap are the same as those for any myocutaneous flap. The disadvantages of the trapezius flap include the limited distance that it can be moved from the donor site, the fact that the donor site requires a split-thickness skin graft, the possible necessity of a planned temporary orocutaneous fistula, and a loss of trapezius function.

STERNOCLEIDOMASTOID

The blood supply to the sternocleidomastoid comes from three sources: (1) superiorly, from a branch of the occipital artery; (2) inferiorly, from a branch of the thyrocervical trunk; and (3) medially, from the inferior and superior thyroid arteries. The source for the skin paddle may be inferiorly from the supraclavicular area or superiorly from the mastoid area. The tumor is resected, and the flap is tunneled under the mandible to the defect.

The clinical uses of the sternocleidomastoid flap include temporal bone and cheek defects and oropharynx dissections.

The advantage of this flap is its easy inclusion in the operative field. There are three main disadvantages: (1) it should not be used in a clinically positive neck, (2) the size of the skin paddle is limited, and (3) a limited arc of rotation results (Fig. 9-8).[14,17]

LATISSIMUS DORSI

The latissimus dorsi is the largest muscle in the human body. The myocutaneous flap is based on the subscapular artery and the thoracodorsal artery, a major branch off the axillary artery. The flap is usually raised from the sixth to the tenth rib area and tunneled through the pectoralis major to the neck.

The advantages of the latissimus dorsi flap are its large skin area, large muscle area, and great length. Disadvantages include difficulty in positioning the patient so that the donor site is within the operative field, and the flap's great size, which may be undesirable (Fig. 9-9).[15]

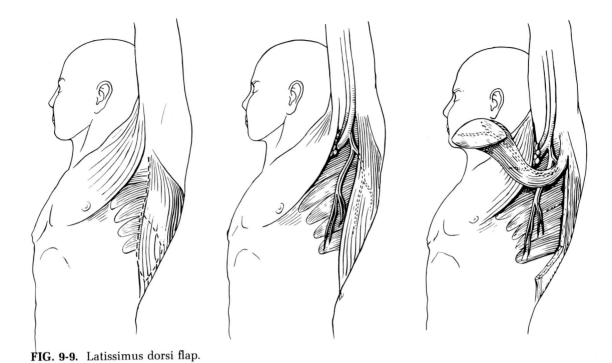

FIG. 9-9. Latissimus dorsi flap.

FREE FLAPS

With recent advances in microsurgical techniques, tissue can be completely severed from its blood supply and connected to a new one. Thus, large amounts of tissue can be moved for reconstruction. The surgeon is not limited to the use of local tissue, so a great deal of variety exists in the type of tissue that can be used.

The disadvantage of these flaps is the need for an artery and a vein that are suitable for anastomosis both on the flap and in the operative field. This procedure is difficult and lengthy, especially when performed after a major tumor resection. It is best carried out by a two-team approach. A common example of this flap is a free jejunal graft to replace the pharynx or cervical esophagus (Fig. 9-10).[1,10,17]

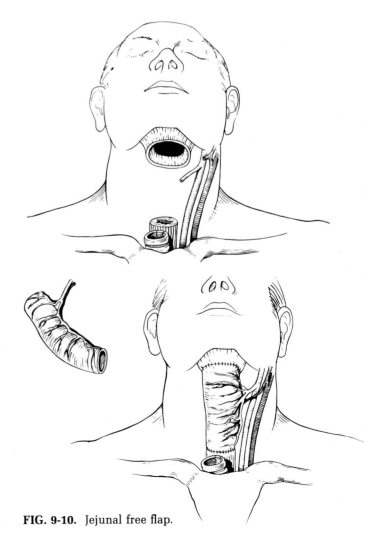

FIG. 9-10. Jejunal free flap.

REFERENCES

1. Alexander JM: Alloplastic augmentation of middle-third facial deformities. J Oral Surg 34:165–172, 1976
2. Ariyan S: The pectoralis major myocutaneous flap: A versatile flap for reconstruction in the head and neck. Plast Reconstr Surg 63:73–81, 1979
3. Bertotti JA: Trapezius-musculocutaneous island flap in the repair of major head and neck cancer. Plast Reconstr Surg 65:16–21, 1980
4. Canalis RF, Saffouri M, Mirra J, Ward PH: The fate of pedicle osteocutaneous grafts in mandibulofacial restoration. Laryngoscope 87:895–908, 1977
5. Clairmont AA, Conley J: The uses and limitations of auricular composite grafts. J Otolaryngol 7:249–256, 1978
6. Converse JM (ed): Reconstructive Plastic Surgery, Principles and Procedures in Correction, Reconstruction, and Transplantation, vol I, pp 152–391. Philadelphia, WB Saunders, 1977
7. Daniel RK, Cunningham DM, Taylor GI: The deltopectoral flap: An anatomical and hemodynamic approach. Plast Reconstr Surg 55:275–282, 1975
8. Demergasso F, Piazza MV: Trapezius myocutaneous flap in

reconstructive surgery for head and neck cancer. An original technique. Am J Surg 138:533–536, 1979

9. Fisch U: Facial nerve grafting. Otolaryngol Clin North Am 7:517–529, 1974

10. Flynn MB, Acland RD: Free intestinal autografts for reconstruction following pharyngolaryngoesophagectomy. Surg Gynecol Obstet 149:858–862, 1979

11. Grabb WC, Smith JW (eds): Plastic Surgery: A Concise Guide to Clinical Practice, 2nd ed, pp 3–130, 423–449, 818–834. Boston, Little, Brown & Co, 1973.

12. Gray H: Anatomy of the Human Body, pp 1105–1115. Philadelphia, Lea & Febiger, 1966

13. Leaf N, Zarem HA: Correction of contour defects of the face with dermal and dermal-fat grafts. Arch Surg 105:715–719, 1972

14. McCraw JB, Magee WP Jr, Kalwaic H: Uses of the trapezius and sternomastoid myocutaneous flaps in head and neck reconstruction. Plast Reconstr Surg 63:49–57, 1979

15. Quillen CG: Latissimus dorsi myocutaneous flaps in head and neck reconstruction. Plast Reconstr Surg 63:664–670, 1979

16. Shapiro MJ: Use of trapezius myocutaneous flaps in the reconstruction of head and neck defects. Arch Otolaryngol 107:333–336, 1981

17. Sharer LA, Horton CE, Adamson JE, Carraway JH, McCraw JB: Intraoral reconstruction in head and neck cancer surgery. Clin Plast Surg 3:495–509, 1976

18. Slanetz CA Jr, Rankow RM: The intraoral use of split-thickness skin grafts in head and neck surgery. Am J Surg 104:721–726, 1962

19. Smithdeal CD, Corso PF, Strong EW: Dermis grafts for carotid artery protection: Yes or no? A ten-year experience. Am J Surg 128:484–489, 1974

Maxillofacial Prosthetics

ALAN C. LEVIN

The importance of maxillofacial prosthetics in the treatment of cancer of the head and neck is intimately related to the quality of the patient's life. "Quality of life" is a many-faceted concept and means different things to different people.

The varying degree of functional and cosmetic success of the prosthesis is illustrated by the histories of two famous people, President Grover Cleveland and Dr. Sigmund Freud (see Chapter 1).[1] Both men had resection of seemingly similar tumors of the hard and soft palate and prosthetic restoration. Both patients survived approximately 15 years following the initial surgery, but with great differences in the prosthetic results. President Cleveland's rehabilitation in 1893 was outstanding; within 2 months of his initial operation (hemimaxillectomy), he spoke in Congress and no one noticed that he had had an operation.

In contrast, Dr. Freud underwent 33 major and minor surgical procedures and several sequences of radiation therapy following the initial removal of the tumor in 1923, which included the right maxilla and hard palate, most of the soft palate, and the anterior border of the ascending ramus of the right mandible. His treatment was complicated by extreme trismus, and Dr. Freud experienced great difficulty with prosthetic rehabilitation, to the extent that he nicknamed his prosthesis "the monster."

PATIENT EDUCATION

The role of maxillofacial prosthodontics occurs mainly during the restorative and rehabilitative phases, but it also occurs in conjunction with and immediately following the cancer therapy.

In order to prepare the patient for the rehabilitative phase, it is necessary to educate him prior to surgery regarding the possibilities and limitations of the restorative phase. This will familiarize the patient with the realities of what is possible functionally and cosmetically and will enable him to gauge what his quality of life will be and to prepare for it. Questions and fears relating to the surgery and rehabilitation should be answered at this stage.

Patient education should start prior to the definitive treatment. This is best accomplished through a multimedia system. Consultation with the various members of the team who will be directly involved in the patient's treatment is essential. Written, illustrated instructions and descriptions should be made available to the patient, as well as material such as slide–tape shows and video cassette tapes that portray the actual results in previously treated patients. Case histories or before-and-after photographs and contact with patients who have had similar treatment are valuable.

The more the patient is educated to realistic expectations, the better his chance will be of having a positive attitude, which is an all-important factor in arriving at a successful end result of rehabilitation.

The patient's pretreatment education should cover the following:

1. The psychological aspects of the treatment as it will affect the patient, the immediate family, and friends. A social worker or counselor is helpful at this time.
2. The functional result, which can best be projected by the prosthodontist and speech pathologist

3. The cosmetic result, which is conveyed best by previously treated patients who can discuss their experiences with the prospective patient, as well as before-and-after photographs, video cassette tapes, and slide–tape shows

4. An explanation by the surgeon of the extent of the planned surgery

The prosthodontist should outline to the patient and the family the approximate number of visits and length of time necessary to carry out the prosthetic restorative procedures. The successive stages in the treatment should be outlined, together with an explanation of the functional and cosmetic results expected at each stage, as well as the duration of its usefulness and any discomfort or pain to which the patient may be subjected.

The necessity of continued maintenance following the definitive treatment must be made clear to the patient, as well as his future dependence on the prosthesis in order to maintain the planned level of rehabilitation.

The patient must be offered encouragement, and the long-term success of the rehabilitative efforts should be stressed. It is important to bear in mind that the patient has been told at this stage that he has "cancer." To many patients this means death is imminent, or, even worse, severe misery followed by death. It is therefore of benefit to the patient to minimize treatment time in the initial phases in order that he may return to familiar surroundings and attempt to pick up his life where it was interrupted by the diagnosis and treatment and to continue in as nearly normal a fashion as possible. The initial treatment should thus be brief, but it must be comprehensive enough to give the optimum function and cosmetic value immediately after the surgery. The more sophisticated and time-consuming definitive restorative techniques can be delayed until the patient is in a better state of health and a more positive frame of mind.

PROSTHETIC RESTORATION AFTER MAXILLECTOMY

Maxillectomy including removal of the hard palate, partial removal of the soft palate, and/or orbital exenteration is the most common operation for cancer that creates an intraoral defect.

This defect has the best prognosis for rehabilitation. The materials that are used, as well as the techniques that are employed, tend to result in the most durable, functionally satisfying, and aesthetically pleasing prostheses. The prosthesis can function and appear in such a manner as to camouflage totally the presence of a surgical defect.

Except in bilateral total maxillectomy, the initial prosthesis should be placed at the time of the operation. The patient is at no time without an intraoral prosthesis and can thus continue swallowing and speaking. The prosthesis used in this situation is termed the *surgical prosthesis*. The surgical prosthesis will be replaced in 7 to 10 days by the interim prosthesis, and when healing is complete, the definitive prosthesis will be constructed.

The main objective of the prosthesis is to seal off the maxillary defect created between the oral and nasal cavities. The quality of the result depends on the size of the defect, the area(s) that have been removed, the prior radiation therapy, the quality of the remaining tissue, the surgical complications, and whether the patient is dentulous.

Preplanning of Surgical Extent and Resulting Defect

Close cooperation between the surgeon and the prosthodontist is necessary for a good result. Preplanning should include a thorough dental evaluation to determine which teeth and structures will be retained after surgery.

Frequently, the surgical procedure can be slightly modified without compromising the surgical result, which can be helpful to the prosthodontist and the patient. As a general rule, the more hard palate and premaxilla that is retained, the better is the prosthetic result. This applies in both dentulous and edentulous situations. The retention of certain key teeth, such as the posterior molar and the anterior canine, can greatly aid rehabilitation, if it can be done without compromising tumor resection. Many seemingly worthless or grossly carious teeth can be restored to health and prove valuable to the retention, support, and stability of a maxillary prosthesis (Fig. 10-1). Patients who have allowed their teeth to get into a poor state of health can be motivated to practice good oral hygiene if they understand the importance of these teeth to the success of the prosthesis. The entire prosthesis should be planned prior to surgical resection, with particular emphasis on the mode of support that the remaining structures will provide for the prosthesis, the amount of stability available for lateral bracing, the amount and mode of gaining retention to resist movement of the prosthesis from the basal seat, and the cosmetic and functional results. The incision can be outlined by the surgeon on a diagnostic cast of the maxilla, from which the extent of the surgical prosthesis can be determined (Fig. 10-2). The initial prosthesis is attached to the patient by wires and when constructing the prosthesis, it is helpful to identify the "wiring in" areas of the prosthesis prior to the time of surgery.

Incision and Surgical Modifications

The bony incision is made along the hard palate. It is advantageous to place the mucosal incision 4 mm to 5 mm lateral to the bony incision to enable the mucosal tissue

FIG. 10-1. Even poor dentition, such as shown here, can be repaired and used for retention of a prosthesis.

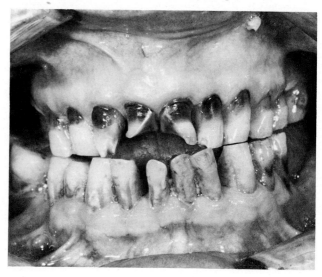

from the hard palate to be used as a rollover flap to close the defect (Fig. 10-3). A defect lined with palatal mucosa is more resistant to abrasion than the nonkeratinized epithelium of the nose. It is essential to have a straight, smooth bony margin to reduce irritation to the mucosa by the prosthesis.

Lining the reflected cheek flap with a split-thickness skin graft also provides some benefits to rehabilitation. This skin graft is more resistant to irritation caused by the prosthesis. In addition, the scar band that forms at the junction of the skin graft and the mucosa tends to contract, leaving a superolateral undercut that can be used in prosthesis construction to aid in retention and lateral stability (see Fig. 10-3).

Retention of the prosthesis in an edentulous patient is a greater challenge. This can usually be managed by a three-point undercut engagement: (1) posteriorly over the cut surface of the soft palate, (2) laterally by the undercut created by the scar band, and (3) anteriorly by the floor of the nose (Fig. 10-4). This engagement can all be buttressed or braced against the medial wall of the defect, which should be covered by palatal mucosa overlying the cut margin of the resected hard palate. The three-point engagement is aided by the retention of as much hard palate and alveolar ridge as possible.

In the dentulous patient, retention of the prosthesis can be attained by use of the remaining teeth. However, these teeth should not be compromised by the surgical procedure. The bony cut through the alveolar ridge should be made as far away from the remaining teeth as possible (see Fig. 10-3). This enhances the bony support important to the retention of a prosthesis. Retaining the canine tooth rather than the central or lateral incisor affords more stability for the prosthesis. If this is not possible, the lateral incisor should be extracted and the bony cut made through the resulting socket. This will allow an adequate buttress of bone next to the central incisor and will improve the clinical prognosis.

In certain situations in which there is a large resection posteriorly and laterally involving the soft palate, it may be advantageous to remove the coronoid process of the mandible in order to avoid possible displacement of the prosthesis as the coronoid process moves upward and forward in its path of closure. However, it should be noted that removal of the coronoid process occasionally results in trismus, which would negate the benefit. The retention of even a small band of soft palate tissue can greatly enhance the posterior retention of the prosthesis (Fig. 10-5).

Special Problems

The problems and difficulties encountered by the dentist in restoring the hard and soft palate may be due to com-

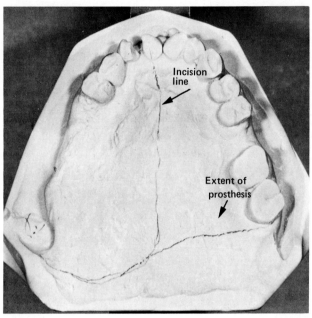

FIG. 10-2. The incision is outlined by the surgeon on a diagnostic cast of the maxilla.

FIG. 10-3. The mucosal incision is placed 4 mm to 5 mm lateral to the bony incision. The bony incision is placed through the socket of the extracted tooth next to the last remaining tooth. The prosthesis should be made so as to be able to engage the undercut on the palatal shelf and the soft tissue of the buccal mucosa above the fibrous scar band.

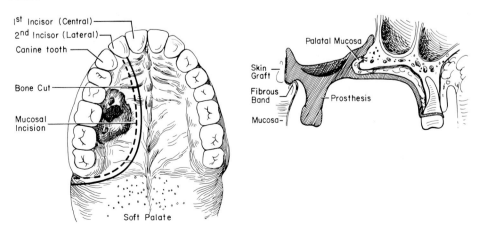

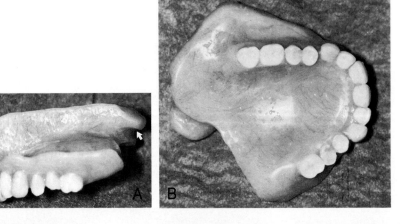

FIG. 10-4. The retention of the prosthesis is managed by a three-point undercut engagement: posteriorly over the cut surface of the soft palate (A), anteriorly by the internal portion of the external nares (*arrows*), and laterally by the undercut created by the soft tissue scar band (B).

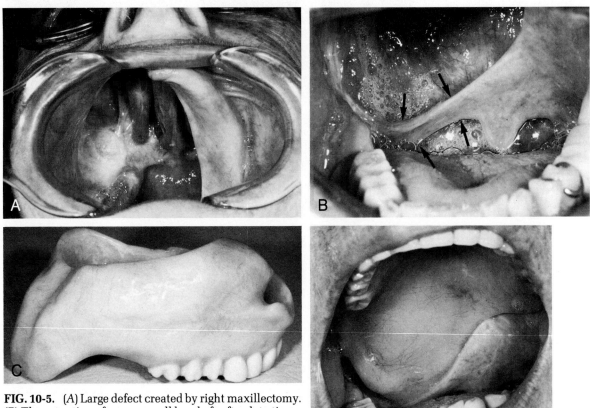

FIG. 10-5. (A) Large defect created by right maxillectomy. (B) The retention of even a small band of soft palate tissue can greatly enhance the posterior retention of the prosthesis (*arrows*). (C) Prosthesis. Note undercuts anteriorly and posteriorly. (D) Prosthesis in place.

plications of surgery (such as trismus), lack of anatomical base, or tissue sensitivity.

The most common problem for the patient is the loss of air, liquids, and solids around the prosthesis into the nose. Leakage results from a faulty obturator seal between the oral and nasal cavities. There will never be a complete seal, since tissues surrounding the obturator move during function and create voids in the seal. Most of the leakage occurs because of the downward movement of the pros-

thesis posteriorly. Liquids are then forced up posteriorly in the swallowing movement, as the tongue closes against the palate in a front-to-back direction. This pumps the liquid up the posterior aspect of the prosthesis and forward, and fluid and air are lost into the nose. This embarassing problem can usually be controlled by making some changes in swallowing and speaking habits. The simplest method is to instruct the patient to swallow with the head tilted slightly backward. In this manner, gravity will force the

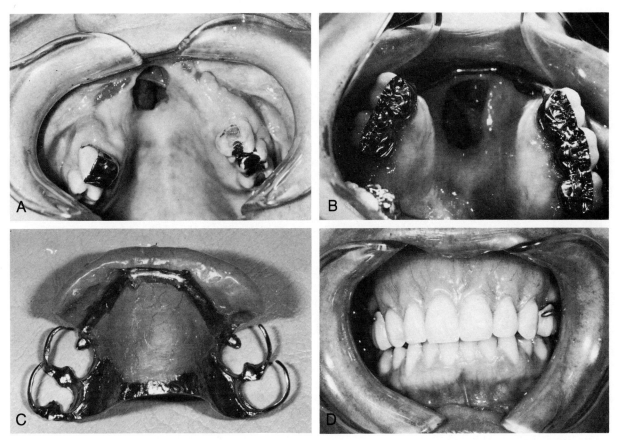

FIG. 10-6. Restoration after anterior maxillectomy. (*A*) Maxillary defect. (*B*) Crowns and bar placed on teeth. (*C*) Removable partial dentures as a prosthesis for anterior maxillectomy. (*D*) Prosthesis in place.

fluids downward and away from the nasal cavity and leakage will be minimized.

The anterior maxillectomy presents a special problem from a restorative point of view (Fig. 10-6*A*). The missing anterior maxilla is replaced by a cantilever prosthesis with no anterior retention or support. Retention is usually obtained by engaging the nasal surface of the residual hard palate and making an extension into the external nares from the inside, in which case *it is essential that the nasal surface of the hard palate be covered by a few millimeters of palatal mucosa.* This is achieved by a soft tissue incision 4 mm to 5 mm toward the defect relative to the bony incision. The internal surface of the nares should be skin lined to resist the abrasive effect of the retentive arm of the prosthesis.

Alternatively, retention is obtained using purely dental means, such as crowns, bars, and a removable partial denture (Fig. 10-6*B–D*).

The cosmetic problems associated with anterior maxillectomy may be compounded by resection and reconstruction of the lip. Use of dentures is also compromised by the lip resection.

In summary, the major complications with prostheses tend to be inadequate retention of the prosthesis and speech problems rather than leakage. Liquids are lost primarily through the posterior portion of the defect rather than the anterior portion, whereas air can be lost at any point. Air loss is greater when retention is poor.

Technical Aspects of Maxillary Obturator Construction

EDENTULOUS MAXILLA

SURGICAL PROSTHESIS

The incision is outlined on the initial cast of the maxilla prior to surgery (Fig. 10-7*A*). The area to be removed is smoothed down, and if the patient has a usable denture, this can be modified for use as the surgical prosthesis. If not, the prosthesis is made from autopolymerizing acrylic resin directly on this modified cast to the outlined extensions (Fig. 10-7*B*). This is a simple 1-hour laboratory procedure. Within the prosthesis are holes for the wires used to retain the prosthesis in place at the time of surgery. These should be located to facilitate removal of the surgical packing. Teeth are not added at this stage. The primary object is to obturate the defect, separate the nasal from the oral cavity, and allow the patient to begin oral feeding early in the postoperative period. This prosthesis remains in place 7 to 10 days, until the packing is removed. The prosthesis is highly polished to facilitate maintenance of oral hygiene.

INTERIM PROSTHESIS

In the edentulous patient, the surgical prosthesis can be readily modified and used as an interim prosthesis. In a

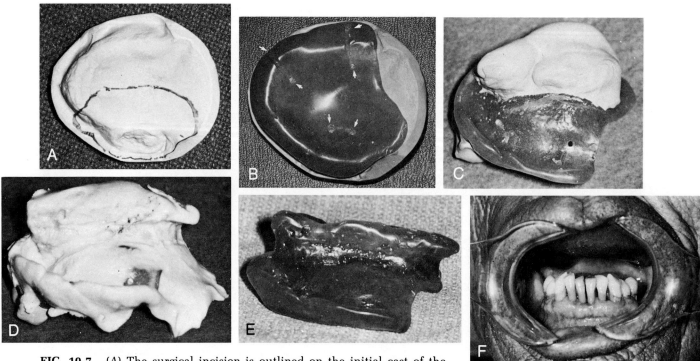

FIG. 10-7. (*A*) The surgical incision is outlined on the initial cast of the maxilla prior to surgery. (*B*) Surgical prosthesis with retention holes (*arrows*). (*C* and *D*) Impression of maxillectomy defect added to surgical prosthesis. (*E*) Interim prosthesis. (*F*) Interim prosthesis in place.

simple clinical procedure, an impression is made of the defect area. The prosthesis is then fashioned using autopolymerizing acrylic resin. It is refinished and polished for use as the interim prosthesis (Fig. 10-7*C–F*). At this stage, it may be necessary to correct the extensions of the prosthesis relative to the borders around the mouth as well as the defect areas. The impression should record all the undercut areas that will be used in the retention of the prosthesis.

The fabrication of the interim prosthesis should be done without delay, since the dimensions of the defect gradually change after removal of the packing. The process should take no longer than 1 hour from the making of the impression to the insertion of the prosthesis. Because of the time element, it is usually not possible to add teeth at this stage.

DENTULOUS MAXILLA

SURGICAL PROSTHESIS

When teeth are present and are to be included in the resection of the tumor, they can be immediately placed onto the surgical prosthesis, thereby simplifying the construction of an interim prosthesis at a later stage. Retention clasps planned for the interim prosthesis are placed on the surgical prosthesis. Holes are placed at strategic points to facilitate wiring of the prosthesis at the time of operation. This immediate placement of the teeth into the surgical prosthesis, although not essential, greatly improves the cosmetic value of the prosthesis as the patient is recovering (Fig. 10-8*A–E*).

The teeth are removed from the cast after the surgical incision has been outlined. The area underlying the teeth must be smoothed and then the artificial teeth added in order to process them to the surgical prosthesis. This process is time consuming, but the benefits outweigh the difficulties.

INTERIM PROSTHESIS

The surgical prosthesis can be converted if retentive clasps have been placed prior to surgery (Fig. 10-8*D–F*). If not, a new interim prosthesis will be needed. An intraoral impression is made that will reflect all teeth and the defect area, including the undercuts that are to be used in retaining the prosthesis. This impression is poured in dental stone and a prosthesis is made, extending to the determined limits, with wire retentive clasps on the key teeth. The speed necessary in making this prosthesis precludes the addition of teeth. It is thus advantageous to have the teeth and clasps placed on the surgical prosthesis. As in the edentulous patient, the prosthesis needs to be placed within 1 to 2 hours of the time that the impression is made. It is important that the patient be comfortable with a prosthesis so that frequent office visits for adjustments are not necessary.

As the patient improves in health and strength and can tolerate longer dental procedures, either a second interim prosthesis can be made with teeth or artificial teeth can be quickly added to the interim prosthesis in order to improve cosmetic value and hasten rehabilitation. It should be emphasized that the placement of teeth on the interim

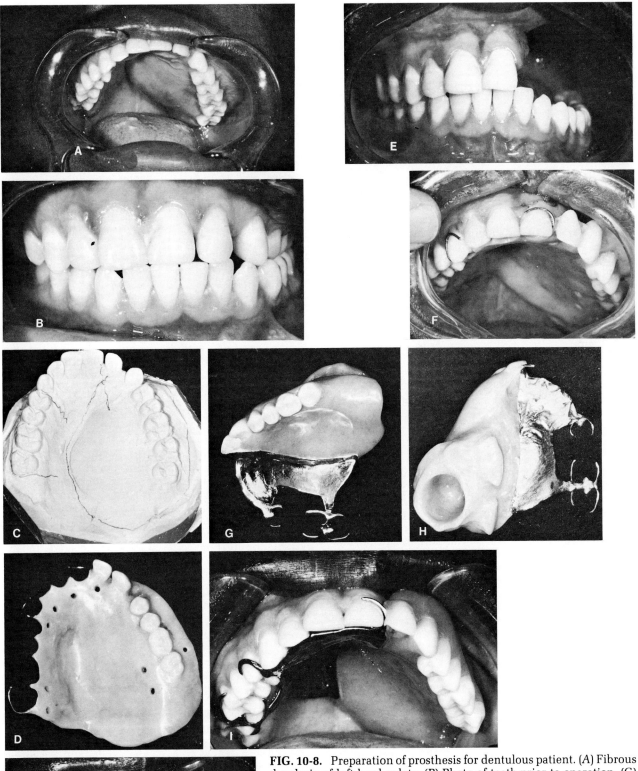

FIG. 10-8. Preparation of prosthesis for dentulous patient. (A) Fibrous dysplasia of left hard palate. (B) Photo of teeth prior to operation. (C) Outline of incision and position for wire clasps. (D) Surgical prosthesis with retention holes; retention clasps are for use on the interim prosthesis. (E) The surgical defect. (F) The interim prosthesis in place. (G) Definitive prosthesis, left lateral view. (H) Definitive prosthesis, nasal view. (I) Definitive prosthesis in place. (J) Definitive prosthesis in place.

prosthesis is for cosmetic value only, since most patients will not chew on the defect side or will find it difficult to do so in an effective manner. As a general rule, the interim prosthesis is used for 4 to 6 months, by which time it may become discolored and begin to cause discomfort. The supporting structures gradually remodel over 4 to 6 months, especially if radiation therapy has been added, and the prosthesis becomes loose and uncomfortable.

DEFINITIVE PROSTHESIS

The definitive prosthesis is made when the healing and remodeling of the defect is stabilized, usually 4 to 6 months after surgery and/or radiation therapy. Dental preparation of the mouth and teeth should be completed or else be planned as an integral part of the fitting of the definitive prosthesis. This treatment plan is carried out so that the prosthesis will restore optimum function and provide a cosmetic result such as has been demonstrated by the interim prosthesis, but on a long-term basis (Fig. 10-8G–J).

It should be emphasized to the patient that the maintenance of good oral hygiene is an important requisite from this point on. The prosthesis can be washed with soap, toothpaste, and water, while the defect should be flushed out twice daily with a Water Pik or similar method. Routine dental care should be maintained throughout the rest of the patient's life. As a general rule, a definitive prosthesis can last 5 to 10 years or longer. If there is difficulty in achieving this goal, reevaluation of the treatment regimen should be considered.

PROSTHETIC RESTORATION AFTER MANDIBULECTOMY

The philosophy in the treatment of patients who have had mandibulectomy must be based on the priorities of function and cosmesis. Even if only the highest priorities can be satisfied by use of a prosthesis, there is significant benefit to the patient. Priorities in order of importance are swallowing and control of saliva, speech, cosmetic result, and masticatory efficiency.

Resection of a portion of the mandible is usually associated with soft tissue defects of the floor of mouth and tongue. The prognosis for prosthetic reconstruction deteriorates rapidly with an increase in the amount of tissue removed. The problems following mandibulectomy without surgical reconstruction include a cosmetic defect, deviation of the mandible to the defect side, and a functional loss proportional to the amount of tongue and soft tissue removed. Surgical reconstruction of the bony mandible is preferable to prosthetic management. Surgical management restores the continuity of the mandible and greatly reduces facial distortion. Removal of a large amount of tongue tissue, however, may not allow restoration of normal speech by either surgical or prosthetic means. Even with greatly reduced tongue tissue, swallowing can be learned by the patient.

When surgical restoration is not planned, prosthetic management must be instituted immediately. Placement of an inclined plane or guide flange prosthesis trains the patient to center the mandible into the previous position of closure, minimizing facial distortion. The inclined plane prosthesis is modified during the healing phase to an interim prosthesis and then, following healing, to a definitive prosthesis, which is used for both cosmetic and functional purposes. This can be carried out for both dentulous and edentulous patients, doing everything necessary to ensure adequate retention of the prostheses.

Patient management and motivation are of great importance in encouraging the patient to use what is essentially a unilateral, lower, removable partial denture. It may present major problems in stability and retention. The limitations of the prosthesis and the expectations of the patient should be honestly evaluated and the patient informed as to its best use. It is essential that the patient exercise and train himself, using a mirror, to close and centralize the mandible properly.

Speech and swallowing problems arise following major tongue resection. A partially successful method of improving tongue function for both speech and swallowing is a palatal-tongue prosthesis. This involves lowering the palate with a thickened prosthesis to enable a resected tongue to touch the palate and aid swallowing. Speech articulation involving the tongue and palate can also be improved in this manner.

In the edentulous patient, the situation must be viewed in perspective: wearing a full lower denture is difficult even for the edentulous patient who has an intact mandible.

The patient who has had a mandibulectomy presents a situation that calls for the construction of a denture on a reduced basal seat with greater potential difficulties (Fig. 10-9A). With marginal resection of the mandible, the superoinferior dimension of the artificial denture is greatly increased. It is therefore potentially unstable, as a result of a poor leverage-to-anchorage ratio. Prosthetic restoration after segmental mandibulectomy requires the construction of a complete denture on the residual mandibular alveolus. The denture should not extend onto the defect area where no bony support is available (Fig. 10-9B).

A patient with a hemimandibulectomy or resection of the arch of the mandible cannot realistically have restoration by means of a prosthesis without surgical augmentation to assist in the retention of the dentures that must be constructed (Fig. 10-9C, D).

A number of dental implants have been proposed as a possible aid in these restorations. These include modifications of the blade vent implant, the staple bone implant, and the subperiosteal implant. Limited experience with these techniques gives reason for caution. There are few documented successful case reports of dental implants.

Edentulous Mandible

There is little chance of regaining the preoperative level of function in the edentulous patient following a mandibulectomy without surgical reconstruction. The reasons for this are the decreased neuromuscular control resulting from denervation of the tissues surrounding the denture, the decreased basal seat to support the denture, the altered mucosal surface as a result of radiation therapy, the altered saliva output with its higher mucin content, and the altered pathway of mandibular closure following a partial mandibulectomy. All these factors, by degree of severity, will influence the prognosis and end result of rehabilitation both cosmetically and functionally.

In summary, to ensure a favorable prognosis for prosthetic reconstruction following mandibulectomy, the following criteria should be present:

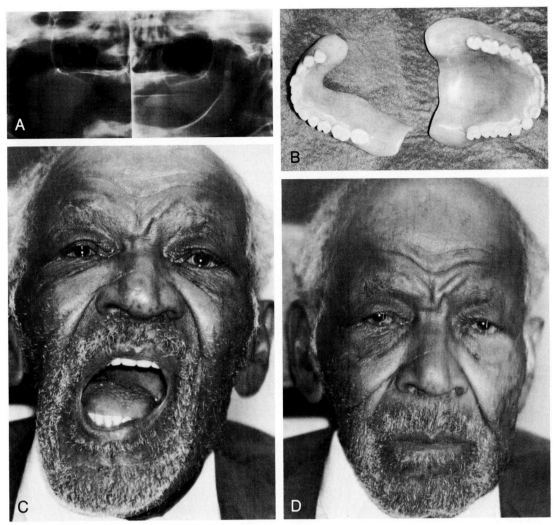

FIG. 10-9. Prosthetic restoration after partial mandibulectomy. (*A*) postoperative roentgenogram. (*B*) Dentures extended for maximum tissue coverage to improve retention and stability. (*C*) Deviation of the mandible on opening the mouth. This may be corrected by designing the dentures so that they guide the mandible into proper position when closing. (*D*) Mandible in proper position when closed.

1. Positive attitude on the patient's part with regard to prosthetic limitations
2. Rim or posterior segmental mandibular resection
3. Minimal soft tissue and tongue resection
4. Minimal deviation of the mandible following surgery
5. No radiation therapy with resulting changes in saliva and mucosa
6. Minimal cosmetic deformation as a result of surgery

The amount and location of the bony resection are probably the most important factors. The more posterior and the smaller the resection, the more favorable is the prognosis.

Dentulous Mandible

The same principles for restoration are used in the dentulous patient as in the edentulous patient, except that retention and stability of the prosthesis are more promising when teeth are present. There are many partially edentulous people who have not had a mandibulectomy yet who cannot or will not wear removable partial dentures.

Although the presence of teeth benefits both the patient and the prosthodontist, the patient must maintain good oral hygiene in a difficult situation. The remaining teeth do not occlude normally and the mouth's self-cleansing mechanism is greatly reduced. When the soft tissues have been resected to a large extent, the self-cleansing mechanisms of the cheeks, floor of the mouth, and tongue are impaired.

To arrive at a realistic prognosis for the dentulous patient, the same criteria are used as for the edentulous patient, except that the prognosis can be improved slightly. It must be remembered, however, that when teeth are present and radiation therapy has been used as a treatment modality, the teeth are subject to more rapid deterioration than under normal circumstances. Preventive measures such as daily topical application of fluoride should be instituted and maintained. The importance of good oral hygiene cannot be emphasized enough to the dentulous patient. This is essential for a favorable prognosis on the life span of his teeth and the prosthesis.

Restoration Using Dental Implants

The dental profession has courted dental implants for many years. The continuing problem with the dental implant, however, is that part of it is embedded in the bone and part extrudes into the oral cavity. Therefore, the possibility of developing periodontal disease or an epithelial downgrowth with a subsequent infection is ever present. When this mode of treatment is considered, it should be kept in mind that patients who have had a mandibulectomy and have teeth remaining will still have cosmetic and functional problems in the restorative phase. Therefore, for a favorable prognosis, one needs to be realistically confident in the planning and placement of the implant in an edentulous patient with a mandibulectomy. If carefully selected and well maintained, a dental implant can be a great aid to an edentulous patient with a mandibulectomy. However, because of the lack of experience in this field, caution is advised, for if an implant is placed and fails, there will be even less residual tissue remaining on which to build a conventional removable prosthesis.

It is better to restore the continuity of the mandible surgically and to place a prosthesis on that base than to place an implant into a segmented mandible.

RESTORATION OF SURGICALLY INDUCED EXTRAORAL DEFECTS

Some basic requirements must be met for any facial prosthesis to be successful. The problems with artificial restoration of facial defects are generally twofold: attachment and camouflage. First, the area where the prosthesis will be attached must be retentive. Retention can be achieved by engaging opposite undercuts with a rubbery type of prosthetic material or by having available a stable skin area to which the prosthesis can be attached by means of an adhesive. Ideally, a stable retentive skin area is an area of skin that is not oily, does not sweat, has no saliva flowing across it, and is not movable. The best method of obtaining such an area is by skin grafting onto a flat bony area.

The second problem is matching colors and camouflaging the borders or edges of the prosthesis. It is easier to restore the entire ear or nose prosthetically rather than a portion of a nose or ear, which is generally unstable and must be overlaid in order to integrate the prosthesis and to ensure stability and retention. This increases the bulk of the prosthesis and interferes with its contour.

Nasal and Auricular Prostheses

Once it has been determined that the defect created by resection of tumor will not be reconstructed surgically, a prosthesis should be constructed.

From a prosthetic viewpoint, it is fortunate that the face has only one nose, which can be of various shapes and sizes. No matching is required (Fig. 10-10). The same is true of ears insofar as it is very rare that both ears are visible at one time to an observer. It is sufficient to create a prosthesis that blends in and matches with the surrounding tissues (Fig. 10-11).

Neither the ear nor the nose moves significantly in the normal situation, and therefore a nonmovable prosthetic ear or nose can appear quite lifelike.

Orbital Prostheses

The restoration of an orbital defect presents an additional problem. The normal eye moves constantly, while the artificial eye has a fixed stare; the eyelids do not move and the gaze does not change direction. The artificial eye must

FIG. 10-10. (A) Nasal defect. (B) Nasal prosthesis in position.

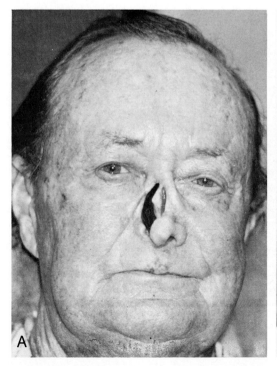
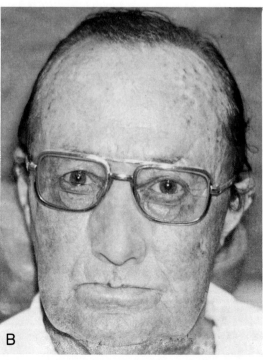

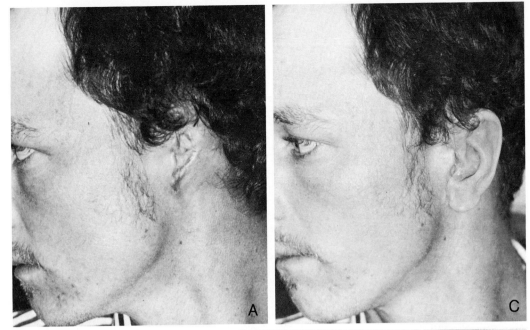

FIG. 10-11. (A) Missing ear. (B) Prosthesis. (C) Prosthetic ear in position.

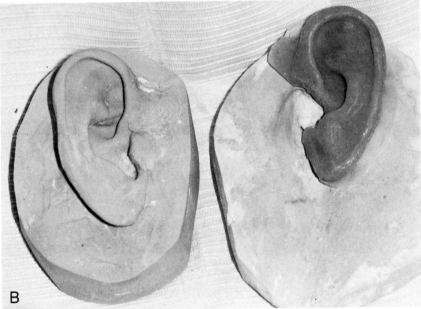

FIG. 10-12. The prosthetic restoration of the orbit following orbital exenteration. (A) Postoperative defect. (B) Prosthesis in place.

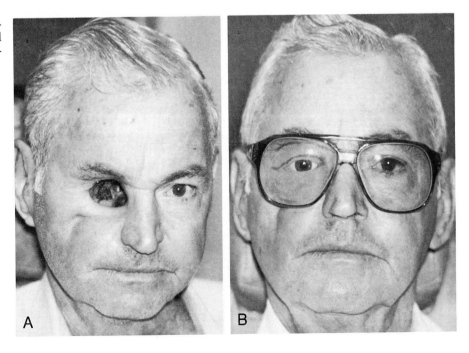

be camouflaged by means of tinted glasses in order to improve the normal appearance. It is necessary to emphasize the difference in cosmetic success of an orbital prosthesis when compared with a nasal or auricular prosthesis, because in a photograph all three appear natural. In reality, however, ear and nasal prostheses appear lifelike, but the orbital prosthesis does not.

The prosthetic restoration of the orbit and its contents is of cosmetic value only (Fig. 10-12). The benefits of this prosthesis should be discussed in advance with the patient. The patient may experience pain when breathing caused by cold air passing through the orbit. A "custom patch" rather than a cloth patch will more effectively seal off the orbit.

The orbital prosthesis should be rigid and securely retained so as not to move in and out of the socket during breathing. This movement is more likely when the nose is blocked, as during a cold.

Before construction of the prosthesis, the patient should understand the cosmetic advantages and disadvantages associated with it. It is helpful if the patient can talk with a patient who has had similar treatment. Demonstrations and audiovisual aids are also of value. The orbital prosthesis is the most difficult to construct and may be poorly accepted by the patient. There are many people who go about their daily business wearing an eye patch as an alternative to a prosthesis.

REFERENCE

1. Curtis TA, Cantor R: The maxillofacial rehabilitation of President Grover Cleveland and Dr. Sigmund Freud. J Am Dent Assoc 76:359–361, 1968

Parenteral Nutritional Management in Patients With Head and Neck Malignancies

EDWARD M. COPELAND III
THOMAS O. RUMLEY

Surveys of protein–calorie malnutrition in major metropolitan hospitals have indicated that 40% of malnourished, hospitalized patients have cancer.[1] Because of this high incidence, the practicing oncologist must recognize the malnourished patient who presents for cancer therapy, must be able to initiate measures for nutritional repletion before proceeding with therapy, and must attempt to prevent further nutritional depletion during treatment. Radiation therapy, chemotherapy, and surgery predictably increase the nutrient requirement and, at the same time, interfere with the patient's ability to eat. Consequently, malnutrition often results from the intensive effort to eradicate the tumor by a combination of these treatment modalities. Each of these therapeutic steps is predicated on recovery from the preceding step. Unless adequate nutrient intake is ensured, the patient is at risk for protein–calorie malnutrition and may lose the benefit of combined effects of radiation therapy, surgery, and chemotherapy.

Patients with malignant neoplasms of the oropharynx present special nutritional problems because they often have a history of smoking, dietary indiscretions, and high intake of alcohol. They may be undernourished and have vitamin deficiencies at the time an oropharyngeal malignancy develops and thus are often malnourished prior to beginning therapy. They then begin a vicious cycle because proper oncologic treatment further impairs optimal oral nutritional repletion. Malnutrition may be potentiated in these patients by the anatomical location of the cancer if it results in obstruction or pain on deglutition.

Protein–calorie malnutrition results in impaired wound healing, reduced immunologic function, increased susceptibility to infection, and decreased tolerance to effective oncologic therapy. Patients with resectable or radio-sensitive neoplasms need to be optimally nourished in order to promote adequate wound healing and to minimize the incidence and severity of complications of surgery and radiation therapy. Clinical and experimental studies have demonstrated that nutritional repletion prior to or during oncologic therapy will restore immunologic function to normal and reduce perioperative mortality and morbidity.[5–7] With the availability of dietary supplements, tube feeding regimens, and intravenous hyperalimentation (IVH), the nutritional needs of patients should not be neglected in the clinical practice of medicine.

The magnitude of therapy that cancer patients are to receive is a major determinant of the degree of metabolic stress the patient will undergo. A set of complex tests is not always necessary for the diagnosis of malnutrition. If the physician knows the initial nutritional state of the patient and the magnitude of the nutritional problem to result from the planned oncologic therapy, then the need for nutritional supplementation can be predicted. Unfortunately, the physician does not always have the luxury of waiting until nutritional repletion is complete before beginning therapy, and the risk of waiting too long to initiate oncologic therapy may negate the benefits of prolonged attempts at nutritional rehabilitation. Although the development

Supported in part by a grant from Home Health Care of America, Inc, Santa Anna, CA.

of tests for nutritional assessment is a major step forward in the management of patients with cancer, these tests do not replace other good surgical, medical, and oncologic judgments. The importance of nutritional rehabilitation cannot be overemphasized, but it must be integrated into the overall management of the cancer patient.

The practicing physician, without the aid of an organized nutritional support service, cannot always perform all available nutritional assessment tests (e.g., anthropometric measurements; creatinine-height indices; and prealbumin, transferrin, and retinol-binding protein serum concentrations). Nitrogen balance as a single test does not assess the nutritional status of the patient. Nitrogen balance studies determine the need for additional protein and calorie intake to offset body protein losses and to meet energy demands. Since amino acids are distinguished from other nutrients by the presence of nitrogen, nitrogen balance is appropriately used as a nutritional index to indicate if the calorie and nitrogen delivery is adequate. A simple way to calculate the calorie and protein needs as an initial starting point is to supply calories at 35 kcal/kg/day if maintenance nutritional levels are necessary or at 45 kcal/kg/day if the patient is malnourished and anabolism should be stimulated. Nitrogen (protein in grams divided by 6.25) should be given at a ratio of approximately 1 g per 120 to 150 nonprotein calories (approximately 1.5 g to 2.0 g/kg/day of protein).

From the standpoint of practicality, a simple definition of malnutrition includes (1) unintentional loss of 10% or more of body weight; (2) a serum albumin concentration of less than 3.4 g/dl, and (3) a negative reaction to a battery of recall skin test antigens. Patients who satisfy two of these three criteria and who have a reasonable chance of responding to appropriate antineoplastic therapy are candidates for aggressive nutritional rehabilitation prior to oncologic therapy. Patients who are incapable of adequate enteral nutrition because of malnutrition imposed by previous oncologic therapy are candidates for nutritional rehabilitation with IVH. Similarly, healthy patients whose treatment plan necessitates multiple courses of chemotherapy, possibly combined with radiation therapy or surgery, and in whom these treatment modalities will predictably result in malnutrition that will either prevent recovery or limit further oncologic treatment should be considered for nutritional supplementation with IVH.

Low serum albumin concentration and loss of delayed cutaneous hypersensitivity are late manifestations of malnutrition. Similarly, the return of these indicators to normal during nutritional rehabilitation is not rapid. For this reason, nutritional support teams have used indices such as serum concentrations of prealbumin, retinol-binding protein, and transferrin, since the half-life of these compounds is shorter than that of albumin. An abnormally low concentration of these compounds may be an early manifestation of undernutrition, whereas a rise during nutritional rehabilitation may indicate the conversion of patients from a catabolic to an anabolic state. For these reasons, the practicing physician should be aware of more specific tests for malnutrition and of the integration of these tests into the overall nutritional management plan for the patient.

The surgeon or radiation therapist who treats patients with head and neck malignancies must attempt to prepare them psychologically, metabolically, and physiologically for the recommended oncologic therapy. The method of feeding patients also depends on the treatment modality to be used and the initial nutritional status of the patient. Attention to nutritional status at presentation and appropriate dietary counseling and vitamin supplementation will result in nutritional rehabilitation of most patients. Ideally, adequate oral feedings should be the ultimate goal in each patient, but often treatment precludes proper oral intake. Also, poor nutritional status may result in lassitude and muscle weakness, further decreasing oral ingestion of nutrients. Basically, standard hospital diets plus oral supplements and/or tube feedings should be ordered for patients who are initially in good nutritional status. Dietary counseling is vital for patients receiving nutritional therapy with oral or tube feedings.

A functional gastrointestinal tract is the best means of ensuring normal digestion and assimilation of foodstuffs; however, delivery of nutriments to the gut does not always result in nutritional restoration of the starving patient because the syndrome of malnutrition may include malabsorption. In severely cachectic patients, the gastrointestinal columnar mucosal cells become cuboidal and the brush border is reduced in height. There is a decrease in production of mucosal cells and a decrease in migration from the crypts. Gastrointestinal motility diminishes, and overgrowth of facultative and anaerobic bacteria results. These morphologic, absorptive, and bacteriologic abnormalities are corrected following protein–calorie replenishment. The process is slow, however, because adequate enteral nutriments are initially partially malabsorbed and the uncomfortable symptoms of nausea, diarrhea, abdominal pain, and bloating limit the patient's desire to eat.[16]

Senyukov reported an evaluation of the efficacy of IVH used perioperatively in malnourished patients with carcinoma of the larynx.[14] Seventy patients received IVH and 90 patients were fed with the use of nasogastric feeding tubes. The two groups of patients were selected carefully to be matched for stage of disease and for dose of preoperative radiation therapy. Primary wound healing occurred in 75% of the IVH-fed group versus 40% of the enterally fed group. Ten percent of patients in the parenteral group developed pharyngeal fistulas compared with 29% of the patients in the enteral group. It appears from this study that malnourished patients who were given the nutrient mixture intravenously, and thereby guaranteed a certain calorie intake, had significantly better postoperative wound healing than did a comparative group who were fed by the gastrointestinal tract and, no doubt, partially malabsorbed enterally ingested nutrients.

Nevertheless, if time permits, restoration of good nutritional status may be possible by tube feeding maneuvers. Short-term nutritional repletion of the moderately malnourished patient or nutritional maintenance of the previously healthy patient who cannot swallow is quite satisfactory with a nasogastric or nasoduodenal feeding tube. Indwelling nasogastric tubes are unsatisfactory for long-term use because they often cause nasopharyngeal ulcerations and esophagogastric reflux around the tube. For those patients whose gastrointestinal tract is unavailable for nutriment administration or who need rapid nutritional repletion in order to initiate antineoplastic therapy quickly, IVH, properly applied, has allowed appropriate cancer treatment to be administered and, in some cases, has been lifesaving.

INTRAVENOUS HYPERALIMENTATION: TECHNIQUES

Solutions for IVH generally contain 3.5% to 5% amino acids and 20% to 30% dextrose. The osmolarity of this solution is between 1800 mOsm and 2400 mOsm, necessitating infusion by way of a large-bore catheter into a central vein rather than a peripheral vein. Most often, the subclavian vein is catheterized percutaneously by the infraclavicular approach so that the tip of the feeding catheter can be placed in the middle of the superior vena cava. Nutriments delivered through this catheter are diluted rapidly in the vena cava, resulting in less risk of inducing thrombophlebitis than if the infusion were into a smaller vessel, such as the internal jugular vein. Accurate positioning of the catheter tip within the middle of the superior vena cava is verified by obtaining a chest roentgenogram prior to beginning infusion of the hypertonic IVH solution.

The IVH delivery system should not be used indiscriminately. Blood, blood by-products, and medication should be infused into an alternate vein, usually a peripheral vein, whenever possible. A simultaneous peripheral intravenous infusion is often necessary to administer antibiotics, supplemental fluids, or chemotherapeutic agents.

The incidence of catheter-related sepsis in our series of patients ranges from 1% to 6%; the highest rate of sepsis occurs in patients with oropharyngeal cancers because they often have open wounds or tracheostomy stomas nearby that constantly contaminate the catheter dressing. Recently, long silastic catheters that can be inserted into the middle of the superior vena cava by way of the antecubital vein have been introduced. If these catheters are properly managed, IVH can be infused safely through them, thereby eliminating the problem of local dressing contamination that is encountered when the subclavian route is employed in patients with oropharyngeal cancers.

Reports of long-term venous catheterization of cancer patients using catheters permanently placed in the superior vena cava are appearing frequently.[3,13] The attainment of venous access is becoming more difficult because sclerosing agents used to treat solid tumors eliminate peripheral veins. Many of these reports indicate that blood may be withdrawn and blood products administered through the permanently placed catheters and that the catheter may also be used for infusion of IVH. The reader should be cautioned that such reports come from medical units having physicians, nurses, and technicians highly skilled in the method of using such catheters for multiple purposes. To generalize the use of central venous feeding catheters for multiple purposes in the head and neck cancer patient population would be disastrous because of the predictable increase in septic complications.

The nurse assigned to the hyperalimentation team changes the patient's catheter dressing and IVH delivery tubing three times a week, each time repreparing the skin with ether or acetone and an antiseptic solution. An antimicrobial ointment and a sterile dressing are reapplied to cover the catheter-skin entrance site. Proper technique must be used always, and in doing so a single feeding catheter can remain in place for prolonged periods of time without complications.

The patient who develops a fever during IVH is presumed to have catheter-related sepsis unless another focus of infection is found. Diagnosis of catheter-related sepsis is confirmed by a blood culture and a catheter culture that are positive for the same organism. The catheter should be removed immediately, and the temperature usually returns to normal within 24 to 48 hours after catheter removal if the catheter was the source of infection. If a primary focus of infection other than the catheter is found and results of blood cultures are negative, the primary focus should be treated appropriately and the catheter left in place. A positive finding on blood culture is an unequivocal indication for catheter removal. Twenty-four to 48 hours after the temperature has returned to normal and results of blood cultures have become negative, the feeding catheter can be reinserted into the superior vena cava, usually through the opposite subclavian or antecubital vein.

A constant rate of infusion of the hypertonic IVH solutions is necessary to promote proper utilization of the administered glucose, amino acids, minerals, and vitamins. Initially, 1000 ml is delivered in 24 hours to confirm the patient's ability to metabolize the infused glucose effectively. In the absence of glycosuria and hyperglycemia, the flow rate may be increased to 1000 ml every 12 hours. Pancreatic islet cells will again need the opportunity to adapt with an increase in insulin output in response to the increased glucose infusion, but within the first 3 to 5 days, the average adult usually will tolerate a daily ration of 3000 ml of IVH. Extremely cachectic patients, however, may tolerate only 2000 ml/day until partial nutritional rehabilitation has been attained.

The abrupt cessation of IVH may lead to insulin shock or reactive hypoglycemia. For this reason, IVH should be tapered off during the 24- to 48-hour period prior to completely discontinuing it. Certainly, prior to the administration of any general anesthetic, IVH should be tapered and discontinued the preceding 24 hours to prevent insulin hypoglycemia from going unrecognized while the patient is asleep, resulting in subsequent permanent brain damage.

The formulation of IVH for daily infusion into a patient with normal levels of sodium, chloride, potassium, magnesium, inorganic phosphorus, and calcium is presented in Table 11-1. Administration of amino acids and hypertonic dextrose without the proper quantity of any one of these necessary elements will significantly impair the patient's ability to achieve positive nitrogen balance and tissue synthesis. The degree of depletion of potassium, phosphorus, and magnesium often parallels the extent of

TABLE 11-1. Solutions for Intravenous Hyperalimentation (500 ml 50% Glucose Plus 500 ml 8.5%–10% Amino Acid Solution)

Additive	Quantity
Sodium chloride	40–50 mEq
Potassium acetate	20–30 mEq
Potassium acid phosphate	10–15 mEq
Magnesium sulfate	10–15 mEq
Multivitamins*	5 ml†
Calcium gluconate*	1 g

* Added to only 1 unit of solution daily.
† M.V.I.—USV Pharmaceutical Corporation, Tuckahoe, NY.

protein–calorie malnutrition, but it is not necessarily reflected by their serum concentration in the cachectic patient. Not until adequate intravenous nutritional replacement of amino-acid building blocks and energy stores has begun do the serum concentrations of these elements diminish and reflect more accurately the true magnitude of the total body deficit. As anabolism progresses and protein synthesis returns to normal, requirements for these elements will be reduced. The reason for the increased need during anabolism in the malnourished patients is unclear; however, potassium, phosphorus, calcium, and magnesium have a much higher concentration in the intracellular compartment than in the extracellular compartment, and loss of body mass probably results in a relative total body deficiency of these elements, which is unmasked when lean tissue replenishment begins.

Generally, the patient can be expected to gain 2 kg to 4 kg during a 3-week interval of IVH; the initial 1- to 2-kg weight gain will be rehydration, but then the patient should gain lean body mass at a rate of 0.25 kg/day. Body weight gain greater than 0.5 kg/day should be considered fluid retention, and the IVH delivery rate should be slowed or a diuretic should be administered.

If, during infusion of IVH, glycosuria is encountered in a patient with a continuously elevated blood glucose concentration, then the patient's capacity for metabolizing the administered glucose has been exceeded, and exogenous crystalline insulin may be supplied or the glucose delivery rate must be reduced. If this situation is encountered in a patient who is receiving inadequate calories, then insulin must be added to ensure adequate metabolism of the needed glucose. When additional insulin is necessary, we recommend that it be added directly to the IVH solutions rather than be given subcutaneously. We recognize that some of the crystalline insulin adheres to the bottle and the administration tubing; however, the amount of insulin lost in this manner is insignificant. If insulin is within the IVH bottle and the infusion stops, then insulin administration also stops. If insulin has been administered subcutaneously, however, and the infusion stops, marked hypoglycemia with its potential adverse clinical results might occur. The initial insulin dose should be 5 to 10 units/1000 ml, and the amount should be increased gradually until the blood glucose level returns to within 120 mg to 180 mg/dl.

Whole blood, plasma, and albumin are often necessary in cachectic patients with oropharyngeal malignancies prior to a major surgical procedure and contain trace elements such as copper, manganese, iodine, chromium, and zinc. Trace elements are not present, however, in the highly purified amino acid solutions. If a course of IVH is to last for more than 3 weeks, the addition of trace elements should be made to the nutritional solutions. Folic acid, vitamin K, and vitamin B_{12} should be administered on a routine basis or as regularly as necessary.

In the preoperative patient who is severely anemic, the normal red cell volume should be corrected by whole blood or packed cell transfusions. Often, hypoalbuminemia must be treated early in the course of parenteral alimentation. From 12.5 g to 50 g of albumin given daily during the first few days of treatment should restore colloid osmotic pressure toward normal. In the vast majority of patients, the serum albumin concentration will increase sufficiently within approximately 14 days of beginning IVH, and exogenous serum albumin will be necessary for only a short interval of time. It should be emphasized that serum albumin is expensive and is used only to increase colloid osmotic pressure when the patient's symptoms dictate that a rise in colloid osmotic pressure is necessary. Exogenous serum albumin is not used as a nutritional substance; the half-life of albumin is too long for it to be an efficient nutrient.

Intravenous fat solutions are now available for parenteral use in the United States. They are isotonic, 290 mOsm/liter, and can be infused by way of a peripheral vein without fear of inducing thrombophlebitis. To date, the primary role of intravenous fat supplementation has been to provide the essential fatty acid, linoleic acid, by the thrice-weekly administration of one 500-ml bottle of the 10% fat solutions. More recently, research has indicated that 40% of the nonprotein calories supplied as fat might be more beneficial to the cancer patient than supplying all nonprotein calories as glucose. Such information comes from the study of tumor-bearing rodents,[2] and similiar observations have yet to be made in humans.

CLINICAL EXPERIENCE WITH IVH IN PATIENTS WITH OROPHARYNGEAL MALIGNANCIES

During a 3-year period at the M. D. Anderson Hospital and Tumor Institute, 70 patients with oropharyngeal malignancies received IVH in order to prepare, maintain, and/or rehabilitate them nutritionally and metabolically so that surgery, chemotherapy, or radiation therapy could be tolerated with maximum safety and efficacy.[4]

Twenty-nine patients received IVH perioperatively. Laryngopharyngectomy was done in 19 patients, radical neck dissection was done in 16 patients, and 10 patients had reconstruction with thoracoacromial flaps. The patients required IVH for an average period of 36.6 days, and in the 15 patients who received IVH both preoperatively and postoperatively, the average weight gain was 5.1 kg. IVH was used preoperatively for an average of 16.1 days and was continued postoperatively for an average period of 20.3 days until adequate nutrition could be maintained enterally. Fourteen patients received IVH only postoperatively for an average period of 36.8 days. The usual indications for IVH postoperatively were complications of malnutrition, such as pneumonia, poor wound healing, or malabsorption of enterally administered nutrients. Possibly, these complications could have been avoided if proper attention had been given to preoperative nutritional repletion. As a rule, it is much easier to promote return of muscle strength, weight gain, significant rise in secretory protein concentration, and improvement of immune function by preoperative nutritional repletion rather than by waiting until malnutrition has become a severe problem postoperatively. Nevertheless, in those patients in this series in whom IVH was used only postoperatively, weight gain was achieved, pneumonia and wound infection resolved, healthy granulation tissue appeared, and skin grafts and flaps could be used to cover denuded surfaces and to close fistulous openings.

Six patients developed pharyngocutaneous fistulas after radical head and neck surgery. Two fistulas closed spontaneously after 17 and 20 days of IVH. The remaining four fistulas were closed surgically after 21 to 47 days of IVH, and the average weight gain for these patients during this time period was 6.8 kg. Attempts at surgical closure had failed prior to beginning IVH in three patients. Fistula management was easier after beginning IVH because salivary and mucosal secretions decreased when the nasogastric feeding tubes were removed.

Three patients had pharyngeal incompetence after a partial glossectomy, a posterior pharyngeal wall resection, or a resection of the tongue and mandible. Enough of the muscles of mastication remained so that pharyngeal incompetence was thought to be secondary to muscle weakness and reversible muscle injury. Weight gain of between 3.6 kg and 11.8 kg was accomplished in these patients, and, concomitant with return of general body muscle strength and tone, swallowing function returned after 18 to 48 days of IVH.

Nine patients were nutritionally maintained and rehabilitated with IVH during treatment with radiation therapy. In two patients, radiation therapy initially was contraindicated because of severe malnutrition; consequently, each patient was begun on IVH 7 to 10 days prior to beginning radiation therapy and was continued on IVH throughout therapy. The remaining seven patients developed severe pharyngitis and stomatitis while receiving radiation therapy, and anorexia and malnutrition ensued. Because radiation therapy otherwise would have been discontinued before a therapeutic or palliative dose was delivered, these patients were admitted to the hospital, rehydrated, and begun on IVH. The planned course of radiation therapy was continued and completed in all but one patient, who died of aspiration pneumonia while receiving treatment for recurrent squamous cell carcinoma of the tongue and floor of the mouth. IVH was used for an average period of 34.8 days, average weight gain was 3.4 kg, and the average dose delivered during IVH was 3250 rad. The average age of these patients was 51.2 years, and the average total dose delivered was 4900 rad. Eight of the nine patients had lesions that were evaluable for therapeutic response, and greater than 50% tumor reduction occurred in five patients. All patients gained strength and experienced improvement in the symptoms of stomatitis and pharyngitis during radiation therapy.

Rehabilitation after radiation therapy is important to strengthen the muscles of mastication and to prevent temporomandibular joint fibrosis. If the latter ensues, eating may become progressively more difficult and painful as joint function becomes limited. This situation was encountered in five patients who received IVH for nutritional support while rehabilitation of joint function was attempted. It was psychologically easier for these poorly motivated patients to be rehabilitated if they were not burdened by nasogastric feeding tubes.

Ten patients were admitted to the hospital for nutritional supportive care after operation or radiation therapy. These patients received IVH for an average period of 25.1 days and achieved an average weight gain of 4.0 kg. One patient died of pneumonia while receiving IVH; two patients required insertion of gastrostomy feeding tubes for long-term ambulatory nutritional maintenance; four patients were eventually discharged from the hospital on nasogastric tube feeding regimens; and three patients who responded favorably to head and neck muscular rehabilitation were able to ingest food orally at discharge.

Sixteen patients received IVH as nutritional support in order to receive intensive chemotherapy with multiple combined chemotherapeutic drug regimens. These patients were severely malnourished secondary to cancer or previous oncologic therapy when they were evaluated by the IVH team, and none was considered a candidate for subsequent chemotherapy without IVH because of the anticipated complications secondary to the combined effects of chemotherapy and malnutrition. With IVH, each patient tolerated chemotherapy, and nausea, vomiting, stomatitis, and diarrhea were minimized. Weight gain during IVH and chemotherapy was 4.5 kg in an average of 27 days of nutritional therapy. Thirty percent of the patients responded with a 50% or greater reduction in measurable tumor volume, and responding patients survived an average period of 6 months compared with an average survival of only 1 month for nonresponding patients.

CONCLUSIONS

Mullen and co-workers have shown by the use of a prognostic nutritional index that malnourished cancer patients have a much higher morbidity and mortality rate from a surgical procedure when nutritional repletion is neglected preoperatively.[6] Müller and co-workers conducted a randomized study of patients with gastrointestinal tract cancer by comparing the results of 10 days of IVH versus those of conventional fluid management.[7] Equal numbers of malnourished patients were in each group. The control group had significantly more deaths and major complications, particularly pneumonia and anastomotic breakdown. Skin test reactivity and retinol-binding protein, prealbumin, and transferrin serum concentrations improved in the IVH group and declined in the control group. This randomized prospective study clearly demonstrates the value of preoperative nutritional repletion and maintenance in the surgery patient population.

Malnutrition is a poor prognostic indicator for response to chemotherapy. Whether or not nutritional repletion, either by enteral or parenteral methods, can reverse malnutrition and convert a predictably poor responder to chemotherapy into a good responder remains unknown. Unfortunately, many of the randomized, prospective trials do not equate response of the cancer to chemotherapeutic drugs to the host response to attempts at nutritional repletion. In fact, host weight gain in these studies is often composed predominantly of an increase in total body water and fat mass with very little documentation of an increase in lean body tissue.[8-10,12] It is important to know if a previously malnourished patient who has been nutritionally replenished with IVH is a better candidate for response to chemotherapy or radiation therapy than is his malnourished counterpart. Such studies are extremely necessary since overinterpretation of the data or bias for or against the use of IVH in the cancer patient population could result in its being withheld when needed or used when unwarranted. Review of the data available indicates that IVH should be reserved for truly malnourished cancer patients for whom there is available oncologic therapy. The well-nourished patient or the malnourished patient for whom there is no available antineoplastic therapy have benefited little or not at all from the use of IVH. The nutritionally intact patient gains weight primarily as water and fat and would be subjected unnecessarily to the inherent complications of IVH. Intravenous hyperalimentation should seldom be used for treatment of the patient who has failed all available methods of cancer therapy. Terminally ill patients may feel somewhat better during the IVH infusion, but this effect ceases rapidly once IVH is discontinued. Prolongation of pain for the patient and anguish for the family are not justifiable indicators for the use of IVH in cancer patients.

Rickard and co-workers did sequential nutritional assessment while using IVH during the treatment of children with advanced neoplastic diseases.[11] A period of 9 to 14 days of IVH was often inadequate to result in a net increase in synthesis of either skeletal or visceral proteins, whereas 28 days of IVH did result in such anabolic changes. Spanier and co-workers correlated change in body composition with change in delayed cutaneous hypersensitivity reactions during IVH.[15] Those patients who converted skin-test reactions from negative to positive also had a significant increase in lean body tissue, thereby indicating a nutritional response to IVH. Those patients who failed to convert skin-test reactions from negative to positive also failed to increase lean body mass in response to IVH.

The data of Rickard and Spanier are important to understand because they imply that just because IVH is used the patient may not necessarily become replenished nutritionally. The induction of anabolism depends on the time, content, and method of administration of IVH solutions, the degree of initial malnutrition, the initial and continuing catabolic response of the patient, the energy expenditure required during oncologic therapy, and the expertise of the physician in the techniques of IVH.

Malnutrition is harmful to cancer patients because the cachectic patient has a narrower safe therapeutic margin for most oncologic therapy. In the malnourished patient, the increased risks of complications secondary to undernutrition can limit the dose of oncologic therapy, and the patient may not be classified as a reasonable treatment candidate even though he has a potentially responsive malignant lesion. Based on retrospective and prospective studies, IVH should be used in cancer patients as a means of nutritional rehabilitation when such a goal is desirable to optimize response to antineoplastic therapy and to minimize complications from such treatment and when this goal cannot be obtained by using the gastrointestinal tract.

REFERENCES

1. Bistrian BR, Blackburn GL, Hallowell E, Heddle R: Protein status of general surgical patients. JAMA 230:858–860, 1974
2. Buzby GP, Mullen JL, Stein P, Miller EE, Hobbs CL, Rosato EF: Host-tumor interaction and nutrient supply. Cancer 45:2940–2948, 1980
3. Copeland EM III: Catheter care and intravenous hyperalimentation. J Parenter Ent Nutr 6:93–94, 1982
4. Copeland EM III, Daly JM, Dudrick SJ: Nutritional concepts in the treatment of head and neck malignancies. Head Neck Surg 1:350–363, 1979
5. Daly JM, Dudrick SJ, Copeland EM III: Intravenous hyperalimentation: Effect on delayed cutaneous hypersensitivity in cancer patients. Ann Surg 192:587–592, 1980
6. Mullen JM, Buzby GP, Matthews DC, Smale BF, Rosato EF: Reduction of operative morbidity and mortality by combined preoperative and postoperative nutritional support. Ann Surg 192:604–613, 1980
7. Müller JM, Brenner U, Dienst C, Pichlmaier H: Preoperative parenteral feeding in patients with gastrointestinal carcinoma. Lancet 1:68–71, 1982
8. Nixon DW, Moffitt S, Lawson D, Ansley J, Lynn MJ, Kutner MH, et al.: Total parenteral nutrition as an adjunct to chemotherapy of metastatic colorectal cancer. Cancer Treat Rep 65(Suppl 5):121–128, 1981
9. Popp MB, Fisher RI, Simon RM, Brennan MF: A prospective randomized study on adjunct parenteral nutrition in the treatment of diffuse lymphoma: Effect on drug tolerance. Cancer Treat Rep 65(Suppl 5):129–135, 1981
10. Popp MB, Fisher RI, Wesley R, Aamodt R, Brennan MF: A prospective randomized study of adjuvant parenteral nutrition in the treatment of advanced diffuse lymphoma: Influence on survival. Surgery 90:195–203, 1981
11. Rickard KA, Grosfeld JL, Kirksey A, Balentine TVN, Baehner RL: Reversal of protein-energy malnutrition in children during treatment of advanced neoplastic disease. Ann Surg 190:771–781, 1979
12. Samuels ML, Selig DE, Ogden S, Grant C, Brown B: IV hyperalimentation and chemotherapy for stage III testicular cancer: A randomized study. Cancer Treat Rep 65:615–624, 1981
13. Sanders JE, Hickman RO, Aker S, Hersman J, Buckner CD, Thomas ED: Experience with double lumen right atrial catheters. J Parenter Ent Nutr 6:95–99, 1982
14. Senyukov MV, Khmelevski IM, Zubov OG, Sloventantor VI, Kaplan NA: Parenteral feeding of patients with cancer of the larynx undergoing combination therapy. Vestn Otorhinolaryngol 2:66–74, 1978
15. Spanier AH, Pietsch JB, Meakins JL, MacLean LD, Shizgal HM: The relationship between immune competence and nutrition. Surg Forum 27:332–336, 1976
16. Viteri FE, Schneider RE: Gastrointestinal alterations in protein-calorie malnutrition. Med Clin North Am 58:1487–1505, 1974

Dental Management
for the Irradiated Patient

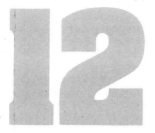

ALAN C. LEVIN

Radiation therapy affects the oral cavity, its contents and its surrounding structures, in a dramatic fashion. Some of the changes occur early and may be reversible, while others occur later and are more permanent. Initially, after the first few radiation treatments, mucositis occurs, which may be followed by ulceration and secondary infection of the mucosa. There is a loss of taste sensation, which may lead to loss of appetite, and there is usually a change in the patient's diet as a result of the pain experienced on swallowing. The result may be severe weight loss during the period of radiation treatment. Dietary supplements can be helpful at this time.

The effect of radiation on the salivary glands is to decrease the output of the serous cells, resulting in a viscous, often ropy saliva with a high mucin content. Bone tends to become less vital due to decreased vascularity following irradiation and will not respond normally to surgical or other injuries.

These changes in the oral cavity impair the patient's ability to maintain good oral hygiene and render the teeth more susceptible to caries and periodontal disease, even if the teeth were not included in the actual radiation field. Root sensitivity may occur following irradiation. This is more marked if there has been gingival recession or recent periodontal treatment with exposure of the root surface. However, gross caries, even with pulpal exposure or teeth broken off at the gingival margin, produces remarkably little pain unless abscess develops.

Osteoradionecrosis is a serious side-effect of radiation therapy, and all possible measures must be taken to reduce the risk of its occurrence. With this in mind, patients must be evaluated prior to radiation treatment. The areas of highest risk are points of underlying bone having a sharp bony exostosis or a sharp ridge covered by a thin layer of oral mucosa, such as the mylohyoid ridge.

DENTULOUS PATIENTS

Pretreatment Evaluation

Prior to radiation treatment, patients must be examined to determine the risk they face for developing bone exposure or full-blown osteoradionecrosis in the future. Dentulous patients have a higher risk of developing osteoradionecrosis than edentulous patients. It must be determined whether the teeth that are present can be maintained. If they cannot, then it must be decided whether to do the extractions before the radiation therapy, thereby delaying the start of treatment, or to attempt to maintain the teeth and extract them later. Both policies may be used, according to the clinical situation.

Patients who have all or most of their natural teeth present, in reasonably good condition, should not be considered candidates for extractions. They should be motivated to raise their level of oral hygiene to prevent any further loss of teeth and so greatly reduce the chance of developing osteoradionecrosis.

In patients with teeth in fair or poor condition or with many missing teeth, many factors must be evaluated before a decision can be made. A

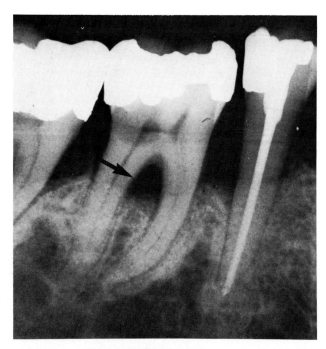

FIG. 12-1. Roentgenogram of molar showing bone destruction in area of bifurcation.

dentition in poor periodontal condition presents a greater risk than one with many carious lesions but with acceptable periodontal condition. The carious lesions can generally be restored, whereas gross periodontal deterioration generally cannot. Lower molars in the radiation field represent a high-risk area. The roots of the lower molars are bifurcated, and an infection located in this crotch is especially difficult to eradicate; the diagnosis is established by periodontal probing and roentgenographic evaluation (Fig. 12-1).

The factors to be considered in deciding to extract teeth before irradiation include the following:

1. The condition of the dentition as a whole, that is, the general condition of the mouth and teeth, as well as the specific condition of each individual tooth must be considered. Particular attention should be paid to teeth that will be in the radiation field.
2. *The patient's level of oral hygiene will be the major factor determining the ultimate condition of the teeth after radiation therapy.* Patients who place a low value on their teeth, particularly those who think that complete dentures would serve them better, are unlikely to maintain their teeth and will invariably have their teeth extracted later on.
3. Mandibular teeth should be scrutinized more closely than maxillary teeth, since osteoradionecrosis occurs almost exclusively in the mandible and rarely in the maxilla.
4. Factors relating to the tumor are important. In consultation with the radiation therapist, the rate of growth of the tumor, the prognosis for tumor control, the size of the radiation field, and the dosage and mode of application of the radiation all must be considered. If the tumor is rapidly growing, delay for dental treatment may not be in the patient's best interest and may compromise the chance of curing

the tumor. The technical factors of the treatment determine the severity of the changes in the oral environment (e.g., the amount of salivary glands to be irradiated and the dose prescribed).

Extractions Prior to Irradiation

When it is determined that extractions are needed prior to the radiation therapy, the teeth should be extracted in groups and radical alveolectomy should be performed to attain primary closure over a smooth bony surface. The surgery should be carried out with as little trauma to the soft tissue as possible. Flaps should be treated gently and closed without tension.

Extractions may delay the start of radiation treatment by 7 to 21 days, depending on the rate of healing and development of any complication such as infection, wound dehiscence, or bone exposure. Immediate scheduling of the extractions will eliminate one source of delay.

The advantage of preirradiation extractions is that a group of teeth can be extracted at one sitting, an alveolectomy can be performed, and healing will occur in 1 to 3 weeks, usually 7 to 10 days. Postirradiation extractions are generally limited to removing one tooth at a time. One avoids the more difficult challenge of obtaining primary closure with single tooth extraction. Postirradiation extractions run an increased risk of delayed healing, bone exposure, and osteoradionecrosis.

Preventive Protocol

If the teeth are to be maintained, a preventive protocol is instituted. The patient must be educated and trained to maintain excellent oral hygiene and to visit his dentist regularly. Daily application of fluoride to the teeth reduces the rate of caries and the incidence of periodontal disease. Many methods of fluoride application have been used, but the method of preference is a daily, 5-minute, self-application by the patient in a custom-made vinyl fluoride carrier (Figs. 12-2 through 12-5). The most effective agent is acidulated phosphate fluoride, 1.23%. However, a neutral fluoride must be used in patients who have porcelain-faced crowns to avoid the surface etching (removal of glaze

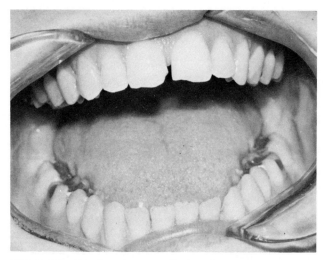

FIG. 12-2. Teeth prior to radiation therapy.

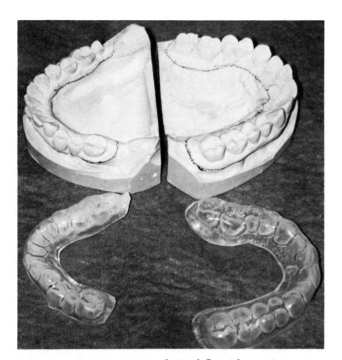

FIG. 12-3. Custom-prepared vinyl fluoride carriers.

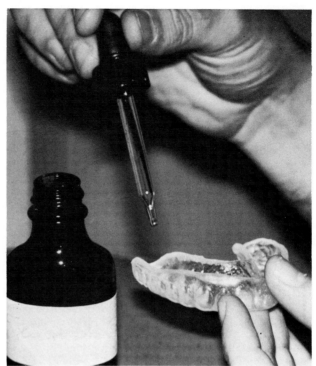

FIG. 12-4. Placing fluoride in carriers.

and shine) that occurs when acidulated phosphate fluoride touches the porcelain.

The fluoride treatment is started during the radiation therapy and continued for the rest of the patient's life. Some patients cannot tolerate the fluoride during the course of radiation therapy and start only after the mucosa is healed, 3 to 4 weeks after completion of treatment. Written instructions are supplied to the patient, since many do not remember the instructions or do not understand the importance of the situation at this time. Reinforcement is needed at follow-up visits. The daily fluoride treatment is continued indefinitely unless the saliva returns and the teeth remain healthy. In these cases we have reduced the applications to two or three times a week, and some patients are weaned entirely from self-application if their saliva is adequate and their dentition is sound. Only a few patients reach this stage of therapy.

The following instructions are given to the patient at the start of fluoride therapy:

1. Remove and clean the prosthesis. Brush and floss the teeth.
2. Place 6 to 8 drops of the gel in each fluoride carrier.
3. Place the carriers with gel onto the teeth and allow them to remain in place for 5 minutes.
4. Remove the carriers and empty the mouth. *Do not rinse, eat, or drink for 30 minutes.*
5. Repeat the procedure once a day *for the rest of your life.*

Restorative Protocol

Prior to the start of radiation therapy or during the first 2 weeks of treatment, routine care such as repair of caries and cleaning may be done, but it should not delay the start of treatment. During the radiation treatment period,

FIG. 12-5. Fluoride carriers in place.

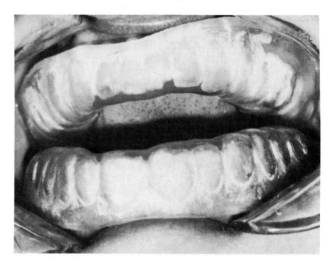

only emergency dental care is done because of the oral discomfort. Definitive restorative treatment is delayed until the radiation treatment is completed and all inflammatory changes have subsided. This will reduce the patient's discomfort during the dental treatment and facilitate the dentist's work.

Postirradiation Care

It is important to restore the teeth so that they are comfortable and nonsensitive, to make it easy for the patient to maintain excellent routine oral hygiene.

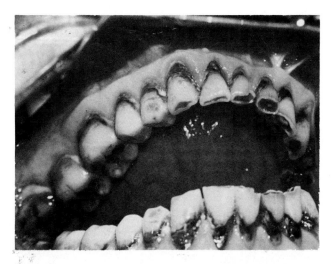

FIG. 12-6. Severe cervical and incisal radiation caries.

All routine dental procedures can be undertaken without unusual precautions except radical periodontal treatment and extractions, which may lead to osteoradionecrosis if undertaken without special care. There is no concern regarding the additional x-ray exposure for dental films, since the dose is miniscule compared with the therapeutic dose given for cancer.

When extreme root sensitivity occurs following radiation treatment, burnishing fluoride onto the exposed root surfaces can decrease the pain or sensitivity to some extent.

There is considerable controversy regarding extractions after irradiation; the published incidence of osteoradionecrosis following extractions ranges from 0 to 100%. Buemer, in 1972, concluded that it was best to defer extraction of teeth as long as possible after irradiation in the hope of reducing the risk of necrosis.[1] He suggested that, when at all possible, endodontics should be attepted before extractions were considered.

When extractions are required, it is best to remove one tooth at a time with as little trauma to adjacent tissues as possible and to obtain complete healing before proceeding to further extractions. Prophylactic antibiotic coverage is started 1 day prior to extractions and continued until the site is healed. Tetracycline, 2 g/day, is the usual adult treatment. Primary closure of the wound should be carried out over a smoothed-down bony surface, and no sharp spicules or ridges should be left under the mucosa. Postirradiation extractions carried out in this manner have a good chance of complete healing without the development of necrosis.

Complications

The most common complications are caries (Fig. 12-6), fracture or amputation of a crown, periapical abscess, periodontal abscess, bone exposure, and osteoradionecrosis.

Periapical abscess can be treated under antibiotic coverage by conservative endodontic therapy. Periodontal abscess can lead to osteoradionecrosis if an infection becomes established in the bone. A protracted period of antibiotic treatment with debridement may be necessary. Should extraction of the tooth become necessary, it should be carried out as described above, with minimal trauma, but with alveolectomy as needed to obtain primary closure.

Treatment of bone exposure and osteoradionecrosis has been controversial. In any case the treatment is a lengthy procedure; many weeks to months or even years may be required to resolve the problem or completely exfoliate the necrotic bone. A conservative approach should be the treatment of choice. Patients having exposed bone or osteoradionecrosis only rarely have extreme pain. In the absence of pain, treatment consists of local irrigation of the exposed bone, packing with local topical antibiotics, and occasionally the use of systemic antibiotics.

Hyperbaric oxygen has been used for the treatment of osteoradionecrosis. It seems to improve the rate of healing, but this is difficult to document since other local procedures are occurring simultaneously. Currently, the expense precludes its use on a routine basis. (See Chapter 14, the Effects of Radiation on Normal Tissues, for further discussion of radiation effect on normal bone.)

EDENTULOUS PATIENTS

If the patient has been edentulous for some time, the risk of developing osteoradionecrosis is minimal. Most edentulous patients who develop osteoradionecrosis had extractions immediately before or after irradiation.

In patients who were edentulous long before irradiation, the wearing of well-made comfortable complete dentures is not contraindicated.

Patients who have preirradiation extractions can have dentures made immediately for the maxilla and occasionally for the mandible. For example, a patient receiving radiation therapy for oropharyngeal cancer might have very little of the denture-bearing mandible in the radiation portal and could have dentures inserted even during the course of therapy. However, a patient with cancer of the floor of the mouth would have the entire denture-bearing mandible irradiated, and insertion of dentures would best be delayed 6 to 12 months or until healing is secure.

It has been reported that when bone exposure exists in small, well-defined areas, complete dentures may be inserted over these areas without harm if the denture is relieved or enlarged over the necrosis. It is advisable in this situation to monitor the patient's progress closely for possible enlargement of the necrotic area.

REFERENCE

1. Beumer J, Silverman S, Benak SB: Hard and soft tissue necroses following irradiation for oral cancer. J Prosthet Dent 27:640–644, 1972

Time–Dose–Volume Relationships in Radiation Therapy

JAMES T. PARSONS

Treatment planning is now structured on the application of the basic radiobiological parameters relative to the risk of infestation around the primary tumor and regional lymphatics and the probability of control with specific doses of irradiation. This approach has made radiotherapy an intellectually gratifying medical discipline.[36]

—GILBERT H. FLETCHER

The goal in treating cancer with irradiation is tumor control with a minimum of treatment complications. In trying to achieve this goal, various treatment schedules have evolved through the years; while many schedules were developed through a rational stepwise progression of science and accumulated clinical experience, many others developed through a process of trial and error. It is now known that optimum control of cancer with a minimum of complications is best achieved by techniques that fractionate the irradiation dose. There is no single method of dose fractionation that has been proven best, and there is not one that will be right for all situations. In most therapy departments, treatments are administered once daily, 5 days a week.

THE SIGMOID DOSE-RESPONSE CURVE

In its early years, radiation therapy was dominated by the concept of an "all or none" dose. Cancers and normal tissues were classified according to the number of "threshold erythema doses" that were necessary to produce cures or complications. In the 1930s and 1940s, Miescher,[73] Holthusen,[50] and Strandquist[103] provided evidence that changed this concept; they produced sigmoid dose-response curves of the general form shown in Figure 13-1 for human skin cancer and normal tissue damage. For homogeneous groups of tumors, such curves have now been shown for many sites other than the skin. These curves demonstrate the probablistic nature of cancer control and normal tissue damage. For any given dose there is a corresponding tumor control probability and a corresponding complication probability. Tissue damage cannot be completely avoided since those doses expected to bring about cure overlap those that can cause complications. However, by manipulating the total dose, the total time over which the dose is administered, the fraction size, and the volume irradiated, an attempt is made to vary the relationship between these two curves in a favorable way, that is, to improve the therapeutic ratio.

CONTROL OF TUMORS BY IRRADIATION

Radiosensitivity and Radiocurability

Following irradiation, cells die when they attempt to undergo mitotic division. A population of proliferative cells that has a long cell cycle may be depleted very slowly by irradiation, while the cells of a rapidly cycling tumor are more quickly eliminated. By the same token, a cell that never divides will not be killed by irradiation, but it would not be of consequence since it would not contribute to tumor growth.

The response of tumors to irradiation is commonly described in terms of *radiosensitivity*, *radioresistance*, and *radiocurability*. The terms *radiosensitivity* and *radioresistance* are imprecisely defined, loosely used, and a source of great confusion to clinicians. The term *radiosensitive* is commonly applied to tumors that regress rapidly under treatment, while *radioresistant* refers to tumors that regress slowly. These definitions have an unfortunate

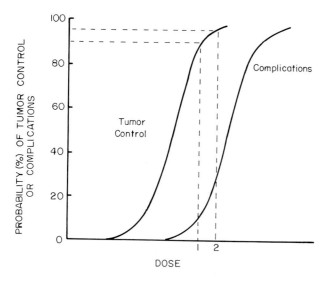

FIG. 13-1. Dose-response curves for control of a hypothetical tumor and for normal tissue damage. Treatment to dose level 1 results in a 90% probability of cure and 10% probability of complications. Because of the shape of the sigmoid response curves, if the dose is increased to level 2, the control rate increases by only 5% but the rate of complications increases more dramatically to 28%. By manipulation of factors other than dose (e.g., time, fraction size, and treatment volume), the actual separation between the two curves may also be varied; for some treatment regimens or tumor types, the complication curve lies to the left of the control curve so that for any chosen dose, the complication rate exceeds the cure rate.

connotation, since many clinicians have tended to equate a slow rate of regression with incurability. A *radioresistant* cancer, such as a slowly regressing adenocarcinoma of the prostate, might in fact be highly *radiocurable*; such lesions often show little or no size reduction at the completion of a 7-week course of therapy, but they gradually shrink and eventually disappear over a period of several months and then remain permanently controlled.

There is no essential difference in the radiocurability of carcinomas arising from the various epithelial cell types. Squamous cell carcinoma, basal cell carcinoma, muco-epidermoid carcinoma, and adenocarcinoma are apparently, size for size, equally radiocurable.[34] The probability of tumor control also does not depend on tumor cell differentiation; although highly differentiated cancers may regress more slowly than poorly differentiated ones, ultimate control rates are similar. A possible exception to this rule is the lymphoepithelioma, for which control is achieved at lower doses than squamous cell carcinomas of equal size.[35]

Soft tissue sarcomas have traditionally been regarded as incurable by irradiation. Many of these cancers are locally advanced when first detected and would predictably do poorly if treated with radiation alone; however, when such lesions receive 5000 rad preoperatively, regression is often dramatic. Small or moderate-sized sarcomas (<5 cm) in sites where the use of high-dose irradiation is feasible are sometimes cured by irradiation alone. In fact, there is

no convincing evidence that, size for size, they are less radiocurable than squamous cell carcinomas. Twenty-two of Cade's soft tissue sarcoma patients could not undergo operation because of unresectability, medical inoperability, patient refusal, and so on; six of the 22 remained disease free 5 to 26 years following irradiation alone.[15] Similar results were noted at 7 to 10 years in a small series of patients after irradiation alone at Memorial Sloan-Kettering Hospital.[64] At Massachusetts General Hospital, local control at 4 years following radiation therapy alone in 26 patients was 61%.[89] While irradiation alone is not advocated for sarcomas that are surgically removable, it is useful to remember that worthwhile results may be achieved in patients who cannot or will not undergo operation or when irradiation is combined with conservative surgery.

Several benign histologies can be controlled with moderate dose irradiation. Chemodectomas of the temporal bone structures and juvenile angiofibromas are two benign conditions for which irradiation is frequently chosen when the lesions are advanced or recurrent after surgery. Chemodectomas that have received greater than 4000 rad are almost all controlled if the treatment volume is adequate (see Chapter 31, Chemodectomas [Glomus Body Tumors]).[22] Juvenile angiofibromas require even lower doses (3000 rad to 3500 rad). Benign mixed salivary tumors infrequently require irradiation since they are usually controlled by surgery alone; a small number of patients at the University of Florida have received high doses (usually 6000 rad to 6500 rad) for recurrent or residual disease. Results have been good (see Chapter 28, Major Salivary Gland Tumors).

For squamous cell carcinomas, it was common practice until the mid 1960s to base the total tumor dose on rate of regression during therapy.[8] As a result, some rapidly responding lesions were underdosed, leading to tumor recurrence. For the majority of squamous cell primary lesions, modification of total dose according to regression rate is probably not a good idea. *Instead, at the outset of treatment, a dose is prescribed that is based on the initial volume of tumor; even if the lesion regresses rapidly, the full dose is administered.* Most squamous cell primary carcinomas regress by at least 20% to 30% by 2 weeks, 50% to 60% by 4 weeks, and 80% to 100% by 6 weeks; completely exophytic lesions regress faster, and deeply infiltrative lesions regress slower. Although there are no specific data to prove the point, one cannot help but believe that at the extremes of responsiveness, ultimate control can be predicted by the regression rate. It is quite rare to see

| TABLE 13-1. | The Influence of Tumor Status at the End of Treatment on Local Control Following Irradiation of Head and Neck Squamous Cell Carcinomas at Various Sites |

Tumor Status at End of Treatment	Local Control Following Irradiation Alone
No tumor clinically present	
M. D. Anderson Hospital[8]	72/88 (82%)
Strong Memorial Hospital[100]	48/68 (71%)
Tumor clinically present	
M. D. Anderson Hospital[8]	15/37 (41%)
Strong Memorial Hospital[100]	23/78 (29%)

recurrence of a squamous cell carcinoma that has completely disappeared 2 to 4 weeks into a 7-week course of therapy. On the other hand, lesions that show only 20% to 30% regression by 5 to 6 weeks are noted to recur with greater frequency. This is the basis for using a trial of irradiation for certain moderately advanced cancers. If the response at 5000 rad has been good, a full course of irradiation is administered; if there has been only minimal regression, an operation is performed.

Although the correlation of tumor control with the rate of regression during therapy remains controversial, most observers agree that tumor status at the completion of treatment correlates with ultimate control. Data on 146 patients with squamous cell carcinoma of the oral cavity, oropharynx, and hypopharynx following radical irradiation at the Strong Memorial Hospital[100] and 125 patients with oropharyngeal cancers treated at the M. D. Anderson Hospital from 1966 through 1970[8] are shown in Table 13-1. In both series, the recurrence rate was significantly higher when there was clinical evidence of residual tumor on the last day of treatment than when complete regression had occurred. *When persistent tumor is noted at or near the end of therapy, a "boost" dose above the initially planned tumor dose is often added.*

THE SIGNIFICANCE OF POSITIVE BIOPSY FINDINGS FOLLOWING IRRADIATION

Even when cancer persists in the follow-up period, 1 to 3 months after treatment, lesions may continue to regress and be permanently controlled. Suit showed in animal tumors that the persistence of histologically intact tumor cells 3 to 6 weeks after irradiation did not indicate the probability of local recurrence, since such cells may be nonviable.[105] The cells may still be capable of diverse metabolic activities, and some may even be able to divide a limited number of times before their progeny die; however, if their capacity for sustained proliferation is lost, they are biologically "dead." Biopsy before 3 months after treatment is generally not recommended unless there is definite progression of cancer, which is a sure sign of treatment failure.

Tumor Size

The probability of tumor control depends on cancer size or, more precisely, on the number of clonogenic cells* present. Cell kill is exponential; that is, each increment of radiation kills the same proportion of cells, not the same absolute number of cells. This is illustrated in the hypothetical situation shown in Figure 13-2. Assume that 500 rad is sufficient to reduce a malignant cell population by 90%. It takes the same dose of irradiation to reduce the cell population from 10^8 to 10^7 cells (i.e., to kill 90,000,000 cells) as it does to reduce the population from 1000 to 100 cells, or 100 to 10 cells (i.e., to kill 900 or 90 cells). Obviously, the larger the volume of cancer, the greater the required dose to achieve tumor control. While this may not seem too difficult a concept, it is one that was disregarded by physicians for many years and continues to be ignored even today by some surgical, medical, and radiation oncologists. A "debulking" of 90%, or even 99%, of gross cancer by either preirradiation surgery or preirradiation chemotherapy may produce an impressive volume reduc-

* A clonogenic cell is one that is capable of regenerating a tumor, that is, of forming a clone.

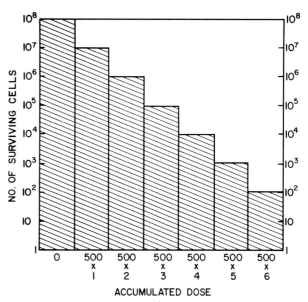

FIG. 13-2. Hypothetical tumor for which a dose of 500 rad is capable of killing 90% of the surviving cells. Since cell killing is exponential, it takes the same dose of irradiation to reduce the population from 10^8 to 10^7 or from 10^7 to 10^6, as it does to reduce the number of surviving cells from 100 to 10, or 10 to 1. A surgical or chemotherapeutic "debulking" that removes 90% (e.g., from 10^{10} down to 10^9 cells) or even 99% (e.g., from 10^{10} down to 10^8 cells) of a gross tumor mass may look impressive clinically but has accomplished little from a radiobiologic standpoint since the population has been reduced by only one or two decades.

tion but achieves little from a radiobiologic standpoint, since it reduces the tumor population by only 1 or 2 decades. In fact, a surgical "debulking" that leaves behind macroscopic disease probably lessens the chance of cure by irradiation. The precise mechanism by which "debulked" cancers are made more difficult to control by irradiation is unknown. At least two possible explanations exist: (1) When a cancer is cut across, tumor cells are disseminated throughout the surgical bed and may be implanted in relatively hypoxic scar tissue where they are less sensitive to irradiation. (2) Alternatively, the remaining cells may find themselves in an environment favorable to growth and begin to proliferate rapidly. The rapidity with which some recurrences are seen following surgery and irradiation in this situation fits well with the latter hypothesis.

Radiation therapists who prescribe a particular tumor dose based on tumor site rather than tumor size also disregard the dose–volume relationship. Such dose prescriptions are still used in some major treatment centers and clinical trials.[65]

The notion that different volumes of cancer require different doses is the basis for the shrinking-field concept of irradiation (Fig. 13-3). The initial treatment volume depends on the tumor size and its regional extensions; all gross and microscopic cancer must be included within the original field(s) if control is to be achieved. After a certain dose, the fields may be reduced in size, since microscopic extensions require less total dose than gross cancer. That

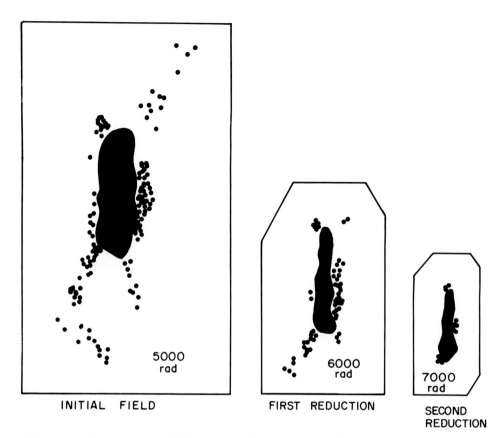

INITIAL FIELD   FIRST REDUCTION   SECOND REDUCTION

FIG. 13-3. The shrinking-field concept of irradiation used in the treatment of gross cancer (*black*) and its microscopic extensions (*dots*). The initial treatment volume covers all gross cancer and generously treats any suspected microscopic extensions. Because small volumes of cancer require less dose to achieve control than larger tumor volumes, the initial fields may be reduced, often at 5000 rad, as in this hypothetical case. The area of moderate tumor infestation receives 6000 rad, then a final reduction is made to boost the gross cancer to 7000 rad or higher. The same concept of applying the greatest amount of treatment to the greatest bulk of cancer is used when combining irradiation and surgery, in which the operation serves as the "boost" treatment to the gross mass and the radiation sterilizes the peripheral tumor aggregates.

is, the dose is distributed in accordance with the number of cancer cells present.

Control of Subclinical Disease

The term *subclinical cancer* refers to tumor deposits that are too small to be detected clinically, despite being present in sites accessible to examination. Such deposits may actually be several millimeters in size but are by definition neither visible nor palpable on physical examination. The existence of subclinical lymph node metastasis has been well documented by the observation that many patients with clinically negative necks will be found to have histologically positive neck specimens if an elective neck dissection is performed or to develop regional nodal recurrence despite control of the primary lesion if no neck treatment is administered. Other patients present with squamous cell carcinoma metastatic to neck lymph nodes and no detectable primary site of origin. If such patients are treated by radical neck dissection alone, the primary site may become apparent after variable amounts of time (see Chapter 16, The Unknown Primary).

ELECTIVE IRRADIATION OF SUBCLINICAL NECK DISEASE

The proportion of patients with squamous cell carcinoma of the head and neck who have cancer in clinically negative necks depends on the tumor site, size, morphology (infiltrative vs. exophytic), histologic grade, and relative density of capillary lymphatics at that site. For most head and neck sites, the incidence is at least 20% and may be as high as 60% to 70% in certain situations (see Table 2-1 in Chapter 2). The usual given dose (5000 rad/5 weeks at D_{max}) for elective lower neck irradiation with cobalt-60 produces a minimum lymph node dose of about 4000 rad to 4500 rad (Fig. 13-4).

Analysis of treatment results of regional lymphatics following irradiation or surgery is complicated by possible further seeding of the neck in patients with uncontrolled primary disease. If the primary lesion does not remain controlled, one cannot distinguish failure of initial neck treatment from failure that is due to further seeding of the lymphatics. At the University of Florida for patients with lesions of the oral cavity, oropharynx, hypopharynx, supraglottic larynx, and nasopharynx who received elective neck irradiation, there were no in-field lymph node failures following 4500 rad to 5000 rad when the primary lesion was controlled.[82] Rarely, patients with very short, thick necks received 6000 rad given dose since it was felt that in these difficult-to-examine patients a small (0.5 cm to 1.0 cm) positive node might escape detection.

Control of subclinical disease by irradiation is not an all or none phenomenon. As in the case of gross cancer, a sigmoid dose-response relationship is apparent for subclinical disease. Following low-dose preoperative irradiation (3000 rad midplane at 200 rad/day, usually from a single ipsilateral field) for squamous cell carcinoma of the pyriform sinus, Marks and co-workers noted a substantial number of failures in the contralateral, initially clinically negative neck that had received a low dose of irradiation.[68] Similar results were noted by Perez and associates in the treatment of tonsillar fossa lesions with preoperative irradiation (Table 13-2).[86] Of 77 patients with T1–T4, N0–N2 disease who received 3000 rad/3 weeks by way of an ipsilateral portal followed by an en bloc radical tonsillectomy and ipsilateral neck dissection, 7 patients (9%) developed failures in the contralateral neck. They estimated that the contralateral neck received 1800-rad tumor dose. In 69 similarly staged patients treated by irradiation alone, the contralateral neck received approximately 5000 rad and no neck failures were observed.

The relationship between probability of control of subclinical metastasis and dose is shown in Table 13-3.[32,51,70] Approximately 70% of subclinical deposits are controlled by 3000 rad to 4000 rad; higher doses control a greater proportion. There is a plateau at approximately 5000 rad, a dose at which failures are exceptional and usually related to geographic miss.[10,32,39,76] Doses higher than 5000 rad are unnecessary.

Control of Gross Cancer

The sigmoid dose-response curve means that a certain dose of irradiation has a certain probability of controlling a lesion of a given size. For example, 2-cm neck nodes are controlled approximately 50% of the time by 5000 rad.[35] Since the shape of the sigmoid curve is steep in its midportion, an increment of only 1500 rad is capable of increasing the

control rate of such nodes to approximately 90%. Further increases to 7000 or even 8000 rad will probably not control 100% of the cancers because the plateau portion of the curve has been reached. Attempts to achieve 100% control by using very high doses will be futile and result in unacceptably high complication rates.

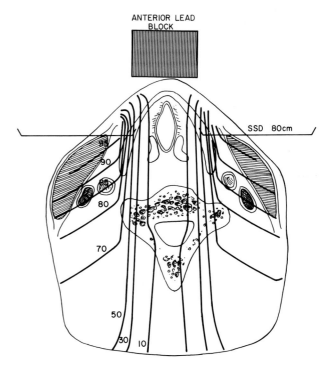

FIG. 13-4. Isodose distribution for cobalt-60 lower neck irradiation. Contour is through the level of the true vocal cords. The SSD is placed on the anterior surface of the sternocleidomastoid muscle opposite the cricoid cartilage. The jugular chain lymph nodes receive a minimum dose that is 80% to 85% of the maximum dose. When 5000 rad is administered to D_{max}, these nodes receive more than 4000 rad. The larynx and spinal cord are shielded by an anterior lead block.

TABLE 13-2. Carcinoma of the Tonsil (T1–T4): Incidence of Failure in the Initially Clinically Negative Contralateral Neck According to Treatment Technique–Mallinckrodt Institute of Radiology

	Failures in Contralateral N0 Neck			
	Irradiation Alone*		Preoperative Irradiation†	
N Stage of Ipsilateral Neck	No. Patients	No. Failures	No. Patients	No. Failures (%)
N0	33	0	34	3 (8%)
N1	23	0	30	3 (10%)
N2	13	0	13	1 (7%)
Total	69	0	77	7 (9%)

* 5000 rad estimated dose to neck.

† 1800 rad/3 weeks estimated dose to neck.

(Adapted from Perez CA, Lee FA, Ackerman LV, Ogura JH, Powers WE: Non-randomized comparison of preoperative irradiation and surgery versus irradiation alone in the management of carcinoma of the tonsil. Am J Roentgenol 126:248–260, 1976. Copyright © 1976, American Roentgen Ray Society)

TABLE 13-3. Efficiency of Elective Neck Irradiation (ENI) for Subclinical Disease by Dose of Irradiation

| Author | Tumor Site | No. Patients | Dose to Neck | Percentage of Patients With N0 → N+ Conversion Following Treatment | | Efficiency* |
				No ENI	ENI	
Fletcher[32]	Oral cavity with N1–N2 ipsilateral neck disease	99	3000–4000 rad/3–4 weeks to contralateral neck	35%†	10%†	71%
Horiuchi[51]	Oral tongue	37	4000 rad/3½–4 weeks	37%	5%	86%
Mendenhall[70]	Oral cavity	40	4500–5000 rad/5 weeks	26%	0‡	100%
Fletcher[32]	Faucial arch with N1–N2 ipsilateral neck disease	82	5000 rad/5 weeks to contralateral neck	30%†	0†	100%

* Efficiency (%) = (1.00 − [failure rate following ENI/failure rate without ENI]) × 100%.

† Failure rate in contralateral N0 neck.

‡ Excludes 1 out-of-field failure.

THE EFFECT OF TISSUE HYPOXIA

The ability of x-rays to kill cells is reduced under conditions of hypoxia. Since tumors tend to outgrow their blood supply, they contain hypoxic areas that may limit the success of radiation therapy.[108] The magnitude of the problem of hypoxia in clinical practice using fractionated therapy is not well known; even large, infected, necrotic tumors may be cured in substantial numbers, suggesting that the problem may be overcome by conventional therapy. During fractionated treatment of most animal tumors, the absolute number of hypoxic cells is not static. Reoxygenation occurs after successive doses.[45] A similar situation likely pertains in human tumors.

Anemia is potentially deleterious.[45] Several observers have noted that anemic patients have a decreased probability of cure following irradiation of squamous cell cancers of the larynx or uterine cervix.[13,30,106] Whether this is secondary to an increased hypoxic cell fraction or is merely due to more advanced cancers in the anemic patients remains controversial. At least two studies suggest that correction of anemia prior to treatment may improve local control.[13,30]

TUMOR RECURRENCE TIMES

Between September 1964 and August 1976, 468 patients with previously untreated squamous cell carcinoma of the oral cavity, oropharynx, nasopharynx, supraglottic larynx, or hypopharynx were treated with curative intent at the University of Florida by external-beam irradiation alone or by external-beam irradiation plus an interstitial radium boost. One hundred sixty-one patients developed in-field primary recurrences following treatment; 155 (96%) of the local recurrences occurred within 24 months after treatment (Fig. 13-5). The greater the tumor volume, the shorter was the median time to recurrence (9 months for T1–T2 and 4½ months for T3–T4 lesions). By 24 months, the cumulative recurrence curve for all stages asymptotically approaches 100%. Two years is therefore an adequate in-

terval of time to assess local control in squamous cell carcinomas of head and neck sites exclusive of the true vocal cord. True glottic lesions tend to recur later than squamous cell carcinomas at other head and neck sites. Fletcher and co-workers, in analyzing 65 recurrent T1–T2 glottic cancers, noted that by 3 years only 74% of the recurrences had appeared; by 7 years 94% of the recurrences were observed, but even at 10 years occasional patients continued to experience failure.[38] It is not possible to distinguish true local recurrence from new primary cancers in such instances; all such late cancers are therefore classified as local recurrence, that is, treatment failure, regardless of when they occur.

Two years is clearly inadequate follow-up for some histologies, especially adenoid cystic carcinoma. All four patients with adenoid cystic carcinoma of the nasal cavity and ethmoid/sphenoid sinuses treated by radical irradiation alone at the University of Florida between 1965 and 1968 developed late recurrences (3½, 4, 5, and 12½ years after treatment).

THE CONCEPT OF LOCAL CONTROL

The practice of using local control as a parameter to assess the efficacy of treatment, either surgery or irradiation, has achieved its greatest popularity only since the 1960s. Prior to that time, 5-year survival was usually regarded as the measure of treatment success. While improved survival is certainly the ultimate goal of therapy, there are so many factors that influence survival rates (e.g., death due to intercurrent disease, second malignancy, distant metastasis, nodal recurrence) that analysis of this factor alone does not adequately gauge the effect of a local treatment. In recent years, analyses of local treatment results have provided considerable insight into the reasons for local failure; such analyses have led to a steady improvement in patient care. Of particular significance have been time–dose analyses, an area in which much work remains to be done.

There remains considerable confusion in the literature

as to what exactly constitutes "local control." The difficulty arises mainly in the interpretation of follow-up intervals. Just because a patient was treated 2 or 5 years before the data were analyzed does *not* mean that the patient has a minimum 2- or 5-year follow-up for local control analysis. Perhaps an example can best illustrate the point: The local control rate with a minimum 2-year follow-up for six patients who received radiation (or surgery) 3 to 9 years ago is presented in Table 13-4; the six patients, how long ago

they were treated, and the end results are listed. There were two local failures (patients 2 and 6), one before and one after 2 years. Patients 1 and 3 are not evaluable for local control with 2-year minimum follow-up since they survived only 1 and 23 months, respectively; they can be scored neither as "local controls" nor "local failures." Patients 4 and 5 were the only patients who were locally controlled for a 2-year minimum. The initial local control rate with 2-year minimum follow-up is, therefore, 2/4 or

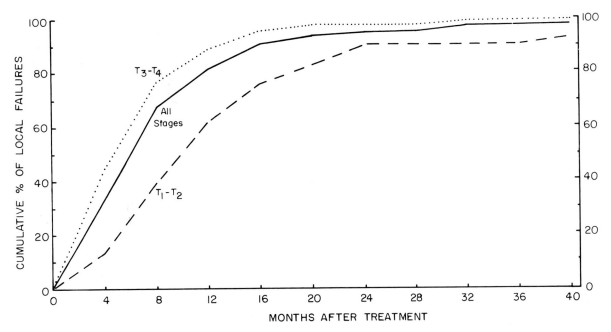

FIG. 13-5. Cumulative recurrence rates plotted as a function of time after treatment. Ninety-six percent (155/161) of all local recurrences became manifest by 2 years after treatment. The median recurrence time for advanced lesions is less than for early ones. (Data from Parsons JT, Bova FJ, Million RR: A reevaluation of split-course technique for squamous cell carcinoma of the head and neck. Int J Radiat Oncol Biol Phys 6:1645–1652, 1980)

TABLE 13-4.	Method of Calculation of Initial Local Control Rate* With 2 Years Minimum Follow-up	
Patient	**Treated (Years Ago)**	**Results**
1	3	Dead due to myocardial infarction at 1 month; no local recurrence.
2	3	Local failure at 3 months; tumor resected; no evidence of disease at 2 years, 9 months.
3	4	Dead of distant metastasis at 23 months; no local recurrence.
4	6	Dead due to cerebrovascular accident at 3 years; no local recurrence.
5	9	No evidence of disease at 9 years.
6	7	Local recurrence at 2½ years; dead of cancer.

* Local control with minimum 2-year follow-up is 2/4 (50%). Although only two patients had local treatment failures the local control rate is *not* 4/6 (66%). See text for discussion.

50% (patients 4 and 5/patients 2, 4, 5, and 6). To count patients 1 and 3 as "local controls," as is frequently done in the medical literature, falsely elevates the local control rate to 4/6 or 66%. It is critical that people involved in data interpretation be aware of these differences in reporting since it is the latter method of calculation, which is not recommended, that is used most commonly.

TIME–DOSE (ISOEFFECT) DATA FOR SQUAMOUS CELL CARCINOMA OF VARIOUS HEAD AND NECK SITES

It is well known that when the treatment time is prolonged, the total dose must be increased to produce the same effect. A popular means of presenting complex clinical time–dose relationships is with isoeffect curves or lines. For each tumor (patient) within a homogeneous group of cancers, one displays on a two-dimensional graph the tumor dose in rad (ordinate) versus the overall treatment time in days or number of fractions in which the treatment was given (abscissa); a log–log scale is generally used. If treatment is administered 5 days per week, then the total treatment time is closely related to the number of fractions. For some fractionation schemes, however, there is little correlation between the fraction number and the overall treatment time. When trying to demonstrate a time–dose relationship, it is essential that lesions be grouped according to tumor volume, since larger tumors require progressively higher doses. Generally, separate analyses are performed for each T stage.

Equal tumor effect may be obtained by a variety of combinations of total dose and overall treatment time, and the line that connects these points of equal effect on the graph is the iso-, or equal, effect line. Theoretically, one can draw lines that describe treatment schedules likely to yield control rates ranging anywhere from 0 to over 90%. Effects other than tumor control (e.g., acute normal tissue reactions or late complications) can also be expressed on these time–dose plots; the curves that describe these effects may or may not be parallel to each other or to the tumor effect curves. A treatment plan is generally chosen by weighing the probability of tumor control against the probability of producing a serious complication.

Time–dose data are now available for a number of tumor systems and are helpful in the formulation of treatment plans. It is important to recognize that the data are generally available over rather narrow ranges of time and dose; attempts to extrapolate the isoeffect lines beyond the zones for which there are available clinical data are unjustified and, as will be seen in succeeding sections, unsafe.

In the time–dose scatter distributions that follow, patients who had treatment fail because part of the tumor was not within the treatment volume (geographic miss) have been excluded, since treatment of these patients would fail no matter what the dose. A true geographic miss is often difficult to identify; although clinical charts, port films, photographs of the patient in treatment position, anatomical diagrams, and pretreatment photographs of the lesion are all helpful on retrospective review, they do not completely

FIG. 13-6. Time–dose scatter distribution for 13 patients with T1 squamous cell carcinoma of the supraglottic larynx treated at the University of Florida (UF) between October 1964 and November 1977 by continuous-course (9 patients) or split-course (4 patients) irradiation. Superimposed on the figure are solid lines that divide the time–dose plot into several dose ranges (I–V) for which data are available from the M. D. Anderson Hospital (MDAH).[95] The inset to the figure combines the University of Florida and M. D. Anderson Hospital time–dose information and shows that there is a generally increasing rate of control within successive dose ranges. Doses on the order of 6000 rad/6 weeks to 6500 rad/6½ to 7 weeks will control nearly all T1 lesions. The only recurrence in the University of Florida patients occurred after a very protracted split-course treatment.

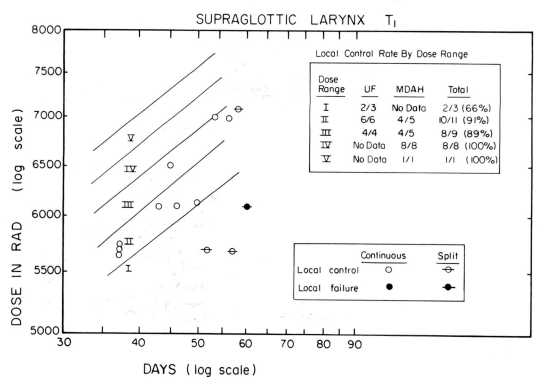

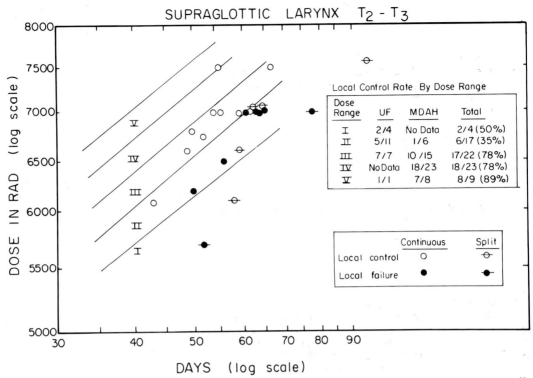

FIG. 13-7. Time–dose scatter distribution for 23 patients with T2–T3 squamous cell carcinoma of the supraglottic larynx treated at the University of Florida (UF) between October 1964 and November 1977 by continuous-course (16 patients) or split-course (7 patients) irradiation. Superimposed on the figure are solid lines that divide the time–dose plot into several dose ranges (I–V) for which data are available from the M. D. Anderson Hospital (MDAH).[95] The inset to the figure combines the University of Florida and M. D. Anderson Hospital time–dose information and shows generally increasing rates of control within successive dose ranges. Doses on the order of 7000 rad to 7500 rad/7 to 8 weeks will control approximately 85% of the lesions for which radiation has been selected as the primary modality. See text for a discussion of selection factors.

rule out the possibility of geographic miss due to unsuspected, subclinical extensions of cancer or errors in actual day-to-day delivery of the treatment.

SUPRAGLOTTIC LARYNX

Time–dose data for T1 lesions of the supraglottic larynx treated at the University of Florida between October 1964 and November 1977 are shown in Figure 13-6. The figure also incorporates data from the M. D. Anderson Hospital, where a clear-cut dose-response curve was elicited for supraglottic larynx cancers.[95] The data from both institutions indicate that a high percentage of cases will be controlled by 6000 rad/6 weeks to 6500 rad/6½ to 7 weeks.

University of Florida time–dose data for T2–T3 lesions of the supraglottic larynx are shown in Figure 13-7; also shown are the dose ranges for which local control data are available from M. D. Anderson Hospital. Although the control rates appear rather high following irradiation alone, it is important to realize that those cancers on which the data are based represent a select subset of the entire population of T2–T3 cases. At both institutions, those lesions that have been treated by irradiation alone have generally been exophytic. Many of the deeply infiltrative cancers and locally advanced T2–T3 lesions are treated by an op-

eration.[44] In some cases, the patient is reevaluated after 5000 rad; if a deeply infiltrative or ulcerative tumor component persists, then radiation therapy is stopped and operation is undertaken. These selection processes eliminate some unfavorable cases from the group of patients receiving irradiation alone. If one so selects T2–T3 cases for radical irradiation, then control rates of approximately 85% are obtained by doses of 7000 rad to 7500 rad/7 to 8 weeks. Occasional patients with unfavorable lesions who either refuse surgery or who cannot undergo an operation for medical reasons are irradiated by default, tending to somewhat offset the selection of a favorable subgroup.

GLOTTIC LARYNX

Most investigators have not been able to demonstrate the sought-for relationship between time and dose for control of early vocal cord cancer. This is partly because the individual stage groupings comprise patients with considerable heterogeneity. (See Chapter 19, Larynx). A small-volume T2 lesion on one cord with minimal extension to the ventricle and false cord and normal mobility has a much better control rate following irradiation than a bulky T2 lesion that involves both cords, with extensive subglottic and supraglottic extension and partial cord fixation. The vocal cord lesions have been separated into prognostic groups based on extent of tumor in order to analyze time–dose relationships.[21]

Minimum tumor dose versus number of treatments for vocal cord cancers with similar tumor volume is analyzed in Figures 13-8 through 13-11. There is a trend in all groups toward improved local control with higher daily fraction size and shorter overall time.

A relationship between fraction size and rate of control of vocal cord cancer has been observed by others. For stage I cancers of the larynx, Kok, in The Hague, delivered a minimum tumor dose of 6300 rad, 5 fractions/week, but

FIG. 13-8. Scatter distribution of minimum dose versus number of fractions (5 fractions/week, continuous-course irradiation) for 85 T1 "nonbulky" carcinomas of one or both vocal cords. Excluded are "bulky" (large exophytic and/or infiltrative) lesions. The dashed lines represent treatment schemes at 215 rad and 225 rad/day, respectively. These lines have been added for ease of interpretation of the data and are not meant to represent isoeffect lines. The two open circles indicated by arrows represent clusterings of 38 and 14 locally controlled patients, respectively, who received the same dose and fraction number. The shorter treatment schemes (using larger daily fractions) tended to produce the best results. The control rate was 35/35 patients (100%) among patients who received greater than or equal to 225 rad/fraction. In the 215 rad to 224 rad/fraction group, 41/44 patients (93%) had local control of their disease, and in the group receiving less than or equal to 214 rad/fraction, control was achieved in 5 of 6 patients (83%). The total doses in the three groups were similar. (University of Florida data; patients treated 10/64–10/77; analysis 10/79)

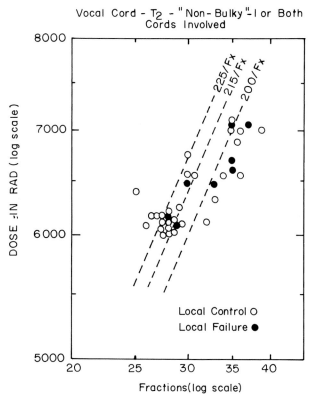

FIG. 13-9. Scatter distribution of minimum dose versus number of fractions (5 fractions/week, continuous-course irradiation) for 36 T2 "nonbulky" vocal cord carcinomas with one or both cords involved. Excluded are T2 "bulky" lesions. The dashed lines have been added for ease of interpretation of data and are not meant to represent isoeffect lines. Protracted treatment schedules using small doses/fraction produced poor results despite the fact that these patients generally received higher total doses. Local control was achieved in 6/6 patients (100%) who received greater than or equal to 225 rad/fraction; 11/13 patients (85%) in the 215 rad to 224 rad/fraction range; 4/6 patients (66%) with 200 rad to 214 rad/fraction; and 7/11 patients (63%) with less than 200 rad/fraction. (University of Florida data; patients treated 10/64–10/77; analysis 10/79)

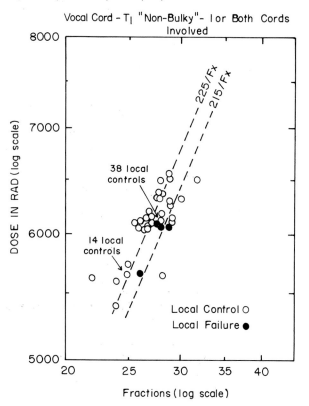

varied the daily dose (and thus the overall treatment time) from 175 rad (×36 fractions) to 190 rad (×33 fractions) to 210 rad (×30 fractions). The 175 rad/fraction treatment was abandoned after treating only 3 patients since only one tumor was controlled. The control rate in the 190 rad/fraction group was 12/14 (86%) and was 4/4 (100%) in the 210 rad/day group. I agree with his conclusion that "a difference in fraction-dose of only 10% can be decisive whether or not there will be a lethal effect on tumor."[59] It is probable that in the more protracted treatment schemes, tumor cell repopulation was significant.

At the University of California, San Francisco, in the late 1950s, emphasis was placed on low daily doses for early vocal cord cancer in order to avoid acute mucosal reactions.[12,109] In general, 180 rad/fraction to total doses of 5500 rad to 7000 rad were administered,[119] but in many cases the daily dose was closer to 160 rad.[12] With these protracted treatment schedules, the local failure rates for T1 (20%) and T2 (48%) lesions were substantial.

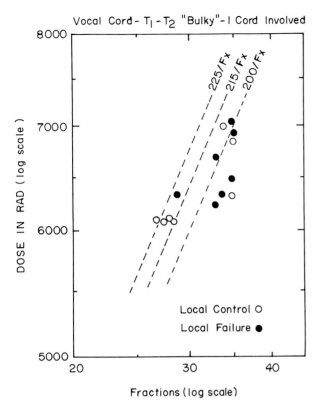

of larger fields often meant that the 4- or 5-week treatment schemes were not practical because of marked acute reactions and late fibrosis, but even so, published time–dose data indicate that many T3–T4 lesions received more than 1000 rad/week. Their control rates following irradiation alone for oropharyngeal lesions have been excellent; a substantial number of the patients in whom treatment was successful received treatment in a short overall time at greater than 1000 rad/week. It is of particular interest to examine the treatment results in two patient groups: one that received high doses per fraction for early lesions (approximately 6000 rad/4 to 5 weeks) and the other that received high-dose treatments for T3 and T4 lesions at weekly dose rates of greater than 1000 rad. Treatment results at the M. D. Anderson Hospital (1954–1973) in patients who received 5500 rad to 6500 rad/<5 weeks for early carcinomas of the oropharynx are given in Table 13-5.[6,43,96,97,102] Although no time–dose analysis is available for the soft palate group, the T1–T2 patients generally received 5500 rad to 6000 rad/4 to 5 weeks;[35] there were no failures in 48 T1–T2 palate lesions.[43] Admittedly, the patients in Table 13-5 had mostly early lesions, and often the smallest lesions within a stage were chosen for short treatment courses.[102] Notwithstanding this fact, the control results (99/103 or 96%) are exceptional. The factors of selection (i.e., general medical condition, amount of neck disease, primary tumor volume, and gross characteristics of the primary lesion) contribute to the probability of local control and therefore 5500 rad to 6500 rad/<5 weeks will *not* produce this high rate of control across the board, although the control rate will be good.

For the more advanced cancers, 5500 rad to 6500 rad/5 weeks will generally not produce satisfactory rates of control;[97,102] higher doses are required. The M. D. Anderson Hospital data suggest that fraction sizes greater than 200

FIG. 13-10. Scatter distribution of minimum dose versus number of fractions (5 fractions/week, continuous course irradiation) for 14 T1–T2 "bulky" (large exophytic and/ or infiltrative) carcinomas of the true vocal cord with only one cord involved. The dashed lines have been added for ease of interpretation of data and are not meant to represent isoeffect lines. Protracted treatment schedules using small doses/fraction produced poor results despite the fact that these patients generally received higher total doses. Local control was achieved in 4/5 patients (80%) who received greater than or equal to 215 rad/fraction; 1/3 patients (33%) in the group receiving 200 rad to 214 rad/fraction; and in 2/6 patients (33%) receiving less than 200 rad/day. (University of Florida data; patients treated 10/64–10/77; analysis 10/79)

FIG. 13-11. Dose versus number of fractions (5 fractions/ week) for 12 patients with T3 squamous cell carcinoma of the true vocal cord treated at the University of Florida between October 1966 and May 1978. The solid lines represent treatments at 180 and 200 rad/fraction, respectively, and have been added for ease of interpretation of data; they are not meant to represent isoeffect lines. For each range of total dose, the time factor is seen to be important. There were no instances of chondronecrosis or severe edema among cured patients.

The treatment of T3 vocal cord cancer is highly individualized (see Chapter 19, Larynx); at the Princess Margaret Hospital, Harwood and co-workers have shown a clear dose-response relationship.[47] The University of Florida data for a small number of patients are shown in Figure 13-11.

OROPHARYNX

In the treatment of oropharyngeal cancers in the early megavoltage years at M. D. Anderson Hospital, the generally recommended plan was 6000 rad/4 weeks when field sizes were less than 50 sq cm, 6000 rad/5 weeks when 50- to 80- sq cm portals were used, and 6000 rad/6 weeks plus a boost when portals were over 80 sq cm.[102] As the irradiation technique evolved through the years, larger treatment portals were used, since there were some marginal recurrences with the small fields and more generous coverage of the subdigastric nodes was desired. The use

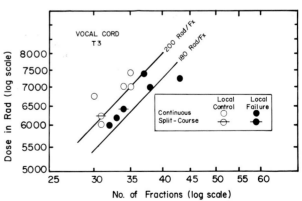

TABLE 13-5. Local Control Following Megavoltage Irradiation of Early Oropharyngeal Carcinomas Receiving Approximately 5500 rad to 6500 rad/<5 Weeks—M. D. Anderson Hospital

T Stage	Glossotonsillar Sulcus[96] (1954–1972)	Base of Tongue[102] (1954–1971)	Tonsillar Fossa[97] (1954–1968)	Anterior Tonsillar Pillar/Retromolar Trigone[6] (1954–1973)	Soft Palate[43] (1954–1967)	Total All Sites (%)
T1		5/6	5/5		18/18	28/29 (97%)
T2		2/3	4/4		30/30	36/37 (97%)
T3		4/4				4/4 (100%)
T2–T3	3/3					3/3 (100%)
T1–T3				28/30		28/30 (93%)

Note: No time–dose scatter distribution for soft palate lesions has been published. Patients generally received 5500 rad to 6000 rad/4 to 5 weeks.[35]

TABLE 13-6. Local Control of T3–T4 Squamous Cell Carcinomas of the Tonsillar Fossa (1954–1968)* and Base of Tongue (1954–1971)† Treated With High-Dose Megavoltage Irradiation at ≧1000 rad/Week —M. D. Anderson Hospital

T Stage	Tonsillar Fossa Lesions Receiving >6500 rad at ≧1000 rad/wk	Base of Tongue Lesions Receiving ≧7000 rad at ≧1000 rad/wk
T3		10/12 (83%)
T4		2/2 (100%)
T3–T4	14/16 (88%)	
Total	14/16 (88%)	12/14 (86%)

* Data from Shukovsky LJ, Fletcher GH: Time–dose and tumor volume relationships in the irradiation of squamous cell carcinoma of the tonsillar fossa. Radiology 107:621–626, 1973.

† Data from Spanos WJ Jr, Shukovsky LJ, Fletcher GH: Time, dose, and tumor volume relationships in irradiation of squamous cell carcinomas of the base of the tongue. Cancer 37:2591–2599, 1976.

rad/day will control a higher proportion of T3 and T4 lesions than slower fractionation schemes. The use of large daily fractions is a double-edged sword, and one must balance the higher control rate against acute reactions and late complications, which are also more severe. Very high rates of control for T3–T4 lesions of the tonsillar fossa and base of the tongue that receive greater than 6500 rad and greater than or equal to 7000 rad, respectively, at weekly dose rates of greater than or equal to 1000 rad are shown in Table 13-6. Few clinical data at these ranges of time and dose are available from the University of Florida. Only three patients with T3–T4 tonsillar fossa or base of tongue lesions have received treatment to these doses at greater than 1000 rad/week; two of three were controlled.

TONSILLAR REGION

University of Florida time–dose data for T1 and T2 squamous cell carcinomas of the tonsillar region, respectively, following continuous-course external beam irradiation are shown in Figures 13-12 and 13-13. In general, the doses have been lower and/or the treatment times longer than those employed at M. D. Anderson Hospital. The only T1 failure occurred after a dose less than 5000 rad.

In Figure 13-13, it is seen that only one University of

Florida T2 lesion was treated at a dose above the M. D. Anderson Hospital 100% exclusion line, where control was achieved in 9/9 patients. A line has been drawn below all the University of Florida data points. For patients treated in the time–dose ranges between the two lines, the University of Florida control rate was 71%, which is very close to the M. D. Anderson Hospital control rate (73%) in this same range of time and dose. This is what would be expected from the shape of the sigmoid dose-response curve.

For T3 lesions of the tonsillar region treated with continuous-course external-beam irradiation alone at the University of Florida, all patients were treated in times and doses below the M. D. Anderson Hospital exclusion line; the University of Florida local control was poor (40%), but as was seen for T2 lesions, the control rate did not differ greatly from the M. D. Anderson Hospital control rate (53%) for T3–T4 lesions treated in the same range of time and dose as University of Florida patients.[97] The overall better results in T3–T4 lesions at M. D. Anderson Hospital were due to more aggressive therapy.

BASE OF TONGUE

University of Florida time–dose data for 22 T2–T3 squamous cell carcinomas of the base of tongue are given in

Figure 13-14.[83] All plotted points lie below the M. D. Anderson Hospital 86% isoeffect line, but the control rates are still quite good for continuous-course irradiation (12/13 or 92%). Split-course irradiation produced poor results, despite doses similar to those given by continuous course.

SOFT PALATE

University of Florida time–dose data for 27 T1–T3 soft palate patients following irradiation are shown in Figure 13-15.

PYRIFORM SINUS

Time-dose data for T1 and T2–T3 pyriform sinus patients, respectively, who received radical irradiation at the University of Florida are presented in Figures 13-16 and 13-17.[75] There is a factor of selection in some T2–T3 patients accepted for radical irradiation; exophytic lesions, especially those of the upper hypopharynx, were often chosen for irradiation, while many infiltrative lesions, and particularly those involving the inferior recess, were treated by operation. A few patients whose tumors showed little response at 5000 rad underwent operation. An understanding of these selection factors is important in the interpretation of the dose-response data. In Figure 13-16, a line has been arbitrarily drawn between 6000 rad/45 days (6½ weeks) and 6500 rad/54 days (7½ weeks), a range in which a high control rate was observed. In Figure 13-17, the solid line is drawn between 6500 rad/7 weeks and 7000 rad/8 weeks; there were no failures in the time–dose range above the line. The dashed line on Figure 13-17 is the line for T1 cancer and is approximately 400 rad lower than the T2–T3 line.

POSTERIOR PHARYNGEAL WALL

Time–dose data for patients treated at the University of Florida for T2–T3 squamous cell carcinomas of the posterior pharyngeal wall are shown in Figure 13-18.

ALTERED FRACTIONATION SCHEMES

The relationship between time and dose may be altered by (1) changing the instantaneous dose rate (i.e., the rad/minute during an individual treatment); (2) varying the overall treatment time (i.e., the number of days between the first and last treatment); or (3) varying the time (hours or days) between successive doses of irradiation. Despite considerable preoccupation with time–dose relationships in radiation therapy, there are still no generally accepted optimum treatment schedules. The literature is replete with clinical trials, retrospective reviews, and experiments in which nonstandard fractionation schemes have been used in the treatment of malignancy. The data are confusing and often conflicting. In order to understand the rationale for altering a fractionation scheme, one must first have some appreciation of the radiobiologic basis for using fractionated treatment.

When treatment is given in many fractions over a few weeks, a higher dose is necessary to accomplish a given effect than when treatment is given in a few fractions in a few days. The increase is due to the following factors:

1. *Repair of sublethal injury*, which has been demonstrated in a wide variety of *in vivo* and *in vitro* sys-

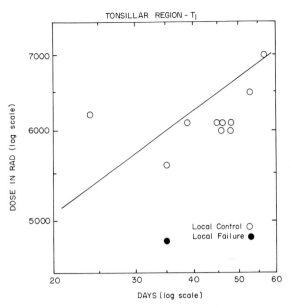

FIG. 13-12. Time–dose scatter distribution for 11 patients with T1 squamous cell carcinoma of the tonsillar region treated with continuous-course external-beam irradiation at the University of Florida between October 1964 and August 1976. The line represents the line above which M. D. Anderson Hospital had 100% local control. The patients at the University of Florida received similar total doses, but the overall treatment times have been longer.

FIG. 13-13. Time–dose scatter distribution for 15 patients with T2 tonsillar lesions treated with continuous-course external-beam irradiation at the University of Florida (UF) between October 1964 and January 1978. The top line (*dotted*) is the M. D. Anderson Hospital (MDAH) exclusion line above which local control was obtained in 9/9 of their patients.[97] The solid line is drawn just below all the University of Florida successes and failures. In the region between the dotted and solid lines, local control was achieved in 10/14 (71%) University of Florida patients, which corresponds closely to the result at the M. D. Anderson Hospital where 14/19 (73%) patients had their disease controlled within the same time–dose range.

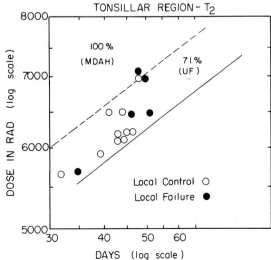

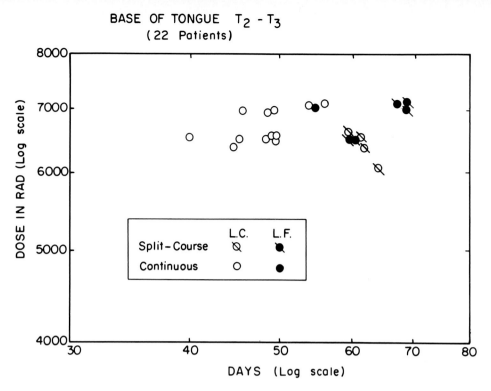

FIG. 13-14. Time–dose scatter distribution for 22 T2–T3 squamous cell carcinomas of the base of the tongue treated at the University of Florida between September 1964 and September 1977. The results of split-course treatment were poor. (*L.C.*, local control; *L.F.*, local failure)

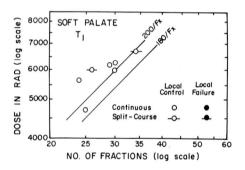

A

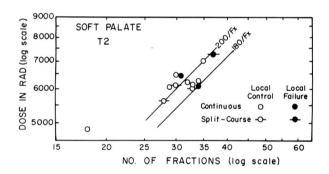

B

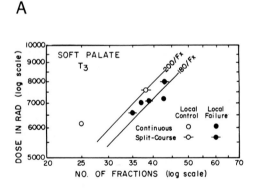

C

FIG. 13-15. Dose versus number of fractions for squamous cell carcinoma of the soft palate treated at the University of Florida between October 1964 and April 1979. The solid lines represent treatments administered at 180 or 200 rad/fraction and have been added for ease of interpretation of the data; they are not meant to be isoeffect lines. (*A*) Stage T1. (*B*) Stage T2. (*C*) Stage T3.

tems. The characteristic shape of a survival curve for mammalian cells is shown in Figure 13-19. Cell death following radiation is believed to be due to the inactivation of certain "targets" within cells; the shape of the curve is usually explained on the basis of two different mechanisms of cell killing. Death that occurs on the initial (shallow slope) part of the curve (*i.e.,* the "shoulder") is generally believed to be due to a single lethal "hit" of a nonrepairable target within the cell. At greater fractional doses, a major cause of cell death is the accumulation of damage to a critical number of repairable targets; until a sufficient number of such targets within the cell have been inactivated, damage by the latter mechanism may be "sublethal" and repairable by cellular processes. Nonrepairable single-hit injury continues at all doses but is largely overshadowed by multiple-hit killing at higher doses. The final (steep) slope of the survival curve represents the sum of both modes of killing.[117]

2. The effect of *repopulation* of cells is important during fractionated treatment. Repopulation may be espe-

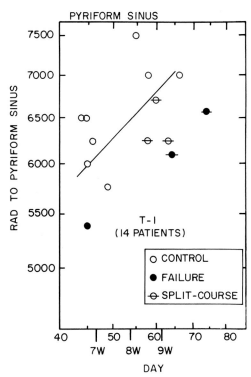

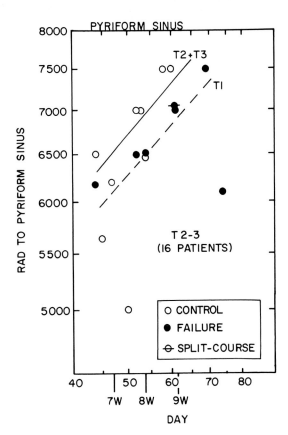

FIG. 13-16. Time–dose scatter distribution for 14 T1 squamous cell carcinomas of the pyriform sinus treated at the University of Florida between October 1964 and April 1978 (analysis, April 1980). An arbitrary line has been drawn between 6000 rad/6½ weeks and 6500/7½ weeks; all three local failures were at least 500 rad below this line, one after a dose of only 5300 rad and the other two following very protracted (>9 weeks) split-course treatments. (Million RR, Cassisi NJ: Radical irradiation for carcinoma of the pyriform sinus. Laryngoscope 91:439–450, 1981)

FIG. 13-17. Time–dose scatter distribution for 10 T2 and 6 T3 squamous cell carcinomas of the pyriform sinus treated at the University of Florida between October 1964 and April 1978 (analysis, April 1980). The solid line connects 6500 rad/7 weeks and 7000 rad/8 weeks. There were no local failures above this line. The dashed line is the line from Figure 13-16 for T1 pyriform sinus lesions; it is approximately 400 below the T2 and T3 line. See text for important discussion of patient selection factors and suitability for radical irradiation. (Million RR, Cassisi NJ: Radical irradiation for carcinoma of the pyriform sinus. Laryngoscope 91:439–450, 1981)

cially significant under certain conditions, such as when using very small fractions that lead to unduly prolonged overall treatment times; when intervals between treatments are prolonged; or during the rest interval of a split-course regimen.[117] Tumors that are rapidly growing are more apt to undergo repopulation during treatment and justify the use of shortened treatment schedules (*e.g.*, by twice-daily fractionation).

Other factors tend to offset 1 and 2:

3. *Redistribution.* Cells in different phases of the cell cycle differ in their sensitivity to radiation (Fig. 13-20). Each dose fraction kills sensitive-phase cells preferentially, leaving behind a relatively resistant subpopulation. Fractionation gives these relatively resistant surviving cells opportunity to pass into more sensitive phases of the cell cycle, thereby sensitizing cycling tissues such as the tumor.

4. *Reoxygenation.* In the absence of oxygen, it is necessary to give a higher dose of radiation to produce the same amount of cell kill as when oxygen is present. During a fractionated course of treatment, hypoxic cells (presumably present in or near necrotic

FIG. 13-18. Dose versus number of fractions for 19 patients with T2–T3 squamous cell carcinomas of the posterior pharyngeal wall treated at the University of Florida between October 1964 and March 1980. Reference lines for treatments administered at 180 and 190 rad/fraction have been added for ease of interpretation of the data. These lines are not isoeffect lines. The best results were obtained in continuous-course patients who received treatment at greater than 190 rad/fraction. More protracted continuous-course treatments and split-course treatments produced poor results.

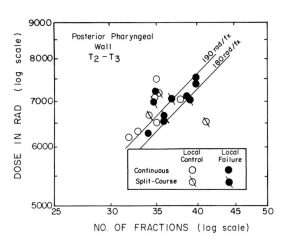

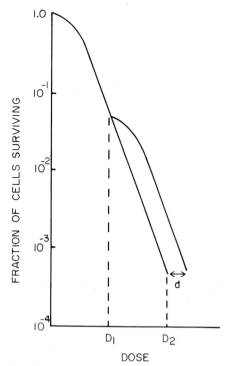

FIG. 13-19. Mammalian cell survival curve on a semilog plot. On the "shoulder" portion of the curve, sublethal injury is being accumulated; this irradiation is less efficient on a rad for rad basis than irradiation on the steep portion of the curve. If, instead of dose D_2, one gives D_1 and waits a sufficient amount of time (a few hours) before again irradiating the tumor, the shoulder must be repeated. To produce the same surviving fraction as produced by D_2, an additional amount of irradiation (d) is required. Dose d is the amount of irradiation that is "wasted" by fractionation.

tumor areas) become better oxygenated secondary to tumor shrinkage, alterations in the metabolic requirements that occur after a dose or radiation, and possibly other factors; this results in sensitization of cells that were previously relatively resistant. The degree to which hypoxic tumor cells impose limits on our ability to cure human cancers with irradiation is unknown; it may be that reoxygenation during fractionated irradiation is sufficient to overcome the problem in most instances.

Manipulation of time–dose relationships is usually done for one of two reasons:

1. *Convenience.* From a practical standpoint, both patient and physician would like for treatment to be completed in as short a time as is consistent with good results. Most clinical investigations have involved delivery of a reduced number of high-dose fractions, or occasionally even single-dose therapy. Such treatment is less expensive, there is less interruption of normal daily activities, and the work load in a busy radiation therapy department is reduced. A few high-dose fractions are also frequently used in experimental trials with hyperbaric oxygen or hypoxic cell sensitizers such as misonidazole. Since the hyperbaric tank is cumbersome in clinical practice, limitation of the number of treatments is a practical (but not necessarily therapeutic) advantage. Since

misonidazole has its greatest sensitizing effect when present in high concentration, and such drug doses cannot be given daily because of neurotoxicity, treatment with fewer fractions is also common when this agent is used.

2. *Improvement in the therapeutic ratio.* The fractionation schedule used in most departments consists of five 180-rad to 200-rad treatments per week. Such treatment may be suitable in many clinical circumstances but is probably not optimum for every cancer. Altered treatment schemes have been devised in order to increase the number of treatment fractions so that the probability of irradiating tumor cells in a sensitive phase is increased. Other schedules attempt to minimize the effect of hypoxia by improving tissue oxygenation or by decreasing the oxygen enhancement ratio (OER)*. Shortening the overall treatment time may offset the effect of tumor cell proliferation during a course of treatment, thereby improving control rates of rapidly growing tumors. Decreasing the size of each fraction decreases the incidence of late complications.

The Calculation of "Biologically Equivalent" Treatment Schedules

Radiation therapists have for many years sought to devise abbreviated treatment schedules that would produce end results "equivalent" to conventional fractionation schemes that use 5 fractions per week. A number of methods have been developed to predict these equivalent doses, the best known of which is the nominal standard dose (NSD) formula of Ellis.[29] Although the NSD concept has never been used at the University of Florida, I will discuss here its

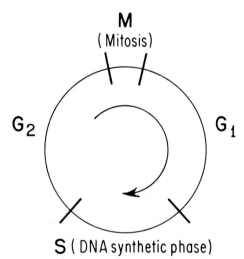

FIG. 13-20. Cell cycle for mammalian cells. G2 and M are most sensitive to irradiation. Late S is most resistant, while G1 to early S are intermediate in sensitivity. (Hall EJ: Radiobiology for the Radiologist, 2nd ed, p 114. Hagerstown, MD, Harper & Row, 1978)

* The oxygen enhancement ratio (OER) is the ratio of doses required to produce the same biologic effect under conditions of hypoxia and aeration. For x- and γ-rays, the value of the OER is 2.5 to 3.0.[45]

utility and associated problems because it has achieved considerable popularity; the treatment of thousands of patients has been altered by use or misuse of the Ellis NSD equation.

The NSD equation is itself mathematically and conceptually complex. It has been estimated that, in the hands of clinicians, it is misused about half the time.[80] Because of its complexity, Orton and Ellis produced tables based on a mathematical simplification of the NSD concept.[81] These tables contain TDF (time, dose, fractionation) factors whereby various fractionation schemes might be compared or equated. By using these tables, clinicians no longer had to perform complex mathematical manipulations. In principle, one could devise any number of treatments that would result in the "same biologic endpoint." For instance, 6300 rad/28 fractions/5½ weeks (5 fractions/week) should, according to the TDF tables, be equivalent to 3720 rad/4 fractions/4 weeks (1 fraction/week), or to 4600 rad/10 fractions/3½ weeks (3 fractions/per week). As we shall see, such extrapolations beyond the range of available clinical data are ill advised and dangerous.

Consequences of Altered Dose Fractionation: The Dissociation Between Acute and Late Effects

In 1962, at the M. D. Anderson Hospital, the treatment schedule for breast cancer was changed from 5 fractions/week to 3 fractions/week; cobalt-60 was used in both patient groups. By adjusting the number of treatments given with bolus, it was possible to produce identical acute skin reactions in the two treatment groups. Despite equal acute reactions, the late effects for the two regimens differed markedly. Late complications in the 3 fraction/week group were "horrendous".[107] Subseqently, a number of other clinical investigators have shown a large increase in late complications, with little or no difference in acute reactions, when treatment regimens were changed to fewer, larger-dose fractions.[107]

The consequences of altered-dose fractionation have also been studied in the laboratory. Withers and co-workers performed fractionation studies on pig skin,[118] which qualitatively and quantitatively responds to radiation in a manner similar to human skin.[45] Treatments were with cobalt-60; one group of animals received 2 and the other received 5 fractions per week. Acute reactions were subjectively graded (0–10) and ranged from no reaction to dry

desquamation, moist desquamation, or frank ulceration; late response was physically measured based on the degree of skin contraction produced by the irradiation. The fact that acute and late reactions are dissociated is shown in Table 13-7. The 5 fraction/week group had more severe acute reactions, but considerably less severe late change than the 2 fraction/week group. Because of the dissociation between acute and late sequelae, the NSD formula obviously cannot be simultaneously applied to both, as has sometimes been assumed.

The possibility of exceeding normal tissue tolerance must always be recognized when using a few high-dose fractions. Abbreviated treatment schedules are best suited for palliation of advanced cancers in patients whose expected survival time is short.

Treatment With 1 or 2 High-Dose Fractions

The idea of treating cancers with a single massive dose of irradiation was developed in the early years (1900–1920s) of radiation therapy;[4] the largest possible dose in the shortest time was administered in hopes of producing a caustic effect or slough of tissues analogous to a surgical excision. Although the technique was generally abandoned, there have been sporadic reports through the years by therapists who have continued to experiment with the technique. In 1965, Andrews reported results of large single-dose treatment in 20 patients with head and neck squamous cell carcinomas.[1] Most (16/20) of the patients had stage I through III disease. The dose varied from 2000 to 2750 R (mode 2500 R) and was administered with megavoltage (2 MeV) equipment. Six of the 20 patients were cured (4 of the 6 had T1–T2 N0 lesions of the buccal mucosa, tonsil, or glottic larynx), but complications were frequent, severe, and sometimes fatal (Table 13-8). Maintenance of adequate nutrition was difficult in all of the patients because of extraordinarily severe acute reactions.

Rubenfeld, at Bellevue Hospital, New York City, reported a similar negative experience with rapid fractionation for head and neck cancer.[90] He gave 3000 R in 2 fractions, administered on consecutive days, with orthovoltage x-rays. The patients developed very severe skin and mucosal reactions that often failed to heal. Treatment complications resulted in the death of two patients and led to abandonment of the technique.

Rapid fractionation schemes in other tumor systems have also produced unexpected, severe complications.[2,26]

TABLE 13-7. Dissociation Between Acute and Late Response of Pig Skin to Cobalt-60 Irradiation.

6½-Week Treatment Schedules With Equivalent TDF		Acute Response		Late Response	
5 Fx/Week*	2 Fx/Week†	5 Fx/Week (grade)‡	2 Fx/Week (grade)‡	5 Fx/Week (grade)‡	2 Fx/Week (grade)‡
32 × 180 rad	13 × 360 rad	4.3 ± 0.45	2.4 ± 0.24	2.6 ± 1.2	5.1 ± 0.75
32 × 200 rad	13 × 385 rad	4.3 ± 0.98	2.5 ± 0.13	3.0 ± 0.21	5.0 ± 0.30
32 × 220 rad	13 × 435 rad	4.8 ± 0.88	2.7 ± 0.17	3.4 ± 0.41	5.5 ± 1.1

* TDF values for 5 fractions/week treatment: 90, 105, 122.

† TDF values for 2 fractions/week treatment: 92, 102, 123.

‡ See text for explanation of grade (0 = least response, 10 = greatest response).

(Modified with permission from Withers HR, Thames HD Jr, Flow BL, Mason KA, Hussey DH: The relationship of acute to late injury in 2 and 5 fraction/week gamma-ray therapy. Int J Radiat Oncol Biol Phys 4:595–601, 1978. Copyright © 1978, Pergamon Press, Ltd.)

TABLE 13-8. Complications Following Single-Dose Megavoltage Treatment (2000–2750 R) of 20 Patients With Head and Neck Squamous Cell Carcinoma—National Cancer Institute

Severe Complications	No. Patients
Soft tissue necrosis, hemorrhage	2
Laryngeal edema	4
Cartilage necrosis	2
Tracheostomy	4
Dysphagia/cachexia	7
Pharyngostomy/gastrostomy	2
Osteoradionecrosis	2
Trismus	3

(Andrews JR: Dose–time relationships in cancer radiotherapy: A clinical radiobiology study of extremes of dose and time. Am J Roentgenol Radium Ther Nucl Med 93:56–74, 1965. Copyright © 1965, American Roentgen Ray Society)

TABLE 13-9. Local Control Following Irradiation of Oropharyngeal Cancer With 3 Versus 5 Fractions/Week With Equivalent NSD—Medical College of Wisconsin

	Local Control	
T Stage	3 Fractions/Week*	5 Fractions/Week†
T1–T2	3/10 (30%)	17/19 (89%)
T3	0/5	6/11 (55%)
T4	0/11	5/13 (38%)

* 3 fractions/week group: 9/26 (35%) were base of tongue or pharyngeal wall primary lesions.

† 5 fractions/week group: 27/43 (63%) were base of tongue or pharyngeal wall primary lesions.

(NSD, nominal standard dose)

(Reprinted with permission from Byhardt RW, Greenberg M, Cox JD: Local control of squamous carcinoma of the oral cavity and oropharynx with 3 versus 5 treatment fractions per week. Int J Radiat Oncol Biol Phys 2:415–420, 1977. Copyright © 1977, Pergamon Press, Ltd.)

TABLE 13-10. Local Control Following Irradiation of Oral Cavity Cancer With 3 Versus 5 Fractions/Week With Equivalent NSD—Medical College of Wisconsin

	Local Control	
T Stage	3 Fractions/Week	5 Fractions/Week
T1–T2	1/1 (100%)	5/7 (71%)
T3	0/2	1/5 (20%)
T4	0/2	3/8 (38%)

(Reprinted with permission from Byhardt RW, Greenberg M, Cox JD: Local control of squamous carcinoma of the oral cavity and oropharynx with 3 versus 5 treatment fractions per week. Int J Radiat Oncol Biol Phys 2:415–420, 1977. Copyright © 1977, Pergamon Press, Ltd.)

Treatment With 1 or 2 Fractions Per Week

There is little clinical information on the treatment of head and neck cancer patients with 1 or 2 fractions/week.

Singh, in India, used once-weekly fractionation in the treatment of stage IIIB cervix cancer because it was so difficult to get his village patients to come for daily treatments.[99] Treatment was calculated to be "equivalent" to their usual 5 fraction/week treatment (4000 rad/20 fractions to the whole pelvis plus an intrauterine radium application, followed by 1000 rad/5 fractions to the pelvic wall), based on NSD and TDF concepts. The alternative schedule consisted of 580 rad × 5 fractions administered once weekly to the pelvis, followed by standard radium treatment, then 670 rad/1 fraction to the pelvic side walls. Cobalt-60 was used in both patient groups. The NSD formula was fairly accurate in predicting acute effects, since the frequency of diarrhea and the acute tumor response (both at the end of treatment and at 3 months) were similar to what had been observed with standard therapy. However, the Ellis equation was found to be a very poor predictor of late reactions: all survivors of the once-weekly treatment regimen developed severe rectal injuries.

In Cape Town, South Africa, Bennett used the NSD concept of biologic equivalence to devise an alternative fractionation schedule for stage III cervix cancer.[9] One patient group received 5 fractions/week and the other 2 fractions/week; "disastrously high morbidity" was found in the 2 fraction/week group.

Dische and associates treated advanced lung cancer with 3400 rad to 3600 rad/6 fractions (twice weekly) in an overall treatment time of 18 days.[23] Of 70 patients who survived a minimum of 6 months, 8 (11%) developed progressive myelopathy.

Treatment With 3 Fractions Per Week

Between 1965 and 1975 at the Medical College of Wisconsin, two different dose schedules, using either 3 or 5 fractions/week, were used in the treatment of patients with squamous cell carcinomas of the oral cavity and oropharynx.[14] Treatments were equated by the NSD formula or TDF factors and delivered 6000 rad to 7200 rad/30 to 36 fractions (5 fractions per week) versus 5400 rad to 7200 rad/18 to 24 fractions (3 fractions per week); the higher total doses were used in the more advanced lesions. Local treatment results for 69 patients with oropharyngeal cancers are given in Table 13-9. Despite equivalent NSDs and a higher proportion of unfavorable tumor sites (base of the tongue and pharyngeal walls) in the 5 fraction/week group, local control was much better when 5 fractions/week were used. The Wisconsin results for oral cavity lesions are shown in Table 13-10. Superior results were achieved in the 5 fraction/week group.

Kok, in The Hague, experimented with a variety of fractionation schemes for stage I carcinoma of the larynx.[59] His results for patients receiving 3 fractions/week versus 5 fractions/week are summarized in Table 13-11. All patients received the same minimum tumor dose of 6300 rad. Despite lower TDFs, the 5 fraction/week group had a higher rate of tumor control.

In Kok's series, the acute reactions (fibrinous exudate) were less severe in the higher TDF, 3 fraction/week group. Conversely, above a certain fraction size, the late effects were much more severe in the 3 fraction/week group. Of

TABLE 13-11. Treatment of Stage I Larynx Cancer With 3 Versus 5 Fractions/Week—The Hague, The Netherlands

Treatment Group	TDF (range)	Local Control (3 years)
5 fractions/week*	100–107	16/18 (89%)
3 fractions/week†	105–133	26/42 (62%)

* 6300 rad/30 to 33 fractions (190–210 rad/fraction).
† 6300 rad/16 to 26 fractions (240–385 rad/fraction).
(Adapted from Kok G: The influence of the size of the fraction dose on normal and tumour tissue in cobalt-60 radiation treatment of carcinoma of the larynx and inoperable carcinoma of the breast. Radiol Clin Biol 40:100–115, 1971)

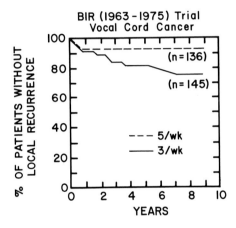

FIG. 13-21. Local recurrence-free rates for 281 patients with cancer of the true vocal cord randomized between 3 versus 5 fractions/week in the British Institute of Radiology trial, 1963–1975. The recurrence-free rate at 8 years is 91% for the 5 fraction/week group versus 75% for the 3 fraction/week group. This difference is statistically significant ($p = 0.026$). (Redrawn from Wiernik G, Bleehen NM, Brindle J, Bullimore J, Churchill-Davidson IFJ, Davidson J et al: Sixth interim progress report of the British Institute of Radiology fractionation study of 3 fractions/week versus 5 fractions/week in radiotherapy of the laryngopharynx. Br J Radiol 51:241–250, 1978)

14 patients who received 320 rad × 20 or 385 rad × 16 fractions thrice weekly, all developed late edema. Kok concluded that increasing the interval between fractions to 48 hours resulted in sparing of both the normal epithelium and the tumor because of cell repopulation but did not spare the connective tissues when large-dose fractions were administered.

Between 1963 and 1975, the British Institute of Radiology conducted a randomized trial of 3 fractions/week versus 5 fractions/week for 732 patients with cancers of the laryngopharynx. A number of different dose schedules were employed. Total doses were 11% to 13% higher in the 5 fraction/week group, but TDF values were nearly identical in the two treatment arms. For tumors of the vocal cord, the local recurrence-free rate at 8 years was significantly better ($p = 0.026$) for the group receiving 5 weekly treat-

ments (Fig. 13-21). No differences in acute and late reactions were noted.[115]

Treatment With Very Prolonged Fractionation Schemes

In 1965, Andrews reported the National Cancer Institute treatment results in 43 patients with head and neck squamous cell carcinomas who received 8,000 R to 10,000 R (mode 9000 R) with 2-MeV x-rays.[1] The overall treatment time was usually 14 weeks with 3 fractions/week. Despite these very substantial doses, only 9 patients were cured (5 of the 9 had early cancers of the vocal cord or nasopharynx and predictably would have done well with lower doses); failure to control moderately advanced and advanced cancers was almost uniform at this extreme degree of fractionation. Regeneration of clonogenic cells during the excessively prolonged treatment period apparently exceeded the ability of these high doses to produce cures.

The smallest daily fraction that is likely to control a high percentage of head and neck squamous cell carcinomas is not precisely known. For very radiocurable cancers, such as Hodgkin's disease or seminoma, fraction sizes as low as or lower than 100 rad/day will produce control. Coutard thought that the "cellucidal threshold" for squamous cell cancers of the larynx never appeared below a daily dose of 150 R with orthovoltage x-rays.[19] Correcting for roentgen to rad conversion and for the difference in radiobiologic effect, this would be approximately 165 rad with megavoltage therapy. We do not recommend daily doses of less than 175 rad for squamous cell carcinoma.

Occasionally, one notes that a lymph node within the treatment field continues to enlarge at 180 rad tumor dose/day. Whether the growth of such nodes is due to tumor cell proliferation during treatment is not known. Sometimes the enlargement occurs rather abruptly, suggesting that it is due to necrosis, with edema or hemorrhage into the tumor-bearing node. Under these circumstances we have sometimes increased the daily fraction size, if this can be tolerated by the volume being irradiated. Alternatively, one can give additional (field-within-a-field) treatment to the node by tangential portals or a small electron boost. Regression of the lesion generally resumes after the daily dose rate is increased. Similar growth of primary lesions during courses of irradiation at 180 rad to 200 rad/day has not been observed. Since regeneration of malignant clonogens during a course of irradiation is a likely cause of failure in rapidly growing tumors, the use of very small daily doses is discouraged.

Split-Course Irradiation

A variety of split-course techniques have been devised by radiation therapists and largely popularized by Sambrook,[91] Holsti,[49] Marcial and co-workers,[65] and Scanlon;[94] many patients in the United States currently receive split-course treatments. Most commonly there is a planned 2- to 3-week rest period, roughly midway through a treatment course that is otherwise conventional, or nearly so, in terms of total dose and daily fraction size. Some split-course proponents arbitrarily increase the total dose by 5% to 10% in order to adjust for any loss in therapeutic efficacy that might result from the treatment interruption. At the University of Florida, where split-course irradiation was used almost routinely from mid-1969 through June 1974, no conscious attempt was made to increase the total dose of irradiation to offset the split. Other investigators have kept the total dose the same but increased the daily fraction size. Some use 3 instead of 5 fractions/week and occasionally more than one split is introduced into the treatment course.

Sambrook, prompted by the wish to spare frail and elderly patients with advanced head and neck cancers the discomfort caused by high-dose, continuous-course irradiation, began to use the split-course technique in 1953 in Wales.[91] By stopping the irradiation when local reactions were commencing, mucosal reactions quickly cleared and treatment could be restarted in 2 to 4 weeks. Therapy could be nearly completed by the time significant reactions reappeared, and the patient thus was relieved of a sustained period of moderately severe discomfort and instead had two shorter periods of milder discomfort. Noticeable tumor shrinkage during the rest interval was consistently observed. This observation raised hope among some therapists that the technique might actually improve local control over standard treatment, because if hypoxic cells were really responsible for failure to control some cancers, then as the tumor shrank during the rest period the remaining cells might become better vascularized and therefore better oxygenated and more sensitive.

Sambrook thought that his technique, which frequently employed two or three rest intervals, resulted in fewer late complications.[92] With multiple splits, he was able to administer 7000 R to 9000 R to the skin with orthovoltage apparatus without producing more than mild mucosal and skin reactions acutely, and he felt that late fibrosis was decidedly less following a split-course regimen.

Scanlon, too, regards the split-course technique as a "safety factor" capable of reducing late morbidity and has even recommended the use of larger treatment fields than would ordinarily be used with conventional therapy.[93] Scanlon analyzed treatment results of 50 patients with a wide variety of head and neck neoplasms including squamous cell carcinomas, lymphoepitheliomas, lymphomas, and adenocarcinomas at 15 different tumor sites. Although he concluded that late sequelae were less frequent than with conventional therapy, no analysis of treatment complications was undertaken and there was no group of conventionally irradiated patients presented for comparison.

Split-course treatment using otherwise standard fractionation probably results in lower rates of tumor control than can be achieved with conventional treatment. Holsti used a split-course technique similar to that employed at the University of Florida except that total doses for the split-course therapy exceeded those used for continuous-course therapy by 5% to 10%.[49] Despite a higher proportion of unfavorable cases in the continuous-course group and the lower doses used in their treatment, survival in the two groups was equal at 2 years. There has been no subsequent update of these results.

Lindberg and Fletcher used split-course irradiation in 23 patients with advanced squamous cell carcinoma of the upper respiratory and digestive tracts.[62] Patients were treated sequentially with 3000 rad tumor dose/15 fractions/3 weeks, a 3-week rest, then another 3000 rad/3 weeks. A 1000-rad to 2000-rad boost was delivered in 1 to 2 weeks, using smaller fields. Because the split-course group had a much lower rate of disease control than a similar group of patients treated by conventional techniques, the split-course scheme was abandoned.

The University of Florida has had considerable experience with split-course irradiation of head and neck cancers[77,82] Between September 1964 and August 1976, 468 patients with previously untreated squamous cell carcinoma of the oral cavity, oropharynx, nasopharynx, supraglottic larynx, or hypopharynx received curative courses of external-beam irradiation to their primary lesion; some patients received a radium implant boost following external irradiation. Two hundred and fourteen patients received treatment by split-course technique and 254 by continuous-course technique. There was no attempt to randomize patients between split- versus continuous-course irradiation. During the first 5 years of the study, almost all of the patients received continuous-course irradiation; in the succeeding 5 years, the split-course technique was used almost exclusively; then during the last 2 years of the study continuous-course irradiation was used. Patients in the split-course group were placed on planned 14- to 16-day rest intervals after 2800 rad to 3000 rad/15 fractions external irradiation to the primary lesion. Patients in both the split-course and continuous-course groups generally received five 180- to 200-rad fractions per week to the primary lesion. Our observations regarding tumor regression and the subsidence of acute reactions during the rest period were in agreement with those of Sambrook.[91] Primary lesions always regressed or stabilized; no tumor was observed to enlarge. Metastatic neck nodes usually stabilized but occasionally regressed during the 2-week split; none enlarged. Patients in the split-course group reported alleviation of acute symptoms 10 to 12 days into the split; mucous membranes appeared normal when the patients returned to resume therapy.

Local treatment results in patients with early, moderately advanced, and advanced lesions are summarized in Tables 13-12 through 13-14, respectively. For all stages of disease, local control was better when continuous-course irradiation was used. The differences between split- versus continuous-course irradiation were greatest for moderately advanced and advanced lesions. Although none of the differences were statistically significant, those for T3 ($p = 0.07$) and T4 ($p = 0.08$) lesions were close to significance levels; that is, there is only a 1/14 or 1/12 chance, respectively, that the observed differences were due to chance.

Analysis of regional nodal control was also undertaken. The control of neck disease by irradiation alone with split- versus continuous-course techniques is shown in Table 13-15. Three marginal (not dose-related) recurrences are excluded. Subclinical disease was controlled in all instances by both techniques, but a significantly greater proportion of N1 ($p = 0.02$) and N2 ($p = 0.05$) neck disease was controlled by continuous-course irradiation. Only 21 N3A necks were treated by irradiation alone; there were insufficient numbers to make valid statistical comparisons in this group.

Differences in survival were also noted. In Figures 13-22 through 13-24 survival data are shown for stages I–II, III, and IV, respectively. There were approximately 10% survival differences at 5 years in favor of the continuous-course group. For stages III and IV the differences were statistically significant ($p = 0.02$ and $p = 0.03$, respectively); for stage IV, the 5-year survival rate of the split-course group is only half that of the continuous-course group.

Soft tissue necroses and bone exposures were graded in severity and analyzed for the 468 patients. Mild complications were those that required conservative management for less than 6 months. Moderately severe injuries required

TABLE 13-12. Split-Course Versus Continuous-Course Irradiation: Local Control by Tumor Site and Treatment Technique: T1–T2* (University of Florida)

Disease Site	External Beam		External Beam + Radium	
	Split Course (6200 rad)†	Continuous Course (6100 rad)†	Split Course (4700/2600 rad)‡	Continuous Course (5000/2500 rad)‡
Oral cavity§	4/8	2/5	8/11	8/13
Oropharynx	17/24	39/45	5/6	6/8
Nasopharynx	4/4	3/3	NA	NA
Hypopharynx	2/4	10/17	NA	NA
Supraglottic larynx	4/6	11/12	NA	NA
Total‖	31/46 (67%)	65/82 (79%)	13/17 (76%)	14/21 (67%)

* 25/63 split-course patients (40%) had T1 lesions versus 36/103 continuous-course patients (35%) with T1 lesions.

† Median dose of external-beam irradiation.

‡ Median dose of external-beam irradiation and calculated interstitial radium dose.

§ Patients with oral cavity primary lesions who received all or more than half of the total tumor dose from interstitial irradiation were excluded.

‖ Total local control: split course 44/63 (70%) versus continuous course 79/103 (77%); $p = 0.20$.

(NA, no data available)

(Reprinted with permission from Parsons JT, Bova FJ, Million RR: A reevaluation of split-course technique for squamous cell carcinoma of the head and neck. Int J Radiat Oncol Biol Phys 6:1645–1652, 1980. Copyright © 1980, Pergamon Press, Ltd.)

TABLE 13-13. Split-Course Versus Continuous-Course Irradiation: Local Control by Tumor Site and Treatment Technique: T3 (University of Florida)

Disease Site	External Beam		External Beam + Radium	
	Split Course (6600 rad)*	Continuous Course (6600 rad)*	Split Course (5600/2600 rad)†	Continuous Course (5600/2600 rad)†
Oral cavity	2/5	1/3	3/10	10/17
Oropharynx	9/22	8/15	3/6	10/19
Nasopharynx	5/6	3/3	NA	NA
Hypopharynx	2/11	5/7	NA	NA
Supraglottic larynx	4/4	4/7	NA	NA
Total‡	22/48 (46%)	21/35 (60%)	6/16 (38%)	20/36 (56%)

* Median dose of external-beam irradiation.

† Median dose of external-beam irradiation and calculated interstitial radium dose.

‡ Total local control: split course 28/64 (44%) versus continuous course 41/71 (58%); $p = 0.07$.

(NA, no data available)

(Reprinted with permission from Parsons JT, Bova FJ, Million RR: A reevaluation of split-course technique for squamous cell carcinoma of the head and neck. Int J Radiat Oncol Biol Phys 6:1645–1652, 1980. Copyright © 1980, Pergamon Press, Ltd.)

TABLE 13-14. Split-Course Versus Continuous-Course Irradiation: Local Control by Tumor Site and Treatment Technique: T4 (University of Florida)

Disease Site	External Beam		External Beam + Radium	
	Split Course (6600 rad)*	Continuous Course (6600 rad)*	Split Course (6600/1400 rad)†	Continuous Course (6100/2300 rad)†
Oral cavity	NA	NA	NA	1/3
Oropharynx	1/18	2/7	0/2	1/2
Nasopharynx	2/6	6/10	NA	NA
Hypopharynx	1/8	0/6	NA	0/1
Supraglottic larynx	1/2	0/2	NA	NA
Total‡	5/34 (15%)	8/25 (32%)	0/2 (0%)	2/6 (33%)

* Median dose of external-beam irradiation.

† Median dose of external-beam irradiation and calculated interstitial radium dose.

‡ Total local control: split course 5/36 (14%) versus continuous course 10/31 (32%); $p = 0.08$.

(NA, no data available)

(Reprinted with permission from Parsons JT, Bova FJ, Million RR: A reevaluation of split-course technique for squamous cell carcinoma of the head and neck. Int J Radiat Oncol Biol Phys 6:1645–1652, 1980. Copyright © 1980, Pergamon Press, Ltd.)

TABLE 13-15. Neck Control in Heminecks Treated by Split-Course Versus Continuous-Course Irradiation Alone (University of Florida)

Neck Stage	Split Course (No. Heminecks [%])	Continuous Course (No. Heminecks [%])
N0	108/108 (100)	158/158 (100)
N1	11/16 (69)	35/37 (95)*
N2A–2B	11/23 (48)	25/34 (74)†
N3A	4/14 (29)	2/7 (29)

* $p = 0.02$, Fisher's exact test.[71]
† $p = 0.05$, χ^2 test.[71]

(Reprinted with permission from Parsons JT, Bova FJ, Million RR: A reevaluation of split-course technique for squamous cell carcinoma of the head and neck. Int. J. Radiat Oncol Biol Phys 6:1645–1652, 1980. Copyright © 1980, Pergamon Press, Ltd.)

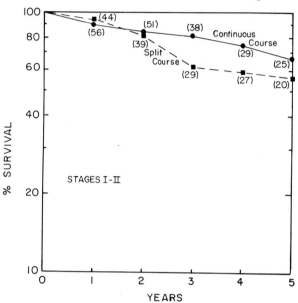

FIG. 13-23. Survival (actuarial method)[20] on semilog plot for patients with stage III squamous cell carcinoma of the head and neck following treatment by continuous-course or split-course irradiation ($p = 0.02$).[42] The number of patients at risk for each succeeding interval is shown. (Modified with permission from Parsons JT, Bova FJ, Million RR: A reevaluation of split-course technique for squamous cell carcinoma of the head and neck. Int J Radiat Oncol Biol Phys 6:1645–1652, 1980. Copyright © 1980, Pergamon Press, Ltd.) ▼

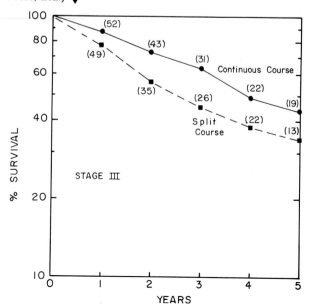

◄ **FIG. 13-22.** Survival (actuarial method)[20] on semilog plot for patients with stage I–II squamous cell carcinoma of the head and neck following treatment by continuous-course or split-course irradiation ($p = 0.2$).[42] The number of patients at risk for each succeeding interval is shown. Nineteen of 47 split-course patients (40%) had stage I disease versus 24 of 63 continuous-course patients (38%) with stage I disease. (Modified with permission from Parsons JT, Bova FJ, Million RR: A reevaluation of split-course technique for squamous cell carcinoma of the head and neck. Int J Radiat Oncol Biol Phys 6:1645–1652, 1980. Copyright © 1980, Pergamon Press, Ltd.)

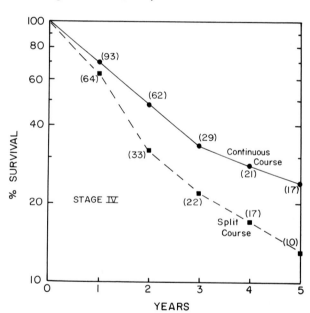

FIG. 13-24. Survival (actuarial method)[20] on semilog plot for patients with stage IV squamous cell carcinoma of the head and neck following treatment by continuous-course or split-course irradiation ($p = 0.03$).[42] The number of patients at risk for each succeeding interval is shown. (Modified with permission from Parsons JT, Bova FJ, Million RR: A reevaluation of split-course technique for squamous cell carcinoma of the head and neck. Int J Radiat Oncol Biol Phys 6:1645–1652, 1980. Copyright © 1980, Pergamon Press, Ltd.)

TABLE 13-16. Complications of Split-Course Versus Continuous-Course Irradiation—Oral Cavity/Oropharynx (315 Patients)* (University of Florida)

Treatment Technique (No. Patients)	Patients (%) With Soft Tissue Necrosis			Patients (%) With Bone Exposure		
	Mild	Moderate	Severe	Mild	Moderate	Severe
External-beam irradiation						
Split course (104)	4 (4%)	4 (4%)	0	4 (4%)	2 (2%)	0
Continuous course (94)	6 (6%)	5 (5%)	1 (1%)	3 (3%)	1 (1%)	2 (2%)
External-beam irradiation and radium implant						
Split course (40)	5 (13%)	4 (10%)	0	5 (13%)	1 (3%)	2 (5%)
Continuous course (77)	13 (17%)	3 (4%)	1 (1%)	8 (10%)	7 (9%)	1 (1%)

* Eighty-two complications occurred in 74 patients. Eight patients who developed both bone exposure and soft tissue necrosis are scored twice.

(Reprinted with permission from Parsons JT, Bova FJ, Million RR: A reevaluation of split-course technique for squamous cell carcinoma of the head and neck. Int J Radiat Oncol Biol Phys 6:1645–1652, 1980. Copyright © 1980, Pergamon Press, Ltd.)

longer periods of conservative treatment, while severe complications required an operation or prolonged hospitalization. Complications arising in the 315 patients with squamous cell carcinoma of the oral cavity and oropharynx are shown in Table 13-16. No significant differences in rate of occurrence of either soft tissue necrosis or bone exposure were noted.

No transverse myelitis or fatal complications of irradiation were observed among the 468 patients.

In summary, the split-course technique as used at the University of Florida resulted in lower rates of primary control, regional control, and survival with no reduction in late complications. The University of Florida series was not randomized, and the results must therefore be interpreted with caution. However, the way in which the treatment was administered eliminates some of the undesirable variables that are inherent in large, multi-institutional randomized trials. All University of Florida patients were subjected to the same therapeutic guidelines, and the technical aspects of irradiation in both the split- and continuous-course groups were identical. The doses in both patient groups were similar and varied according to T stage. All treatments were administered by a single therapist at a single institution. Routine use of the split-course technique has been abandoned at the University of Florida. A rest period is used only in those instances in which clinical judgment dictates a rest. The rest period is as short as possible, and it is started as late as possible in the course of treatment.

The likely explanation for lower control rates following split-course irradiation is repopulation of clonogenic cells during the rest interval. Tumor cell repopulation during a rest interval may actually occur at an accelerated rate. Such an effect may be demonstrated following noncurative doses of irradiation administered to some animal tumors.[48] Regeneration of clonogenic cells may not be reflected in volume changes in the tumor; although dead tumor cells continue to be removed and the tumor continues to regress during a split in therapy, there may in fact be considerable simultaneous proliferation of surviving cells, which may lead to treatment failure.[116] Only small differences in local control were noted between split-course versus continuous-course techniques for T1–T2 lesions. For these small tumors, which are usually readily controlled by irradiation,

one can probably afford repopulation of a few clonogens during the rest period. For T3–T4 lesions, control is difficult to achieve with irradiation; tumor cell proliferation during the rest interval may be responsible for the lower rate of control following split-course treatment of these lesions.

It is customary to think that the effects of a rest period can be overcome by merely increasing the total dose by 5% to 10%. However, analysis of time–dose data for each site and stage provides no evidence that one can compensate for the effects of the split in this manner. Although there was never a conscious attempt to raise the doses at the University of Florida to offset the split, through the years there has been a gradual upward adjustment of the dosage schedules for many tumor sites. Since the split-course technique was used in 5 of the last 7 years of the study, the overall effect was higher doses in many of the split-course patients compared with continuous-course patients who received treatment in the earlier years. Even when higher doses were used, the results of split-course irradiation have been poor (see Fig. 13-14). This suggests a subpopulation of tumors that show little or no repopulation during the rest interval and are cured by conventional total doses and another group of tumors that proliferate to such an extent during the rest interval that they are no longer curable by slightly increased doses. The dose required to compensate for the rest interval is not known; our own time–dose data suggest that a 5% to 10% increase may be insufficient.

Multiple Daily Fractionation

Although once-a-day treatment has been the mainstay of most radiation therapy departments, the idea of giving more than one treatment per day is not new in head and neck cancer management. Coutard often delivered two daily fractions when treating patients with laryngeal and hypopharyngeal cancers.[18] In the past several years, there has been considerable interest in multiple daily fractionation schemes. Most of the interest has been stimulated by an ever-increasing interaction between radiobiology and clinical radiation therapy. There are several reasons why multiple daily fractionation schedules might, in some situations, be more efficacious than conventional techniques:

1. By increasing the number of fractions, one increases the probability that redistributing tumor cells (and also actively proliferating normal tissue cells, such as those of the skin and mucous membrane) will be irradiated during a sensitive phase of the cell cycle. Since the fibrovascular connective tissues responsible for late radiation damage are relatively nonproliferative, they will be less affected by redistribution between treatments.[116] This may result in less severe late normal tissue injury for a given rate of tumor control.

2. Most multiple daily fractionation schemes for head and neck carcinomas have used doses in the range of 110 rad to 120 rad/fraction. Cell death after these doses occurs by the single-hit mechanism, which is less dependent on the presence of molecular oxygen than multiple-hit killing. The effect of hypoxic areas within tumors might, therefore, be reduced.

3. If one allows sufficient time between successive doses (110 rad to 120 rad), sublethal injury in both tumor and normal tissue can be repaired and very little of the cell killing will occur by accumulation of sublethal damage. The repair of accumulated sublethal damage is believed to occur exponentially with a half-time of approximately 1 hour.[24] Thus, if the interval between two treatments is 1 hour, approximately 50% of sublethal damage is repaired; if the interval is 2 hours, 75% is repaired; if 3 hours, 87.5%; and so on. There is some evidence to indicate that the rate of repair of sublethal damage is faster in normal tissues than in hypoxic tumor cells. By varying the time interval between fractions, it may be possible to exploit this difference in repair rate. Knowledge of how best to exploit this difference (if, indeed, it even exists) is lacking.

4. It has become apparent that the tissues responsible for late effects consistently show a greater sparing effect from dose fractionation than do the tissues responsible for acute effects.[107,116] If, as is suspected, most tumors behave like acute-responding tissues, then a favorable differential between tumor response and late normal tissue response is to be expected by using a larger number of smaller-than-conventional dose fractions (*i.e.*, hyperfractionation).

Since 1977, at the University of Florida, 120 rad twice daily to total doses of 7440 rad to 7920 rad has been given to some patients with moderately advanced and advanced primary lesions of the head and neck. The mucosal reactions produced by this therapy are similar to those produced by large-volume irradiation at 200 rad/fraction/day. It appears that 120 rad twice daily is right on the edge in terms of what can be tolerated by the majority of head and neck cancer patients treated by a continuous course of irradiation. Wang and co-workers have used 160 rad twice a day, but patients require at least a 7- to 10-day break after 4000 rad because acute reactions have been severe.[113]

As employed at the University of Florida, multiple daily fractionation using 120 rad fractions generally shortens the overall treatment time by 1½ to 2 weeks (e.g., from 7500 rad/8 to 8½ weeks to 7440 rad to 7680 rad/6 to 6½ weeks). This shortening may provide an additional advantage to hyperfractionation by limiting the potential for regeneration by the tumor during treatment. It is not possible to further diminish the overall treatment time even

in rapidly growing tumors because the acute response of the mucosa will not permit it. In a series of 22 patients who received 200 rad three times daily to 4800 rad to 5400 rad/8 to 12 days, mucositis often took several months to subside, and 9 patients died as a result of necrosis without evidence of tumor recurrence;[85] such very abbreviated schedules may also be disadvantageous in terms of tumor control because of the lower total doses used and, theoretically, because reoxygenation may be less effective than with longer courses of therapy. An advantage of compressing the overall treatment time in rapidly proliferating tumors was observed clinically at M. D. Anderson Hospital in the treatment of inflammatory breast cancer by irradiation alone: by using twice-daily treatments (5100 rad/4 weeks, prior to the "boost" treatment), the overall treatment time was reduced to approximately half that of the once-daily treatment schedule (6000 rad/8 weeks, prior to the "boost" treatment). The rate of failure to control local breast disease dropped from 38% to 9%.[7] A similar improvement in local results was obtained in the treatment of another rapidly growing tumor, Burkitt's lymphoma, when thrice-daily fractionation replaced conventional treatment, reducing the treatment time from 3 weeks to 2 weeks.[78]

Whether twice- or thrice-daily fractionation in head and neck cancer will improve therapeutic results over conventional once-daily treatment is not clear. A number of centers have reported encouraging preliminary impressions,[54,98] but no randomized trials or retrospective analyses have yet documented clearly improved results. The EORTC is comparing multiple daily fractionation to once-a-day treatment in randomized trials. The University of Florida results are also preliminary but quite encouraging. Twice-a-day therapy is being used with increasing frequency at the University of Florida.

The observations regarding twice-a-day treatment at the University of Florida are as follows:

1. The rate of local and regional control following 7440 rad to 7680 rad/62 to 64 fractions is at least as good as and possibly better than the control rate following 7000 rad to 7500 rad by once-a-day (approximately 180 rad/fraction) techniques.

2. Resection of the primary lesion has been safely accomplished after 5000 rad/4 weeks and neck dissection safely performed after 7680 rad/6½ weeks.

3. An implant boost of 1500 rad has been added in four patients after 7680 rad without complication.

4. No significant soft tissue necrosis, bone necrosis, or persistent severe edema has been observed.

5. The soft tissues of the neck generally feel less indurated at 2 to 5 years' follow-up than after once-a-day treatment.

6. Acute and late skin reactions are similar to those seen in patients who received once-a-day therapy.

7. Radiation myelitis has not been observed in 22 patients who received approximately 4600 rad to the spinal cord and who have been free of disease for over 2 years.

Summary of External-Beam Time–Dose Recommendations for Primary Lesions

The best local control rates for several head and neck sites have been obtained with daily fractions of greater than

200 rad (e.g., 210 rad to 225 rad/day), 5 fractions/week (see Figs. 13-8 through 13-11 and Tables 13-5 and 13-6). The advantages of delivering greater than 1000 rad/week and using short overall treatment times must be balanced against the disadvantages, which include greater acute mucosal reactions, which some patients are unable or unwilling to accept, and more severe late effects on normal tissues. In past years at the University of Florida 200 rad/day was generally not exceeded except in the treatment of vocal cord cancer. The usual approach has been to administer treatment to initial large portals at 180 rad to 190 rad/fraction, then to increase the dose/fraction to 200 rad to 225 rad/fraction to reduced portals during the last 1 or 2 weeks of treatment. Interstitial implantation or use of an intraoral cone are other means of delivering a boost dose to a limited volume in a short overall time. Attempts to treat large volumes to high doses using daily fractions in excess of 200 rad may result in interrupted (split) treatment courses in some patients because of severe acute reactions, and consequently diminished local control, and/or excessively severe late reactions, which largely defeat the purpose of radiation therapy in head and neck cancer. One must remember that for many head and neck sites, surgical salvage is feasible after failure of radiation therapy; efforts to push for the highest control rates attainable are

not warranted if the complication rate exceeds an acceptable level. The treatment schedules adopted at the University of Florida for each anatomical site are listed in the appropriate chapter; the schedules are constantly being reviewed and revised to improve the therapeutic ratio. The use of multiple daily fractions is being explored as one means of improving the ratio.

Continuous Low-Dose-Rate Irradiation

Continuous low-dose-rate irradiation may be likened to fractionated irradiation with an infinite number of very small individual doses. The continuous low-dose-rate technique is commonly used in head and neck cancer therapy since this is the method of dose delivery by interstitial implants. There is little experience with continuous low-dose-rate irradiation by external beam.[87] The dose-rate effect is illustrated in Figure 13-25. Continuous low-dose-rate and multiple daily fractionation schemes presumably share the same potential radiobiologic advantages. Experimental data suggest that cells exposed to continuous low-dose-rate irradiation tend to accumulate or "pile up" in the G2-M (sensitive) phase of the cell cycle.[57]

CONTINUOUS LOW-DOSE-RATE IRRADIATION BY INTERSTITIAL IMPLANTATION

Pierre and Marie Curie discovered radium in 1898, and in 1904 it was applied to exposed surfaces of the body to treat lesions of the skin, accessible mucous membranes, and uterus. Early success was observed in the treatment of these lesions, even though the methods were crude. Interestingly, the idea of increasing the dose to deep cancers by using radium interstitially appears to have come from educator and inventor of the telephone Alexander Graham Bell:[101]

Dear Dr. Sowers:

I understand from you that the Röntgen rays, and the rays emitted by radium, have been found to have a marked curative effect upon external cancers, but that the effects upon deep-seated cancers have not thus far proved satisfactory.

It has occurred to me that one reason for the unsatisfactory nature of these latter experiments arises from the fact that the rays have been applied externally, thus having to pass through healthy tissues of various depths in order to reach the cancerous matter.

The Crookes' tube, from which the Röntgen rays are emitted, is of course too bulky to be admitted into the middle of a mass of cancer, but there is no reason why a tiny fragment of radium sealed up in a fine glass tube should not be inserted into the very heart of the cancer, thus acting directly upon the diseased material. Would it not be worth while making experiments along this line?

Alexander Graham Bell

Many early therapists acquired considerable skill in implant therapy, but when supervoltage equipment became generally available, interest in interstitial treatment declined in many centers. Implant therapy is an art in which many of today's therapists have not been adequately trained. There are certain situations in which interstitial implantation, either alone or in combination with external-beam irradiation, is more appropriate than external irra-

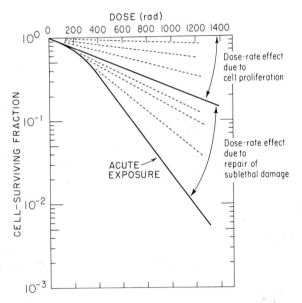

FIG. 13-25. Dose-rate effects due to repair of sublethal damage and cell proliferation. The lower solid line illustrates the dose-response curve for cells following a single x-ray exposure. Note the broad initial shoulder on the curve. As the dose rate (*i.e.,* rad/hour) is reduced (*lower dotted lines*), repair of sublethal damage may take place during the exposure. If the dose rate is low enough, all sublethal damage is repaired and the survival curve assumes the shape of the upper solid line, with all damage being due to single hits. If the dose rate is sufficiently low (*upper dotted lines*), a critical level may be reached where cell proliferation continues during the radiation exposure. At the dose rates (30 rad to 100 rad/hour) generally used clinically in low-dose rate continuous therapy, a dose-rate effect due to cell proliferation is probably not very important. (Hall EJ: Radiobiology for the Radiologist, 2nd ed, p 146. Hagerstown, MD, Harper & Row, 1978)

diation alone.[11] An implant is capable of delivering a very high dose of radiation in a short time to a limited volume of tissue with very rapid decrease in dose outside the implant volume. For some very limited lesions, implant therapy is the only treatment necessary. In other situations when external-beam irradiation constitutes the main treatment, the implant is used to "boost" the dose to the bulky central portion of the tumor, thereby limiting the volume of high-dose irradiation. In still other circumstances, the implant is the main treatment, but moderate dose (3000 rad/2 weeks) external irradiation is given prior to the implant to compensate for any areas of localized underdosage ("cold spots") within the implanted volume, to reduce the tumor size (e.g., for bulky lip cancer) to facilitate the implant, or electively to irradiate the lymph nodes (e.g., oral tongue carcinoma). Interstitial dose rates are low and continuous, and treatment is delivered in a short overall time. For instance, 6000 rad to 6500 rad may be administered to an implanted volume in 6 to 8 days, while a similar dose delivered by external-beam irradiation would typically require 6 to 7 weeks of therapy.

Potential disadvantages of interstitial irradiation include the following:

1. The dose throughout the implanted volume is inhomogeneous. Areas of localized underdosage ("cold spots") may result in local recurrence of tumor. Conversely, bunching of sources may produce areas of overdosage ("hot spots") that cause necrosis.
2. Hospital admission is required, and general anesthesia is usually necessary.
3. Technical and conceptual skills are required to achieve a good dose distribution. Some of the problems of achieving a good geometric distribution have been overcome by using preloaded implant devices[27,67] or afterloading techniques, but it is still not possible to achieve a textbooklike distribution every time. On the other hand, Martin and Martin, who had a vast experience in treating cancers by radium implantation, noted that some deviation from perfect was acceptable, as long as the overall pattern of the implant covered the desired volume.[69] Slight variations seemed to make little difference in their treatment results, and the University of Florida experience is in agreement: the most perfect-appearing implant may be unsuccessful while the one that looks geometrically poor may control the cancer.
4. Therapists and operating room personnel are exposed to irradiation. While the problem of exposure cannot be entirely eliminated, it can be reduced by using either preloaded implant devices that can be rapidly positioned[27,67] or afterloading techniques. Compared with a typical gynecologic radium case, in which 65 mg or more of radium is loaded into a tandem and ovoid system, only about 10 mg of radium is used in a typical head and neck implant case, and therefore personnel exposure is relatively low.

The relative disadvantages of implant therapy can generally be overcome by careful treatment planning. For lesions of the oral tongue and floor of the mouth, interstitial treatment is indispensable, whether it is used alone or in combination with external-beam irradiation. It is a rare patient in whom an interstitial implant cannot be used when such therapy is clearly indicated.

Mendenhall and co-workers retrospectively analyzed the University of Florida treatment results for carcinoma of the oral tongue and floor of the mouth in 1981.[72] Between October 1964 and December 1977, 74 patients with squamous cell carcinoma of the oral tongue and 73 patients with lesions of the floor of the mouth received radical irradiation; all patients had a minimum 2-year follow-up. Patients who died before 2 years with their primary lesions still controlled were excluded from the local control analysis. Until approximately the end of 1969, early (T1–T2) lesions were most often treated with radium alone or with preneedling low-dose external-beam irradiation (2000 rad/1 week or 3000 rad/2 to 3 weeks) followed by an implant. The external-beam treatment volume was usually limited to the primary lesion alone or to the primary lesion and first-echelon nodes. After 1969, more comprehensive neck treatment was emphasized and the dose schedule was modified to deliver 4500-rad to 6000-rad external-beam irradiation to the primary site and draining nodes, followed by a 1500- to 3000-rad implant. During both time periods, moderately advanced lesions (T3) usually received 4700-rad to 6000-rad external-beam irradiation followed by a 2000- to 3000-rad implant.

It is difficult to make dose comparisons between patients treated by external-beam, interstitial, or a combination of both types of irradiation, since the dose distributions and the time over which the dose is administered differ greatly for the various techniques. While it may be argued that a mere addition of the dose delivered by external beam to the dose delivered by an implant is to take too great a radiobiologic liberty, such additions must be performed almost routinely in the clinic whenever one combines external-beam and interstitial irradiation; it therefore makes some sense to combine the doses when reviewing the data. The University of Florida data on oral tongue carcinoma suggest that the greater the proportion of the total dose given by radium as opposed to external beam, the higher is the rate of local control (Table 13-17). The difference for T2 lesions was statistically significant and occurred in spite of the fact that the patients who received a greater proportion of their treatment with radium actually received lower total doses (see Fig. 17-29 in Chapter 17).

There was no trend toward higher control with more radium in T1 or T3 lesions, since there was only one T1 failure, and the T3 lesions all received about the same treatment.

The University of Florida results for lesions of the floor of the mouth are shown in Table 13-18. The rate of control versus the proportion of dose delivered by radium did not differ significantly for T1 or T2 lesions because of the paucity of failures in early cases. Local control for T3 lesions following external-beam irradiation alone was poor (3/10) compared with the rate achieved when all or part of the dose was administered by radium implant (9/15).

The contention that carcinomas of the oral tongue are more readily controlled by implantation than by external beam irradiation is not new. Martin and Martin observed that oral tongue lesions "responded quite well" to a 6000 R/7 day radium implant, but 7000 R/5 to 7 weeks with a cobalt bomb was generally incapable of producing cure.[69] Several authors have published data showing improved local control for cancer of the oral tongue and floor of the mouth treated by implant alone or implant plus external-beam irradiation versus external-beam irradiation alone.[17,40,41,51,53,61,72] There are some differences when considering individual T stages, and the reader is urged to individually review the cited papers. The current approach for cancers of the oral tongue and floor of the mouth is to

TABLE 13-17. Oral Tongue Carcinoma: Local Control Versus Proportion of Dose Delivered by Radium Implant (University of Florida)

Stage	Radium Alone or Radium + Low-Dose (<3000 rad) External Beam	Radium + High-Dose (≧3000 rad) External Beam	External Beam Alone	No. Controlled/ No. Treated	No. Salvaged/ No. Attempts	No. Ultimately Controlled/No. Treated
T1	5/5	2/2	0/1	7/8	1/1	8/8
T2	*10/11	*7/15	1/1	18/27	4/7	22/27
T3	0/2	7/20	0	7/22	5/10	12/22

* Significance level = 0.02, Fisher's exact test.[71]
(Reprinted with permission from Mendenhall W, VanCise WS, Bova FJ, Million RR: Analysis of time-dose factors in squamous cell carcinoma of the oral tongue and floor of mouth treated with radiation therapy alone. Int J Radiat Oncol Biol Phys 7:1005–1011, 1981. Copyright © 1981, Pergamon Press, Ltd.)

TABLE 13-18. Carcinoma of the Floor of the Mouth: Local Control Versus Proportion of Dose Delivered by Radium Implant (University of Florida)

Stage	Radium Alone or Radium + Low-Dose (<3000 rad) External Beam	Radium + High-Dose (≧3000 rad) External Beam	External Beam Alone	No. Controlled/ No. Treated	No. Salvaged/ No. Attempts	No. Ultimately Controlled/No. Treated
T1	8/8	4/5	2/3	14/16	0/1	14/16
T2	1/1	9/12	3/4	13/17	3/4	16/17
T3	1/2	*8/13	*3/10	12/25	5/9	17/25
T4		1/3		1/3	0/1	1/3

* Significance level = 0.11, Fisher's exact test.[71]
(Reprinted with permission from Mendenhall W, VanCise WS, Bova FJ, Million RR: Analysis of time-dose factors in squamous cell carcinoma of the oral tongue and floor of mouth treated with radiation therapy alone. Int J Radiat Oncol Biol Phys 7:1005–1011, 1981. Copyright © 1981, Pergamon Press, Ltd.)

administer as much of the treatment by interstitial therapy as is reasonable.

DOSE SPECIFICATION

Dosimetry for all except the simplest implants is done by computer. At various points within the implanted volume, the doses contributed by each radioactive source are summed; points of equal dose are then connected by lines, called "isodose curves." Although computer dosimetry provides a large amount of dose information, including information regarding "hot" and "cold" areas that would not be readily available with conventional methods of calculation, there is still the problem of where to specify the dose. In the early years of computer dosimetry, the tendency was to be overgenerous in selecting minimum tumor doses, often resulting in higher doses to larger volumes than had previously been given when calculations were made by the Paterson–Parker method. At M. D. Anderson Hospital, where computer dosimetry became available in January 1961, overdosage led to low recurrence rates (3/30 or 10%) in lesions of the oral tongue and floor of the mouth treated in 1961–1962, but 77% of the patients developed soft tissue necrosis and 13% required surgical treatment of bone necrosis.[16] No general rule can be stated regarding the choice of the isodose line with which one specifies the minimum tumor dose. The rapid change in dose surrounding an implant makes dose specification somewhat arbitrary. Comparisons of interstitial dose between two institutions may be meaningless, since the technique of dose specification varies from center to center; indeed, the selection may vary within a single institution by a single physician. At the University of Florida, an isodose line 3 mm to 5 mm outside a multiple-plane or volume implant and about 5 mm from a single-plane implant is usually chosen. However, depending on the physician's clinical judgment (i.e., whether he thinks a tumor will be difficult or easy to control), there is always a "fudge factor" whereby a little higher or lower total dose than usual may be administered by merely selecting a slightly more or less generous isodose line. For both cases, the "tumor dose" that is said to have been delivered would be identical even though the actual doses may differ by 10% to 15% or more. The technique routinely adopted by Martin of leaving a full-intensity implant in place for 7 days can hardly be criticized considering his results and the lack of consistency in today's methods of dose specification.[69] Isodose curves through several levels of the tumor should be reviewed, and at least two planes of calculation, generally at right angles to each other, should be viewed.

Paterson[84] and Ellis[28] both recommended adjustment of the total interstitial dose according to dose rate (Fig. 13-26). Paterson used as his reference a 7-day implant and set out the doses that, when given in 5 to 10 days, would be equivalent to the 7-day dose. As an example, suppose one desired an effect equivalent to 6000 rad/7 days (36 rad/hour). If the geometric arrangement of sources is such that a higher dose rate (e.g., 46 rad/hour) is achieved, then according to Paterson's recommendations the total dose should be reduced to approximately 5500 rad/5 days. Conversely, if a dose rate lower than 36 rad/hour is obtained, then a total dose higher than 6000 rad should be administered in an overall time of greater than 7 days.

The initial Paterson curve "owed more to inspiration than to science" but was said to have been gradually corrected over a period of time to match his actual experience. Since no data were ever published to substantiate either the Ellis or Paterson curves, one cannot assess their degree of accuracy.

The curves of Paterson and Ellis have not been verified by available clinical data. The data of Pierquin and associates on interstitial treatment of cancer of the floor of

the mouth and oral tongue indicate that for the same tumor dose of 7000 rad, the treatment time may vary from 3 days (approximately 90 rad/hour) to 9 days (approximately 30 rad/hour) without affecting the rates of necrosis or tumor recurrence (Table 13-19)[88] For 3- to 9-day treatments, he concluded that one need not adjust the total dose to compensate for different dose rates. Awwad and co-workers, in treating T1–T2 tongue cancers by interstitial radium, usually adjusted the total dose according to dose rate so that "biologically equivalent" doses would be achieved.[3] When the total dose was lowered to correct for higher dose rates, local control was poor. At the University of Florida, no adjustment in total dose is recommended for implant therapy in the 30-rad to 80-rad/hour range; we generally attempt to maintain the rate as close to 40 rad/hour as possible, thereby largely eliminating dose rate as a variable in our implant patients.

We usually choose low-intensity (0.33 mg/cm or 0.66 mg/cm) radium needles so that the dose rate falls in the 35-rad to 60-rad/hour range. Very small-volume implants (e.g., T1 cancers of the floor of mouth) often require 0.66 mg/cm needles, while large volume two- or three-plane implants usually require 0.33 mg/cm needles. Very high-intensity implants (e.g., 6300 rad/20 hours at 315 rad/hour with 5 mg/cm radium needles for oral tongue cancer) may result in a high rate of necrosis,[25] but this has not been noted in all centers; at the Radium Center in Aarhus, Denmark, 766 lip cancers were treated between 1946 and 1966 with a very short (4 hours), high-intensity (10 mg radium/cm) needle technique with a high rate of tumor control and acceptable cosmetic results and complication rates.[56] At the other extreme of very low dose rate, patient discomfort becomes a problem because the implant times are very long; of even greater importance, at sufficiently low dose rates, tumor cell proliferation may continue during therapy.

In the early years of radiation therapy with kilovoltage apparatus, it was observed that the x-ray dose that the skin would tolerate was a function of the area (sq cm) irradiated. The same principle applies today to supervoltage therapy: the greater the volume (cc), the lower the dose that can be safely delivered. Applying the same principle to interstitial therapy, Paterson recommended that the total dose be reduced when large volumes were implanted. For a single-plane implant to the tongue, 6750 rad/7 days was permissible; a small volume (cylindrical) implant to a tongue lesion might safely deliver 6300 rad/7 days while

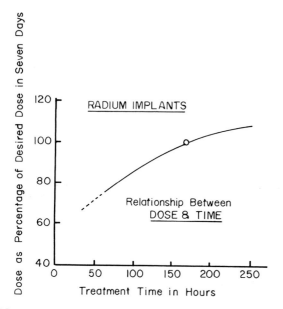

FIG. 13-26. Paterson's recommended relationship between time and dose for radium implants. The curve shows the variation of total dose with treatment time to produce the same (iso-) effect in 5 to 10 days as that produced by a 7 day implant. (Redrawn from Paterson R: Studies in optimum dosage. The Mackenzie Davidson Memorial Lecture. Br J Radiol 25, No. 298:505–516, 1952)

T Stage*	Treatment Time 3–4 Days Necrosis	Treatment Time 3–4 Days Local Control	Treatment Time 5–6 Days Necrosis	Treatment Time 5–6 Days Local Control	Treatment Time 7–8 Days and Over Necrosis	Treatment Time 7–8 Days and Over Local Control
T1	ND	ND	ND	ND	0/2	2/2 (100%)
T2	ND	ND	2/11 (18%)	10/11 (90%)	0/15	15/15 (100%)
T3	1/8 (13%)	8/8 (100%)	6/25 (24%)	20/25 (80%)	4/16 (25%)	12/16 (75%)
T4	0/1	0/1	1/3 (33%)	1/3 (33%)	ND	ND

TABLE 13-19. Carcinomas of the Anterior Tongue and Floor of Mouth Treated with Interstitial Iridium-192: 7000 rad Tumor Dose (Institut Gustav-Roussy and Hôpital Henri Mondor)

* T stages differ from AJCC staging system: T1: <1 cm; T2: 1–3 cm; T3: 3–5 cm; T4: >5 cm.
(ND, no data)

(Modified from Pierquin BM, Chassagne D, Baillet F, Paine CH: Clinical observations on the time factor in interstitial radiotherapy using iridium-192. Clin Radiol 24:506–509, 1973) large volume implants should be limited to 5850 rad/7 days. "As a result, the tumors of larger volume with, for that reason, the poorer prognosis, tend to get lower dose than those of smaller size".[84] This approach ignores the fact that the greater the number of malignant clonogens, the higher is the dose necessary to achieve tumor control. A dose reduction in interstitial implant therapy is not recommended when treating large tumors. The dose in such cases is, in fact, generally higher than in small implants. Pierquin's experience with carcinomas of the floor of the mouth and oral tongue justifies this approach (see Table 13-19).[88] When patients are grouped according to overall treatment time, one notes that as the T stage (and thus the implanted volume) increases, there is a trend toward higher rates of necrosis. The increased rate of necrosis is, however, not so great that one should risk underdosage of tumor.

There is no reported experience with fractionated implant therapy, that is, implant therapy divided into two or more treatment sessions, as is standard for cancers of the uterine cervix.

PLANNED COMBINED TREATMENT

Planned combined surgery and irradiation is useful in the treatment of certain large tumors in which treatment by a single modality would likely be unsuccessful. When irradiation is the only treatment, failure to control large masses is frequent. On the other hand, surgery is quite good for large, resectable disease, but even very radical procedures frequently do not remove all microscopic tumor in the presence of extensive infiltration. Either preoperative or postoperative irradiation may be employed, and each has certain advantages and disadvantages.

Time–Dose Data for Postoperative Irradiation

In undissected tissues, 5000 rad/5 weeks produces a high rate of control of subclinical squamous cell carcinoma in both primary and lymph node sites. Following surgical interruption of the normal vasculature and scarring in the tumor bed of advanced head and neck cancers, 5000 rad is incapable of producing control of residual disease in a substantial number of patients; the failure rate following this dose is 40% to 50% for some tumor sites. At the M. D. Anderson Hospital, control above the clavicles following postoperative irradiation for advanced lesions of the supraglottic larynx and pyriform sinus was good—87% and 89%, respectively.[37,44] For advanced lesions of the oral cavity and oropharynx, however, treatment failed in more than half of the patients because of disease recurrence above the clavicles following 5000 rad to 6000 rad (Table 13-20).[46] Although some of the failures were in untreated areas of the neck, the failure rate at the primary site alone was 31%. The results of modest-dose (4500 rad to 5400 rad) postoperative irradiation for a variety of tumor sites at Memorial Sloan-Kettering, New York City, are also shown in Table 13-20.[111] The failure rate is 50% for patients who have a minimum of 2 years' follow-up.

The M. D. Anderson Hospital and Memorial Sloan-Kettering postoperative irradiation series for oral cavity–oropharynx lesions have recently been updated.[31,112] At M. D. Anderson Hospital, 81 evaluable patients had 2 years' minimum follow-up. Postoperative doses were 6000 rad to 6500 rad in 61 (75%) of 81 patients, and 5000 rad to 5500 rad in the remainder. Thirty-eight percent (31/81) developed in-field (dose-related) failures above the clavicles. When surgical margins at the primary site were positive, doses in the 6000-rad to 6600-rad range controlled the primary lesion in only 3 (33%) of 9 patients; in some instances, the dose to the site of failure was actually lower than the dose specified since several failures occurred near the field edge. In the Memorial Sloan-Kettering series, when one excludes from analysis those patients who died of intercurrent disease or distant metastasis alone, the failure rate was 14/35 (40%) following 4500 rad/4½ weeks to 6000 rad/6 weeks.

Combined treatment of tongue lesions presents three special problems: (1) the surgeon often has difficulty at the operating table in judging adequate margins; (2) the entire organ is not removed; and (3) local control by external-beam irradiation alone is worse, stage for stage, than for other sites within the oral cavity, oropharynx, or larynx.[74] Bamberg and co-workers found that very substantial doses

TABLE 13-20.	Results of Postoperative Treatment for Advanced Squamous Cell Carcinomas of the Head and Neck			
Institution	**Tumor Sites**	**Dose (rad/Weeks)**	**No. Evaluable Patients***	**Failure Above the Clavicles (%)**
M. D. Anderson Hospital	Oropharynx, oral cavity	5000/5 to 6000/6	39	20 (51%)
Memorial Sloan-Kettering	Oral cavity, oropharynx, supraglottic larynx, hypopharynx, salivary gland	4500–5400/5–5½	14	7 (50%)

* Patients who died with less than 2 years' minimum follow-up of intercurrent disease, distant metastases, or complications with disease controlled above the clavicles are excluded from analysis.

(Data from Hamberger AD, Fletcher GH, Guillamondegui MD, Byers MD; Advanced squamous cell carcinoma of the oral cavity and oropharynx treated with irradiation and surgery. Radiology 119:433–438, 1976, and Vikram B: The importance of the time interval between surgery and postoperative radiation therapy in the combined management of head and neck cancer. Int J Radiat Oncol Biol Phys 5:1837–1840, 1979

of external-beam irradiation were required postoperatively in order to obtain satisfactory control rates for oral tongue carcinoma managed by very conservative resections.[5]

At the University of Florida, postoperative irradiation is used in preference to preoperative radiation therapy (see Chapter 7, General Principles for Treatment of Cancers in the Head and Neck: Combining Surgery and Radiation Therapy). In 1979, Marcus and associates performed a retrospective dose-response analysis on postoperatively irradiated patients.[66] In 1981, the data were reanalyzed with a larger number of patients and longer follow-up.* In contrast to the 1979 analysis, only patients who received a continuous course of irradiation were analyzed because the rate of failure above the clavicles for split-course patients was high (11/19 or 58%) compared with those treated by continuous-course technique (10/55 or 18%). Between October 1964 and December 1979, 74 patients with advanced squamous cell carcinomas of the oral cavity, oropharynx, glottic larynx, supraglottic larynx, or pyriform sinus were treated at the University of Florida by radical surgery and postoperative continuous-course irradiation with cobalt-60 or 2 MeV. Sixty-nine of 74 patients had AJCC stage III or IV disease. The decision to give postoperative irradiation was based on the preoperative evaluation, the findings at surgery, and the pathology report from the resected specimen. All patients had a minimum 2-year follow-up. None had evidence of gross cancer at the time of irradiation. Irradiation was begun in all patients within 3 months of surgery; in most patients, irradiation was started 2 to 4 weeks after operation. Nineteen patients were excluded from the control analysis because they died of intercurrent disease (9) or distant metastasis (10), with disease controlled above the clavicles, before 2 years had elapsed; 55 patients were therefore evaluable for control above the clavicles.

Most patients were irradiated with parallel opposed fields to the primary lesion and upper neck; the low neck and supraclavicular areas were treated with a single anterior field. Scars were bolused to ensure adequate dosage to these high-risk sites. Portals were reduced off the spinal cord at 4700 rad to 5000 rad. Electrons were not available during the study period so the dose to the neck behind the plane of the spinal cord was generally 5000 rad or less, depending on the relative weighting of the fields. In the early years, a small number of patients (13) with laryngeal or hypopharyngeal primary lesions were treated with a single anterior field that encompassed the primary site and both the upper and the lower neck.

Ten patients developed failures above the clavicles, eight in the primary field alone, one in both the primary and low neck fields, and one out of the treatment field. The low neck failure occurred after 5000 rad given dose; although a wide range of doses was used for the lower neck, a time–dose analysis is pointless since there was only one failure. The current University of Florida recommendation is 5000 rad to 6000 rad to the lower neck, depending on the presence or absence of subglottic extension and the number of nodes involved.

Although four failures occurred on mucosal surfaces, most of the recurrences were located in the soft tissues of the neck, in or about the surgical scar. These recurrences apparently stemmed from wound implantation, tumor at the deep surgical margins of the primary lesion, positive lymph nodes left behind after radical neck dissection, or

* Jacobson HM: Unpublished data, 1982.

perinodal extensions. Since it is impossible to accurately categorize many failures as either *primary* or *nodal* in origin, it is easier to lump both types of failure together under a single term, *failure above the clavicles.*

There was little correlation between the failure rate and the T or N stages. Failures correlated best with dose. The time–dose analysis for the primary lesion and upper neck field is complex because not all points within the field received the same dose. Reductions were made off the spinal cord at 4700 rad to 5000 rad, so that the posterior upper neck always received a lower dose than the tissues anterior to the spinal cord. Because the relative weights of the portals were not always equal, the dose to the right and left necks was frequently different. Dose calculations have been made for each posterior neck region (posterior to the plane of the cord) as well as for the primary region (anterior to the plane of the cord). For the patients who received treatment by way of an anterior field alone, the dose to the primary lesion was taken at 4 cm depth. There were six failures anterior to the plane of the spinal cord, three posterior to the cord, and one out of the radiation field. Failure in the primary and upper neck regions versus dose for sites that were histologically proven to have contained disease (i.e., the primary site and pathologically positive necks) is analyzed in Table 13-21. Below 5750 rad, there was a 16% failure rate, while above this dose only 3% developed in-field failures. For sites that were clinically and/or pathologically negative, 5000 rad is generally sufficient (Table 13-22).

Postoperative dose versus overall treatment time (days) is plotted in Figure 13-27 for areas that were histologically proven to have contained disease (i.e., primary sites and posterior upper necks of patients with pathologically positive nodes). Clinically and/or pathologically negative necks are excluded in order to gain a better appreciation of the dose required to produce control of subclinical cancer in surgically dissected tissues. There was only one failure at or above 6000 rad (a patient with a T3N3B tonsillar lesion who had positive margins at the primary site). Unless the margins of resection are positive, it can be concluded that 6000 rad/6 to 6½ weeks will produce a high rate of control for most primary sites. For patients with positive or questionable margins at any site, no less than 6500 rad is recommended, and if the site of positive margins is the oral cavity or oropharynx, 7000 rad/8 weeks is delivered through reducing portals. For lesions of the tongue, less than 6500 rad/7 weeks is never administered, even if margins are negative. Patients with tumors at any site who have more than one indication for postoperative irradiation (e.g., close margins plus perinodal tumor extension or cartilage invasion plus multiple positive nodes) receive 6500 rad/7 weeks to the areas of highest risk. There is a great need for more time–dose information in the postoperative setting. The dose recommendations at the University of Florida are based on a limited number of failures; these recommendations will no doubt continue to be revised as more data are accumulated and a better appreciation is gained of the risks as they relate to tumor site and various pathologic features.

Complications of the soft tissue and bone did not strongly correlate with dose (Table 13-23). The complications analyzed in Table 13-23 (laryngeal edema, stricture, soft tissue and bone necrosis, and painful fibrosis) are those secondary to combined therapy; complications of surgery that healed before irradiation are not included. Five patients (9%) had severe complications. There were no deaths related to

TABLE 13-21. Number (%) of Patients With Primary and/or Upper Neck Failure According to Postoperative Dose to Areas Pathologically Proven to Have Contained Cancer (University of Florida)

Dose Range (rad)	Primary Field (Anterior to Spinal Cord)	Posterior Upper Neck Field (N⁺ Pathologically)	Other Field Arrangement*	Total
≦4750	0/1	0/16	1/1	1/18 (6%)
4751–5250	0/1	2/6	3/7	5/14 (36%)
5251–5750	1/8		0/3	1/11 (9%)
5751–6250	0/8†	0/6	0/1	0/15
6251–6750	1/17†		0/1	1/18 (6%)
≧6751	0/5			0/5

* Mostly anterior field alone.

† Two patients are excluded who died before 2 years due to failure elsewhere in the treatment volume without evidence of recurrence in the primary field of irradiation.

Note: University of Florida data; patients treated 10/64–12/79; minimum 2-year to unlimited follow-up; analysis 12/81 by H. M. Jacobson, MD.

TABLE 13-22. Number (%) of Patients With Posterior Upper Neck Failure According to Postoperative Dose to Pathologically and/or Clinically Negative Areas (University of Florida)

Dose Range (rad)	Posterior Upper Neck Field		Total
	N− (Pathologically)	N− (Clinically)	
≦4750	0/6	0/22	0/28
4751–5250	0/2	1/11	1/13 (8%)
5251–5750		0/1	0/1
5751–6250	0/2	0/1	0/3
6251–6750			
≧6751			

Note: University of Florida data; patients treated 10/64–12/79; minimum 2-year to unlimited follow-up; analysis 12/81 by H. M. Jacobson, MD.

FIG. 13-27. Time–dose scatter distribution for control following continuous-course postoperative irradiation. The points plotted are for sites contained in Table 13-21, that is, sites known to have contained disease (primary sites and/or pathologically positive necks). (University of Florida data; patients treated 10/64–12/79; analysis 12/81 by H. M. Jacobson, MD)

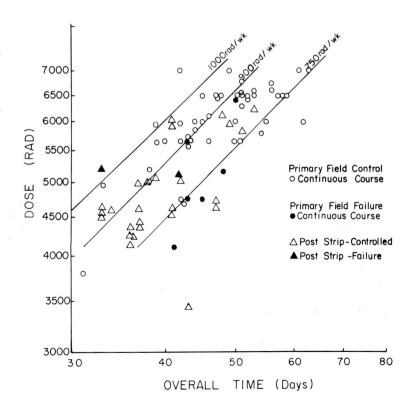

TABLE 13-23. Postoperative Dose Versus Soft Tissue and Bone Complications

Dose Range (rad)	Oral Cavity—Oropharynx			Supraglottic and Glottic Larynx, Pyriform Sinus		
	No. Patients	Moderate*	Severe†	No. Patients	Moderate*	Severe†
≦5750	3	0	1 (33%)	21	2 (10%)	1 (5%)
5751–6250	1	1 (100%)	0	6	1 (17%)	1 (17%)
6251–6750	6	0	0	13	2 (15%)	1 (8%)
≧6751	5	0	1 (20%)			

* Persistent problem (*e.g.,* stricture) that required only conservative treatment or a single simple procedure to correct.
† Required operation.

Note: University of Florida data; patients treated 10/64–12/79; minimum 2-year to unlimited follow-up; analysis 12/81 by H. M. Jacobson, MD.

TABLE 13-24. Prospective Randomized Trials of Low-Dose (1000–2000 R) Preoperative Irradiation for Head and Neck Squamous Cell Carcinomas

	Memorial Sloan-Kettering Hospital[104]		Medical College of Virginia[60]		National Cancer Institute[58]	
	2000 R/5 Days to Neck Then Operation as Soon as Possible*	Neck Dissection Alone*	700 rad × 2, 24 and 48 Hours Preoperatively†	Operation Alone†	1000 R 24 Hours Preoperatively‡	Operation Alone‡
Recurrence above clavicles	Not applicable; primary site not always irradiated		15/63 (24%)	24/63 (38%)	12/60 (20%)	6/18 (33%)
			($p = 0.13$)		($p = 0.14$)	
Neck recurrence with primary controlled	52/181 (17.6%)	23/131 (28.7%)	Not given		Not given	
	($p = 0.032$)					
Distant metastasis	Not given		12/63 (19%)	11/63 (17%)	36%	30%
Major complications	No difference		No difference		21%	0
Survival	No difference		No difference		Not given	

* One year minimum follow-up. † Six months minimum follow-up. ‡ No minimum period of follow-up.

postoperative irradiation. Although subcutaneous fibrosis is possibly greater after 6500 rad to 7000 rad than after 6000 rad, such a subjective judgment is difficult to make; there has not been a major difference in symptomatology among the higher dose versus the lower dose patients, and the prospects of increased local-regional control seem to outweigh the problem of fibrosis, especially in patients with positive margins.

Preoperative Irradiation

LOW-DOSE (≦3000 RAD) PREOPERATIVE IRRADIATION

It has been theorized by several investigators and shown for some animal tumors that low doses of irradiation may diminish the ability of cancer cells to implant in surgical wounds or distant sites.[52,79] A number of preoperative irradiation trials have tested this hypothesis in head and neck cancer patients.[58,60,104] The results are summarized in Table 13-24. In the Medical College of Virginia and Memorial Sloan–Kettering Hospital trials, the local results are given with minimum 6- and 12-month follow-up, respectively; that is, patients who died of other causes before 6 or 12 months with disease still controlled are excluded from analysis. There was no period of minimum follow-up in the National Cancer Institute study, so some of the patients who lived for only a short time postoperatively were scored as "controlled." All of the trials showed modest reductions in the frequency of local-regional recurrence but not enough difference to affect survival rates significantly.

At M. D. Anderson Hospital, 2000 rad/5 fractions was

TABLE 13-25. Randomized Trial of Preoperative Versus Postoperative Irradiation for Carcinoma of the Pyriform Sinus, Arytenoid, or Aryepiglottic Fold (Gustave-Roussy Institute and Henri Becquerel Center)

Treatment	No. Patients Randomized	No. Patients Who Completed Intended Therapy	5-Year Survival (%)	No. (%) Carotid Artery Ruptures	No. (%) Treatment-Related Deaths
Preoperative irradiation (5500 rad/5½ weeks—2-week delay—operation)	25	16	28%	6 (38%)	5 (31%)
Postoperative irradiation (operation—<4-week delay—5500 rad/6 weeks)	24	23	56%	0 (0%)	0 (0%)

(Data from Vandenbrouck C, Sancho H, LeFur R, Richard JM, Cachin Y: Results of a randomized clinical trial of preoperative irradiation versus postoperative irradiation in treatment of tumors of the hypopharynx. Cancer 39: 1445–1449, 1977)

used preoperatively for ten stage III–IV squamous cell carcinomas of the oral cavity.[46] Five (63%) of eight evaluable patients developed treatment failures above the clavicles. Because of these poor results, the technique was quickly abandoned. It was concluded that this schedule was particularly inefficacious when there was perinodal tumor extension into the connective tissues of the neck.

At Washington University in St Louis, medium-dose irradiation (3000 rad/3 weeks to the midline, usually from a single ipsilateral field) followed by resection was for many years a frequently employed treatment strategy for head and neck cancers. In an analysis of 137 patients with carcinoma of the pyriform sinus who were treated by preoperative irradiation followed by either partial laryngopharyngectomy or total laryngectomy–partial pharyngectomy and ipsilateral neck dissection, Marks and co-workers were disappointed by the significant numbers of failures at the primary site and ipsilateral neck.[68] (See Chapter 21, Hypopharynx: Pharyngeal Walls, Pyriform Sinus, and Postcricoid Pharynx.) Fixed lymph nodes rarely (2/11 or 18%) became resectable after this dose, nor did low-dose treatment of the contralateral neck (approximately 2500 rad/3 weeks) prevent the growth of subclinical disease since 20/137 patients (15%) developed contralateral neck failure following surgery. My colleagues and I agree with their conclusions:

1. The preoperative doses were too low.
2. Operation and high-dose postoperative irradiation for advanced lesions would likely result in fewer recurrences above the clavicles and would be safer than a switch to high-dose preoperative irradiation.

HIGH-DOSE (4500 RAD TO 5500 RAD)
PREOPERATIVE IRRADIATION

In terms of local and regional control, it seems that 5000 rad preoperatively is as efficacious as 5000 rad to 6000 rad postoperatively. For advanced oral cavity and oropharyngeal squamous cell carcinomas at M. D. Anderson Hospital, 32% and 31% of patients developed recurrences at the primary site when given preoperative or postoperative irradiation, respectively.[46] Whether neck dissection is preceded or followed by such doses, Lindberg and Fletcher observed very low failure rates in the operated neck.[63]

A major difference between high-dose preoperative and postoperative irradiation, for most head and neck sites, is that postoperative irradiation generally results in a lower immediate complication rate.[55] In general, 5000 rad is the upper limit that can be given preoperatively to the entire treatment volume when composite resection is to follow; occasionally a small-field boost can be given for an additional 1000 rad to an area of heavy tumor infestation where there will be no closing sutures.[33] When a composite resection is done after preoperative irradiation, the incidence of fistulization, carotid artery rupture, and skin sloughs is higher than after operation alone.[114] When neck dissection is the only operative procedure to be performed, 6000 rad to 8000 rad may have been delivered to the primary lesion and upper neck. With a small primary lesion and large node, only the lymph node mass(es) receive the higher doses (see Chapter 7, General Principles for Treatment of Cancers in the Head and Neck: Combining Surgery and Radiation Therapy). The complication rate from neck dissection after high-dose irradiation is acceptable.

The more extensive the surgical procedure and the higher the preoperative dose, the more frequent and severe are the complications. Between May 1967 and February 1969, a randomized trial between 5500 rad preoperatively or postoperatively for pyriform sinus, aryepiglottic fold, or arytenoid carcinomas was conducted in France.[110] The operation was the same in both groups: total laryngectomy, partial pharyngectomy, and ipsilateral radical neck dissection. Results of the trial, which favor postoperative irradiation both in terms of survival and morbidity, are shown in Table 13-25.

REFERENCES

1. Andrews JR: Dose–time relationships in cancer radiotherapy: A clinical radiobiology study of extremes of dose and time. Am J Roentgenol Radium Ther Nucl Med 93:56–74, 1965
2. Atkins HL: Massive dose technique in radiation therapy of inoperable carcinoma of the breast. Am J Roentgenol Radium Ther Nucl Med 91:80–89, 1964
3. Awwad HK, Burgers JMV, Marcuse HR: The influence of tumor dose specification on the early clinical results of in-

terstitial radium tongue implants. Radiology 110:177–182, 1974

4. Baclesse F: Clinical experience with ultra-fractionated roentgen therapy. In Buschke F (ed): Progress in Radiation Therapy, vol I, pp 128–143. New York, Grune & Stratton, 1958

5. Bamberg M, Schulz U, Scherer E: Postoperative split-course radiotherapy of squamous cell carcinoma of the oral tongue. Int J Radiat Oncol Biol Phys 5:515–519, 1979

6. Barker JL, Fletcher GH: Time, dose, and tumor volume relationships in megavoltage irradiation of squamous cell carcinomas of the retromolar trigone and anterior tonsillar pillar. Int J Radiat Oncol Biol Phys 2:407–414, 1977

7. Barker JL, Montague ED, Peters LJ: Clinical experience with irradiation of inflammatory carcinoma of the breast with and without elective chemotherapy. Cancer 45:625–629, 1980

8. Barkley HT, Fletcher GH: The significance of residual disease after external irradiation of squamous cell carcinoma of the oropharynx. Radiology 124:493–495, 1977

9. Bennett MB: The treatment of stage III squamous carcinoma of the cervix in air and hyperbaric-oxygen (abstr). Br J Radiol 51:68, 1978

10. Berger DS, Fletcher GH, Lindberg D, Jesse RH: Elective irradiation of the neck lymphatics for squamous cell carcinomas of the nasopharynx and oropharynx. Am J Roentgenol Radium Ther Nucl Med 111:66–72, 1971

11. Bloedorn FG, Cuccia CA, Mercado R: The place of interstitial gamma-ray emitters in radiation therapy: Indications—technique—examples. Am J Roentgenol Radium Ther Nucl Med 85:407–447, 1961

12. Buschke F, Vaeth JM: Radiation therapy of carcinoma of the vocal cord without mucosal reaction. Am J Roentgenol Radium Ther Nucl Med 89:29–34, 1963

13. Bush RS, Jenkin RDT, Allt WEC, Beale FA, Bean H, Dembo AJ, Pringle JF: Definitive evidence for hypoxic cells influencing cure in cancer therapy. Br J Cancer 37:302–306, 1978

14. Byhardt RW, Greenberg M, Cox JD: Local control of squamous carcinoma of the oral cavity and oropharynx with 3 versus 5 treatment fractions per week. Int J Radiat Oncol Biol Phys 2:415–420, 1977

15. Cade S: Soft tissue tumours: Their natural history and treatment. Proc R Soc Med 44:19–36, 1951

16. Castro JR, Lindberg RD, Fletcher GH: Clinical application of computer dosimetry in interstitial radium therapy. Am J Roentgenol Radium Ther Nucl Med 105:165–171, 1969

17. Chu A, Fletcher GH: Incidence and causes of failures to control by irradiation the primary lesions in squamous cell carcinoma of the anterior two-thirds of the tongue and floor of mouth. Am J Roentgenol Radium Ther Nucl Med 117:502–508, 1973

18. Coutard H: Roentgen therapy of epitheliomas of the tonsillar region, hypopharynx, and larynx from 1920–1926. Am J Roentgenol Radium Ther 28:313–331, 1932

19. Coutard H: X-ray treatment of inoperable carcinoma of the larynx. Surg Gynecol Obstet 68:467–471, 1939

20. Cutler SJ, Ederer F: Maximum utilization of the life table method in analyzing survival. J Chron Dis 8:699–712, 1958

21. Dickens WJ, Cassisi NJ, Million RR, Bova FJ: Treatment of early vocal cord carcinoma: A comparison of apples and apples. Laryngoscope 93:216–219, 1983

22. Dickens WJ, Million RR, Cassisi NJ, Singleton GT: Chemodectomas arising in temporal bone structures. Laryngoscope 92:188–191, 1982

23. Dische S, Martin WMC, Anderson P: Radiation myelopathy in patients treated for carcinoma of the bronchus using a six fraction regime of radiotherapy. Br J Radiol 54:29–35, 1981

24. Dutreix J, Wambersie A, Bounik C: Cellular recovery in human skin reactions: Application to dose fraction number overall time relationship in radiotherapy. Eur J Cancer 9:159–167, 1973

25. Eberhard TP: Radium in the treatment of cancer of the tongue. Am J Roentgenol Radium Ther Nucl Med 69:789–791, 1953

26. Edelman AH, Holtz S, Powers WE: Rapid radiotherapy for inoperable carcinoma of the breast: Benefits and complications. Am J Roentgenol Radium Ther Nucl Med 93:585–599, 1965

27. Ellingwood KE, Million RR, Mitchell TP: A preloaded radium needle implant device for maintenance of needle spacing. Cancer 37:2858–2860, 1976

28. Ellis F: The relationship of biological effect to dose–time–fractionation factors in radiotherapy. Curr Top Radiat Res 4:357–397, 1968

29. Ellis F: Dose, time, and fractionation: A clinical hypothesis. Clin Radiol 20:1–7, 1969

30. Evans JC, Bergsjø P: The influence of anemia on the results of radiotherapy in carcinoma of the cervix. Radiology 84:709–717, 1965

31. Feldman M, Fletcher GH: Analysis of the parameters relating to failures above the clavicles in patients treated by postoperative irradiation for squamous cell carcinomas of the oral cavity or oropharynx. Int J Radiat Oncol Biol Phys 8:27–30, 1982

32. Fletcher GH: Clinical dose-response curves of human malignant epithelial tumors. Br J Radiol 46:1–12, 1973

33. Fletcher GH: Indications for combination of irradiation and surgery. J Radiol Electrol 57:379–390, 1976

34. Fletcher GH: Basic principles of the combination of irradiation and surgery. Int J Radiat Oncol Biol Phys 5:2091–2096, 1979

35. Fletcher GH: Textbook of Radiotherapy, 3rd ed, pp 180–219. Philadelphia, Lea & Febiger, 1980

36. Fletcher GH: Pierluigi Nervi International Award acceptance speech. Int J Radiat Oncol Biol Phys 8:87, 1982

37. Fletcher GH, Jesse RH: The place of irradiation in the management of the primary lesion in head and neck cancer. Cancer 39:862–867, 1977

38. Fletcher GH, Lindberg RD, Hamberger A, Horiot J-C: Reasons for irradiation failure in squamous cell carcinoma of the larynx. Laryngoscope 85:987–1003, 1975

39. Fletcher GH, Shukovsky LJ: The interplay of radiocurability and tolerance in the irradiation of human cancers. J Radiol Electrol 56:383–400, 1975

40. Fu KK, Chan EK, Phillips TL, Ray JW: Time, dose and volume factors in interstitial radium implants of carcinoma of the oral tongue. Radiology 119:209–213, 1976

41. Fu KK, Ray JW, Chan EK, Phillips TL: External and interstitial radiation therapy of carcinoma of the oral tongue: A review of 32 years' experience. Am J Roentgenol 126:107–115, 1976

42. Gehan EA: A generalized Wilcoxon test for arbitrarily comparing single-censored samples. Biometrika 52:203–223, 1965

43. Gelinas M, Fletcher GH: Incidence and causes of local failure of irradiation in squamous cell carcinoma of the faucial arch, tonsillar fossa, and base of tongue. Radiology 108:383–387, 1973

44. Goepfert H, Jesse RH, Fletcher GH, Hamberger A: Optimal treatment for the technically resectable squamous cell carcinoma of the supraglottic larynx. Laryngoscope 85:14–32, 1975

45. Hall EJ: Radiobiology for the Radiologist, 2nd ed. Hagerstown, MD, Harper & Row, 1978

46. Hamberger AD, Fletcher GH, Guillamondegui MD, Byers MD: Advanced squamous cell carcinoma of the oral cavity and oropharynx treated with irradiation and surgery. Radiology 119:433–438, 1976

47. Harwood AR, Beale FA, Cummings BJ, Hawkins NV, Keane TJ, Rider WD: T3 glottic cancer: An analysis of dose time-volume factors. Int J Radiat Oncol Biol Phys 6:675–680, 1980

48. Hermens AF, Barendsen GW: Changes of cell proliferation characteristics in a rat rhabdomyosarcoma before and after x-irradiation. Eur J Cancer 5:173–189, 1969

49. Holsti LR: Clinical experience with split-course radiotherapy: A randomized clinical trial. Radiology 92:591–596, 1969

50. Holthusen H: Erfahrungen über die Verträglichkeitsgrenze für Röntgenstrahlen und deren Nutzanwendung zur Verhütung von Schäden. Strahlentherapie 57:254–269, 1936

51. Horiuchi J, Adachi T: Some considerations on radiation therapy of tongue cancer. Cancer 28:335–339, 1971

52. Hoye RC, Smith RR: The effectiveness of small amounts of preoperative irradiation in preventing the growth of tumor cells disseminated at surgery: An experimental study. Cancer 14:284–295, 1961

53. Inoue T, Fuchihata H, Wada T, Shigematsu T: Local prognosis after combined external and interstitial radiation therapy for carcinoma of the tongue. Acta Radiol Ther Phys Biol 15:315–320, 1976

54. Jampolis S, Pipard G, Horiot J-C, Bolla M, Le Dorze C: Preliminary results using twice-a-day fractionation in the radiotherapeutic management of advanced cancers of the head and neck. AJR 129:1091–1093, 1977

55. Jesse RH, Lindberg RD: The efficacy of combining radiation therapy with a surgical procedure in patients with cervical metastasis from squamous cancer of the oropharynx and hypopharynx. Cancer 35:1163–1166, 1975

56. Jørgensen K, Elbrønd O, Andersen AP: Carcinoma of the lip: A series of 869 cases. Acta Radiol Ther Phys Biol 12:177–190, 1973

57. Kal HB, Barendsen GW: Effects of continuous irradiation at low dose-rates on a rat rhabdomyosarcoma. Br J Radiol 45:279–283, 1972

58. Ketcham AS, Hoye RC, Chretien PB, Brace KC: Irradiation twenty-four hours preoperatively. Am J Surg 118:691–697, 1969

59. Kok G: The influence of the size of the fraction dose on normal and tumour tissue in ^{60}Co radiation treatment of carcinoma of the larynx and inoperable carcinoma of the breast. Radiol Clin Biol 40:100–115, 1971

60. Lawrence W, Terz JJ, Rogers C, King RE, Wolf JS, King ER: Preoperative irradiation for head and neck cancer: A prospective study. Cancer 33:318–323, 1974

61. Lees AW: The treatment of carcinoma of the anterior two-thirds of the tongue by radiotherapy. Int J Radiat Oncol Biol Phys 1:849–858, 1976

62. Lindberg RD, Fletcher GH: Clinical experiences with altered fractionation. Rev Interam Radiol 7:15–21, 1972

63. Lindberg RD, Fletcher GH: The role of irradiation in the management of head and neck cancer: Analysis of results and causes of failures. Tumori 64:313–325, 1978

64. McNeer GP, Cantin J, Chu F, Nickson JJ: Effectiveness of radiation therapy in the management of sarcoma of the soft somatic tissues. Cancer 22:391–397, 1968

65. Marcial VA, Hanley JA, Chang C, Davis LW, Moscol JA: Split-course radiation therapy of carcinoma of the nasopharynx: Results of a national collaborative clinical trial of the Radiation Therapy Oncology Group. Int J Radiat Oncol Biol Phys 6:409–414, 1980

66. Marcus RB Jr, Million RR, Cassisi NJ: Postoperative irradiation for squamous cell carcinomas of the head and neck: Analysis of time–dose factors related to control above the clavicles. Int J Radiat Oncol Biol Phys 5:1943–1949, 1979

67. Marcus RB Jr, Million RR, Mitchell TP: A preloaded, custom-designed implantation device for stage T1–T2 carcinoma of the floor of mouth. Int J Radiat Oncol Biol Phys 6:111–113, 1980

68. Marks JE, Kurnik B, Powers WE, Ogura JH: Carcinoma of the pyriform sinus: An analysis of treatment results and patterns of failure. Cancer 41:1008–1015, 1978

69. Martin CL, Martin JA: Low Intensity Radium Therapy. Boston, Little, Brown & Co, 1959

70. Mendenhall WM, Million RR, Cassisi NJ: Elective neck irradiation in squamous cell carcinoma of the head and neck. Head Neck Surg 3:15–20, 1980

71. Mendenhall W, Ott L, Larson RF: Statistics: A Tool for the Social Sciences, p 336. North Scituate, MA, Duxbury Press, 1974

72. Mendenhall WM, Van Cise WS, Bova FJ, Million RR: Analysis of time–dose factors in squamous cell carcinoma of the oral tongue and floor of mouth treated with radiation therapy alone. Int J Radiat Oncol Biol Phys 7:1005–1011, 1981

73. Miescher G: Erfolge der Karzinombehandlung an der Dermatologischen Klinik Zurich: Einzeitige Höchstdosis und frakionierte Behandlung. Strahlentherapie 49:65–81, 1934

74. Million RR: Squamous cell carcinoma of the head and neck: Combined therapy: Surgery and postoperative irradiation. Int J Radiat Oncol Biol Phys 5:2161–2162, 1979

75. Million RR, Cassisi NJ: Radical irradiation for carcinoma of the pyriform sinus. Laryngoscope 91:439–450, 1981

76. Million RR, Fletcher GH, Jesse RH: Evaluation of elective irradiation of the neck for squamous-cell carcinoma of the nasopharynx, tonsillar fossa, and base of tongue. Radiology 80:973–988, 1963

77. Million RR, Zimmerman RC: Evaluation of the University of Florida split-course technique for various head and neck squamous cell carcinomas. Cancer 35:1533–1536, 1975

78. Norin T, Onyango J: Radiotherapy in Burkitt's lymphoma, conventional or superfractionated regime: Early results. Int J Radiat Oncol Biol Phys 2:399–406, 1977

79. Olch PD, Eck RV, Smith RR: An experimental study of the effect of irradiation on the dissemination of cancer. Cancer Res 19:464–467, 1959

80. Orton CG: Errors in applying the NSD concept. Radiology 115:233–235, 1975

81. Orton CG, Ellis F: A simplification in the use of the NSD concept in practical radiotherapy. Br J Radiol 46:529–537, 1973

82. Parsons JT, Bova FJ, Million RR: A reevaluation of split-course technique for squamous cell carcinoma of the head and neck. Int J Radiat Oncol Biol Phys 6:1645–1652, 1980

83. Parsons JT, Million RR, Cassisi NJ: Carcinoma of the base of tongue: Results of radical irradiation with surgery reserved for irradiation failure. Laryngoscope 92:689–696, 1982

84. Paterson R: Studies in optimum dosage: The Mackenzie Davidson Memorial Lecture. Br J Radiol 25:505–516, 1952

85. Peracchia G, Salti C: Radiotherapy with thrice-a-day fractionation in a short overall time: Clinical experiences. Int J Radiat Oncol Biol Phys 7:99–104, 1981

86. Perez CA, Lee FA, Ackerman LV, Ogura JH, Powers WE: Non-randomized comparison of preoperative irradiation and surgery versus irradiation alone in the management of carcinoma of the tonsil. Am J Roentgenol 126:248–260, 1976

87. Pierquin B, Mueller WK, Baillet F: Low dose rate irradiation of advanced head and neck cancer: Present status. Int J Radiat Oncol Biol Phys 4:565–572, 1978

88. Pierquin B, Chassagne D, Baillet F, Paine CH: Clinical observations on the time factor in interstitial radiotherapy using iridium-192. Clin Radiol 24:506–509, 1973

89. Rosenberg SA, Suit HD, Baker LH, Rosen G: Sarcomas of the soft tissue and bone. In DeVita VT Jr, Hellman S, Rosenberg SA: Cancer: Principles and Practice of Oncology, pp 1036–1093. Philadelphia, JB Lippincott, 1982

90. Rubenfeld S: Experiences with a rapid irradiation technic in oral carcinoma. Radiology 60:724–731, 1953

91. Sambrook DK: Clinical trial of a modified ("split-course") technique of x-ray therapy in malignant tumors. Clin Radiol 13:1–18, 1962

92. Sambrook DK: Split-course radiation therapy in malignant tumors. Am J Roentgenol Radium Ther Nucl Med 91:37–45, 1964

93. Scanlon PW: Split-dose radiotherapy: Followup in 50 cases. Am J Roentgenol Radium Ther Nucl Med 90:280–293, 1963

94. Scanlon PW: Radiotherapeutic problems best handled with split-dose therapy. Am J Roentgenol Radium Ther Nucl Med 93:639–650, 1965

95. Shukovsky LJ: Dose, time, volume relationships in squamous cell carcinoma of the supraglottic larynx. Am J Roentgenol Radium Ther Nucl Med 108:27–29, 1970

96. Shukovsky LJ, Baeza MR, Fletcher GH: Results of irradiation in squamous cell carcinomas of the glossopalatine sulcus. Radiology 120:405–408, 1976

97. Shukovsky LJ, Fletcher GH: Time–dose and tumor volume relationships in the irradiation of squamous cell carcinoma of the tonsillar fossa. Radiology 107:621–626, 1973

98. Shukovsky LJ, Fletcher GH, Montague ED, Withers HR: Experience with twice-a-day fractionation in clinical radiotherapy. Am J Roentgenol 126:155–162, 1976

99. Singh K: Two regimes with the same TDF but differing morbidity used in the treatment of stage III carcinoma of the cervix. Br J Radiol 51:357–362, 1978

100. Sobel S, Rubin P, Keller B, Poulter C: Tumor persistence as a predictor of outcome after radiation therapy of head and neck cancers. Int J Radiat Oncol Biol Phys 1:873–880, 1976

101. Sowers ZT: The uses of radium. Am Med 6:261, 1903

102. Spanos WJ Jr, Shukovsky LJ, Fletcher GH: Time, dose, and tumor volume relationships in irradiation of squamous cell carcinomas of the base of the tongue. Cancer 37:2591–2599, 1976

103. Strandquist M: Studien über die kumulative wirkung der röntgenstrahlen bei fraktionierung. Erfahrungen aus dem Radiumhemmet an 280 haut- und lippenkarzinomen. Acta Radiol [Suppl] (Stockh) 55:245–300, 1944

104. Strong EW: Preoperative radiation and radical neck dissection. Surg Clin North Am 49:271–276, 1969

105. Suit HD, Gallager HS: Intact tumor cells in irradiated tissue. Arch Pathol 78:648–651, 1964

106. Taskinen PJ: Radiotherapy and TNM classification of cancer of the larynx: A study based on 1447 cases seen at the Radiotherapy Clinic of Helsinki during 1936–1961. Acta Radiol [Suppl] (Stockh) 287, 121 pages, 1969

107. Thames HD Jr, Withers HR, Peters LJ, Fletcher GH: Changes in early and late radiation responses with altered dose fractionation: Implications for dose-survival relationships. Int J Radiat Oncol Biol Phys 8:219–226, 1982

108. Thomlinson RH, Gray LH: The histological structure of some human lung cancers and the possible implications for radiotherapy. Br J Cancer 9:539–549, 1955

109. Vaeth JM, Buschke F: Radiation therapy of carcinoma of the vocal cord wthout mucosal reaction. Am J Roentgenol Radium Ther Nucl Med 97:931–932, 1966

110. Vandenbrouck C, Sancho H, Le Fur R, Richard JM, Cachin Y: Results of a randomized clinical trial of preoperative irradiation versus postoperative in treatment of tumors of the hypopharynx. Cancer 39:1445–1449, 1977

111. Vikram B: The importance of the time interval between surgery and postoperative radiation therapy in the combined management of head and neck cancer. Int J Radiat Oncol Biol Phys 5:1837–1840, 1979

112. Vikram B, Strong EW, Shah J, Spiro RH: Elective postoperative radiation therapy in stages III and IV epidermoid carcinoma of the head and neck. Am J Surg 140:580–584, 1980

113. Wang CC: Twice daily radiation therapy for carcinomas of the head and neck (abstr). Int J Radiat Oncol Biol Phys 7:1261–1262, 1981

114. Weichert KA, Aaron BS, Maltz R, Shumrick D: Carcinoma of the tonsil: Treatment by a planned combination of radiation and surgery. Int J Radiat Oncol Biol Phys 1:505–508, 1976

115. Wiernik G, Bleehen NM, Brindle J, Bullimore J, Churchill-Davidson IFJ, Davidson J et al: Sixth interim progress report of the British Institute of Radiology fractionation study of 3 fractions/week versus 5 fractions/week in radiotherapy of the laryngopharynx. Br J Radiol 51:241–250, 1978

116. Withers HR: Cell renewal system concepts and the radiation response. In Vaeth JM (ed): Frontiers of Radiation Therapy and Oncology, vol 6, pp 93–107. Baltimore, University Park Press, 1972

117. Withers HR, Peters LJ: Basic principles of radiotherapy: Biologic aspects of radiation therapy. In Fletcher GH: Textbook of Radiotherapy, 3rd ed, pp 103–180. Philadelphia, Lea & Febiger, 1980

118. Withers HR, Thames HD Jr, Flow BL, Mason KA, Hussey DH: The relationship of acute to late skin injury in 2 and 5 fraction/week gamma-ray therapy. Int J Radiat Oncol Biol Phys 4:595–601, 1978

119. Woodhouse RJ, Quivey JM, Fu KK, Sien PS, Dedo HH, Phillips TL: Treatment of carcinoma of the vocal cord: A review of 20 years' experience. Laryngoscope 91:1155–1162, 1981

The Effect of Radiation on Normal Tissues of the Head and Neck

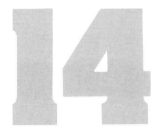

JAMES T. PARSONS

INTRODUCTION

Acute Versus Late Injury

For convenience, the effects of irradiation on normal tissues are usually divided into (1) acute effects, which are present both during a course of irradiation and in the immediate postirradiation period, and (2) late effects, which become manifest months to years following treatment. While patients are generally most concerned about acute side-effects, clinicians mainly fear late sequelae since the latter may be chronic and progressive, as opposed to acute effects, which are generally self-limited. Most acute effects (e.g., mucositis and loss of taste) are temporary; others, such as xerostomia, which develops early during a course of irradiation, may be permanent if a substantial dose has been administered. Late injuries may be nonhealing (e.g., radiation myelitis), or they may spontaneously heal, such as in many instances of soft tissue and bone necrosis.

There is little correlation between the occurrence of acute and late effects of irradiation on normal tissues. The severity of one does not necessarily predict the other; a patient with moderately or very severe acute side-effects may suffer no late injury, while another patient with very little acute reaction may develop a severe or even fatal late complication. Numerous radiation trials using altered fractionation schemes have demonstrated this dissociation between acute and late reactions (see Chapter 13, Time–Dose–Volume Relationships in Radiation Therapy).

More is known about the mechanism of acute than late injury. In general, tissues with a rapidly dividing cell population (e.g., mucous membrane and skin epithelium) respond acutely and those with slowly proliferating or nonproliferating cells (e.g., connective tissue or spinal cord) are affected late.

While there is sometimes an obvious precipitating cause of late complications, such as trauma or thermal injury, the exact mechanism of most late injuries is incompletely understood; there are two major schools of thought. One theory states that irradiation injury of the microvasculature is responsible; the other holds that late damage results from parenchymal and/or stromal cell death. According to the second theory, late damage would differ from acute damage only in that the cells of late-responding tissues or organs do not divide rapidly and therefore cell death is not quickly expressed. The latter theory considers the microvasculature itself to be a late-responding tissue that, when injured, further contributes to late injury. Fibroblast dysfunction may also be important.[58]

Late complications are, in part, dependent on the total dose and volume of tissue irradiated. Since large tumors require both higher total doses and larger treatment volumes than smaller lesions, a certain percentage of complications may be accepted when one attempts to control advanced cancers by irradiation alone. At times, it is preferable to treat advanced cancers by a combination of surgery and irradiation, in order to lessen the complications of very radical therapy by either modality alone. As discussed elsewhere (see Chapter 13, Time–Dose–Volume Relationships in Radiation Therapy), daily fraction size is another important factor in the production of late injury. Also important is homogeneity of dose. A simple but useful way of thinking about tumor control and treatment complications is to remember that the probability of tumor control is largely dependent on the minimum dose that any portion of the cancer receives and that complications are usually dependent on the maximum dose. Ideally, whether using external-beam or interstitial therapy, one tries to make the dose within the tumor volume as homogeneous as possible, to minimize the risks of localized underdosage or overdosage.

Treatment of All Portals at Each Therapy Session

When treating head and neck cancers by irradiation, two or more treatment portals are usually employed. While it is expedient to treat only one field at each therapy session, ideally all fields should be treated daily. In a multiportal setup, the technique of treating only one portal daily results in an increased biologic effect on the normal tissues, as discussed by Wilson and Hall.[107]

This concept is illustrated in Fig. 14-1. The plan is to deliver 6000 rad/30 fractions to the midplane with cobalt-60 by a two-field technique. The patient thickness is 16 cm, and field sizes are 10 × 10 cm. In plan A, only one field is treated each day. The daily midplane dose is 200 rad; point P, lateral to the midplane, receives 290 and 130 rad on alternating days. In plan B, both fields are treated daily. The daily midplane dose, 200 rad, is the same as that in plan A; point P receives 210 rad on each of the 30 treatment days.

The total absorbed dose at point P, 6300 rad, is identical for the two plans (290 rad × 15 treatments plus 130 rad × 15 treatments in plan A versus 210 rad × 30 treatments in plan B). Wilson and Hall showed that the biologic consequences at point P of the one field per day technique (plan A) are more severe than the effects of the two-field per day technique (plan B).[107] This difference has been observed among patients who received pelvic irradiation by a four-field box technique; subcutaneous changes have been more severe in patients who received treatment to only one field per day versus those who received treatment to two of the four fields daily. In Figure 14-1, if point P happens to represent an important structure (e.g., the spinal cord or pterygoid musculature), then plan A is more likely to cause a late treatment complication. The same concept probably applies to tumor cells: cancer in a lymph node at point P would receive a biologically higher dose when one field is treated per day. There are no formulas to convert these differences to rad units, but the differences may be observed clinically.

For very small field separations, such as in the treatment of early vocal cord cancer, there is little biologic difference between treating one versus two fields per day, and the one field per day scheme is acceptable.

ACUTE EFFECTS

Mucous Membranes

ORAL CAVITY, PHARYNX, AND LARYNX

The mucous membranes of the upper aerodigestive tract respond early during a course of fractionated external-beam irradiation. With five 200-rad fractions per week, mucosal erythema develops within 1 week. At approximately 2 weeks, the reddened mucous membrane develops small white or slightly yellow patches, 2 mm to 3 mm in diameter, called "mucositis" or "false membrane" formation. Mucositis represents caking of dead surface epithelial cells, fibrin, and polymorphonuclear leukocytes on a moist background. Patients usually note a sore throat at 2 weeks. In many patients, the patches of mucositis become confluent by the third week.

Mucositis is sensitive to changes in daily dose of radiation. At 170 rad to 180 rad five times weekly, the maximal reaction is usually only intense erythema, with an occasional patch of mucositis, even when large volumes are irradiated (e.g., for cancer of the nasopharynx or advanced cancer of the oral cavity); in this situation, the cell-killing and repopulation of mucous membrane stem cells are essentially in equilibrium. If the daily dose is more than 200 rad and the treatment volume is large, cell-killing exceeds the proliferative capacity of the mucous membrane stem cells; almost all patients develop confluent mucositis by the third week, producing severe discomfort and often limiting adequate nutrition. At the University of Florida, doses of 225 rad/fraction are used only for very limited fields (e.g., early vocal cord cancer or "boost" fields).

The soft palate, tonsillar pillars, buccal mucosa, lateral border of the tongue, pharyngeal walls, and portions of the larynx readily develop mucositis. Other sites, such as the hard palate, gingival ridges, dorsum of the tongue, and the true vocal cords, may either develop no mucositis during a treatment course or develop it only after very high doses.[18] Coutard noted that mucositis often first appears over the tumor itself, sometimes as early as 5 to 7 days into treatment (i.e., a week before the appearance of mucositis over the normal mucous membranes).[19] This early reaction is frequently dubbed "tumoritis" and is observed most often when treating tumors of the soft palate and anterior tonsillar pillar.

Symptoms of sore throat are usually maximal 2½ to 3 weeks into therapy; thereafter, the symptoms usually diminish, even though therapy is continued. While the patient is under treatment, the mucous membranes should be examined at least weekly since the distribution of the mucosal reaction confirms adequate coverage of the tumor.

Patients with metallic dental restorations (e.g., gold crowns) develop a pronounced mucositis on the adjacent buccal mucosa, secondary to backscattered low-energy electrons. Since the range of these electrons is short, excessive mucositis can be prevented by placing a few millimeters of moistened gauze or paraffin between the mucosa and the teeth.

Following external therapy, the mucous membranes normally heal rather dramatically at 2½ to 3 weeks, although an occasional patient requires longer. Up until that time, there is usually little obvious change, either objectively or subjectively; the sore throat then suddenly subsides and, over the next 2 to 3 days, improves rapidly. After a month the mucosa is healed in 90% to 95% of patients and sore throat is absent or minimal.

The mucositis produced by a 7-day radium implant appears 7 to 10 days after removal and is maximal approximately 2 weeks after its removal. The reaction generally subsides by 6 weeks, unless the implanted volume was large, in which case complete healing sometimes requires several months.[66]

NASAL CAVITY

High-dose irradiation of the anterior nares produces a brisk mucosal reaction. The moist mucosal surfaces tend to ad-

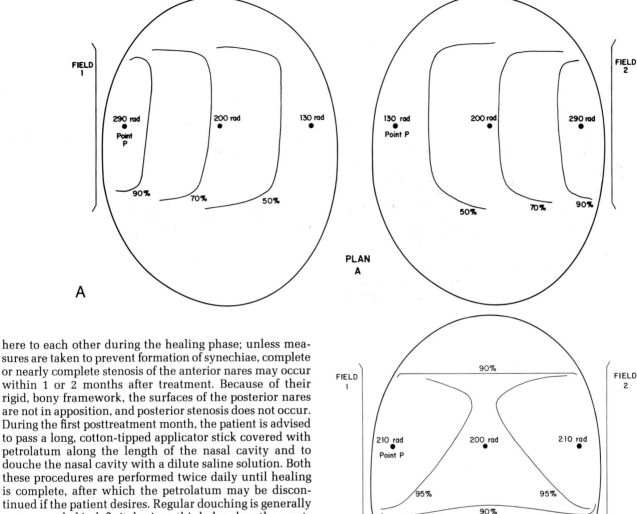

here to each other during the healing phase; unless measures are taken to prevent formation of synechiae, complete or nearly complete stenosis of the anterior nares may occur within 1 or 2 months after treatment. Because of their rigid, bony framework, the surfaces of the posterior nares are not in apposition, and posterior stenosis does not occur. During the first posttreatment month, the patient is advised to pass a long, cotton-tipped applicator stick covered with petrolatum along the length of the nasal cavity and to douche the nasal cavity with a dilute saline solution. Both these procedures are performed twice daily until healing is complete, after which the petrolatum may be discontinued if the patient desires. Regular douching is generally recommended indefinitely since this helps clear the crusts and debris that tend to collect on the dry membranes. If at the time of the first follow-up the patient is already developing stenosis, the synechiae can generally be lysed with the use of topical cocaine anesthesia; the patient is then asked to use the applicators more frequently and to return to the clinic on a weekly basis until the problem is resolved. If complete stenosis develops, surgical division may be necessary.

Conjunctiva

During a course of cobalt-60 irradiation for cancers of the paranasal sinuses, patients typically develop mild or moderate symptoms of conjunctivitis (foreign body sensation and occasionally photophobia) and lid irritation. Unless all of the lacrimal tissue has received a high dose, these symptoms generally resolve within 4 to 6 weeks after treatment.

Sense of Taste

Taste buds are numerous on the circumvallate papillae. They are found in moderate numbers on the fungiform papillae, which are scattered all over the anterior two thirds of the tongue, and on the foliate papillae along the pos-

FIG. 14-1. The importance of treating all fields at each therapy session. The dose is 6000 rad/30 fractions delivered to the midplane by a two-field technique with cobalt-60, 80 cm SSD. (A) Treatment plan A: Fields 1 and 2 are treated on alternate days. For a daily dose of 200 rad at midplane, point P receives 290 rad and 130 rad in alternation. (B) Treatment plan B: Fields 1 and 2 are both treated each day. For a daily midplane dose of 200 rad, point P receives 210 rad daily. Although the total dose, 6300 rad, to point P is identical for plans A and B, the biologic effects produced by 290 rad × 15 fractions plus 130 rad × 15 fractions are more severe than those produced by 210 rad × 30 treatments.

terolateral surfaces of the tongue. Additional taste buds are located on the tonsillar pillars, base of the tongue, soft palate, and laryngeal surface of the epiglottis, and a few are on the posterior pharyngeal wall. The filiform papillae of the tongue possess no taste buds. Taste buds atrophy with age; those on the posterior one third of the tongue and on the epiglottis usually disappear early in life.[105]

The taste buds that mediate each of the four primary taste sensations tend to be localized to special areas of the tongue: sweet on the anterior surface and tip, sour on the lateral sides, bitter on the circumvallate papillae, and salty all over the tongue.[41]

Loss of taste occurs rapidly and exponentially near the beginning of a radiation treatment course. Some patients report a bitter taste during the early part of their treatment course, but most simply state that their taste is diminished. The higher the pretreatment taste acuity, the more rapid is the loss.[15] Acuity is essentially absent by the end of the third treatment week, although a few patients report minimal changes even by the end of therapy. The mechanism by which taste is impaired is unknown. Conger suggests that taste loss is secondary to radiation-induced damage to the microvilli of the taste cells and has performed electron microscopic studies in mice that show loss of microvilli following irradiation.[15]

After therapy is finished, acuity of taste is recovered rapidly at first, then more slowly; most patients report some improvement within 20 to 60 days. Full recovery of preirradiation taste acuity is usually reached within 60 to 120 days.[15] Some patients state that their taste is never quite as sharp as before treatment, but it is usually quite adequate. At least part of this subjective loss may be due to xerostomia, which in itself may affect taste acuity. Mossman and Henkin suggest that zinc therapy may be useful in ameliorating symptoms in some patients whose taste does not completely return to normal after therapy; the University of Florida has no experience with this approach, and these tentative results require verification by other investigators.[72]

Salivary Tissue

The normal human salivary glands produce 1000 ml to 1500 ml/day of saliva, most of which is recycled by the gut.[27] The major salivary glands account for 70% to 80% of the salivary flow; the remaining flow comes from minor salivary glands that are scattered throughout the mouth. Under resting conditions, the flow from the submandibular glands is at least as great as that from the parotids or possibly greater;[32,90] the sublingual glands contribute only 2% to 5% to the flow rate.[68] Under conditions of stimulation (e.g., eating or drinking), the parotid glands become the main contributors. In humans, the parotids consist entirely of serous acini. The submandibular glands contain both mucous and serous acini;[85] the minor salivary glands are predominantly mucus secretors.

XEROSTOMIA

If only the submandibular and sublingual glands are included in the treatment area, and not both parotids, most patients note little or no difference in the quality and quantity of their saliva. If one or both parotids are irradiated, along with the submandibular glands, some dryness is noted after only a few treatments. If the parotids are irradiated and the submandibular glands spared, moisture may be preserved.[68,90]

A few patients report little subjective change, even after radical courses of irradiation, but the vast majority note partial to complete loss of salivary function. If both parotids, both submandibular glands, and a large number of minor salivary glands are included in the treatment area, severe dryness results (e.g., as in cancer of the nasopharynx). Presumably because the serous acini are affected earlier than the mucous acini, the saliva first becomes thick, sticky, and ropy. Patients often have considerable difficulty handling these tenacious secretions in their dry mouths. Continued use of tobacco and alcohol produces an additional drying effect. The patient is instructed to use salt-and-soda mouthwash or gargle several times daily, both during the course of irradiation and until mucosal healing is complete. This solution, which consists of a teaspoon each of table salt and baking soda in a quart of water, serves to refresh the mouth, decrease the pain from mucositis, and loosen the thick, tenacious saliva. Commercial preparations of artificial saliva are available, but few patients will use them because they often state that the solutions produce an unpleasant taste.

SIALADENITIS

Within 12 hours after the first treatment, about 5% of patients develop a transient, usually painless, enlargement of one or more of the salivary glands within the treatment portal. Occasionally, there is mild pain and tenderness, but usually symptoms are limited to a "tight" sensation. In contrast to acute suppurative parotitis, systemic symptoms are minimal or nonexistent. The patient is oten quite alarmed and may call his physician just after having eaten supper, thinking that his cancer is growing rapidly in his neck. The swelling has been noted more frequently in the submandibular than in the parotid glands, but either may occur; one or both sides may be affected. The swelling is transient and usually disappears within 1 or 2 days despite continuation of treatment. Coincidental with the swelling and its resolution is a transient rise and fall in the serum amylase level.[54] The proper management is to anticipate the problem and warn the patient in advance.

Skin and Subcutaneous Tissues

The skin consists of two layers, epidermis and dermis, beneath which is a subcutaneous layer containing varying amounts of adipose tissue. The epidermis is a stratified squamous epithelium, entirely devoid of blood vessels; its deepest cells constitute the basal layer, which, in the head and neck area, is at an average depth of 0.03 mm to 0.05 mm.[106] Mitotic activity in the basal layer forms new cells to replace the superficial keratinized cells that are continually exfoliated from the skin surface. Melanin granules are formed by melanocytes in the deep layers of the epidermis and are transferred into neighboring epidermal cells. Tubular invaginations of the epidermis (called hair follicles) surround each hair shaft and extend deep into the dermis.

The dermis consists mostly of dense connective tissue and contains nerve endings, blood and lymph vessels, and sweat and sebaceous glands. The ducts of sweat glands discharge onto the epidermal surface, and those of sebaceous glands discharge into hair follicles. It is difficult to measure precisely the thickness of the dermis, since its boundary with the subcutaneous layer is indistinct; it is 1 mm to 2 mm thick in the head and neck area.[94]

In the orthovoltage era, treatment plans were dictated by the limits of skin tolerance. Essentially never, in the modern era of supervoltage therapy, is the skin *per se* a major dose-limiting tissue. High energy x-rays are "skin-sparing;" that is, the buildup characteristics of the absorbed dose are such that the skin receives a low dose relative to the deeper structures. Skin-sparing is lost or reduced when tissue-equivalent material, called bolus, is placed on the skin; when the beam enters the body tangentially, rather than perpendicular to the skin surface; or when the lead blocks and blocking tray used to shape the x-ray fields are too close to the patient (see Chapter 15, Treatment Planning for Irradiation of Head and Neck Cancer). Under certain conditions, when tumor actually invades the skin and subcutaneous tissues, or when tumor cells may have been seeded in surgical scars, skin-sparing is undesirable and steps are taken to ensure an adequate skin dose.

When parallel-opposed cobalt-60 fields are treated to tumor doses in the range of 7000 rad to 7500 rad (five 180-rad to 200-rad fractions/week), acute skin effects are limited to erythema, peeling, and tanning. These changes are reversible. Erythema is often noted first around hair follicles since the invaginations of epidermis receive a higher dose than cells on the skin surface; follicular erythema is seen more often in the lower neck fields than in the primary fields. Peeling (or "dry desquamation") of the skin results from radiation-killing of basal cells in the epidermis. Scales of skin (which are sometimes dark because radiation stim-ulates melanin production) result from caking of dead cells, a situation analogous to that seen on the mucous membranes (mucositis). As with a sunburn, the patient notes increased sensitivity to touch and may complain of itching and drawing until healing is complete, 2 to 3 weeks after completion of therapy.

If the skin has been bolused or tangentially irradiated, then the capacity of the basal cell layer to repopulate the epidermis may be exceeded and the patient develops areas of complete epidermal denudation, called "moist desquamation," a medical euphemism for a "radiation burn." The dermis is exposed and oozes serum. Although the appearance may alarm those unfamiliar with the reaction, healing generally occurs spontaneously within 2 to 4 weeks depending on the area involved and unless infection supervenes. Areas of moist desquamation should be kept clean; crusts may be removed by soaking with a dilute hydrogen peroxide solution. Reepithelialization occurs from the periphery of the field and, if the dose has not been too great, from single surviving cells in the middle of the field. In Figure 14-2, which is reproduced from a classic paper by Coutard,[17] the healing phase after a reaction produced by orthovoltage irradiation is shown.

Epilation of the beard usually begins during the third week of treatment. Sweat and sebaceous glands cease to function.

Acute skin reactions vary with the size of the area irradiated, dose, overall treatment time, number of fractions, quality of radiation, and a number of patient-related variables, including degree of pigmentation, age, and site irradiated. For orthovoltage irradiation, recommended dose schedules below a level that would produce moist desquamation in most patients are shown in Table 14-1;[23] the schemes shown are primarily for palliation.

For the same dose, the face reacts less vigorously than the upper neck, and the upper neck reacts less than the lower neck and supraclavicular area. The skin response is thus related to the relative exposure to sun.

The severity of acute skin reactions is not a predictor of late changes.

LATE EFFECTS

Salivary Tissue

Xerostomia causes discomfort, alters taste acuity, contributes to deterioration of oral hygiene, and promotes dental decay. The remaining saliva has an altered electrolyte content and reduced pH. Histologically, the heavily irradiated gland is obliterated and largely replaced by collagen.

Loss of salivary function is usually complete and permanent after doses above approximately 3500 rad. In patients with very low preirradiation flow rates, lesser doses may cause permanent dryness. Marks and co-workers found that only one fifth of those patients whose parotid glands had received 4000 rad to 6000 rad had any measurable parotid flow following salivary stimulation; above 6000 rad, none of 24 parotid glands had measurable flow.[65] Although occasional patients report subjective improvement in the sensation of dryness several years after treatment, objective recovery of salivary flow has not been documented in such cases. If salivary tissue receives less than 3000 rad to 3500 rad, there is often some return of function during the 6 months following therapy. Young

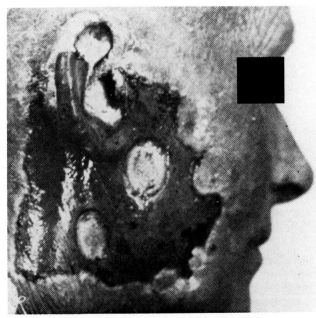

FIG. 14-2. The repair of radioepidermitis following orthovoltage irradiation. Repair occurs from the field edge, by proliferation of peripheral epithelial cells, and assumes a typical polycyclic appearance. When not all of the epidermal cells within the field have been destroyed, repair also occurs from central islands and from squamous epithelial cells of the lumina of the sebaceous and sweat glands. (Coutard H: Roentgen therapy of epitheliomas of the tonsillar region, hypopharynx, and larynx from 1920–1926. Am J Roentgenol Radium Ther 28:313–331, 1932)

patients are more likely than older patients to recover salivary flow.

During treatment planning, one should attempt to limit the volume of salivary tissue irradiated and the dose delivered, whenever practical to do so. Minor changes in field size and shape may preserve some salivary flow (see Fig. 17-18 in Chapter 17). If over half of the parotid tissue receives a high dose along with the rest of the major salivary glands, significant xerostomia usually results. Patients with high pretreatment salivary flow rates develop less dryness following a particular dose[68] or treatment volume[10] than those with low pretreatment flow rates. The decrease in flow after irradiation follows an exponential decay curve. A certain dose reduces flow by approximately the same percentage, not by the same absolute amount, in two patients. A patient whose initial salivary flow rate is 0.2 ml/minute would require a reduction by only 50% to reach a minimal flow rate (0.1 ml/minute), while a patient whose flow rate is 1.0 ml/minute would require a 90% reduction to reach the same level of flow. The latter patient would require approximately three times as much irradiation as the former to reach 0.1 ml/minute. Based on resting collections from all of the salivary glands, Mira and co-workers showed that during courses of irradiation that included almost all of the salivary tissue, 3500 rad to 4000 rad was capable of inducing minimal flow ($\leqq$0.1 ml/minute) in patients with high initial flow rates (0.9 ml to 1.5 ml/minute); 500 rad to 1500 rad resulted in minimal flow in patients with low (0.15 ml to 0.40 ml/minute) initial flow rates. Patients in whom minimal flow rate was induced during irradiation showed no recovery of flow in samples taken 1 to 17 months after treatment. Although Mira and co-workers have suggested that split-course irradiation might protect salivary tissue, such a protective effect has not been observed at the University of Florida.[68]

Patients with significant xerostomia may get some symptomatic relief by using one of the commercially available artificial saliva preparations. These solutions have a pH of about 7 and a consistency similar to saliva. Some patients carry a bottle of artificial saliva with them at all times; others use plain or flavored glycerin to lubricate their mouth, but the majority use water.

Teeth

The pathologic changes that occur in the teeth secondary to irradiation are mainly due to diminished salivary flow, rather than a direct effect on teeth or surrounding bone.

Whether the teeth are inside or outside of the irradiation field, they are similarly affected. If the salivary glands are not irradiated, caries does not occur as a result of treatment, even if the teeth and jaw receive high-dose irradiation.

During and immediately after treatment, the patient suffers from a sore throat and a dry, sticky mouth; he stops eating a rough diet and changes to a soft, high-carbohydrate diet that has little detergent value and favors the growth of plaque. There is a tendency to stop routine dental care because the tissues are tender. In association with radiation-induced xerostomia, there are pronounced shifts from the normal oral microflora to a highly cariogenic microbial population.[5] Unless stringent measures are taken to protect the teeth, rampant dental caries may begin to develop as early as 3 to 6 months after treatment and progress to complete destruction of all the teeth over a period of 3 to 5 years.

The histologic character of radiation caries is similar to that of dental caries; the two lesions differ, however, in several important aspects. The lesions that develop after irradiation are more widespread; there is frequently a generalized attack on enamel, beginning as fine, punctate defects that progress to larger lesions. Patients complain of hot–cold hypersensitivity and sensitivity to sweet foods.[36] Typical dental caries occurs mainly on the proximal surfaces and fissures, sites not easily reached by saliva, and therefore prone to food retention. The lesions induced by irradiation occur mostly on the buccal, palatal, or lingual surfaces and on the incisal and occlusal edges of the teeth. All of these surfaces are normally readily bathed by saliva[36] and are usually resistant to caries development. The edges of the teeth may appear as though they have been finely sanded or filed; the concentric layers around the pulp may sometimes be seen in cross section.[24]

As the late effects of irradiation progress over several months, there is shrinkage of the periodontal tissues, leading to exposure of cementum. Decay occurs at the exposed cervical portion of the tooth, usually beginning on the labial or buccal surfaces, then extending superficially around the neck of the tooth to produce an annular lesion that may eventually result in complete amputation of the crown. The root remains in the alveolar cavity and is slowly eliminated.[24]

Before irradiation, the dentulous patient must be evaluated by a dentist; together with the radiation therapist a decision is made to perform extractions or keep the teeth. The important considerations regarding this decision are discussed elsewhere (see Chapter 12, Dental Management for the Irradiated Patient).

TABLE 14-1.   Suggested Maximum Skin Doses (rad) for Palliation With Orthovoltage* Irradiation (Below Moist Desquamation Level for Average Patient)

| No. Fractions | No. Days | Small Field | | Medium Field | | Large Field | |
		10 sq cm	50 sq cm	100 sq cm	150 sq cm	200 sq cm	300 sq cm
1	1	2000	1750	1500	1250	1000	
2	2	2750	2500	2000	1750	1500	
4	4	3500	3250	2500	2250	2000	
5	5	3750	3500	2750	2500	2250	2000
10	14	5000	4500	3750	3250	3000	2750
15	21	5500	5000	4250	3750	3500	3250
25	35	6000	5500	5000	4500	4250	4000

* 250 kV, HVL 1.5 mm to 3.0 mm copper filtration.

(Delclos L, Johnson GC: Palliative irradiation in breast cancer. Radiology 83:272–276, 1964)

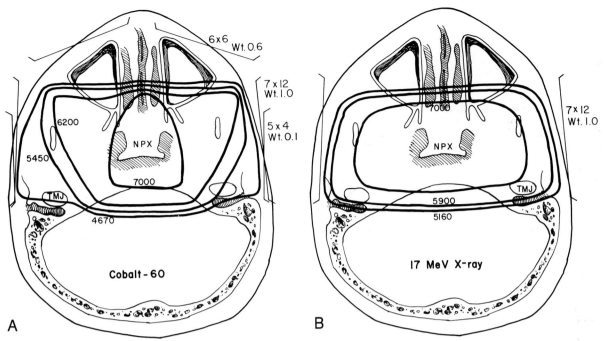

FIG. 14-3. Comparison of dose distribution from (A) four-field technique with cobalt-60 to (B) two-field technique with 17-MeV x-rays for irradiation of nasopharyngeal (NPX) cancer. For a tumor dose of 7000 rad, the four-field technique delivers a dose to the temporomandibular joint (TMJ), tympanic cavity, and pterygoid musculature that is 500 rad to 600 rad less than that delivered by the high-energy two-field technique. Weights (Wt.) refer to the relative given dose (at D_{max}) to each field.

Masticatory Muscles and Temporomandibular Joint

High-dose irradiation to voluntary muscles may produce fibrosis, particularly when cancer has invaded and partially destroyed the muscles. Fibrosis of the muscles of mastication (temporalis, masseter, and pterygoid muscles) may cause trismus. Many patients with advanced head and neck cancer have trismus at the time of diagnosis, secondary to local tumor extension into the pterygoid musculature. Although this symptom often disappears during a course of irradiation, it may gradually reappear in the postirradiation period if significant pterygoid muscle fibrosis develops. The temporomandibular joint itself is reasonably resistant to ankylosis secondary to irradiation; the risk of injury increases if the joint has been invaded by tumor. Patients may complain of clicking, crackling noises and pain associated with motion at the temporomandibular joint; on examination, the exact site of injury, joint versus masticatory muscles, may not be obvious.

Radiation-induced trismus occurs most often after irradiation of cancer of the nasopharynx, tonsil, retromolar trigone, or paranasal sinuses. The use of large daily fractions increases the risk of impairment of motion at the temporomandibular joint.[69] In the treatment of nasopharyngeal cancers, many centers use a two-field technique that delivers 7000 rad or more to the temporomandibular joint and masticatory muscles. One report cites a 10% incidence of temporomandibular joint complications following treatment by opposed lateral fields with 4-MeV to 6-MeV x-rays.[46] Even if one uses high-energy x-rays (e.g., 17 MeV), the two-field technique delivers a dose to the joint and

muscles that is substantially higher than that delivered by the four-field technique with cobalt-60 (Fig. 14-3). Trismus has not been observed with the four-field technique. There are some situations in which the four-field technique is inappropriate, and two fields must then be used.

Since there is no simple treatment of severe trismus, attempts should be made to avoid the problem by careful treatment planning. At the University of Florida no patient has developed severe enough masticatory muscle fibrosis to require specific therapy unless the problem was present before irradiation. If severe trismus develops, dental extractions might be necessary for purposes of feeding.

Patients who have received both surgery and irradiation are at greater risk of developing trismus than patients treated by either modality alone. High-risk patients, and especially those in whom trismus is already beginning to develop, should perform exercises several times daily in an attempt to increase the interarch distance; exercises should begin as soon as practical in the postoperative period, and should continue both during and after irradiation. One technique is to have the patient insert a number of stacked tongue blades between the teeth, then successively wedge additional blades into the stack until slight pain is encountered. Alternatively, a tapered cork can be inserted between the teeth to a point where minimal discomfort is reached; over a period of days to weeks, the patient attempts to place the cork farther and farther into his mouth. Another technique uses a clothespin onto which a rubber band is tightly wound so as to open the mouth forcibly (Fig. 14-4). The exercises are usually done for about 30 seconds every 2 hours. The distance between the upper and lower incisors should be measured and the patient

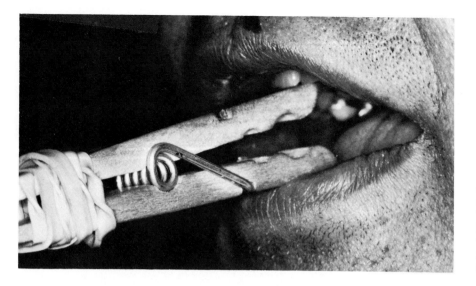

FIG. 14-4. Trismus secondary to extensive squamous cell carcinoma of paranasal sinuses, with invasion of pterygoid musculature. During the course of irradiation, the patient used a clothespin, onto which a rubber band had been tightly wound, in order to exercise and gradually increase the interincisor distance. Conscientious efforts should be made to reverse existing trismus or prevent its occurrence after irradiation, since it is difficult to manage once established.

continually urged to increase this distance by gradually breaking down existing fibrosis. Most patients will function quite well if an interincisor distance of 35 mm (dentulous patients) or interalveolar distance of 50 mm (edentulous patients) is achieved. Early evaluation by a dentist is helpful in preventing or solving these problems.

Soft Tissue and Bone Necrosis

Radiation necrosis is simply a destruction of normal tissue. It is most commonly thought that necrosis is due to the avascular effect of radiation. Following healing of the acute reaction of the mucous membrane, the epithelium is thinner than normal. The clinical appearance is that of a pale, hypotrophic epithelium through which telangiectatic vessels may be seen. Such mucosa is more susceptible than normal to mechanical injury and to the noxious effects of alcohol and tobacco. Necrosis usually begins with breakdown of this damaged mucosa, leaving a small ulcer.

If ulceration occurs on soft tissues that have no underlying bone, the result is a "soft tissue necrosis". If it occurs on soft tissues of the gingiva and there is no obvious sequestration or bone necrosis, the ulcer is called "bone exposure"; if there is serious injury to the underlying bone, "bone necrosis" or "osteoradionecrosis" is said to be present. Although the terms *bone exposure* and *osteoradionecrosis* are frequently used indiscriminately, it is important to realize that few exposures progress to severe bone necroses.

BONE EXPOSURE/OSTEORADIONECROSIS OF THE MANDIBLE/MAXILLA

If the area of exposure is less than 1 cm, actual necrosis of the underlying bone and sequestration may not occur or may be minimal; roentgenograms appear normal. Small exposures generally heal spontaneously after a period of weeks to months. On the other hand, if the bone exposure enlarges and persists for a long period, bone necrosis followed by sequestration may occur. A segment of mandible or, rarely, maxilla is exposed, with dead-appearing bone. Histologically, true osteoradionecrosis is characterized by damage to the cellular elements of bone, as well as vascular

changes. The marrow space is infiltrated by inflammatory cells and loose connective tissue.[73] Such bone may become infected, after which the infectious, necrotic process may extend for a considerable distance in the involved bone. Roentgenograms show an irregular lytic defect that frequently extends beyond the clinically apparent area of destruction. Very severe necroses may lead to orofacial fistulas and pathologic fractures.

While there is a direct effect of radiation on bone itself, most bone, including the mandible, will tolerate rather high doses of radiation without serious problems so long as the tissues overlying the bone remain intact and the bone is not subjected to excessive stress or trauma. Although occasional patients develop mandibular necroses beneath normal-appearing mucous membranes, 95% of necroses are associated with soft tissue necrosis. Compared with the maxilla, the gingiva of the mandible has a rather tenuous blood supply. The mucosal covering is thin and constantly traumatized (by eating and dentures, for example). Once mandibular necrosis occurs, it is difficult to obtain healing. Necroses of the maxilla occur less often and heal more easily.

Most bone problems first appear 3 to 12 months after irradiation, but there is some risk for many years, especially if the patient undergoes dental extractions at some time in the future.

The mylohyoid ridge, which is normally prominent and covered by a thin gingival mucosa, and the anterior arch of the mandible are favorite sites of bone exposure. Posterior exposures, at the angle or ascending ramus of the mandible, sites that are well covered by muscle, are rare. If posterior necrosis does occur, it may result in severe infection and trismus.[24]

Although the patient who has been edentulous for many years is still at risk of developing mandibular necrosis, his overall risk is less than in the dentulous patient. According to a number of practitioners with a great deal of clinical experience, patients who have undergone extractions just prior to irradiation are not at increased risk[71,73,74] if healing is adequate before irradiation is begun. If the patient has teeth, radiation caries that develops in teeth that were within the field of irradiation may instigate a secondary radiation necrosis, particularly if it later becomes necessary to extract these teeth. Necrosis is most likely following extraction of mandibular teeth; although there may be some delay in healing following maxillary extractions, necroses are infrequent if special precautions are taken. Radiation caries in teeth that are outside the field of irradiation does not predispose to osteoradionecrosis since the bone at these sites has not received high-dose irradiation; healing is usually normal after extraction.

Occasional patients have unerupted teeth in the molar area when they present for treatment. If well-covered, these teeth usually cause no problem in the postirradiation period. If a tooth is partially erupted, it should generally be extracted if high-dose irradiation is anticipated.[74] In actual practice, most partially erupted third molars occur in younger patients whose tumors, usually lymphomas, require lesser doses of irradiation so that postirradiation surgery can be accomplished at a later date with little risk. Impacted third molars are not extracted prior to irradiation, since a prolonged period of healing may be required when the bony defect is large.

Destruction of tissue by tumor increases the likelihood of necrosis; patients whose tumors involve the gingiva are at increased risk for bone exposure following irradiation. Patients who continue to smoke and drink after irradiation are also at increased risk. High doses, large treatment volumes, large fractions, and probably the addition of a radical neck dissection all place the patient at greater risk. Patients whose treatment includes an interstitial implant are also more likely to develop necroses. Of 315 patients who received irradiation for carcinomas of the oral cavity/oropharynx at the University of Florida between September 1964 and August 1976, approximately 5% of the 198 patients whose treatment was by external-beam irradiation alone developed bone necrosis of mild or moderate severity (i.e., healed spontaneously in less than 6 months or greater than 6 months, respectively); 1% developed severe osteoradionecrosis requiring mandibular resection. Of 117 patients whose treatment consisted of external-beam irradiation plus a radium implant, the rate of development of mild or moderately severe necrosis was 18%. Severe necroses occurred in 3%.[81]

MANAGEMENT

In the 1960s, it was common practice to perform mandibulectomies on patients with bone exposure. From experience it is now known that most bone exposures will heal spontaneously following conservative treatment (see Table 13-16 in Chapter 13, which shows that 86% of bone exposures at the University of Florida healed after conservative treatment). Even large, moderately severe necrosis may eventually heal.

The key to the treatment of minor bone exposures is patience. Both the patient and physician must understand that several months may be required before healing occurs and that the area may enlarge before it starts to heal. A number of conservative measures may be tried in order to promote healing and keep the patient comfortable. If the bone is rough or protrudes above the level of the gingiva, the oral surgeon files it down to promote healing and prevent irritation of the tongue. If the patient wears a denture, it should either be discontinued or, at the very least, relieved over the site of exposure so that it will cause no further trauma. If the exposure is greater than 1 cm, it is preferable to discontinue the denture until healing is complete.

Surprisingly, the majority of these patients do not have major discomfort; pain is usually controlled with analgesics such as aspirin and local care. In some patients, continued alcohol ingestion no doubt is contributory to the analgesia, although it retards healing. A 2- to 3-week course of antibiotics frequently reduces discomfort within a few days. A local anesthetic such as viscous lidocaine, applied with a cotton-tipped applicator, helps to control the pain. Under conservative management, most small areas of exposure eventually heal with little or no loss of bone. Local debridement of moderate-sized necroses is done by the oral surgeon if and when it becomes necessary. Small sequestra can be removed in the office. It is not unusual for patients to report that a sequestrum was spontaneously extruded while at home and, when next examined, the area is completely healed.

Hyperbaric oxygen at 2.4 atmospheres absolute pressure, 2 hours/day for 60 days, along with antibiotic therapy and local debridement, may increase the healing rate.[21] Those patients treated by hyperbaric oxygen at the University of Florida have been closely followed by an oral surgeon, sometimes on a daily or every-other-day basis, with meticulous local care and frequent debridement until improvement is noted. The relative importance of hyperbaric oxygen therapy is difficult to assess, since most necroses heal spontaneously; it is mainly used for difficult cases. The University of Florida hyperbaric unit is shown in Figure 14-5.

For the patient who has intractable pain, recurrent severe infections, or trismus, surgical treatment is necessary. Localized curettage of devitalized bone and coverage with an island pedicle flap may allow preservation of continuity of the mandible.[77] Mandibular resection should be undertaken only as a last resort; the intraoral route is recommended. If external fistulization has occurred, there is usually little hope of averting mandibulectomy. When the posterior mandible requires resection, functional and cosmetic losses are usually not severe. Anterior arch resections, on the other hand, are functionally and cosmetically debilitating and difficult to reconstruct because of previous high-dose radiation.

TEMPORAL BONE NECROSIS

Osteoradionecrosis of the temporal bone is an unusual complication that may occur after high-dose irradiation of carcinomas of the middle ear, auditory canal, or mastoid. Incidental irradiation of the normal external auditory canal and temporal bone (e.g., in the treatment of the nasopharynx or parotid tumors) rarely produces necrosis. In 1976, Wang and Doppke reported seven bone necroses in patients who were irradiated postoperatively for ear tumors.[102] Patients typically developed pain, nausea, vertigo, and ataxia. Clinical findings are those of chronic infection (i.e., otitis media, mastoiditis, foul discharge from the ear canal) and exposed, devitalized bone. Fistulization may lead to meningitis or brain abscess.

Temporal bone necrosis is usually related to technical factors in the treatment. Orthovoltage irradiation, with its high bone absorption, increases the risk. Total dose and fraction size are important; the complications in Wang and Doppke's patients all occurred after temporal bone doses calculated to be greater than or equal to 7600 rad at 200 rad/fraction with megavoltage apparatus. At the University of Florida there has been one case (Fig. 14-6) that occurred after 6850 rad/32 fractions (215 rad/fraction) delivered to a parotid tumor. Osteonecrosis following irradiation of

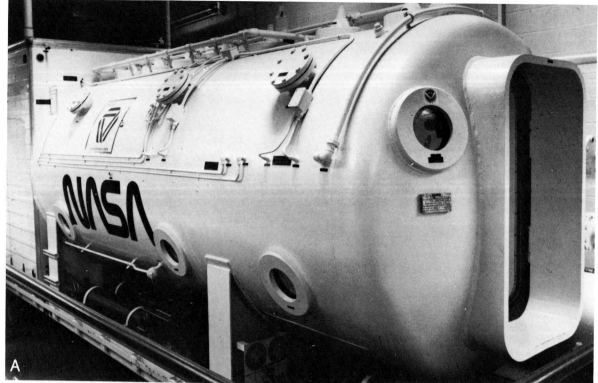

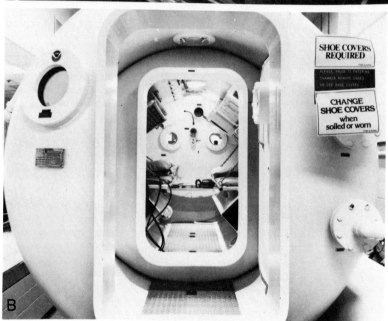

FIG. 14-5. University of Florida hyperbaric treatment facility. (*A*) External view of chamber, which is on long-term loan to Shands Teaching Hospital from the National Aeronautics and Space Administration (NASA). (*B*) Up to 3 patients may be treated simultaneously in the 10-foot-long main compartment.

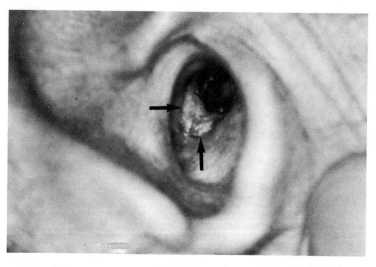

FIG. 14-6. Osteoradionecrosis of external auditory canal in a 55-year-old white woman 3½ years after superficial parotidectomy and postoperative irradiation of an adenoid cystic carcinoma of the parotid gland. Examination of the resected specimen revealed positive margins and extensive perineural spread. The dose to the temporal bone was 6850 rad/32 fractions by a continuous course. At 3½ years, the patient complained of pain and drainage from the right ear. There was exposed bone on the inferior and posterior walls of the external auditory canal (*arrows*). Infection and pain have been controlled with antibiotics, and there has been no evidence of extension of the osteoradionecrosis to surrounding structures. There is no tumor recurrence at 4 years; the bone exposure persists.

chemodectomas of the temporal bone structures has occurred in one patient at the University of Florida. The patient received 4200 rad to treat a postsurgical recurrent lesion and required revision mastoidectomy to remove a bony sequestrum 10 years after successful irradiation.

MANAGEMENT

Management of necrosis consists of antibiotics, local care, and surgical debridement when necessary.

SOFT TISSUE NECROSIS

Atrophy of the mucosa and its supporting stroma, reduced tissue vascularity, and tissue destruction by tumor all predispose the patient to soft tissue necrosis. The risk of necrosis is increased by continued alcohol and tobacco consumption.

The vast majority of pure soft tissue necroses occur within 2 years. Soft tissue necrosis in association with bone exposure may occur at any time. Following interstitial therapy, the majority of necroses appear within 5 to 8 months. Occurrence after 2 years is generally preceded by trauma to the mucosa.

Soft tissue necroses are most common following irradiation of lesions within the oral cavity or oropharynx; they are unusual after treatment of cancers of the nasopharynx and larynx. Following successful irradiation of cancers of the posterior pharyngeal wall, an occasional patient is noted to have persistent soft tissue ulceration. Necrosis is related to fraction size, total dose, volume, and use of interstitial treatment. Of 315 patients with squamous cell cancers of the oral cavity/oropharynx who received radical irradiation at the University of Florida between 1964 and 1976, mild (spontaneously healed within 6 months) or moderately severe (spontaneously healed, but required longer than 6 months) soft tissue necroses were observed in approximately 10% of patients following external-beam irradiation alone and in approximately 20% of those who received a combination of external-beam and interstitial irradiation; severe soft tissue necroses (requiring an operation or prolonged hospitalization) were rare, occurring in 1 of 198 (0.5%) of patients treated by external-beam therapy alone and 1 of 117 (1%) after external-beam plus interstitial irradiation.[81]

MANAGEMENT

Necrosis must first be distinguished from recurrent cancer. While both conditions frequently ulcerate the mucosa, there are some clinical parameters that help distinguish between the two. Recurrence of the primary cancer after irradiation almost always occurs at the center of the initial lesion. Ulceration outside the original cancer area is usually due to necrosis. Most cancer ulcers have a rolled margin, as opposed to the nearly flat, more sharply demarcated margins of necroses. The induration around a tumor recurrence is usually a little more pronounced than around a necrosis. Both kinds of ulcer may enlarge, but a cancer ulcer rarely decreases in size.

If one cannot decide whether the ulcer represents tumor recurrence or necrosis, the patient may be asked to return every 2 weeks for reexamination. If soft tissue necrosis is the most likely cause of the ulcer, it is not biopsied, since this may cause the necrosis to enlarge. If recurrent tumor is likely, biopsy is mandatory, since the chance to perform surgical salvage may be lost if one procrastinates too long;

it is better to err on the side of biopsy when there is doubt. Our batting average on the clinical diagnosis of necrosis versus recurrence is only fair, approximately 70%. In some areas, particularly the tongue, biopsy may have to be done under anesthesia since a deep biopsy may be necessary to show recurrence. A negative biopsy should be viewed with suspicion if there is a strong likelihood of recurrence, and repeat biopsies are in order.

The management of soft tissue necrosis depends on the site involved and severity of pain produced. Tiny necroses may be asymptomatic, but in certain sites (e.g., the lateral tongue or floor of the mouth) even a 1-mm to 2-mm superficial ulcer may be painful. A topical anesthetic such as lidocaine viscous, 2%, may make the patient comfortable enough to eat normally. Antibiotics such as tetracycline hydrochloride, 250 mg orally four times a day, often produce dramatic relief of pain, particularly when the ulceration is deep and infected. It is essential that the patient discontinue the use of alcohol and tobacco. If the area of necrosis is constantly traumatized by dentures, they should not be worn until healing has occurred. Over 95% of soft tissue necroses heal with conservative treatment, although many months and great patience on the part of both physician and patient may be required. Cases that fail to respond to more conservative means may benefit from a course of hyperbaric oxygen, but such therapy has the disadvantage of being time consuming and expensive. Once healing has occurred, the scar appears pale and thin and often is slightly depressed below the level of the surrounding mucosa; reappearance of necrosis at the same site is unusual.

Cartilage Necrosis

Adult cartilage has no blood vessels and contains a large amount of interstitial substance with only a few cells of low mitotic activity. Numerous normal cartilaginous structures in the head and neck area, including the larynx, trachea, external ear, eustachian tube, and nose, are incidentally or intentionally irradiated to a high dose. The often-voiced fear of cartilage necrosis arose from the orthovoltage days when vocal cord and skin cancers were treated with large daily fractions; cartilage necrosis was a constant worry of therapists in that era. It is now known that cartilage that is covered by a normal mucous membrane or skin usually tolerates conventionally fractionated high-dose irradiation quite well. Although cartilage that has been compromised by tumor invasion, infection, or prior surgery is somewhat more vulnerable to radiation injury, these conditions themselves constitute no contraindication to irradiation since the risk of cartilage necrosis is still very low. At the University of Florida, there have been numerous uncomplicated cures following irradiation of moderately advanced cancers of the suprahyoid and infrahyoid epiglottis (see Chapter 19), nose (see Chapter 23), and skin (see Chapter 26), in which cartilage invasion was present.

Chondronecrosis generally occurs within the first posttreatment year, but it can be precipitated by trauma many years after treatment. Like bone exposure, it probably starts with necrosis of the soft tissues (skin or mucous membrane) overlying cartilage.

LARYNGEAL CHONDRONECROSIS

Chondronecrosis of the larynx is rare, occurring in approximately 1% of patients who receive doses in the range of 6000 rad to 7000 rad at 200 rad to 225 rad/fraction. The risk increases with larger daily fractions (Table 14-2)[7,35,43,55,96] and large treatment volumes; the risk is greater for supraglottic than for vocal cord carcinoma. Cartilage that has been compromised by partial laryngectomy would seem more likely to develop necrosis after irradiation, but in practice it is rarely seen. Patients who continue to smoke or drink alcohol after treatment are at increased risk.

The symptoms and signs of cartilage necrosis (hoarseness, pain, edema, and foul breath) mimic those of recurrent cancer. Aspiration pneumonia or lung abscess may result. Since most necroses and many recurrences occur within 1 year after treatment, time to onset is not helpful in distinguishing the two. Tumor recurrence is many times more common than cartilage necrosis, and deep biopsy is therefore recommended. There are recognized problems with this approach, since deep biopsy may exacerbate necrosis and may fail to obtain representative tissue in some recurrent cancers. Tracheotomy may be necessary for aspiration or edema. Antibiotic therapy is begun. If conservative measures are unsuccessful in relieving the signs and symptoms, laryngectomy is recommended because the problem is more apt to be tumor recurrence than necrosis.

CHONDRONECROSIS OF THE NOSE AND EAR

In treating cancers of the nasal cavity and paranasal sinuses, the normal nasal ala frequently receive 7000 rad/7 weeks; at the University of Florida, no chondronecrosis has been observed in this patient group. Skin cancers on the nose or ear also require high-dose cartilage irradiation. Even when such lesions invade cartilage, necrosis is rare after well-fractionated therapy.[25,80] (See Chapter 23, Nasal Vestibule, Nasal Cavity, and Paranasal Sinuses, and Chapter 26, Carcinoma of the Skin.) If necrosis does occur, it may require debridement and grafting.

Skin and Subcutaneous Tissues

Since modern radiation therapy is generally conducted with supervoltage equipment, severe late skin changes are infrequent. Today, the only common indication for orthovoltage irradiation is skin cancer. Following orthovoltage treatment, there is usually epidermal atrophy and sometimes telangiectasis. The skin is hairless and dry because function of sweat and sebaceous glands ceases. Some patients find it necessary to regularly apply petrolatum in order to keep the skin pliable and prevent fissuring. Acne does not occur in the irradiated field. Pigment changes may also occur; if the treatment was not well fractionated, a thin, achromic, and telangiectatic scar develops. Achromia results from melanocyte destruction. Such areas readily sunburn. If the skin is severely damaged, it may ulcerate, especially after trauma; sometimes grafting is required. With the regimens outlined in the chapter on skin cancer, skin necrosis following initial healing has not been seen.

SUBCUTANEOUS FIBROSIS

Although skin injury is rarely a major problem in modern-day therapy, late effects on subcutaneous tissues are still important. Subcutaneous fibrosis usually appears within 6 to 12 months after treatment and is slowly progressive. There is decreased pliability of the subcutaneous tissues. In severe cases, the tissues may have a woody texture and become fixed into a single hard mass in which the subcutaneous tissue is not separable from overlying skin or underlying muscle or bone. If the radiation entered the patient tangential to the skin, then skin and subcutaneous changes occur simultaneously. Patients with a great amount of adipose tissue in the subcutaneous layer tend to develop the most severe changes. Fibrosis is rarely painful.

TABLE 14-2. Chondronecrosis Following Irradiation of Laryngeal Cancer: Time–Dose Relationships

Study	Primary Site	Tumor Dose (rad/No. Weeks)	Fraction Size (rad)	No. Patients	No. (%) With Necrosis
University of Florida*	Glottis (T1–T3)	5400 rad to 7000 rad/ 4½ to 7 weeks	180–255	156	1 (0.6%)
Princess Margaret Hospital[43]	Glottis (T1)	5500 rad/5 weeks	210–230	283	0
M. D. Anderson Hospital[35]	Glottis and supraglottis	6000 rad to 7000 rad/ 5½ to 7 weeks	200–225	503	6 (1%)
Rush Presbyterian-St. Lukes[55]	Glottis (T1–T2)	6500 rad/5 to 5½ weeks	225–250	135	1 (0.7%)
Liverpool[96]	Glottis and supraglottis	5500 rad/3 weeks	344	129	9 (7%)
Penrose[7]	Glottis (T1–T2)	6100 rad to 6600 rad/ 3½ to 4 weeks	~300	16	1 (6%)

* University of Florida data; patients treated 10/64–10/77; analysis 4/80.

After high-dose treatment of vocal cord cancer with a single ipsilateral 4 × 4- to 5 × 5-cm field, the only change is an unsightly puckered area with subcutaneous plaque-like thickening in the center of the field, and extending posteriorly into the leading edge of the sternocleidomastoid muscle. The thickened area is occasionally confused with an enlarged lymph node by the inexperienced clinician. Lesser subcutaneous changes are noted in the anterior half of the field and in the anterior midline. The maximum dose (at 5 mm) is related to the incidence of subcutaneous fibrosis for cobalt-60 in Table 14-3. There were no detectable subcutaneous changes below 6850 rad, even with many years of follow-up. When parallel opposed cobalt-60 portals are used to treat vocal cord cancer, late changes in the skin and subcutaneous tissues are minimal.

Large areas of fibrosis may be accompanied by a "tight" constrictive sensation. Obstructive lymphedema may be associated with fibrosis and produce intermittent episodes of erysipelas.

High-dose irradiation of metastatic lymphadenopathy results in greater subcutaneous fibrosis in the neck than does a comparable dose to a neck that has no palpable adenopathy; apparently the fibrous stroma that replaces the tumor mass contributes to the reaction. Large daily fractions also increase the risk of subcutaneous fibrosis. Although fat necrosis is a potential risk following high dose irradiation, this condition has rarely been observed at the University of Florida.

The Eye

Because of the thinness of its medial wall and floor, the orbit is frequently secondarily invaded by cancers of the paranasal sinuses. Among University of Florida patients with carcinomas of the nasal cavity and ethmoid/sphenoid sinus who received radical irradiation, one half had demonstrable orbital invasion; in one fourth of the patients, invasion was extensive enough to produce blindness, proptosis, or a palpable orbital mass. Although tumor invasion of the eyeball itself is rare, the eye is frequently incidentally irradiated in order to ensure adequate coverage of the orbit and adjacent sinuses.

Depending on how extensively carcinoma invades the orbit, varying amounts of the eye receive high-dose irradiation (Fig. 14-7), thereby producing a variety of ophthalmologic syndromes:[82]

1. When orbital invasion is extensive, all of the orbital contents are irradiated, including the eyeball and lacrimal tissue (Fig. 14-7A). A dry eye results, and usually within the first 6 to 10 months after treatment, there is visual loss secondary to degeneration of the anterior segment of the eye (corneal ulceration and opacification).
2. If orbital invasion is present but not extensive, then most of the lacrimal tissue may be spared high-dose irradiation (Fig. 14-7B, C). Severe dry eye problems do not occur. However, if the dose to the eyeball itself has been high, visual loss secondary to posterior segment degeneration occurs, usually after a 2- to 3-year latency period; the most frequent manifestation is radiation retinopathy.
3. If there is no orbital invasion at all, a portion of the ipsilateral orbit still must receive irradiation, including approximately the medial one fourth to one third

TABLE 14-3.	Dose to Produce Subcutaneous Fibrosis Following Irradiation of T1 and T2 Vocal Cord Cancer With a Single Open Field (Cobalt-60, SSD 80 or 100 cm, 25 to 28 Fractions)
Maximum Dose at 5 mm*	**Subcutaneous Fibrosis**
6350 rad to 6850 rad	0/6
6900 rad to 7100 rad	3/12
7150 rad to 7540 rad	4/4

* Collimation with penumbra trimmers or 3-cm thick lead blocks on wire mesh tray.

Note: University of Florida data; patients treated 10/64–12/74; analysis 3/77; minimum 2-year follow-up.

of the eyeball (Fig. 14-7D). Although visual loss secondary to eyeball injury is rare in this setting, there is still a risk of blindness due to optic nerve injury, usually after a 1- to 6-year latency period; the risk depends on the daily fraction size and total dose.

Certain tumors (e.g., lymphomas) require low- or moderate-dose irradiation (usually <5000 rad), compared with the doses used for squamous or other carcinomas of the paranasal sinuses. Visual loss may occur secondary to cataract formation, without retinal or optic nerve injury. This form of visual loss may be reversible by cataract extraction if necessary.

Preirradiation assessment of the patient who is about to receive eye or optic nerve irradiation by an ophthalmologist who is knowledgeable and interested in radiation complications is mandatory. In general, the dose of irradiation that is to be administered depends on the histology (i.e., lymphoma vs. carcinoma) and tumor size, while the volume of the eye and optic nerve that is treated depends on the tumor distribution. Most potential visual complications can be anticipated during the treatment planning stage, and the patient should be apprised of the risks. Continued follow-up in the posttreatment period should be routine. Frequently, there are a number of problems occurring simultaneously, making ophthalmologic assessment confusing and management difficult. Before undertaking any specific treatment, the ophthalmologist should discuss the situation with the radiation therapist and thoroughly familiarize himself with the details of the prior radiation treatment, since there are some potential pitfalls that can be avoided. Anterior segment disease should be managed early and intensively to avoid corneal complications. Visual symptoms and ocular pain require individualized care.

The following data are based on observations made in 74 patients who received irradiation to the eye and/or optic nerves with 2-MeV x-rays or cobalt-60 at the University of Florida between October 1964 and March 1979. Included are patients with tumors of the paranasal sinuses, orbit, nasopharynx, and eyeball.

Dose calculations were made at each area of interest as follows:

1. The dose to the lacrimal apparatus was calculated at a depth of 1 cm from the anterior skin surface.

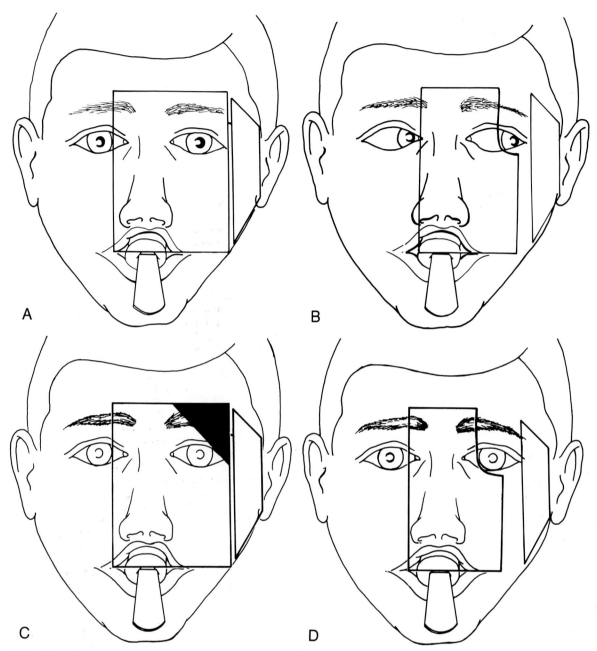

FIG. 14-7. Anterior portals used to treat tumors of nasal cavity and paranasal sinuses. (A) Extensive orbital invasion (e.g., palpable orbital mass, proptosis, or blindness). No lacrimal shielding. (B) Limited orbital invasion present. The major lacrimal gland is shielded. Patient is instructed to gaze laterally to displace lens from portal. This technique was discontinued at the University of Florida after 1970. (C) Limited orbital invasion present. The major lacrimal gland is shielded. This technique has been used at the University of Florida since 1971. (D) No orbital invasion. (Reprinted with permission from Parsons JT, Fitzgerald CR, Hood CI, Ellingwood KE, Bova FJ, Million RR: The effects of irradiation on the eye and optic nerve. Int J Radiat Oncol Biol Phys 9:609–622, 1983. Copyright © 1983, Pergamon Press, Ltd.)

2. Retinal doses were calculated only for those patients in whom half or more of the posterior pole of the eye was encompassed by the high-dose region. The specified dose is the minimum dose received by the majority of the retina.
3. Optic nerve doses are the maximum dose to any portion of the nerve.

Not all patients had all of these structures irradiated.

LACRIMAL APPARATUS

THE LACRIMAL GLANDS

The tears are composed of secretions from the following:

1. The major lacrimal gland, which is closely applied to the globe in the superior temporal quadrant of the orbit

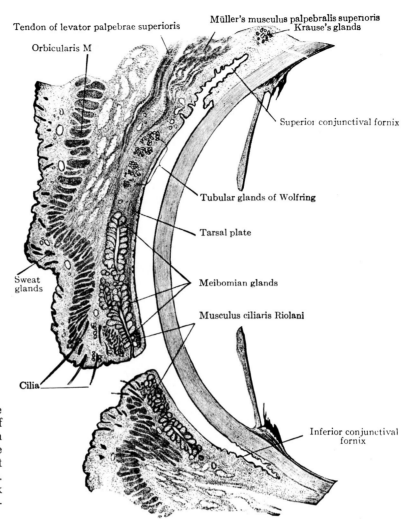

Tendon of levator palpebrae superioris

Orbicularis M

Müller's musculus palpebralis superioris

Krause's glands

Superior conjunctival fornix

Tubular glands of Wolfring

Tarsal plate

Sweat glands

Meibomian glands

Musculus ciliaris Riolani

Cilia

Inferior conjunctival fornix

FIG. 14-8. Sagittal section through the eyelids and eyeball. Note the location of the accessory lacrimal glands of Krause in the superior conjunctival fornix and the accessory lacrimal glands of Wolfring at the superior margin of the tarsal plate. (Scheie HG, Albert DM: Adler's Textbook of Ophthalmology, 8th ed., p 44. Philadelphia, WB Saunders, 1969)

2. The accessory lacrimal glands of Krause, which are located in the conjunctival fornices, mainly the superior fornix
3. The accessory lacrimal glands of Wolfring, which are located at the superior margin of the upper tarsal plate
4. The sebaceous meibomian glands, which are somewhat more plentiful in the upper than the lower lid
5. The accessory sebaceous glands of Zeis and the glands of Moll, which lie near the lid margins
6. The goblet cells, which are distributed throughout the conjunctiva

Although their mass is small in relation to the major lacrimal gland, the accessory lacrimal glands are believed to be responsible for the basal secretion of tears (Fig. 14-8).[87] Reflex secretion is from the main lacrimal gland.[51]

Under normal conditions, the tears form a thin layer that wets, lubricates, and flushes the corneal and conjunctival surfaces and tends to improve the optical properties of the cornea by smoothing any existing surface irregularities. The fluid flows to the lacrimal puncta, especially the lower one, thence through the canaliculi, lacrimal sac, nasolacrimal duct, and into the nose beneath the inferior turbinate.

The tear film consists of three layers: (1) a superficial lipid layer, derived from meibomian and Zeis gland se-

cretions, which helps retard evaporation; (2) a middle aqueous layer, produced by the major and accessory lacrimal glands; and (3) a deep mucinous layer, which serves to wet the relatively hydrophobic corneal and conjunctival epithelium. The mucin of the deep layer is elaborated by conjunctival goblet cells. Deficiency of any of the three components may result in loss of tear film stability, with the result being dry spots due to rapid breakup of the tear film. A dry eye (keratoconjunctivitis sicca) is the result, and this in turn leads to damage of the conjunctival and corneal epithelium. Corneal epithelial defects stain with fluorescein. Because the corneal epithelium is endowed with numerous nerves, pain from a dry eye is often marked.

In a histopathologic study of eight eyes that were exenterated 5 days to 16 years following irradiation (mostly using cobalt-60 for tumors of the paranasal sinuses), Karp and colleagues demonstrated diffuse involutional atrophy of the meibomian glands in all eight specimens; in three there was total loss of meibomian glands and ducts.[53] In six, no accessory lacrimal tissue could be identified. In one patient from whom the entire lacrimal gland was available for study, the gland was diffusely atrophic. In three of seven specimens where it could be determined, the sebaceous glands of Zeis were absent. Although the glands of Moll could usually be identified, they were frequently atypical.

Since most of the basal secretion of tears comes from

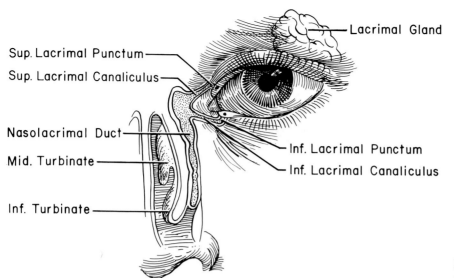

FIG. 14-9. The major lacrimal gland and lacrimal drainage system.

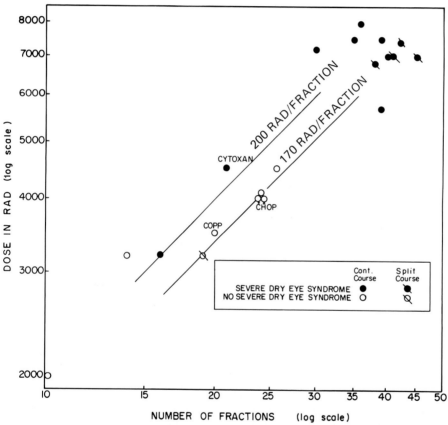

FIG. 14-10. Dose to the lacrimal tissue versus the number of fractions for production of severe dry-eye syndrome (corneal opacification, vascularization, or ulceration sufficient to cause visual loss). Included are data on 20 eyes in 19 patients following continuous- or split-course irradiation with cobalt-60 or 2-MeV x-rays for a variety of head and neck tumors. The dose to the lacrimal tissue is regarded as the dose at 1.0-cm depth (*i.e.*, at approximately the major lacrimal gland). The exact dose received by the accessory lacrimal tissue in the eyelids is difficult to estimate because the lid is so thin; however, in the eye-open position, which was used in all patients, one would not expect significant sparing of the lacrimal tissue (located mainly in the superior conjunctival fornix and tarsal portion of the upper lid), since it would be bolused by the soft tissues of the orbital portion of the lid. Three patients (four eyes) who received chemotherapy in addition to irradiation are so designated. Length of follow-up on the eight eyes that did not develop severe dry-eye syndrome was 2½ to 12 years (mean 6.2 years, median 5 years). Reference lines have been added for ease of interpretation of the data and represent treatments administered at 170 and 200 rad/fraction, respectively; they are not isoeffect lines. (Reprinted with permission from Parsons JT, Fitzgerald CR, Hood CI, Ellingwood KE, Bova FJ, Million RR: The effects of irradiation on the eye and optic nerve. Int J Radiat Oncol Biol Phys 9:609–622, 1983. Copyright © 1983, Pergamon Press, Ltd.)

the accessory lacrimal glands, which are most plentiful in the upper lid and superior conjunctival fornix, efforts should always be made to shield some of the upper lid in addition to the major lacrimal gland; because tumors most frequently invade the orbit through its floor (maxillary sinus) or medial wall (ethmoid sinus), one can usually shield the superolateral orbit (Fig. 14-9) unless orbital invasion is extensive. During treatment, the eye is locally anesthetized and a lid retractor is inserted so that part of the upper lateral eyelid is displaced from the treatment field; maintenance of the open eye position during treatment also prevents bolus effect by the lids on the cornea and conjunctiva.

When the orbit is extensively invaded by carcinoma, high-dose irradiation of the entire orbit is necessary and generally results in a severe "dry eye syndrome." If the dose to the entire eye and lacrimal tissue exceeds 5000 rad, prospects of maintaining vision are poor. The patient develops a red, painful, scratchy eye (foreign body sensation) and photophobia. The drying effects of wind are particularly bothersome. Although the majority of patients suffered moderate to severe pain, two had very little pain and little or no conjunctival reaction during the first few posttreatment months, but eventually they lost sight due to corneal injury.

A time–dose scatter distribution for the production of severe dry-eye syndrome (corneal opacification, ulceration, or vascularization sufficient to cause visual loss) is shown in Figure 14-10.[82] Included are data on 20 eyes in 19 patients following irradiation with cobalt-60 or 2-MeV x-rays to the entire orbit. Whenever portal reductions were made to exclude the major lacrimal gland, the dose shown is that prior to reduction. All eyes that received greater than or equal to 5700 rad became severely affected by keratoconjunctivitis sicca within 1 to 2 months after treatment; frequently, the cornea was opaque by 1 year. The 2 eyes that were injured after lower doses (3200 and 4500 rad) suffered slowly progressive corneal opacification and vascularization. Enucleation was eventually required at 4 and 8 years, respectively, because of moderately severe symptoms and visual acuity of only "hand motion" in both eyes. Symptoms in "uninjured eyes" ranged from none to occasional mild photophobia and mild foreign body sensation. Although additional data are needed, it would appear that the majority of patients tolerate doses in the range of 3000 rad to 4000 rad to the entire orbit with cobalt-60 without developing severe symptoms of a dry eye (Fig. 14-11).[82]

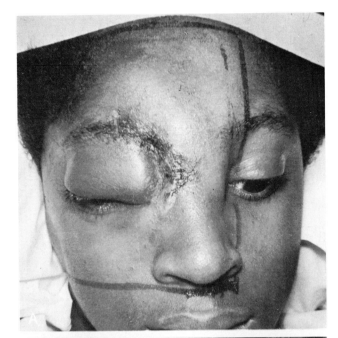

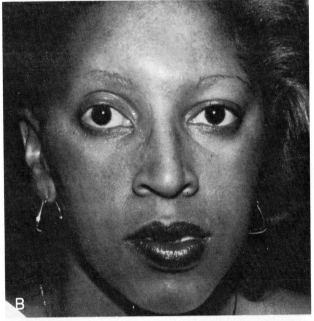

FIG. 14-11. (A) Fifteen-year-old black female with an extensive orbital lymphoma. There were enlarged right preauricular and right jugulodigastric nodes. The right eye and entire lacrimal apparatus received 4000 rad/24 fractions/34 days with cobalt-60. (B) There was no evidence of disease at 12 years. A cataract was extracted at 4 years. The patient tolerates a hard contact lens over the right eye (visual acuity 20/30), and has spectacle correction over the left eye (visual acuity 20/20). (C) The right fundus appears normal. (Photograph was made at 8 years.) (Reprinted with permission from Parsons JT, Fitzgerald CR, Hood CI, Ellingwood KE, Bova FJ, Million RR: The effects of irradiation on the eye and optic nerve. Int J Radiat Oncol Biol Phys 9:609–622, 1983. Copyright © 1983, Pergamon Press, Ltd.)

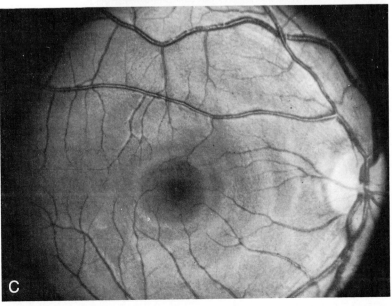

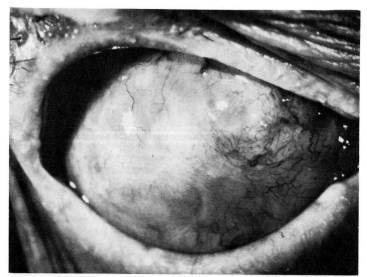

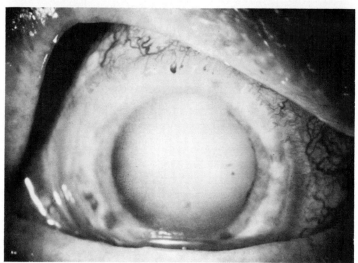

FIG. 14-13. Right eye of a 59-year-old white woman, 18 months after treatment of an advanced squamous cell carcinoma of the ethmoid sinus, which had extensively invaded the right orbit, producing proptosis and ophthalmoplegia. The eye and lacrimal gland received 7000 rad/ 40 fractions/71 days by split-course irradiation, following which the patient suffered from keratitis and conjunctivitis. Nine months after treatment, she was treated for iridocyclitis and had intermittently elevated intraocular pressures that were believed secondary to the anterior uveitis. Over the next month, vision decreased from 20/40 to 20/ 200 and by 15 months was "light perception" only. Retrobulbar injections of alcohol failed to relieve pain, except for brief periods. At 18 months there was a further exacerbation of pain, plus lid swelling, chemosis, and a slightly purulent conjunctival discharge; there was considerable loss of corneal epithelium. Severe rubeosis iridis occurred, and the anterior chamber was filled with pus. The patient was believed to have endophthalmitis, and evisceration was performed. Cultures of the intraocular contents, cornea, and conjunctiva all grew β-hemolytic streptococci. The pathologic specimen revealed numerous gram-positive cocci within the corneal stroma. There was no tumor recurrence at 3½ years. (Reprinted with permission from Parsons JT, Fitzgerald CR, Hood CI, Ellingwood KE, Bova FJ, Million RR: The effects of irradiation on the eye and optic nerve. Int J Radiat Oncol Biol Phys 9:609–622, 1983. Copyright © 1983, Pergamon Press, Ltd.)

FIG. 14-12. Eye of a 57-year-old white man 3 years and 10 months after treatment of an advanced adenoid cystic carcinoma of the ethmoid sinus, which extensively invaded the orbit and base of the skull. The entire eye and orbital contents received 6800 rad/38 fractions/66 days by split-course irradiation. At the end of treatment, the patient had a severe dry-eye syndrome with keratitis and conjunctivitis. By 9 months, the cornea was scarred and there was pannus formation. The patient developed rubeosis iridis and neovascular glaucoma (intraocular pressure, 60 mm Hg). Attempts to control pain by cyclocryotherapy were unsuccessful and enucleation was recommended. (Parsons JT, Fitzgerald CR, Hood CI, Ellingwood KE, Bova FJ, Million RR: The effects of irradiation on the eye and optic nerve. Int J Radiat Oncol Biol Phys 9:609–622, 1983)

High-energy x-rays (e.g., 17 to 20 MeV) would be more sparing of the lacrimal tissue owing to the buildup characteristics of the beam, but they would create other undesirable technical problems.

In association with corneal ulceration, five patients developed an acute anterior uveitis; pain was often severe, sometimes requiring hospitalization and intensive medical management with cycloplegics, mydriatics, narcotic analgesics, tranquilizers, and antibiotic therapy as indicated.

Treatment of a dry eye is symptomatic. For mild or moderate dry-eye syndrome, artificial tears are used during the day and a sterile ophthalmic lubricating ointment is applied at night. Hydrophilic soft contact lenses are sometimes used as a protective bandage for corneal epithelial defects and may serve as a tear reservoir, but they are not always well tolerated by patients who have severe dry eyes secondary to irradiation; one patient developed a spontaneous corneal perforation while using a soft contact lens over a centrally thinned cornea. In two other patients, a full conjunctival flap was used to cover corneal epithelial defects in an attempt to control severe pain; pain relief was complete in one, but incomplete in the second patient. In the early stages of the dry-eye syndrome, visual acuity is usually only slightly impaired. If severe dry-eye syndrome develops, then corneal stromal edema, clouding, and eventually corneal scarring and vascularization occur (Fig. 14-12).[82] Vision deteriorates rapidly. The entire eye becomes vulnerable to bacterial infection (Fig. 14-13).[82] Treatment of a painful, nonseeing eye is by evisceration or enucleation.

THE NASOLACRIMAL DRAINAGE SYSTEM

The nasolacrimal duct is usually not affected by high-dose irradiation unless it has been disrupted by tumor or prior surgery. Only one patient is known to have developed epiphora secondary to obstruction of a previously normal nasolacrimal duct in the presence of normal puncta and canaliculi; he was offered treatment by dacryocystorhinostomy, but declined. Since ductal patency was not routinely evaluated, possibly other injuries escaped detection. In one patient whose nasolacrimal duct was obstructed by tumor prior to treatment, a small plastic tube was passed through the inferior canaliculus, through the entire nasolacrimal drainage system, and out the nose; the tube was left in place for the entire treatment course and was maintained until 1 month posttreatment (Fig. 14-16A). Permanent obstruction was not prevented.

Stenosis of the lacrimal puncta or canaliculi following high-dose irradiation was more common. Efforts to correct obstruction in the postirradiation period by conjunctivodacryocystorhinostomy were unsuccessful in two patients.

THE RETINA

When the lacrimal apparatus is shielded from high-dose irradiation, permanent visual loss secondary to degeneration of the anterior segment of the eye is usually preventable; there is still, however, a risk of radiation injury to the retina. The retina is unique in that its small blood vessels are readily accessible to examination by ophthalmoscopy. Study of the retinal vasculature is aided by fluorescein angiography. By using appropriate filters, it is possible to photograph the retinal vessels, including the capillary system, which one cannot visualize with an ophthalmoscope. The retina has one of the highest oxygen consumptions in the body and is supplied by an end-arterial system. Branches of the central retinal artery supply the inner retina, while the outer retina is supplied by the choroidal circulation by way of the posterior ciliary arteries; irradiation may affect the vessels of both systems.[30] The retina is highly vulnerable to vascular insults and has little capacity for regeneration; repair of injury results in a mixed glial and collagenous scar.

MANIFESTATIONS OF RADIATION RETINOPATHY

Radiation retinopathy presents a clinical picture similar to that seen in diabetic retinopathy. Retinal injury following high-dose irradiation is usually not expressed clinically for 1½ to 3 years following irradiation, during which time visual acuity often remains normal. Subsequent deterioration is thought to occur because of progressive obliteration of small retinal vessels, resulting in retinal ischemia, edema, capillary microaneurysm formation, hemorrhage, and retinal neovascularization. Retinal hemorrhages in the nerve fiber layer appear flame shaped, while deep retinal hemorrhages are round. Capillary microaneurysms are seen most readily on fluorescein angiograms and are usually located near areas of capillary nonperfusion; although the precise pathogenesis of the microaneurysms is unclear, they are generally associated with vascular occlusive disease and retinal ischemia. Retinal ischemia is also the likely cause of neovascularization: it is theorized that the hypoxic retina may elaborate a vasoproliferative factor similar to that thought responsible for new vessel formation in diabetic retinopathy. New vessels are situated on the retina, the optic disc, or both. As neovascularization progresses, the vessels may invade the plane between the vitreous and retina, and eventually the vitreous itself. Detachment of the sensory retina from the retinal pigment epithelium may result. Hemorrhage into the vitreous is another common sequela, since the new vessels are generally quite fragile.

Fluorescein angiography often delineates focal retinal capillary nonperfusion or occluded branch arterioles; central retinal artery occlusion has been described[45,92] but has not been observed in patients at the University of Florida. It seems that the capillaries are most susceptible to obliteration, followed by the smaller branch arterioles, with the main arterioles being least susceptible. Histologically, affected vessels have thick and hyalinized walls and the lumens may be occluded by a fine fibrillary material.[30]

Leakage of plasma from damaged vessels, microaneurysms, or areas of neovascularization can be seen by fluorescein study (Fig. 14-14).[45,82]

Some patients with radiation retinopathy develop a neovascular proliferation on the anterior surface of the iris, called rubeosis iridis. The cause of anterior segment neovascularization may be the same as for posterior segment neovascularization (i.e., a vasoproliferative factor produced by the hypoxic retina). Whether direct irradiation of the iris plays any role in producing rubeosis iridis is unknown. New blood vessels usually appear first at the pupillary margin, then progress to the angles, resulting in peripheral anterior synechiae and secondary angle closure (neovascular) glaucoma (Figs. 14-14 and 14-15).[82] The vessels are also very prone to hemorrhage, leading to hyphema. Rubeosis was preceded by ischemic optic neuropathy and central retinal vein occlusion in one patient (Fig. 14-16).[82]

"Cotton-wool" exudates are frequently seen on ophthalmoscopic examination and are apparently a direct result of retinal ischemia. Such lesions are not true exudates, but are instead infarcts in the nerve fiber layer. They usually appear round and are seldom wider than the optic disc. True retinal exudates (also called "hard" or "waxy" exudates) may also be seen and are presumably due to extravasation of fluid from abnormally permeable vessels. They are most common near microaneurysms and have a particular predilection for the region of the macula. With time, the fluid is resorbed, leaving behind a protein- or lipid-rich residue.[57]

Most commonly, there is a 2- to 3-year period during which the visual acuity remains normal or near normal; then, over several months, the vision progressively deteriorates. If the dose to the retina was only 5000 rad to 5500 rad, there may be a longer latent period (e.g., 5 to 6 years). Visual loss is usually painless unless neovascular glaucoma develops, as it did in ten patients at the University of Florida. Pain from the latter condition has not been controlled by medical means, retrobulbar injections of alcohol, or cyclocryotherapy (cryotherapy applied to the ciliary body in an attempt to decrease aqueous production); enucleation or evisceration of the glaucomatous eye was necessary for pain relief in eight patients and was recommended, but not undertaken, in another. It is unclear from the medical records of the tenth patient whether there was significant pain secondary to glaucoma or whether enucleation was recommended; his eye was not removed.

TIME–DOSE ANALYSIS FOR RETINAL INJURY

A log–log plot of dose versus number of fractions for retinal injury sufficient to produce visual loss following irradiation of the entire or almost the entire retina is shown in Figure 14-17.[82] The major lacrimal gland in these patients was shielded throughout treatment (21 eyes), most commonly with field arrangements as shown in Fig. 14-7B and 14-7C, or it was shielded after it had received less than or equal to 4500 rad (7 eyes); patients who lost sight secondary to anterior segment degeneration are excluded. Patients in whom the central retina was shielded by a cylindrical lead corneal block on the anterior field, with the patient gazing straight ahead, are also excluded since determination of the retinal dose is not possible in this situation.

The shape of the sigmoid dose-response curve is apparently steep between 5000 and 6000 rad. There was only one instance of clinically detectable retinal injury at or below 5000 rad (a 10-year-old patient who suffered a vit-

(Text continues on p. 194.)

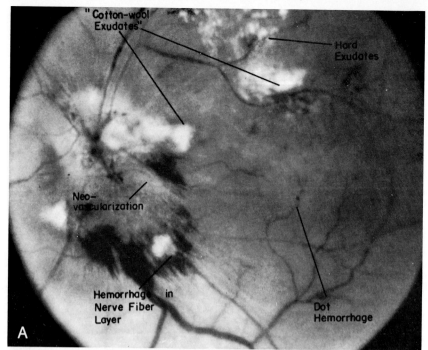

"Cotton-wool Exudates"

Hard Exudates

Neo-vascularization

Hemorrhage in Nerve Fiber Layer

Dot Hemorrhage

A

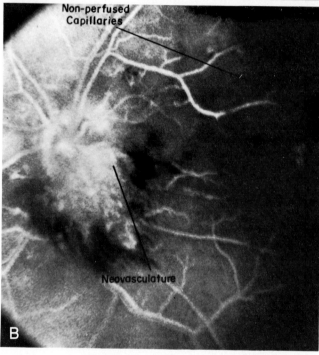

Non-perfused Capillaries

Neovasculature

B

FIG. 14-14. (*A*) Appearance of left eye on ophthalmoscopic examination 2 years, 8 months after irradiation of a low-grade fibrosarcoma of the left nasal cavity, paranasal sinuses, and orbit in a 42-year-old woman. The dose to the left retina was 6000 rad/ 32 fractions/61 days by split-course technique; the lacrimal gland was shielded. Visual acuity remained 20/20 in the left eye for 2 years following irradiation, but by 2 years and 7 months she had developed an edematous, congested optic disc; her visual acuity was 20/300. One month later, at the time of this photograph, there was a Marcus-Gunn pupil and vision was "counts fingers"; the disc margins were hazy and there were cotton-wool spots, hard exudates, intraretinal and preretinal hemorrhages, and irregular, tortuous branch retinal arterioles. (*B*) Fluorescein angiography showed irregular fluorescence of the large vessel walls superiorly, compatible with damage to these structures. There was an extensive fluorescein leak from neovascular tissue over the disc, and an area of retinal capillary nonperfusion superior to the fovea. Several months later, the patient presented to her local ophthalmologist with severe pain secondary to neovascular glaucoma (40 mm Hg). Enucleation was performed. In addition to rubeosis iridis, the surgical specimen showed neovascular tissue arising from the surface of the nerve head and extending into the vitreous. (Reprinted with permission from Parsons JT, Fitzgerald CR, Hood CI, Ellingwood KE, Bova FJ, Million RR: The effects of irradiation on the eye and optic nerve. Int J Radiat Oncol Biol Phys 9:609–622, 1983. Copyright © 1983, Pergamon Press, Ltd.)

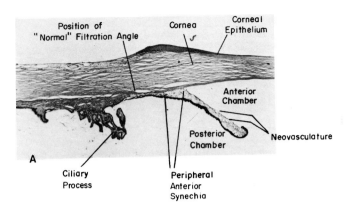

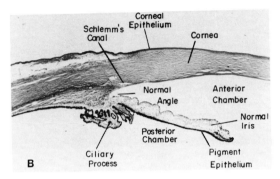

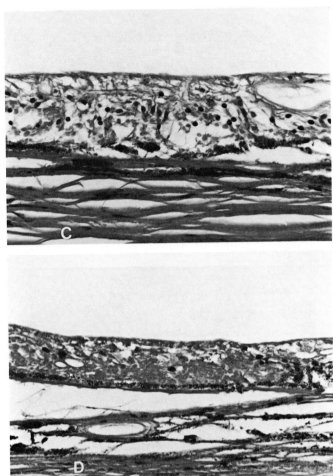

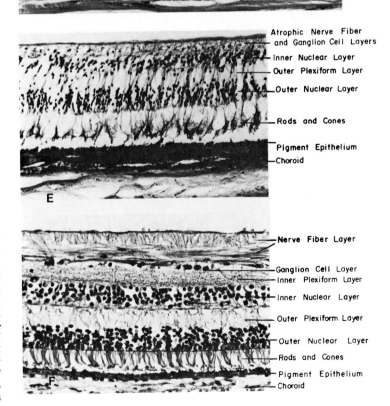

FIG. 14-15. A 47-year-old white man received 6500 rad/ 32 fractions/44 days to the nasal half of his right eye for a poorly differentiated cancer involving the ethmoid sinus and orbit. The position of the eye during treatment was "lateral gaze." Until 14 months after treatment, he noted only epiphora, which had been present before treatment, and occasional "flashes of light" in the right eye; visual acuity remained 20/40. Three months later, there was severe sheathing of retinal arterioles and declining visual acuity. At 22 months, vision was "counts fingers" and the patient complained of ocular pain. Ocular tension was 44 mm Hg. Pain was progressive and unrelieved by narcotic analgesics and carbonic anhydrase inhibitors. Blood in the anterior chamber (hyphema) was noted. Enucleation was required. (A) The surgical specimen showed rubeosis iridis (note numerous dilated vessels on the anterior surface of the iris), ectropion uveae, and a broad, peripheral anterior synechia, which obliterated the filtration angle. (B) Normal iris and normal filtration angle for comparison with A. (C) The retina was in place. Retinal changes were most severe in those portions of the retina that received the highest dose. Microscopic section shows severe atrophy and disorganization of the nasal (irradiated) retina. (D) Microscopic section from another area of the nasal retina showed full-thickness retinal necrosis. (E) The temporal retina, which received a low dose of irradiation, showed only the effects of elevated intraocular pressure, rather than effects due to a direct action of irradiation. The nerve fiber layer was atrophic and the ganglion cells absent. Nuclei of the inner nuclear layer were decreased in number, while those of the outer layer were preserved. (F) Appearance of normal retina for comparison with C through E. It should be noted that the histologic changes secondary to irradiation are nonspecific. (Reprinted with permission from Parsons JT, Fitzgerald CR, Hood CI, Ellingwood KE, Bova FJ, Million RR: The effects of irradiation on the eye and optic nerve. Int J Radiat Oncol Biol Phys 9:609–622, 1983. Copyright © 1983, Pergamon Press, Ltd.)

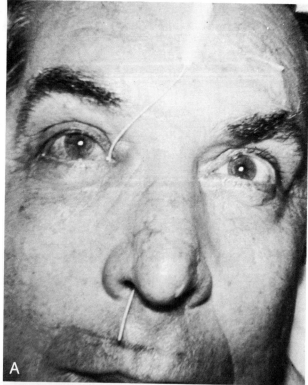

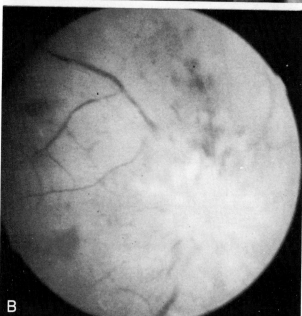

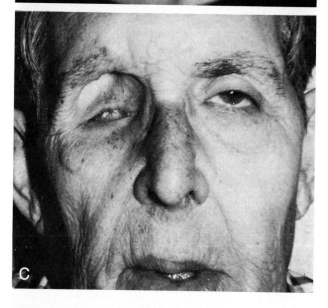

◀ **FIG. 14-16.** (A) A 54-year-old white man presented with a several year history of right-sided epiphora and chronic dacryocystitis. A dacryocystorhinostomy (note scar and subcutaneous soft tissue mass in right medial canthal and infraorbital region) temporarily relieved his epiphora, but 4 months later "respiratory mucosa" was noted to have grown over the surgically created ostium. A new opening was made and a polyethylene tube was passed through the inferior canaliculus into the nose. Biopsy at that time showed squamous cell carcinoma; further evaluation revealed tumor in the ethmoid and maxillary sinuses, nasal cavity, and medial orbit. During the course of irradiation, the right eye received 6100 rad/32 fractions/57 days by split-course irradiation; the lacrimal gland was shielded. The polyethylene tube was left in place until 1 month after treatment. Following irradiation, both lacrimal puncta were progressively obliterated, and at 25 months the patient underwent a conjunctivocystorhinostomy with insertion of a Jones tube in an attempt to alleviate his epiphora. There was good function for 1 month, but the tube was subsequently dislodged by a vigorous sneeze. It was replaced but was similarly dislodged 1 week later. The patient refused replacement. (B) Between 32 and 36 months, the patient developed painless visual loss and was noted to have ophthalmoscopic findings of central retinal vein occlusion, with venous engorgement, scattered retinal hemorrhages, and edema of the optic disc. The clinical picture was felt to be compatible with ischemic optic neuropathy, with secondary disc edema leading to venous stasis. One month later, severe pain developed secondary to neovascular glaucoma. Retrobulbar injection of alcohol gave only temporary relief, and evisceration was required. (C) There has been no evidence of cancer recurrence for 12 years. The patient is unable to keep an ocular prosthesis in place because of progressive contraction of the orbital soft tissues. (Reprinted with permission from Parsons JT, Fitzgerald CR, Hood CI, Ellingwood KE, Bova FJ, Million RR: The effects of irradiation on the eye and optic nerve. Int J Radiat Oncol Biol Phys 9:609–622, 1983. Copyright © 1983, Pergamon Press, Ltd.)

reous hemorrhage 13 months after 4500 rad plus cyclophosphamide). Above 5000 rad, only one retina was not severely injured and this case was equivocal. The retina of this patient received 6000 rad/35 fractions, following which vision was lost at 2½ years secondary to a dense cataract. Because of moderate dry-eye symptoms in a nonseeing eye, enucleation was undertaken at 4 years and 2 months. Although retinal function could not be assessed, the retina and retinal vessels were normal on histologic examination. The analysis of risk of injury versus time–dose factors is difficult because there are few data between 5000 rad and 5500 rad. Of the four patients whose eyes received these doses, one also received multiagent chemotherapy (the interaction between irradiation and chemotherapy almost certainly increases the risk of injury[8,40]), and two were treated with large-dose fractions (305 rad to 325 rad/fraction). The best estimate at this time from the available data is that one begins to run a significant risk of severe injury after delivery of retinal doses that exceed 5000 rad (at 180 rad to 200 rad/fraction).

MANAGEMENT OF RADIATION RETINOPATHY

Often, when there is severe retinal injury, the goal is simply to maintain a comfortable, cosmetically acceptable eye. Since the only effective treatment of neovascular

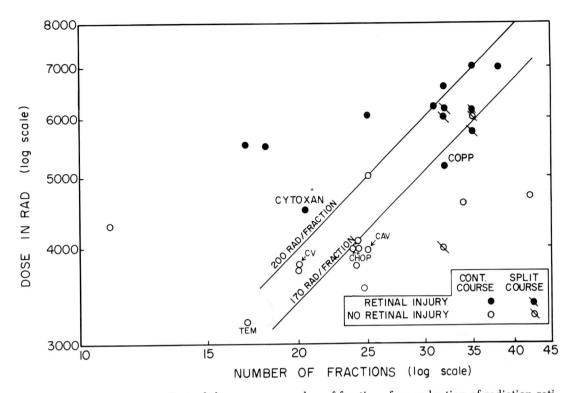

FIG. 14-17. Retinal dose versus number of fractions for production of radiation retinopathy. Included are data on 28 eyes (27 patients) following continuous- or split-course irradiation (cobalt-60 or 2 MeV) of a variety of head and neck tumors at the University of Florida (10/64–3/79). All patients have been followed for a minimum of 3 years and the maximum follow-up is 16 years; patients who died within 3 years without developing retinal injury are not included. Reference lines for treatments administered at 170 rad/ fraction and 200 rad/fraction have been added for ease of interpretation of the data; these lines are not isoeffect lines. There is a mean follow-up of 6.6 years and a median follow-up of 5.5 years in the 15 uninjured eyes. Severe injury was documented in the remaining 13 eyes at 1 to 6½ years after treatment; mean and median times to injury were both 2.5 years. Ten of the 13 injuries were detected within 3 years. Six patients (7 eyes) who received single-agent or multiagent chemotherapy in addition to irradiation are so designated. Visual acuity in the injured eyes was 20/200 in one eye, "counts fingers" at 1 or 2 feet in 2 eyes, "hand motion" in one eye, "light perception" in 3 eyes, and "no light perception" in 6 eyes. (Reprinted with permission from Parsons JT, Fitzgerald CR, Hood CI, Ellingwood KE, Bova FJ, Million RR: The effects of irradiation on the eye and optic nerve. Int J Radiat Oncol Biol Phys 9:609–622, 1983. Copyright © 1983, Pergamon Press, Ltd.)

(closed angle) glaucoma is removal of the eyeball, efforts should be made to prevent this complication. In diabetic patients who have proliferative retinopathy, there is evidence that suggests that panretinal laser photocoagulation may eliminate the stimulus to new vessel formation in the anterior and posterior segments and thus prevent or at least reduce the risk of developing glaucoma.[101] The rationale for such treatment rests on the laser's ability to destroy hypoxic areas of the retina that are believed to produce a vasoproliferative factor. Whether neovascular glaucoma can be prevented in the severely damaged eye following irradiation is an unanswered question. The laser has been used in only one patient at the University of Florida who had early neovascularization; he has had no further neovascularization for 3 years and has not developed evidence of rubeosis iridis. Chaudhuri and colleagues have reported regression of neovascularization on the optic disc and retina within 2 weeks of panretinal laser photocoagulation in a patient who received irradiation for a carcinoma of the paranasal sinuses.[9] No direct treatment of the new vessels was performed; there was no recurrence of the neovascularization at 4 months.

PREVENTION OF RADIATION RETINOPATHY

All fields should be treated daily. The dose per fraction generally should not exceed 180 rad to 190 rad/day. If feasible, fields should be reduced to limit the retinal dose to 5000 rad. Computed tomographic (CT) scanning is thought to improve our ability to judge the degree of orbital involvement compared with conventional tomography and therefore allows tighter treatment planning near the eye.

When only a portion of the eye is irradiated, its position during treatment is important. Until 1970, patients at the University of Florida with ethmoid sinus carcinomas were instructed to gaze laterally to displace the ipsilateral crystalline lens from the treatment field (see Fig. 14-7B); the field edge was at or near the medial limbus. This position rotates the posterior pole, and thus most of the sensory retina, into the treatment field. Currently, patients are instructed to gaze straight ahead with the lids open during treatment, the latter in order to prevent bolus effect.

Ten patients who had no evidence of orbital invasion were treated with an anterior field that transected the eyeball at the medial limbus, with straight-ahead gaze (see Fig. 14-7D). These patients have been followed for 3.5 to 10 years (mean 5.5 years, median 6 years). It is impossible to gauge the dose to the medial one third of the eye since it lies in the penumbra of the anterior portal. There has been no detectable retinopathy, but three eyes lost sight due to retrobulbar optic nerve injury.

There is no answer to the question of how best to protect the retina during irradiation. On the anterior portal, many centers use a "corneal cylinder" on a blocking tray that is located 15 cm to 20 cm from the patient. For the past 12 years at the University of Florida it has been generally preferred to use no cylinder and, instead, reduce the portals after a "safe" dose whenever possible. Use of a long cylinder that allows little transmission of x-rays has the undesirable effect of shielding areas potentially involved by tumor. If a short cylinder were used (e.g., 1 HVL or less), then the dose to the retina might be limited to 5000 rad for a 7000-rad treatment course. The two techniques whereby one might limit the retinal dose (i.e., portal reduction vs. a short corneal cylinder) would produce a different effect on the retina; although the total retinal doses for the two techniques might be nearly the same, the former delivers 5000 rad/27 to 28 fractions/5½ weeks before fields are reduced, while the dose from the latter technique would be spread out over the entire treatment course (e.g., 5000 rad/38 fractions/7½ weeks). The latter technique, which has not been tried, would be more sparing to the eye, but also more sparing to cancer in the orbit.

THE OPTIC NERVE

On ophthalmoscopic examination, the optic nerve head normally looks orange red. Following ganglion cell death, the nerve head looks pale secondary to loss of small blood vessels and glial proliferation of the disc; this condition is called optic atrophy. *Optic atrophy* is a descriptive term that does not imply a specific etiology or mechanism of injury. Symptoms include loss of visual acuity, visual field defects, or both. Atrophy may be initiated by a lesion anywhere from the ganglion cell bodies in the retina to the synapses of their axons in the lateral geniculate bodies (on the inferior aspect of the thalamus). The entire disc may be pale, or there may be pallor of only one sector. Fluorescein angiography reveals a loss of vessels in both the superficial and deep vascular networks.

Two types of optic nerve injury are seen clinically: (1) injury at the distal end of the nerve (i.e., at the disc) producing a condition called ischemic optic neuropathy, the postulated mechanism of which is occlusion of the posterior ciliary arteries that supply the optic nerve and choroid, and (2) more proximal injury to the nerve, producing retrobulbar optic neuropathy. Infarction secondary to small vessel injury is also believed responsible; patients with preexisting small vessel occlusive disease are probably at increased risk.

ISCHEMIC OPTIC NEUROPATHY

Ophthalmoscopic findings in ischemic optic neuropathy are those of disc pallor and edema with splinter hemor-

rhages on or adjacent to the disc; the clinical picture may be similar to that seen in patients with papilledema. Although it might be possible for only one sector of the disc to be involved, this was not observed in the University of Florida series. Five eyes in four patients developed such injury; there was a 2-year latent period in three eyes, a 3-year latent period in one eye, and a 4-year latent period in the fifth eye. Treatment of three patients (four optic nerves) with orally administered corticosteroids failed to halt progressive loss of vision over a period of several months. Visual acuity in two eyes became 20/400; the other three had "no light perception." Disc pallor is permanent.

RETROBULBAR OPTIC NEUROPATHY

Seven eyes in five patients developed visual loss secondary to proximal injury to the nerve, without evidence of disc edema or hemorrhage. Time to onset of injury in the University of Florida patients was sometimes shorter than in the M. D. Anderson Hospital series, in which Shukovsky and Fletcher noted a 4- to 5-year latent interval.[92] Visual difficulties were first noted at 11, 12, 14, 28, 42, 72, and 100 months and were thought by the patients to have occurred quite suddenly in all seven instances.

In three patients there was associated ocular pain and unilateral headache at the time of visual loss; I have no ready explanation for the pain in this setting.

Three eyes initially lost vision in all fields at the onset of injury. In the other four eyes, the initial visual symptom was a field cut. Within 2 weeks to 2 months after losing a portion of their visual field, the remaining field of vision also abruptly became affected in three of the four eyes; follow-up in the fourth patient is only 1 month. Ophthalmoscopic examinations shortly after the onset of symptoms usually revealed a normal-appearing disc or a disc with pallor of only one sector. There was eventual progression to a chalk white disc in six cases; in the seventh (recently injured) case, fluorescein angiography reveals a paucity of capillaries over one half the disc. Visual acuity became "counts fingers at 1 or 2 feet" in two eyes, "light perception" in the third, and "no light perception" in the other four eyes.

TIME–DOSE ANALYSIS FOR OPTIC NERVE INJURY

The risk of injury correlates best with daily fraction size for patients who received greater than 5500 rad (Fig. 14-18).[82] At approximately 165 rad to 190 rad/fraction, 6000 rad to 7300 rad produced injuries in 8% (2/24) of long-term survivors. Following daily doses of 195 rad or greater, the risk within the same dose range was substantially greater (41%, or 7/17). Some series have reported optic nerve injuries after doses as low as 5000 rad, generally in patients with pituitary adenomas who commonly present with optic nerve deficits secondary to mass effect. Previous compromise of the nerve almost certainly increases the risk of injury; patients with pituitary adenoma were excluded from the present series.

THE LENS

The crystalline lens is avascular, biconvex, and almost completely transparent. The most anterior and posterior parts of the lens are termed the *anterior* and *posterior poles*, respectively; the peripheral portion is called the equator. The lens is entirely surrounded by a highly refractile capsule. Under the anterior capsule, there is a layer of epithelial cells. Under the posterior capsule, there is no epithelium. Toward the equator of the lens, the epithelial cells become progressively elongated and are transformed into lens fibers; the fibers are 7 mm to 10 mm in length and contain a flattened nucleus, located near the lens equator. Subcapsular epithelial cells are capable of reproduction; most of the dividing cells are located in the anterior equatorial region. It is generally thought that it is these dividing pre-equatorial cells that are susceptible to the effects of ionizing radiation. Since the number of mitotic cells decreases with age, the lenses of adults are somewhat less susceptible to radiation than those of infants and children.

Strictly, any opacity in the normally transparent crystalline lens constitutes a cataract. The earliest changes are detectable only on slit-lamp examination, at a time when the patient is still asymptomatic. As a cataract progresses, it may cause visual disturbances, including glare secondary to light scattering, image blur, and eventually blindness. If vision in the opposite eye is normal, some patients are not aware of the presence of a unilateral cataract, even though vision in the affected eye may be severely impaired.

RADIATION CATARACTS

The morphology of radiation cataracts has been well described.[67] The initial change is vacuole formation in the equatorial region, secondary to injury to the dividing epithelial cells.[63] These opacities (composed of degenerate fibers and cell debris) slowly migrate posteriorly to the posterior subcapsular zone. Ophthalmoscopically, the opacity initially appears as a dot at the posterior pole of the lens, then gradually enlarges to 1 mm to 2 mm. Scattered granules and vacuoles may be seen around the central opacity. With further enlargement, the opacity develops a clear center so that it assumes a doughnut shape. At about the same time, granular opacities appear in the anterior subcapsular zone. Depending on the radiation dose and its fractionation, the cataract may remain stationary at any stage of development and produce little or no visual impairment; conversely, it may become a nonspecific mature cataract, indistinguishable from other types of cataract, resulting in complete blindness.

The time to onset of clinically detectable lenticular opacities is inversely related to dose. Fractionation lengthens the latent period. Following low-dose irradiation, the latent period may be many years, while very intense exposures may result in a progressive cataract within 6 months. Several University of Florida patients have not developed cataracts until 3 to 3½ years after 4000 rad to 7000 rad to the lens with external-beam irradiation.

TIME–DOSE ANALYSIS FOR CATARACT FORMATION

The largest body of clinical data relating cataract formation to dose comes from Merriam and Focht.[67] In 1957, they published data on 173 patients from the Memorial Center and the Radiotherapy Department of the Institute of Ophthalmology, Columbia Presbyterian Medical Center, New York City. Patients were treated for a wide variety of benign and malignant conditions by a variety of techniques, including low-dose-rate continuous irradiation from gold seeds or radium plaques; orthovoltage external-beam irradiation alone was used in only 16 adult patients.

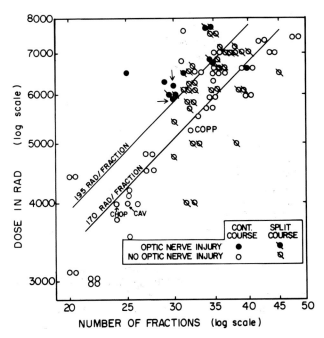

FIG. 14-18. Dose versus number of fractions for optic nerve injury secondary to irradiation. Included are data on 92 optic nerves in 55 patients following continuous or split-course irradiation (cobalt-60 or 2 MeV) of a variety of head and neck tumors at the University of Florida (10/64–3/79). All patients had a minimum of 3 years follow-up and the maximum is 14 years; patients who died within 3 years without developing optic nerve injury are excluded. Eyes that lost sight due to severe retinal injury are also excluded. There is mean follow-up of 6.35 years and a median follow-up of 6.5 years for the 80 optic nerves that showed no clinical evidence of injury following irradiation. Eight of 12 injuries were detected by 3 years. Reference lines for treatments administered at 170 rad/fraction and 195 rad/fraction have been added for convenience of interpreting the data; these lines are not isoeffect lines. Two optic nerves (*arrows*) received an additional small dose from a radium implant (approximately 200 rad to the optic nerves) following external irradiation. Three patients who received concomitant chemotherapy are so designated. (Reprinted with permission from Parsons JT, Fitzgerald CR, Hood CI, Ellingwood KE, Bova FJ, Million RR: The effects of irradiation on the eye and optic nerve. Int J Radiat Oncol Biol Phys 9:609–622, 1983. Copyright © 1983, Pergamon Press, Ltd.)

Treatments were reconstructed as accurately as possible on a phantom skull, and dose measurements were made at the lens with a small ionization chamber. Irrespective of the degree of fractionation, all patients who received at least 1150 R to the lens developed some degree of cataract; above 1450 R, all the cataracts were progressive. The work of Merriam and Focht is in general agreement with that of Cogan and Dreisler, who noted radiation cataracts in three of five adult patients whose lenses had received 600 R to 1000 R fractionated external-beam orthovoltage irradiation for orbital or conjunctival lymphomas; the two cataract-free patients had been followed for only 2½ and 3 years, respectively, so were still at risk.[12] Other investigators suggest that somewhat higher doses may be given without producing clinically significant cataracts.[4,79] The University of Florida data do not readily lend themselves to a time–dose analysis of radiation cataractogenesis, since all patients who received high doses developed cataracts while those who received low doses had their lenses protected by eye shields or corneal cylinders, making dose determination impossible.

MANAGEMENT OF RADIATION CATARACTS

Some radiation cataracts produce few or no symptoms and require no treatment. Even if a cataract impairs vision, it may not require removal if the patient has good vision in the other eye. If cataract extraction is performed, visual rehabilitation may be more difficult than in unirradiated patients. It is not possible to use spectacles with an aphakic lens over only one eye, since the thick aphakic lens will produce a 30% to 35% magnification of objects in the field of view, with resultant image size discrepancy and diplopia. Although a contact lens largely avoids the problems of image magnification and image size diplopia, it is not likely to be well tolerated if the eye is dry from prior irradiation (i.e., if the dose to the whole eye and lacrimal apparatus was greater than 4000 rad) (see Fig. 14-11). If the patient will not be able to wear a contact lens after extraction, he will generally function better if the cataract is not removed (assuming that he has good vision in the contralateral eye). If cataract extraction becomes necessary because of severe glare or another problem, surgery can usually be accomplished without a greatly increased risk of operative complications. One should always evaluate retinal function with bright flash electroretinography and transscleral visual evoked response prior to cataract extraction, since there will be little or no improvement after extraction if radiation retinopathy is also present. Probably, if the retinal dose was greater than 5500 rad, extraction is pointless in terms of restoration of vision. In two recent patients, cataract extractions were performed about 2 years after retinal doses of approximately 7000 rad; although the prospects of maintaining useful vision are essentially zero in these patients, it is hoped that the extractions will allow the ophthalmologist to closely observe the retina and apply the laser as necessary should neovascularization occur.

The University of Florida has had limited experience (three patients) with intraocular lens implantation in heavily irradiated eyes; the procedure is generally not recommended, since the operation requires greater intraocular manipulation than routine extraction, with an increased risk of complications. The implants were performed at 2, 2½, and 4 years after 5100, 3500, and 6000 rad, respectively, to the entire eye; in all three patients, the major lacrimal gland had been shielded. The first patient required reoperation to replace a dislocated lens. Postoperatively, she developed uveitis and severe corneal edema, leading to aphakic bullous keratopathy with severe pain and irritation; a conjunctival flap was required to relieve pain from the keratopathy, and all useful vision was lost. Visual acuity in the second patient returned to 20/15, and there were no operative complications. The third patient never achieved better than 20/200 visual acuity in the operated eye and also suffered from keratopathy in the postoperative period.

THE ORBIT

Ten University of Florida patients who received high-dose irradiation to the eye underwent evisceration or enucleation to relieve pain caused by neovascular glaucoma and/ or corneal complications. In three patients, a glass or silicone orbital implant was sutured in place in an attempt to take up the orbital dead space and thereby improve cosmesis. In all three patients, the implants were spontaneously extruded 1 to 5 months postoperatively because of progressive fibrosis and contraction of the orbital soft tissues. Several patients were fitted with ocular prostheses but were often dissatisfied with them since they were frequently irritating or would "pop out" when the patient blinked or sneezed. Most patients prefer to wear a patch full time and wear the prosthesis for only a few hours each day.

The Ear

SEROUS OTITIS MEDIA

Serous otitis media is a frequent complication of irradiation of cancers of the paranasal sinuses and nasopharynx, occurring in at least 15% to 20% of patients. Patients with nasopharyngeal cancer often present with otitis because of obstruction of the eustachian tube by tumor. When tubal patency is compromised, oxygen in the middle ear is absorbed by the blood vessels of the mucous membrane, resulting in a relative negative pressure; the tympanic membrane becomes retracted and an effusion results. Patients whose tumors involve the eustachian tube are at greater risk of developing posttreatment otitis than patients with normal ears, which suggests that fibrosis of previously damaged tissue may be contributory. However, one or both ears may develop otitis even when uninvolved by tumor.

Usually otitis is transient and results from desquamated cells and debris and edema of the mucous membrane lining the eustachian tube. Patients complain of a stuffy feeling in their ear and conductive hearing loss. Some cases resolve when oral decongestants are administered, but others require myringotomy, usually within the first year after treatment. It is rarely necessary to perform myringotomy during a course of irradiation, except in the unusual circumstance when the patient has pain. Bacterial infection rarely supervenes.

SENSORINEURAL HEARING LOSS

Sensorineural hearing loss is a rarely reported complication of ear irradiation; its incidence is unknown, but it may be more common than generally thought. Of 137 patients who underwent nasopharyngeal irradiation at the Massachusetts General Hospital between 1961 and 1969, 7 of 13 patients who had pretreatment and posttreatment audiometric evaluation were noted to have developed sensorineural hearing loss.[70] Since there was a selection factor (i.e., those patients evaluated were the ones who were having problems), the incidence of injury could not be established. Hearing losses ranged from 10 dB to almost total deafness; the most profound losses occurred after very high-dose treatment (greater than 20,000 rad). Small sensorineural hearing losses were noted during the first few years, but the onset of severe losses was gradual and occurred 3 to 6 years after treatment. Small losses had flat audiometric patterns, while the more profound losses were most severe in the high-frequency range. The risk may be greater in older patients.[61,70]

There are few reports of histologic studies of irradiated temporal bone. In a patient autopsied at 1 year posttreatment, Leach noted absence of the organ of Corti and atrophy of the spiral ganglion and cochlear nerve. Schuknecht and Karmody described a patient who suffered temporal bone radionecrosis 8 years after irradiation; autopsy at 12 years showed atrophy of the organ of Corti, loss of some hair cells, atrophy of the basilar membrane, and loss of some of the cells of the spiral ganglion.[88]

VESTIBULAR DISORDERS

Little is known about the effects of conventional fractionated radiation on vestibular function. Leach described several patients who complained of vertigo in the postirradiation period, some of whom had abnormal results of ice-water caloric tests.[61] In one patient, 1 year after treatment, absence of the macula (of the utricle) and cristae (of the semicircular canals), the structures whose hair cells transmit sensory information by way of the vestibular nerve to the central nervous system, was noted at autopsy. Vestibular dysfunction has not been reported by any patient receiving incidental irradiation of the semicircular canals at the University of Florida.

The Spinal Cord

LHERMITTE'S SYNDROME

A transient radiation myelopathy, manifested by Lhermitte's or the "barber chair" sign, is a fairly frequent occurrence in patients whose spinal cords are incidentally irradiated. The syndrome consists of a momentary, but very disturbing, electriclike shock that is triggered by flexion of the cervical spine. The sensation may be limited to the spine, but more commonly it radiates into the extremities, particularly the backs of the thighs. The distribution of the sensation does not correspond with the finite territory of any dermatome. The distribution is usually symmetrical and equal on both sides of the body. Symptoms usually appear 1 to 3 months following completion of irradiation and last from 1 to as long as 8 to 9 months, with an average duration of 3 to 4 months. The symptoms usually subside gradually. The syndrome produces no symptoms of muscle weakness or sphincter disturbance, and there are no accompanying neurologic signs. The character, latency period, and duration of symptoms in this radiation syndrome are identical to those that have been described following traumatic injury to the neck.

Lhermitte's syndrome is an early-appearing, benign form of myelopathy and should be distinguished from later-occurring, progressive radiation myelopathy. Lhermitte's syndrome rarely leads to progressive cord degeneration and transverse myelopathy. When the syndrome arises fairly soon after completion of irradiation, healing almost always occurs without permanent damage. However, when the syndrome appears late (9 to 12 months), radiation myelitis may follow.[50]

Damage to the posterior columns is though to be a prerequisite for Lhermitte's syndrome.[6] Jones attributes the transient myelopathy to temporary demyelination.[50] I am unaware of autopsy data that prove or disprove this concept. The minimum dose of radiation that will produce Lhermitte's syndrome has not been clearly identified, but a spinal cord dose as low as 3000 rad/25 fractions/7 weeks by split-course irradiation to the Hodgkin's mantle field, with both fields treated daily, may produce mild symptoms.

The syndrome is self-limited, reversible, and generally requires no specific therapy. In two patients who were extremely symptomatic, a cervical collar was used for several months until symptoms resolved. Patients should be warned about the syndrome so as to avoid unnecessary alarm should symptoms occur.

TRANSVERSE MYELITIS

Radiation-induced transverse myelitis is a rare complication of brain stem and spinal cord irradiation. The process is almost always irreversible and no effective therapy is known. Symptoms and signs of partial or complete transection of the cord usually appear 6 months to 2 years after irradiation. Typically, patients first develop paresthesias, followed by steadily progressive sensorimotor disturbances, bowel and bladder dysfunction, and paraplegia. Symptoms progress at a variable rate. Complete transverse myelitis at the level of the upper cervical cord or brain stem results in death, usually secondary to bronchopneumonia. A number of reported patients with myelopathy developed the Brown-Séquard syndrome, with loss of voluntary movements and Babinski's sign on one side and loss of pain and temperature sensations on the opposite side. Since the differential diagnosis of cord injury includes extramedullary compressive lesions (which are considerably more common than radiation-induced transverse myelopathy), myelography should be performed. Cervical spine films rule out cord injury secondary to severe bony changes.

The white matter seems more susceptible to radiation injury than the gray matter. A notable manifestation of myelopathy is demyelination, which may be due to injury to the oligodendrogliocyte (the myelin-forming cell of the central nervous system), obliterative changes in small blood vessels, or both.

With conventional fractionation at 180 rad to 200 rad/day, 5 fractions/week, the risk of a cord lesion at 5000 rad total dose is nearly zero if only a short segment of the upper cord is irradiated. The longer is the length of cord irradiated, the greater is the likelihood of myelitis. Those centers that extend the lateral portals to cover the entire neck irradiate long lengths of cord and increase the risk of damage. The risk of myelitis after 6000 rad/7 weeks is probably around 5%. Many of the myelitis cases reported in the literature were the result of technical errors in patient positioning and field arrangement[56] or of unconventional fractionation schemes.[1,83] Fractionation has a great sparing effect on the spinal cord. The daily dose should probably not exceed 170 rad if doses in the 6000-rad range must be delivered to the cord. The effect of overall treatment time is less important than that of fraction size;[47] split-course schemes probably do not significantly reduce the risk of injury.[100] Lhermitte's syndrome has been observed in about 15% of patients treated twice a day to 4600-rad cord dose at the University of Florida; myelitis has not been observed in 22 University of Florida patients at risk for 2 years nor in those patients reported by Horiot.*

The Brain

TRANSITORY CENTRAL NERVOUS SYSTEM SYNDROME

Following irradiation of advanced tumors of the ethmoid/sphenoid sinuses or nasopharynx, about 10% of patients develop a clinically recognizable syndrome characterized

---

* Horiot JC: Personal communication, May 1982.

by lethargy, nausea, occasional vomiting, headache, and dizziness; rarely, transient cranial nerve palsies or ataxia develop. The syndrome typically appears 2 to 3 months after treatment, lasts 2 to 4 weeks, then disappears spontaneously. Patients should be forewarned of this alarming problem, since it appears about the time that they are beginning to recover from the acute effects of radiation.

The syndrome is believed to result from transient demyelination, secondary to incidental brain irradiation. The latent period corresponds to the turnover time for myelin; it is speculated that the syndrome is similar in etiology to Lhermitte's syndrome of the spinal cord.[60,91] With the irradiation technique used for tumors of the nasal cavity and ethmoid/sphenoid sinuses, the given dose (at Dmax) to the anterior portal is high, frequently on the order of 7000 rad. A substantial volume of brain is incidentally irradiated. In the treatment of advanced nasopharyngeal cancers, portions of the base of the brain, particularly the temporal lobes, may receive very high doses; the antral fields add lesser doses to other areas of the brain.

The differential diagnosis is usually recurrent tumor versus delayed transient central nervous system syndrome. The symptoms and signs of both may be similar. The time course for the central nervous system syndrome is fairly characteristic and helps one arrive at the correct diagnosis. Although usually no specific therapy is required, corticosteroids have been reported to relieve signs and symptoms in severe cases.[29,91]

BRAIN NECROSIS

Brain necrosis is a rare complication of irradiation. Most reported cases have followed treatment with large daily fractions or multiple courses of therapy. There have been only about 25 reported cases following single courses of irradiation to doses less than 7250 rad to 7500 rad at 200 rad/fraction.[91] Nevertheless, the fact that there has been a handful of well-documented cases following 5000 rad to 6000 rad, at 170 rad to 200 rad/day, means that there is some risk of its occurrence following radical treatment of cancers of the temporal bone, nasopharynx, paranasal sinuses, or advanced skin lesions on the scalp. The incidence of the complication is difficult to determine because literature reports are anecdotal.

Symptoms and signs depend on the site of necrosis. The injury tends to be most severe in white matter. Pathologic changes include obliteration of small blood vessels, demyelination, loss of oligodendrogliocytes, and coagulation necrosis.

The Ellis formula underestimates the importance of fraction size on the production of central nervous system injury; furthermore, the formula does not take into account the volume of tissue irradiated. When treating large volumes of the central nervous system to high doses, 180 rad/day is rarely exceeded.

There is no specific therapy for radiation-induced brain necrosis. Some necrotic foci act like mass lesions; resection of necrotic tissue may be lifesaving in this circumstance. Corticosteroids may relieve surrounding cerebral edema.[29] The differential diagnosis includes recurrent cancer or other central nervous system disease that produces a similar clinical picture.

Cranial and Peripheral Nerves

The cranial and peripheral nerves are seldom regarded as major dose-limiting tissues in treatment planning. Injury is uncommon, even after high-dose therapy. This is in contrast to the brain stem and spinal cord, which are frequently the major dose-limiting tissues within a treatment volume. High-dose treatment to the latter structures may cause major morbidity. The reason for these differing susceptibilities to injury is unknown.

The most frequent cranial nerve deficit that follows high-dose treatment of cancers of the nasopharynx, tonsillar fossa, and base of the tongue is palsy of the hypoglossal nerve. Palsy is most likely when tumor lies near the nerve or when necrosis develops in the glossotonsillar sulcus area. The commonly postulated mechanism of injury is entrapment of the nerve by posttreatment fibrosis; proof of this concept by autopsy or surgical pathologic studies is, however, lacking, and it is possible that the damage is due to direct nerve injury. Most such injuries appear 3 or more years after treatment; time to onset is inversely related to dose.[3] Often the patient is unaware of a deficit of the hypoglossal nerve. Speech is usually not greatly affected except in the rare circumstance of bilateral palsy.

Soft tissue necrosis in the glossotonsillar sulcus may lead to an early-appearing hypoglossal nerve deficit, as observed in two patients with cancer of the base of the tongue at the University of Florida. Necroses occurred at 5 and 7 months and were followed within 1 month by hypoglossal nerve palsy in both patients; although the necroses spontaneously healed, the nerve deficits persisted. The patients died without evidence of tumor recurrence at 6½ and 8 years, respectively.

Any of the nerves in the parapharyngeal space may be affected, with the vagus and the spinal accessory being next in frequency after the hypoglossal. All three nerves may be involved in the same patient. Recurrent tumor may produce a similar syndrome, and the differential diagnosis may be difficult; both the timing of the deficit and the absence of other symptoms of tumor recurrence help establish the diagnosis. Although the facial nerve rather routinely receives 7000 rad to 8000 rad, injury to this nerve has not been observed at the University of Florida; nor has injury to the olfactory, oculomotor, trochlear, or trigeminal nerves been observed in the University of Florida series. One patient developed an abducens nerve palsy 10 years after high-dose treatment of an advanced nasopharyngeal carcinoma. There is no reason to believe that any of the cranial nerves could not be affected.

Five of 118 patients treated for T1–T2 cancers of the glottic larynx who had normal pretreatment cord mobility and no evidence of tumor recurrence, developed ipsilateral cord palsies in the posttreatment period. All were treated by a single ipsilateral portal that delivered a very high dose to the normal tissues lateral to the cancer. The palsies, which were possibly due to injury to the recurrent laryngeal nerve, occurred at 7, 8, 9, 42, and 42 months; complete cord fixation, without evidence of tumor recurrence or significant edema, was noted in all cases. Mobility returned after a few weeks to a few months in the three cords that became immobile at 7, 8, and 9 months; the other two cords never regained mobility. All five patients have been followed for 8 to 12½ years without developing cancer recurrence.

The brachial plexus is included within the treatment volume when the lower neck is irradiated. Brachial plexus neuropathy is exceedingly rare following standardly fractionated therapy and has been observed at the University of Florida in only one head and neck cancer patient, who underwent a second course of irradiation for a late supraclavicular nodal failure. The total dose was greater than

13,000 rad. The patient developed marked fibrosis in the supraclavicular fossa with limitation of shoulder and neck motion, painless motor and sensory deficits in the affected arm, diminished brachial and radial pulses, and ipsilateral phrenic nerve palsy, with elevation of the hemidiaphragm.

Most reported cases of radiation-induced brachial plexus neuropathy developed 6 to 24 months following postoperative irradiation of women with breast cancer. Such injuries are quite rare following treatment at less than or equal to 200 rad/day. In the largest reported series, Stoll and Andrews reported on 117 postoperatively irradiated patients who received nonstandard fractionation (480 rad to 525 rad three times weekly to 5775 rad to 6300 rad total dose); 32% of their patients developed neurologic symptoms attributable to brachial plexus neuropathy.[97] The most common symptom was paresthesia; hypesthesia and hand weakness were also common. Examination usually revealed mixed sensory, motor, and reflex changes. This is merely another example of the danger of treatment with large fractions to high doses.

The Anterior Lobe of the Pituitary Gland

The pituitary and hypothalamus are incidentally irradiated during treatment of tumors of the paranasal sinuses and nasopharynx. Pituitary dysfunction following irradiation was, for many years, regarded as a rather rare phenomenon. In 1966, Tan and Kunaratnam reported an unusual case of pituitary dwarfism in a young woman who had received two courses of irradiation (total dose greater than 9000 rad) for a T4N3 squamous cell carcinoma of the nasopharynx at age 12.[98] The patient stopped growing almost immediately, compared with her two sisters; she developed amenorrhea, hoarseness, and became intolerant of cold weather. Examination 11 years after treatment revealed no evidence of tumor recurrence, but a number of abnormalities were present. The genitalia were small, the breasts were underdeveloped, and pubic and axillary hair was completely absent. Her height was 4 feet, 6 inches. There was no evidence of diabetes insipidus. This is the first well-documented case of hypopituitarism secondary to irradiation of an extracranial neoplasm.

Most of the early observations on pituitary function after irradiation relied on the detection of gross clinical abnormalities.[26] Lederman, in reviewing the treatment results in 241 patients with nasopharyngeal cancer treated by irradiation at the Royal Marsden Hospital between 1933 and 1958, found no evidence of pituitary dysfunction in any patient.[62] There also was no suggestion of pituitary dysfunction among 830 nasopharynx patients irradiated in Singapore between 1954 and 1962.[98] With the advent of sophisticated testing (e.g., determination of hormone levels by radioimmunoassay and tests employing synthetic hypothalamic hormones) that was unavailable to early investigators, pituitary dysfunction following irradiation has been shown to be more common than appreciated in the past. Its exact incidence is still unknown, since many of the patients who have been evaluated were selected for study because of some clinical abnormality such as short stature. The pituitary of the child may be more sensitive than that of the adult.[37]

The most extensive data on the effects of irradiation on pituitary and hypothalamic function come from the M. D. Anderson Hospital, where Samaan and colleagues studied 110 patients with tumors of the nasopharynx or paranasal sinuses 1 to 26 years following radiation therapy.[86] None of the patients had roentgenographic evidence of tumor invading the pituitary fossa, and all were free of disease at the primary site. Seventy-six patients showed one or more features suggestive of hypothalamic lesions, and 43 had evidence of primary pituitary deficiency. The percentage of patients with clinical and biochemical abnormalities increased as a function of time up to 10 years after treatment.

GROWTH HORMONE

It has been suggested that growth hormone may be the hormone most frequently affected by hypothalamic-pituitary irradiation.[37,103] Its secretion is episodic, and its serum concentration is affected by sleep, eating, stress, exercise, and various other stimuli. Demonstration of a low serum level is not sufficient to make a diagnosis of growth hormone deficiency; one must demonstrate inability of the pituitary to respond to one of various stimuli, including insulin-induced hypoglycemia, L-dopa, or arginine. Samaan and colleagues detected subnormal serum growth hormone levels during insulin-induced hypoglycemia in 56 M. D. Anderson Hospital patients; 21 prepubertal patients showed growth failure and delayed bone age.[86] At the University of California, San Francisco, 9 patients who had received incidental pituitary irradiation (3850 rad to 5700 rad) during childhood were referred for evaluation of growth retardation.[103] All nine demonstrated growth hormone deficiency after provocative stimulation testing; the intervals between irradiation and evaluation ranged from 1 to 7½ years.

Establishing the diagnosis of growth hormone deficiency in an adult is of academic interest only since the hormone need not be replaced. In children, growth hormone deficiency results in retardation of growth and bone age; the deficiency is correctable with intramuscular injections of human growth hormone, which should be continued throughout puberty. Annual assessment of function should be routine following pituitary irradiation in children.

CORTICOTROPIN

The seemingly obvious way to detect corticotropin (ACTH) deficiency would be to measure its plasma concentration; however, such a determination is not useful since the levels fluctuate markedly throughout the day and night. Even normal patients may have ACTH levels that are below the level of detectability of the assay. Likewise, single determinations of plasma cortisol are of little help; although the cortisol level may be low, it is frequently in the normal range even in patients with pituitary insufficiency.[52] Detection of ACTH deficiency requires stimulation testing with metapyrone (followed by measurement of plasma ACTH, 11-deoxycortisol, and/or 24-hour urinary 17-hydroxycorticosteroid levels) or insulin (measuring ACTH or cortisol levels).

Thirty of the M. D. Anderson Hospital patients showed a subnormal rise of plasma cortisol during insulin hypoglycemia. Twenty-two of these patients complained of general weakness and extreme fatigue, and 8 others showed signs of severe cortisol deficiency as evidenced by epigastric pain, diarrhea, hypotension, and drowsiness, which responded promptly to cortisol administration.[86] The basal levels of cortisol are usually normal in such patients. Wara and co-workers found a subnormal cortisol response to insulin hypoglycemia in 1 of 7 patients who received pituitary irradiation in childhood.[103]

While detection of Addisonian crisis is usually not a great diagnostic dilemma, early detection of corticotropin deficiency may be quite difficult, unless one keeps the possibility of its occurrence in mind. Complete correction of the metabolic derangement is readily achieved with replacement therapy by mouth with a glucocorticoid hormone. Mineralocorticoid hormone therapy is rarely necessary.

GONADOTROPINS

The anterior pituitary secretes two gonadotropins, follicle stimulating hormone (FSH) and luteinizing hormone (LH), which regulate the development, reproductive functions, and hormonal secretions of the testicle and ovary. The screening tests for gonadotropin insufficiency measure the products of the target organs: testosterone in the male, and estradiol in the female. Once it has been established that serum testosterone or plasma estradiol is low, gonadotropin levels are measured. If the gonadotropins are also low, the deficiency is due to a hypothalamic or pituitary problem. If one wishes to further establish the site of injury, this can be done by administering gonadotropin-releasing hormone: If the FSH and LH levels rise, the problem resides in the hypothalamus. If no rise occurs, the pituitary itself is implicated.

Thirty-three M. D. Anderson Hospital patients showed subnormal LH and FSH levels before and after administration of LH-releasing hormone, indicating a primary pituitary deficiency.[86] Signs and symptoms included amenorrhea, impotence, absence of pubic and axillary hair, and testicular atrophy; decreased libido may also occur.

Replacement therapy in the male consists of testosterone to improve libido and problems with impotence. Estrogen replacement in the premenopausal female may return menstrual function, improve secondary sexual characteristics such as skin texture and breast development, increase libido, and help prevent osteoporosis.[52] Because of associated risks of estrogen administration, the minimum effective dose should be used, and the patient should receive an annual pelvic examination. Infertile young women with potentially normal-functioning ovaries who desire pregnancy may be treated with gonadotropins; there is a high likelihood of multiple births following such therapy.[52] Similarly, the infertile male may be chronically treated with an LH–FSH combination.

THYROTROPIN

Hypothyroidism occasionally results from incidental irradiation to the thyroid gland (primary hypothyroidism) or pituitary (secondary hypothyroidism). Twenty-one M. D. Anderson Hospital patients had low thyroid function, and thyrotropin levels that were not elevated and failed to rise after administration of thyrotropin-releasing hormone (TRH), indicating pituitary deficiency.[86] Nine other patients with low thyroid function had low thyrotropin levels that showed a delayed rise after TRH administration, suggesting a hypothalamic problem. If there had been primary hypothyroidism, one would have expected high thyrotropin levels due to loss of the normal feedback mechanism. Symptoms and signs in these patients included cold intolerance, dry skin, constipation, and slow relaxation of tendon jerks. Hypothyroidism is readily controllable with replacement therapy.

PROLACTIN

Prolactin secretion from the anterior pituitary gland is under hypothalamic control with production of a prolactin-inhibiting factor. In the presence of a hypothalamic lesion, the basal serum prolactin level is elevated. Forty-three of the 100 M. D. Anderson Hospital patients showed hyperprolactinemia, presumably as a result of a hypothalamic lesion.[86] One 25-year-old woman developed amenorrhea-galactorrhea 2 years after radiation therapy for an esthesioneuroblastoma; anterior pituitary function and sella turcica tomograms were normal, indicating that the lesion was in the hypothalamus. Following administration of bromocriptine, which inhibits release of prolactin from the anterior pituitary gland, regular menses resumed and she had a normal pregnancy and delivery.

The Posterior Lobe of the Pituitary Gland

Diabetes insipidus has been reported after deliberate pituitary ablation by transsphenoidally implanted yttrium-90 pellets, which deliver tens of thousands of rad to the pituitary gland. I am not aware of this complication following standardly fractionated radiotherapy.

Thyroid Gland

Clinical hypothyroidism develops after lower neck irradiation in approximately 5% of adults and a somewhat higher proportion of children. Signs and symptoms may be classic but are often nonspecific, subtle, and readily attributable to other causes. The chemical detection of hypothyroidism can be made some weeks before clinical symptoms or signs develop. Onset of hypothyroidism may occur within weeks of the completion of treatment but more often occurs months or years later. Frequency of development appears to be dose- as well as volume-related;[38] it is worthwhile to shield the isthmus of the gland during lower neck irradiation if practical to do so. The addition of a hemithyroidectomy after irradiation increases the risk of subsequent hypothyroidism.[78]

The screening test is the serum thyroxine (T_4) level. Serum triiodothyronine (T_3) resin uptake is also usually measured in order to exclude abnormal binding of thyroxine to plasma proteins; patients with hypothyroidism have low or low-normal uptake. A high serum thyrotropin level confirms the diagnosis of primary hypothyroidism.

Glatstein and co-workers found a number of patients, most of whom had received incidental thyroid irradiation during therapy for lymphomas, who had elevated thyrotropin but normal T_4 levels.[38] This may indicate mild or developing hypothyroidism that has been compensated by increased thyrotropin secretion. In some patients, the thyrotropin levels are only transiently elevated and return to normal; other patients may remain euthyroid for long periods during which the serum thyrotropin level is persistently high, while still others develop frank hypothyroidism.

For the patient with hypothyroidism, the management is straightforward and consists of thyroid hormone replacement. Patients with compensated hypothyroidism (elevated thyrotropin, normal T_4 levels) present a management question since the long-term effects of this condition are unknown. As a minimum, such patients should have their thyrotropin and T_4 levels checked at regular intervals; some authors advocate replacement therapy. The possibility that thyroid neoplasia may be induced in such patients secondary to prolonged thyrotropin stimulation, as has been observed in some animals, has been mentioned.[37]

Parathyroid Glands and Parafollicular Cells

Serum calcium concentration is maintained in part by the interaction of parathormone (which is secreted by the parathyroid glands) and calcitonin (which is secreted by the parafollicular cells of the thyroid gland). I am unaware of disorders of calcium and phosphorus homeostasis secondary to irradiation of these structures. Detailed preirradiation and postirradiation chemical studies, which might detect subtle changes, are lacking.

The Lung

Following lower neck irradiation, fibrosis of the apical segments of the lungs is frequently seen on routine follow-up chest roentgenograms, beginning 6 to 12 months after treatment. Fibrosis of the apices is of little consequence and produces no dyspnea, since these areas of the lung are poorly perfused and ventilated.

Chronic Lymphatic Obstruction, Lymphedema, and Erysipelas

Irradiation or neck dissection may produce chronic obstructive lymphedema that predisposes the patient to erysipelas. Erysipelas follows large-field irradiation of nasopharynx cancer in approximately 10% of long-term survivors. It develops months or years after treatment. At the University of Florida this condition has been observed less commonly after treatment of other head and neck primary cancers, usually after combined radiation therapy and surgery. Similar infections occur in edematous extremities after axillary or inguinal lymphadenectomy; irradiation increases the risk. Some patients have repeated exacerbations of erysipelas. Group A β-hemolytic *Streptococcus* is usually considered the responsible organism, although cultures were not performed on patients at the University of Florida.

The onset of the skin infection is abrupt; a history of a preceding upper respiratory tract infection is sometimes obtained. Both irradiated and unirradiated skin may be affected. The skin is hot, bright red, tense, and slightly raised. There may be fever, chills, and, rarely, severe toxemia. The infection spreads rapidly behind a well-demarcated border. Appropriate antibiotics are started without delay and reverse the situation in short order.

For a detailed discussion of the acute and subacute effects of radiation on the lymphatics, see Chapter 4, General Principles for Treatment of Cancers in the Head and Neck: Selection of Treatment Modality.

Paranasal Sinuses

Following high-dose irradiation of cancers of the nasal cavity and ethmoid/sphenoid sinuses, 5 of 37 patients at the University of Florida had one or more episodes of purulent sinusitis, unassociated with tumor recurrence. One patient required nasal antrostomy at 16 months, after antibiotics failed to control infection. Another who had intermittent episodes of purulent sinusitis developed meningitis 4½ years after treatment. A third developed a 3-mm, asymptomatic fistula between the ethmoid sinus and anterior facial skin 7 years after treatment. A fourth underwent a negative Caldwell-Luc procedure to rule out recurrence 2 years after treatment, while the fifth was readily managed by antibiotics alone.

The patient typically presents with a purulent nasal discharge, headache, tenderness and pain over the sinus area, facial edema, conjunctival edema, and low-grade fever. The sinus does not transilluminate. Roentgenograms and CT scan show opacity. The differential diagnosis is recurrent cancer. Exploration may be required for diagnosis and drainage if response to antibiotics is incomplete.

When the sinuses are uninvolved by neoplasm, it is distinctly unusual for the patient to develop radiation-induced sinusitis.

Large Arteries

Radiation-induced carotid artery disease is generally regarded as a rare phenomenon and its incidence is unknown for the following reasons

1. There are very few case reports that have clinico-pathologic correlation.
2. Irradiation is delivered at an age when atherosclerotic disease of carotid arteries is common.
3. Most reported cases of radiation-induced injury have occurred after a latent interval of 5 to 10 years or more, making an extended period of followup mandatory in order to assess the risk.
4. Carotid narrowing may be clinically silent in the presence of good collateral flow.

Eldering and colleagues found a nonsignificant ($p = 0.39$) trend toward an increased risk of stroke in 910 patients who had received irradiation to at least one entire side of the neck and who survived for a minimum of 5 years following treatment of lymphoma or primary head and neck cancer.[31] There was no apparent correlation between dose and incidence of injury.

Histologic changes that have been described include intimal thickening with or without superimposed thrombus, fragmentation of the internal elastic membrane, atheroma formation, fibrosis of the media, and adventitial fibrosis. Atheromatous narrowing may involve portions of the great vessels not usually involved with atherosclerosis.[93]

Possible mechanisms of radiation injury to large arteries include direct large vessel damage; damage to small nutrient vessels (vasa vasorum); fibrosis of adjacent tissues, leading to arterial constriction; and acceleration of naturally occurring atherosclerosis.

Vascular reconstruction may be undertaken when indicated. Following moderate doses (4500 rad to 5500 rad) at Stanford University, carotid endarterectomy was technically more difficult than in unirradiated patients, but it was accomplished without increased morbidity or mortality.[93] Although one might suspect that higher doses would significantly increase the operative risk, several University of Florida patients have undergone endarterectomy in heavily irradiated necks without serious complications.

In one heavily irradiated patient (dose unknown), Levinson and co-workers at the University of California, San Francisco, performed bilateral carotid endarterectomies and successfully bypassed both common carotid arteries from the level of the clavicle to the bulb by means of saphenous vein grafts.[64] The only bypass reported by the Stanford group (after 12,000-rad skin dose) was unsuccessful due to clot formation.

Radiation-Induced Neoplasia Following Therapeutic Irradiation

The carcinogenic effect of ionizing radiation has long been recognized. The first case of a radiation-induced malignancy was reported in 1902 and was an epidermoid carcinoma on the hand of a radiation technician. Despite extensive use of therapeutic irradiation for head and neck cancers, induction of malignancy is, fortunately, quite rare. Most reported cases have been sarcomas, usually osteogenic sarcomas or fibrosarcomas of bone, less often soft tissue sarcomas.

The latent interval between irradiation and the development of cancer varies from several to many years. In order to qualify as a radiation-induced cancer, there must be histologic proof of a new cancer and the lesion must be within the prior field of irradiation. Three aspects of the problem of radiation-induced neoplasia will be briefly explored: (1) the risk of inducing new mucosal lesions, primarily squamous cell carcinomas, by therapeutic irradiation; (2) radiation-induced sarcomas; and (3) thyroid neoplasia.

RADIATION-INDUCED MUCOSAL CANCER

At the M. D. Anderson Hospital, Kögelnik, Fletcher, and Jesse reviewed the late clinical courses of a large number of patients who had received head and neck cancer therapy at their institution and who had lived for a minimum of 5 years following treatment without developing recurrence of cancer within that 5-year period.[59] The clinical occurrences subsequent to 5 years were recorded in 1163 patients

who had received curative therapy (surgery, irradiation, or combined treatment) for squamous cell carcinomas of the upper respiratory and digestive tracts; the follow-up intervals for these patients ranged from 7½ to 25½ years. The incidence of new cancers developing in the original disease site, the immediate vicinity of the original lesion, or sites remote from the primary lesion but still within the oral cavity and pharynx is shown in Table 14-4. In order to determine if irradiated patients had a greater incidence of new cancers than patients treated by surgery alone, the patients are grouped according to their treatment by surgery alone or by irradiation with or without an operation. The incidence of new mucosal cancers was not higher in the irradiation group within the study period. It was concluded that irradiation did not produce any new squamous cell carcinomas of the mucous membrane that had received either high- or modest-dose irradiation during treatment of the original lesion. Data from the Fox Chase Cancer Center, Philadelphia, on almost 2000 patients who were operated on or irradiated for cancers of the oral cavity or oropharynx showed a slightly higher incidence of new upper aerodigestive cancers in the surgery group.[89]

RADIATION-INDUCED SARCOMA

The rarity of radiation-induced sarcomas, the long latent period to their development, and the difficulty in obtaining reliable long-term follow-up data make the task of estimating the true risk of cancer induction difficult.[13] Most series report one or two cases of radiation-induced bone sarcoma per 1000 five-year survivors.[44,84,89,95] If one assumes malignant induction in 1 patient of every 500 long-term survivors, then with an estimated 5-year survival rate of 40% for all irradiated head and neck cancer patients, one case would be induced per 1250 patients treated. The younger the patient, the greater would be the risk of developing a new cancer since the at-risk period would be longer; whether children are generally more susceptible than adults to neoplastic induction, as is suspected by many authors, remains unproved but seems likely (see Chapter 33, Pediatric Tumors of the Head and Neck).

Data on second malignancies following radiation therapy of Hodgkin's disease have been compiled by investigators at Strong Memorial Hospital and five treatment centers in

TABLE 14-4. Incidence of New Head and Neck Cancers Developing 5 Years or More After Treatment of First Head and Neck Squamous Cell Carcioma

	Modality of Treatment of Original Lesion	
Location of New Lesion	Surgery (337 Patients)	Irradiation ± Operation (826 Patients)
Same site	6 (1.8%)	22 (2.7%)
Vicinity	14 (4.2%)	26 (3.1%)
Remote sites in oral cavity or pharynx	16 (4.7%)	47 (5.7%)

Note: M. D. Anderson Hospital data; patients treated 1/48–12/65; analysis 8/73

(Kögelnik HD, Fletcher GH, Jesse RH: Clinical course of patients with squamous cell carcinoma of the upper respiratory and digestive tracts with no evidence of disease 5 years after initial treatment. Radiology 115:423–427, 1975)

Italy; follow-up for the two series was 2 to 19 years and 2 to 10 years, respectively.[2,76] Information on these patients is of more than passing interest to the head and neck specialist, since doses used to treat Hodgkin's disease (3500 rad to 4500 rad) are similar to those used to treat juvenile angiofibromas and chemodectomas. Combining data from the two Hodgkin's disease series, only 1 of 225 patients developed a second cancer within a radiation field, and it is doubtful whether this tumor (a malignant melanoma) was related to radiation since it arose less than 1 year after treatment, an extremely short latent interval for a radiation-induced solid malignancy. Thus, the following can be concluded:

1. The risk of radiation-induced cancer following treatment of juvenile angiofibroma or chemodectoma is real;[20] several cases have been reported.[16,33,39,48]
2. The risk is low; none of the 47 angiofibroma patients irradiated at the Radiumhemmet who were followed for over 10 and up to 40 or more years developed a radiation-induced cancer,[49] nor were there any instances among 45 irradiated patients at Princess Margaret Hospital with 2 to 20 years of follow-up.[33,34]
3. The risk of malignant induction must be weighed against risks of operation; in many large surgical series in which an analysis of complications was undertaken, operative deaths have been reported.[11,16,42,75,104]

It is often conjectured that megavoltage irradiation, which produces equal absorption of energy on a gram-for-gram basis in bone and soft tissue, induces fewer bone sarcomas than orthovoltage irradiation, which has a high absorption in bone compared with soft tissue. This may be true, but it is probably premature to draw firm conclusions about the risk of malignant induction following supervoltage irradiation, since such equipment has been in use in most therapy departments for less than 30 years. The nature of the relationship between dose of radiation and the risk of sarcomatous transformation in bone is also controversial.[89,99]

Most authors concur that previously abnormal bone, such as that affected by fibrous dysplasia, is more prone to sarcomatous change than normal bone.[14,22,99] Whether the addition of chemotherapy to irradiation increases the risk is unknown; the fact that the only two cases of sarcoma following irradiation of nasal cavity/sinus cancer at Thomas Jefferson University developed in patients who had received concomitant chemotherapy is suggestive, but certainly inconclusive, of an increased risk from combined therapy.[14]

RADIATION-INDUCED THYROID CANCER

An association between radiation and thyroid neoplasia has long been recognized.[28] The latent period is usually 10 to 30 years. Almost all the reported cases have followed doses (<6 rad to 1500 rad) of radiation that are well below the levels delivered for squamous cell carcinomas (5000 rad to 7000 rad). Doses above 2000 rad are associated with a very low risk of induction of thyroid neoplasia compared with lower doses of radiation. This is probably because higher doses either completely destroy the follicular cells or, at least, render the surviving cells incapable of division. Such a situation is seen following iodine-131 therapy for hyperthyroidism; many patients become hypothyroid but very few develop thyroid cancer.

REFERENCES

1. Abbatucci JS, Delozier T, Quint R, Roussel A, Brune D: Radiation myelopathy of the cervical spinal cord: Time, dose, and volume factors. Int J Radiat Oncol Biol Phys 4:239–248, 1978
2. Baccarani M, Bosi A, Papa G: Second malignancy in patients treated for Hodgkin's disease. Cancer 46:1735–1740, 1980
3. Berger PS, Bataini JP: Radiation-induced cranial nerve palsy. Cancer 40:152–155, 1977
4. Britten MJ, Halnan KE, Meredith WJ: Radiation cataract: New evidence on radiation dosage to the lens. Br J Radiol 39:612–617, 1966
5. Brown LR, Dreizen S, Handler S, Johnston DA: Effect of radiation-induced xerostomia on human oral microflora. J Dent Res 54:740–750, 1975
6. Butler WM, Taylor HG, Diehl LF: Lhermitte's sign in cobalamin (vitamin B12) deficiency. JAMA 245:1059, 1981
7. Chahbazian CM, Del Regato JA; Cobalt-60 teletherapy of early carcinoma of the vocal cords. Am J Roentgenol Radium Ther Nucl Med 99:333–335, 1967
8. Chan RC, Shukovsky LJ: Effects of irradiation on the eye. Radiology 120:673–675, 1976
9. Chaudhuri RP, Austin DJ, Rosenthal AR: Treatment of radiation retinopathy. Br J Ophthalmol 64:623–625, 1981
10. Cheng VST, Downs J, Herbert D, Aramany M: The function of the parotid gland following radiation therapy for head and neck cancer. Int J Radiat Oncol Biol Phys 7:253–258, 1981
11. Christiansen TA, Duvall AJ III, Rosenberg Z, Carley RB: Juvenile nasopharyngeal angiofibroma. Trans Am Acad Ophthalmol Otolaryngol 78(ORL):140–147, 1974
12. Cogan DG, Dreisler KK: Minimal amount of x-ray exposure causing lens opacities in the human eye. Arch Ophthalmol 50;30–34, 1953
13. Coleman CN: Adverse effects of cancer therapy. Am J Pediatr 4:103–111, 1982
14. Coia LR, Fazekas JT, Kramer S: Postirradiation sarcoma of the head and neck: A report of three late sarcomas following therapeutic irradiation for primary malignancies of the paranasal sinus, nasal cavity, and larynx. Cancer 46:1982–1985, 1980
15. Conger AD: Loss and recovery of taste acuity in patients irradiated to the oral cavity. Radiat Res 53:338–347, 1973
16. Conley J, Healey WV, Blaugrund SM, Perzin KH: Nasopharyngeal angiofibroma in the juvenile. Surg Gynecol Obstet 126:825–837, 1968
17. Coutard H: Roentgen therapy of epitheliomas of the tonsillar region, hypopharynx, and larynx from 1920–1926. Am J Roentgenol Radium Ther 28:313–331, 1932
18. Coutard H: Principles of x-ray therapy of malignant diseases. Lancet 227:1–8, 1934
19. Coutard H: X-ray treatment of inoperable carcinoma of the larynx. Surg Gynecol Obstet 68:467–471, 1939
20. Cummings BJ: Relative risk factors in the treatment of juvenile nasopharyngeal angiofibroma. Head Neck Surg 3:21–26, 1980
21. Davis JC, Dunn JM, Gates GA, Heimbach RD: Hyperbaric oxygen: A new adjunct in the management of radiation necrosis. Arch Otolaryngol 105:58–61, 1979
22. DeLathouwer C, Brocheriou C: Sarcoma arising in irradiated jawbones: Possible relationship with previous nonmalignant bone lesions. J Maxillofac Surg 4:8–20, 1976
23. Delclos L, Johnson GC: Palliative irradiation in breast cancer: The place of radiotherapy in the palliation of local recurrences and distant metastases. Radiology 83:272–276, 1964
24. Del Regato JA; Dental lesions observed after roentgen therapy in cancer of the buccal cavity, pharynx, and larynx. Am J Roentgenol Radium Ther 42:404–410, 1939
25. Del Regato JA, Vuksanovic M: Radiotherapy of carcinomas of the skin overlying the cartilages of the nose and ear. Radiology 79:203–208, 1962

26. DeSchryver A, Ljunggren JG, Båryd: Pituitary function in longterm survival after radiation therapy of nasopharyngeal tumors. Acta Radiol (Ther) 12:497–508, 1973

27. Dreizen S, Brown LR, Handler, S, Levy BM: Radiation-induced xerostomia in cancer patients: Effect on salivary and serum electrolytes. Cancer 38:273–278, 1976

28. Duffy BJ, Fitzgerald PJ: Thyroid cancer in childhood and adolescence: A report on 28 cases. Cancer 3:1018–1032, 1950

29. Edwards MS, Wilson CB: Treatment of radiation necrosis. In Gilbert HA, Kagan AR (eds): Radiation Damage to the Nervous System: A Delayed Therapeutic Hazard, pp 129–144. New York, Raven Press, 1980

30. Egbert PR, Fajardo LF, Donaldson SS, Moazed K: Posterior ocular abnormalities after irradiation for retinoblastoma: A histopathological study. Br J Ophthalmol 64:660–665, 1980

31. Eldering SC, Fernandez RN, Grotta JC, Lindberg RD, Causay LC, McMurtrey MJ: Carotid artery disease following external cervical irradiation. Ann Surg 194:609–615, 1981

32. Enfors B: The parotid and submandibular secretion in man: Quantitative recordings of the normal and pathological activity, 67 pages. Acta Otolaryngol [Suppl] (Stockh) 172, 1962

33. Fitzpatrick PJ, Briant DR, Berman JM: The nasopharyngeal angiofibroma. Arch Otolaryngol 106:234–236, 1980

34. Fitzpatrick PJ: The nasopharyngeal angiofibroma. Can J Surg 13:228–235, 1970

35. Fletcher GH, Barkley HT, Shukovsky LJ: Present status of the time factor in clinical radiotherapy: II. The nominal standard dose formula. J Radiol Electrol 55:745–751, 1974

36. Frank RM, Herdly J, Philippe E: Acquired dental defects and salivary gland lesions after irradiation for carcinoma. J Am Dent Assoc 70:868–883, 1965

37. Fuks Z, Glatstein E, Marsa GW, Bagshaw MA, Kaplan HS: Longterm effects of external radiation on the pituitary and thyroid glands. Cancer 37:1152–1161, 1976

38. Glatstein E, McHardy-Young S, Brast N, Eltringham JR, Kriss JP: Alterations in serum thyrotropin (TSH) and thyroid function following radiotherapy in patients with malignant lymphoma. J Clin Endocrinol Metab 32:833–841, 1971

39. Gisselsson L, Lindgren M, Stenram U: Sarcomatous transformation of a juvenile nasopharyngeal angiofibroma. Acta Pathol Microbiol Scand 42:305–312, 1958

40. Griffin JD, Garnick MD: Eye toxicity of cancer chemotherapy: A review of the literature. Cancer 48:1539–1549, 1981

41. Guyton AC: Textbook of Medical Physiology, 4th ed, p 641. Philadelphia, WB Saunders, 1971

42. Härma RA: Nasopharyngeal angiofibroma: A clinical and histopathological study, 74 pages. Acta Otolaryngol [Suppl] (Stockh) 146, 1958

43. Harwood AR, Hawkins NV, Rider WD, Bryce DP: Radiotherapy of early glottic cancer: I. Int J Radiat Oncol Biol Phys 5:473–476, 1979

44. Hatfield PM, Schulz MD: Postirradiation sarcoma: Including 5 cases after x-ray therapy of breast carcinoma. Radiology 96:593–602, 1970

45. Hayreh SS: Post-radiation retinopathy: A fluorescence fundus angiographic study. Br J Ophthalmol 54:705–714, 1970

46. Hoppe RT, Goffinet DR, Bagshaw MA: Carcinoma of the nasopharynx: Eighteen years' experience with megavoltage radiation therapy. Cancer 37:2605–2612, 1976

47. Hornsy S, White A: Isoeffect curve for radiation myelopathy. Br J Radiol 53:168–169, 1980

48. Hudson WR: Discussion (pp 17–18) following Sessions RB, Wills PI, Alford BR, Harrell JE, Evans RA: Juvenile nasopharyngeal angiofibroma: Radiographic aspects. Laryngoscope 86:2–18, 1976

49. Jereb B, Änggård A, Båryd I: Juvenile nasopharyngeal angiofibroma: A clinical study of 69 cases. Acta Radiol (Ther) 9:302–310, 1970

50. Jones A: Transient radiation myelopathy (with reference to Lhermitte's sign of electrical parasthesia). Br J Radiol 37:727–744, 1964

51. Jones LT: The lacrimal secretory system and its treatment. Am J Ophthalmol 62:47–60, 1966

52. Jubiz W: Endocrinology: A Logical Approach for Clinicians, pp 10–32, 276. New York, McGraw-Hill, 1979

53. Karp LA, Streeten BW, Cogan DG: Radiation-induced atrophy of the meibomian glands. Arch Ophthalmol 97:303–305, 1979

54. Kashima HK, Kirkham R, Andrews JR: Postirradiation sialadenitis: A study of the clinical features, histopathologic changes and serum enzyme variations following irradiation of human salivary glands. Am J Roentgenol Radium Ther Nucl Med 94:271–291, 1965

55. Kim JC, Elkin D, Hendrickson FR: Carcinoma of the vocal cord: Results of treatment and time-dose relationships. Cancer 42:1114–1119, 1978

56. Kim YH, Fayos JV: Radiation tolerance of the cervical spinal cord. Radiology 139:473–478, 1981

57. Klintworth GK, Landers MB III: The Eye: Structure and Function in Disease, pp 56–58. Baltimore, Williams & Wilkins, 1976

58. Kögelnik HD, Kärcher KH: Radiobiological considerations of late effects arising from radiotherapy. In Radiobiological Research and Radiotherapy, vol I, pp 275–286. Vienna, International Atomic Energy Agency, 1977

59. Kögelnik HD, Fletcher GH, Jesse RH: Clinical course of patients with squamous cell carcinoma of the upper respiratory and digestive tracts with no evidence of disease 5 years after initial treatment. Radiology 115:423–427, 1975

60. Kramer S, Southard ME, Mansfield CM: Radiation effect and tolerance of the central nervous system. Front Radiat Ther Oncol 6:332–345, 1972

61. Leach W: Irradiation of the ear. J Laryngol Otol 79:870–880, 1965

62. Lederman M: Cancer of the Nasopharynx: Its Natural History and Treatment, p 95. Springfield, IL, Charles C Thomas, 1961

63. Leinfelder PJ, Evans TC, Riley E: Production of cataracts in animals by x-rays and fast neutrons. Radiology 65:433–438, 1955

64. Levinson SA, Close MB, Ehrenfeld WK, Stoney RJ: Carotid artery occlusive disease following external cervical irradiation. Arch Surg 107:395–397, 1973

65. Marks JE, Davis CC, Gottsman VL, Purdy JE, Lee F: The effects of radiation on parotid salivary function. Int J Radiat Oncol Biol Phys 7:1013–1019, 1981

66. Martin CL, Martin JA: Low Intensity Radium Therapy, p 53. Boston, Little, Brown, & Co, 1959

67. Merriam GR, Focht EF: A clinical study of radiation cataracts and the relationship to dose. Am J Roentgenol Radium Ther Nucl Med 77:759–785, 1957

68. Mira JG, Wescott WB, Starcke EN, Shannon IL: Some factors influencing salivary function when treating with radiotherapy. Int J Radiat Oncol Biol Phys 7:535–541, 1981

69. Moench HC, Phillips TL: Carcinoma of the nasopharynx: A review of 146 patients with emphasis on radiation dose and time factors. Am J Surg 124:515–518, 1972

70. Moretti JA: Sensorineural hearing loss following radiotherapy to the nasopharynx. Laryngoscope 85:598–602, 1976

71. Morrish RB, Chan E, Silverman S Jr, Meyer J, Fu KK, Greenspan D: Osteonecrosis in patients irradiated for head and neck carcinoma. Cancer 47:1980–1983, 1981

72. Mossman KL, Henkin RI: Radiation-induced changes in taste acuity in cancer patients. Int J Radiat Oncol Biol Phys 4:663–670, 1978

73. Murray CG, Herson J, Daly TE, Zimmerman S: Radiation necrosis of the mandible: A 10 year study: I. Factors influencing the onset of necrosis. Int J Radiat Oncol Biol Phys 6:543–548, 1980

74. Murray CG, Herson J, Daly TE, Zimmerman S: Radiation necrosis of the mandible: A 10 year study: II. Dental factors:

Onset, duration, and management of necrosis. Int J Radiat Oncol Biol Phys 6:549–553, 1980

75. Neel HB, Whicker JH, Devine KD, Weiland LH: Juvenile angiofibroma: A review of 120 cases. Am J Surg 126:547–556, 1973

76. Nelson DF, Cooper S, Weston MG, Rubin P: Second malignant neoplasms in patients treated for Hodgkin's disease with radiotherapy or radiotherapy and chemotherapy. Cancer 48:2386–2393, 1981

77. Nickell WB, Vasconez LO, Jurkiewicz MJ, Salyer KE: One stage surgical repair of mandibular osteoradionecrosis with jaw preservation. Am J Surg 126:502–504, 1973

78. Palmer BV, Gaggar N, Shaw HJ: Thyroid function after radiotherapy and laryngectomy for carcinoma of the larynx. Head Neck Surg 4:13–15, 1981

79. Parker RG, Burnett LL, Wooton P, McIntyre DJ: Radiation cataract in clinical therapeutic radiology. Radiology 82:794–799, 1964

80. Parker RG, Wildermuth O: Radiation therapy of lesions overlying cartilage: I. Carcinoma of the pinna. Cancer 15:57–65, 1962

81. Parsons JT, Bova FJ, Million RR: A reevaluation of split-course technique for squamous cell carcinoma of the head and neck. Int J Radiat Oncol Biol Phys 6:1645–1652, 1980

82. Parsons JT, Fitzgerald CR, Hood CI, Ellingwood KE, Bova FJ, Million RR: The effects of irradiation on the eye and optic nerve. Int J Radiat Oncol Biol Phys 9:609–622, 1983

83. Phillips TL, Buschke F: Radiation tolerance of the thoracic spinal cord. Am J Roentgenol Radium Ther Nucl Med 105:659–664, 1969

84. Phillips TL, Sheline GE: Bone sarcomas following radiation therapy. Radiology 81:992–996, 1963

85. Reith EJ, Ross MH: Atlas of Descriptive Histology. pp 100–103. New York, Harper & Row, 1969

86. Samaan NA, Vieto R, Schultz PN, Maor M, Meoz RT, Sampiere VA, Cangir A, Ried HL, Jesse RH: Hypothalamic, pituitary, and thyroid dysfunction after radiotherapy to the head and neck. Int J Radiat Oncol Biol Phys 8:1857–1867, 1982

87. Scheie HG, Albert DM (eds): Adler's Textbook of Ophthalmology, 8th ed, p 43. Philadelphia, WB Saunders, 1969

88. Schuknecht HF, Karmody CS: Radionecrosis of the temporal bone. Laryngoscope 76:1416–1428, 1966

89. Seydel HG: The risk of tumor induction in man following medical irradiation for malignant neoplasm. Cancer 35:1641–1645, 1975

90. Shannon IL, Trodahl JN, Starcke EN: Radiosensitivity of the human parotid gland. Proc Soc Exp Biol Med 157:50–53, 1978

91. Sheline GE, Wara WM, Smith V: Therapeutic irradiation and brain injury. Int J Radiat Oncol Biol Phys 6:1215–1228, 1980

92. Shukovsky LJ, Fletcher GH: Retinal and optic nerve complications in a high dose irradiation technique of ethmoid sinus and nasal cavity. Radiology 104:629–634, 1972

93. Silverberg GD, Britt RH, Goffinet DR: Radiation-induced carotid artery disease. Cancer 41:130–137, 1978

94. Southwood WFW: The thickness of the skin. Plast Reconstr Surg 15:423–429, 1954

95. Steeves RA, Bataini JP: Neoplasms induced by megavoltage radiation in the head and neck region. Cancer 47:1770–1774, 1981

96. Stell PM, Morrison MD: Radiation necrosis of the larynx: Etiology and management. Arch Otolaryngol 98:111–113, 1973

97. Stoll BA, Andrews JT: Radiation-induced peripheral neuropathy. Br Med J 1:834–837, 1966

98. Tan BC, Kunaratnam N: Hypopituitary dwarfism following radiotherapy for nasopharyngeal carcinoma. Clin Radiol 17:302–304, 1966

99. Tountas AA, Fornasier VL, Harwood AR, Leung PMK: Post-irradiation sarcoma of bone: A perspective. Cancer 43:182–187, 1979

100. Van der Kogel AJ: Radiation tolerance of the spinal cord: The dependence on fractionation and extended overall times. In Radiobiological Research and Radiotherapy, vol I, pp 83–90. Vienna, International Atomic Energy Agency, 1977

101. Wand M, Dueker DK, Aiello LM, Grant WM: Effects of pan-retinal photocoagulation on rubeosis iridis, angle neovascularization, and neovascular glaucoma. Am J Ophthalmol 86:332–339, 1978

102. Wang CC, Doppke K: Osteoradionecrosis of the temporal bone: Consideration of nominal standard dose: Int J Radiat Oncol Biol Phys 1:881–883, 1976

103. Wara WM, Richards GE, Grumbach MM, Kaplan SL, Sheline GE, Conte F: Hypopituitarism after irradiation in children. Int J Radiat Oncol Biol Phys 2:549–552, 1977

104. Ward PH, Thompson R, Calcaterra T, Kadin MR: Juvenile angiofibroma: A more rational therapeutic approach based upon clinical and experimental evidence. Laryngoscope 84:2181–2194, 1974

105. Warwick R, Williams PL (eds): Gray's Anatomy, 35th British ed. Philadelphia, WB Saunders, 1973

106. Whitton JT: New values for epidermal thickness and their importance. Health Phys 24:1–8, 1973

107. Wilson CS, Hall EJ: On the advisability of treating all fields at each radiotherapy session. Radiology 97:419–424, 1971

Treatment Planning for Irradiation of Head and Neck Cancer

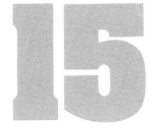

FRANCIS J. BOVA

The planning procedures that are implicit in the treatments described in this text are explained in this chapter. It is assumed that the reader has a fundamental understanding of medical physics as it applies to radiation therapy.

POSITION

The selection of treatment position depends on the beam-shaping system, the location of the lesion, and the extent of the treatment portals. A single position (supine, lateral, sitting, prone) or a combination of two or more positions may be used. The supine position is the most comfortable and is easily reproduced. The sitting position, while used successfully in some departments, must be used with caution; patients may slump during treatment if not properly stabilized. Both the supine and the sitting position require the use of beam-shaping techniques with the treatment unit in a horizontal orientation. The lateral or "chicken wing" position, while slightly uncomfortable, permits the treatment unit to be oriented vertically during the treatment of lateral portals. This allows the use of free-standing or stacked beam-shaping blocks (BSB). The prone position is used occasionally for a posteroanterior boost portal to a neck mass.

Whatever the position, it is important for the patient to achieve the same alignment each day and hold that alignment throughout the time required to treat all portals. It is preferable to treat all portals without having to shift position for each treatment.

In the lateral position, there are two techniques for positioning the head. The simpler is the use of two foam wedges, one with an indentation for the head, the other to adjust the height (Fig. 15-1). If this technique cannot be used, the alternative is a universal adjustable head holder, which allows the head to be leveled after the patient has been positioned (Fig. 15-2). For patients who have problems maintaining the lateral position, sandbags or straps of Velcro hook-and-loop fasteners at the chest and abdominal levels can help stabilize the position.

If the supine position is adopted, a neck support and bite block aid repositioning (Fig. 15-3). With the adjustable bite block and a set of neck supports, the apparatus can easily be adjusted to fit a wide variety of patients.

Customized semirigid positioning aids are used in many clinics; they are being used for 80% of all head and neck treatments at the University of Florida beginning in 1983 (Fig. 15-4).

SHIELDING MASKS

For orthovoltage and small-field electron-beam treatments, it is often advantageous to place the final collimation at or near the skin surface in order to improve dose distribution at the periphery of the portal. The process is explained in Figure 15-5A through D. The entire procedure requires approximately 1½ hours and can be performed by one person. It should be noted that adult contours do not vary appreciably, and two or three universal positives can be cast in metal (e.g., Lipowitz's metal) and used in almost all routine cases (Fig. 15-5E).

(Text continues on p. 215.)

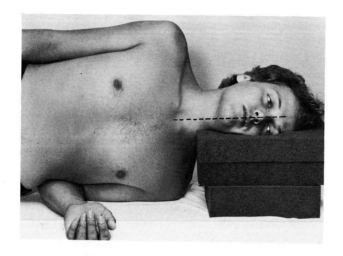

FIG. 15-1. An assortment of foam headholders are stacked to adjust the height of the head and neck in the lateral position. If the patient has a tendency to roll, supports can be added anteriorly or posteriorly or a table strap can be placed at midchest level. Tape is usually placed over the head to help prevent movement. The elbow is tucked under the rib cage in order to lower the underneath shoulder out of the exit irradiation. Large or obese patients may find this position difficult. The patient is aligned visually and with laser lights.

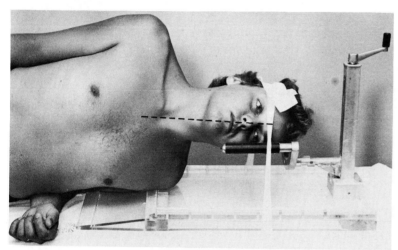

FIG. 15-2. The universal headholder is easily adjusted to level the head. Tape is used to reduce head movement. The acrylic base has a tunnel that holds a cassette for localization films. During routine use, a thin foam pad is placed between the patient and the acrylic base for patient comfort. The tip of the nose, the chin, and the suprasternal notch are aligned, usually with the aid of laser lights.

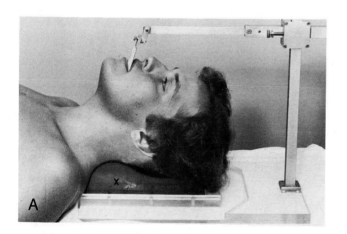

FIG. 15-3. (A) A contoured head and neck support (x) slides into the base of the bite-block apparatus. The bite-block apparatus has calibrated vertical and horizontal adjustments, although the daily positioning is usually achieved by visual adjustment. The bite pads originally were coated with dental impression material and custom-formed for each patient. The current technique uses universal bite-blocks, coated with a $\frac{3}{16}$-inch foam pad and covered with a finger cot. (B) The bite block is an aluminum base with a foam cover. (C) A finger cot is used to prevent the foam from absorbing saliva. A second cot is stretched over the first for daily use. (D) The bite block is easily mounted to the hinged support by a single thumbscrew. The patient is placed in position and the bite block is inserted, the head is adjusted, and the thumbscrews are tightened on the vertical upright.

FIG. 15-3 (continued)

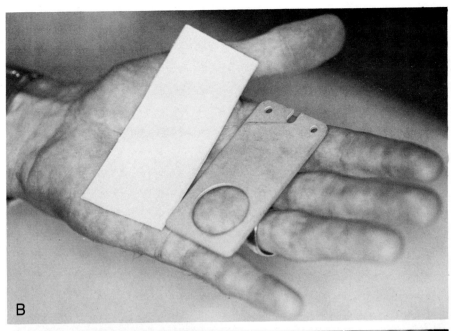

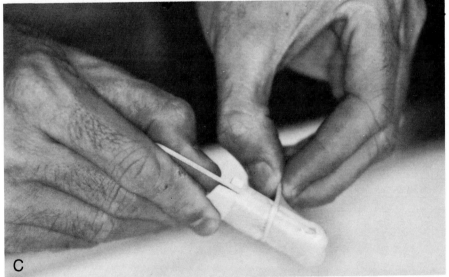

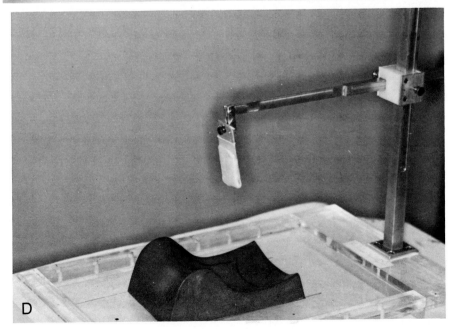

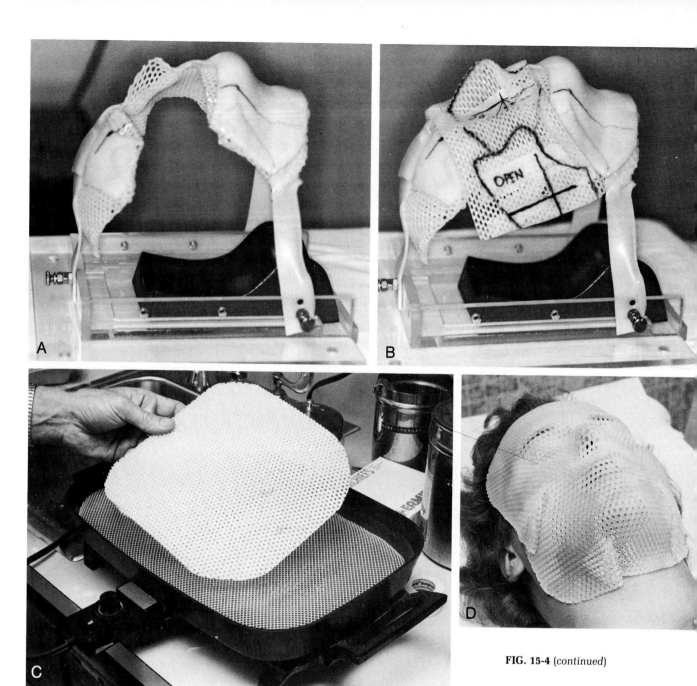

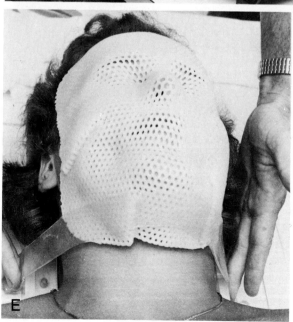

FIG. 15-4 (continued)

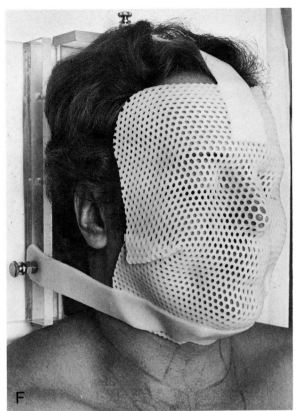

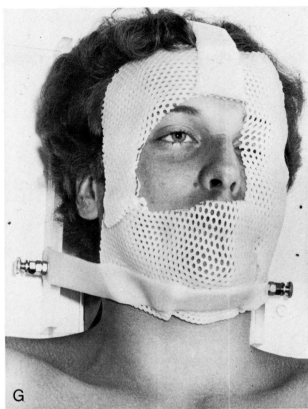

FIG. 15-4. (*A*) Customized Aquaplast mask and acrylic base plate. (*B*) A second mask may be made to aid in beam positioning. The portals are inked on the mask rather than on the patient. This mask is removed prior to treatment. (*C*) Fabrication of an Aquaplast mask. Aquaplast is cut and placed into a water bath (~140°F). When the Aquaplast becomes translucent and pliable, it is removed from the bath and placed on a towel to dry. Aquaplast will adhere to itself while in the pliable translucent state, and care must be taken not to let the sheet fold onto itself. If a larger water bath is used, a full sheet of Aquaplast can be heated. The larger sheet extends to the base plate, eliminating the need for the fastening strips shown in E. (*D*) The patient is placed on the head/neck support and aligned. A ¼-inch spacer is placed under the head/neck support to compensate for a 7% shrinkage of the Aquaplast. (This shrinkage occurs in the final stages of cooling and involves the mask and connecting strips. The spacer is removed only after fabrication is complete and the mask has fully cooled.) The heated Aquaplast is removed from the water bath, patted dry, and applied to the patient and pressed to fit. Aquaplast cools quickly and can easily be applied to the skin without discomfort. It takes approximately 5 minutes for the material to return to its hard, opaque form. (*E*) Once the mask has cooled and hardened, 1-inch Aquaplast strips are heated and permanently attached to the original mask by firmly pressing together the warm and the cold Aquaplast. The acrylic base plate has been drilled and tapped. Pressing the end of the strip against the acrylic with the fingers (as shown here) produces an indentation on the Aquaplast. The connecting straps are pressed firmly against the screw holes to identify the spot to be punched. If a full sheet of Aquaplast is used, it is similarly extended to the base plate and pressed against the screw holes. (*F*) The holes are made in the strips with a ¼-inch hole punch. The process requires about 20 minutes to this point. The patient is then ready for simulation. (*G*) After the treatment portals have been decided and the beam-shaping block fabricated, the portals are transferred back to the patient's surface and the mask is cut away to preserve skin-sparing.

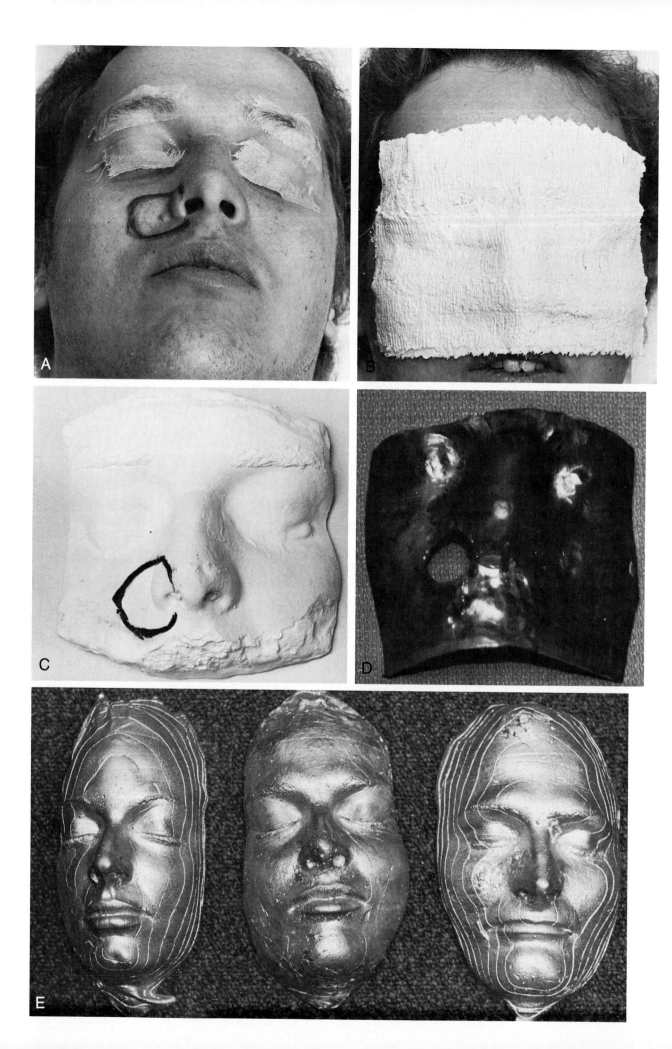

FIG. 15-5. Fabrication of a lead mask. (A) Step 1. Petrolatum-coated gauze is placed over the eyebrows and eyelashes to prevent plaster from sticking to the hair. The remainder of the skin is covered with a light coat of petrolatum to ease separation of the mask. Cotton may be placed in the nostrils. The treatment portal is outlined in ink and will transfer to the plaster. (B) Step 2. Moistened plaster strips are applied to the skin and allowed to harden. (C) Step 3. A hard stone positive is then prepared, using a material such as white Castone (manufactured by Ranson and Randolf), and the portal is transferred to the positive. Sheet lead (thick enough to reduce transmission to 5% or less) is then formed onto the stone positive with a hammer and the portal is cut out. (D) A completed lead mask. (E) A set of face casts made of low melting-point alloy. These three casts can be used to prepare lead masks in 95% of cases.

SIMULATION

To design treatment portals from planning films, areas of clinical interest are outlined or marked with radiopaque material. Solder wire can be used to mark lymph nodes of interest, the skin surface, or the location of a portal border that must be determined by physical examination rather than from the roentgenogram. For example, the match line between the low-neck portals and the lateral face portals or the posterior neck border of the primary portal can be located and marked. The location of tumor in the tongue, floor of the mouth, or oropharynx can be indicated by stainless-steel pins (Fig. 15-6).

FIG. 15-6. (A) Simulation film with radiopaque markers to show pertinent anatomy. A lead marker is placed at each external ear canal to gauge rotation of the head as well as to locate the canals. (B) Stainless-steel wire is cut into short segments. Following topical anesthesia, a 20-gauge spinal needle is used to insert the pins. The water-soluble lubricant is placed on the pins to help hold them in the tip of the needle. (C) Insertion of needle under local anesthesia into the anterior border of an oral tongue lesion.

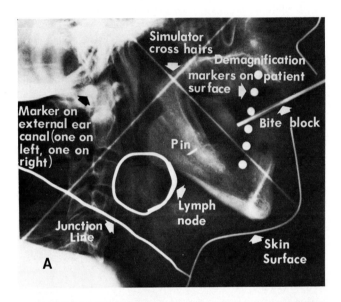

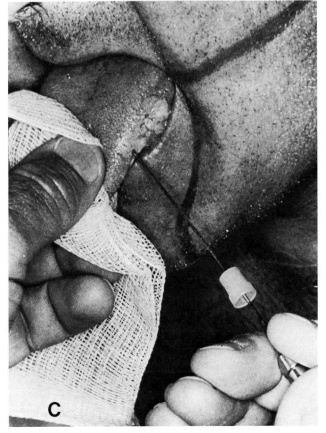

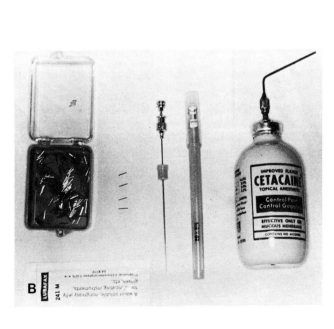

BEAM SHAPING

Rectangular beams emanating from the treatment units must be converted into irregular shapes in order to shield normal tissues. Beam shaping is achieved by two basic techniques: (1) free style, using stacked lead blocks, and (2) custom designed, using low-melting-point alloy shields. The advantage of free-style hand blocking is that the set of lead blocks can be used for all patients, reducing costs and simulation time. This system works well for almost all situations but requires the treatment unit to be in a vertical orientation. There are methods available to hold a single layer of lead blocks sandwiched between two acrylic plates or bolted to a single plate for lateral mounting; except for simple corner blocking, these methods have limited application and are not recommended. Disadvantages of free-style blocking include lack of easy reproducibility and inability to obtain complex free-form portal shapes. These problems are eliminated when custom-designed BSB are used. The custom-designed BSB have three major advantages: (1) more normal tissues can be shielded; (2) the patient can easily be treated in the supine position, since the BSB can be mounted with the treatment unit at any angle; and (3) the portal outline is reproduced precisely

each day (although this does not guarantee that errors in daily alignment may not occur). There is a temptation to design the BSB with narrow margins, which then requires greater precision in alignment. Use of custom-designed BSB also adds to the cost of the treatment, and their fabrication often delays the start of treatment.

One difference between the custom block and the stacked block is the sloping divergent side on the custom BSB versus the vertical side on the stacked BSB. While the correct divergence is appealing, for small fields (<80 sq cm) there exists little physical difference in the resulting

FIG. 15-7 (continued)

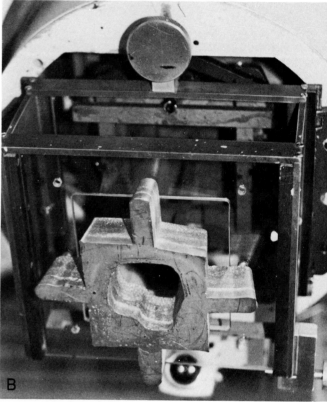

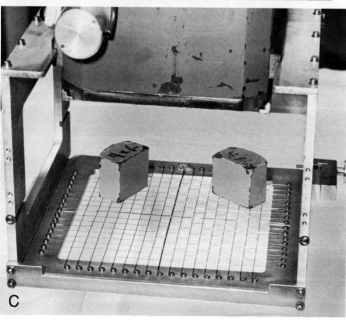

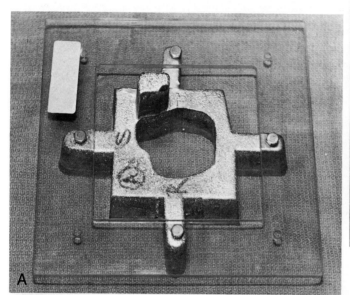

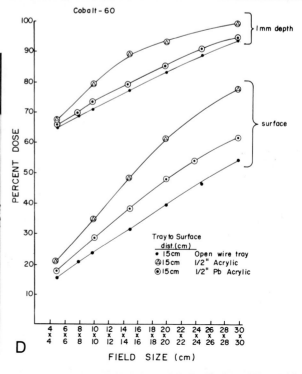

penumbra and no clinical difference. It should be remembered that the physical penumbra (the dose gradient at the edge of the portal) as measured by isodose scanning and demonstrated by isodose distribution is substantially altered by minor daily alignment errors and patient motion.

The goal in beam shaping is to reduce the transmitted beam to 5% or less of its unattenuated intensity. The thickness of the BSB is usually a compromise between this goal and a practical size for routine use. For cobalt-60, the standard lead blocks for free-style stacking have been 3 cm thick, which transmits 15% of the beam. However, since the blocks are used mainly to collimate the edge of the beam, this is a satisfactory compromise. In many situations, lead blocks are stacked in two or three tiers to achieve the proper shape. Blocks that are thicker than 3 cm will not work very well in the space available. Critical areas are double blocked (e.g., 6 cm).

Stacked blocks for 8-MV and 17-MV x-rays are 8 cm thick (5% transmission), which limits the number of tiers that can be stacked. Extra shielding may be added to reduce the dose to a critical structure such as an uninvolved eye. For example, the dose to the eye under a 5-cm alloy block is 10% at 5 mm depth for cobalt-60. This is partly from transmitted beam (~5%) and partly scattered from the treated volume (~5%). For 6000 rad given dose (D_{max}), the eye would receive 600 rad from the anterior portal alone. If a 10-cm thick BSB is used, the eye receives only 6% of the given dose to the anterior portal. Similar dose reductions are seen with 8-MV and 17-MV x-ray beams, which give an eye dose of 9% with 7.5 cm of low-melting-point alloy shielding and 6% with 15 cm of shielding. This reduction may be critical in preventing cataract formation (Fig. 15-7A).

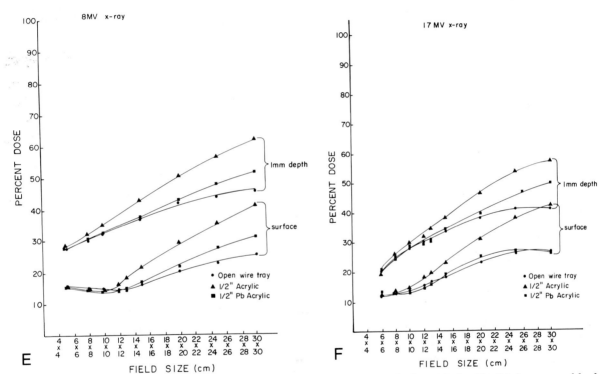

FIG. 15-7. (A) Head and neck block (3 inches thick) with double-thickness eye block for 8- or 17-MV x-ray. This can reduce the dose to the eye by 3% to 5% compared with single thickness. For 7000-rad tumor dose, this is a reduction of 200 rad to 350 rad. (B) Head and neck block mounted to a treatment unit. The central portion of the Lucite mounting tray has been removed to reduce low-energy scatter to the skin. (C) Wire tray for free-hand blocking. Stainless-steel wires, 0.02 inches diameter, on 1-cm centers are used. (D) Doses at the surface and at 1 mm for a Picker C-9000, cobalt-60 teletherapy unit. The blocking tray is 65 cm from the source, surface of phantom at 80 cm SSD. *The doses for the wire tray are the same for a 10- to 25-cm tray to surface distance.*

For example, when parallel opposed cobalt-60 portals are used to deliver a 7000-rad midline tumor dose (separation 14 cm), the wire tray would deliver approximately 500 rad less at 1 mm depth and approximately 700 rad less at the surface compared with an acrylic tray. These differences are thought to be clinically significant. (E) Doses at the surface and at 1 mm depth for a Philips SL75-20, 8 MV x-rays. Blocking tray is 65 cm from target, surface of phantom at 100 cm SSD. (F) Doses at the surface and at 1 mm depth for a Philips SL75-20, 17 MV x-rays. Blocking tray is 65 cm from target, surface of phantom at 100 cm SSD. (E and F from Bova FJ, Hill LW: Surface doses for acrylic vs. lead blocking trays for cobalt-60, 8 MV, and 17 MV photons. Med Phys 10:254–256, 1983)

There is a difference in skin-sparing depending on the tray used to hold or mount the blocks (Fig. 15-7B, C). Secondary scatter from an acrylic tray increases the surface dose and the dose at 1 mm (dermis). The buildup of surface dose versus field size for cobalt-60, 8-MV x-ray, and 17-MV x-ray beams is shown in Figure 15-7D and E.[1] For free-hand blocks the standard acrylic tray can be replaced with a wire tray (Fig. 15-7F), while for custom blocks an acrylic tray is used with its central portion removed (see Fig. 15-7B). The advantage of the wire tray or the acrylic tray with the center removed for high energies and a 35-cm tray-to-surface distance begins at fields 15 cm in diameter. For cobalt-60, however, savings can be experienced at 15 cm tray-to-surface distance for all field sizes. Lead acrylic is similar to the wire tray until very large field sizes are used and can be used if the strength of a full sheet of acrylic is required (see Fig. 15-7C–E).

The BSB is aligned to the patient by mounting the block on the simulator. The BSB is quickly adjusted under fluoroscopy and a double-exposure roentgenogram taken (one exposure with and one without the BSB). If the simulator cannot accept the weight of the blocks, then a lead template (cut from 0.03-inch lead sheet) may be used in place of the BSB. A third technique is to use the Styrofoam mold that was used to cast the custom blocks: the inside of the mold is brushed with barium, which projects a thin radiopaque line around the proposed portals.

PREPARATION OF CROSS-SECTIONAL OUTLINE

The methods of transferring the patient's cross-sectional outline onto paper ("contouring") use stiff wire, plaster strips, molding rods or, more recently, the computed tomographic (CT) scan. The contouring procedure is shown in Figure 15-8. A small error in reproducing the surface shape results in an error that is small compared with errors in diameter. *Attention should be given to anteroposterior, lateral, and triangulation distances.* The levels at which the contours are taken should receive careful thought. For example, the treatment field shown in Figure 15-9 is studied through levels A and B, and two substantially different isodose distributions are obtained. These differences are greater for low-energy photon beams than for high-energy beams and are even greater for electron beams. It is therefore advantageous to study several levels through the tumor volume when the treatment portals are altered in shape or where the patient's thickness varies. Additional sections in the coronal or sagittal planes may be useful (see section on treatment planning in Chapter 24, Nasopharynx).

BEAM CHARACTERISTICS

The characteristics of the available photon and electron beams must be known before treatment planning is started. These characteristics include the buildup region as well as the falloff regions at the edges and deep margins. The buildup region for photons and electrons is highly machine dependent. The primary collimator and the type of tray used to support collimator blocks affect the surface dose. The buildup curves for cobalt-60 and 8-MV and 17-MV photon beams are shown in Figure 15-10A; the buildup curves for 6-MeV through 18-MeV electron

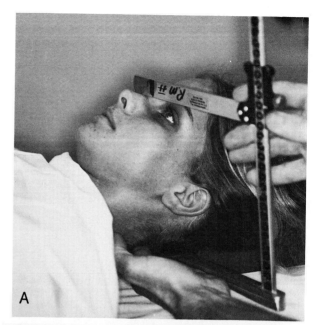

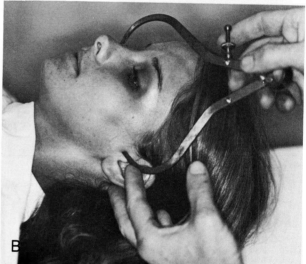

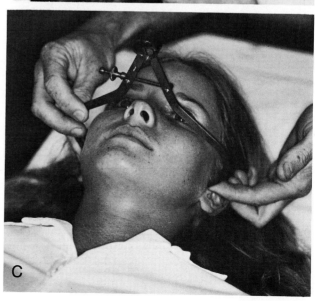

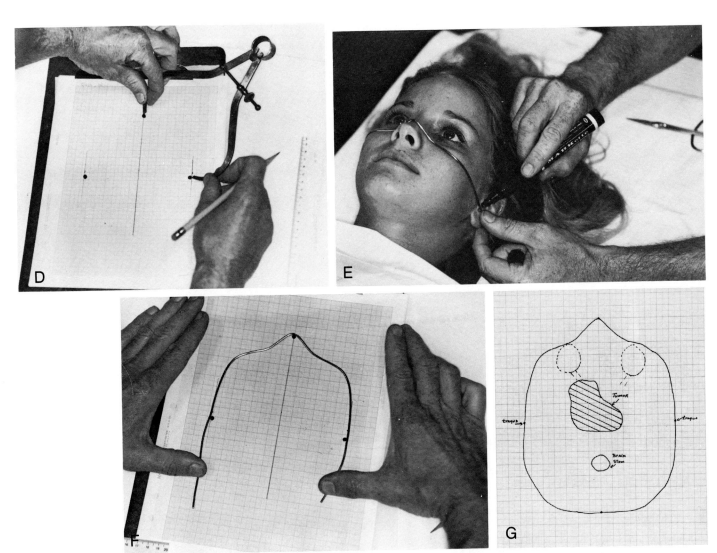

beams are shown in Figure 15-10B.[4] For photon beams, the buildup region extends to greater depths as energy increases, while the surface dose decreases with increasing photon energy. Electron beams exhibit just the opposite behavior, with the surface dose increasing as beam energy increases.

Photon beams are routinely specified by manufacturers by a percentage depth dose at a depth of 10 or 20 cm. For electron beams, either the extrapolated range method or the depth of the 50% ionization point is used to designate beam energy. The buildup region is disregarded for photons and electrons. It is therefore possible and likely that two beams of similar energies can differ in surface dose by 10% to 20%. A 17-MeV electron beam from a Philips SL75-20 and a 17-MeV electron beam from a Therac 20 are shown in Figure 15-10C. The surface doses are 87% and 82%, respectively. For a tumor dose of 6000 rad at the 90% depth dose, the surface dose with the Philips SL75-20 would be 5800 rad and for the Therac 20, 5460 (a difference of 340 rad). This might be advantageous or disadvantageous, depending on the tumor location. The depth contained in the 90% to 100% depth dose is also different: Philips SL75-20, 0.3 cm to 3.9 cm; Therac 20, 0.8 cm to 5.6 cm. Therefore, it is important when comparing techniques from one facility to another or one accelerator to another to examine

FIG. 15-8. Procedures for manual contouring. Step 1. Measurements are taken (anteroposterior, lateral, and one or more points of triangulation) and transferred to paper. (A) Anteroposterior diameter measured with calipers. (B) Measurement from midline to tragus. (C) Lateral diameter measured with calipers. (D) Transfer of diameters to paper. (E) Step 2. A solder wire is molded to the plane of the contour, and the three points of triangulation are marked onto the wire. (F) Step 3. The contour is transferred to paper, making sure to align the triangulation points. (G) Cross section with critical structures identified. The position of the radiation portals is then added, and the contour is entered into the treatment planning computer along with the critical structures and the position of the radiation portals.

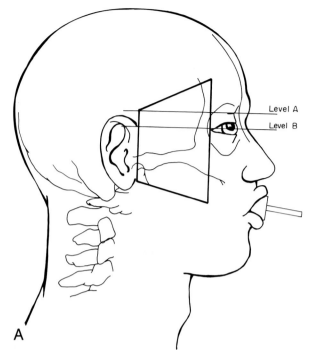

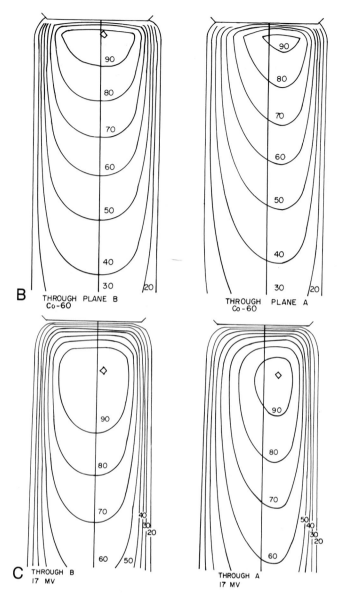

FIG. 15-9. (A) The routine contour through a lateral face field is either through the central axis or through a critical organ such as the eye. The extension superior to the eye, where the field begins to taper (level A), shows a decreased dose due to decreased scatter. The dose distribution through planes A and B are shown for cobalt-60 (B) and 17-MV x-rays (C). In both cases, the distribution through plane A is substantially altered. This lateral field is often combined with an anterior field, both with wedges. The dose to the posterior portion at level A can be much lower than can be appreciated by dosimetry through level B.

the beam characteristics and not simply to use similar nominal energies.

CORRECTIONS FOR INHOMOGENEITY (CT TREATMENT PLANNING)

Routine dosimetry is performed assuming homogeneous tissues; structures such as the mandible are ignored. If a dose of 7000 rad is computed to the tonsillar pillar at 4 cm (assuming homogeneity), the actual dose after correction for 1.5 cm of mandible is as follows:

Cobalt-60	6700 rad
8-MV x-rays	6900 rad
17-MV x-rays	6900 rad
17-MeV electrons	6550 rad
20-MeV electrons	6700 rad

The difference between the 20-MeV and 17-MeV electron beams is the position at which the initial dose is specified. For the 17-MeV beam, the 4-cm depth is equal to the 93% isodose line. Any shift will therefore occur along the steep falloff region of the depth-dose curve. For the 20-MeV beam, the 4-cm depth corresponds to a plateau of the depth-dose curve. A similar shift in depth therefore results in a smaller change in dose value.

The correction for bone and air gaps, based on "normal anatomy atlases" with assumed normal densities, can lead to inaccuracies as large as the assumption of homogeneity. However, CT scanning can yield not only a precise contour but also an accurate map of the electron density relative to water. The CT treatment planning technique involves marking the field edges to allow their position to be easily located on the CT slice, reproducing the treatment geometry within the restraints of the CT table and aperture, and being able to remove the artificially imposed CT numbers if a contrast medium has been introduced. Other problems involve attempting to design treatment portals from CT scout views that may not have the correct divergence. The design of a portal from a nondivergent scout view can result in the inclusion in the final portal of critical structures adjacent to the field. However, if allowance is made for these problems, a more accurate dose estimate can be achieved and adjustments made for inhomogeneity. CT-based treatment planning systems are just becoming generally available and will undergo considerable inves-

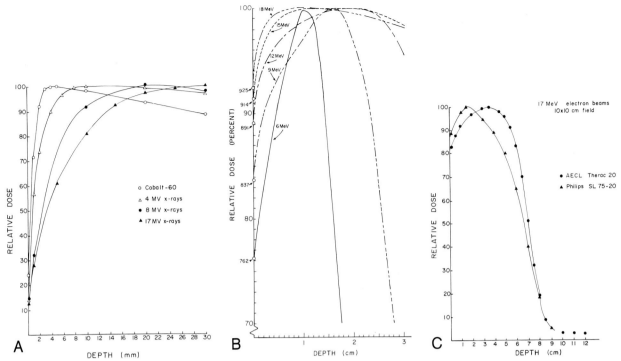

FIG. 15-10. (*A*) Buildup curves for 10 × 10-cm field for cobalt-60 (Picker C-9000, SSD = 80 cm) and 4-MV (SSD = 80 cm), 8-MV, and 17-MV x-rays (Philips SL75-20, SSD = 100 cm). (*B*) Buildup curves for 6-, 9-, 12-, 15-, and 18-MeV electron beams.[4] Cone size is 10 × 10 cm; SSD = 100. (*C*) Electron central axis depth dose curves for 17 MeV 10 × 10-cm fields for a Philips SL75-20 scattering foil system and a Therac 20 scanning beam system. (*B* from Turner AP: Surface dose measurements of Clinac 18 electron beams. In Proceedings of the Eighth Varian Clinac Users Meeting, January 31 through February 2, 1980, Kauai, Hawaii)

tigation in attempts to improve the delivery of radiation therapy to head and neck neoplasms.

ELECTRON-BEAM DOSIMETRY

The early use of electron-beam treatment routinely used the 80% isodose level for prescribing the tumor dose. However, this should not be considered optimal. If a tumor dose is prescribed to the 80% isodose value, there will be a 20% gradient of dose across the tumor. This is in marked contrast to acceptable external-beam treatment planning, where the tumor volume should be no worse than 90% to 95% of the maximum dose, resulting in a 5% to 10% dose gradient. Although prescribing to the 90% to 95% isodose level will result in a slightly higher dose to tissue beyond the depth of the tumor, this tissue is still in the declining dose region. This slight increase in dose to the deeper tissue may be a small price to pay for the ability to decrease the given dose by 12.6%; as always, each clinical situation must be evaluated separately.

Prescribing to the 90% to 100% isodose line requires consideration of the surface dose. If there is frank tumor at the skin surface or if a surgical scar is present, it may be necessary to bolus either the entire surface or simply the region at risk to obtain a 95% to 100% depth dose. This usually requires 3 mm to 5 mm of tissue-equivalent bolus. If the region of compensation or bolus is large, the effect on the depth of coverage must be considered. Due

to the rapid falloff of electron beams with depth, a small amount of bolus can significantly shift the depth-dose distribution. A second consideration is the size of the radiation portal. If the 90% isodose line is prescribed, the field size must be increased to compensate for the constriction of the 90% and 100% isodose lines that lie inside the physical edge of the beam.

Two or more adjacent electron portals or an adjacent electron and photon portal may be selected in certain situations. The easiest solution is to treat to a common match line and vary the position of the match line one or two times during the treatment course. However, there are common situations when electron portals are used for only 500 rad to 1000 rad, and moving match lines is not practical. A common clinical situation is the use of a posterior electron strip to boost the neck nodes behind the plane of the spinal cord. Three examples of the dose distribution for adjacent photon and electron portals are given in Figure 15-11. A small area of high dose is created by using a common junction line. The general rule is to use a common match line between photon and electron fields and to treat the line with *both* the photon and the electron beam.

It is important to ensure that the treatment planning system properly predicts the electron-beam isodose distribution for the specific treatment parameters used. For example, the dose distribution for an electron field blocked on the surface as opposed to one blocked 6 cm from the surface should be properly predicted by the electron-beam algorithm (Fig. 15-12). If the algorithm cannot predict such

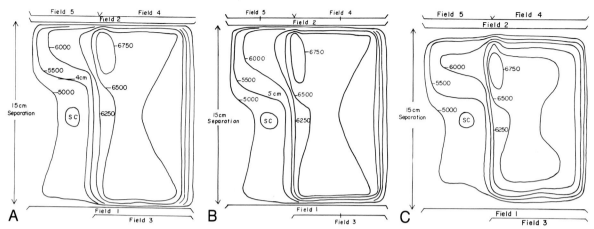

FIG. 15-11. Isodose distribution for parallel opposed photon portals plus one posterior electron strip. When treating a primary lesion to high doses, a reduction is usually planned at 4500 rad to 5000 rad to exclude the spinal cord from the field. The dose to the primary lesion is then raised to the final dose (6500 rad in this example). The dose to the posterior cervical lymph nodes or large lymph node mass is approximately 5000 rad at this point. Electron fields can be used to increase the dose to these lymph nodes or a mass without increasing the spinal cord dose. (A) Cobalt-60 parallel opposed beams (weighted 1:1) and 10-MeV electron beam posterior strip.

Fields 1 and 2: Cobalt-60, 12 × 12 cm, SSD = 80 cm, 3495 rad given dose
Fields 3 and 4: Cobalt-60, 8 × 12 cm, SSD = 80 cm, 1067 rad given dose
Field 5:   10-MeV electrons, 5 × 12 cm, SSD = 100 cm, 1000 rad given dose

The electron field is butted against the edge of the photon field (i.e., no gap). A small area receives 6750 rad, which is clinically acceptable. The treatment volume under the electron portal extends from 0.5 cm to 4.0 cm to a minimum of 5500 rad, while the spinal cord dose is approximately 5200 rad. (B) In this example, the electron-beam energy is increased to 12 MeV and the 5500 rad lymph node dose is extended to 5 cm, with the spinal cord dose essentially unchanged.

Fields 1 and 2: Cobalt-60, 12 × 12 cm, SSD = 80 cm, 3495 rad given dose
Fields 3 and 4: Cobalt-60, 7 × 12 cm, SSD = 80 cm, 1067 rad given dose
Field 5:   12-MeV electrons, 5 × 7 cm, SSD = 100 cm, 1000 rad given dose

(C) Eight MV x-rays are substituted for cobalt-60 in this example. There is a reduced skin dose, but the distribution is otherwise similar to B.

Fields 1 and 2: 8-MV x-ray, 12 × 12 cm, SSD = 100 cm, 2985 rad given dose
Fields 3 and 4: 8-MV x-ray, 7 × 12 cm, SSD = 100 cm, 900 rad given dose
Field 5:   12-MeV electrons, 5 × 12 cm, SSD = 100 cm, 1000 rad given dose

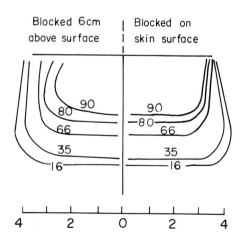

FIG. 15-12. A 10-MeV electron-beam portal. A 10 × 10-cm beam is reduced to a 7 × 7-cm field by a lead block. Isodose distribution with block placed on skin surface and 6 cm above the surface (i.e., in the electron cone). Note that the effective width for the 90% isodose is 5 cm to 6 cm for the block on the surface and is reduced to 4 cm to 5 cm if blocked at 6 cm above the surface.

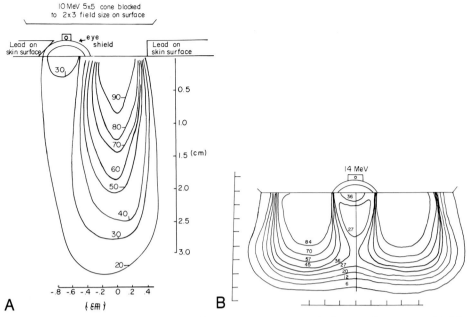

FIG. 15-13. (A) Isodose distribution for a 2 × 3-cm 10-MeV electron-beam portal with eye shield (e.g., for treatment of a lower eyelid lesion). Energies of approximately 10 MeV and higher can penetrate the shield and give substantial doses to the eye. For the case shown, a 5000-rad tumor dose would deliver 1000 rad to 1500 rad to parts of the shielded eye. (B) A 14-MeV electron-beam portal; 10 × 10-cm cone blocked to 7 cm diameter, 6 cm above surface. Eye shield on central axis. The combined effect of scatter plus beam penetration of the shield results in a high dose to the entire eye. In certain clinical situations this might be acceptable.

changes in dose distribution, then the clinical parameters routinely used should be measured and modeled individually.

Skin cancer has historically been treated with orthovoltage units. Many of these treatments are now being carried out with electron beams. There are several problems involved in this transition that must be examined to avoid underdosing the lesion or overdosing a normal structure (e.g., the eye). The output (rad/minute) for small electron fields (1 cm to 3 cm diameter) is dependent on beam energy and the position of the BSB. The problem of field uniformity is critical, and for small fields, acceptable flatness can be achieved only by placing the final collimation on the skin surface. There is also the problem of side scatter under lead shields. Eye shields are particularly susceptible to this problem because of their small diameter. For low electron energies (5 MeV to 8 MeV) the beam scatter under the shield can result in unexpected doses to the eye. Higher-energy beams can also penetrate standard-thickness eye shields (Fig. 15-13).

To compound these problems, the relatively low surface dose (70% to 80%) of low-energy (5 MeV to 8 MeV) electron beams must be taken into account. If gross tumor lies at the surface, bolus must be used, in which case the field size (to allow for constriction of the 90% isodose lines), the given dose, or the energy must be increased to achieve the desired tumor dose. Orthovoltage energies remain the technique of choice in my clinic for many skin cancers.

COMPARISON OF PARALLEL OPPOSED PORTAL TECHNIQUES

The maximum dose and target tumor depth for a single portal will occur at the same point only for relatively superficial lesions. An optimum treatment plan, one with a maximum tumor dose and a minimum dose to normal tissues, is usually achieved by a multiple portal arrangement. The most common arrangement in the irradiation of head and neck cancer involves parallel opposed lateral portals. Varying amounts of normal tissue are treated to doses as high as or higher than the prescribed tumor dose. *With modern-day equipment, the dose to tissues outside the tumor volume should seldom be more than 5% to 10% above the prescribed tumor dose.*

The ability to localize and create a homogeneous tumor dose is optimized by the choice of the correct beam energy and beam weight. Cobalt-60, 6-MV beams, and 17-MV beams for parallel opposed fields that are 5 cm, 10 cm, and 15 cm apart are compared in Figure 15-14. When the separation is increased from 5 cm to 15 cm, several interesting phenomena occur. First, at the small separations, the extensive buildup region of the higher-energy photon beam causes reduced doses near the skin surfaces. If desired, a greater uniformity across the separation is achieved with the cobalt-60 beam. However, when a 15-cm separation is reached, the lack of dose at depth for cobalt-60 beams begins to create an area of low dose at mid-depth

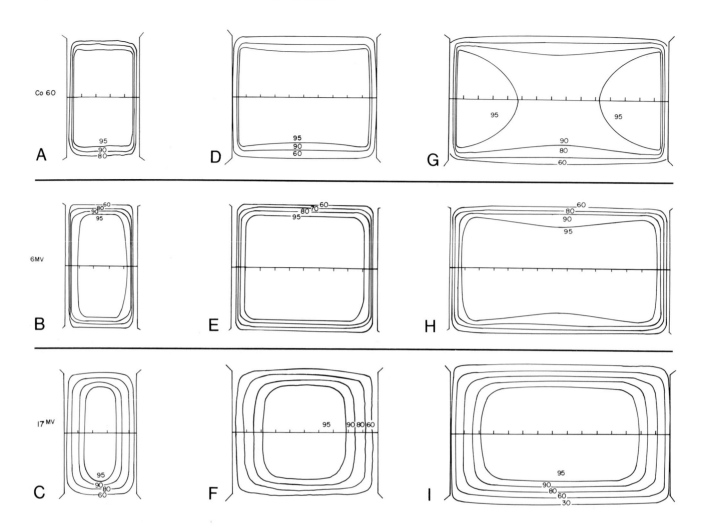

FIG. 15-14. Comparison of the isodose distributions for cobalt-60, 6-MV x-rays, and 17-MV x-rays for parallel opposed equally weighted 8 × 8-cm portals. Cobalt-60: SSD = 80 cm; 6 MV and 17 MV: TSD = 100 cm. (*A–C*) 5-cm separation. (*D–F*) 10-cm separation. (*G–I*) 15-cm separation.

separations. At this point, the depth dose from the higher-energy photon beams may offer a substantial advantage in certain clinical situations and a disadvantage in others.

There is a popular misconception that the falloff in dose near the edge of the portal is much greater with cobalt-60 than with linear accelerators; examination of the isodose distributions shows a small difference for the first 1 cm to 2 cm inside the geometric edge of the portals. The major advantage of higher-energy photons is the increased percentage depth dose and, in some instances, the decrease in the skin and subcutaneous dose. The edges of the portal are usually aimed at subclinical disease so that a slightly reduced dose is acceptable, if not desirable. However, when gross disease occurs near the edge of the portal (e.g., carcinoma of the posterior pharyngeal wall), there are advantages to beams with less falloff near the beam edge.

A COMPARISON OF TECHNIQUES FOR LATERALIZED LESIONS

A frequent situation in head and neck radiation therapy is a well-lateralized lesion to be managed mainly by external-beam irradiation. The following examples (Figs. 15-15 through 15-19) compare possible techniques for a carcinoma of the retromolar trigone/anterior tonsillar pillar.

A single ipsilateral cobalt-60 field enters the tumor region at the 93% isodose level and exits at the 80% isodose level, a gradient of 13% (Fig. 15-15). The normal tissue at 5-mm depth receives a dose 20% greater than the minimum tumor dose. If a set of equally weighted, parallel opposed lateral cobalt-60 fields is used, the gradient across the region is 5% (90% to 95%) (Fig. 15-16A). The maximum dose to

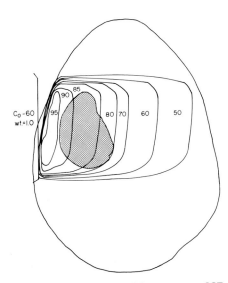

FIG. 15-15. Single cobalt-60 field, 7 × 7 cm, SSD = 80 cm.

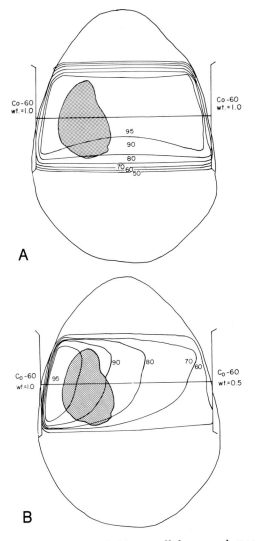

FIG. 15-16. Cobalt-60 fields, parallel opposed, 7 × 7 cm, SSD = 80. (A) Weighted given dose 1.0 to 1.0. (B) Weighted given dose 1.0 to 0.5.

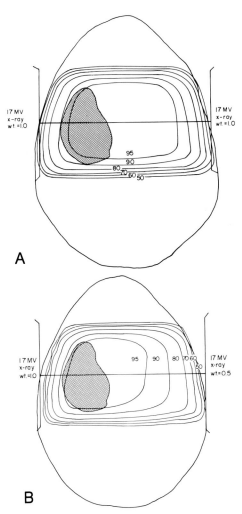

FIG. 15-17. A 17-MV x-ray beam, field size 7 × 7 cm, SSD = 80. (A) Weighted given dose 1.0 to 1.0. (B) Weighted given dose 1.0 to 0.5.

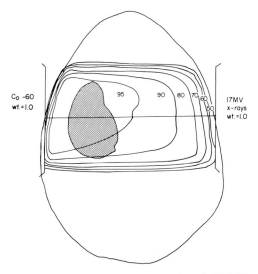

FIG. 15-18. Cobalt-60 (SSD = 80 cm) and 17-MV x-rays (SSD = 100 cm), parallel opposed fields, field size 7 × 7 cm. Weighted given dose, cobalt-60 to 17-MV x-ray, is 1.0 to 1.0.

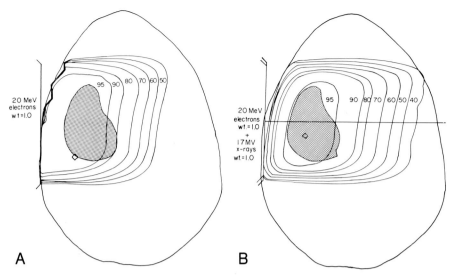

FIG. 15-19. (A) 20-MeV electrons, field size 8.5 × 8.5 cm, SSD = 100 cm. (B) 20-MeV electrons, field size 8.5 × 8.5 cm, and 17-MV x-rays, field size 7 × 7 cm. SSD = 100 cm for both. Weighted given dose is 1.0 to 1.0. The addition of the 17-MV x-ray beam reduces the surface dose and gives a dose distribution that is affected less by bone.

normal tissue is only 10% greater than the minimum tumor dose, but a much larger volume of normal tissue is exposed to a high dose. If the portals are weighted 2:1, there is still a 5% gradient across the tumor (Fig. 15-16B). The maximum dose is 10% greater only on the ipsilateral side, and the high-dose volume is reduced. There would still be sufficient dose to deliver 4500 rad to 5000 rad to the contralateral lymph nodes. If the tissues extending to the right and left skin surfaces are at risk, the parallel opposed cobalt-60 fields are satisfactory. However, if the cervical lymph nodes are not clinically involved, a high-energy (6 MV to 17 MV) photon beam can adequately cover the region and reduce the volume of superficial normal tissue exposed and still deliver an acceptable dose (e.g., 4500 rad) for subclinical disease in the lymph nodes. There is at least 1 cm of skin and subcutaneous tissues overlying the lymph nodes at risk, and they would fall within the 70% to 95% depth dose (Fig. 15-17). A combination of cobalt-60 and 17-MV x-rays can improve the distribution in certain situations (Fig. 15-18). This combination may be used when there is a requirement for only 4500 rad to 5000 rad to the contralateral upper neck lymph nodes, 5000 rad to 5500 rad to cover possible mucosal spread near the midline (7 cm), and 7000 rad or more to the tonsillar area (3.5 cm) and ipsilateral neck.

A third or fourth portal may be added in certain clinical situations to further localize the high-dose volume to the area of interest (e.g., see Chapter 24, Nasopharynx; section on base of the tongue in Chapter 18, Oropharynx; Chapter 23, Nasal Vestibule, Nasal Cavity, and Paranasal Sinuses; and section on vocal cord carcinoma in Chapter 19, Larynx).

A common technique for lateralized or superficial lesions is a combination of electron and photon beams, or only electrons (e.g., parotid gland, early anterior tonsillar pillar/retromolar trigone, buccal mucosa, nasal vestibule, and skin).

If a tumor volume extends from 1.0 cm to 4.5 cm in depth from the skin surface, a simple ipsilateral 20-MeV electron beam adequately covers the region (e.g., carcinoma of the retromolar trigone and anterior tonsillar pillar). This volume would include the ipsilateral lymph nodes at risk in the upper neck. Due to the rapid falloff of the electron beam, the dose 3 cm to 4 cm past the tumor volume is usually less than 50% of the tumor dose. There are two

disadvantages to using only electrons in this situation: (1) high skin dose and (2) differential absorption by the mandible. The use of a single high-energy electron field can often result in a dose at 5 mm of 95% to 100%. Although this dose may be acceptable, it may be advantageous to lower it at the price of a slight increase in the dose at depths beyond the tumor.

The use of a single 20-MeV electron beam (uncorrected for bone absorption) to treat a bulky retromolar trigone or anterior tonsillar pillar lesion is shown in Figure 15-19A. The surface dose is 90% and the dose at 5 mm is 95%, while the dose 3 cm past the tumor volume is at the 50% isodose line. The addition of a 17-MV x-ray beam would result in the distribution shown in Figure 15-19B. The dose to the subcutaneous tissues at 5 mm is decreased to 50%, the tumor is confined to a 6% gradient, and the tissues 3 cm beyond the tumor volume are at the 70% depth dose line. The overall effect is the reduction of the high dose to the subcutaneous tissues and an elevation of dose to tissues beyond the tumor, but not beyond acceptable levels. One critical organ in this example would be the contralateral parotid; if the dose is limited to 3000 rad, then there is usually an approximately 50% recovery of saliva on one side. The addition of a high-energy photon beam also decreases the effect of inhomogeneities such as the mandible.

The combination of photons and electrons offers a simple alternative to ipsilateral angled wedge portals. Advantages of the combined beam compared with angled wedge portals include the ability to tailor the entrance beam to fit the tumor volume, the ease of reduction of portals, and the relatively simple inclusion of contiguous lymph node groups.

The mixture of the electrons and photons is usually straightforward. The combined depth dose generally moves the 90% depth dose less than 1 cm compared with electrons alone. When the beams are weighted equally, the choice of electron beam is therefore similar to that for the single beam case. For maximum skin-sparing, the highest available photon beam is usually the best choice. However, if the dose at the surface must be relatively high (e.g., carcinoma of the skin or postoperative radiation therapy for parotid neoplasms), then cobalt-60 or 4-MV x-rays will yield a better distribution. Multiple energies (>2) may sometimes be combined to develop the best distribution.

COMPENSATION FOR SURFACE CONTOURS

Irregular surface contours can be compensated by wedges or full, individually tailored compensators.[3] One of the technical difficulties is the proper alignment of the compensating device with the surface. However, a small misalignment usually does not result in large inaccuracies. An exception to this rule would be the four-field box technique for treatment of the cervical esophagus (see Chapter 22, Carcinoma of the Cervical Esophagus). There is a sharp change in diameter of the lateral fields, and a small misplacement of the compensator in either direction would result in an incorrect dose. To eliminate this possible error, a large wax surface compensator is used. The disadvantage of this technique is the loss of skin sparing, although this has not presented a serious clinical problem in the esophagus technique; this disadvantage is offset by the simplicity of compensator fabrication and the ease of daily treatment alignment.

INTRAORAL BLOCKING

A beam absorber can sometimes be inserted intraorally for both photon and electron therapy to reduce transit irradiation. For example, if a simple orthovoltage treatment is to be given to the lower lip, a lead shield can easily be fabricated to spare the underlying structures from the transmitted radiation. When such shields are used, a thin (1 mm to 2 mm) coat of wax is necessary to protect the inner lip from backscatter dose from the lead shield. (See section on the lip in Chapter 17, Oral Cavity.)

If higher-energy photon or electron beams are used to treat lateralized lesions in the oral cavity or oropharynx, an intraoral shield can be of use. This shield is usually several centimeters thick (Fig. 15-20). Due to the variation from patient to patient, a variety of shapes and sizes are useful. Care must be given to the fabrication of the intraoral shield to avoid excessive backscatter from the lead to the adjacent tissue. The increase in dose due to backscatter is well documented for both gamma and electron radiation. Backscatter measurements from a lead surface for 250-kVp through 17-MV photons and 5-MeV through 20-MeV electrons are presented in Table 15-1.

For 250-kV photons and cobalt-60, a thin coat of wax over the lead is sufficient to absorb all of the backscattered beam. However, when the photon energy is increased to 8-MV or 17-MV x-rays, or when 5 MeV to 20 MeV electrons are used, a composite of 3 mm aluminum and 1 mm wax is required to reduce the backscatter dose from the electron beams. All intraoral blocks are fabricated with aluminum and beeswax, which eliminates the potential error of using the wrong shield for the high-energy photon beams. (See Fig. 17-52 in Chapter 17 for an example.)

FIG. 15-20. Intraoral block for high-energy photon and electron-beam treatment. The lead shield is covered with aluminum and wax to absorb extensive backscatter. Thin electron shields are coated with aluminum and wax for use behind a lip or ear.

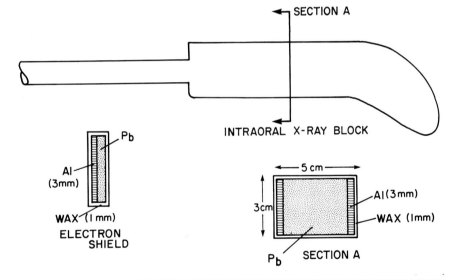

Millimeters of Absorber Placed Over 3 cm of Lead	250 kVp*	Cobalt-60*	8 MV*	17 MV*	5 MeV†	10 MeV†	20 MeV†
None	730	110	100	90	70	50	30
0.4 mm wax	0	50	60	70	ND	ND	ND
3.0 mm wax	0	0	20	30	ND	ND	ND
3.0 mm Al	ND	ND	20	30	10	10	20
3.0 mm Al + 1 mm wax	0	0	10	10	10	10	20

TABLE 15.1   Backscatter Measurements: Increase Above Homogeneous Dose (%)

* Relative ionization.

† Relative TLD response (Harshaw TLD–100 chips), measurements at a depth equal to D_{max}.

(ND = no data)

TABLE 15-2 Commonly Used Isotopes

Source	Half-Life	HVL (Pb)	Source Type	Type of Loading	Inventory	Sterilization	Dosimetry
Radium	1629 years	7.4 cm	Needles 0.51–6.0 cm A.L.	See Chapter 17, Oral Cavity. Afterloading not generally available; may be preloaded	Usually purchased	Generally not sterilized	Relatively simple due to rigid source lines
Cesium-137	30 years	5.3 cm	Needles 1–6 cm A.L.	Afterloading possible	Purchased or leased	Afterloading sheaths can be autoclaved	Same as radium
Iridium-192	72 days	0.3 cm	Seeds or wire	Routine afterloading	Usually ordered for each case	Nylon sheaths must be gas sterilized and allowed to vent for 24 to 48 hr	May be difficult when definable planes do not exist
Gold-198	2.7 days	0.3 cm	Seeds	Individual seed usually loaded into preloaded cartridges for use with implant gun	Ordered for each case	Generally not sterilized	Generally single plane, relatively simple
Iodine-125	60.2 days	0.025 mm	Seeds	Individual seed and preloaded	Ordered for each case	Flash sterilize prior to implantation	Volume implants have problems similar to iridium-192

(HVL, half-value layer; Pb, lead; A.L., active length)

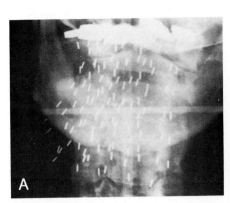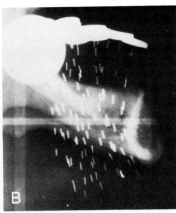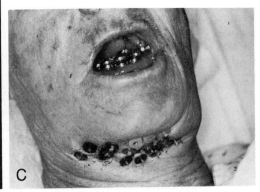

FIG. 15-21. (A) Anteroposterior roentgenogram of an iridium-192 implant in the floor of the mouth. The ability to use long, flexible sources is of substantial aid in implantation of large lesions. (B) Lateral roentgenogram. (C) For implants of the floor of the mouth, it is advantageous to shield the structures superior to the implant by capping the nylon afterloading tubes with gold or stainless-steel shields. Either crimping the ends of the source with metal buttons or melting the ends against nylon buttons secures the source in the nylon tubes. The small diameter and flexibility of the source result in little edema compared with a radium or cesium implant of the same volume.

INTERSTITIAL THERAPY

Interstitial therapy has undergone significant improvements in technique and dosimetry over the past few decades. As recently as the late 1960s, it was common to implant head and neck lesions free-hand with radium needles and compute the dose distribution with the Paterson-Parker or Quimby systems. This procedure did not allow a precise dose–volume computation. The Paterson-Parker tables were constructed to give an "effective minimum dose." This effective minimum dose was a dose 10% above the absolute minimum for a plane or volume. For planar implants, the point of specification was a plane 5 mm from the implant, while for multiple planes it was the midpoint between planes. For volume implants, the point of dose specification was 2 mm to 3 mm outside the circumference of the implant with a dose variation of 10% to 25% across the volume. These calculations did not identify regions of dose inhomogeneity.

The adoption of computer-based treatment planning systems in the 1960s allowed reconstruction of implants from orthogonal or stereo-shift roentgenograms for routine clinical use. Dose computations in planes of interest allowed the therapist to consider the dose inhomogeneity in prescribing the duration of the implant.

The choice of isotopes for implantation has also expanded from radium-226 (and radon-222) to include cesium-137, iridium-192, iodine-125, and gold-198 (Table 15-2).

Cesium-137

Cesium-137 needles are commonly used as a replacement for radium and are usually calibrated in milligrams of radium equivalent. The photon spectrum for cesium-137 is different from radium, but the dose distribution near the sources is similar due to the more important effect of inverse square.

The half-life of cesium-137 (30 years) is long enough to be ignored during a single implant. The entire inventory, however, must be decayed at the rate of 2% per year. This decay is the only disadvantage of cesium-137 when compared with radium-226. After 10 years the dose rate from an interstitial implant will be decreased by 20%. The biologic importance of dose rates is discussed in Chapter 13, Time–Dose–Volume Relationships in Radiation Therapy.

There is an advantage in radiation protection with cesium-137. The problem of leakage as experienced with radium is reduced. Cesium-137 can be effectively shielded with lesser thicknesses of lead or concrete.

Cesium-137 needles are of a smaller diameter than radium needles and can be obtained in an afterloading form. It may, however, be difficult to afterload the rigid needles in certain clinical situations.

While the use of cesium-137 addresses some of the problems of radiation protection, the problems of source lengths (<6 cm active length) and inability to implant along curved lines remain.

Iridium-192

Iridium-192 is usually obtained as seeds loaded into a flexible nylon sheath or thin, flexible wire sources used in the form of a "hairpin." The strength and interspacing of the sources can be altered to suit individual case requirements. For example, if an implant requires linear sources spanning 6 cm to 8 cm, the use of iridium-192 allows one source to span this length instead of using two cesium or radium sources in tandem.

The short half-life of iridium-192 (72 days) is both an advantage and a disadvantage. It usually requires the iridium to be ordered individually for each case, 4 to 5 workdays prior to the scheduled implant. However, this also allows the specification of source strength to be adjusted for each implant.

There are several techniques for implanting iridium-192. They all have the common advantage of afterloading.

This is a substantial advantage in large implants, for which the dose rate at 1 meter from the patient is often in excess of 100 mRem/hr. This high dose rate can pose a substantial protection problem in postoperative recovery. The ability to afterload the implant in the patient's room significantly reduces the problem of exposure of personnel; however, the high dose rates often require shielding of the hospital room.

While the flexibility of iridium sources enables complex implants to be performed, it also makes dosimetry substantially more complex. The location of 100 to 200 iridium seeds on orthogonal or stereo-shift roentgenograms is more difficult than the entry of linear sources. The matching of the dosimetry with the patient's anatomy is also difficult because of the absence of the plane that would have been created by rigid linear sources (Fig. 15-21).

Seed Implants

For areas where temporary implants are difficult to use, such as the soft palate and posterior pharyngeal wall, permanent seed implants have been used. They have also been used for molds and for palliative treatment of lymph node metastases. The isotopes currently available are radon-222, gold-198, and, more recently, iodine-125. Whereas radon-222 and gold-198 have similar time-dose schemes, iodine-125 is substantially different. The clinical effect of this difference is not known. While radon seeds are usually handled individually in the operating room, gold has the advantage of preloading into a cartridge (Fig. 15-22). Iodine also has similar devices available for implantation.

TREATMENT PLANNING FOR IMPLANTS

The preplanning of implants is particularly advantageous if custom preloaded devices are used or if isotope strength must be determined, such as for iridium-192, radon-222, and gold-198 implants. The best dose estimate is obtained by mocking up the implant and computing the dose distribution.

The reconstruction of the actual implant from either stereo shifts or orthogonal radiographs, while relatively simple for planar implants, is complex for volume implants. Seed identification becomes difficult and error checking is a necessary part of the reconstruction algorithm. When

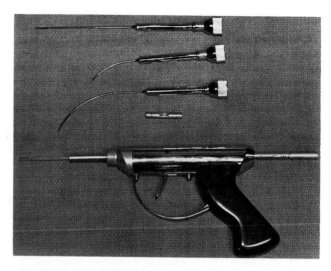

FIG. 15-22. Gold implant gun. Seeds are preloaded into the cartridges, which eliminates the individual handling of seeds during the procedure.

a large number of sources are to be matched, it is tempting to use stereo views and small shift distances (*i.e.*, 100-cm tube to implant distance ± 15-cm shifts). These small shifts may, however, result in large errors in source placement.[2] To minimize such errors, a shift distance should be used that is two thirds the tube-to-implant distance.

REFERENCES

1. Bova FJ, Hill LW: Surface doses for acrylic vs. lead acrylic blocking trays for cobalt-60, 8 MV, and 17 MV photons. Med Phys 10:254–256, 1983
2. Fitzgerald LT, Mauderli W: Analysis of errors in three-dimensional reconstruction of radium implants from stereo radiographs. Radiology 115:455–458, 1975
3. Sampiere VA: Radiation measurements and dosimetric practices. In Fletcher GH (ed): Textbook of Radiotherapy, 3rd ed, pp 1–40. Philadelphia, Lea & Febiger, 1980
4. Turner AP: Surface dose measurements Clinac 18 electron beams. Proceedings of the Eighth Varian Clinac Users Meeting, January 31 through February 2, 1980, Kauai, Hawaii, pp 13–17

The Unknown Primary

RODNEY R. MILLION
NICHOLAS J. CASSISI

"The Unknown Primary" sounds like the title for a whodunit rather than a medical treatise. In fact, the search for the site of origin of metastatic neck disease does resemble detective work, and the riddle is not always solved. Failure to detect the primary tumor site in patients presenting with metastatic cancer in neck lymph nodes represents 2% to 3% of the total head and neck cancer cases.[6]

Spontaneous remission of the primary site is assumed to have occurred in a portion of squamous cell carcinoma cases, since successful treatment of the neck and long-term follow-up may never reveal the site of origin.

At one time, many of these unknown primary neck masses were thought to arise from branchial cleft epithelial remnants in the soft tissue of the lateral neck, but current opinion argues against this site of origin.[7] Spontaneous remission is also occasionally reported for the primary site in breast cancer, testicular tumors, malignant melanoma, neuroblastoma, and others.

PATHOLOGY

The histology reflects the possible site of origin, but all too often the biopsy reveals a poorly differentiated carcinoma, which does not exclude much of anything. Poorly differentiated lymphomas and poorly differentiated carcinomas occur in the same age-group and histologically may appear similar.

Two neoplasms may coexist in the same node, such as chronic lymphocytic leukemia and metastatic squamous cell carcinoma.

Adenocarcinoma almost always originates from below the clavicles, but if it occurs in the upper neck a search for a major or minor salivary gland tumor, thyroid cancer, or the rare parathyroid cancer is required.

Metastatic melanoma may be particularly difficult to diagnose in the absence of melanin and with no obvious skin lesion.

Fishkin and Spiegelberg reported two cases in which plasmacytoma was diagnosed in cervical lymph nodes 2 years prior to the discovery of the primary lesions in the epiglottis and nasopharynx;[2] we have observed a similar case presenting in a supraclavicular lymph node with a primary site not discovered.

PATTERNS OF SPREAD

Squamous Cell Carcinoma

If only the metastatic neck masses are treated, the primary lesion may either never appear or appear later over a wide time range. The incidence of the primary lesion becoming manifest depends on the initial treatment. When only the neck is treated by surgery, the eventual appearance of a primary lesion in the head and neck region was reported as only 20% (Table 16-1).[4] This figure is low, since many patients die of regional persistence, distant metastasis, or intercurrent disease without a sufficient interval of observation. When the high-risk mucosal sites are irradiated, only 6% developed a head and neck primary lesion and these were all outside the radiation portals.[4] This 6% incidence is also probably low due to insufficient follow-up of many

TABLE 16-1. Location of Primary Lesion Appearing After Treatment (184 Patients)

Location	Surgery	Radiation Therapy	Combination Therapy
Hypopharynx	6	1	1
Tonsil or faucial arch	4	0	1
Base of tongue, vallecula	4	0	0
Oral cavity, salivary glands	2	2	0
Nasopharynx	2	0	0
Maxillary antrum	0	0	1
Aryepiglottic fold, epiglottis	1	0	1
Cervical esophagus	1	0	0
Thyroid	1	0	0
Total head and neck	21/104 (20%)*	3/52 (6%)†‡	4/28 (16%)‡
Below clavicle	5	3	1

* Primary lesion was controlled in 14/21 (8 by radiation therapy, 6 by surgery).
† Portals covered Waldeyer's ring in 45/52 patients.
‡ Primary lesion was controlled in 2/7 (by surgery).
(Jesse RH, Perez CA, Fletcher GH: Cervical lymph node metastasis: Unknown primary cancer. Cancer 31:854–859, 1973)

cases. Appearance of a mucosal lesion after 3 years may actually represent a new and totally unrelated problem and should be treated as such. The unknown primary site is only occasionally found at autopsy.[3]

Upper Neck

A solitary upper jugular chain mass is the most common situation, since virtually all head and neck cancers spread first to this area. Solitary upper neck lymph nodes uncommonly originate from below the clavicle. If the mass is high in the upper neck, between the angle of the mandible and the tip of the mastoid, it suggests origin in the nasopharynx, oropharynx, or occasionally malignant melanoma or other skin cancer. If the mass is a bit lower in the upper neck, the oral cavity, larynx, and hypopharynx must also be included as likely sites. Bilateral upper neck nodes point to the nasopharynx, base of the tongue, soft palate, supraglottic larynx, and pyriform sinus as sites of origin.

A solitary submaxillary mass suggests a site of origin in the oral cavity, lip, or nasal vestibule or a primary submaxillary gland salivary tumor.

A solitary submental mass is rare; lymphoma and sarcoma are considered along with carcinoma in the differential diagnosis.

Midneck

A solitary midneck mass favors a primary tumor of the larynx, hypopharynx, or, less commonly, the thyroid or cervical esophagus or disease originating below the clavicle.

Lower Neck

The solitary lower neck mass is most often metastatic from the chest or abdomen, but thyroid and cervical esophagus must be considered. Rarely, a primary lesion of the head and neck will present in the low jugular or low posterior cervical region, having skipped the upper neck nodes; thus the head and neck examination should not be overlooked for these presentations.

Miscellaneous Sites

A solitary spinal accessory mass suggests a nasopharyngeal primary site. A preauricular node mass of squamous cell carcinoma is almost always from a skin cancer and not a primary parotid neoplasm.[1] When multiple nodes are present, the location of the largest mass gives the same clue as a solitary mass.

Lymphoma and Leukemia

The distribution of the lymph nodes is a hint to the histology. Non–Hodgkin's lymphoma tends to involve the upper neck nodes, including the preauricular, mastoid, submental, and occipital lymph nodes. A careful search should be made for a mucosal primary lesion. Hodgkin's disease most often involves the lower neck nodes; a mucosal primary lesion is rare in Hodgkin's disease. Lymph nodes in patients with leukemia tend to be multiple, discrete, and bilateral.

CLINICAL PICTURE

The hallmark of the unknown primary syndrome in 75% of cases is a painless, solitary neck mass that is usually discovered by the patient. About 15% will have multiple ipsilateral masses, and the remaining 10% will have bilateral neck lymph node metastases.[4] The mass is usually a minimum of 2 cm to 3 cm, but often it is enormous. Since most benign neck masses also present as a solitary, painless mass, this history is of little help in the differential diagnosis. The patient often reports that the mass "suddenly appeared" overnight. Mild discomfort in a carcinomatous lymph node usually indicates pockets of necrosis. Large, fixed, upper neck lymph nodes produce pain in the temporal area. Huge neck masses result in lymphatic obstruction, and the resulting lymphedema may bulge the lateral pharyngeal wall and tonsillar area. A localized area of erysipelas may appear proximal to the lymphatic blockage. Palsy of the facial, glossopharyngeal, vagus, spinal accessory, and hypoglossal nerves and the sympathetic nerve chain may occur.

Physical Examination

Routine head and neck examination must include inspection of the scalp, skin, and ear canal. A surgical or radiation scar may indicate prior treatment for a skin neoplasm. The clinical impression may be enhanced by the physical characteristics of the mass; soft, rubbery, matted nodes suggest lymphoma and leukemia, while rock-hard or fixed masses are more often carcinoma. Invasion of the skin may occur with any histology, including lymphomas.

DIFFERENTIAL DIAGNOSIS AND STAGING

A list of the seemingly endless possibilities in the differential diagnosis is provided below:

Benign

Developmental
  Inclusion cysts (sublingual and submaxillary salivary glands)
  Thyroglossal duct cysts
  Congenital arteriovenous fistulas or aneurysms
  Branchial cleft cysts
  Cystic hygromas
  Laryngocele
  Teratomas
Inflammatory
  Benign reactive hyperplasia
  Lymphadenitis (associated with upper respiratory tract infections, dental disease, cat-scratch fever, infectious mononucleosis, dermatitis, and others)
  Infected sebaceous cyst
Benign neoplasms
  Hemangioma, lymphangioma
  Thyroid nodules or goiter
  Parathyroid adenomas
  Lipoma
  Fibroma
  Neurofibroma

Malignant

Metastatic carcinoma, sarcoma, or melanoma in lymph node
Lymphoma or leukemia
Carotid body tumor
Glomus jugulare tumor
Soft tissue, bone, or cartilage sarcoma
Primary major salivary gland tumor
Malignant melanoma
Adnexal carcinoma of the skin
Thyroid cancer
Parathyroid cancer
Direct extension of a head and neck neoplasm into the neck
Histiocytosis
Plasmacytoma
Carcinoid

The diagnosis by neck location for 207 patients who presented with cervical adenopathy and had a biopsy is shown in Table 16-2.[5] Only 10 (6%) were found to have squamous cell carcinoma without a demonstrable primary lesion. The most common diagnosis was a benign condition, except for supraclavicular lymph nodes. The age of the patient, the position of the mass, and the history will quickly narrow the possibilities. The vast majority of small lymph nodes in children are inflammatory or reactive nodes. Midline masses are usually benign, with the exception of those in the thyroid gland.

A malignant supraclavicular mass usually represents lymphoma or metastatic disease from below the clavicle, but in the odd case it may represent a regional metastasis from the cervical esophagus, a thyroid carcinoma, or even a primary sarcoma. If the histologic diagnosis is adenocarcinoma, then the search for the primary lesion is directed toward those primary sites for which specific therapy may be recommended: the thyroid, breast, endometrium, prostate, and the rare adrenal cortex carcinoma. All of these tumors may respond to specific hormonal or chemical treatment. The only lesion considered curable would be a carcinoma of the thyroid. It is usually fruitless and expensive to search for primary lesions in the lung, gastrointestinal tract, pancreas, ovary, and kidney, since there is no good specific treatment available for these malignancies. In any event, the primary lesion is found in less than 10% of patients in this situation.[9]

The remainder of this section will deal with the patient who presents with disease predominantly in the middle and upper neck; supraclavicular masses usually represent lymphoma or metastatic disease from below the clavicle.

The patient presenting with a neck mass is a common problem, and so are the errors surrounding the approach to diagnosis. An estimated 10% to 15% of patients with squamous cell carcinoma of the head and neck will present

TABLE 16-2. Diagnosis for 207 Patients Presenting With Cervical Lymphadenopathy

Location	Patients	Squamous Cell Carcinoma	Infraclavicular Metastasis	Lymphoma	Thyroid Carcinoma	Benign
Submental	15	0	0	13%	0	87%
Anterior cervical	25	12%	0	8%	20%	60%
Jugulodigastric	36	19%	14%	8%	8%	51%
Supraclavicular	49	0	39%	31%	2%	28%
Low postcervical	37	0	9%	39%	5%	47%

(Reprinted with permission from Johnson JT, Newman RK: The anatomic location of neck metastasis from occult squamous cell carcinoma. Otolaryngol Head Neck Surg 89:54–58, 1981)

because of a neck mass, and for carcinoma of the naso-pharynx it represents the most common presenting complaint. Unless a clinical diagnosis of benign disease is quite certain, the diagnosis must be pursued according to the age of the patient, the location of the mass, and the remainder of the history and physical examination. A trial of antibiotics may seem harmless but may dangerously delay the diagnosis and treatment, and the patient may not return for follow-up if the mass "gets a little smaller." In fact, lymphomatous masses, both Hodgkin's and non-Hodgkin's, will sometimes show a temporary decrease in size as part of their natural behavior. If the mass is probably a lymph node and lies in the upper two thirds of the neck, the most crucial part of the initial workup is a thorough search for a head and neck mucosal lesion.

In about 90% of cases, the primary lesion will be found by physical examination. It has often been our experience on several occasions to find the lesion after several previous thorough examinations, including an examination with the patient under anesthesia. *Repeated examinations and examinations by several physicians are the key to finding the primary lesion—not examination with the patient under anesthesia, random biopsies, or exotic roentgenographic studies.*

If the primary focus is not found by physical examination, then the workup depends on the age of the patient and the location of the mass. If lymphoma is suspected, the pathologist requires either a whole node or a generous portion of a large node for examination. This is especially true for Hodgkin's disease, and one of the largest accessible nodes should be excised, since smaller adjacent nodes are often not diagnostic (see Chapter 35, Lymphomas and Related Diseases Presenting in the Head and Neck). If carcinoma is suspected, a fine-needle aspiration biopsy will expedite the diagnosis with the least likelihood of disseminating tumor cells.[8] The histologic type (squamous cell carcinoma or adenocarcinoma) can often be determined and influences the direction of the workup. Needle biopsy is not done if the pathologist is unwilling to interpret the specimens obtained by needle, if lymphoma or leukemia is suspected, or if the mass is small and would be difficult to needle. If the result of the needle biopsy is negative, one should proceed to roentgenographic studies, including chest roentgenogram, barium examination of the esophagus, and computed tomographic (CT) scan of the nasopharynx and paranasal sinuses. The next step is examination with random biopsies with the patient under anesthesia; bronchoscopy and esophagoscopy are done at the same time. An excisional or incisional biopsy of the neck mass is done if a primary lesion is not found. Examination under anesthesia and roentgenographic studies uncommonly find the primary lesion. Fitzpatrick and Kotalik report that they did not find a single primary site by examination with the use of anesthesia and random biopsies in 86 patients;[3] our experience is similar. The biopsy of the neck mass is frequently done at the time of examination of the patient under anesthesia if results of prior needle biopsy were negative or confusing and if no primary site is found. The incision should be planned to facilitate either radical neck dissection or radiation therapy. Frozen section ensures that proper tissue is obtained.

Physicians unfamiliar with head and neck cancer diagnosis and treatment will frequently go directly to incisional biopsy of the neck mass after cursory or no examination of the mucous membranes. Although this approach does not exclude a curative result, it probably reduces the chance of cure and certainly increases the mor-bidity associated with treatment. If it is not malpractice, it is certainly poor practice, and patients are not amused by the physician who did not bother with a thorough head and neck examination.

TREATMENT

This section will deal only with those situations in which a primary focus is not found, the histologic diagnosis is squamous cell carcinoma, and *the location of the lymph node(s) favors a head and neck mucous membrane site of origin.*

Selection of Treatment Modality

It is clear that some patients will be cured by therapy confined to the neck, particularly the group with a solitary, well-differentiated subdigastric mass. However, should the primary lesion subsequently appear in the head and neck, many patients are unsuccessfully managed and the 3-year survival rate is reduced by one half.[4] For this reason, nearly every patient in our clinic receives elective irradiation of the nasopharynx, oropharynx, supraglottic larynx, pyriform sinus, and both sides of the neck as the initial therapy. An appropriate neck dissection is then added, as outlined in Chapter 4, General Principles for Treatment of Cancers in the Head and Neck: Selection of Treatment for the Primary Site and for the Neck. This approach represents a certain amount of overkill. It has the advantage of complete treatment at the first instance with a small risk of a primary lesion subsequently appearing and an excellent chance of neck control with combined therapy. The major disadvantage is the sequela of xerostomia after 5500 rad to 6000 rad/7 weeks.

If the patient has a solitary, well-differentiated, mobile, low subdigastric node, then neck dissection alone may be sufficient according to some authors, and the primary lesion is treated if it appears.[4] Our own practice is to irradiate electively most of these patients.

The neck control according to the treatment plan is shown in Table 16-3. If the lymph node has been excised, then radiation therapy alone (with a boost to the scar) is sufficient. In the early years, we treated the neck for cure with radiation therapy alone if the lymph nodes regressed completely during therapy, and the results for N2A–N2B disease were good. However, we now prefer to reduce the radiation dose to the neck and add a neck dissection, since the ultimate control rate is better and the neck fibrosis is less after 1 year. It is a moot point whether to do the neck dissection prior to radiation therapy or afterward for stages N2A and N2B disease, and it probably makes little difference. However, for N3A disease we prefer to start with radiation therapy because the lymph node is usually fixed. Treatment of N3B disease must be individualized.

LOW NECK DISEASE

Supraclavicular node(s) usually represent metastasis from the chest, abdomen, or breast and therefore are an incurable situation.

If the patient is otherwise in excellent condition, an attempt should be made to control the supraclavicular disease, as a few patients live quite a long time before other disease becomes manifest; an occasional patient with either squamous cell carcinoma or adenocarcinoma is reported

TABLE 16-3.   Unknown Primary Lesion: Control in Treated Necks*

Stage	Radiation Therapy	Surgery + Radiation Therapy	Radiation Therapy + Surgery
NX–N1	6/6	0/0	0/0
N2A	3/3	0/0	1/1
N2B	4/4	0/1	0/0
N3A	1/2	1/4	3/5
N3B	0/2	1/1	1/1
Total	14/17	2/6	5/7

* Six patients are excluded from analysis who died of intercurrent disease or distant metastases with less than 2 years' survival with no *known* neck disease at the time of death.

Note: University of Florida data; patients treated 10/64–2/80; analysis 2/82 by T. A. Brant, MD.

to live over 5 years with a primary focus never being observed. Radical neck dissection is seldom recommended. Those patients who are pursuing a downhill course are either given a short course of palliative radiation therapy (e.g., 1000 rad × 2, 1 week apart) or just observed.

Surgical Treatment

A discussion of neck dissection is provided in Chapter 5, General Principles for Treatment of Cancers in the Head and Neck: Surgery.

Irradiation Technique

Treatment planning depends on the location of the lymph nodes. Upper and midjugular lymph nodes indicate elective irradiation of the nasopharynx, oropharynx, supraglottic larynx, hypopharynx, and both sides of the neck to the level of the clavicles. A solitary submaxillary lymph node is preferably treated by neck dissection and observation, since irradiation of the entire oral cavity plus the neck causes major morbidity. A preauricular lymph node (or nodes) containing squamous cell carcinoma almost always represents metastasis from a skin cancer and is treated by a combination of parotidectomy and radiation therapy or radiation therapy alone (See Chapter 26, Carcinoma of the Skin.) Supraclavicular nodes are irradiated through a generous regional portal, which should include the adjacent apex of the axilla.

An analysis of the dose for control at the primary site revealed an in-field failure rate of 2 of 13 with 5000 rad/ 5 to 6 weeks and 0 of 8 for 5500 rad to 6000 rad/6 to 7 weeks. There have been two in-field failures (base of the tongue) with continuous therapy, one at 5000 rad/6 weeks and another at 5000 rad/5 weeks. The recommended dose is 5500 rad/6 weeks to 6000 rad/7 weeks, 180 rad/fraction. It is probably safe to insert a 2-week split midway in the therapy without risking mucosal recurrence. If there is a suspicion of a primary focus, but no proof, an extra 500 rad may be added to a specific site, especially if a total dose of 5000 rad is selected. It is important to spare a midline strip of neck skin to avoid lymphedema. An individualized treatment plan for a patient with bilateral neck disease is shown in Figure 16-1.

The neck is usually thinner than the head, and this difference must be adjusted by compensators or portal reductions at appropriate times.

Management of Recurrence

If a head and neck primary lesion appears, management is individualized. If radiation therapy has not been used, the treatment decisions are governed by the anatomical site. If the new lesion is well outside a prior irradiation field and unsuitable for operation, irradiation may be considered. Limited recurrence in the neck may be suitable for radical re-treatment by surgery, radiation therapy, or both. The appearance of a new lymph node in the neck requires repeat workup for a primary site.

RESULTS OF TREATMENT

Fitzpatrick and Kotalik, at Princess Margaret Hospital, Toronto, reported 233 patients presenting with an unknown primary lesion.[3] The 5-year absolute survival rate was 18%. Among 68 patients with disease limited to the upper neck and midneck treated by irradiation to the neck and suspected primary sites and receiving a minimum dose of 4500 rad/4 weeks, the 5-year survival rate was 44%. The recurrence rate in the neck was 26% (18 of 68). The results were the same for squamous cell carcinoma and anaplastic carcinoma.

Jesse and co-workers reported the M. D. Anderson Hospital experience for 184 patients with disease limited to neck nodes (excluding supraclavicular presentations).[4] Treatment was individualized. The 3-year absolute survival rate was 53%, and the 5-year absolute survival rate was 43% of 151 patients. The survival by N stage and therapeutic category is shown in Table 16-4. The location of the primary lesion appearing after initial treatment is given in Table 16-1. There were no new mucosal lesions appearing within the irradiated areas. Although many of the patients were said to have had successful local treatment when the primary lesion finally appeared, the eventual result was poor due to reseeding of the neck or to distant metastases. The 3-year survival rate was 31% for those in whom a primary focus appeared, compared with 58% for those who never developed a primary lesion. Since the

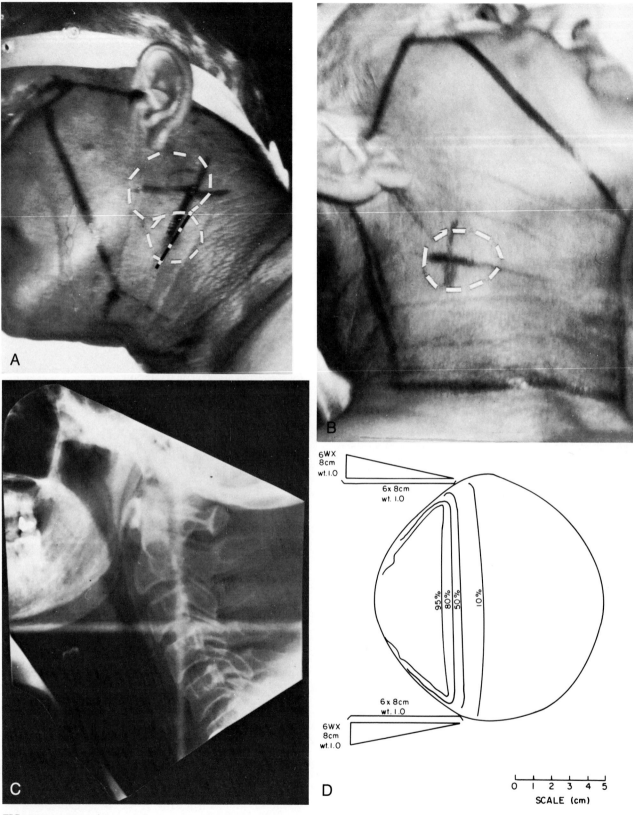

FIG. 16-1 (continued)

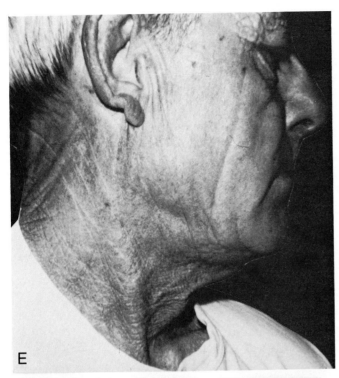

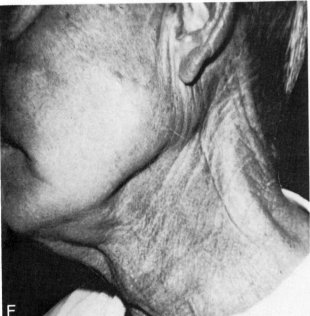

FIG. 16-1. A 51-year-old white male patient presented with a 3-month history of a mass in the left neck. Multiple physical examinations and endoscopy with random biopsies of the nasopharynx, tonsillar fossae, base of the tongue, and pyriform sinuses revealed no mucosal primary lesion. An incisional biopsy was used to obtain tissue from the left neck node. Poorly differentiated carcinoma was reported. (A) The left neck contained a 5.3 × 3.0-cm high subdigastric node and an immediately subjacent 3 × 3-cm area of induration beneath the surgical scar (*dashed line*). No mucosal primary lesion was apparent. (B) There was a 4 × 5-cm right subdigastric node (*dashed line*). (C) Five thousand rad in 30 fractions was administered to the "unknown primary" treatment volume shown, including the nasopharynx, oropharynx, hypopharynx, and supraglottic larynx. The lower border includes the cricoid cartilage (C6). Note sparing of an anterior skin strip. The lower neck was treated with an anterior field (5000 rad given dose/ 25 fractions). (D) The right neck node was boosted by an additional 2000-rad tumor dose specified at the 95% normalized isodose line, cobalt-60, with a combination of anterior and posterior open and wedge fields. Weights (*wt.*) refer to the relative given doses to each of the four fields. The total tumor dose to the right neck node was 7000 rad/ 8 weeks. The medial field edge was placed 2 cm off the midline. For the posterior field, the patient was prone. The dose to the spinal cord from the tangential fields was less than 10% of the tumor dose. Because of the large volume of disease in the left neck, a radical neck dissection was performed 6 weeks after irradiation. No tumor was found in 38 nodes. (E and F) The patient was asymptomatic 6 years after treatment except for moderate xerostomia. He was using fluoride daily, and his teeth remained in good condition.

subsequent appearance of a primary lesion halves the survival rate, our practice has been to use elective mucosal and neck irradiation at the time of initial neck treatment for most cases, including solitary subdigastric nodes. The absolute and determinate 2-year and 5-year survival rates by stage and treatment for 36 cases are shown in Table 16-5.

FOLLOW-UP POLICY

Follow-up includes a thorough head and neck examination at monthly intervals for 2 years and less frequently thereafter. Routine head and neck roentgenograms are not obtained unless indicated by the history.

COMPLICATIONS OF TREATMENT

The operative complications are essentially those associated with neck dissection.

The main radiation therapy complication is xerostomia. If the mucosal dose is 5000 rad/6 weeks to 6000 rad/7 weeks, there should be no persistent edema even though the entire supraglottic larynx and hypopharynx are included and a neck dissection is added. There has been one minor bone exposure in 36 cases.*

* Brant TA: Unpublished data, 1982.

TABLE 16-4. Three-Year Absolute Survival, Free of Cancer

Stage	Surgery		Radiation Therapy		Combination Therapy	
NX	31/39	(79%)	8/9	(89%)	3/3	
N1	4/6	(67%)	1/3		1/3	
N2	10/22	(45%)	3/4	(75%)	5/9	(55%)
N3	14/37	(38%)	13/36	(36%)	4/13	(31%)
Total	59/104*	(57%)	25/52†	(48%)	13/28†	(47%)

* Salvage in eight patients by radiation therapy and six patients by surgery.
† Salvage in one patient by surgery.
Note: M. D. Anderson Hospital data; 184 patients treated 7/48–6/68.
(Jesse RH, Perez CA, Fletcher GH: Cervical lymph node metastasis: Unknown primary cancer. Cancer 31:854–859, 1973)

TABLE 16-5. Absolute Survival

Stage	Radiation Therapy Alone		Radiation Therapy + Surgery		Total	
	2-Year	5-Year	2-Year	5-Year	2-Year	5-Year
NX-N1	6/6	5/6	0/0	0/0	6/6	5/6
N2A	3/3	2/2	1/1	1/1	4/4	3/3
N2B	4/5	2/4	0/2	0/2	4/7	2/6
N3A	1/2	0/2	6/11	2/8	7/13	2/10
N3B	0/2	0/2	2/4	2/3	2/6	2/5
Total					23/36 (66%)	14/30 (48%)

Note: Determinate survival: 2-year, 23/33 (70%); 5-year, 14/27 (52%).
Note: University of Florida data; patients treated 10/64–2/80; analysis 2/82 by T. A. Brant, MD.

REFERENCES

1. Cassisi NJ, Dickerson DR, Million RR: Squamous cell carcinoma of the skin metastatic to parotid nodes. Arch Otolaryngol 104:336–339, 1978
2. Fishkin BG, Spiegelberg HL: Cervical lymph node metastasis as the first manifestation of localized extramedullary plasmacytoma. Cancer 38:1641–1644, 1976
3. Fitzpatrick PJ, Kotalik JF: Cervical metastases from an unknown primary tumor. Radiology 110:659–663, 1974
4. Jesse RH, Perez CA, Fletcher GH: Cervical lymph node metastasis: Unknown primary cancer. Cancer 31:854–859, 1973
5. Johnson JT, Newman RK: The anatomic location of neck metastasis from occult squamous cell carcinoma. Otolaryngol Head Neck Surg 89:54–58, 1981
6. Nordstrom DG, Tewfik HH, Latourette HB: Cervical lymph node metastases from an unknown primary. Int J Radiat Oncol Biol Phys 5:73–76, 1979
7. Shaw HJ: Metastatic carcinoma in cervical lymph nodes with occult primary tumours—diagnosis and treatment. J Laryngol Otol 84:249–265, 1970
8. Simpson GT II: The evaluation and management of neck masses of unknown etiology. Otolaryngol Clin N Am 13:489–498, 1980
9. Templer J, Perry MC, Davis WE: Metastatic cervical adenocarcinoma from unknown primary tumor: Treatment dilemma. Arch Otolaryngol 107:45–47, 1981

Oral Cavity

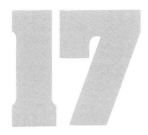

RODNEY R. MILLION
NICHOLAS J. CASSISI

The oral cavity consists of the lip, floor of the mouth, oral tongue (the anterior two thirds of the tongue), buccal mucosa, upper and lower gingiva, hard palate, and retromolar trigone. The relative frequency of involvement by cancer for the various oral cavity sites is shown in Table 17-1.[28] The asymptomatic, early, red lesions are most often diagnosed on the floor of the mouth and the lateral surface of the oral tongue in the oral cavity and the soft palate in the oropharynx.[32]

Asymptomatic, red lesions 1 mm to 5 mm in diameter have an equal chance of being carcinoma in situ or invasive carcinoma; lesions measuring 6 mm to 2 cm are more likely (3:1) to be invasive, and nearly all red lesions over 2 cm in diameter are invasive.[32]

The squamous mucosa of the oral cavity consists for the most part of a thick layer of squamous cells with rete pegs and a keratin layer. However, the floor of the mouth and the undersurface and lateral sides of the tongue have a thin mucosa with little surface keratin; coincidentally, these are the most frequent sites of cancer.

Squamous cell carcinomas of the oral cavity occur mostly in men after the age of 45 and are associated with the use of tobacco and alcohol.

The American Joint Committee (AJCC) staging system for all primary tumors of the oral cavity is listed below.[1]

TX   Minimum requirements to assess the primary tumor cannot be met.

T0   No evidence of primary tumor

Tis   Carcinoma in situ

T1   Greatest diameter of primary tumor 2 cm or less

T2   Greatest diameter of primary tumor more than 2 cm but not more than 4 cm

T3   Greatest diameter of primary tumor more than 4 cm

T4   Massive tumor more than 4 cm in diameter with deep invasion to involve antrum, pterygoid muscles, base of the tongue, or skin of the neck

LIP

Cancer of the lip occurs more often in men (50:1). People with light-colored skin or with prolonged exposure to sunlight are most prone to develop lip carcinoma. Cigarette smoking is probably a causative agent; the relationship of the development of the disease to pipe smoking is undecided. Most cases appear after age 40, but about 10% occur before age 40 and a few cases are seen before age 30. The disease is uncommon in blacks.

Anatomy

The lips are composed of the orbicularis muscle, with skin on the external surface and mucous membrane on the internal surface. The transition from skin to mucous membrane of the oral cavity is the dry lip vermilion, where the muscle is covered by a very thin layer of squamous epithelium that allows the underlying vasculature to show, thus giving the lips their reddish color. The blood supply is the labial artery, a branch of the facial artery. The motor nerves are branches of the facial nerve. The sensory nerve to the lower lip is the mental nerve, which is a branch of the inferior alveolar nerve. The commissure is supplied in part by the buccal branch of the

239

TABLE 17-1. Distribution of Oral Cavity Cancer: 1717 Total Cases (M. D. Anderson Hospital)

Location	Percentage
Lip	44.9%
Oral tongue	16.5%
Floor of mouth	12.1%
Gingiva, lower	12.1%
Palate/upper gingiva	4.7%
Buccal mucosa	9.7%

(Data from MacComb WS, Fletcher GH, Healey JE Jr: Intra-oral cavity. In MacComb WS, Fletcher GH [ed]: Cancer of the Head and Neck, pp 89–151. Copyright © 1967, the Williams & Wilkins Co., Baltimore)

mandibular nerve. The sensory nerve to the upper lip is the infraorbital branch of the maxillary nerve.

Pathology

The most common neoplasms are low-grade squamous cell carcinomas; about 5% are high grade. Basal cell carcinomas arise from the skin of the lip and may invade the vermilion, but do not arise from the vermilion. Verrucous carcinomas are rare. Benign lesions such as hemangiomas, fibromas, and cysts may involve the lips.

Severe dysplasia and leukoplakia are common problems on the lower lip and may precede the appearance of carcinoma by many years. Keratoacanthoma may occur and be mistaken for squamous cell carcinoma. Primary lesions arising from the moist mucosa of the lip are considered in the section on buccal mucosa.

Patterns of Spread

Squamous cell carcinomas start on the vermilion of the lower lip, rarely on that of the upper lip. They usually appear on the sun-exposed vermilion between the commissures. The commissure is rarely the site of origin. Early lesions first invade adjacent skin and the orbicularis muscle, which lies very near the surface.

Advanced lesions invade the adjacent commissures of the lip and buccal mucosa, the skin and wet mucosa of the lip, the adjacent mandible, and eventually the mental nerve. Perineural invasion occurred in 2% of the cases reported by Byers and co-workers and was related to recurrent lesions, large tumor size, mandibular invasion, and poorly differentiated histology.[7] Lymphatic spread from the lower lip is to the submental, submaxillary, and subdigastric lymph nodes and rarely to a facial node. Lesions located near the midline may spread to either side, and when the skin of the lip is invaded the spread pattern may be erratic owing to lack of valves in the dermal lymphatic vessels. The lymphatic drainage of the upper lip is primarily to the submaxillary lymph nodes, but occasionally the preauricular and parotid lymph nodes may be involved. Lymph node involvement occurs in 5% to 10% on admission, but in 19% for commissure lesions because of asso-

ciated mucosal involvement. Five to 10% of patients with a clinically negative neck will subsequently develop lymph node metastasis.[30] The risk of lymphatic involvement is increased by high-grade histology, large lesions, spread to involve the wet mucosa of the lip and buccal mucosa, and invasion of the dermis; it is especially increased in patients with recurrent disease. Although the lymph node metastases are relatively uncommon for early, low-grade lesions, they may be missed because they may not become evident for 3 to 4 years.

Clinical Picture

Asymptomatic, red lesions are sometimes seen and resemble other red lesions of the oral cavity. Carcinoma of the lip may present as an enlarging, exophytic lesion that is nontender unless it ulcerates and becomes infected. Occasionally there will be minor bleeding. These lesions are easily diagnosed by their appearance. However, some lesions develop very slowly on a background of leukoplakia and present as superficially ulcerated lesions with little or no bulk and a history of repeated episodes of scab formation without complete healing. These lesions are not so easy to diagnose clinically, and only excisional biopsy provides the answer.

Erythema of the adjacent skin suggests dermal lymphatic invasion. Palpation of the lip will reveal the extent of induration. Anesthesia or paresthesia of the skin of the lip indicates mental nerve invasion; however, nerve invasion may be encountered at operation in the absence of symptoms.

Methods of Diagnosis and Staging

The differential diagnosis includes actinic cheilitis, leukoplakia, herpes simplex, keratoacanthoma, keratosis, syphilitic chancre, cysts, fibromas, myeloblastomas, benign mixed tumors, hemangiomas, pyogenic granulomas, and papillomas.

The diagnosis is readily established by biopsy, or, if the lesion is not discrete, a cheiloplasty (lip shave) may be done. Mandible films are requested when bone or mental nerve involvement is suspected. The mental foramen may be enlarged in patients with nerve invasion.

The AJCC staging for oral cavity cancer (presented earlier in this chapter) includes only the lesions arising from those portions of the lips that oppose each other (i.e., the dry vermilion).

Treatment

SELECTION OF TREATMENT MODALITY

LEUKOPLAKIA, HYPERKERATOSIS, CHEILITIS, CARCINOMA *IN SITU*

These superfical lesions are managed by vermilionectomy ("lip shave") with or without a small cuff of muscle, depending on the thickness of the lesion.

SQUAMOUS CELL CARCINOMA

Early Lesions (0.5 cm to 1.5 cm)
The majority of the early lesions are surgically excised and closed primarily, either as outpatient procedures or

with a short inpatient stay. The excision may be combined with a cheiloplasty.

Radiation therapy produces equal cure rates. Implantation with gold or radon seeds is a short outpatient procedure that is performed with the use of local anesthesia and is equivalent in cure rate, time, and cost to an excision. A removable interstitial implant requires a 7-day hospitalization, and external-beam therapy requires several outpatient visits. In order to produce long-term cosmetic results comparable to excision of small lesions, external-beam therapy is preferably protracted over 3 to 5 weeks; shorter courses cure the patient, but many will develop progressive radiation changes with the passing years.

Irradiation would be selected for lesions involving excision of the commissure, for lesions greater than 1.5 cm on the lower lip, and for all but the smallest lesions of the upper lip, since the cosmetic and functional result would be better (Figs. 17-1 and 17-2). The occasional poorly differentiated lesion is preferably treated by radiation therapy in order to cover a more generous treatment volume and perhaps include the first-echelon lymph nodes. (See also section on skin of the upper lip and lip commissure in Chapter 26, Carcinoma of the Skin.)

Moderately Advanced Lesions (1.5 cm to 5.0 cm)

The length of the lower lip is 4 cm to 5 cm; it may be shorter in edentulous patients or in those who have had prior surgery. Removal of greater than 2 cm (40%) of the lower lip followed by simple closure often produces a relatively poor cosmetic and functional result and therefore requires a reconstructive procedure. If reconstruction will be required, radiation therapy has the advantage of a relatively better functional and cosmetic result with intact muscle and skin innervation. These larger lesions are managed by interstitial implantation, external-beam irradiation, or both (Fig. 17-3).

Advanced Lesions

Advanced lesions may have extensive infiltration of neighboring skin and muscle, involvement of the labial commissure and buccal mucosa with extension to the upper lip, or invasion of the mandible and nerve. Lesions with invasion of bone and/or nerve invasion are selectively managed by resection and postoperative radiation therapy. Skin involvement is best managed initially with radiation therapy, since the dermal lymphatics are involved (inflammatory carcinoma) and wide coverage of the primary lesion is indicated (Fig. 17-4). Surgical resection may or may not be added depending on the response to radiation therapy. Most of these advanced lesions can be cured with careful planning.

SURGICAL TREATMENT

VERMILIONECTOMY

There are three basic types of vermilionectomy or lip shave. A simple excision of the vermilion to the orbicularis muscle is used for very superficial lesions such as hyperkeratosis and leukoplakia, when there is no underlying induration (Fig. 17-5, *left*). A modified vermilionectomy includes a transverse wedge of the underlying orbicularis muscle and is usually used for carcinoma *in situ*, very early superficial multicentric lesions, chronic cheilitis with some thickening of the vermilion, persistent noncancerous ulcers, and even a redundant lip (Fig. 17-5, *center*). In

(Text continues on p. 245.)

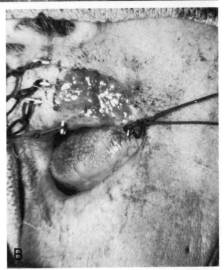

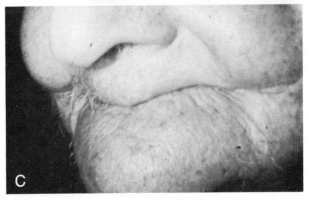

FIG. 17-1. An 88-year-old woman presented with a lesion on the upper lip that she had had for 10 years. (A) Squamous cell carcinoma of the upper lip with involvement of the vermilion and skin. The lesion measured 2.5 × 1.5 × 1.0 cm. The patient was admitted for excision, but owing to "poor risk for surgery," it was elected to use radiation therapy. (B) A single-plane radium needle implant was performed with the use of local anesthesia, 7000 rad specified at 0.5 cm. The crusts were removed prior to implant. The implant area was 4 × 2 cm. (C) Eight months after treatment. The patient died 3 years later of intercurrent disease with no evidence of recurrence.

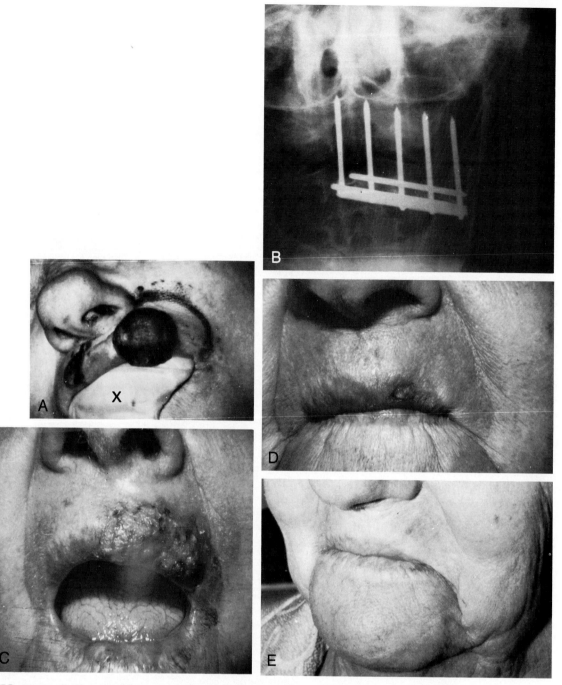

FIG. 17-2. A 72-year-old woman presented with a rapidly growing, moderately differentiated squamous cell carcinoma of the left upper lip. The globular lesion was 2.5
cm in diameter with induration in the lip extending to 3 cm maximum diameter. The
maximum thickness was 1.5 cm. Radiation therapy was selected because of the large
size and the extensive reconstruction that would be required after excision. (*A*) External-
beam irradiation was used initially to flatten the lesion to facilitate the placement of
an implant (3000 rad/3½ weeks, 170 rad/day, 250 kV, Thoreus III). A lead shield
(covered with a condom) was inserted under the upper lip (*X*). There was complete
flattening of the very bulky lesion prior to radium implant with only residual induration
and superficial ulceration remaining in the lip. The ink marks outline the external-
beam portal, which included part of the columella and lateral ala nasi. (*B*) A single-
plane implant was done using five, 2-cm active length needles held in a bar; two crossing
needles were attached to the bar. A cylindrical pack was sutured behind the upper lip
to displace the lip and radium from the upper gum; another pack was tied to the bar
to space the lower lip away from the needles. (*C*) Moist desquamation 2 weeks following
the implant. (*D*) Nearly complete healing at 5 weeks. (*E*) Two years following treatment
and free of disease.

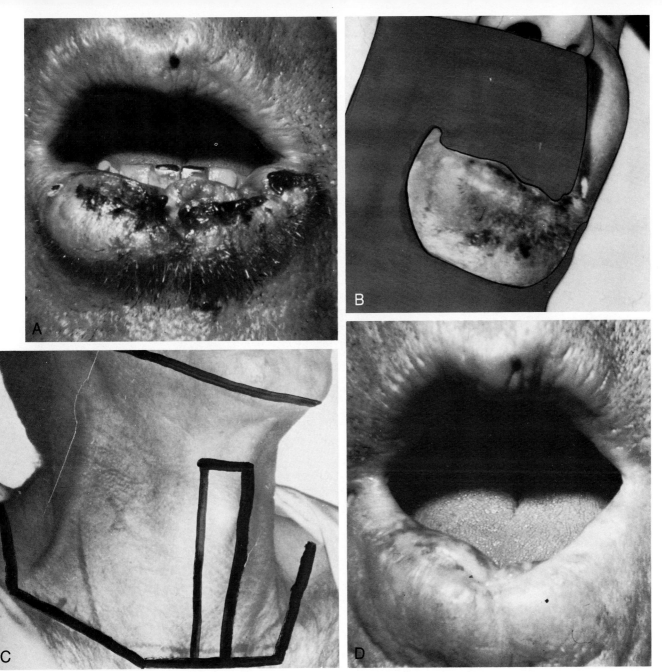

FIG. 17-3. A 46-year-old commercial fisherman presented with a lesion that was first noted 14 months prior to treatment. Nine months before treatment, a biopsy proved negative. A rebiopsy 7 months prior to treatment again showed no tumor. A third biopsy revealed well differentiated epidermoid carcinoma of the lip. (*A*) The lesion was large and infected, involving the left commissure and three fourths of the lower lip. The induration extended from commissure to commissure and 2 cm beyond the gross lesion. There were small, mobile, firm submaxillary nodes that were considered positive. The lesion was staged T3N3B. Radiation therapy was elected because of the extent of disease. (*B*) The initial treatment consisted of 5000 rad/4½ weeks with orthovoltage (250 kV, Thoreus III). A lead shield was fashioned to outline the portal. An extension of the lead fits behind the lower lip to reduce transit irradiation. (*C*) The entire neck was irradiated using a single anterior cobalt-60 field, 5000 rad/5 weeks; the larynx was shielded. Treatment to the lip was completed with a single-plane radium implant using six vertical needles; 1500 rad was added at 0.5 cm. The patient underwent bilateral supraomohyoid neck dissection because of the clinically positive nodes. Metastatic squamous cell carcinoma was found in one right neck node adjacent to the submaxillary gland; there were no positive nodes in the left neck. A biopsy of the lip at the time of neck dissection showed no residual tumor. (*D*) Appearance 2½ years after treatment. Patient is free of disease at 6 years and has been encouraged to wear a surgical mask while fishing.

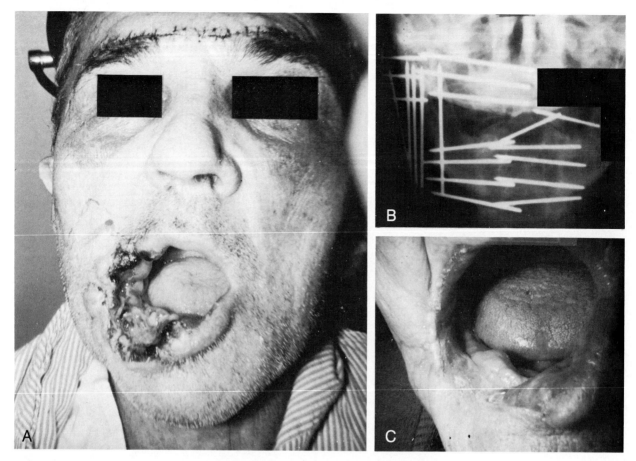

FIG. 17-4. A 66-year-old man presented with a progressively enlarging ulcer of the lip. He refused to seek medical help until his neighbors reported him to the local health department. (*A*) The patient was admitted for surgical resection and repair and actually underwent the elevation of a forehead flap before the decision was made to treat him with radiation therapy. The lesion occupied two thirds of the lower lip, the commissure, and one third of the right upper lip. There was obvious gross tumor extending along the cheek for 5 cm; the diameter of the lesion was 8 × 6 cm. There were no clinically positive nodes. The patient received 6000 rad, split course, over 7½ weeks, 250 kV, Thoreus III. (*B*) A large single-plane radium implant added 2500 rad. (*C*) There was nearly complete healing by 3 months and no obvious tumor; at 9 months there was only smooth induration and no obvious tumor. Reconstruction was offered, but the patient declined.

FIG. 17-5. Vermilionectomy. (*Left*) Superficial lesion. Dry vermilion is excised down to muscle and wet mucosa is advanced. Muscle is not removed. (*Center*) A small cuff of muscle is included if the lesion is suspicious for early invasion. (*Right*) The hair shafts are removed at the vermilion/skin junction to avoid annoying hair growth that accompanies the superior movement of skin.

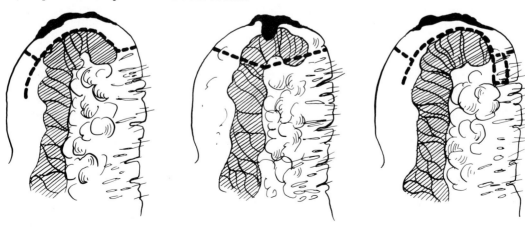

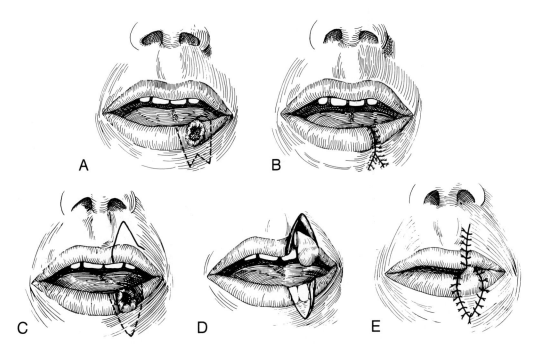

FIG. 17-6. Small lip lesions not involving the oral commissure can be removed using a W excision (*A*) and closed primarily (*B*). Larger lesions of the lip may be removed in a V fashion (*C*) and the defect closed using an Abbe flap from the upper lip (*D*), with a second procedure to release the flap 2 weeks later (*E*). (Million RR, Cassisi NJ, Wittes RE: Cancer in the head and neck. In DeVita VT Jr, Hellman S, Rosenberg SA [eds]: Cancer: Principles and Practice of Oncology, pp 301–395. Philadelphia, JB Lippincott, 1982)

many patients who have a squamous cell carcinoma of the lip, there are associated changes on the remainder of the lower lip, and an excision of the lip lesion may be combined with a vermilionectomy.

Vermilionectomy is done with the use of either a local infiltration anesthetic or a general anesthetic. The wet mucosa is then advanced and sutured to the skin anteriorly. Initially there is no sensation to the lip, and patients must be aware of the potential for burning the lip until sensation returns. In some cases, the procedure causes the skin edge to be everted toward the oral cavity and the hair on the skin grows at such an angle that it causes an irritation of the upper lip or tongue when the lips are wetted. One or 2 mm of the deep layer of the dermis, which contains the hair follicles, can be excised at the time of lip shave to avoid this aggravation (Fig. 17-5, *right*).

The complications of this procedure are usually minor and uncommon, and the cosmetic result is good. It would be quite rare to have a carcinoma develop on a resurfaced lip, unless carcinoma had been present at the time of the resurfacing. One patient was seen who had developed a lip cancer 20 years after lip shave.

EXCISION

Surgical treatment for early lesions (0.5 cm to 1.5 cm) involves a W- or U-shaped excision (Fig. 17-6).[38] V-shaped excisions may be used for very small lesions but do not give as good a margin for the larger tumors. Larger lesions (over 1.5 cm) may be closed with a full-thickness pedicle flap from the upper lip to reconstruct the lower lip defect. If the vermilion is diffusely involved, with little or no involvement of the muscle, then a cheiloplasty (lip shave)

may be done and the wet mucosa from the oral cavity advanced to cover the defect. If the commissure must be sacrificed, it must be reconstructed in order to prevent microstomia and also to allow the edentulous patient enough opening to insert dentures.

RESECTION OF ADVANCED LESIONS OF THE LIP

Surgical resection of large lesions of the upper or lower lip is generally reserved for radiation failure or for lesions that involve bone or nerve. A variety of flaps are available for reconstruction, depending on the extent of tissue to be replaced. If the superior or anterior margin of the arch of the mandible is involved, a rim resection may be added.

IRRADIATION TECHNIQUE

Lip cancer may be successfully treated by external-beam irradiation, interstitial implants, or a combination of both (see Figs. 17-1 through 17-4 and 17-7 through 17-9).

Interstitial implants may be accomplished with removable sources such as radium needles or iridium-192. Gold or radon seeds may be permanently implanted as an outpatient procedure with the use of a local anesthetic and the patient sent home the same day, radiation exposure permitting.

External-beam techniques use orthovoltage or electrons with lead shields behind the lip to limit exit irradiation. The dose schemes are similar to those used for skin cancer. (See Chapter 26, Carcinoma of the Skin.) Fractionation schemes of 4 to 6 weeks are preferred over the shorter regimens in order to diminish the late effects of atrophy, telangiectasis, fibrosis, and ulceration. Bulky lesions may be first treated with external-beam irradiation, 3000 rad to 5000 rad, and treatment completed by interstitial therapy (see Figs. 17-2, 17-4, and 17-7).

The regional lymphatics are not electively treated for early cases. Advanced lesions, poorly differentiated lesions, and especially recurrent lesions should have either elective neck irradiation or elective neck dissection, depending on the treatment selected for the primary lesion. Clinically positive nodes are managed according to policies outlined in Chapter 4, General Principles for Treatment of Cancers in the Head and Neck: Selection of Treatment for the Primary Site and for the Neck.

MANAGEMENT OF RECURRENCE

Although the overall cure rate for lip cancer is quite high, the patient with a recurrence is at significant risk to die of the disease, and treatment must be carefully planned. Most surgical failures are managed by radiation therapy since a large amount of lower lip would need to be resected (Fig. 17-8). A combination of surgery and radiation therapy may be selected in certain situations (Fig. 17-9). The regional lymph nodes in particular are more apt to be involved, and elective neck treatment is advised along with re-treatment of the primary lesion.

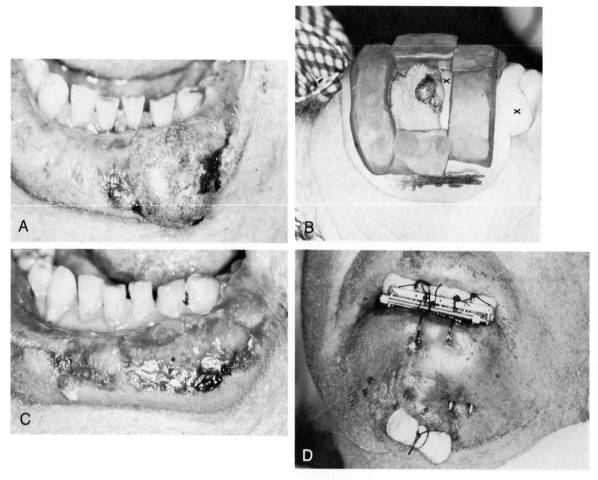

FIG. 17-7. A 67-year-old man presented with a T2N0 squamous cell carcinoma of the lower lip. (*A*) The lesion measured 3.0 × 2.0 × 1.5 cm. Radiation therapy was elected because of the functional deficit likely to result from excision of the large lesion. (*B*) A 2-mm thick, lead mask was designed to outline the portal. A separate lead shield covered with beeswax was inserted behind the lower lip (*X*). He received 3000 rad/2 weeks, 300 rad/fraction, 250 kV (0.5 mm Cu). Lead putty has been added to the shield to reduce transit irradiation to less than 1%. (*C*) By the completion of 3000 rad, he had a brisk mucositis of the lip and 60% to 70% regression of the obvious tumor. (*D*) A single-plane radium needle implant with double crossing. A pack was tied to the top of the bar to displace the upper lip away from the radiation. A chin pack was used to anchor the gingivolabial pack in place (see *E*). (*E*) A gauze pack was sewn into the gingivolabial gutter to displace the radium from the mandible, teeth, and gums. (*F* and *G*) Roentgenograms of implant. The implant added 3500 rad at 0.5 cm. (*H*) At 2½ weeks after implantation, there was superficial ulceration. (*I*) At 3 years and 8 months there was no evidence of disease and the lip was completely healed.

(continued)

Results of Treatment

MacKay and Sellers reviewed 2854 patients with all stages of lip cancer, of whom 92% were managed initially by radiation therapy.[30] All patients had a minimum 5-year follow-up. The primary lesion was controlled by the initial treatment in 84% of cases, and an additional 8% were saved by later treatment, for an overall local control rate of 92%. Fifty-eight percent of those who presented with clinically involved nodes had control of disease, but the rate was only 35% when neck nodes appeared later. The determinate 5-year survival rate was 89% and the absolute 5-year survival rate was 65%. Death due to intercurrent disease occurred in 17%.

Jørgensen and co-workers in Denmark reported the results for 869 cases of squamous cell carcinoma of the lip, managed initially by irradiation in all but 29 patients.[25] Seven hundred and sixty-six of the patients were managed by a rather unique radium implantation technique that required only 4 hours to deliver the dose. In 90% of the patients the lesions measured 2 cm or less. The recurrence rate for the 766 patients treated by the special radium technique was 7.4% for stage T1, 12.7% for stage T2, and 24.6% for stage T3 lesions. Eventually, after using every therapeutic modality available, it was possible to control the primary lesion in all but 7 of the 869 cases, a rather remarkable feat. Twenty-nine of the irradiated patients were said to have had a complication, many of which were

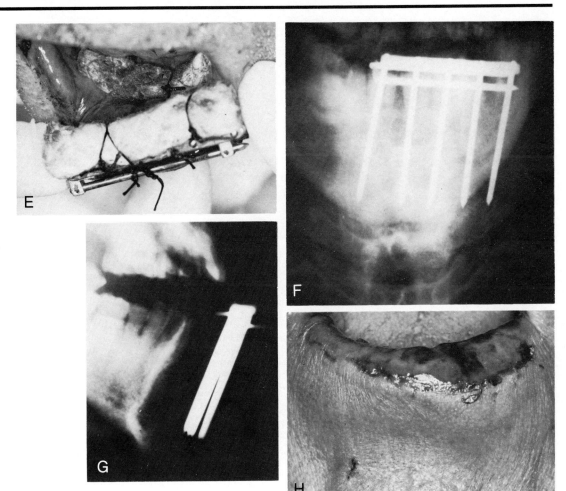

FIG. 17-7 (continued)

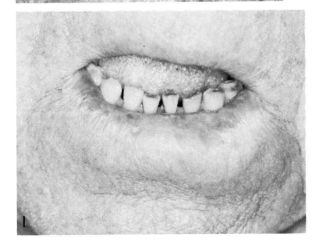

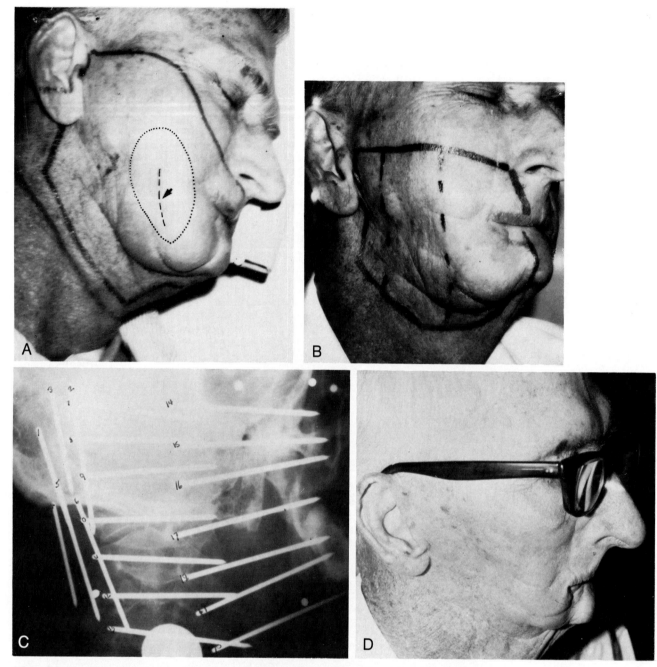

FIG. 17-8. A 64-year-old man was first treated in 1969 by electrocautery and wedge resection for squamous cell carcinoma of the right lower lip. Four years later he had a recurrence that required a right hemimandibulectomy with flap reconstruction. He had two more reconstructive procedures the same year. In 1974 he was admitted for a bone graft to bridge the right mandibular defect. At the time of surgery, recurrent epidermoid carcinoma was noted. (*A*) The arrow indicates the site of positive biopsy. The dotted line indicates the area of palpable recurrent disease. The solid line is the outline of the radiation therapy portal. The entire neck was electively irradiated. The patient received 5000 rad tumor dose, split course, for 8½ weeks, cobalt-60. (*B*) A large single-plane implant was planned to deliver 1500 rad at 0.5 cm. The solid lines outline the borders for the radium needle implant. (*C*) Roentgenogram of implant. (*D*) Patient was free of disease 8 years following treatment. (Appearance at 7 years.) Long-term salvage in this type of recurrence is unusual.

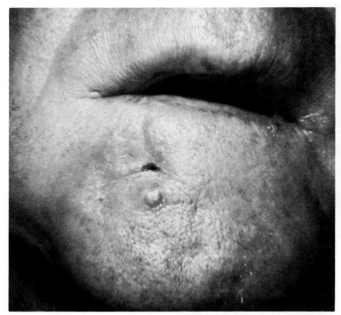

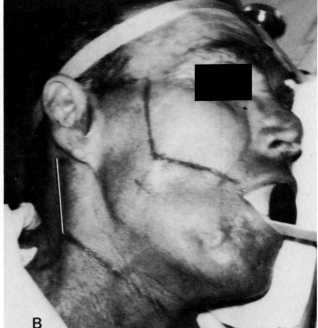

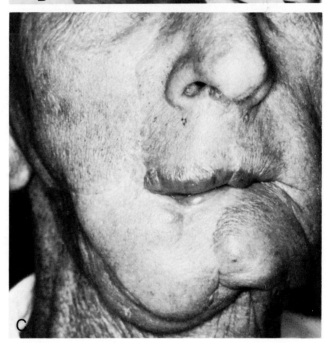

judged to be mild. Seventeen had scarring with tissue loss, nine had chronic ulceration that required a wedge excision, and another five had chronic ulceration that went untreated. Two patients had bone necrosis. After correction for mortality from other causes, the 5-year survival rate for the entire group was 96.7%, with only 4% dying of lip cancer. Only a small number of patients had primary lesions on the upper lip, but the results were similar.

The M. D. Anderson Hospital local control rates for 444 previously untreated patients are shown in Table 17-2; 83% were managed initially by excision.[28] The 3- and 5-year determinate survival rate was 94%.

Baker and Kraus reported the treatment results from the University of Michigan; 47% of patients were treated by irradiation and 53% by operation.[4] Excision with primary closure of the wound was the surgical management in 153 patients, while excision and a local flap was necessary in only 6 patients. Radiation therapy was used more commonly in the advanced lesions. The results of treatment are given in Table 17-3. The 5-year determinate and absolute survival rates for *in situ*, T1, and T2 tumors were essentially identical when comparing surgery and radiation therapy. Cervical metastasis occurred in approximately one third of the patients who developed local recurrence, indicating a need for elective neck treatment at the time of management of local recurrence.

Follow-up Policy

Patients with recurrence are often salvaged by secondary attempts. About 20% of local and regional recurrences appear after 5 years, and approximately 5% of the patients develop completely new lip cancers.

FIG. 17-9. Carcinoma of the right lower lip treated initially by local excision. (A) Six months after excision the patient developed recurrence at the inferior border of the incision with a 4 × 5-cm area of palpable induration in the skin of the right chin with fixation to the mandible; there was anesthesia of the right side of the chin. There were two small submaxillary lymph nodes. (B) The treatment plan was preoperative radiation therapy, 5000 rad tumor dose, to include the area of involvement and the inferior alveolar nerve to the base of the skull. There was a boost to the base of the skull area to 7000 rad because of the nerve involvement. (C) The lesion was resected and repaired with a flap. However, the patient developed extensive local recurrence and eventually died of disseminated disease 3 years after his treatment for recurrent disease.

TABLE 17-2. Cancer of the Lip: Previously Untreated Patients (M. D. Anderson Hospital)

Size of Lesion	Treatment	No. Patients	No. With Local Recurrence	No. Salvaged
0–1 cm	RT	30	0	
	S	239	6	6
1–2 cm	RT	36	2	1
	S	116	3	1
>2 cm	RT	7	0	
	S	7	3	0
Massive	RT	1	0	
	S	8	1	0

(RT, radiation therapy; S, surgery)

(Adapted from MacComb WS, Fletcher GH, Healey JE Jr: Intra-oral cavity. In MacComb WS, Fletcher GH [ed]: Cancer of the Head and Neck, pp 89–151. Copyright © 1967, the Williams & Wilkins Co., Baltimore)

TABLE 17-3. Squamous Cell Carcinoma of the Lip: 1953–1973 (University of Michigan)

Size of Lesion	No. Patients	Local Recurrence*	5-Year Survival Determinate	5-Year Survival Absolute
<1 cm	85	10.6%	100%	76%
1–3 cm	154	9.1%	92%	71%
>3 cm	29	20.7%	71%	52%
Bone invasion	11	90.9%	50%	45%

* Treated by radiation therapy, 47%; treated by surgery, 53%.

(Modified from Baker SR, Kraus CJ: Carcinoma of the lip. Laryngoscope 90:19–27, 1980)

Complications of Treatment

SURGICAL TREATMENT

Microstomia and drooling secondary to oral incompetence may occur when a large flap reconstruction is necessary, especially if the commissure is resected. If the oral opening is too small, the patient may not be able to insert a denture. Speech is not often affected. The cosmetic result is usually good after excision of small lesions or after small flap reconstruction of lesions not involving the commissure, but the appearance is impaired with reconstruction of larger lesions, particularly those previously irradiated.

RADIATION THERAPY

There will be some atrophy of the irradiated tissues, and this progresses with time. Continued exposure to the elements may result in a soft tissue necrosis; this problem is reduced by treatment schemes that prolong the treatment. The irradiated lip must be carefully protected from sun exposure by use of hats and ultraviolet protectants. Fishermen and boaters must wear a surgical face mask while on the water, since the various ultraviolet protectants are insufficient. (See Chapter 26, Carcinoma of the Skin.)

The anterior teeth and gingiva are protected by lead shields when treatment is given by external-beam irradiation. Radiation caries, bone exposure, and rarely osteoradionecrosis are uncommon late sequelae of interstitial therapy.

FLOOR OF THE MOUTH

Anatomy

The floor of mouth is a U-shaped area bounded by the lower gum and the oral tongue; it terminates posteriorly at the insertion of the anterior tonsillar pillar into the tongue. The paired sublingual glands lie immediately below the mucous membrane. The glands are separated by the paired midline genioglossus and geniohyoid muscles. Bony protuberances, the genial tubercles, occur at the point of insertion of these two muscle groups on the symphysis. They may be quite prominent and easily palpable in some patients and interfere with the placement of interstitial sources. The mylohyoid muscle arises from the mylohyoid ridge of the mandible and is the muscular floor for the oral cavity. The mylohyoid muscle ends posteriorly at about the level of the third molars. The normal submaxillary gland is about the size of a walnut. Most of the gland rests on the external surface of the mylohyoid muscle in the niche between the mandible and the insertion of the mylohyoid. A tonguelike process wraps around the posterior border of the mylohyoid muscle and extends forward on the internal surface of the mylohyoid. This process is absent in 10% to 20% of cases. The submaxillary duct (Wharton's duct) is about 5 cm long. It courses between the sublingual gland and the genioglossus muscle and exits in the anterior floor of mouth near the midline. The relationships of the lingual nerve, hypoglossal nerve, and submaxillary duct are shown in Figure 17-10.[38] The lingual nerve provides the sensory pathway to the floor of the mouth. The arterial supply is through the lingual artery, the second branch of the external carotid.

Pathology

The majority of neoplasms are squamous cell carcinoma, usually of moderate grade. Adenoid cystic and mucoepidermoid carcinomas account for 2% to 3% of malignant tumors in this area.

Patterns of Spread

PRIMARY

Approximately 90% of neoplasms originate within 2 cm of the anterior midline floor of the mouth. They penetrate quite early beneath the mucosa into the sublingual gland and the midline genioglossus and geniohyoid muscles. The mylohyoid muscle acts as an effective barrier until the lesion becomes very advanced. Extension toward the gingiva and periosteum of the mandible occurs early and frequently. Even small lesions become attached to the periosteum. The periosteum is an effective barrier to mandibular invasion; when tumor reaches the periosteum, the tumor first spreads along the periosteum rather than through it. Mandible invasion is usually a late manifestation. The tumor will often grow along or over the alveolar ridge before it grossly invades bone. The skin of the lower lip may be involved in advanced cases. Posterior extension occurs into the muscles of the root of the tongue; this pattern of extension is usually associated with ulceration of the floor of the mouth and undersurface of the tongue.

One or both submaxillary ducts are frequently obstructed by a tumor, and the enlarged duct may be palpated through the floor of the mouth. It is difficult to distinguish between tumor extension and low-grade infection in an obstructed duct. A tumor rarely grows inside the duct but may grow along the path of the duct. The submaxillary gland will frequently enlarge and become quite firm and occasionally painful when the duct is obstructed. It is impossible to distinguish between tumor involving the gland and chronic infection related to obstruction.

Tumors arising in the lateral floor of mouth are less common but have the same general spread patterns. Extensive lesions may escape the oral cavity by following the anatomical plane of the mylohyoid muscle to its posterior extremity, emerging in the neck near the angle of the mandible.

LYMPHATICS

Approximately 30% of patients will have clinically positive nodes on admission; 4% will have bilateral nodes. The distribution of nodal metastases on admission is shown in Figure 17-11.[27] Southwick reported 50% pathologically positive nodes after elective neck dissection.[45] The reported incidence of conversion from N0 to N+ with no neck treatment varies from 20% to 35%.[3,9,12,36]

The first nodes involved are the submaxillary and the subdigastric nodes. The submental nodes are bypassed; Lindberg reported 2% clinically positive submental nodes in 258 cases.[27] Since most lesions either approach or cross the midline, the risk for bilateral spread is fairly high. Fletcher reports that 47% of patients (9 of 19) with ipsilateral positive lymph nodes (N1 or N2) developed contralateral neck disease if no elective neck treatment was given. This rate was reduced to 10% (3 of 28) after 3000 rad to 4000 rad was given to the upper neck.[16]

Clinical Picture

PRESENTING SYMPTOMS

Early carcinomas are asymptomatic, red, slightly elevated mucosal lesions with ill-defined borders. A background of leukoplakia may be present. White lesions (leukoplakia) are less likely to be malignant, but 5% to 10% are said to become cancer. These lesions are usually diagnosed by the dentist or physician on routine oral examination.

T1–T2 tumors are first noticed when the patient feels a lump in the floor of mouth with the tip of his tongue. There

FIG. 17-10. Anatomical relationships of the floor of the oral cavity. (Million RR, Cassisi NJ, Wittes RE: Cancer in the head and neck. In DeVita VT Jr, Hellman S, Rosenberg SA [eds]: Cancer: Principles and Practice of Oncology, pp 301–395. Philadelphia, JB Lippincott, 1982)

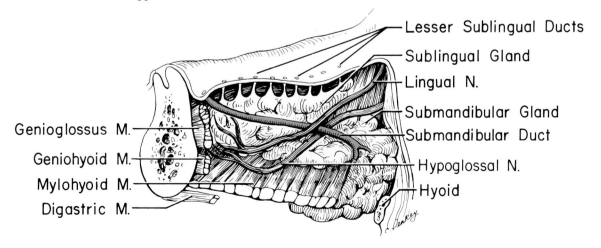

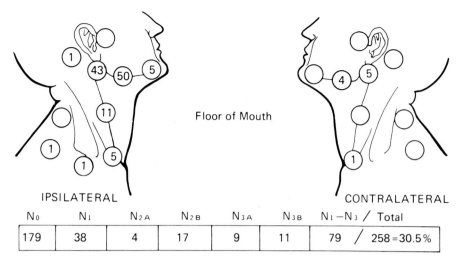

Floor of Mouth

IPSILATERAL   CONTRALATERAL

N₀	N₁	N₂ₐ	N₂ᵦ	N₃ₐ	N₃ᵦ	N₁–N₃ / Total
179	38	4	17	9	11	79 / 258 = 30.5%

FIG. 17-11. Nodal distribution on admission, M. D. Anderson Hospital, 1948–1965. (From Lindberg RD: Distribution of cervical lymph node metastases from squamous cell carcinoma of the upper respiratory and digestive tracts. Cancer 29:1446–1450, 1972)

FIG. 17-12. Pathways for referred pain to the ear. The auriculotemporal nerve (*left*) supplies the skin covering the front of the helix and tragus, the skin of the anterior wall of the external auditory canal, the tympanic membrane, and the skin of the temple. The tympanic nerve of Jacobson (*center*) supplies the tympanic cavity and produces a constant, deep-seated earache. The auricular nerve (*right*) is sensory to the skin of the back of the pinna and posterior wall of the external auditory canal. (Million RR, Cassisi NJ, Wittes RE: Cancer in the head and neck. In DeVita VT Jr, Hellman S, Rosenberg SA [eds]: Cancer: Principles and Practice of Oncology, pp 301–395. Philadelphia, JB Lippincott, 1982)

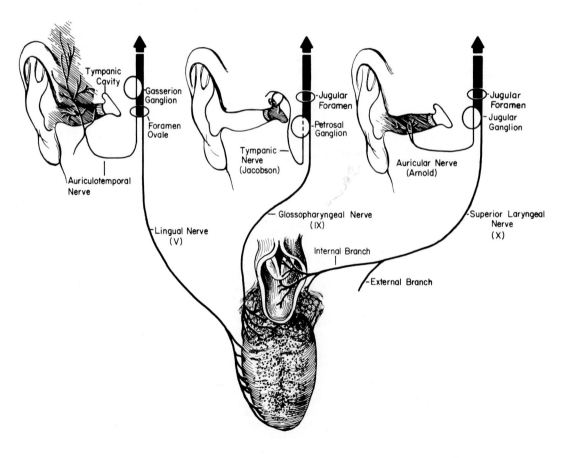

is mild soreness when eating or drinking that is usually thought by the patient (and sometimes the physician) to be due to a canker or denture sore. Advanced lesions produce increased pain, bleeding, foul breath, loose teeth, change in speech due to fixation of the root of the tongue, and a submaxillary mass, which is often painful. Pain may be referred to the ear (Fig. 17-12).

PHYSICAL EXAMINATION

The earliest lesions appear as a red area, slightly elevated, with ill-defined borders and very little induration. As the lesion enlarges, the edges of the tumor become distinct, elevated, and "rolled" with a central ulceration and induration.

Some lesions start with a background of leukoplakia. If the leukoplakia is extensive, it is difficult to know where or when to biopsy.

Bimanual palpation will determine the extent of the induration and the degree of fixation to the periosteum. Large lesions bulge into the submental space and rarely grow through the mylohyoid muscle into the soft tissues of the neck and even the skin. The submaxillary duct and gland are evaluated by bimanual palpation.

Methods of Diagnosis and Staging

BIOPSY TECHNIQUE

Small (5 mm) discrete lesions may be excised for diagnosis and cure; the margins of the resected lesion must be tagged by sutures and carefully examined for adequate margins. The deep margin is the one that is most often positive. For larger lesions an incisional or punch forceps biopsy is used.

STAGING PROCEDURES

The occlusal view (dental film) of the arch or ramus of the mandible is the best technique for determining early invasion. Oblique mandible views and a Panorex view are not useful for determining early bone invasion, but they may be obtained to evaluate the teeth and to determine the extent of invasion if extensive bony destruction is obviously present. These latter views also assist the surgeon in evaluating whether enough mandible exists in edentulous patients for a rim resection.

Submaxillary gland sialograms are not useful in determining the presence or absence of cancer in the gland.

The AJCC staging given earlier in this chapter was developed for all oral cavity lesions. No specific consideration is given to fixation to the periosteum of the mandible or bone invasion, and even small lesions may invade the periosteum. Fixation of the tongue, growth through the mylohyoid muscle to the skin in the submental area, or bone invasion should qualify for T4 status.

Treatment

SELECTION OF TREATMENT MODALITY

LEUKOPLAKIA

Patches of thin leukoplakia are usually observed and no biopsy or treatment is done. Biopsy is done if the area becomes symptomatic or if the appearance changes and malignancy is suggested. Localized areas of leukoplakia may be excised, but many patients have extensive or scattered areas that preclude complete excision.

Radiation therapy is not recommended for treatment of leukoplakia. When leukoplakia is inadvertently irradiated along with an adjacent carcinoma, the leukoplakia may disappear, but in most cases it will reappear at a later time.

EARLY LESIONS

Operation and radiation therapy produce similar cure rates for T1 and early T2 lesions, and therefore treatment decisions are based on rather subtle differences in expected functional result, the management of the neck, and the estimated risk of radiation necrosis.

A few patients are seen after excisional biopsy of a tiny lesion, and the only finding is a surgical scar with varying degrees of induration or nodularity under the scar (TX). The margins are stated to be free, close, or positive. If the excisional biopsy is judged to be inadequate, these patients are usually treated with an interstitial implant alone, since the surgeon has difficulty knowing where to start and stop the reexcision. The use of margin checks for reexcision is essentially useless under these conditions since there are very few tumor cells present and the pathologist is "looking for a needle in a haystack." Additionally, a few tumor cells may be spread at some distance from the excision site by way of the hematoma. The radiation therapist can be slightly generous with the treatment volume and cover potential spread without functional loss. The neck is usually observed. A review of six patients treated in this manner at M. D. Anderson Hospital revealed a 100% local control rate,[2] and similar patients treated at the University of Florida have a 100% local control rate. None of the patients developed neck nodes. If the margins of the excisional biopsy are free or close and there is little or no induration or nodularity, 5000 rad to 5500 rad is delivered by implant. If the margins are positive or if there is slight induration or nodularity, the dose is raised to 6000 rad to 6500 rad. In cases where gross cut-through is suspected, one may wish to use external-beam irradiation, 5000 rad, to include regional nodes prior to the interstitial implant.

Small lesions, up to 5 mm in diameter, may be excised transorally if there is a margin of normal mucosa between the lesion and the gingiva. If the excision includes the submaxillary duct, then the submaxillary gland and duct are also removed in continuity.

A common presentation is an anterior midline lesion, 1 cm to 3 cm in diameter, with a clinically negative neck; there is a risk for subclinical disease in one or both sides of the neck in 20% to 30% of cases. If the lesion is not attached to the periosteum, our preference is to recommend radiation therapy, since it has the added advantage of electively treating the nodes as well as the primary lesion. If the nodes are clearly positive on one side, elective neck irradiation also sterilizes any subclinical disease on the opposite side, and a neck dissection to the clinically positive neck follows the radiation therapy. Anterior midline lesions that are 1 cm to 3 cm in size and firmly attached to the periosteum are best managed by a rim resection and either observation of the neck or bilateral elective supraomohyoid neck dissections. The indication for rim resection may be the presence of mandibular tori that make an interstitial implant more difficult and the risk of bone exposure greater. If the lesion encroaches on the tongue and a significant amount of tongue would need to be resected, preference is given to radiation therapy because of the better functional result and possibly the better local control rate.

The less common lesions in the narrow lateral floor of the mouth fall into two general categories. One presentation involves the floor of the mouth and extends toward the mandible with little or no tongue invasion. These lesions are best managed by excision, including either a rim of mandible or mandibulectomy and neck dissection. A second presentation involves the floor of the mouth with extension toward the undersurface of the tongue. These lesions are usually managed by radiation therapy, including an interstitial implant.

MODERATELY ADVANCED LESIONS

An operation for moderately advanced cancers of the floor of the mouth can produce major cosmetic and functional disability, especially if the arch of the mandible is removed ("Andy Gump" deformity). Rim resection, which preserves continuity of the mandible, produces a good cure rate with acceptable speech and swallowing. Success with irradiation varies widely, but the highest rate of local control occurs when interstitial irradiation is used either alone or as part of the treatment. The local control rate by T stage for three different radiation series is compared in Table 17-4.[10,19,35] The local control rates increase with increasing doses and a greater proportion of treatment given by interstitial implant; these high control rates are accompanied by a progressively higher risk of a complication.

The undesirable aspect of radical irradiation is simply the risk of soft tissue and bone necrosis with the doses required for a high rate of control. The risk of a serious complication has decreased over the past 10 years at the University of Florida due to changes in management of the teeth and improved interstitial technique. However, the risk of a minor necrosis or bone exposure remains unchanged and a nagging, but tolerable problem.[31] (See Chapter 14, The Effect of Radiation on Normal Tissues of the Head and Neck.)

Extension of tumor to the periosteum or gingiva does not exclude the use of radiation therapy. The results of treatment according to the degree of gingival/periosteal involvement for 25 T2–T3 lesions are shown in Table 17-5. The control rate is 56% and independent of the extent of periosteal fixation, but the incidence of major complications in the patients with large, fixed lesions is quite high. If the operative alternative for the large, fixed lesion is a resection of the mandibular arch, floor of the mouth, and anterior tongue, which produces major disability, then radiation therapy is frequently chosen as the initial treatment. However, if rim resection can be done, that is the preferred plan of management, with irradiation added postoperatively.

ADVANCED LESIONS

Patients who have T4 lesions only because of bone invasion have a small chance of cure with combined surgery and radiation therapy (Fig. 17-13). Only palliation can be offered to those who have extensive tongue invasion with fixation, extension to submental skin, or massive neck disease.

TABLE 17-4.   Carcinoma of the Floor of the Mouth: Local Control With Primary Radiation Therapy

Institution	Type of RT	Stage T1		Stage T2		Stage T3		
		RT Alone	Ultimate Control	RT Alone	Ultimate Control	RT Alone	Surgical Salvage	Ultimate Control
M. D. Anderson Hospital[10]	Mixed	48/49 (98%)	100%	68/77 (88%)	93%	46/60 (73%)	11/14	95%
University of Florida[35]	Mixed	14/16 (88%)	88%	13/17 (76%)	94%	12/25 (48%)	5/9	68%
University of California, San Francisco[19]	External beam	29/38 (76%)	90%	21/39 (54%)	70%	8/32 (25%)	3	34%

(RT, radiation therapy; mixed = external-beam irradiation + interstitial implant)

(Million RR, Cassisi NJ, Wittes RE: Cancer in the head and neck. In DeVita VT Jr, Hellman S, Rosenberg SA [eds]: Cancer: Principles and Practice of Oncology, pp 301–395. Philadelphia, JB Lippincott, 1982)

TABLE 17-5.   Carcinoma of the Floor of the Mouth: Local Control (Radiation Therapy Alone) Related to Gingival Extension (Stage T2–T3)

Extent of Disease	Local Control	Surgical Salvage	Ultimate Local Control	Complications Requiring Surgery
Minimal gingival/periosteal extension	4/8	3/4	7/8	1
Tethered to gingiva/periosteum	4/6	1/2	5/6	0
Fixed to gingiva	6/11	1/2	7/11	4
Total			19/25 (76%)	

Note: University of Florida data; patients treated 10/64–12/77; analysis 12/79 by W. M. Mendenhall, MD.

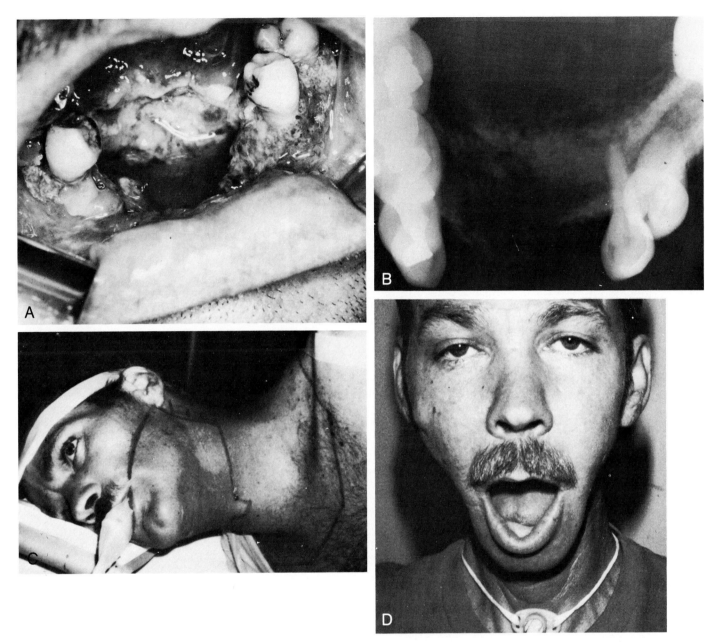

FIG. 17-13. (*A*) Advanced squamous cell carcinoma of the floor of the mouth with invasion of the tongue, gingiva, mandible, and skin of chin. (*B*) Roentgenogram of mandible showing extensive bone destruction and penetration through the outer cortex. (*C*) Preoperative radiation therapy portals. Note bulging of skin of chin due to tumor in subcutaneous tissues. Skin was red and warm over the mass. The patient received 6000 rad/5 weeks, 120 rad twice a day. The low neck received 5000 rad/5 weeks. (*D*) Appearance 6 months following bilateral hemimandibulectomy, resection of the floor of mouth, oral tongue, and adjacent soft tissues. Specimen was negative for tumor. Patient had no evidence of disease at 4½ years.

SURGICAL TREATMENT

WIDE LOCAL EXCISION

Small, superficial lesions, 5 mm to 6 mm or less in size, may be excised transorally with a 1-cm margin and primary closure. If the duct is involved, the submaxillary gland and duct are removed in continuity.

RIM RESECTION

Rim resection removes the mandible and periosteum adjacent to the tumor but does not remove the full thickness of the mandible, and therefore leaves the bone intact while providing an adequate surgical margin (Figs. 17-14 and 17-15). If the edge of the carcinoma is within 1 cm of the bone, then rim resection should be considered. In some

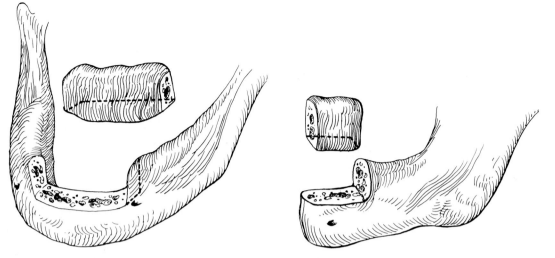

FIG. 17-14. Schematic of rim resection for early carcinoma of the floor of the mouth. (Million RR, Cassisi NJ, Wittes RE: Cancer in the head and neck. In DeVita VT Jr, Hellman S, Rosenberg SA [eds]: Cancer: Principles and Practice of Oncology, pp 301–395. Philadelphia, JB Lippincott, 1982)

FIG. 17-15. Schematic for rim resection of the arch of the mandible. (Million RR, Cassisi NJ, Wittes RE: Cancer in the head and neck. In DeVita VT Jr, Hellman S, Rosenberg SA [eds]: Cancer: Principles and Practice of Oncology, pp 301–395. Philadelphia, JB Lippincott, 1982)

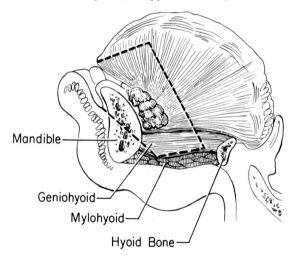

instances, only the periosteum is removed to provide the margin. The most common indication is for carcinoma either growing onto the gingiva or attached to the periosteum with a normal roentgenogram (occlusal view).

The defect may be covered with a split-thickness skin graft in most unirradiated cases. If adequate floor of the mouth mucosa remains, the mandible may be covered with floor of the mouth mucosa and buccal/labial mucosa. A tongue flap is used when the lingual nerve has been sacrificed, since that portion of the tongue is numb and easily traumatized. The same flaps are used in the irradiated as the unirradiated cases, but skin grafts have a lower rate of take; a flap may be necessary if the graft does not work.

Rim resection is most commonly employed for lesions in the anterior floor of mouth, but it is also applied successfully to selected lesions in the lateral floor of the mouth.

Postoperative radiation therapy may be used after a rim resection that is repaired by a split-thickness graft. Rim resection has been used for four radiation therapy failures, but bone exposure and necrosis occurred in all four patients. A split-thickness skin graft will usually take over the irradiated bed. Patients who have been edentulous for a long time may have a thin, atrophic mandible and are not suitable for rim resection since the mandible is likely to fracture.

Full or partial dentures may be used in most cases after rim resection.

MANDIBULECTOMY ("JAW-NECK")

The indications for mandibulectomy include roentgenographic evidence of bone invasion, extensive deep infiltration of the floor of the mouth adjacent to the mandible, tumor growth into the dental sockets, and a thin mandible unsuitable for rim resection. A neck dissection is almost always added, since the neck is entered to perform the mandibulectomy.

Lateral Floor of the Mouth

A neck dissection is performed and the specimen remains attached to the mandible.

Partial mandibulectomy with resection of the floor of mouth is done through a lip-splitting incision. A cheek flap is elevated to the level of the mandibular condyle to provide exposure. The mandible is separated at the mental foramen anteriorly and the neck of the condyle posteriorly. The primary lesion and neck specimen are then removed in continuity. Primary closure is usually feasible, unless a sizable portion of the oral tongue must be removed, in which case a myocutaneous flap is necessary to repair the defect.

The cosmetic and functional result is acceptable to patients, and very few request mandibular reconstruction. The mandible shifts to the opposite side, and if the patient has teeth, chewing may be impaired but may be corrected with a glide plane. (See Chapter 10, Maxillofacial Prosthetics.) Edentulous patients cannot wear a lower denture.

Anterior Floor of the Mouth

Lesions requiring full-thickness resection of the anterior mandible (arch) usually require removal from mental foramen to mental foramen. A spacer, such as a K wire or a cobalt-chromium alloy (Vitallium) tray, is necessary to maintain separation of the remaining mandible. This operation results in major cosmetic and functional loss and is usually reserved for advanced lesions with bone invasion or for irradiation failures. New techniques for reconstruction include the use of a trapezius myocutaneous flap with a portion of the scapular spine to bridge the bony gap or a free flap. Results are available for relatively few patients. These reconstructive efforts require extensive tissue dissection at the donor site and immobilization to promote healing. Moreover, there is still a significant failure rate of these flaps.

IRRADIATION TECHNIQUE

PRIMARY LESION

The availability of interstitial therapy is essential if maximum local control rates are to be obtained. External-beam irradiation alone gives inferior local control results even to T1N0 lesions (Tables 17-6 and 17-7).[10,19] Local control rate is related to total dose and the use of interstitial therapy; the overall time does not seem to be as critical as that for cancer of the oral tongue (Figs. 17-16 and 17-30).[35]

The dose schemes prescribed at the University of Florida are shown in Table 17-8. Doses are actually based on volume of tumor rather than diameter or T stage. A lesion may be 5 cm in total length and be very superficial and easily cured, while a 2- to 3-cm lesion may be 2- to 3-cm thick and invade the tongue and periosteum and require higher doses.

External-Beam Irradiation

External-beam portals for carcinoma of the anterior floor of the mouth are usually opposed lateral portals. The tongue

TABLE 17-6. Local Control of Lesions of the Oral Tongue and Floor of Mouth as a Function of Radiation Modality Employed

	Oral Tongue			Floor of the Mouth		
Study	E + R vs E	R vs E	E + R vs R	E + R vs E	R vs E	E + R vs R
Chu and Fletcher[10]	E + R > E	R > E	No difference	E + R > E	R > E	No difference
Fu and co-workers[18]			No difference*			
Fu and co-workers[20]	E + R > E	R > E	E + R < R†			
Inoue and co-workers[24]			No difference			
Horiuchi and Adachi[23]	E + R > E	R > E	E + R > R‡			
Lees[26]	E + R > E	R > E	No difference			
Mendenhall and co-workers[35]			E + R < R§	E + R > E‖		No difference

* External plus more than 4000 rad radium produced significantly better results than external plus less than 4000 rad radium.

† Local control alone not reported by T stage.

‡ Difference noted primarily in T3 and T4.

§ T2 lesions.

‖ T3 lesions.

(E, external beam; R, radium)

(Reprinted with permission from Mendenhall WM, Van Cise WS, Bova FJ, Million RR: Analysis of time-dose factors in squamous cell carcinoma of the oral tongue and floor of mouth treated with radiation therapy alone. Int J Radiat Oncol Biol Phys 7:1005–1011, 1981. Copyright © 1981, Pergamon Press, Ltd.)

TABLE 17-7. Carcinoma of the Floor of the Mouth: Local Control Versus Proportion of Dose Delivered by Radium Implant

Stage	Radium or Radium + <3000 rad	Radium + ≥3000 rad	External Beam	No. Controlled/No. Treated	No. Salvaged/No. Attempts	No. Ultimately Controlled/No. Treated
T1	8/8	4/5	2/3	14/16	0/1	14/16
T2	1/1	9/12	3/4	13/17	3/4	16/17
T3	1/2	*8/13	*3/10	12/25	5/9	17/25
T4		1/3		1/3	0/1	1/3
Total	10/11	22/33	8/17	40/61	8/15	48/61

* Significance level = 0.11, Fisher's exact test[33,34]

(Reprinted with permission from Mendenhall WM, VanCise WS, Bova FJ, Million RR: Analysis of time-dose factors in squamous cell carcinoma of the oral tongue and floor of mouth treated with radiation therapy alone. Int J Radiat Oncol Biol Phys 7:1005–1011, 1981. Copyright © 1981, Pergamon Press, Ltd.)

TABLE 17-8. Carcinoma of the Floor of the Mouth: Dose Schemes Currently Prescribed at the University of Florida

	Interstitial Only (rad)	External Beam + Interstitial (rad)
TX—No visible or palpable tumor	5500	Not recommended
TX—Palpable induration or nodularity	6500	Not recommended
TX—Tumor at margins, gross residual	Not recommended	5000 + 2500
Early (<1 cm)	6500	6000–6500 (external only)
Early (1 cm to 3 cm)	7000	5000 + 2500
Moderately advanced (3 cm to 5 cm)	Not recommended	5000 + 3000
Advanced	Not recommended	6000–7000 ± implant
Postoperative radiation therapy	Not recommended	6500/7 weeks
Preoperative radiation therapy	Not recommended	5000/6 weeks

(Million RR, Cassisi NJ, Wittes RE: Cancer in the head and neck. In DeVita VT, Hellman S, Rosenberg SA [eds]: Cancer: Principles and Practice of Oncology, pp. 301–395. Philadelphia, JB Lippincott, 1982)

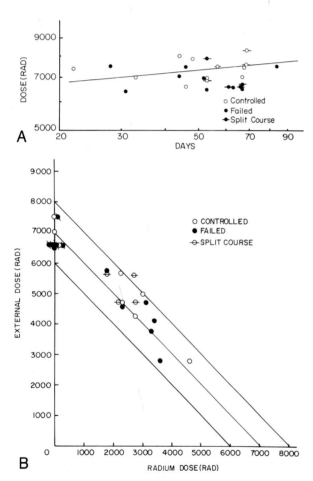

FIG. 17-16. (*A*) T3 floor of mouth carcinoma: time–dose analysis. The interstitial dose is added to the external-beam irradiation dose. (*B*) T3 floor of mouth carcinoma: interstitial versus external-beam irradiation dose. (Reprinted with permission from Mendenhall WM, VanCise WS, Bova FJ, Million RR: Analysis of time–dose factors in squamous cell carcinoma of the oral tongue and floor of mouth treated with radiation therapy alone. Int J Radiat Oncol Biol Phys 7:1005–1011, 1981. Copyright © 1981, Pergamon Press, Ltd.)

is positioned by use of rubber corks taped to a wooden tongue blade (Fig. 17-17). If the lesion is small and confined to the floor of the mouth, the tip of the tongue is elevated out of the portal and the lip is pressed outward. The dotted lines show the borders of the portal. If the lesion has grown into the tongue, the tongue is depressed or flattened to reduce the superior border. The entire width of the arch of the mandible is included in the portal. The superior border is shaped when possible in order to spare part of the parotid and minor salivary glands (Fig. 17-18). A stainless-steel pin is inserted into the posterior border of the tumor as a marker for external-beam therapy and for confirmation of coverage at the time of implant. The submaxillary and subdigastric nodes are included to the level of the thyroid notch if the neck is clinically negative. The submental nodes are included coincidentally, although they are uncommonly involved. Note the sparing of about 1 cm of skin and subcutaneous tissue in the submental area. If the neck is clinically positive, the portals are enlarged to include all of the upper neck nodes, and an en *face* lower neck field is added.

Interstitial Irradiation

Small lesions confined to the floor of the mouth with minimal extension to the mucosa of the tongue or minimal extension to the gingiva or periosteum can be managed by interstitial irradiation.

A preloaded, custom-designed, metal or plastic implant device for radium needles has been in use at the University of Florida since 1976. It holds the radium needles in a fixed position. The location of the needles relative to the gingiva can be tailored. Homogeneity of dose is improved as the implant is checked by computer calculations prior to implantation. This device avoids piercing and unnecessarily irradiating the tongue, as was required with free-hand techniques. The entire implant is completed in an instant with minimal exposure and minimal implant trauma. The custom holder is suitable only for T1–T2 lesions. The arrangement of the needles for early lesions is usually a modified, curved, teardrop-shaped, two-plane implant with a single needle crossing the top of the implant (Fig. 17-19). The use of the implant holder for an early lesion of the floor of mouth is shown in Figure 17-20.

Implants for late T2 and T3 lesions are usually modified volume or multiplane arrangements. Radium needles or iridium-192 wires are inserted through the tongue. Sources at least 4.0 to 4.5 cm in active length are required (Fig. 17-21).

Intraoral Cone Irradiation

An intraoral cone can be used for small anterior superficial lesions in the edentulous patient with a low alveolar ridge. The major advantages of this technique are less dose to the adjacent bone and avoidance of an implant. Lesions that extend to involve the tongue are not suitable since the tongue is mobile. Lesions more than 1 cm thick are less suitable for orthovoltage intraoral cone therapy because of the rapid fall-off in depth dose. The orthovoltage cones in use at the University of Florida are 2 cm to 6 cm in diameter; they are poured from lead and can be individually trimmed to adapt the cone to the anatomy.

Electron-beam cones can be individually fabricated as described by Tapley.[48] *Intraoral cone therapy requires careful daily positioning by the physician.*

Doses vary from 5000 rad/15 fractions/3 weeks to 5500 rad/20 fractions/4 weeks, depending on the size of the lesion.

Intraoral cone therapy may also be considered as a reduced field treatment in which only 1000 rad to 2000 rad is given in conjunction with external-beam portals. It is preferable to give the intraoral cone therapy prior to the external-beam therapy because the mouth becomes sore and the lesion disappears.

(Text continues on p. 263.)

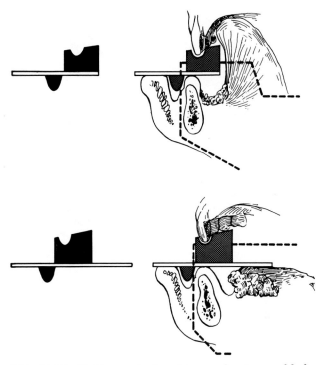

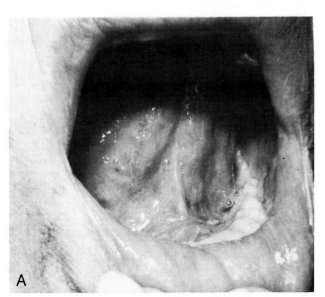

FIG. 17-17. Rubber corks taped to wooden tongue blade.

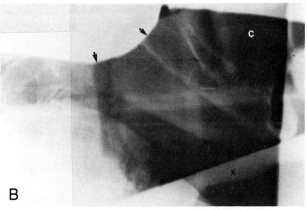

FIG. 17-18. (*A*) A 55-year-old woman presented with a 2.2 × 1.5 × 1.0-cm squamous cell carcinoma in the left anterior floor of the mouth that was slightly tethered to the periosteum; the majority of the lesion was submucosal. The lesion extended to the midline. The roentgenographic appearance of the mandible was normal. The lower teeth showed marked periodontal disease. The neck was negative (T2N0). The patient was offered surgery or radiation therapy and elected irradiation. The remaining teeth were extracted prior to start of treatment. (*B*) Roentgenogram of external-beam portal. Stainless-steel pin represents posterior border of lesion. A cork (c) displaces the tip of the tongue superiorly. The superior margin of portal (*arrows*) is shaped to spare part of the parotid and other normal structures. Approximately 1 cm of submental skin and subcutaneous tissues is shielded (*X*). The tumor dose was 5000 rad/5 weeks to the floor of the mouth and lymph nodes. (*C*) Radium needle implant—2000 rad tumor dose. (*D*) The mucosa healed initially, but a 7-mm area of bone exposure developed at 7 months. (*E*) At 1 year, bone exposure persisted. Symptoms were mild and intermittent. The exposed bone was smoothed with a file; 3 months later, the gingiva appeared nearly healed. (*F*) Three small areas of bone exposure are shown at 2 years. (*G*) At 2½ years a 5-mm area of bone exposure appeared; it was associated with a small abscess that extended lateral to the mandible and seemed to communicate with the bone exposure. The abscess disappeared in 1 week with antibiotics. (*H*) No evidence of tumor at 5 years and no new necroses after 3½ years.

(continued)

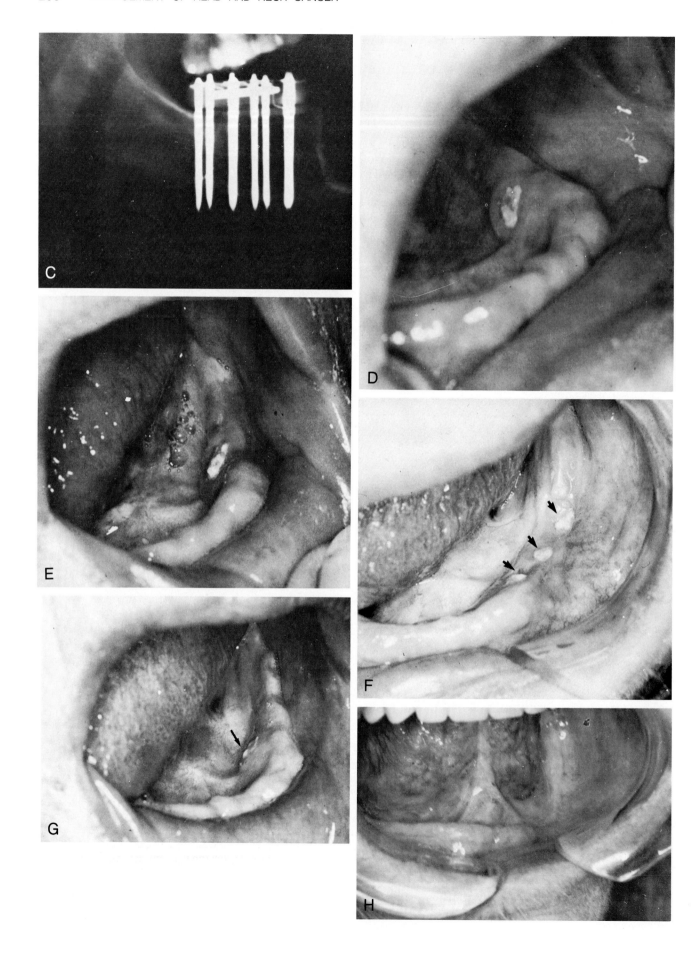

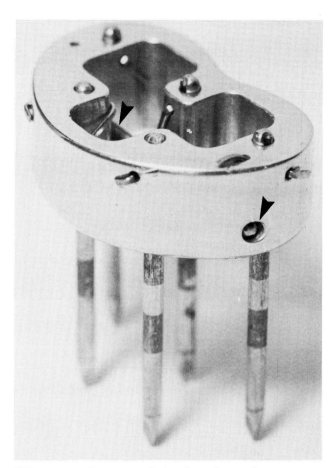

FIG. 17-19. Custom-made implant device for stage T1–T2 carcinomas of the floor of the mouth. Note single crossing needle through center of device (*arrowheads*). The device is now machined from nylon. (Reprinted with permission from Marcus RB Jr, Million RR, Mitchell TP: A preloaded, custom-designed implantation device for stage T1–T2 carcinoma of the floor of the mouth. Int J Radiat Oncol Biol Phys 6:111–113, 1980. Copyright 1980, Pergamon Press, Ltd.)

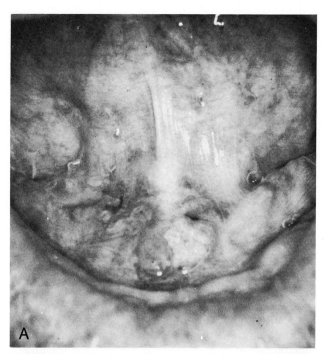

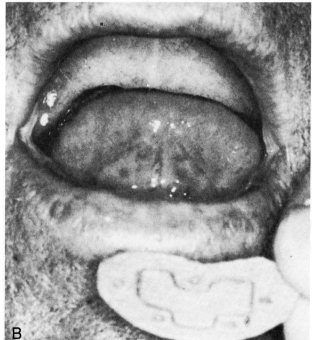

FIG. 17-20. (*A*) Squamous cell carcinoma of the floor of the mouth (T2N0). The lesion measured 2.5 × 2.5 cm, including the induration, and was tethered to the periosteum in the midline. The treatment plan was 5000 rad/5 weeks with parallel opposed portals that included the submaxillary and subdigastric lymph nodes. The midjugular lymph nodes were treated with an anterior portal. An implant was planned to add 1500 rad. (*B*) Cardboard template used for design of the radium needle holder. (*C*) Implant in position. Device was secured with two sutures from the submental skin. There were five, 2.0-cm active length, full-intensity needles without crossing. (*D*) Sagittal isodose distribution. The 50 rad/hour line was selected for specification of dose, and the implant remained in place for 30 hours. Stippled area represents the implant device. (*E*) Midplane isodose distribution. The 50 rad/hour isodose line is approximately 1 mm outside the needles. The highest dose rate to the anterior lingual gingiva would be about 30 rad to 35 rad/hour or at least 450 rad lower than the minimum tumor dose. (*F*) The patient was free of disease at 4 years with no complications.

(continued)

FIG. 17-20 (continued)

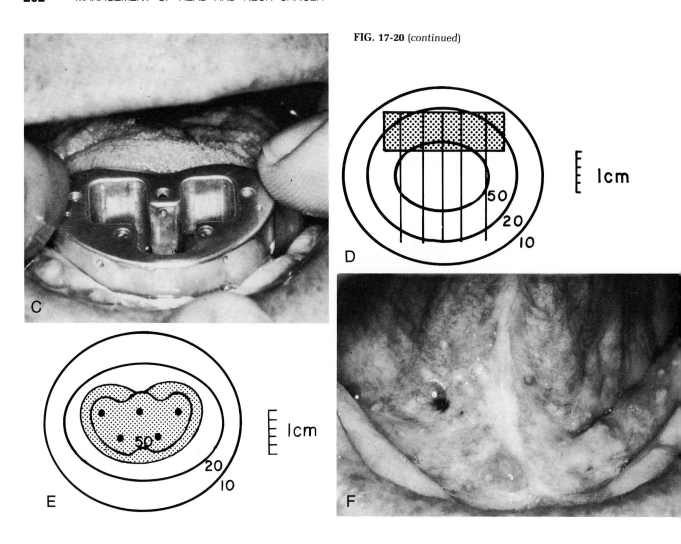

FIG. 17-21. (*A*) Radium implant for extensive squamous cell carcinoma of the floor of mouth and undersurface of the tongue (T3N0). Each rack of needles was sutured to the tongue with two 3-0 silk ligatures. (*B*) Lateral roentgenogram of implant using eleven, 4.5-cm active length (6.2-cm overall length) needles. (Ellingwood KE, Million RR, Mitchell TP: A preloaded radium needle implant device for maintenance of needle spacing. Cancer 37:2858–2860, 1976)

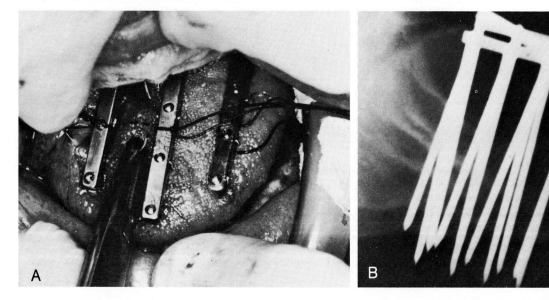

MANAGEMENT OF THE NECK (PRIMARY LESION TREATED BY IRRADIATION ALONE)

N0

Small superficial lesions, 1 cm or less in diameter, are treated by interstitial irradiation alone; the neck is not treated unless the histology is poorly differentiated, in which case the neck and the primary lesion are treated to 5000 rad by way of external-beam irradiation followed by interstitial implant. Patients with lesions more than 1 cm in size receive radiation therapy (4500 rad to 5000 rad) to the primary lesion and the upper neck on both sides to include the submental, submaxillary, and subdigastric nodes to the level of the thyroid notch; treatment of the primary lesion is completed by an interstitial implant.

N+

All patients receive bilateral whole-neck irradiation, 5000 rad minimum. If the neck mass is large and fixed, the dose to the mass is increased to 6000 rad to 8000 rad through reduced fields and an implant is then placed in the floor of the mouth. An appropriate neck dissection is performed 4 to 6 weeks later. If the patient cannot have a neck dissection, the dose to the clinically positive node(s) is boosted by additional external-beam treatment or an interstitial implant.

COMBINED TREATMENT POLICIES

The results of combined surgery and irradiation may be better than those for sequential therapy in the large, infiltrative, ulcerative lesions. Surgical resection and postoperative irradiation is the preferred sequence, but preoperative irradiation may be used if the patient has a large fixed node (5 cm or larger in size) or if a trial of radiation therapy is desired to evaluate response before the final decision on an operation. Advanced lesions that extend anteriorly to the skin of the lip are irradiated preoperatively in order to gain control of tumor in the dermal lymphatics and because the extensive reconstruction might delay start of radiation therapy (Fig. 17-13). If rim resection is possible, postoperative irradiation is preferred, since the risk of bone

complications and fistulas is higher with preoperative irradiation. Surgical clearance is most difficult in the tongue, and preoperative irradiation further obscures the borders of the disease. Postoperative irradiation portals usually include the entire oral tongue and the floor of the mouth. The daily dose is 180 rad and the tumor dose is 6500 rad. If the tongue margins were close or positive, the dose may be 7000 rad.

MANAGEMENT OF RECURRENCE

Radiation failures are treated by an operation. The salvage rate is quite high for patients with early lesions and moderately good for the more advanced lesions (see Table 17-7). Rim resection may be used for selected radiation therapy failures.

Surgical failures may be treated by a repeat operation, radiation therapy, or both on an individual basis. Radiation therapy is not likely to salvage surgical failures except with limited recurrences that can be implanted as all or part of their treatment.

Results of Treatment

Survival rates at 2 and 5 years for patients initially treated with radiation at the University of Florida are shown in Table 17-9. Survival rates for surgical series are similar. The local control rates for patients with stage III–IV disease treated by combined surgery and radiation therapy are given in Table 17-10.

Guillamondegui and Jesse report 20 patients treated by rim resection.[22] All patients had invasion of the periosteum and 7 had early bone invasion on pathologic examination of the specimen. With 1-year minimum follow-up, there was only one local recurrence. Four patients, however, failed in the neck, and for this reason the authors recommend postoperative radiation therapy.

Atkins and Cassisi reviewed the University of Florida experience for rim resection in 20 patients with squamous cell carcinoma of the floor of the mouth (Table 17-11).

TABLE 17-9. Carcinoma of the Floor of the Mouth: Survival for Patients Treated Initially by Irradiation ± Radical Neck Dissection With Surgery for Salvage

Stage	Absolute Survival		Determinate Survival*	
	2 Years	5 Years	2 Years	5 Years
I	14/17 (82%)	6/8 (75%)	14/14 (100%)	6/6 (100%)
II	11/14 (78.5%)	4/7 (57%)	11/13 (85%)	4/4 (100%)
III	20/28 (71%)	11/27 (41%)	20/24 (83%)	11/19 (58%)
IV	4/14 (28.5%)	0/7	4/11 (36%)	0/6
Total	49/73 (67%)	21/49 (43%)	49/62 (79%)	21/35 (60%)

* Excludes patients who died of intercurrent disease.

Note: University of Florida data; patients treated 10/64–12/77; analysis 12/79 by W. M. Mendenhall, MD.

(Million RR, Cassisi NJ, Wittes RE: Cancer in the head and neck. In DeVita VT Jr, Hellman S, Rosenberg SA [eds]: Cancer: Principles and Practice of Oncology, pp 301–395. Philadelphia, JB Lippincott, 1982)

TABLE 17-10. Carcinoma of the Floor of the Mouth: Stage III–IV, Local Control With Primary Combined Treatment (Surgery Plus Radiation Therapy)

Study	Local Control	Ultimate Control
University of Louisville[17]	13/15	13/15 (87%)
University of California, San Francisco[19]	9/10	9/10 (90%)
University of Florida[35]	5/11	5/11 (46%)

(Million RR, Cassisi NJ, Wittes RE: Cancer in the head and neck. In DeVita VT Jr, Hellman S, Rosenberg SA [eds]: Cancer: Principles and Practice of Oncology, pp 301–395. Philadelphia, JB Lippincott, 1982)

TABLE 17-11. Carcinoma of the Floor of the Mouth: Results of Treatment by Rim Resection in 20 Patients

Stage	No. Patients	Local Recurrence	No. Salvaged/ No. Attempted	Ultimate Control
T2	11	3	1/2	9/11 (81%)
T3	8	4	2/2	6/8 (75%)
T4	1	1	0/0	0/1 (0%)

Note: University of Florida data; patients treated 6/73–6/81; analysis 3/83 by J. S. Atkins, Jr., MD, and N. J. Cassisi, MD.

Postoperative radiation therapy was added in three patients and preoperative radiation therapy was used in one. Two of the patients had evidence of bone invasion on examination of the specimen, and treatment failed locally in both, in spite of postoperative irradiation. Four rim resections were attempted in patients who had a recurrence after radiation therapy; the disease was controlled in three of four patients, but all developed a bone complication and loss of mandibular continuity. The local control and salvage rates are nearly identical to those shown in Table 17-7 for irradiation.

Follow-up Policy

Patients are seen at 4- to 6-week intervals for the first 2 years.

There are two major diagnostic difficulties in follow-up after irradiation: soft tissue ulcer and enlarged submaxillary gland. A bone exposure is almost always a necrosis and not due to cancer.

The appearance of an ulcer in the floor of the mouth within 2 years of treatment can be either recurrence or necrosis. If the lesion appears to be a soft tissue necrosis, a trial of conservative therapy and observation at close intervals is adequate. The soft tissue necroses are notoriously slow to heal. Failure to stabilize or show some indication of healing is an indication for biopsy. A negative biopsy does not rule out recurrence, and if the lesion remains suspicious, repeat deep biopsies are in order.

An enlarged submaxillary gland(s) is a common sequel to obstruction of the submaxillary duct. The gland may be enlarged on initial examination or it may enlarge during or after treatment. Since it is difficult to distinguish between an enlarged submaxillary gland and tumor in a lymph node, only removal will clarify the situation.

Follow-up for cases treated by an operation is complicated by the normal postoperative induration, which persists for several months. Large split-thickness skin grafts and myocutaneous flaps increase the difficulty in distinguishing normal scar from recurrent tumor.

Complications of Treatment

RADIATION COMPLICATIONS

A small soft tissue necrosis may develop in the floor of the mouth, usually in the site of the original lesion where the dose is highest. These ulcers are moderately painful and respond to local anesthesia, antibiotics, and time. A decision regarding biopsy depends on the clinical course.

If the ulceration develops on the adjacent gingiva, then the underlying mandible is exposed. These areas are mildly painful. They are managed by discontinuing dentures, using a local anesthetic, administering antibiotics, and smoothing of the bone by filing if needed. These small bone exposures do not often progress to full-blown osteonecrosis. They either sequestrate a small piece of bone or are simply re-covered by mucous membrane. Healing is slow, and the patient requires constant reassurance that the discomfort and ulcer are not due to cancer. (See section on complications of radiation therapy in treatment of cancer of the oral tongue later in this chapter.)

SURGICAL COMPLICATIONS

Surgical complications include bone exposure and orocutaneous fistula. The mandible may fracture after rim resection. Salvage procedures after radiation therapy are associated with an increased risk of mandible complications. Removal of the oral tongue may produce a speech defect and difficulty in swallowing. Mandibulectomy of the arch is often associated with oral incompetence and disfigurement.

ORAL TONGUE

Anatomy

The muscular anatomy of the tongue is shown in Figure 17-22.[11] The circumvallate papillae locate the division between oral tongue and base of tongue. The papillae foliatae may be recognized as 2 mm to 4 mm, slightly elevated, irregular areas on the dorsum at the junction with the anterior tonsillar pillar. There are mucous and serous glands beneath the squamous epithelium, particularly of the tip and ventrolateral surfaces.

The arterial supply is mainly from paired lingual arteries, which are branches of the external carotid. The midline fibrous septum of the tongue is quite complete and restricts anastomosis between the vessels except near the tip of the oral tongue. One lingual artery may be sacrificed without

danger of necrosis, but sacrifice of both lingual arteries results in an increased risk for loss of the oral tongue and almost certain loss of the base of tongue.

The sensory pathway is by way of the lingual nerve to the gasserian ganglion (see Fig. 17-12). The motor nerve is the hypoglossal nerve. The taste buds are supplied by the chorda tympani, a branch of the sensory root of the facial nerve.

The lymphatic pathways of the tongue are shown in Figure 17-23.[41]

Pathology

More than 95% of lesions of the oral tongue are squamous cell carcinomas. Coexisting leukoplakia is common. Verrucous carcinoma and minor salivary gland tumors are quite uncommon. Granular cell myoblastoma is a benign tumor of uncertain origin that commonly occurs on the dorsum of the tongue and may be confused histologically with carcinoma because of the associated pseudo-epitheliomatous hyperplasia.

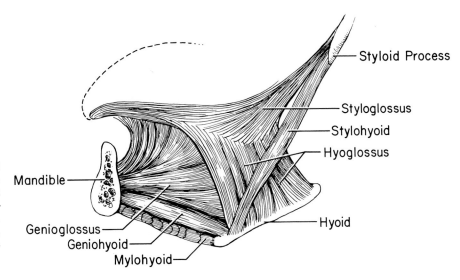

FIG. 17-22. Musculature of the tongue and floor of the oral cavity. (Redrawn from Sabotta drawings in Clemente CD: Anatomy: A Regional Atlas of the Human Body. Philadelphia, Lea & Febiger, 1975. Copyright 1975, Urban & Schwarzenburg, München–Berlin–Wien)

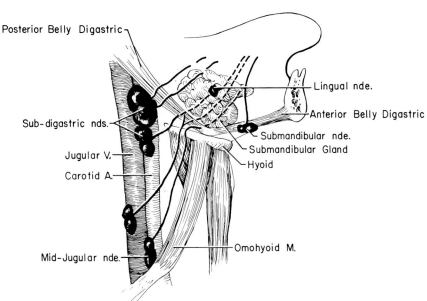

FIG. 17-23. Lymphatics of the tongue. (Modified from Rouvière H: Anatomy of the Human Lymphatic System, pp 44–56. Ann Arbor, Edwards Brothers, 1938)

Patterns of Spread

PRIMARY

Nearly all squamous cell carcinomas of the oral tongue occur on the lateral and undersurfaces of the tongue. Rarely, lesions appear on the dorsum, usually in the posterior midline. Most of the lateral border lesions occur on the middle and posterior thirds, with a few on the anterior third. Oral tongue carcinomas tend to remain in the tongue until quite large.

Anterior third (tip) lesions are usually diagnosed early. Advanced lesions invade the floor of mouth and root of tongue, producing ulceration and fixation.

Middle third lesions invade the musculature of the tongue and later invade the lateral floor of the mouth.

Posterior one-third lesions grow into the musculature of the tongue, the floor of the mouth, the anterior tonsillar pillar, the base of the tongue, the glossotonsillar sulcus, and the mandible. Posterior one-third lesions behave more like cancer of the base of the tongue with a higher incidence of lymph node metastasis.

LYMPHATICS

The first-echelon nodes are the subdigastric and submaxillary nodes. The submental and spinal accessory lymph nodes are seldom involved. Rouvière describes lymphatic trunks that bypass the subdigastric and submaxillary nodes and terminate in the midjugular lymph nodes (see Fig. 17-23).[41] One seldom sees this pattern clinically. The lymphatic vessels of the tongue anastomose freely, allowing contralateral lymph flow, usually under conditions of partial obstruction by tumor or operation. Thirty-five percent of patients with cancer of the oral tongue have clinically positive nodes on admission, and 5% are bilateral. The distribution of nodal metastases on admission is shown in Figure 17-24. The incidence of subclinical disease is approximately 30% (see Table 2-1, Chapter 2, The Natural History of Squamous Cell Carcinoma). The incidence of positive nodes increases with T stage.[27]

Patients with N1–N2 ipsilateral nodes have a 27% risk of developing node metastasis in the opposite neck.[16]

Clinical Picture

PRESENTING SYMPTOMS

Mild to moderate irritation and the sensation of a lump in the tongue are the most frequent complaints. The patient may present because he thinks he has bitten his tongue. The pain may occur only during eating or drinking. As ulceration develops, the pain becomes progressively worse and may be referred to the external ear canal (see Fig. 17-12). Extensive infiltration of the muscles of the tongue affects speech and swallowing. Patients with advanced lesions have a foul odor. Hemorrhage is uncommon.

PHYSICAL EXAMINATION

The extent of disease is easily determined by visual examination and palpation. The tongue protrudes incompletely and toward the side of the lesion as fixation develops. Posterior lesions of the oral tongue may grow inferiorly, behind the mylohyoid, and present as a mass in the neck at the angle of the mandible; the mass may be confused with an enlarged lymph node. Invasion of the hypoglossal nerve is rare and may cause atrophy. Posterolateral lesions may be difficult to evaluate because of pain, and examination using an anesthetic is often required. An enlarged submaxillary gland may be due to cancer involving the gland or to inflammation due to obstruction of the submaxillary duct.

Methods of Diagnosis and Staging

The differential diagnosis includes granular cell myoblastomas, which are usually 0.5-cm to 2.0-cm slow-growing, nontender masses. The lesions are well circumscribed, firm, and slightly raised, and they may be multiple. Malignant behavior is either nonexistent or rare, and wide local excision is the treatment of choice. Pyogenic granulomas mimic small exophytic carcinomas. The papillae foliatae may be hypertrophied secondary to chronic inflammation and be confused with a carcinoma starting at the junction of the anterior tonsillar pillar and tongue. Tuberculous ulcer and syphilitic chancre are rare considerations.

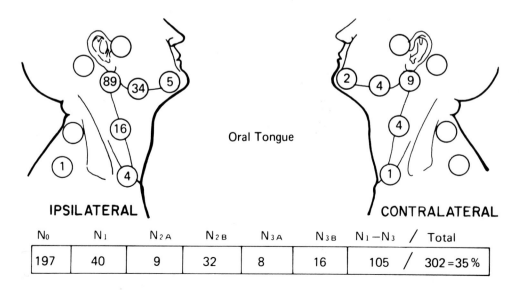

FIG. 17-24. Nodal distribution on admission, M. D. Anderson Hospital, 1948–1965. (Lindberg RD: Distribution of cervical lymph node metastases from squamous cell carcinoma of the upper respiratory and digestive tracts. Cancer 29: 1446–1450, 1972)

N0	N1	N2A	N2B	N3A	N3B	N1–N3 / Total
197	40	9	32	8	16	105 / 302 = 35%

BIOPSY TECHNIQUE

Biopsy is by punch forceps or incisional biopsy performed with the use of a local anesthetic. Small superficial lesions, less than 1 cm in size, may be excised and margins carefully examined.

STAGING PROCEDURES

Staging is by physical examination. Roentgenograms of the mandible are indicated only when the growth is tethered to the bone.

The AJCC staging for oral cavity carcinoma presented earlier in this chapter is reasonably good for staging lesions of the oral tongue. However, a superficial lesion that measures more than 4 cm will have a prognosis more like a T1 or T2 lesion than a T3 lesion. Mandible invasion or fixation of the oral tongue would place the lesion in the T4 category.

Treatment

SELECTION OF TREATMENT MODALITY

Both glossectomy and irradiation are curative for cancer of the oral tongue, and the reported cure rates are similar for similar stages. However, for irradiation to produce satisfactory control rates, the availability of interstitial therapy is essential. If hemiglossectomy is the surgical option, a degree of speech impediment and difficulty in swallowing is produced, and irradiation is usually selected as the initial treatment with glossectomy reserved for recurrence. Surgical salvage of irradiation failures is fairly successful for early lesions, but drops to a 50% success rate for larger lesions. For this reason, glossectomy and radiation therapy are often advised as initial therapy for the more advanced lesions, although many patients refuse glossectomy because of the anticipated morbidity.

The neck is managed according to the guidelines in Chapter 4, General Principles for the Treatment of Cancers in the Head and Neck: Selection of Treatment for the Primary Site and for the Neck. When irradiation is selected for the primary lesion, elective neck irradiation is given for patients with a clinically negative neck except in the case of a small, superficial lesion. When an operation is selected for the primary lesion, functional elective neck dissection may be added for the clinically negative neck, or the neck may be observed for the appearance of metastatic disease.

EXCISIONAL BIOPSY (TX)

Excisional biopsy of a small lesion may show inadequate margins. An interstitial implant, 5500 rad to 6000 rad, will produce a high rate of control and is favored over reexcision.[2] (See section on treatment of early lesions of the floor of the mouth.)

EARLY LESIONS (T1–T2)

Operation and irradiation produce similar local control rates, and treatment decisions must be based on functional and cosmetic loss and patient preference.

Wide local excision is the treatment of choice for small, well-circumscribed lesions that can be excised transorally, small lesions on the tip of the tongue, and the rare lesion on the dorsum of the tongue. Irradiation is usually selected for larger T1 lesions and for T2 lesions to preserve normal speech and swallowing (Fig. 17-25).

Glossectomy may result in speech impediment and difficulty swallowing, and it is hard to predict which patients will have trouble. The surgeon has difficulty in determining the extent of tumor invasion into the tongue at the time of the operation; for this reason, preoperative irradiation should be avoided, since it further obscures the margins and compounds the problem.

MODERATELY ADVANCED LESIONS (T2–T3)

Lesions that have a large surface involvement, but minimal infiltration, are favorable lesions and can be cured with radiation therapy alone; glossectomy is reserved for radiation failure. Those lesions that are deeply infiltrative (more than 2 cm in depth) will have a higher control rate with combined surgery and radiation therapy, but the patient must be willing to accept glossectomy and possibly mandibulectomy (Fig. 17-26).

ADVANCED LESIONS (T4)

Combined treatment with surgery and radiation therapy will cure a few patients, especially those with minimal neck disease. Most patients in this category will receive palliative irradiation.

SURGICAL TREATMENT

EARLY LESIONS (T1–T2)

Examples of two lesions and the amount of tongue to be removed are shown in Figure 17-27. Speech impediment or difficulty in swallowing would be unlikely in either case. Glossectomy offers the advantage of a short treatment time. Primary closure is generally done (Fig. 17-28), although with large resections a flap may be necessary.

MODERATELY ADVANCED LESIONS (T2–T3)

Deeply infiltrative lesions not suitable for irradiation alone are managed by glossectomy followed by postoperative radiation therapy. It is difficult when cutting the tongue to judge projections of tumor, and the likelihood of cutting across a tumor is greater than for the other head and neck sites. It is an advantage to the surgeon to be able to feel the tumor mass in order to obtain a wide margin. This is not easy if radiation therapy has preceded the glossectomy. Finally, if the mandible must be sacrificed after preoperative radiation therapy, the likelihood of fistula, exposed bone, and radionecrosis is increased.

ADVANCED LESIONS (T4)

Advanced lesions require either a total glossectomy/laryngectomy or total glossectomy with myocutaneous flap reconstruction; postoperative radiation therapy would usually be recommended. Total glossectomy is only offered to patients in good general condition and with minimal neck disease.

IRRADIATION TECHNIQUE

The treatment plans are given in Table 17-12.

The ability to control the primary lesion is enhanced by giving all or part of the treatment by interstitial radiation therapy (see Table 17-6).[10,20,23,26,35] The local control rate by T stage and the rate of salvage by operation are shown

(Text continues on p. 270.)

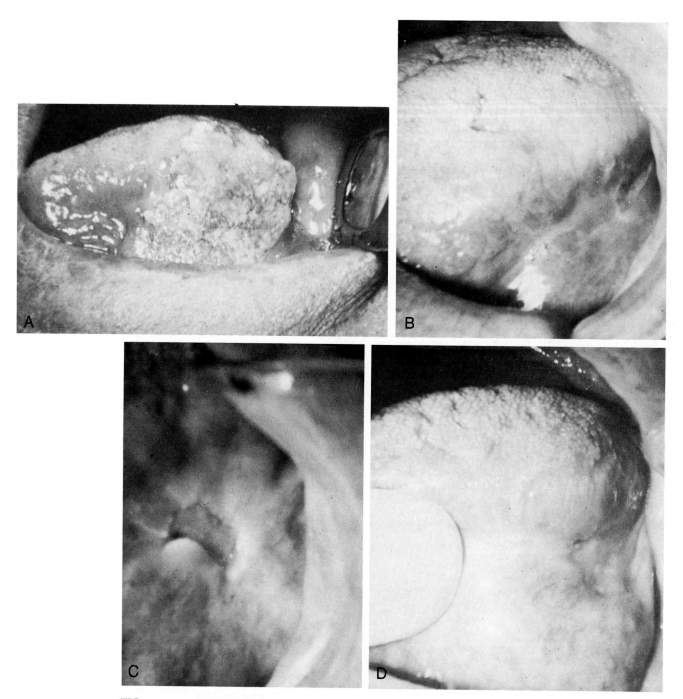

FIG. 17-25. (A) Squamous cell carcinoma of the oral tongue (T2N0) treated with a single lateral portal, 3000 rad/2 weeks, 2-MV x-rays, followed by a single-plane needle implant, 5000 rad at 0.5 cm. (B) Appearance 1 month after completion of treatment. (C) The patient developed a small, painful ulceration on the lateral border of the tongue 1 year after treatment. (D) Complete healing 1 month later. There were no further complications. This would be an example of a 1+ soft tissue necrosis. The patient died 10 years later of a cerebrovascular accident.

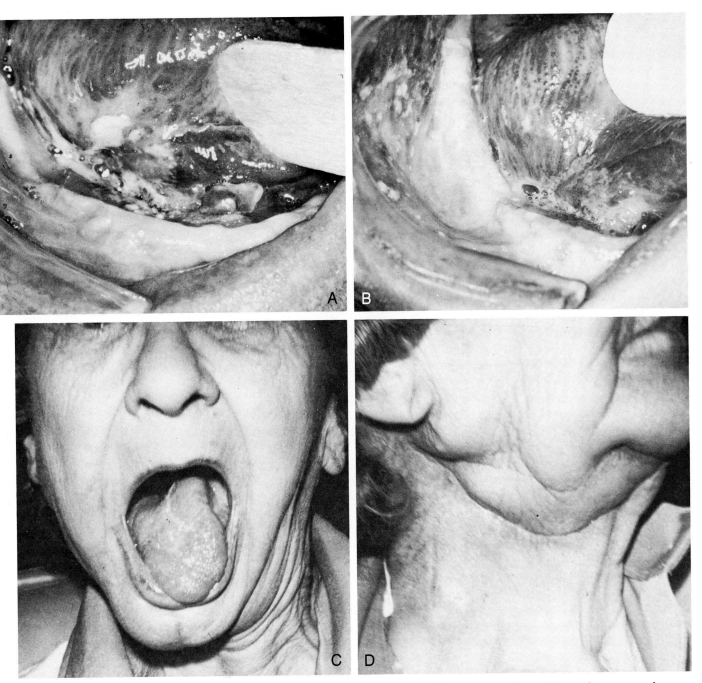

FIG. 17-26. (A) Squamous cell carcinoma of the undersurface of the oral tongue and floor of the mouth with multiple right upper neck nodes, all mobile and small (T3N2B). The lesion was tethered to the mandible, and the tongue could not be fully protruded. The patient received 5000 rad/4 weeks, 120 rad twice a day, to the primary lesion and upper neck nodes and 4050 rad/3 weeks to the lower neck nodes. (B) At completion of radiation therapy, tumor regression was estimated at 60%. Partial glossectomy, mandibulectomy, and right neck dissection were performed 4 weeks after radiation therapy. Fourteen nodes were positive for disease. The submandibular gland was noted to have tumor that extended into the soft tissue adjacent to the gland. Margins were clear. (C and D) Anterior and lateral views 6 weeks following operation. The patient was free of disease at 4 years; the only complaint was persistent right shoulder pain. Speech was altered but understandable. Swallowing was not impaired.

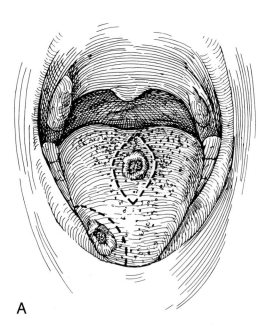
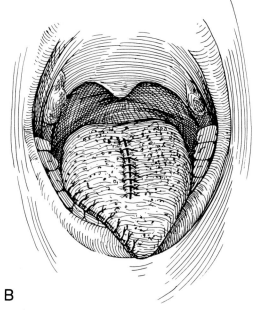

A   B

FIG. 17-27. Small lesions on the anterior free margin of the tongue or in the midline of the tongue can be excised (A) and the defect closed primarily (B). (Million RR, Cassisi NJ, Wittes RE: Cancer in the head and neck. In DeVita VT Jr, Hellman S, Rosenberg SA [eds]: Cancer: Principles and Practice of Oncology, pp 301–395. Philadelphia, JB Lippincott, 1982)

TABLE 17-12. Irradiation Policies for Carcinoma of the Oral Tongue at the University of Florida		
Criteria	Interstitial Alone (rad)	External Beam + Interstitial (rad)
TX—No visible or palpable tumor	6000	Not recommended
TX—Palpable induration or nodularity	7000	Not recommended
TX—Tumor at margins; gross residual	7500	5000 + 3000
Early (<1 cm)	6500	Not recommended
Early (1 cm to 3 cm)	Not recommended	3000/2 weeks + 3500
Moderately advanced (3 cm to 5 cm)	Not recommended	3000/2 weeks + 4000
Advanced	Not recommended	5000 + 3500
Postoperative radiation therapy	Not recommended	6500–7000/7–8 weeks
Preoperative radiation therapy (fixed nodes)	Not recommended	5000/6 weeks

(Million RR, Cassisi NJ, Wittes RE: Cancer in the head and neck. In DeVita VT Jr, Hellman S, Rosenberg SA [eds]: Cancer: Principles and Practice of Oncology, pp 301–395. Philadelphia, JB Lippincott, 1982)

in Table 17-13. Treatment of the neck is an integral part of the treatment plan and is outlined in Chapter 4, General Principles of Treatment of Cancers in the Head and Neck: Selection of Treatment for the Primary Site and for the Neck. We favor elective neck irradiation for almost all lesions over 1 cm in size.

INTRAORAL CONE IRRADIATION

Intraoral cone therapy is generally unsatisfactory because it is difficult to immobilize the tongue. It may be used in the cooperative patient with a small anterior lesion who cannot have interstitial therapy. Fayos and Lampe

reported a local control rate of 82% for lesions 1 cm to 3 cm and 58% for lesions 3 cm to 5 cm in diameter.[15]

INTERSTITIAL IRRADIATION

Interstitial therapy is essential if maximum local control is to be obtained; external-beam therapy alone gives inferior cure rates even for T1 lesions (see Table 17-6). That control of T2 oral tongue lesions is improved if a greater proportion of the treatment is by interstitial therapy is shown in Figure 17-29. A time–dose analysis for T2 lesions is presented in Figure 17-30; the time factor is shown to be critical in predicting success. A time–dose analysis for T3 lesions is

TABLE 17-13.   Carcinoma of the Oral Tongue: Local Control

| | No. of Patients With Local Control/No. Treated | | | | No. Salvaged/ No. Attempts | No. Ultimately Controlled/No. Treated |
Stage	Radium or Radium + <3000 rad	Radium + ≧3000 rad	External Beam	Radiation Therapy Alone (Total)		
T1	5/5	2/2	0/1	7/8	1/1	8/8
T2	*10/11	*7/15	1/1	18/27	4/7	22/27
T3	0/2	7/20	0	7/22	5/10	12/22
Total	15/18	16/37	1/2	32/57	10/18	42/57

* Significance level = 0.02, Fisher's exact test[33,34].

Note. University of Florida data; patients treated 10/64–12/77; analysis 12/79.

(Reprinted with permission from Mendenhall WM, VanCise WS, Bova FJ, Million RR: Analysis of time–dose factors in squamous cell carcinoma of the oral tongue and floor of mouth treated with radiation therapy alone. Int J Radiat Oncol Biol Phys 7:1005–1011, 1981. Copyright © 1981, Pergamon Press, Ltd.)

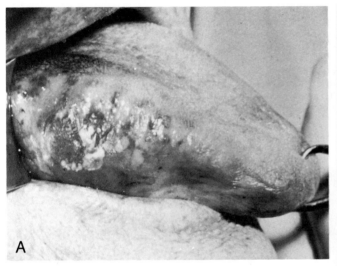

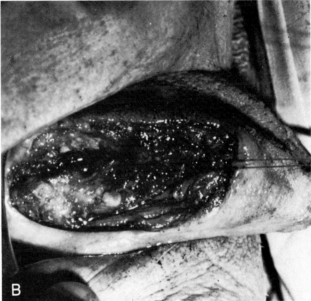

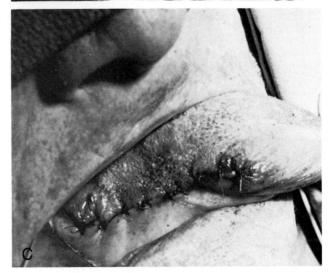

FIG. 17-28.   (*A*) Squamous cell carcinoma of the right lateral oral tongue (T1N0). (*B*) Wide local excision. (*C*) Primary closure.

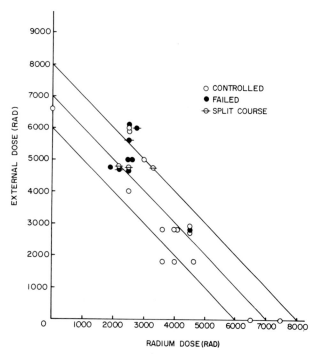

FIG. 17-29. T2 oral tongue carcinoma: comparison of local control according to proportion of dose by external-beam and interstitial therapy. Control increases with greater proportion of interstitial treatment even though the summed doses were often less. (Reprinted with permission from Mendenhall WM, VanCise WS, Bova FJ, Million RR: Analysis of time–dose factors in squamous cell carcinoma of the oral tongue and floor of mouth treated with radiation therapy alone. Int J Radiat Oncol Biol Phys 7:1005–1011, 1981. Copyright © 1981, Pergamon Press, Ltd.)

given in Figure 17-31. Local control increased with increasing dose and with decreased overall time. Either radium or iridium sources may be used. The implant is done within 1 week of completion of the external-beam therapy. Implants are usually arranged in planes or modified planes. A single plane is adequate for lesions up to 1.0 cm thick. A two-plane implant is used for lesions 2.0 cm to 2.5 cm thick, and a volume or three-plane implant is used for larger lesions. The implant covers the gross extent of the lesion plus a margin of normal tongue.

Radium needles may be mounted in a holder to maintain proper spacing and improve alignment (Figs. 17-32 and 17-33).[13] The technique is easy to apply for a single lateral tongue plane, but it requires some dexterity and maneuvering to insert the medial plane, particularly if the oral cavity is small or the tongue is large.

The dose to the mandible/gingiva may be significantly reduced by inserting a pack into the floor of the mouth, as shown in Fig. 17-34.

The majority of implants are done with the patient under general anesthesia. Nasotracheal intubation gives added working space. Tracheostomy is not done routinely, but it is advised for appropriate cases. The tongue may become quite large during or immediately after the implant; methylprednisolone sodium succinate (Solu-Medrol) may be given intravenously in the recovery room with rapid reduction of tongue size.

All needles are sutured in placed with 2-0 silk. The sutures are cut long enough to exit the mouth and sutured to the skin of the cheek; this aids in finding the knots when it comes time to remove the implant.

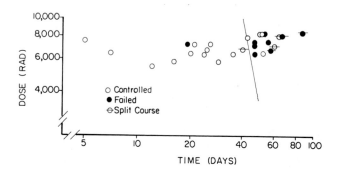

FIG. 17-30. Control of T2 oral tongue carcinoma: time–dose analysis. The data were analyzed using a discriminant analysis technique to provide an optimal line to separate successes from failures. (Reprinted with permission from Mendenhall WM, VanCise WS, Bova FJ, Million RR: Analysis of time–dose factors in squamous cell carcinoma of the oral tongue and floor of mouth treated with radiation therapy alone. Int J Radiat Oncol Biol Phys 7:1005–1011, 1981. Copyright © 1981, Pergamon Press, Ltd.)

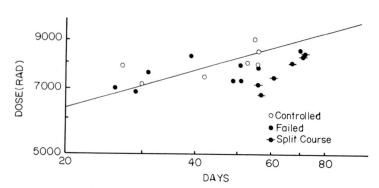

FIG. 17-31. T3 oral tongue lesions: time–dose analysis. The data were analyzed using a discriminant analysis technique to provide an optimal line to separate successes from failures. (Reprinted with permission from Mendenhall WM, VanCise WS, Bova FJ, Million RR: Analysis of time–dose factors in squamous cell carcinoma of the oral tongue and floor of mouth treated with radiation therapy alone. Int J Radiat Oncol Biol Phys 7:1005–1011, 1981. Copyright © 1981, Pergamon Press, Ltd.)

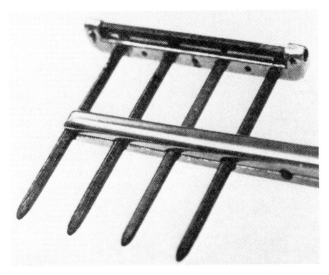

FIG. 17-32. Radium needles mounted in a rigid device for implantation of oral tongue cancer. The holders were originally fashioned from stainless steel or aluminum, but more recently nylon has proved more satisfactory. The needles are secured to the bar with half-hard stainless steel wire passed through the eyelets. An Allen forceps has been drilled to grasp the needles. Crossing needles may be attached to bar or inserted separately. (Ellingwood KE, Million RR, Mitchell TP: A preloaded radium needle implant device for maintenance of needle spacing. Cancer 37:2858–2860, 1976)

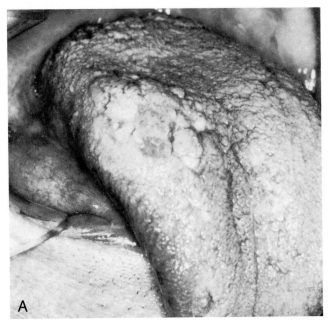

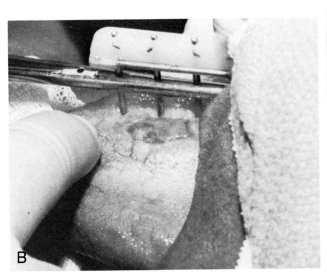

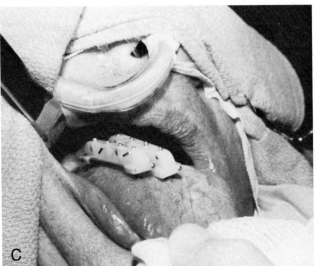

FIG. 17-33. A 51-year-old man presented with a 3-month history of a painful sore on the right dorsum of the tongue. The lesion measured 3 × 2 cm and extended near the midline. Biopsy revealed squamous cell carcinoma (T2N0). The patient refused glossectomy. Treatment plan: (1) Opposed lateral portals, 3000 rad/2 weeks, cobalt-60. (2) Radium needle implant, 4500 rad. (A) Squamous cell carcinoma on dorsum of oral tongue. (B) Insertion of lateral row of radium needles. The needles were mounted in a nylon bar. There were two crossing needles in the lateral bar and one crossing needle in the medial bar. The nylon holder assisted in maintaining the active portion of the needles above the lesion in order to give an adequate dose to the dorsum of the tongue. (C) Radium implant in place. (D) Mucositis at 2 weeks. (E) Complete healing at 3 months. There was no evidence of disease at 21 months.

(continued)

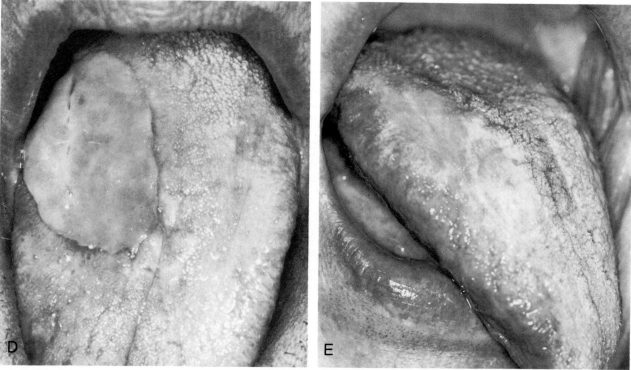

FIG. 17-33 (continued)

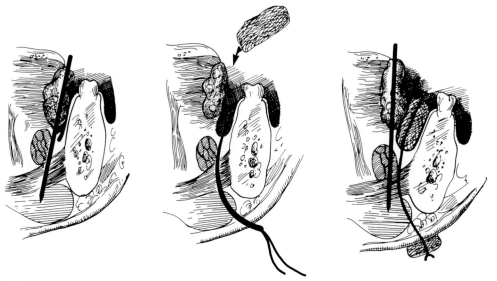

FIG. 17-34. Use of packing to reduce dose to mandible. (*Left*) Implant without packing. (*Center*) Large curved needle inserted through skin to floor of the mouth. (*Right*) Gauze pack tied to suture and secured between mandible and tongue after implant is completed.

EXTERNAL-BEAM IRRADIATION

A single ipsilateral portal or parallel opposed fields are used depending on the size of the primary lesion, the presence or absence of nodes, and the proportion of the dose planned by external-beam therapy. The portal includes the submaxillary and subdigastric lymph nodes if the neck is clinically negative. If the neck is clinically positive, the contralateral neck and lower neck lymph nodes on both sides are included. If an implant or operation is to be performed at a later date, an India ink tattoo(s) will assist in location of the initial borders. If the patient has teeth with metal fillings that lie against the tongue or buccal mucosa, a thin layer of cotton or gauze is inserted between the teeth and tongue or buccal mucosa to prevent a high-dose effect. The anterior skin and subcutaneous tissues of the submental area should be shielded when possible to reduce submental edema and late fibrosis. The preinterstitial dose of 3000 rad/2 weeks is preferred because of a higher success rate compared with other plans.[35] However, for the more advanced oral tongue lesions or when the neck is clinically positive and requires a higher dose prior to radical neck dissection, then the external-beam dose is usually 5000 rad/5 weeks prior to implant.

COMBINED TREATMENT POLICIES

When glossectomy is selected for large lesions, the operation is performed first. Even without previous irradiation, the surgeon has a difficult time estimating tumor extent in the tongue. The major indication for preoperative irradiation is a large node, in which case it is hoped that the irradiation will reduce the size and allow surgical clearance. An interstitial implant may be used to deliver a portion of the dose to the tongue if radiation therapy is given before an operation. Postoperative irradiation should begin within 4 to 6 weeks. Since most of the oral cavity is irradiated, the dose per fraction is 180 rad/day, with a total dose of 6500 rad. Interstitial implants are not usually employed in postoperative radiation therapy because recurrences may appear at any point along the surgical dissection. If the margins in the tongue are close or positive, 7000 rad is preferred because of the difficulty of eradicating even small amounts of tumor in the tongue after glossectomy.[5,37] (See Chapter 13, Time–Dose–Volume Relationships in Radiation Therapy.)

MANAGEMENT OF RECURRENCE

Most recurrences appear in the first 2 years. Local recurrence after radiation therapy or surgery is heralded by ulceration, pain, increased induration, or obvious exophytic cancer. A trial of antibiotics such as tetracycline will often reduce the pain of either radiation necrosis or recurrent tumor. Recurrences have a slightly elevated or rolled border, while radiation necroses usually have minimal or no elevation of the border. The induration associated with necrosis is usually less than with recurrence. Contrary to the situation with lesions of the floor of the mouth, biopsy should be done as soon as ulceration appears if the ulcer occurs within the original cancer site, since little or no increased morbidity is likely from the biopsy. Ulcers that appear on adjacent normal tissues (e.g., the gingiva) are due to radiation effect and not to cancer. Outpatient biopsies performed using a local anesthetic may miss the tumor. If suspicion remains high for local recurrence after a negative biopsy, deep, generous biopsies using a general anesthetic are required, and even this maneuver will occasionally miss persistent tumor.

Irradiation failure is managed by glossectomy (Fig. 17-35). Surgical failure is occasionally salvaged by radiation therapy or an operation, if the recurrence is limited to the mucosa. Recurrence in soft tissues of the neck is rarely eradicated by any procedure.

Lymph nodes appearing in a previously untreated neck are managed by neck dissection with or without postoperative radiation therapy.

Results of Treatment

The local control rates for a series of 57 patients treated initially with or without radical neck dissection and the absolute and determinate 2- and 5-year survival rates are shown in Tables 17-13 and 17-14, respectively. Approximately 20% of patients will die of intercurrent disease and 10% will die of distant metastases.

Ange and co-workers reviewed 17 patients treated by irradiation after excisional biopsy.[2] All patients had control of the primary lesion. Two patients subsequently developed disease in the neck and were salvaged by surgery.

Spiro and Strong reported the surgical results for glossectomy during the years 1957 to 1963; 288 patients received surgery only, and 15 additional patients received preoperative irradiation.[46] Overall local control was 122 (48%) of 256 determinate cases. The determinate 5-year survival rate was 69%, stage I; 53%, stage II; 37%, stage III; and 0 of 13 patients, stage IV.

Follow-up Policy

The recurrence rate at the primary site and in the untreated neck is substantial for all but the smaller lesions; early recognition of recurrence leads to an improved chance of salvage.

Surgical failures that occur on the mucosa are easy to detect, but those appearing deep in the operative field initially produce vague induration that is similar to postoperative induration. The appearance of pain should be considered recurrent cancer until proved otherwise.

Radiation failures almost always appear at the site of the original lesion. An ulcer may represent necrosis or recurrence, and biopsy, often performed with the patient under general anesthesia, may be required to establish the diagnosis.

Complications of Treatment

SURGICAL TREATMENT

Orocutaneous fistula, flap necrosis, and dysphagia are the three most common complications of surgery of the tongue. Damage to the lingual nerve or the hypoglossal nerve, although rare, increases the difficulty in swallowing and in speaking.

Fistulas and flap necrosis must be handled judiciously since the danger of carotid artery hemorrhage increases with either of these complications.

Enunciation difficulties occur whenever the tongue is bound down by scarring; it is often difficult to predict which patients will have difficulty. The incidence of complications increases for surgical salvage attempts after irradiation failure; the patient must be willing to accept these risks and must be informed that multiple procedures may be necessary.

RADIATION THERAPY

Many patients will complain of a sensitive tongue for many months after completion of treatment, even when the mucosa is quite well healed. This is hardly surprising since the tongue has been "burned" and, like any other burned area, remains sensitive for a period of time. This effect usually disappears with time.

Taste will reappear from 1 week to several months after treatment. Taste may return to normal, but more frequently it is "not quite as keen" as before. The dryness of the mouth may contribute to the poorer sense of taste.

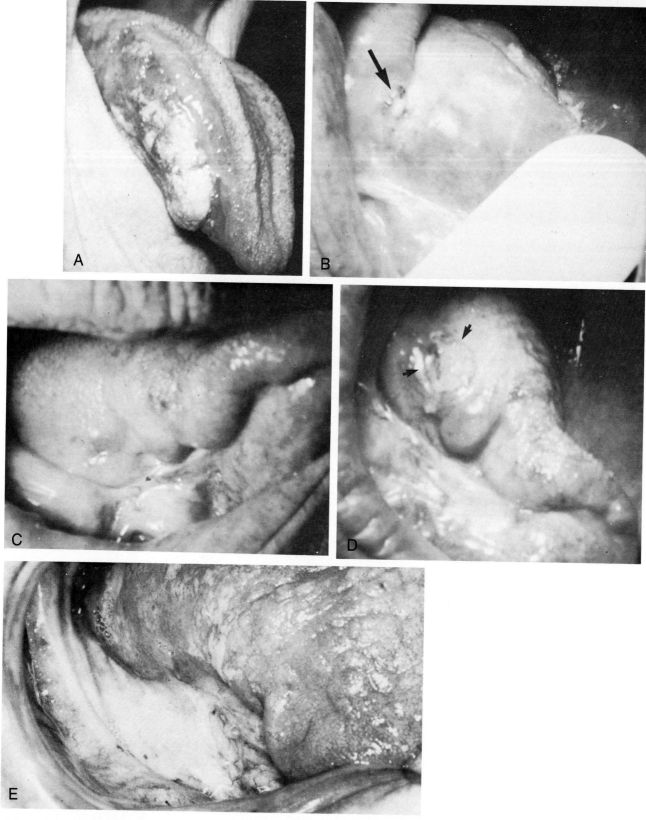

FIG. 17-35. A 73-year-old woman presented with squamous cell carcinoma of the tongue (T2N0). (*A*) The lesion measured 4.0 × 1.5 × 1.5 cm. She received 5000 rad by external-beam irradiation, single lateral portal, followed by 2760 rad from a single-plane radium needle implant. (*B*) Local recurrence (*arrow*) 6 months after radiation therapy was treated by wide local excision. (*C*) Appearance 6 months after wide local excision; there is no evidence of cancer. (*D*) Second recurrence (*arrows*) appeared 8 months after wide local excision; again patient was treated by wide local excision. (*E*) Appearance 10 years following second excision. Patient remained free of cancer at 12 years, and neck remained normal. Speech was minimally affected.

TABLE 17-14. Carcinoma of the Oral Tongue: Survival for Patients Treated Initially by Irradiation ± Radical Neck Dissection With Surgery Reserved for Salvage

Stage	Absolute		Determinate*	
	2 Years	5 Years	2 Years	5 Years
I	7/12 (58%)	5/11 (45%)	7/7 (100%)	5/5 (100%)
II	16/22 (73%)	10/17 (59%)	16/18 (89%)	10/14 (71%)
III	17/24 (71%)	6/20 (30%)	17/24 (71%)	6/17 (35%)
IV	9/16 (56%)	1/12 (8%)	9/10 (90%)	1/2
Total	49/74 (66%)	22/60 (37%)	49/59 (83%)	22/38 (58%)

* Excludes patients dead of intercurrent disease.
Note: University of Florida data; patients treated 10/64–12/77; analysis 12/79 by W. M. Mendenhall, MD.
(Million RR, Cassisi NJ, Wittes RE: Cancer in the head and neck. In DeVita VT, Hellman S, Rosenberg SA [eds]: Cancer: Principles and Practice of Oncology, pp. 301–395. Philadelphia, JB Lippincott, 1982)

Return of saliva is variable, depending on the treatment volume and the dose to the salivary glands. Patients treated with interstitial therapy alone will eventually have nearly normal saliva. Patients treated with 4500 rad external-beam therapy plus interstitial therapy will eventually have 25% to 50% return of saliva if one parotid gland receives 3000 rad or less.

SOFT TISSUE NECROSIS

Soft tissue necrosis is fairly common, although frequently of minor degree. Once recurrence has been ruled out, considerable patience is required for healing. The patient associates pain with recurrence of his cancer, since the original lesion frequently caused a similar pain. He needs to be constantly reassured that the ulcer will heal slowly and that there is no evidence of recurrence. Patients who develop a true necrosis rarely get a recurrence, so in a sense, at least, there is some good news associated with the pain (Fig. 17-36).

The treatment plan for soft tissue necrosis is mainly to rule out recurrent cancer, to provide local and general analgesia, and to reduce local infection. If the ulcerated lesion has all the earmarks of necrosis, a trial of conservative treatment is instituted. The patient is placed on a biweekly or monthly examination schedule, photographs are taken, and precise drawings are made. Broad-spectrum antibiotics (e.g., tetracycline, 1 g/day), local anesthesia to be applied by a cotton-tipped applicator, and analgesics as needed are prescribed. Aspergum will give good analgesia if the patient can chew gum. Frequently, pain will be reduced dramatically in 1 to 3 days after starting antibiotics, but sometimes there is no response. Lidocaine (Xylocaine Viscous) can be applied to the ulcer with a cotton swab for local analgesia. We have had no success with alcohol nerve blocks. Hyperbaric oxygen treatment may be tried in difficult cases, but it is expensive. We have tried local fulguration with silver nitrate to attempt pain relief but have had little success; we have a variable experience with cryotherapy.

When all else fails and the necrosis is persistent and the pain is uncontrollable, the necrosis must be resected (Fig. 17-37). A myocutaneous flap may be needed to fill in the void.

The key word for management of radiation necroses is *patience.*

RADIATION-INDUCED BONE DISEASE

The retromolar trigone and horizontal ramus of the mandible are common sites of radiation-induced bone disease. The ascending ramus of the mandible is uncommonly the site of radiation-induced bone disease. The edentulous person is less likely than is a patient with teeth to develop serious radiation-induced disease of the mandible. There are several ways in which the mandible may be affected.

The most frequent problem involving the mandible is termed *bone exposure.* The onset varies from 4 months to many years following completion of radiation therapy. The gingiva and usually the periosteum disappear, exposing the underlying bone. The exposed area or areas usually vary from 2 mm to 2 cm in diameter. There is either minimal pain or modest discomfort, which is usually intermittent. In fact, if the exposed area is small, the patient is often unaware of the problem. The bone appears intact on roentgenograms. Biopsy is not needed unless there was tumor on the gingiva prior to treatment. If the patient has dentures, they should be discontinued or, in certain cases, altered by the dentist to relieve the denture over the exposed bone. If sharp bony edges appear, they are filed to a smooth contour and the bone edge lowered to speed healing. The bone exposure may become more or less stationary at this point. Healing may require months to even years. Healing occurs when the gingiva regrows over the exposed area; a small piece of bone may sequestrate first, and then the gingiva regrows to cover the exposed area. *Patience* is the major requirement (Fig. 17-38).

In some instances the bone exposure may progress so that a large area of bone is exposed. Pain is usually intermittent and mild to moderate; occasionally it is severe. Antibiotics will usually reduce pain when it does occur. Local care is similar to that used for early bone exposures. It is amazing that rampant osteomyelitis rarely develops in the exposed, relatively avascular bone.

In some cases, the bone becomes frankly necrotic with intermittent sequestration. Hyperbaric oxygen treatment has been used with some success. It is a matter of individualization as to when surgical intervention should be instituted. Conservative measures should be given a fair trial, but if pain becomes a problem, an operative procedure must be considered. In advanced cases, the dead bone is removed and covered with a flap carrying its own blood supply.

(Text continues on p. 281.)

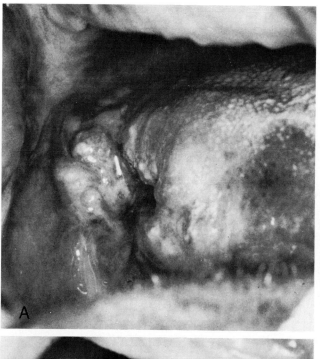

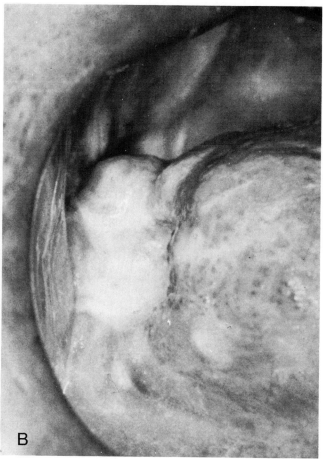

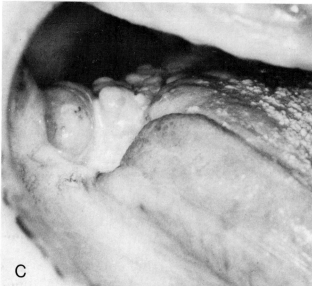

FIG. 17-36. (*A*) Ulcerated squamous cell carcinoma of the posterior lateral oral tongue (T3N2B). Patient refused operation. Treatment was 7000 rad/7 weeks, cobalt-60, plus radium implant, 2000 rad. (*B*) Appearance 3 months after radiation therapy. Soft tissue necrosis was present with pain. There was induration beneath the necrosis. Patient steadfastly refused surgery in case of proven recurrence, so biopsy was not done. (*C*) Appearance 16 months after radiation therapy. Pain persisted intermittently, but healing gradually progressed so that he was free of pain by 1½ years and the ulcer was healed. The patient died of lung cancer 2½ years following treatment of his tongue; there was no recurrence of his tongue cancer.

FIG. 17-37. (*A*) A 60-year-old man presented with carcinoma of the left lateral border of the tongue measuring 3 × 2 cm (T2N0). He was treated with 3000 rad tumor dose/2 weeks followed by a 2-plane radium needle implant delivering 5000 rad. (*B*) There was initial healing of the lesion, but at 4 months the patient returned with a deep ulcer at the site of the primary lesion. This ulcer was biopsied and showed no tumor. It persisted for approximately 1½ years, when it began to heal. He experienced intermittent major pain during this time. (*C*) At 20 months, the soft tissue necrosis of the tongue had healed but a bone exposure (*arrow*) had appeared in the left molar gingiva. (*D*) At 2 years, the bone exposure (*arrows*) had increased to 2 cm in length. (*E*) A submaxillary abscess developed in association with the gingival necrosis. The patient was experiencing major discomfort, and a resection of the involved mandible was done. (*F*) There was complete relief of pain following resection of the osteoradionecrosis. Patient returned 4 years later with a second large primary lesion of the epiglottis; because of his poor general health, only palliation could be offered. He died of the second primary cancer of the epiglottis, 7 years after radiation therapy for the oral tongue lesion.

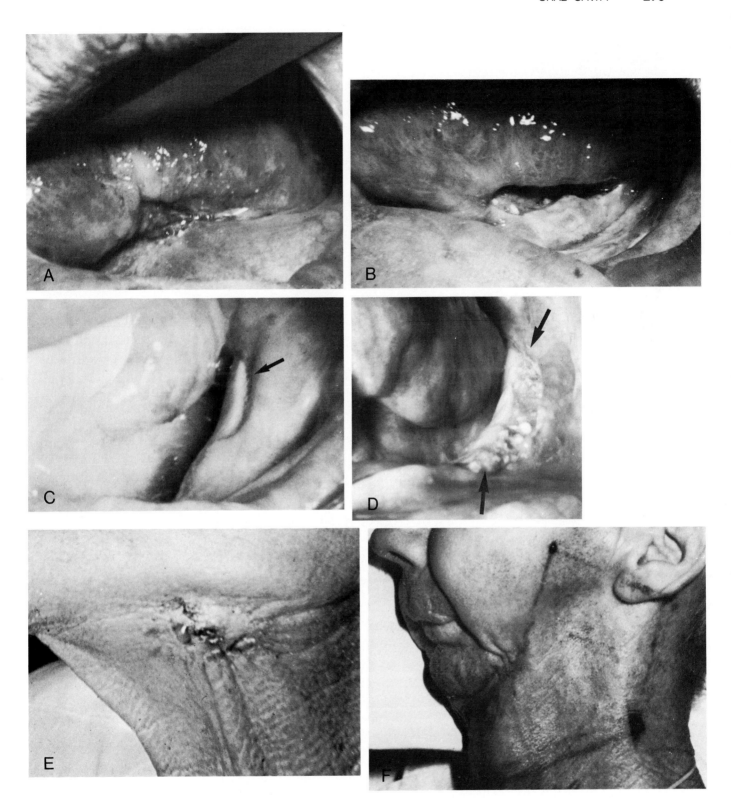

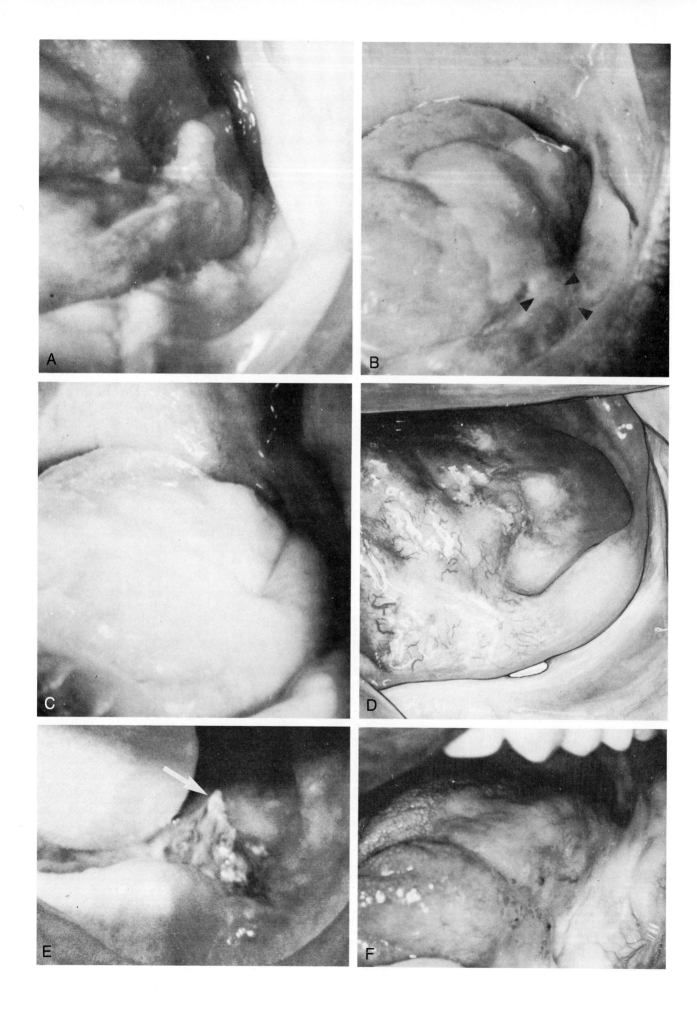

BUCCAL MUCOSA

Carcinoma of the buccal mucosa is associated with the use of snuff and chewing tobacco. The disease is infrequent in the United States.

Anatomy

The buccal mucosa is the mucous membrane covering the inner surface of the cheeks and lips. It ends above and below with a transition to the gingiva. It ends posteriorly at the retromolar trigone. The parotid duct opens into the buccal mucosa opposite the second upper molar. The muscular wall is composed mainly of the orbicularis oris anteriorly and the buccinator muscle posteriorly. The buccinator is covered externally by the buccal fat pad. The masseter muscle lies lateral to the buccinator muscle with its anterior margin opposite the retromolar trigone. The blood supply is a branch of the facial artery. The long buccal nerve, a branch of the mandibular, is sensory to the buccal mucosa and the skin of the cheek, which overlies the buccinator muscle. The facial nerve is the motor nerve to the buccinator muscle.

Pathology

The majority of malignant tumors are low-grade squamous cell carcinoma, and they frequently appear on a background of leukoplakia. This is the most frequent site for verrucous carcinoma to occur. Verrucous carcinoma may be particularly difficult to diagnose histologically because of associated inflammatory changes. An example of a patient who had multiple biopsies interpreted as pseudoepitheliomatous hyperplasia until the tumor grew through the skin and into the temporal fossa is shown in Figure 17-39.

Patterns of Spread

Almost all of the squamous cell carcinomas originate on the lateral walls and rarely on the inside of the lips. Early lesions are usually discrete, elevated tumors and are often exophytic. As they enlarge they penetrate the underlying muscles and eventually penetrate to the skin and infratemporal fossa. Peripheral growth occurs into the gingivobuccal gutters and eventually onto the gingiva and underlying bone. The parotid gland and facial nerve are invaded in advanced lesions.

Squamous cell carcinomas arising from the moist mucosa of the lips are quite uncommon. The three cases observed were all in the midline of the lower lip near the gingivolabial sulcus in the precise area where snuff was held (Fig. 17-40).

The lymphatic spread is first to the submaxillary and subdigastric nodes. Contralateral involvement on admission would be unusual. The incidence of positive nodes on admission is 9% to 31% and the risk of subclinical disease is 16%. (See Table 1 in Chapter 2).

Clinical Picture

Early, asymptomatic lesions may be discovered by the dentist or physician. A background of leukoplakia is common and sometimes quite extensive. Small lesions produce the sensation of a lump that is felt with the tongue. Pain is minimal even when the lesion becomes large, unless there is posterior extension to involve the lingual and dental nerves. Pain may be referred to the ear. Obstruction of Stensen's duct may product parotid enlargement. Extension posteriorly behind the pterygomandibular raphe or into the buccinator and masseter muscles will eventually cause trismus. Intermittent bleeding occurs when the lesion is irritated by chewing or is ulcerated by growing against the teeth. Multiple lesions may be present (Fig. 17-41).

Methods of Diagnosis and Staging

The differential diagnosis includes leukoplakia, lichen planus, lues, and tuberculosis.

If the first biopsy report is chronic inflammation or pseudoepitheliomatous hyperplasia, and there is an obvious neoplasm present, repeat biopsy is in order. Multiple repeat biopsies are often required to establish the diagnosis, and the physician must be skeptical of a benign diagnosis in the face of an obvious neoplasm that is enlarging and not responding to conservative management.

◄ **FIG. 17-38.** (A) A 57-year-old man presented with a 1.0 × 1.5-cm ulcerative lesion of the lateral border of the oral tongue (T1N0). In November 1968 the patient was treated with 3000-rad tumor dose/2 weeks through a single left lateral field that included the submaxillary and subdigastric lymph nodes, followed by a single-plane radium implant to the tongue delivering 5000 rad at 0.5 cm. No packing was placed between the gingiva and tongue. (B) Acute radiation mucositis was noted 3 weeks after radium needle implant. Note the small patch of mucositis extending to adjacent gingiva (*arrowheads*). (C) Complete healing was noted at 6 weeks (photograph at 4 months, March 1969). (D) In January 1970 there was a 1-cm superficial ulceration on the surface of the tongue, which healed in 1 month. The patient was wearing his dentures all the time. In February 1971, a 2-mm, asymptomatic ulcer appeared on the left mandible with bone exposed. In May 1972, the bone exposure had increased in size but was still asymptomatic. Six years following therapy, at the time of this photograph (December 1974), there was a 4 × 12-mm area of bone exposure but the patient was still asymptomatic. (E) The bone exposure remained stable until May 1978 (9½ years), when it was noted to have increased in size to 1.0 × 1.5 cm with a sequestrum (*arrow*) projecting about 1 cm above the gingiva. (F) The sequestrum separated spontaneously, and the gingiva completed covered the defect in the gum, as shown in this photograph of January 1982. The patient remained alive and free of disease at 14 years.

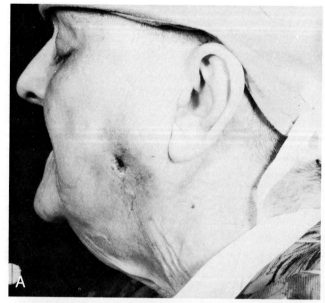

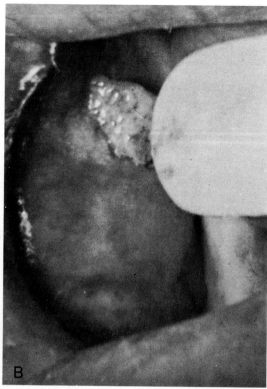

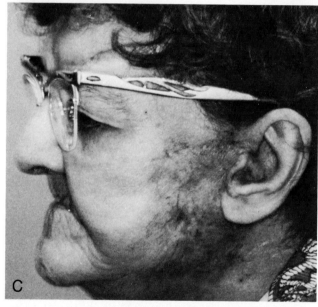

FIG. 17-39. Stage IV (T4N0) verrucous carcinoma of the buccal mucosa. In August 1968, after a 4-month history of pain in the cheek and spontaneous drainage of purulent material through the skin of the left cheek 10 days prior to admission, a biopsy was reported as grade I epidermoid carcinoma of the left buccal mucosa. This diagnosis was revised in 1982 to verrucous carcinoma. Multiple biopsies prior to admission had been reported as "pseudoepitheliomatous hyperplasia and chronic inflammation." (A) Appearance prior to treatment. Physical examination revealed a large subcutaneous mass involving the entire left cheek and extending posteriorly to the level of the tragus, into the temporal fossa, and beneath the mandible. There was ulceration of the buccal mucosa near the retromolar trigone. The neck was negative for disease. Roentgenograms of the mandible showed extensive destruction of the body, angle, and ascending ramus. The initial plan was to resect the lesion and repair with a forehead flap, and a flap was prepared for this procedure; however, the lesion proved to be unresectable owing to invasion into the squamous

portion of the temporal bone, and radiation therapy was elected. The patient received 5450-rad tumor dose, cobalt-60, through superior- and inferior-angled wedge fields. This was followed by a large single-plane radium needle implant for 3500 rad at 0.5 cm. The findings of multiple biopsies are listed below:

6 Months: 2 × 2-cm recurrence buccal mucosa. Local excision—verrucous carcinoma.

1 Year: 1.0 × 1.5-cm recurrence anterior buccal mucosa. Local excision—verrucous carcinoma.

3½ Years: granular lesion of retromolar trigone/glossotonsillar sulcus (B). Local excision—acute and chronic infection, no tumor.

4½ Years: biopsy of retromolar trigone—acute and chronic infection, no tumor.

5 Years: biopsy of retromolar trigone—hyperkeratosis, no tumor.

8½ Years: biopsy of retromolar trigone—hyperkeratosis, no tumor.

9 Years: irregular lesion of retromolar trigone area, 2.5 × 2.5 cm. Biopsy—no tumor.

(C) Appearance 9 years after initial treatment. Note the marked skin and subcutaneous changes from high-dose irradiation to an advanced lesion. Repeat biopsy at 9½ years showed spindle cell carcinoma. Review of two previous biopsies revealed spindle cell carcinoma to be present in all specimens. At 10 years chemotherapy was reported to produce a good response. Patient died of cancer at 10½ years.

This case history emphasizes the difficulties faced by the pathologist and treating physician in the management of very low-grade neoplasms. It is a moot point whether the change to a higher-grade lesion is related to the radiation therapy or is a natural history of the disease.

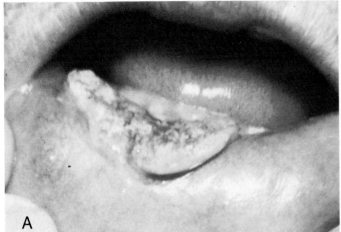

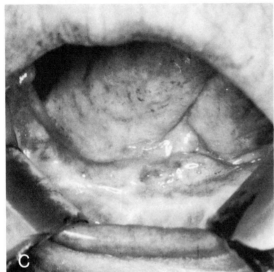

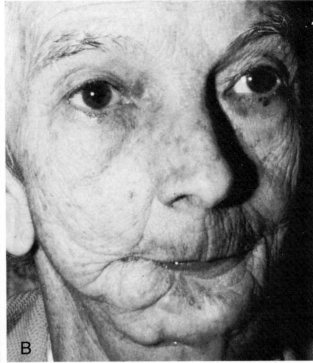

FIG. 17-40. (A) Squamous cell carcinoma of the wet mucosa of the lower lip. Initial treatment was by radium implant; the carcinoma recurred locally 2 years later and was managed by surgical excision. (B and C) There is no evidence of cancer 9 years after surgical resection.

The AJCC staging system was given at the beginning of this chapter. Roentgenograms of the mandible and maxilla are requested when tumor has spread onto these areas and for posterior extension. Extension posterior to the pterygomandibular raphe is often underestimated. A computed tomographic (CT) scan may help define posterior and superior extension.

Treatment

SELECTION OF TREATMENT MODALITY

Small lesions (less than 1 cm) may be simply excised with primary closure; small lesions that involve the oral commissure are best treated by radiation therapy. Lesions that are 1 cm to 3 cm in size are usually treated by radiation therapy (Figs. 17-42 and 17-43). These lesions can be excised and grafted, but the graft tends to shrink and become firm; this makes detection of recurrence difficult, and the lining of the cheek feels tight, rough, and uncomfortable to the patient. Larger lesions are treated by either radical surgical excision, radiation therapy, or a combination of both on an individual basis. Preference is given to radiation therapy when the tumor invades near the commissure. Preference is given to an operation when there is invasion of the mandible or maxilla.

SURGICAL TREATMENT

Lesions that invade the mandible or maxilla require that an appropriate amount of bone be resected along with the

FIG. 17-41. Two discrete verrucous carcinomas occurring in a woman who used snuff for many years. There were multiple other areas of leukoplakia and dysplasia throughout the oral cavity. Treatment was by wide local excision.

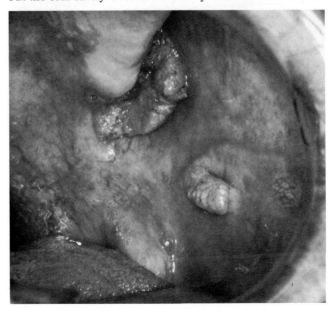

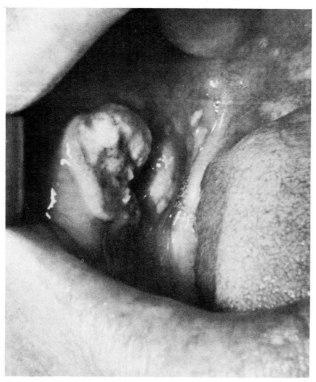

FIG. 17-42. Squamous cell carcinoma of the right buccal mucosa, 3.0 × 2.5 cm (T2N0). Lesions that are 1 cm to 3 cm in size are usually treated by radiation therapy.

soft tissues. Repair may require a maxillary prosthesis. Full-thickness removal of the cheek is repaired by a myocutaneous flap.

IRRADIATION TECHNIQUE

Localized buccal mucosa lesions are suitable for treatment with electrons, intraoral cone, and interstitial techniques in order to spare the contralateral normal tissues. When tumor extends into one of the gingivobuccal gutters or onto bone, treatment must be entirely by external-beam irradiation. A lead block placed in the mouth will help decrease radiation to the opposite side. There are no data on the dose required for control. Marginal failures occur, and the initial treatment area should be a bit more generous than for lesions of comparable size in other sites.

MANAGEMENT OF RECURRENCE

Surgical failures are managed by surgery, radiation therapy, or both. Radiation therapy failures are managed by extensive resection and repair with a flap. Local excision with primary closure or split-thickness skin graft is usually not possible for radiation therapy failures.

Results of Treatment

Ash reported 35% absolute 5-year survival for 374 patients with carcinoma of the buccal mucosa for all stages.[3] The primary lesion was initially controlled in 53% of patients with early lesions and 25% with advanced lesions; salvage

FIG. 17-43. (A) An 87-year-old woman presented with a 2.5 × 3.0-cm squamous cell carcinoma involving the anterior buccal mucosa (arrowheads) with extension of filmy leukoplakia (arrow) to the commissure of the lip. Treatment was a radium needle implant, 6000 rad at 0.5 cm. (B) Appearance at 4 months. The patient died at 21 months of intercurrent disease. The filmy leukoplakia also disappeared.

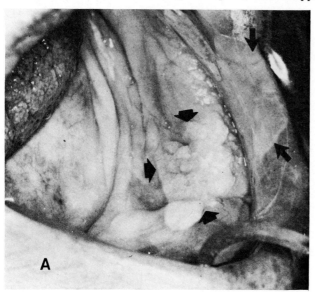

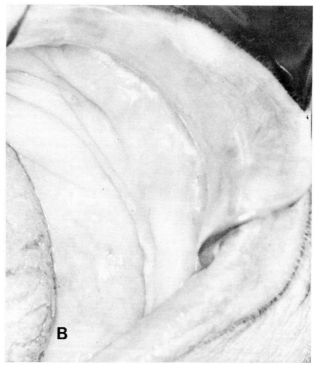

raised the ultimate control rates to 69% and 34%. The initial treatment to the primary lesion was radiation therapy in 97% of the patients.

MacComb and co-workers reported the results for 115 patients treated between 1947 and 1962.[28] Irradiation was the initial treatment in 69 patients, surgery was used in 44 patients, and combined therapy was used in 2 patients. The local recurrence rate was 10% for stage I, 12% for stages II and III, and 38% for stage IV. The 3-year absolute survival rate was 49%, and the 5-year absolute survival rate was 48%. The determinate 3- and 5-year survival rates were 71% and 70%, respectively. The same authors reported a 35% cure rate for 40 patients referred after failure of initial treatment given elsewhere.

Follow-up Policy

Patients who have been treated by surgical excision and split-thickness skin graft are difficult to evaluate because the graft contracts and makes interpretation of physical findings quite difficult.

Complications of Treatment

The buccal mucosa is quite tolerant of high-dose radiation therapy, and complications are uncommon. Bone exposure may appear on the mandible or maxilla. Trismus may develop if the muscles of mastication receive high doses.

Surgical injury of Stensen's duct may cause obstruction and parotitis. The parotid gland will eventually atrophy.

GINGIVA AND HARD PALATE (INCLUDING RETROMOLAR TRIGONE)

Carcinomas arising from the upper and lower gingiva have a similar clinical picture and require a similar approach to diagnosis and management. Primary squamous cell carcinoma of the hard palate is unusual, the majority of hard palate neoplasms being minor salivary gland tumors. (See Chapter 29, Minor Salivary Gland Tumors.) Some authors include the retromolar trigone with the anterior tonsillar pillar, but their anatomical relationships, natural history, and management are closer to lesions of the lower gingiva.

Anatomy

The lower gingiva includes the mucosa covering the mandible from the gingivobuccal gutter to the origin of the mobile mucosa on the floor of the mouth. Behind the third molar is a small triangular surface covering the ascending ramus that is called the retromolar trigone; it is continuous above with the maxillary tuberosity.

Beneath the mucosa of the retromolar trigone is the tendinous pterygomandibular raphe, which is attached to the pterygoid hamulus and the posterior mylohyoid ridge of the mandible and serves as the insertion of the buccinator, orbicular oris, and superior constrictor muscles. Just behind the pterygomandibular raphe and between the medial pterygoid muscle and the ascending ramus is the pterygomandibular space, which contains the lingual and dental nerves. The pterygomandibular space is related posteriorly to the deep lobe of the parotid and the contents of the parapharyngeal space.

There are no minor salivary glands in the "mucous" membrane over the alveolar ridges.

Pathology

The majority of neoplasms are squamous cell carcinoma. Verrucous lesions occur, usually on the lower gingiva. Melanoma is reported. Metastatic lesions to the underlying bone may be confused with primary tumors.

Epidermoid carcinoma may arise within the body of the mandible or maxilla (intra-alveolar epidermoid carcinoma) either from odontogenic epithelium or from epithelium trapped during embryonic development. It is more frequent in the mandible than the maxilla and is most common in the molar regions. It must be distinguished from metastatic squamous cell carcinoma and ameloblastoma.

Ameloblastoma is a rare tumor with an incidence of about 1% of all tumors of the maxilla and mandible. Most patients are in the age range of 20 to 50 years. Eighty percent of these tumors occur in the mandible, with the molar regions most commonly involved. No appreciable differences are found by sex or race.[44]

Histologically, the ameloblastoma is an epithelial tumor. The epithelium forms sheets or islands, and the peripheral layer is formed by atypical columnar cells.[43] The lesion may appear histologically benign, but it is expansive and tends to recur locally.[39] Ameloblastoma is histologically similar to basal cell carcinoma.

Patterns of Spread

LOWER GUM

Squamous cell carcinomas invade the periosteum and adjacent buccal mucosa and floor of the mouth. Slow-growing, low-grade lesions tend to produce atrophy of adjacent bone and cause a smooth, saucerized defect before invading the mandible. Moderate- to high-grade lesions invade the bone directly or through recently opened dental sockets.

Lymphatic spread is to the submaxillary and subdigastric nodes. Eighteen to 52% of patients have clinically positive nodes on admission; subclinical disease occurs in 17% to 19% (see Table 2-1 in Chapter 2). Contralateral lymph node involvement was found in only 2 of 62 cases reported by Byers and associates.[6]

Ameloblastoma is a rather indolent tumor that destroys bone and slowly extends to adjacent areas by continuous growth. Regional and even distant metastasis may occur in a few cases, but even when present it may be compatible with a long natural course. Metastatic disease is usually reported in the lungs, but bone and liver metastases have been reported.[42]

UPPER GUM AND HARD PALATE

Most of the carcinomas originate on the gingiva and spread secondarily to the hard palate, soft palate, buccal mucosa, and underlying bone; the maxillary antrum is invaded quite late unless there are recent extractions that provide an open pathway. Primary carcinoma originating in the maxillary antrum must be excluded since it frequently presents in the upper gum and hard palate. The risk for positive lymph nodes is 13% to 24% on admission, and the incidence of subclinical disease is 22% (see Table 2-1 in Chapter 2).

RETROMOLAR TRIGONE

The retromolar trigone is a small area, and spread to adjacent buccal mucosa, anterior tonsillar pillar, and maxilla occurs quite early. Posterior spread occurs early into the pterygomandibular space and the medial pterygoid muscle. Posterolateral spread occurs into the buccinator muscle and fat pad. Invasion of the periosteum of the mandible occurs early, but invasion of the underlying mandible tends to be a late manifestation. The cortical bone is quite dense, which explains the infrequent bone invasion in the region of the retromolar trigone and the angle of the mandible.

The submaxillary and subdigastric lymph nodes are the first-echelon lymph nodes.

The incidence of clinically positive nodes on presentation is about 40%, and the risk for subclinical disease is about 25% (see Table 2-1 in Chapter 2).

Clinical Picture

The patient with squamous cell carcinoma may present first to the dentist with either ill-fitting dentures, dental pain, loose teeth, or a sore that will not heal. A history of inappropriate dental extractions or root canal therapy is common. Intermittent bleeding and mild pain occur when the lesion is traumatized. Involvement of the inferior dental nerve usually occurs outside the mandible and may produce paresthesias or anesthesia of the lower lip. A background of leukoplakia is frequently present.

Retromolar trigone lesions that involve the lingual and inferior dental nerve cause local pain and pain referred to the external auditory canal and preauricular area (see Fig. 17-12). Invasion of the pterygoid muscle produces trismus, usually accompanied by severe pain. Invasion of the underlying mandible occurs in the advanced lesion, but small lesions show only periosteal invasion.

Intra-alveolar epidermoid carcinoma presents with a submucosal mass and dental symptoms. Roentgenograms show a lytic lesion in the mandible.

Ameloblastoma is a slow-growing neoplasm with few symptoms in the early stages. Patients may notice a gradually increasing facial deformity or loosening of the teeth or denture.[21] On roentgenograms, a radiolucent area is seen with some of the following features: expansion of the overlying cortical plate, a scalloped margin, a multilocular appearance, and resorption of the roots of adjacent teeth.[29]

Methods of Diagnosis and Staging

The differential diagnosis includes denture sore, dental abscess, granuloma, papilloma, and underlying bony cyst or tumor originating in bone, including metastatic tumor.

Roentgenograms, including tomograms when needed, are required for almost all lesions. Dental roentgenograms (occlusal views) should be used when fine detail is needed to look for early invasion. The Panorex and oblique mandible views are useful for determining the extent of invasion where mandible involvement is obvious. Tomograms of the maxilla are required to detect involvement of the alveolus and hard palate. It is difficult to exclude

bone invasion in the presence of severe periodontal and periapical disease or when recent extractions have been done.

The AJCC staging systems for oral cavity lesions is difficult to apply to gum lesions. In fact, the possibility of mandible invasion is not even considered. Evidence of lytic bone invasion should qualify for T4. Since even small lesions (less than 2 cm) may invade bone, there will be a wide prognostic range for T4 tumors. Swearingen and co-workers reported a 56% incidence of mandible involvement for gum lesions and 10% for retromolar trigone lesions.[47]

Treatment

SELECTION OF TREATMENT MODALITY

LOWER GUM

The majority of lesions are managed by operation. Small lesions may be remedied by intraoral resection with or without a rim resection of bone and repaired with a split-thickness skin graft. When bone invasion is present, removal of a segment of mandible is required. An appropriate neck dissection is generally included with segmental mandibulectomy since the neck is entered in order to resect the primary lesion. Large lesions require hemimandibulectomy. Irradiation may be used for small lesions or for those with only a pressure defect in the bone with good curative results, but the overall results are generally better after operation.

RETROMOLAR TRIGONE

Small retromolar trigone lesions may appear innocuous and easily cured, but they are often more extensive than they seem. For early, well-localized lesions without detectable bone invasion, a rim or marginal resection of mandible may be done in order to preserve continuity of the mandible. If rim resection is not feasible, initial treatment with radiation therapy should be considered, with partial mandibulectomy reserved for radiation therapy failure. Radiation therapy is recommended for lesions involving a rather large surface area, such as lesions with extension to the anterior tonsillar pillar, soft palate, and buccal mucosa (Fig. 17-44). Evidence of bone invasion requires partial mandibulectomy. Preference is given to surgical treatment unless the cosmetic and functional result would be unacceptable to the patient, in which case operation is reserved for radiation therapy failure. Moderately advanced and advanced lesions are usually managed by resection followed by postoperative radiation therapy.

UPPER GUM AND HARD PALATE

Squamous cell carcinoma on the hard palate is relatively rare. Surgical resection is the usual treatment for most lesions of the upper gum. Postoperative radiation therapy is added as needed. If the lesion is superficial and extensively involves the hard palate or involves a significant portion of the soft palate, then radiation therapy may be tried as the initial treatment. If the lesion is small and discrete and there is no bone involvement, the resection includes the periosteum or occasionally some underlying bone (Fig. 17-45). Bone invasion requires a partial or total maxillectomy (Fig. 17-46). The defect is reconstructed with a prosthesis.

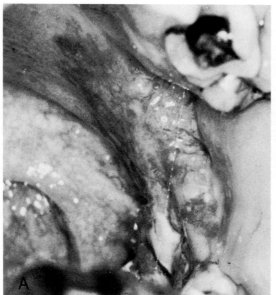

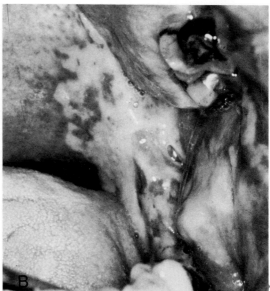

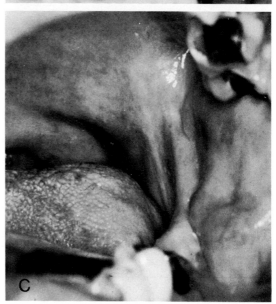

FIG. 17-44. A 57-year-old man presented with a squamous cell carcinoma of the left retromolar trigone and a clinically negative neck (T2N0). (A) The lesion covered the retromolar trigone, extended slightly onto the buccal mucosa, involved the lingual gingiva and the lateral margin of the tongue, and extended onto the soft palate to within 1.5 cm of the midline. Posteriorly the lesion extended nearly to the tonsil. Treatment options included surgical resection followed by postoperative irradiation or irradiation alone. The patient was made aware that there was probably some decreased chance of cure by using radiation therapy as the initial treatment as opposed to combined treatment. He elected to accept the increased risk of recurrence in order to avoid the functional losses associated with surgical excision. (B) After 1800 rad, marked tumoritis and mucositis were present. The patient was treated with parallel opposed fields weighted 2:1 left to right, cobalt-60. The final dose was 7500 rad/8 weeks. (C) Appearance 2½ years after radiation therapy; no evidence of recurrence or necrosis. Patient was living, free of disease, at 3 years.

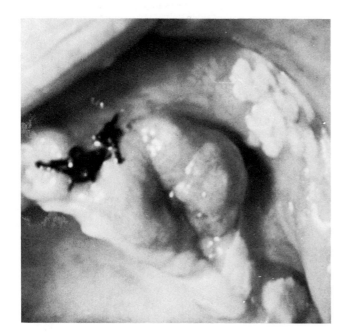

FIG. 17-45. Squamous cell carcinoma of the left upper gingiva. There was no bone involvement. The resection included the periosteum. Note leukoplakia on the buccal mucosa.

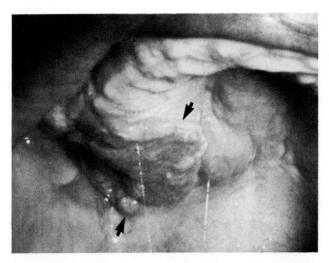

FIG. 17-46. Squamous cell carcinoma of the right upper gingiva/hard palate with extension to the gingivobuccal sulcus. The lesion was fixed to the periosteum. Tomograms suggested early bone invasion. Treatment was partial maxillectomy.

AMELOBLASTOMA

Ameloblastoma occurring in the mandible is best managed by mandibulectomy with adequate margins. Immediate reconstruction of the mandibular defect is usually done because little or no soft tissue is sacrificed, and postoperative radiation therapy is rarely used (Fig. 17-47).

The treatment of choice for ameloblastoma of the maxilla is partial maxillectomy with repair by a prosthesis. Curettage is unacceptable treatment in either the maxilla or mandible because it is accompanied by a very high rate of recurrence.

Ameloblastoma responds readily to radiation therapy in our limited experience (Fig. 17-48). However, irradiation has generally been applied to patients after multiple operative failures or in cases of very advanced disease. Therefore, the curative ability is not entirely clear.

SURGICAL TREATMENT

RIM RESECTION (CORONAL RESECTION)*

Early gingival and retromolar trigone lesions may be resected by an intraoral resection of the tumor that includes a cuff of normal periosteum or bone. Larger lesions of the lower gingiva and retromolar trigone, especially those fixed to the periosteum but with normal roentgenograms, may be managed by rim resection, which allows preservation of the continuity of the mandible (Fig. 17-49).

SEGMENTAL MANDIBULECTOMY

For small lesions with minimal bone invasion, a short section of mandible is removed in continuity with the

* The term *marginal resection* has sometimes been applied to the operation in which only a rim or coronal section of mandible is removed adjacent to the tumor but leaving the contour of the mandible intact. The term *marginal* suggests, however, that the operation gives very close borders to the neoplasm and for this reason it is avoided.

tumor (e.g., removal of the mandible from the angle to the mental foramen).

PARTIAL MANDIBULECTOMY

The mandible and tumor are resected from the mental foramen to the coronoid process; the head of the condyle usually remains intact (Fig. 17-50). If teeth are present in the remaining segment of the mandible, a K wire or cobalt–chromium alloy (Vitallium) mesh spacer with or without bone chips is used for rehabilitation. Otherwise, mandibular shift occurs after resection, which results in poor dental occlusion and difficulty in chewing (Fig. 17-51). In edentulous patients, no spacer is required, since the patient is rarely able to wear a lower denture. The cosmetic and functional loss after partial mandibulectomy is acceptable.

K wires are not often used today because of their tendency to extrude within a short period of time. The cobalt–chromium alloy mesh trays have a 60% to 75% success rate provided there is adequate soft tissue for coverage; postoperative irradiation has been used in some cases without obvious difficulties, but the success rate is probably reduced.

HEMIMANDIBULECTOMY

Extensive lesions may require removal of the mandible from symphysis to condyle on one side. Massive anterior lesions require removal of the mandible from angle to angle. This produces a major cosmetic and functional loss that is reconstructed with myocutaneous flaps, metal trays, and autogenous rib or iliac bone grafts.

PARTIAL MAXILLECTOMY

See Chapter 23, Nasal Vestibule, Nasal Cavity, and Paranasal Sinuses.

IRRADIATION TECHNIQUE

Small lesions of the lower gum and retromolar trigone may be treated by intraoral cone therapy for all or part of their therapy (Fig. 17-52). Well-lateralized lesions of the retromolar trigone may be treated by ipsilateral mixed-beam techniques (Fig. 17-53) or with angled-wedge techniques. A lead intraoral shield reduces contralateral irradiation. Lesions of the anterior gingiva are treated by parallel opposed lateral portals.

The dose for retromolar trigone lesions is 7000 rad/7 weeks for T1–T2 and 7500 rad/7 weeks for T3. The dose for gum lesions is similar.

Local control by radiation therapy alone for lesions with early bone invasion (erosion defect) is reported by Fayos to be approximately 50% (8 of 17) and for extensive invasion about 25% (7 of 25) (Fig. 17-54).[14]† His report included 29 patients with squamous cell carcinoma of the lower alveolus.

MANAGEMENT OF RECURRENCE

Radiation therapy failures may be salvaged by operation. Surgical failures may be salvaged by surgery, radiation therapy, or a combination of both (Tables 17-15 through 17-17).

† Fayos JV: Personal communication, June 7, 1974.

(*Text continues on p. 295.*)

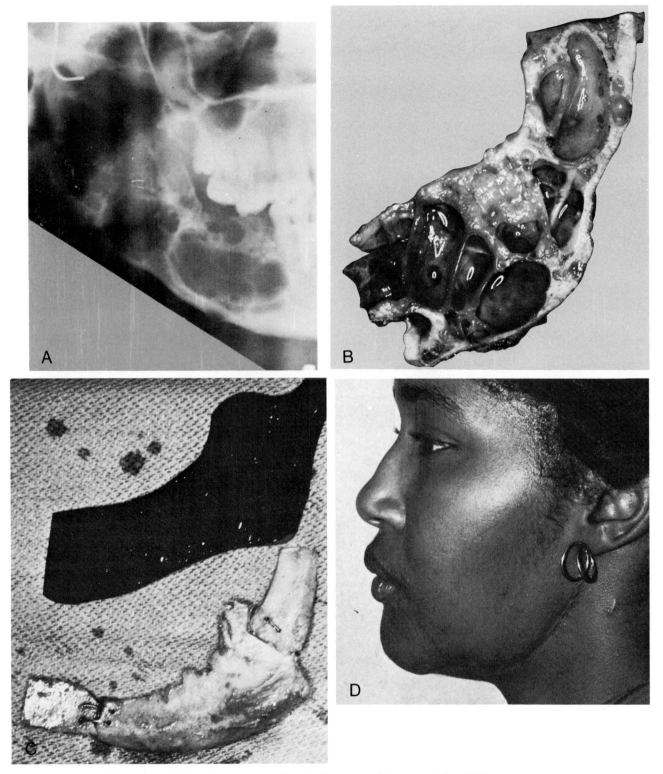

FIG. 17-47. (A) Roentgenogram of ameloblastoma of the mandible. (B) Gross specimen. (C) Silhouette (*above*) of opposite normal mandible obtained from roentgenogram. Three pieces of bone from iliac crest fashioned to size and contour of contralateral mandible (*below*). (D) Postoperative appearance.

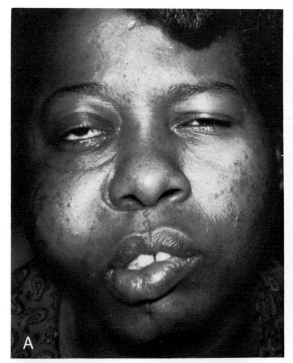

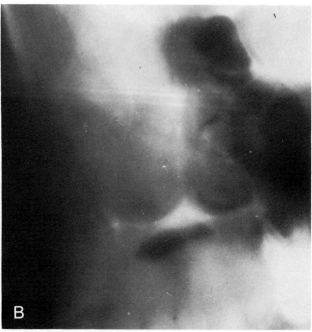

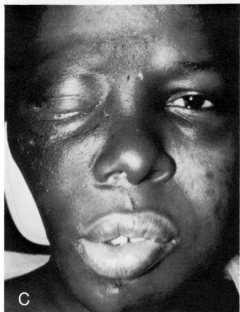

FIG. 17-48. In 1962 an 18-year-old woman had a bone cyst and tooth removed. In 1965 she had a partial right mandibulectomy. Diagnosis: ameloblastoma. In 1967 she had a right submandibular mass excised. Diagnosis: ameloblastoma. In 1968 there was extensive recurrence in the right maxilla with extension to the zygoma, infratemporal fossa, right orbit, and right nostril and erosion into the oral cavity through the right upper posterior alveolar ridge (A). (B) Coronal tomograms revealed destruction of the right maxilla, zygoma, floor of the orbit, and ethmoid sinuses with possible extension to the clivus, sphenoid sinus, and cribriform plate. The patient was treated with 2-MV x-rays, receiving a minimum tumor dose of 5670 rad by an anterior and right lateral wedge technique. (C) Complete regression of tumor was noted within 3 months. In 1970 the patient had facial reconstruction due to oral-antral fistula and bone necrosis. The chest roentgenogram showed lung nodules; biopsy diagnosis: ameloblastoma. In 1976 a small area of local recurrence was noted; biopsy diagnosis: ameloblastoma. A right lower lobectomy was done; diagnosis: ameloblastoma. Local recurrence in right cheek was found in 1980 and wide local excision was done. In 1982 patient was living with local disease; the lung nodules are stable.

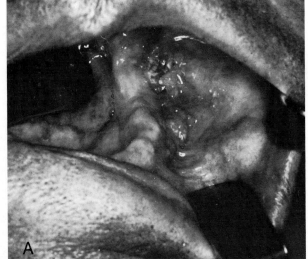

FIG. 17-49. (*A*) Squamous cell carcinoma of the left gingivobuccal sulcus (T2N0). (*B*) The lip was split and a cheek flap elevated, exposing the body of the mandible. Drill holes were placed in the body of the mandible to facilitate a precision cut. (*C*) Rim resection was completed and specimen was removed; 1.0 to 1.5 cm of mandible remained intact. (M, mandible, T, tongue, P, hard palate) (*D*) Intraoral defect after healing. (*E*) Contour of jaw is intact. This patient has an abnormal degree of hypertrophic scarring in the lip incision. For this reason some surgeons prefer a visor-type flap.

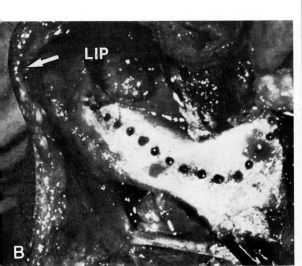

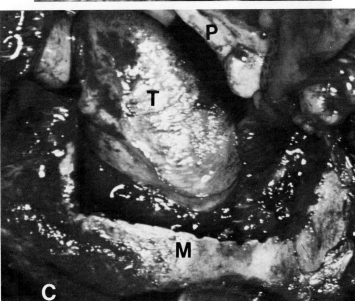

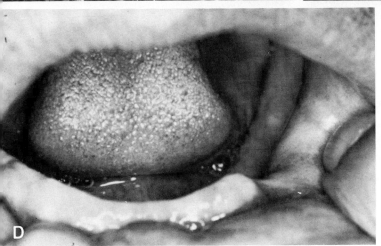

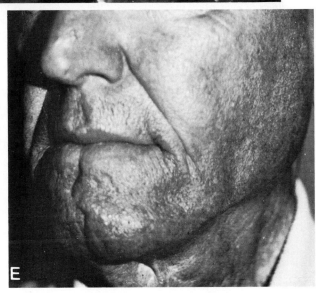

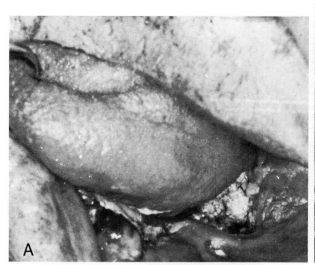

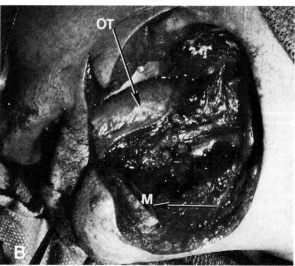

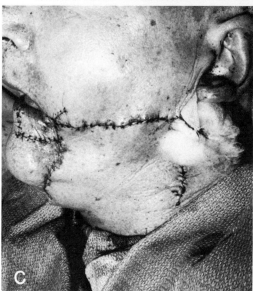

FIG. 17-50. (*A*) Verrucous carcinoma of the alveolar ridge with extension to the floor of the mouth, buccal mucosa, and skin of the cheek. Roentgenograms showed mandible invasion. (*B*) A hemi-mandibulectomy plus resection of the floor of the mouth, buccal mucosa, and involved skin was done. (OT, oral tongue, M, mandible [cut edge]) (*C*) Rotation flaps were used to close the defect. The mandible was not reconstructed because of the large amount of soft tissue resected.

FIG. 17-51. Hemangioendothelioma of the left mandible with soft tissue extension. (*A*) Replacement of left mandible with cobalt-chromium alloy (Vitallium) mesh spacer. (SMX, submaxillary gland) (*B*) Postoperative appearance. Patient received postoperative irradiation, 6500 rad. There was no evidence of disease at 30 months.

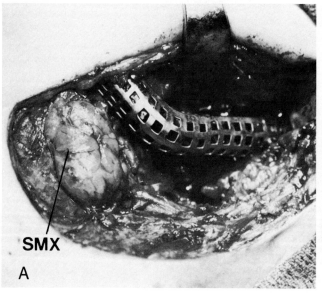

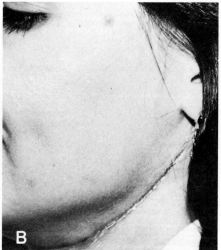

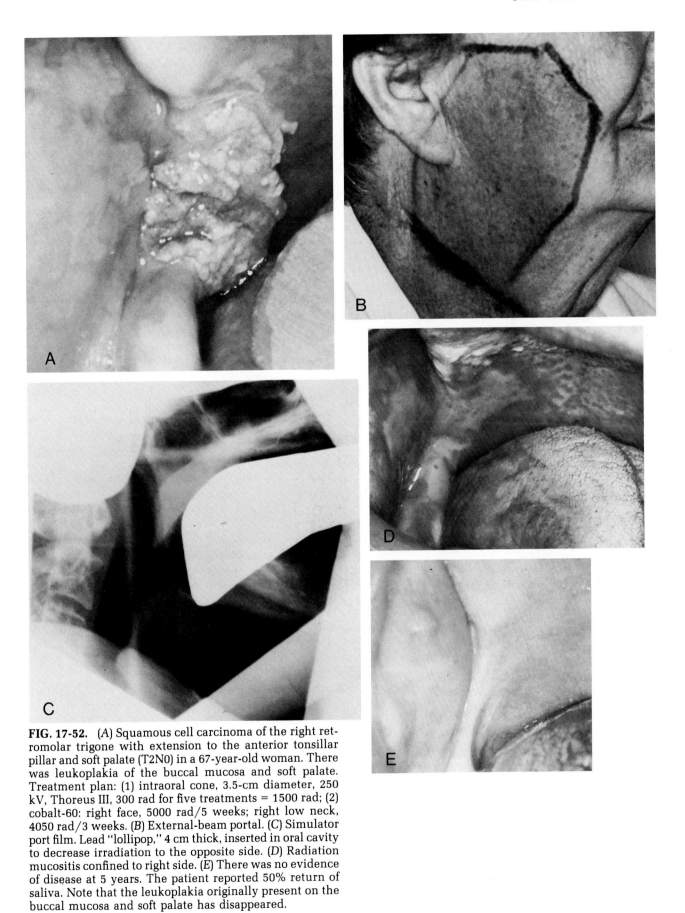

FIG. 17-52. (*A*) Squamous cell carcinoma of the right retromolar trigone with extension to the anterior tonsillar pillar and soft palate (T2N0) in a 67-year-old woman. There was leukoplakia of the buccal mucosa and soft palate. Treatment plan: (1) intraoral cone, 3.5-cm diameter, 250 kV, Thoreus III, 300 rad for five treatments = 1500 rad; (2) cobalt-60: right face, 5000 rad/5 weeks; right low neck, 4050 rad/3 weeks. (*B*) External-beam portal. (*C*) Simulator port film. Lead "lollipop," 4 cm thick, inserted in oral cavity to decrease irradiation to the opposite side. (*D*) Radiation mucositis confined to right side. (*E*) There was no evidence of disease at 5 years. The patient reported 50% return of saliva. Note that the leukoplakia originally present on the buccal mucosa and soft palate has disappeared.

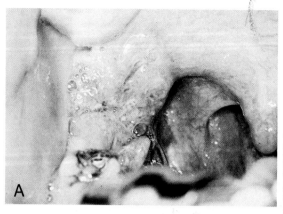

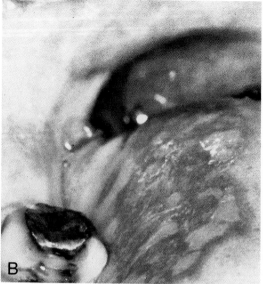

FIG. 17-53. (*A*) Squamous cell carcinoma of the right retromolar trigone with extension to the anterior tonsillar pillar and soft palate; roentgenogram of mandible normal (T2N0). Treatment plan: 7500 rad/8 weeks, mixed beam (20-MeV electrons and 17-MV photons). (*B*) No evidence of tumor at completion of treatment. Recurrence appeared at 5 months and was treated by partial mandibulectomy and palatectomy and by right radical neck dissection. A small rim of bone was saved inferiorly, and the incision was closed primarily. One focus of tumor extended near the deep margin. A second recurrence appeared 1 year later.

FIG. 17-54. (*A*) Squamous cell carcinoma of the left lower gum (T4N0). Patient refused mandibulectomy. (*B*) Erosion (saucerization) of mandible (*arrows*). (*C*) Appearance 6 months following 6500 rad/7 weeks, cobalt-60. Patient was free of disease at 6 years. There were no complications.

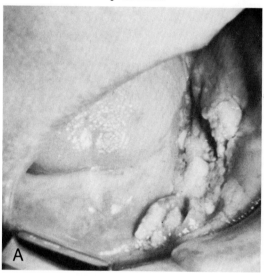

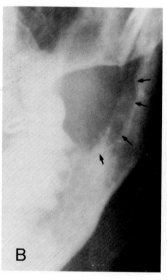

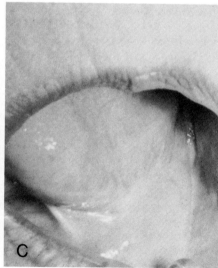

Results of Treatment

CARCINOMA

The analysis of local control for lower gum, retromolar trigone, and upper gum lesions is shown in Tables 17-15 through 17-17. The high rate of local failure with radiation therapy for early retromolar trigone lesions is not explained by low dose or marginal failure. The absolute survival for 43 patients was 56% at 2 years and 34% at 5 years. The local control for both surgery and radiation therapy has improved in recent years.

Cady and Catlin reported an absolute 5-year survival rate of 43% for patients with lower gum lesions and 40% for those with upper gum lesions treated by surgery.[8]

Byers and co-workers reported a 5-year absolute survival rate of 43% for 61 patients with squamous cell carcinoma of the lower gum treated from 1970 to 1975.[6] Fifty-one patients were managed by surgical resection. Intraoral resection including a rim of bone was selected for 28 early lesions. There was only one local failure. Eight patients subsequently developed neck node metastases; all were controlled.

Segmental mandibulectomy and neck dissection were used for 23 patients with more advanced disease; there were no local failures. Three had recurrence in the neck and all were salvaged. Six additional patients were given postoperative radiation therapy for close margins, perineural invasion, or extensive nodal metastasis; one patient had failure in the neck.

The overall rate of control above the clavicle for operation with selected use of postoperative radiation therapy was 95%.

AMELOBLASTOMA

Sehdev and associates reported that curettage was followed by local recurrence in 90% of mandibular and all maxillary ameloblastomas.[42] Subsequent resection controlled 80% of the mandibular tumors but only 40% of the maxillary tumors. The initial use of segmental mandibular resection controlled 78% (18/23), with subsequent resection controlling the treatment failures. The use of partial maxillectomy as the first treatment controlled 100% (7/7) of maxillary ameloblastomas as opposed to only 40% when partial maxillectomy was performed for recurrence. Hemimandibulectomy controlled 100% of curettage failures in one series.[40]

TABLE 17-15.   Carcinoma of the Lower Gum: Local Control (26 Patients)

Stage	Initial Treatment by Radiation Therapy		Initial Treatment by Surgery (No. Controlled/No. Treated)	Initial Treatment by Surgery Plus Radiation Therapy (No. Controlled/No. Treated)
	Initial Control (No. Controlled/ No. Treated)	Surgical Salvage (No. Salvaged/ No. Attempted)		
T1	1/1		2/2	0
T2	1/5	0/2	3/5*	0
T3	0		0	0
T4	1/2	0/1	3/4*	4/7*

* Salvage not attempted in any failures.
Note: University of Florida data; patients treated 10/64–12/80; analysis 4/83 by G. R. Ayers, MD.

TABLE 17-16.   Carcinoma of the Retromolar Trigone: Local Control (42 Patients)

Stage	Initial Treatment by Radiation Therapy		Initial Treatment by Surgery		Initial Treatment by Surgery Plus Radiation Therapy
	Initial Control (No. Controlled/ No. Treated)	Surgical Salvage (No. Salvaged/ No. Attepted)	Initial Control (No. Controlled/ No. Treated)	Radiation Therapy or Surgical Salvage (No. Salvaged/ No. Attempted)	
T1	4/4		1/2	1/1*	0
T2	2/8	0/3	2/2		3/4
T3	2/2		3/4	0/0	2/3†
T4	0/4	0/1	2/3	0/1	3/6†

* Follow-up 10 months after salvage by radiation therapy.
† Salvage not attempted in any failures.

Note: University of Florida data; patients treated 10/64–12/80; analysis 4/83 by G. R. Ayers, MD.

TABLE 17-17. Carcinoma of the Upper Gum: Local Control (9 Patients)

| Stage | Initial Treatment by Radiation Therapy | | Initial Treatment by Surgery (No. Controlled/No. Treated) | Initial Treatment by Surgery Plus Radiation Therapy (No. Controlled/No. Treated) |
	Initial Control (No. Controlled/No. Treated)	Surgical Salvage (No. Salvaged/No. Attempted)		
T1	0		0	1/1
T2	0/2	1/1	0	0
T3	0		0	0
T4	0/1	0	3/5*	0

* Salvage not attempted in any failures.
Note: University of Florida data; patients treated 10/64–12/80; analysis 4/83 by G. R. Ayers, MD.

Follow-up Policy

A high rate of local recurrence indicates careful observation every 4 to 6 weeks for 2 years. Ulceration with persistent recurrent pain may indicate either necrosis or cancer, and biopsy is required to establish the diagnosis.

Complications of Treatment

Surgical complications include orocutaneous fistula, bone exposure with sequestration, and loss of graft or flap.

The complications of radiation therapy include dental caries and soft tissue necrosis, with bone exposure and subsequent osteoradionecrosis. The risk is greatest for patients with advanced lesions of the lower gum and retromolar trigone.

Eight patients in the University of Florida series had attempted surgical salvage, which was successful in four. Complications included fistula, wound infection requiring removal of bone graft, and chronic aspiration requiring a gastric tube. Four patients had attempted salvage by radiation therapy, which was successful in two. There were no complications.

REFERENCES

1. American Joint Committee on Cancer: Manual for Staging of Cancer, 2nd ed., pp 25–30. Philadelphia, JB Lippincott, 1983.
2. Ange DW, Lindberg RD, Guillamondegui OM: Management of squamous cell carcinoma of the oral tongue and floor of mouth after excisional biopsy. Radiology 116:143–146, 1975
3. Ash CL: Oral Cancer: A twenty-five year study. Am J Roentgenol Radium Ther Nucl Med 87:417–430, 1962
4. Baker SR, Kraus CJ: Carcinoma of the lip. Laryngoscope 90:19–27, 1980
5. Bamberg M, Schulz U, Scherer E: Postoperative split course radiotherapy of squamous cell carcinoma of the oral tongue. Int J Radiat Oncol Biol Phys 5:515–519, 1979
6. Byers RM, Newman R, Russell N, Yue A: Results of treatment for squamous carcinoma of the lower gum. Cancer 47:2236–2238, 1981
7. Byers RM, O'Brien J, Waxler J: The therapeutic and prognostic implications of nerve invasion in cancer of the lower lip. Int J Radiat Oncol Biol Phys 4:215–217, 1978
8. Cady B, Catlin D: Epidermoid carcinoma of the gum: A 20-year survey. Cancer 23:551–569, 1969
9. Campos JL, Lampe I, Fayos JV: Radiotherapy of carcinoma of the floor of the mouth. Radiology 99:677–682, 1971
10. Chu A, Fletcher GH: Incidence and causes of failures to control by irradiation the primary lesions in squamous-cell carcinomas of the anterior two-thirds of tongue and floor of mouth. Am J Roentgenol Radium Ther Nucl Med 117:502–508, 1973
11. Clemente CD: Anatomy: A Regional Atlas of the Human Body. Philadelphia, Lea & Febiger, 1975
12. Crissman JD, Gluckman J, Whiteley J, Quenelle D: Squamous-cell carcinoma of the floor of the mouth. Head Neck Surg 3:2–7, 1980
13. Ellingwood KE, Million RR, Mitchell TP: A preloaded radium needle implant device for maintenance of needle spacing. Cancer 37:2858–2860, 1976
14. Fayos JV: Carcinoma of the mandible: Result of radiation therapy. Acta Radiol Ther Phys Biol 12:378–386, 1973
15. Fayos JV, Lampe I: Peroral irradiation of carcinoma of the oral tongue. Radiology 93:387–394, 1969
16. Fletcher GH: Elective irradiation of subclinical disease in cancers of the head and neck. Cancer 29:1450–1454, 1972
17. Flynn MB, Mullins FX, Moore C: Selection of treatment in squamous carcinoma of floor of mouth. Am J Surg 126:477–481, 1973
18. Fu KK, Chan EK, Phillips TL, Ray JW: Time, dose, and volume factors in interstitial radium implants of carcinoma of oral tongue. Radiology 119:209–213, 1976
19. Fu KK, Lichter A, Galante M: Carcinoma of the floor of mouth: An analysis of treatment results and the sites and causes of failures. Int J Radiat Oncol Biol Phys 1:829–837, 1976
20. Fu KK, Ray JW, Chan EK, Phillips TL: External and interstitial radiation-therapy of carcinoma of oral tongue. Am J Roentgenol 126:107–115, 1976
21. Goldberg SJ, Friedman JM: Ameloblastoma: Review of the literature and report of case. J Am Dent Assoc 90:432–438, 1975
22. Guillamondegui OM, Jesse RH: Surgical treatment of advanced carcinoma of floor of the mouth. Am J Roentgenol 126:1256–1259, 1976
23. Horiuchi J, Adachi T: Some considerations on radiation therapy of tongue cancer. Cancer 28:335–339, 1971
24. Inoue T, Fuchihata H, Wada T, Shigematsu Y: Local prognosis after combined external and interstitial radiation therapy for carcinoma of tongue. Acta Radiol Ther Phys Biol 15:315–320, 1976
25. Jørgensen K, Elbrønd O, Andersen AP: Carcinoma of the lip: A series of 869 cases. Acta Radiol Ther Phys Biol 12:177–190, 1973
26. Lees AW: The treatment of carcinoma of the anterior two-

thirds of the tongue by radiotherapy. Int J Radiat Oncol Biol Phys 1:849–858, 1976

27. Lindberg RD: Distribution of cervical lymph node metastases from squamous cell carcinoma of the upper respiratory and digestive tracts. Cancer 29:1446–1449, 1972

28. MacComb WS, Fletcher GH, Healey JE Jr: Intra-oral cavity. In MacComb WS, Fletcher GH (ed): Cancer of the Head and Neck, pp 89–151. Baltimore, Williams & Wilkins, 1967

29. McIvor J: The radiological features of ameloblastoma. Clin Radiol 25:237–242, 1974

30. MacKay EN, Sellers AH: A statistical review of carcinoma of the lip. Can Med Assoc J 90:670–672, 1964

31. Marcus RB Jr, Million RR, Mitchell TP: A preloaded, custom-designed implantation device for stage T1–T2 carcinoma of the floor of mouth. Int J Radiat Oncol Biol Phys 6:111–113, 1980

32. Mashberg A, Meyers H: Anatomical site and size of 222 early asymptomatic oral squamous cell carcinomas: A continuing prospective study of oral cancer. II. Cancer 37:2149–2157, 1976

33. Mendenhall W: Introduction to Probability and Statistics, 4th ed, pp 284–286. North Scituate, MA, Duxbury Press, 1975

34. Mendenhall W, Ott L, Larson RF: Statistics: A Tool for the Social Sciences, p 336. North Scituate, MA, Duxbury Press, 1974

35. Mendenhall WM, VanCise WS, Bova FJ, Million RR: Analysis of time–dose factors in squamous cell carcinoma of the oral tongue and floor of mouth treated with radiation therapy alone. Int J Radiat Oncol Biol Phys 7:1005–1011, 1981

36. Million RR: Elective neck irradiation for T_xN_0 squamous carcinoma of the oral tongue and floor of mouth. Cancer 34:149–155, 1974

37. Million RR: Squamous cell carcinoma of the head and neck: Combined therapy: Surgery and postoperative irradiation. Int J Radiat Oncol Biol Phys 5:2161–2162, 1979

38. Million RR, Cassisi NJ, Wittes RE: Cancer in the head and neck. In DeVita VT Jr, Hellman S, Rosenberg SA: Cancer: Principles and Practice of Oncology, pp 301–305. Philadelphia, JB Lippincott, 1982

39. Pandya NJ, Stuteville OH: Treatment of ameloblastoma. Plast Reconstr Surg 50:242–248, 1972

40. Rankow RM, Hickey MJ: Adamantinoma of the mandible: Analysis of surgical treatment. Surgery 36:713–719, 1954

41. Rouvière H: Anatomy of the Human Lymphatic System, pp 44–56. Ann Arbor, MI, Edwards Brothers, 1938

42. Sehdev MK, Huvos AG, Strong EW: Ameloblastoma of maxilla and mandible. Cancer 33:324–333, 1974

43. Sinclair NA: Cysts and ameloblastomas: Relationship. Aust Dent J 22:27–30, 1977

44. Small IA, Waldron CA: Ameloblastomas of the jaws. Oral Surg 8:281–297, 1955

45. Southwick HW: Elective neck dissection for intraoral cancer. JAMA 217:454–455, 1971

46. Spiro RH, Strong EW: Surgical treatment of cancer of the tongue: Surg Clin North Am 54:759–765, 1974

47. Swearingen AG, McGraw JP, Palumbo VD: Roentgenographic pathologic correlation of carcinoma of the gingiva involving the mandible. Am J Roentgenol Radium Ther Nucl Med 96:15–18, 1966

48. Tapley NduV: Clinical Applications of the Electron Beam, pp 125–129. New York, John Wiley & Sons, 1976

Oropharynx

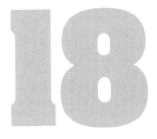

RODNEY R. MILLION
NICHOLAS J. CASSISI

The oropharynx includes four areas: (1) the base of the tongue, (2) the tonsillar region (tonsillar fossa and tonsillar pillars), (3) the soft palate, and (4) that portion of the pharyngeal wall between the pharyngoepiglottic fold and the nasopharynx. The oropharyngeal walls will be considered in Chapter 21, Hypopharynx: Pharyngeal Walls, Pyriform Sinus, and Postcricoid Pharynx.

ANATOMY

The base of the tongue is bounded anteriorly by the circumvallate papillae, laterally by the glossopharyngeal sulci, and posteriorly by the epiglottis. The vallecula is a 1-cm, smooth strip of mucosa that is the transition from the base of the tongue to the epiglottis; it is considered as part of the base of the tongue. The surface of the base of the tongue appears irregular and "bumpy" owing to scattered submucosal lymphoid follicles; the mucous membrane itself is actually smooth compared with the dorsum of the oral tongue. The surface of the base of the tongue lies in a nearly vertical position with the tongue at rest.

The musculature of the base of the tongue is continuous with that of the oral tongue. A midsagittal section through the oropharynx shows important relationships with neighboring sites (Fig. 18-1).[2] A cross section through the oropharynx to demonstrate relationships to the lateral pharyngeal space is shown in Figure 18-2.

The tonsillar area is a triangular region bounded anteriorly by the anterior tonsillar pillar (palatoglossal muscle), posteriorly by the posterior tonsillar pillar (palatopharyngeal muscle), and inferiorly by the glossopharyngeal sulcus and pharyngoepiglottic fold. The palatine tonsil lies within the triangle. The tonsillar region is bounded laterally by the pharyngeal constrictor muscle and its fascia, the mandible, and the lateral pharyngeal space. The external maxillary artery and its tonsillar and associated palatine branches are separated from the tonsil by the constrictor muscle. The internal carotid lies 2 cm to 3 cm lateral and posterior to the tonsil.

The tonsillar area is separated from the base of the tongue by the glossotonsillar sulcus. The narrow sulcus lies in a vertical plane between the anterior tonsillar pillar and the pharyngoepiglottic fold. Beneath the mucous membrane of the sulcus are the styloglossal muscle and the stylohyoid ligament.

The soft palate is a thin, mobile muscle complex that separates the nasopharynx from the oral cavity and oropharynx. The epithelium of the oral surface of the soft palate is squamous and the epithelium of the nasopharyngeal surface is respiratory. The soft palate is continuous laterally with the tonsillar pillars.

PATHOLOGY

Squamous cell carcinoma or one of its variants accounts for 95% of malignant lesions. Lymphoepithelioma occurs in the tonsil and base of the tongue. Verrucous carcinoma occurs rarely. Malignant lymphomas account for

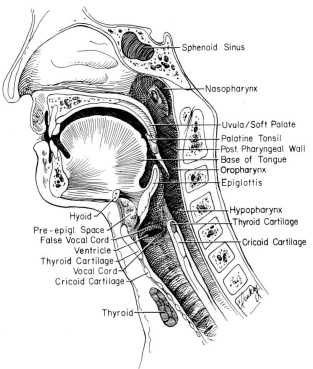

FIG. 18-1. Sagittal section of the upper aerodigestive tract. (Redrawn from Sabotta drawings. In Clemente CD [ed]: Anatomy: A Regional Atlas of the Human Body. Philadelphia, Lea & Febiger, 1975. Copyright © 1975, Urban & Schwarzenberg, Munich)

approximately 5% of tonsillar malignancies and 1% to 2% of malignancies of the base of the tongue. Minor salivary gland malignancies, plasmacytoma, and other rare tumors make up the remainder.

PATTERNS OF SPREAD

Base of the Tongue

PRIMARY

Squamous cell carcinoma of the base of tongue tends to early, silent, deep infiltration, and therefore the extent of tumors of the base of the tongue is usually underestimated by clinical examination. The tumor tends to remain in the base of the tongue unless it begins at the very peripheral margin. Vallecular lesions spread along the mucosa to the lingual surface of the epiglottis, laterally along the pharyngoepiglottic fold, and then to the lateral pharyngeal wall and anterior wall of the pyriform sinus. They frequently penetrate through the thin mucous membrane of the vallecula; tumor spread is contained for a while by the hyoepiglottic ligament, but this thin, often incomplete structure is eventually breached and cancer enters the preepiglottic space (see section on anatomy in Chapter 19, Larynx).

Lesions that begin on the lateral base of the tongue may invade the glossotonsillar sulcus. Deep penetration in the glossotonsillar sulcus allows the tumor to escape into the neck, since there is no effective muscular barrier at this point. The mylohyoid muscle is an effective barrier for oral tongue lesions, but the mylohyoid terminates near

FIG. 18-2. Section at the level of the midoropharynx to show relationships in the parapharyngeal space.

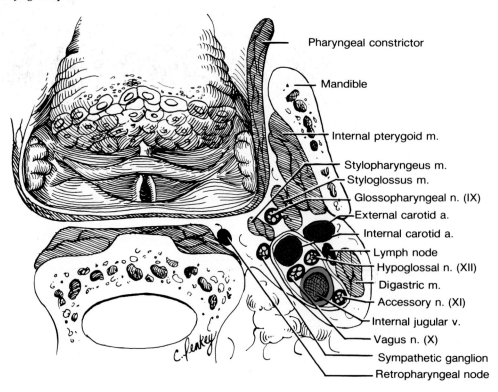

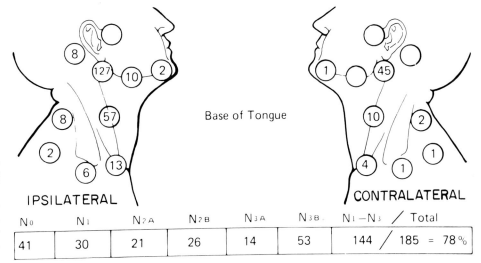

FIG. 18-3. Nodal distribution on admission at M. D. Anderson Hospital, 1948–1965, for carcinoma of the base of tongue. (Lindberg RD: Distribution of cervical lymph node metastases from squamous cell carcinoma of the upper respiratory and digestive tracts. Cancer 29:1446–1450, 1972)

Base of Tongue

IPSILATERAL   CONTRALATERAL

N₀	N₁	N₂ₐ	N₂ʙ	N₃ₐ	N₃ʙ	N₁–N₃ / Total
41	30	21	26	14	53	144 / 185 = 78%

the angle of the mandible. The base of the tongue mass may be palpable below the angle of the mandible and may be confused with an involved lymph node.

Advanced lesions tend to spread toward the larynx or oral tongue; spread into the parapharyngeal space is frequently seen on CT scan, but it is difficult to appreciate on physical examination.

LYMPHATICS

The distribution and N staging on admission prior to treatment for 185 previously untreated patients with squamous cell carcinoma of the base of the tongue is shown in Figure 18-3.[5] The first-echelon nodes are the subdigastric; the path of spread is then along the jugular chain to the midjugular and lower jugular nodes. The submaxillary nodes may become involved if tumor extends anteriorly into the oral tongue or if massive upper neck disease is present. Submental spread is rare. The posterior cervical nodes are involved often enough to be included in treatment plans.

Approximately 75% of patients with cancer of the base of the tongue will have clinically positive neck nodes on admission; 30% will have bilateral nodes. The incidence of occult disease in clinically negative necks is reported at 22%,[9] but this figure is undoubtedly low, considering the selection of smaller lesions for operation and the use of preoperative irradiation. The actual risk for occult disease is estimated to be 50% to 60%.

Tonsillar Area

The tonsillar area includes the anterior and posterior tonsillar pillars and the tonsillar fossa. Some authors group retromolar trigone lesions with the anterior tonsillar pillar lesions (because both areas are often involved simultaneously), but the retromolar trigone lesions are more appropriately considered as oral cavity lesions and grouped with the gingival (gum) lesions.

There are subtle differences in the spread patterns, clinical findings, treatment, and prognosis within the tonsillar area. When the lesions are early, the site of origin may be determined, but the more advanced lesions usually involve most if not all of the tonsillar area.

ANTERIOR TONSILLAR PILLAR

Almost all malignant tumors arising on the anterior tonsillar pillar are squamous cell carcinomas. Asymptomatic mucosal lesions are common and may be red lesions, white lesions, or a mixture. Leukoplakia is frequently of the speckled variety. The borders of early lesions are often indistinct. The early lesions tend to be flat with relatively little bulk or infiltration and therefore prognosis is good. As the lesions progress, they may develop a central ulcer with a rolled margin and infiltrate the palatoglossal muscle. Superomedial spread occurs onto the soft palate, the most posterior hard palate, and the maxillary gingiva, but invasion of the maxilla is uncommon. Anterolateral spread to the retromolar trigone is frequent, with subsequent spread to the posterior gingivobuccal sulcus and buccal mucosa. Once tumor gains access to the buccal mucosa, there is a risk for anterior occult extension in the buccal pouch, as exemplified by anterior marginal failure in patients treated by irradiation or operation.

Invasion of the tongue is frequent; careful palpation is necessary to detect the early submucosal nodule at the junction of the anterior tonsillar pillar and tongue.

As these lesions advance they adhere to the mandible and eventually invade the bone. Extension toward the base of the skull and nasopharynx is a late phenomenon, usually associated with infiltration of the medial pterygoid muscle and possible erosion of the medial pterygoid plate; such lesions produce trismus and marked temporal pain.

TONSILLAR FOSSA

Tonsillar fossa lesions arise either from the remnants of the palatine tonsil or from the mucous membrane within the triangle. There are some differences in development and spread patterns for squamous cell carcinomas of the tonsillar fossa compared with anterior tonsillar pillar lesions. Leukoplakia rarely occurs within the fossa, and asymptomatic red mucosal lesions are infrequently seen. The initial lesions tend to be exophytic. Central ulceration plus an infiltrative component develops as the lesion expands. Extension to the posterior tonsillar pillar and the oropharyngeal wall is common. Invasion into the glossopharyngeal sulcus and the base of the tongue occurs in approximately 25% of cases. As the lesions advance they penetrate to the parapharyngeal space and gain access to the base of the skull superiorly. Cranial nerve involvement, however, is uncommon. Advanced lesions invade the mandible, nasopharynx, and base of the tongue and may extend below the pharyngoepiglottic fold into the pyriform sinus.

POSTERIOR TONSILLAR PILLAR

Discrete lesions arising from the posterior tonsillar pillar are uncommon and for some unknown reason have an evil reputation. The only two lesions we have seen were 1.0-cm to 1.5-cm discrete lesions with a raised border and central ulceration, and both were cured. There are two major differences in their potential spread patterns. They may spread inferiorly along the palatopharyngeal muscle to its three points of insertion: (1) the middle pharyngeal constrictor, (2) the pharyngoepiglottic fold, and (3) the posterior border of the thyroid cartilage. Second, the junctional and spinal accessory lymph nodes are more likely to be involved.

Lymphatics

The distribution and N staging on admission prior to treatment for previously untreated patients with retromolar trigone/anterior tonsillar pillar and tonsillar fossa squamous cell carcinomas are shown in Figure 18-4.[5]

Retromolar trigone/anterior tonsillar pillar lesions have a lower risk of clinically positive lymph nodes (45%) com-

pared with the tonsillar fossa (76%). The distribution for the retromolar trigone/anterior tonsillar pillar on the ipsilateral side is to the internal jugular vein and submaxillary lymph nodes with a very low risk for junctional and spinal accessory lymph nodes. Contralateral spread is uncommon (5%) and is confined to the internal jugular chain. The risk of occult disease in the clinically negative neck (N0) is 10% to 15%.[15] The incidence of positive nodes increases with T stage (see Table 2-2 in Chapter 2).

Tonsillar fossa lesions have a high risk of clinically positive lymph nodes (76%). The lymph node distribution for tonsillar fossa lesions on the ipsilateral side includes the junctional, spinal accessory, and the more posterior submaxillary lymph nodes. Contralateral spread occurs in only 11% of patients and is mainly to the internal jugular vein lymph nodes, but there is some risk for spinal accessory and submaxillary involvement. The risk of contralateral spread is related to invasion of the tongue, spread near or across the midline of the soft palate, and large lymph nodes in the ipsilateral neck that produce lymphatic obstruction; when these features are present, treatment of the opposite neck must be considered. The incidence of occult disease after preoperative irradiation is 22%;[13] the actual risk is probably closer to 50% to 60%.

Discrete lesions of the posterior tonsillar pillar are uncommon, but they should have a pattern of lymph node distribution intermediate between the tonsillar fossa and the nasopharynx with a definite risk for junctional and spinal accessory lymph node involvement.

Advanced lesions of the tonsillar fossa usually involve all three areas, and the distribution of lymph node metastases assumes characteristics of the sites involved.

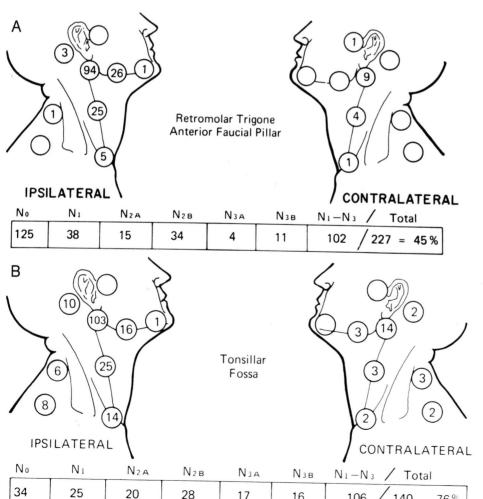

FIG. 18-4. Nodal distribution on admission at M. D. Anderson Hospital, 1948–1965. (A) Carcinoma of the retromolar trigone and anterior tonsillar pillar. (B) Carcinoma of the tonsillar fossa. (Lindberg RD: Distribution of cervical lymph node metastases from squamous cell carcinoma of the upper respiratory and digestive tracts. Cancer 29:1446–1450, 1972)

Retromolar Trigone
Anterior Faucial Pillar

IPSILATERAL

CONTRALATERAL

N_0	N_1	N_{2A}	N_{2B}	N_{3A}	N_{3B}	N_1–N_3 / Total
125	38	15	34	4	11	102 / 227 = 45%

Tonsillar Fossa

IPSILATERAL

CONTRALATERAL

N_0	N_1	N_{2A}	N_{2B}	N_{3A}	N_{3B}	N_1–N_3 / Total
34	25	20	28	17	16	106 / 140 = 76%

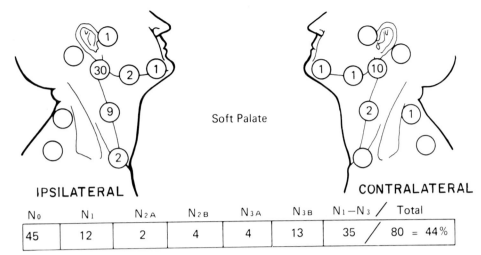

FIG. 18-5. Nodal distribution on admission at M. D. Anderson Hospital, 1948–1965, for carcinoma of the soft palate. (Lindberg RD: Distribution of cervical lymph node metastases from squamous cell carcinoma of the upper respiratory and digestive tracts. Cancer 29:1446–1450, 1972)

N₀	N₁	N₂A	N₂B	N₃A	N₃B	N₁–N₃ / Total
45	12	2	4	4	13	35 / 80 = 44%

Soft Palate

Nearly all soft palate squamous cell carcinomas occur on the oral side of the palate. The nasopharyngeal side seems nearly immune to tumor production. Even large tumors of the nasopharynx seldom invade the soft palate.

The earliest tumors are red lesions with ill-defined borders. White lesions are common on the soft palate and may be leukoplakia, carcinoma *in situ*, or early invasive carcinoma. Multiple sites of involvement with normal-appearing intervening mucosa are common. This finding is dramatically demonstrated during the first week of radiation therapy when the abnormal epithelium at the tumor sites "lights up" (tumoritis).

The majority of soft palate carcinomas are diagnosed while still confined to the soft palate and adjacent pillars. The diameter of the lesions may qualify as T2 (2 cm to 4 cm) or T3 (>4 cm), but the lesions may be rather thin with a relatively small tumor volume compared with a T2 or T3 lesion of the base of the tongue or tonsillar fossa. Spread from the soft palate occurs first to the tonsillar pillars and hard palate. Involvement of the lateral wall(s) of the nasopharynx is common in advanced lesions. Advanced lesions may present with perforation or ulcerative destruction of part of the soft palate. Lateral spread may eventually penetrate the superior constrictor muscle with subsequent invasion of the medial pterygoid muscle and compression or invasion of cranial nerves in the parapharyngeal space. Invasion of bone is rarely detected.

LYMPHATICS

The distribution of neck nodes and N staging for previously untreated patients with squamous cell carcinoma of the soft palate is shown in Figure 18-5.[5]

The spread pattern is first to the subdigastric nodes and then along the jugular chain. The submaxillary, junctional, and spinal accessory lymph nodes are uncommonly involved. Anterior extension along the anterior tonsillar pillar and retromolar trigone increases the risk of submaxillary involvement. Extension to the tonsillar fossa and posterior tonsillar pillar increases the risk of junctional and spinal accessory lymph node involvement.

Approximately 44% of patients will have clinically positive lymph nodes of admission; 16% will have bilateral nodes. The incidence of occult disease is not well established, since the first-echelon nodes are usually irradiated in all but the earliest lesions. Lindberg and co-workers noted approximately a 20% incidence of occult disease following either no or partial neck irradiation and with the primary lesion controlled.[6] The incidence of clinically positive nodes increases with T stage: 8% positive for T1, 36% for T2, and about 66% for T3 and T4.

CLINICAL PICTURE

Base of the Tongue

PRESENTING SYMPTOMS

Asymptomatic lesions are rarely diagnosed, since the base of the tongue is visualized only by indirect mirror examination. Many of the early lesions are relatively silent, and a subdigastric neck mass(es), often quite large, is frequently the first sign. The patient may insist that a 5 cm or larger neck mass "came up overnight." In a sense the patient is correct, since small clinically positive lymph nodes, 1 cm to 4 cm in diameter, are almost always asymptomatic. Sudden enlargement may occur due to necrosis or internal bleeding with rapid increase in size and mild tenderness.

The earliest symptom related to the tongue lesion is often a mild or vague sore throat. The patient may sense a lump in the back of the tongue, and actually feel it by digital palpation; the patient is not amused by the physician who cannot see the lesion with a tongue depressor and fails to palpate the base of the tongue. Difficulty in swallowing, a nasal voice, and deep-seated ear pain occur as the lesion enlarges (see Fig. 17-12 in Chapter 17).

Far-advanced lesions fix the tongue. Deep ulceration and necrosis result in foul breath.

PHYSICAL EXAMINATION

Indirect mirror examination, digital palpation, and a high level of suspicion are the ingredients for diagnosis. Early lesions are often submucosal and relatively soft, and since the base of the tongue is irregular, diagnosis is often a challenge. The rigid and flexible fiberoptic telescopes will allow examination in some patients not easily visualized by indirect mirror examination. Examination may show only a slight bulge in the tongue. A small lesion (<1 cm) originating in the glossotonsillar sulcus area may ulcerate and produce symptoms quite early. It may be overlooked unless the area is examined by separating the tongue from the lateral pharyngeal wall and inspecting the sulcus. Palpation through the lateral floor of the mouth is the best method to detect anterior extension. Inferior penetration through the vallecula produces a fullness in the soft tissues above the hyoid bone. Fixation of the tongue is indicated by incomplete protrusion or protrusion toward the side that is fixed. There is a tendency to underestimate the size of lesions of the base of the tongue.

Lymphomas are usually large, entirely submucosal masses and can be suspected by their appearance. Minor salivary gland tumors are also usually submucosal but more discrete and firm than lymphomas.

Tonsillar Area

ANTERIOR TONSILLAR PILLAR

Asymptomatic lesions are frequently found on routine examination by both dentists and physicians. Early symptoms include sore throat, usually aggravated by food or drink, and ear pain. If the lesion involves the hard palate or posterior upper gum, dentures may fit improperly or cause irritation. Advanced lesions invade the pterygoid or buccinator muscle and produce trismus and temporal pain. Invasion of the tongue will eventually limit tongue mobility and, when accompanied by ulceration at the junction of the anterior tonsillar pillar and oral tongue, causes a great deal of pain.

TONSILLAR FOSSA

Signs and symptoms are similar to those for anterior tonsillar pillar lesions except that the lesions tend to be larger before symptoms develop. Ipsilateral sore throat and ear pain are the hallmark of these lesions. Detection by visual examination with a tongue depressor is sufficient for most lesions of the tonsillar fossa; however, a few cancers arise near the glossotonsillar sulcus or lower pole of the tonsil and are only visible by indirect examination. A few patients will present with a mass in the neck. Lymphomas of the tonsil tend to be large submucosal masses but may ulcerate and appear similar to carcinomas.

Soft Palate

The earliest symptom is usually mild sore throat, which is often aggravated by food or drink. The sore throat is not well localized; discomfort may improve temporarily if antibiotics are given. Advanced lesions interfere with swallowing and may cause a voice change. Regurgitation of food and liquid into the nasopharynx and nose occurs with destruction, perforation, or fixation of the soft palate. Lateral and superior spread to the nasopharynx and parapharyngeal space is associated with trismus, otitis media, temporal headache, and rarely cranial nerve involvement.

Early lesions appear as red, white, or mixed changes in the mucosa; the mucosa may appear roughened. The margins are ill defined. Multiple foci on the soft palate and anterior tonsillar pillars are common. Moderately advanced lesions have rolled edges with central ulceration, or they may be mainly exophytic, particularly around the uvula. The nasopharynx should be inspected and palpated for submucosal extension along the lateral wall; extension along the nasopharyngeal surface of the soft palate is uncommon until the late stages. Extension to the posterior nasal cavity is seen only in advanced lesions that erode the posterior hard palate.

METHODS OF DIAGNOSIS AND STAGING

Biopsy Technique

Most lesions of the oropharynx can be biopsied by incisional or punch forceps biopsy using a local anesthetic in the outpatient clinic. Lesions of the base of the tongue may require a general anesthetic. Frozen section control is helpful in lesions of the base of the tongue, since it is sometimes difficult to obtain representative tissue. Special handling of tissue is required if lymphoma is suspected.

Staging Procedures

Early lesions are staged by physical examination; direct laryngoscopy with the patient under general anesthesia may be required for base of the tongue and vallecular lesions.

Mandible films and tomograms of the base of the skull are obtained when involvement is suspected. A computed tomographic (CT) scan may be useful to determine spread to the lateral pharyngeal space and soft tissue extension in carcinomas of the base of the tongue. A lateral xerogram may show an unsuspected deep ulcer crater.

Staging

All oropharyngeal sites are included in one T-stage system:[1]

- Tis Carcinoma *in situ*
- T1 Tumor 2 cm or less in greatest diameter
- T2 Tumor more than 2 cm but not more than 4 cm in greatest diameter
- T3 Tumor more than 4 cm in greatest diameter
- T4 Massive tumor more than 4 cm in diameter with invasion of bone, soft tissues of the neck, or root (deep musculature) of the tongue

There is a tendency to overestimate the diameter of lesions in the oropharynx; insertion of a measuring device will help judge the maximum diameter. The difference between T3 and T4 is not so easily determined. It is difficult to distinguish between direct invasion of soft tissues of the neck and a deep lymph node mass. Tumors of the tonsillar area or base of the tongue that penetrate the glossopharyngeal sulcus can frequently be palpated as a deep mass just under the angle of the jaw and qualify as stage T4 if the primary is larger than 4 cm in diameter; bimanual palpation and CT scan help outline the continuity of the mass. Fixation of the tongue indicates invasion of the root or deep musculature of the tongue. If cancer of the base of the tongue can be palpated easily through the lateral floor of mouth or in the submentum, then invasion of deep muscle has probably occurred. Tonsillar lesions that produce trismus or cranial nerve palsy or invade the nasopharynx should be classed as T4.

TREATMENT: BASE OF THE TONGUE

Selection of Treatment Modality

Although a few centers continue to recommend glossectomy as the treatment of choice, irradiation is the more commonly prescribed treatment in our clinic. Operation and irradiation produce similar cure rates for early lesions of the base of the tongue, but since excision of the base of the tongue generally causes greater disability, radiation therapy is the treatment of choice for the majority of lesions, with operation reserved for salvage of radiation therapy failures. Radiation therapy automatically encompasses the neck nodes on both sides of the neck.

Extended supraglottic laryngectomy may be used for limited lateralized vallecular lesions, but there are definite criteria that must be satisfied, and this selection limits its usefulness. The following conditions must be met:

1. No gross involvement of the pharyngoepiglottic fold
2. Preservation of one lingual artery
3. Resection of less than 80% of the base of the tongue
4. Pulmonary function suitable for supraglottic laryngectomy
5. Medical condition suitable for a major operation.

At least an ipsilateral neck dissection is indicated, but with the high risk of bilateral neck disease even in the N0 patient, this represents incomplete treatment. Finally, the surgeon has difficulty determining tumor extent in the tongue at the time of excision. Postoperative irradiation may have to be administered in any event for close margins or for fear of recurrence in the neck. Therefore, radiation therapy is usually the treatment of choice for the primary lesion, with neck dissection added as needed.

Surgical Treatment

Operation is best suited for well-lateralized lesions with minimal neck disease. An anterior lesion may be resected leaving the larynx intact, while a posterior lesion may

FIG. 18-6. Portals for irradiation of cancer of the base of tongue. (A) Simulation film. A small stainless-steel pin was inserted to identify the anteriormost portion of the base of the tongue; the pin also indicates the anterior margin of palpable tumor. The amount of oral tongue that is irradiated depends on the anterior extent of disease as determined by palpation. The lower larynx is usually excluded from the primary portals. The superior border is 3 cm above the tip of the mastoid (TM). The vallecula and epiglottis are outlined. (A, arytenoids) (B) Outline of radiation portal. Note sparing of submental skin and subcutaneous tissues in submentum and adequate coverage of internal jugular vein nodes at base of the skull by treating 2 cm to 3 cm above the tip of the mastoid. (Parsons JT, Million RR, Cassisi NJ: Carcinoma of the base of the tongue: Results of radical irradiation with surgery reserved for irradiation failure. Laryngoscope 92:689–696, 1982)

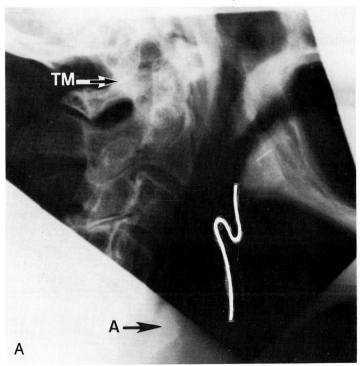

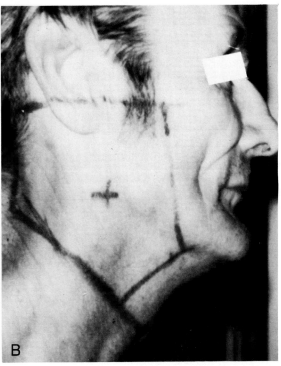

require the addition of supraglottic laryngectomy The surgical approach for small neoplasms of the base of the tongue is either by splitting the lip, mandible, and oral tongue in the midline in order to reach the base of the tongue, or by dividing the mandible near the angle and approaching the base of the tongue from the side. After the tumor has been removed, the mandible is wired together. Only one lingual artery may be sacrificed. A radical neck dissection is done in continuity with excision of the lesion of the base of the tongue. Removal of large tumors requires simultaneous removal of part or all of the larynx. A myocutaneous flap may be used to connect the remaining larynx to the tongue.

Irradiation Technique

The irradiation of cancer of the base of the tongue is basically accomplished by parallel opposed external-beam portals, which also encompass the regional lymph nodes on both sides. The usual initial treatment volume (Fig. 18-6) includes the base of the tongue, valleculae, suprahyoid epiglottis, upper portion of the preepiglottic space, pharyngeal walls, and varying amounts of the oral tongue, depending on the anterior extent of disease; the internal jugular chain and junctional and spinal accessory nodes on both sides are encompassed up to the base of the skull.[10] The lower border of the primary treatment field is the thyroid notch unless tumor extends into the supraglottic larynx, hypopharynx, or preepiglottic space. The skin and subcutaneous tissues in the submental midline are shielded unless the patient is very thin or tumor extends into the submental area. The spinal cord is shielded from the treatment volume at 4500 rad to 5000 rad/5 weeks.

One of the common errors in planning therapy using external-beam portals is failure to recognize anterior growth of the neoplasm as determined by palpation through the lateral floor of the mouth.

Management of the lymphatics is critical. One of the major advantages of radiation therapy is the ease of irradiating the lymph nodes at risk. Even small, well-lateralized lesions of the base of the tongue will spread to the opposite neck, and both sides are always treated. The initial primary portals include the upper internal jugular, posterior submaxillary, junctional, and spinal accessory lymph node(s) (Fig. 18-7). The superior border is approximately 3 cm above the tip of the mastoid to ensure coverage of the nodes near the base of skull. The lower neck nodes on both sides are always treated. (See Chapter 6, General Principles for Treatment of Cancers in the Head and Neck: Radiation Therapy, for discussion of neck management.)

A boost of 500 rad to 1500 rad may be delivered to the base of tongue by way of the submental route. This technique reduces the dose to the mandible. The submental boost may be given with either high-energy electrons or a photon beam aimed superiorly to avoid the previously irradiated spinal cord (Fig. 18-8). The submental boost is selected for those base of the tongue lesions that are central and posterior. Lateralized lesions that involve the glossotonsillar sulcus and lie immediately adjacent to the mandible are not suitable for the submental boost. Large lesions that extend into the oral tongue are not suited for submental boost, since the distance from the skin to the tongue surface is greater than 6 cm and the portal is inefficient; an interstitial boost or reduced lateral portals are used for the final dose in these cases.

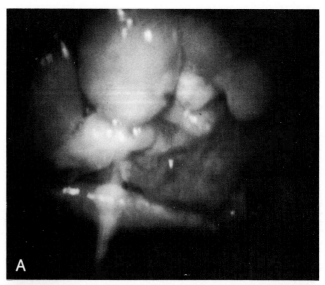

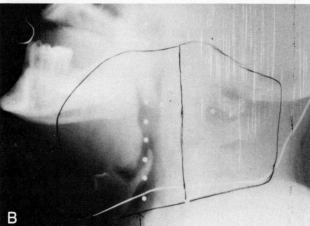

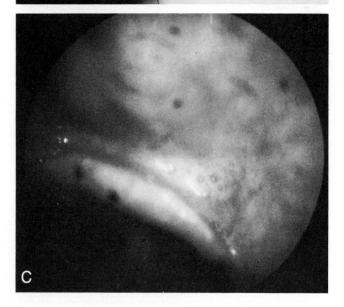

FIG. 18-7. Poorly differentiated squamous cell carcinoma of the base of the tongue. (A) A 2.5 × 2.5-cm midline tumor of the base of the tongue. There was a 3.0-cm right subdigastric positive lymph node. The patient had a short thick neck that was difficult to evaluate (T2N1). (B) Simulator planning film. The base of tongue mass is easily seen; the vallecula is spared. The epiglottis is forced backward by the mass. The initial treatment portal is outlined for preparation of a Cerrobend beam-shaping block. Compare treatment volume with that shown in Figure 18-6. The portal in Figure 18-6 was shaped using rectangular lead blocks stacked on a tray. The Cerrobend beam-shaping technique permits free-form shapes and shielding of some normal tissues not possible with former techniques. After 4500 rad, the portion of the portal behind the cervical bodies is eliminated from the photon fields and a new block is made. Treatment is completed to the posterior section ("posterior strip") with 12-MeV electrons. Five hundred rad was added to the right posterior strip at 3 cm and 1000 rad to the left. Five thousand rad is usually sufficient for subclinical disease, but the neck was difficult to evaluate and neck dissection was not planned. Treatment to the base of the tongue was continued to 7000 rad/7 weeks through lateral portals; a 500-rad submental boost was added with 17-MeV electrons. (C) No disease was evident at 3 years, 6 months.

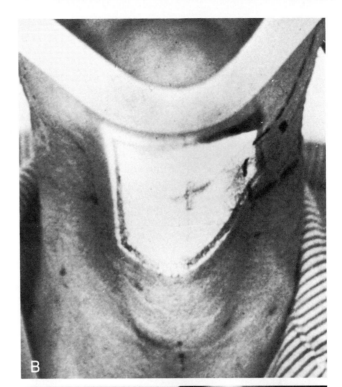

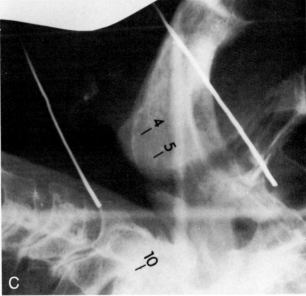

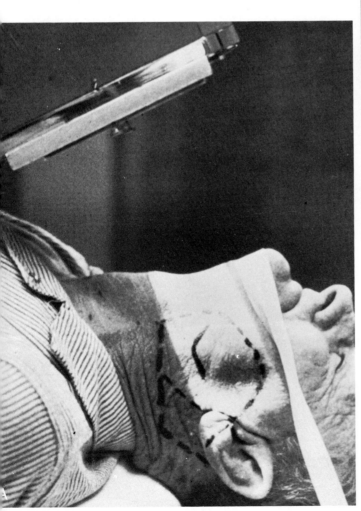

FIG. 18-8. (A) Patient in treatment position for submental boost. The head is lowered below the level of the table. Collimators are opened wide to adjust superior tilt of the field so that no or only slight overlap occurs at that portion of the spinal cord that is irradiated by the lateral portals. Lateral portals are indicated by dashed lines. The lateral portals were reduced at 5000 rad to exclude the spinal cord. The angle of the mandible is marked. (B) The lower border of the submental boost field is near the thyroid notch. The field may be shaped by secondary collimation to include unilateral or bilateral upper neck nodes. (C) Roentgenogram of submental boost anatomy. The base of the tongue lies 4 cm to 5 cm from the skin along the central axis. The spinal cord lies approximately 10 cm from the skin along the lower edge of the portal. (A and B from Parsons JT, Million RR, Cassisi NJ: Carcinoma of the base of the tongue: Results of radical irradiation with surgery reserved for irradiation failure. Laryngoscope 92:689–696, 1982)

Interstitial implants may be used for part of the treatment if the lesion is small, discrete, and located in the antero-lateral base of the tongue. Implants of posterior lesions are technically difficult; these implants are usually accomplished with a flexible source (e.g., iridium-192 ribbons) that allow through-and-through implantation from the base of the tongue to the skin. There is no advantage in our experience in local control for interstitial boost with radium needles as opposed to external-beam treatment alone. Lesions of the base of the tongue have a fairly good local control rate with external-beam therapy alone. The T2–T3 control rate for external-beam therapy alone was 72% compared with 53% when a radium boost was added.[10] The base of the tongue has a good vascular supply and tolerates high doses of radiation with few soft tissue necroses.

The guidelines for doses usually prescribed and the local control rates are outlined in Table 6-10 in Chapter 6 and Fig. 13-14 in Chapter 13. Split-course techniques resulted in poorer local control and are not used. The initial dose per fraction is 180 rad to 200 rad; after 5000 rad the treatment volume is reduced, and the daily fraction is increased to 200 rad to 225 rad if patient tolerance is satisfactory.

See Figures 5-2, 5-6, and 5-7 in Chapter 5 for examples of neck dissection following radical irradiation for base of tongue lesions and Figure 6-2 in Chapter 6 for a discussion of portal arrangement for neck irradiation.

Combined Treatment Policies

Combined treatment is seldom selected since an operation for moderately advanced lesions usually implies major functional loss, and few patients are willing to accept the morbidity and possible immediate mortality. The most common indication for offering glossectomy and laryngectomy is a lesion that is simply failing to respond to irradiation after 5000 rad. However, if the patient is offered and accepts a glossectomy–laryngectomy, we would prefer an immediate operation followed by postoperative radiation therapy.

Management of Recurrence

A painful ulcer must be biopsied to distinguish between recurrence and radiation necrosis; general anesthesia is usually necessary to obtain representative tissue. Radiation failures are treated surgically, but salvage is infrequent. At the University of Florida there have been 36 patients with local failure; 11 had a salvage operation, but it was successful in only 2. Fletcher reports surgical salvage of radiation failures in 2 of 9 patients with T2 disease, 1 of 13 with T3 disease, and 2 of 15 with T4 disease.[4]

Recurrence of a small, discrete primary may be managed by a wide local excision. The remaining recurrences require either a jaw–tongue–neck resection or glossectomy–laryngectomy.

Surgical failures are rarely salvaged by either an operation or radiation therapy, except for the early lesion with a discrete local recurrence.

RESULTS OF TREATMENT: BASE OF THE TONGUE

Surgical Results

Whicker and co-workers at the Mayo Clinic reported 102 patients selected for curative attempts by operation between 1960 and 1967.[19] Of 23 who received preoperative or postoperative radiation therapy, 5 survived for 5 years. Of 11 treated for irradiation failure, 3 survived for 5 years. Twenty-two had radiation salvage attempted after surgical failure, but only 1 survived 5 years. Twenty-three percent required partial or total laryngectomy. Fifty-six percent had positive nodes in the specimen; 22 patients developed delayed appearance of neck metastasis. Only 7% had bilateral pathologically positive nodes at the initial operation. The operative mortality rate was 4%, with a 27% local recurrence rate and 10% neck failure rate with the primary lesion controlled. The 5-year survival rate was 42%.

Irradiation Results

The local control and salvage rates for 89 patients treated for cure by irradiation are shown in Table 18-1. Ten percent had stage I or II disease, 19% had stage III disease, and 71% had stage IV disease. The actuarial survival by stage is shown in Figure 18-9.[3] The 5-year absolute and determinate survival is given in Table 18-2.[10]

FOLLOW-UP POLICY: BASE OF THE TONGUE

Operation or radiation therapy or both will occasionally salvage the failure of treatment of an early lesion. Radiation failures may present as an ulcer and must be distinguished from radiation necrosis. Many radiation necroses appear

---

TABLE 18-1. Carcinoma of the Base of the Tongue: Local Control by Irradiation Alone

T Stage	No. Patients	Excluded*	Local Control With 2-Year Minimum Follow-up	Surgical Salvage	Ultimate Control
T1	11	3	6/8 (75%)	0/2	6 (75%)
T2	21	6	10/15 (67%)	1/3	11 (73%)
T3	30	8	14/22 (64%)	0/11	14 (64%)
T4	27	3	3/24 (13%)	1/5	4 (17%)

* Dead or intercurrent disease or metastases less than 2 years after treatment with primary lesion controlled.
Note: University of Florida data; patients treated 9/64–9/77; analysis 9/79.
(Modified from Parsons JT, Million RR, Cassisi NJ: Carcinoma of the base of the tongue: Results of radical irradiation with surgery reserved for irradiation failure. Laryngoscope 92:689–696, 1982)

in the vallecula or glossotonsillar sulcus, not on the base of the tongue proper. Biopsies performed with the patient under general anesthesia are usually necessary to obtain adequate tissue and control of bleeding.

COMPLICATIONS OF TREATMENT: BASE OF THE TONGUE

Surgical Complications

The complications of surgery include an operative mortality of about 5%; other complications include fistula, mandibular necrosis, dysphagia, hoarseness, trismus, and carotid rupture.

Complications of Irradiation

The risk of radiation therapy complications by boost technique is shown in Table 18-3.[10] Bone exposure and osteoradionecrosis are uncommon. Soft tissue necrosis is the major problem and occurs in 6% to 10% of patients treated solely by external-beam irradiation. Treatment of necrosis requires patience and reassurance to the patient, who assumes the pain is due to cancer. Antibiotics will often reduce pain. The patient will lose weight due to dysphagia and will require nutritional support. A few of the necroses persist for several months. Serious hemorrhage is uncommon.

Hypoglossal nerve palsy occurred in two patients and is reported in other series. It is usually associated with an ulcer in the posterior glossotonsillar sulcus. Unilateral hypoglossal nerve palsy does not produce serious morbidity since the opposite side compensates very nicely.

An occasional patient cured by radiation therapy of advanced cancer of the base of the tongue may have difficulty swallowing solid foods. The action of the base of the tongue is to force the bolus of food into the hypopharynx, and loss of full motion impedes swallowing. This is probably a result of some fibrosis of the base of the tongue, compounded by a dry mouth. Aspiration is unusual, however, even if the tip of the epiglottis has been amputated by tumor.

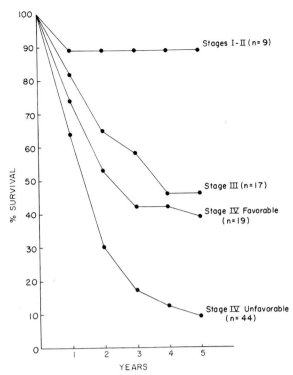

FIG. 18-9. Survival (actuarial method[3]) for 89 patients who received radical courses of irradiation to the base of the tongue. The number of patients within each stage is shown in parentheses. The stage IV favorable subgroup includes those patients with T1–T3 primary lesions and N2A-B or N3A neck disease. The stage IV unfavorable subgroup includes patients with T4 and/or N3B disease. (Parsons JT, Million RR, Cassisi NJ: Carcinoma of the base of the tongue: Results of radical irradiation with surgery reserved for irradiation failure. Laryngoscope 92:689–696, 1982)

TABLE 18-2.	Carcinoma of the Base of the Tongue: Absolute and Determinate 5-Year Survival Following Irradiation Alone to the Primary Lesion (65 Patients)			
Stage	No. Patients	No Evidence of Disease at 5 Years	Died of Intercurrent Disease Within 5 Years	Determinate Survival
I	2	2 (100%)	0	2/2 (100%)
II	2	2 (100%)	0	2/2 (100%)
III	12	6 (50%)	5	6/7 (86%)
IV	49	11 (22%)	4	11/45 (24%)

Note: University of Florida data; patients treated 9/64–9/74; analysis 9/79.
(Parsons JT, Million RR, Cassisi NJ: Carcinoma of the base of the tongue: Results of radical irradiation with surgery reserved for irradiation failure. Laryngoscope 92:689–696, 1982)

TABLE 18-3.   Base of Tongue Carcinoma: Bone Exposure and Soft Tissue Necrosis by Boost Technique

Boost Technique (No. Patients)	Patients (%) With Bone Exposure			Patients (%) With Soft Tissue Necrosis		
	Mild	Moderate	Severe	Mild	Moderate	Severe
Submental (47)	0	1 (2%)*	0	2 (4%)	3 (6%)	0
Lateral (17)	0	0	0	0	1 (6%)	0
Radium (25)	2 (8%)	3 (12%)	0	4 (16%)	2 (8%)	0
Total (89)†	2 (2%)	4 (4%)	0	6 (7%)	6 (7%)	0

* Dental extractions 2 months after radiation therapy.

† Two patients who developed both bone exposure and soft tissue necrosis are scored twice.

Note: University of Florida data; patients treated 9/64–9/77; analysis 9/79.

(Parsons JT, Million RR, Cassisi NJ: Carcinoma of the base of the tongue: Results of radical irradiation with surgery reserved for irradiation failure. Laryngoscope 92:689–696, 1982)

Complications of Combined Treatment

Preoperative irradiation will increase the risk of fistula, delayed healing, and carotid exposure.

Postoperative irradiation increases the amount of fibrosis in the neck. Radiation necrosis of the soft tissues or bone is uncommon. The added effect of xerostomia further worsens the swallowing defect produced by glossectomy.

TREATMENT: TONSILLAR AREA

Selection of Treatment Modality

EARLY LESIONS (T1–T2)

Early lesions are generally treated by irradiation with a high rate of success and relatively low morbidity; a neck dissection may be added after radiation therapy as outlined in Chapter 4, General Principles for Treatment of Cancers in the Head and Neck: Selection of Treatment for the Primary Site and for the Neck, section on management of the neck. An occasional small lesion is cured by wide local excision or tonsillectomy, but surgical excision is usually prescribed only under unusual circumstances, such as prior use of radiation therapy or a very small, discrete lesion on the anterior tonsillar pillar. A surgical attack usually implies removal of the mandible, the tonsillar area including both pillars and part of the soft palate, and perhaps a small amount of the tongue; additionally, an ipsilateral neck dissection is performed even with a clinically negative neck. The functional loss is not justified in view of the high success rate with irradiation, which leaves the patient intact; even a dry mouth may be avoided when well-lateralized lesions are treated by techniques that allow at least partial salivary recovery. An operation will often salvage the few radiation treatment failures.

MODERATELY ADVANCED LESIONS (T2–T3)

The local failure rate with radiation therapy is approximately 20% for T2 and 30% to 50% for T3 when adequate doses are prescribed. Preoperative irradiation followed by an operation has not shown any improvement in the cure rate compared with radical radiation therapy with surgical salvage.[11,16,17] Surgical salvage is better for anterior tonsillar pillar failures than for those of the tonsillar fossa. The major indication for combined treatment is a lesion that is failing to regress after 5000 rad; these patients are offered an operation.

ADVANCED LESIONS (T3–T4)

If the lesion is assigned to stage T4 only because of mandible invasion, then an operation followed by radiation therapy should be advised. However, invasion of the mandible is usually associated with other extensions that contraindicate surgical removal. Radical irradiation will control approximately 25% of these advanced lesions if large doses are applied.

Surgical Treatment

Surgical treatment for very early cancers of the tonsillar area (less than 1 cm in size) consists of a wide local excision through a transoral approach. Larger lesions require removal of the adjacent mandible as well as a portion of the tongue and soft palate. Depending on the size of the defect, a tongue, deltopectoral, or myocutaneous flap may be required to close the defect. Flaps are usually necessary for extensive lesions or after failure of radiation therapy. Deglutition is not generally a problem, but some patients remain on liquid diets. Chewing is difficult since a portion of the mandible has been removed, and the patient will be unable to wear dentures. Speech will probably be impaired if a portion of the tongue or palate has been removed.

Irradiation Technique

The basic portal arrangement depends to a large degree on the extent of the local lesion and presence or absence of positive lymph nodes. The risk for contralateral lymph node metastases is very small unless there is tongue invasion, invasion of the soft palate within 1 cm to 2 cm of the midline, or clinically positive nodes in the ipsilateral neck. If these risk features are absent, an ipsilateral portal with a combination of photons and electrons that spare the contralateral mucosa and salivary glands may be used. The major advantage of these techniques is not a greater cure rate, but a lower incidence of xerostomia secondary to partial preservation of minor and major salivary gland function on the contralateral side. An intraoral lead block may also be added, which further protects the minor sal-

TABLE 18-4.   Carcinoma of the Tonsillar Region: Local Control With Radiation Therapy With or Without Neck Dissection (Continuous Course)—99 Patients

Stage	Excluded*	No. Patients	Local Control		Surgical Salvage	Ultimate Control
			External Beam Alone (53)	External Beam + Radium (23)		
T1	3	14	11/13 (85%)	1/1 (100%)	2/2	14/14 (100%)
T2	8	29	18/23 (78%)	5/6 (83%)	3/4	26/29 (89%)
T3	11	25	6/13 (46%)	9/12 (75%)	0/2	15/25 (60%)
T4	1	8	1/4 (25%)	1/4 (25%)		2/8 (25%)

* Twenty-three patients excluded from analysis of local control who died of intercurrent disease less than 2 years following treatment with no evidence of local recurrence.

Note: University of Florida data; patients treated 10/64–1/81; analysis 2/83 by B. D. Greenberg, M.D.

ivary glands and a portion of the parotid. Since the lesions lie behind the dense mandible, an extra 1.0 cm to 1.5 cm is added to the depth-dose calculations for the electron portion of the treatment. (See Chapter 15, Treatment Planning for Irradiation of Head and Neck Cancer.)

Lesions with a risk for bilateral neck disease are treated with parallel opposed photon portals, usually weighted 2:1 or 3:2 to the involved side; if there are positive contralateral nodes or extension across the midline, the portals are usually equally weighted.

There is frequently invasion of the adjacent tongue, and a boost may be added by a small interstitial implant for an additional 1000 rad to 1500 rad.

The rates of local control by T stage and dose are given in Table 6-10 in Chapter 6, and in Figures 13-12 and 13-13 in Chapter 13, the dose for local control is analyzed. The local control, surgical salvage, and ultimate control rates by T stage for 99 tonsillar area lesions treated by continuous-course radiation therapy are presented in Table 18-4. Tonsillar fossa lesions have a slightly lower recurrence rate than those arising from the anterior tonsillar pillar area when comparing T1–T2 lesions.

The dose prescribed for tonsillar area lesions is critical if a high rate of control is to be achieved. There is a notable improvement in the local control rate by radiation treatment as the dose is increased; the complication rate also increases (Table 18-5).

See Chapter 4, General Principles for Treatment of Cancers in the Head and Neck: Selection of Treatment for the Primary Site and for the Neck, for management of neck node metastases.

Combined Treatment Policies

Patients selected for combined treatment preferably have resection first, followed by postoperative irradiation. A large, fixed node is the most common indication for preoperative irradiation.

Patients whose lesions show a poor response to radiation therapy after 5000 rad are reevaluated and offered an operation.

Management of Recurrence

An operation will salvage a good proportion of T1–T2 radiation therapy failures, but only an occasional advanced

TABLE 18-5.   Carcinoma of the Tonsillar Region: Local Control by Dose (Continuous Course)—Stage T3, 25 Patients

Total Dose (rad)*	Local Control	Complications	
		2+	3+
5500–5900	0/2	0	0
6000–6900	2/5 (40%)	2	0
7000–7900	6/10 (60%)	1	1
≥8000	7/8 (88%)	3	0

* An interstitial implant to the tongue was part of the treatment in 12 patients.

Note: University of Florida data; patients treated 10/64–1/81; analysis 2/83 by B. D. Greenberg, M.D.

lesion is salvaged (see Table 18-4). A neck recurrence after only radiation therapy can occasionally be salvaged by neck dissection.

RESULTS OF TREATMENT: TONSILLAR AREA

The disease-free survival for 99 patients with squamous cell carcinoma of the tonsillar region treated by continuous-course irradiation is given in Table 18-6.[8] There is a high rate of intercurrent death for stages I and II. Fourteen patients were selected for operation and radiation therapy and were usually the less favorable cases. Eight were treated with preoperative radiation therapy; 7 developed a local recurrence, and only 1 has no evidence of disease over 2 years from treatment. Six were treated by resection and postoperative radiation therapy; only 1 developed a local recurrence, and 4 have no evidence of disease over 2 years.

COMPLICATIONS OF TREATMENT: TONSILLAR AREA

The risk of bone and soft tissue complications for 99 patients treated initially by irradiation is outlined in Table 18-7.[8] Four patients required an operative procedure. Improved

TABLE 18-6. Carcinoma of the Tonsillar Region: Disease-Free Survival (Actuarial Method[3]) by Stage—Continuous-Course Irradiation ± Neck Dissection, 99 Patients

	2-Year Survival		5-Year Survival	
AJCC Stage	Absolute	Determinate	Absolute	Determinate
I	75%	100%	42%	100%
II	78%	95%	56%	90%
III	74%	77%	60%	75%
IVA	47%	53%	17%	33%
IVB	28%	29%	18%	22%

Note: University of Florida data; patients treated 10/64–1/81; analysis 2/83 by B. D. Greenberg, M.D.

TABLE 18-7. Carcinoma of the Tonsillar Region: Complications of Radiation Therapy (Continuous Course) ± Neck Dissection—99 Patients

	No. Complications	
Soft Tissue and/or Bone Necrosis*	External Beam Alone (69)	External Beam + Radium (30)
Mild	11 (16%)	10 (33%)
Moderate	3 (4%)	5 (17%)
Severe	2 (3%)	2 (7%)†

*Thirty-three complications in 99 patients (33%); 19 patients had soft tissue necrosis or bone necrosis, 7 patients had soft tissue necrosis and bone necrosis.

† One fatal soft tissue and bone complication.

Note: University of Florida data; patients treated 10/64–1/81; analysis 2/83 by B. D. Greenberg, M.D.

management of the teeth has reduced the incidence of serious complications.

TREATMENT: SOFT PALATE

Selection of Treatment Modality

Very small (2 mm to 5 mm), well-defined lesions may be excised, but the multifocal nature of soft palate lesions predicts marginal recurrence after limited treatment unless patients are very carefully selected. Tiny lesions confined to the uvula may be treated by surgical excision with little morbidity, but the neck must be watched very carefully. Irradiation is the modality most often selected for early and advanced soft palate carcinomas; neck dissection is added as needed. The success rate with irradiation is good, and it leaves the patient functionally intact without the need for a prosthesis or elaborate reconstruction.

Surgical Treatment

Surgical excision for early lesions (<5 mm in size) of the soft palate can achieve a high cure rate with little or no

functional loss. However, if a major resection is required, then a prosthesis is generally required to restore velopharyngeal competence. Surgical salvage of radiation recurrence should include full-thickness removal of the soft palate.

Irradiation Technique

The basic irradiation technique for early and advanced lesions involves parallel opposed external-beam portals that include the primary lesion and the upper neck nodes on both sides, since even patients with very tiny lesions are at some risk for occult lymph node disease. If the primary lesion is discrete, a portion of the treatment may be given by intraoral cone or a single-plane radioactive seed implant. If intraoral cone therapy is to be used, it should be given prior to external-beam therapy when the lesion is clearly visible and the mouth is not yet sore from the radiation reaction. Intraoral cone therapy requires meticulous care to avoid geographic miss.

A small single-plane radioactive seed implant is an effective reduced-field technique. The seeds (radon or gold) are placed on a 1-cm grid to include the gross lesion with a small margin. The implant may be done prior to external beam if the lesion is flat, or after external beam if flattening of the lesion prior to performing implant is preferred.

The major advantage of the seed boost is a reduction of external-beam dose by 1500 rad to 2500 rad with fewer late radiation side-effects and the hope of a better local control rate due to the higher biologic dose. The disadvantages are the added cost and technical requirements for accurate seed placement.

The external-beam technique is usually equally weighted, parallel opposed portals. The minimum treatment volume for early lesions includes the entire soft palate and the adjacent tonsillar areas. If the neck is clinically negative, high-energy photons (10 MeV to 17 MeV) will produce an isodose distribution allowing a tumor dose at the soft palate of 6500 rad to 7000 rad while maintaining the lymph node dose at 5000 rad. If the lymph nodes are clinically positive, then cobalt-60 or 4 MeV to 6 MeV is preferred on the involved side(s).

There is little information on dose for control of soft palate lesions, but schedules similar to those for the anterior tonsillar pillar are used. (See Table 6-10 in Chapter 6 and Fig. 13-15 in Chapter 13.)

Combined Treatment Policies

Combined therapy is rarely planned because of the success rate with radiation therapy and the morbidity associated with resection of the soft palate.

Management of Recurrence

Soft tissue necrosis is uncommon after radiation therapy, so a persistent ulcer is the hallmark of recurrent disease following irradiation. Recurrence following irradiation is treated by surgical removal when feasible, and salvage is achieved in a few patients.

RESULTS OF TREATMENT: SOFT PALATE

Surgical Results

Ratzer and co-workers reported the Memorial Sloan-Kettering results for 299 patients with squamous cell carcinoma of the soft palate.[12] Of these patients, 112 were treated by surgery, 139 by radiation therapy, and 22 by combined treatment. The 5-year absolute survival rate was 21%, and the determinate survival rate was 30%. The determinate survival rate for just the group treated by surgery was 38%. The main cause of failure was recurrence at the primary site.

Irradiation Results

Weller and associates reported a local control rate of 50% in 30 patients with soft palate lesions; only 5 had T1 lesions.[18]

Seydel and Scholl reviewed the results of 41 patients with previously untreated soft palate malignancies, including four nonsquamous carcinomas.[14] Thirty-one patients were treated with doses between 6000 and 7000 rad, and 10 (32%) developed local recurrence.

Parsons analyzed the University of Florida data for 25 patients.* Local control was achieved in all of 4 patients

* Parsons JT: Unpublished data, 1979.

with T1 lesions, in 8 of 10 with T2 lesions, in 2 of 7 with T3 disease, and in 1 of 4 with T4 disease. A time–dose relationship could not be observed.

Lindberg and Fletcher reported a high rate of control for soft palate lesions (T1, 100%; T2, 88%; T3, 77%; and T4, 83%).[7] A few failures were salvaged by operation.

COMPLICATIONS OF TREATMENT: SOFT PALATE

Surgical Complications

Nasal speech and regurgitation of food into the nasopharynx are sequelae of full-thickness resection of the soft palate. A prosthesis is only partially successful in correcting the functional defect.

Complications of Irradiation

Complications are few. Persistent soft tissue necrosis of the soft palate is quite uncommon, and an ulcer must be considered to be a possible recurrence. The soft palate may become retracted following successful treatment of advanced lesions, and this may result in regurgitation into the nasopharynx and slight alteration in speech. Small perforations may persist after successful treatment at sites where tumor has grown through the soft palate. These perforations usually occur far laterally and do not interfere with function.

REFERENCES

1. American Joint Committee on Cancer: Manual for Staging of Cancer, 2nd ed, p 33. Philadelphia, JB Lippincott, 1983
2. Clemente CD (ed): Anatomy: A Regional Atlas of the Human Body. Philadelphia, Lea & Febiger, 1975
3. Cutler SJ, Ederer F: Maximum utilization of the life table method in analyzing survival. J Chronic Dis 8:699–712, 1958
4. Fletcher GH: Oral cavity and oropharynx. In Fletcher GH (ed): Textbook of Radiotherapy, 2nd ed, pp 212–254. Philadelphia, Lea & Febiger, 1975
5. Lindberg RD: Distribution of cervical lymph node metastases from squamous cell carcinoma of the upper respiratory and digestive tracts. Cancer 29:1446–1450, 1972
6. Lindberg RD, Barkley HT Jr, Jesse RH, Fletcher GH: Evolution of the clinically negative neck in patients with squamous cell carcinoma of the faucial arch. Am J Roentgenol Radium Ther Nucl Med 111:60–65, 1971
7. Lindberg RD, Fletcher GH: The role of irradiation in the management of head and neck cancer: Analysis of results and causes of failure. Tumori 64:313–325, 1978
8. Million RR, Cassisi NJ, Wittes RE: Cancer in the head and neck. In DeVita VT Jr, Hellman S, Rosenberg SA: Cancer: Principles and Practice of Oncology, pp 301–395. Philadelphia, JB Lippincott, 1982
9. Ogura JH, Biller HF, Wette R: Elective neck dissection for pharyngeal and laryngeal cancers: An evaluation. Ann Otol Rhinol Laryngol 80:646–651, 1971
10. Parsons JT, Million RR, Cassisi NJ: Carcinoma of the base of the tongue: Results of radical irradiation with surgery reserved for irradiation failure. Laryngoscope 92:689–696, 1981
11. Perez CA, Lee FA, Ackerman LV, Ogura JH, Powers WE: Nonrandomized comparison of preoperative irradiation and surgery versus irradiation alone in the management of carcinoma of the tonsil. Am J Roentgenol 126:248–260, 1976
12. Ratzer ER, Schweitzer RJ, Frazell EL: Epidermoid carcinoma of the palate. Am J Surg 119:294–297, 1970

13. Rolander TL, Everts EC, Shumrick DA: Carcinoma of the tonsil: A planned combined therapy approach. Laryngoscope 81:1199–1207, 1971

14. Seydel HG, Scholl H: Carcinoma of the soft palate and uvula. Am J Roentgenol Radium Ther Nucl Med 120:603–607, 1974

15. Southwick HW: Elective neck dissection for intraoral cancer. JAMA 217:454–455, 1971

16. Strong MS, Vaughan CW, Kayne HL, Aral IM, Ucmakli A, Feldman M, Healy GB: A randomized trial of preoperative radiotherapy in cancer of the oropharynx and hypopharynx. Am J Surg 136:494–500, 1978

17. Weichert KA, Aron BS, Maltz R, Shumrick D: Carcinoma of the tonsil: Treatment by a planned combination of radiation and surgery. Int J Radiat Oncol Biol Phys 1:505–508, 1976

18. Weller SA, Goffinet DR, Goode RL, Bagshaw MA: Carcinoma of the oropharynx: Results of megavoltage radiation therapy in 305 patients. Am J Roentgenol 126:236–247, 1976

19. Whicker JH, DeSanto LW, Devine KD: Surgical treatment of squamous cell carcinoma of the base of the tongue. Laryngoscope 82:1853–1860, 1972

Larynx

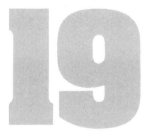

RODNEY R. MILLION
NICHOLAS J. CASSISI

Cancer of the larynx represents about 2% of the total cancer risk and is the most common head and neck cancer (skin excluded). The number of new cases in 1982 in the United States is estimated at 10,900 (9,100 in men and 1,800 in women) with an estimated 3,700 deaths due to laryngeal cancer.[45] Localized cases are estimated at 62%, those with regional spread around 26%, and those with distant metastasis at the time of first diagnosis at 8%.[45] The ratio of glottic to supraglottic carcinoma is approximately 3:1.

A study of trends in cancer incidence in the United States from 1935 to 1970 shows that cancer of the larynx has increased by 33% in white men, but is 3½ times increased in nonwhite men. The incidence in women has shown only a very minimal increase, in spite of the fact that lung cancer in women has quadrupled in the same period.[8]

Cancer of the larynx seems to be primarily related to cigarette smoking. The risk of tobacco-related cancers of the upper alimentary and respiratory tract declines among exsmokers after 5 years and is said to approach the risk of nonsmokers after 10 years of abstention.[52]

A 12-year American Cancer Society study has shown that smoking low-tar and low-nicotine cigarettes (less than 18 mg of tar and less than 1.2 mg of nicotine) results in slightly lower death rates from lung cancer, but whether or not the risk of laryngeal cancer is affected is unknown.[19]

The importance of alcohol in the etiology of laryngeal cancer remains unclear, but it is probably less important than in cancer in other head and neck sites.[50]

The geographic distribution for laryngeal cancer in the United States shows excess occurrence in the Northeast, particularly in northern New Jersey, New York City, and along the Hudson River. The rates are also high along the southeastern Atlantic Coast and the Gulf Coast. This distribution closely resembles the high-risk areas for lung cancer.[15]

ANATOMY

The anatomy of the larynx has been studied in great detail in recent years by whole-organ serial sections. These studies provide the basis for understanding not only the anatomy but also the routes of local tumor spread and the basis for partial laryngectomies, both the vertical hemilaryngectomy and the horizontal supraglottic laryngectomy. Anatomically, the larynx is divided into the supraglottic, glottic, and subglottic regions. The supraglottic larynx consists of the epiglottis, the false vocal cords, the ventricles, and the aryepiglottic folds, including the arytenoids. The glottis includes the true vocal cords and the anterior commissure. The subglottic area is located below the vocal cords (Figs. 19-1 and 19-2 and Plates 10 through 12).[7,31]

The line of demarcation between the glottis and the supraglottic larynx is considered from the clinical viewpoint to be the apex of the ventricle, the point at which the epithelium of the vocal cord turns upward to form the lateral wall of the ventricle. This transition can only be seen by direct laryngoscopy. The demarcation between the glottis and subglottis is also ill defined but is considered to begin 5 mm below the free margin of the vocal cord and to end at the inferior border of the cricoid cartilage.

The vocal cords are about 2.2 cm in length in men and 1.8 cm in women.

They are 3 mm to 5 mm thick, being relatively thin at the anterior commissure, thicker in their midportion, and then slightly thinner at the vocal process. Technically, the vocal cords terminate posteriorly with their attachment to the vocal process. The mucosa between the arytenoids forms the posterior part of the glottis (i.e., the posterior commissure). This posterior commissure area is rarely the site of origin of cancer, but it may be invaded by tumors of the vocal cord, arytenoid, pyriform sinus, and postcricoid pharynx.

Framework

The framework of the larynx is composed of bone and cartilage joined together by numerous ligaments. The outside shell is formed by the hyoid bone, thyroid cartilage, and cricoid cartilage, the cricoid cartilage being the only complete ring. The more mobile interior framework is composed of the heart-shaped epiglottis and the arytenoid, corniculate, and cuneiform cartilages. The corniculate and cuneiform cartilages produce small, rounded bulges at the posterior end of the aryepiglottic folds.

The thyroid, the cricoid, and a portion of the arytenoids are hyaline cartilage and may partially ossify with age, particularly in men. The remaining cartilages are elastic cartilage and do not ossify. Ossification, when it occurs, is patchy and makes interpretation of computed tomographic (CT) scans and other roentgenograms difficult as to whether destruction is present.

The epiglottic cartilage and thyroepiglottic ligament are porous, especially the infrahyoid portion, due to the multiple foramina for the ducts of minor salivary glands (see Plates 10A and 12).

The hyoid bone and various cartilages are joined together by an elaborate system of ligaments and fibroelastic membranes.

The external framework is linked together by the thyrohyoid, the cricothyroid, and the cricotracheal ligaments or membranes (Fig. 19-3). All three of these ligaments are thin, and the thyrohyoid in particular is rather flimsy and a poor barrier to tumor spread. There is a small gap between the middle and inferior pharyngeal constrictor muscles where the neurovascular bundle penetrates the thyrohyoid membrane; this weak point allows ready exit into the neck for tumors involving the lateral pharyngeal wall.

The epiglottis is joined superiorly to the hyoid bone by the hyoepiglottic ligament. The epiglottis is joined to the thyroid cartilage by the thyroepiglottic ligament at a point just below the thyroid notch and above the anterior commissure (see Plate 12). The arrangement of the ligaments that connect the cricoid and arytenoid cartilages and form the vocal ligaments, which are part of the true vocal cords, is shown in Figure 19-2D. The conus elasticus (cricovocal ligament) is the lower portion of the elastic membrane that connects the inferior framework. It connects the upper

(Text continues on p. 320.)

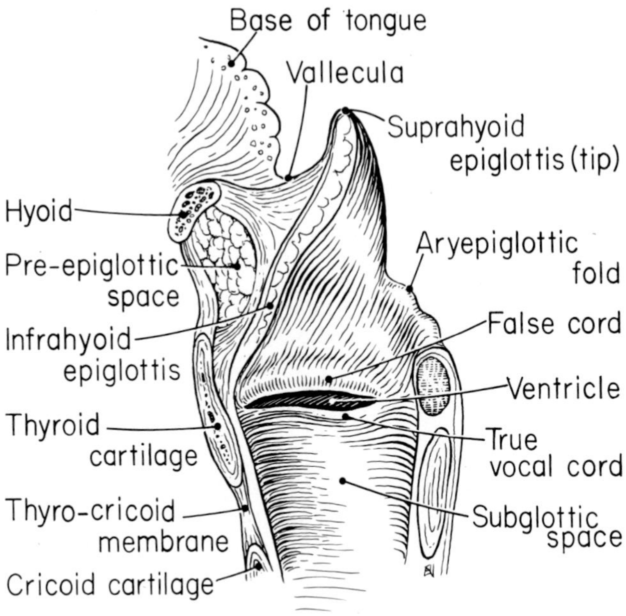

FIG. 19-1. Diagrammatic sagittal section of the larynx. (Redrawn from Sabotta drawings in Clemente CD: Anatomy: A Regional Atlas of the Human Body. Philadelphia, Lea & Febiger, 1975. Copyright © 1975, Urban & Schwarzenberg, Munich)

FIG. 19-2. (A) Larynx. (A, posterior pharyngeal wall; B, arytenoid; C, aryepiglottic fold; D, false vocal cord; E, true vocal cord; F, infrahyoid epiglottis; G, suprahyoid epiglottis; H, pyriform sinus) (B) Cross section of larynx at level of vocal cords. (C) CT scan at the level of the vocal cords. Note the low-density paraglottic space between the margins of the vocal cords and the thyroid cartilage (arrow). (Arrowhead, vocal process of the arytenoid; PS, air in the pyriform sinus) (D) Framework of the larynx. (A from Million RR, Cassisi NJ: The management of local and regional laryngeal cancer. In Carter SK, Glatstein E, Livingston RB [eds]: Principles of Cancer Treatment, pp 633–643. New York, McGraw-Hill, 1981. B and D redrawn from Sabotta drawings in Clemente CD: Anatomy: A Regional Atlas of the Human Body. Philadelphia, Lea & Febiger, 1975. Copyright © 1975, Urban & Schwarzenberg, Munich)

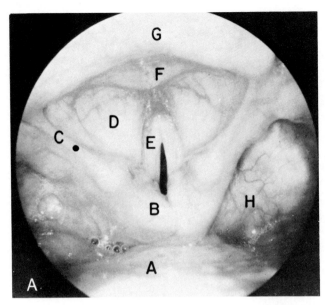

A.

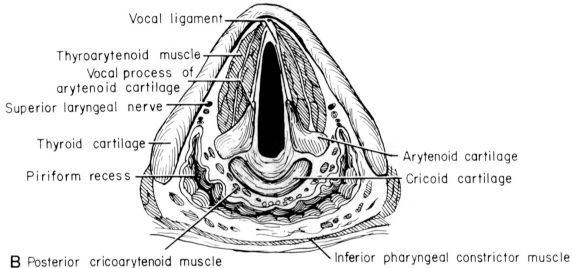

Vocal ligament

Thyroarytenoid muscle

Vocal process of arytenoid cartilage

Superior laryngeal nerve

Thyroid cartilage

Piriform recess

Arytenoid cartilage

Cricoid cartilage

B Posterior cricoarytenoid muscle

Inferior pharyngeal constrictor muscle

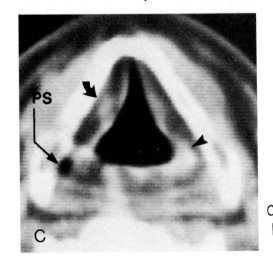

PS

C

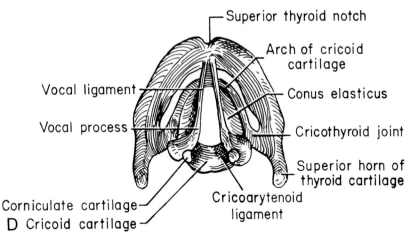

Superior thyroid notch

Arch of cricoid cartilage

Vocal ligament

Conus elasticus

Vocal process

Cricothyroid joint

Superior horn of thyroid cartilage

Corniculate cartilage

Cricoarytenoid ligament

D Cricoid cartilage

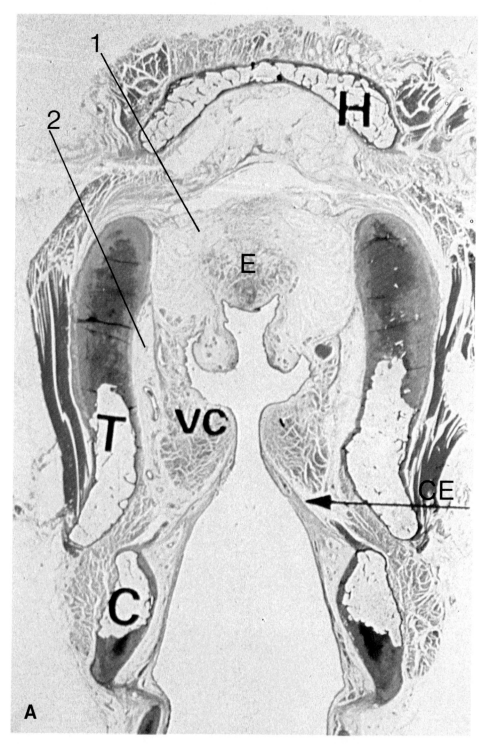

Plate 10. (*A*) Coronal whole-organ laryngeal section near middle third of vocal cord. The conus elasticus (*CE*) extends from the cricoid cartilage (*C*) to the vocal cord (*VC*). The thyroid cartilage (*T*) is partially ossified as is the cricoid cartilage; a CT scan might be interpreted as "cartilage destruction" when, in fact, there is a normal partially ossified cartilage. The epiglottis (*E*) is seen surrounded by the preepiglottic (*1*) and paraglottic (*2*) fat spaces, which extend inferiorly to the conus elasticus. (*H*, hyoid bone) (*B*) Coronal diagram of larynx. (*C*) Normal axial CT scan through the hyoid bone. Note the low-density semilunar preepiglottic fat space. The epiglottis is represented by a thin, patchy density next to the airway. There is air in each pyriform sinus. The hyoepiglottic ligament (*HEL*) can often be identified at this level because it is slightly more dense than the surrounding fat; the HEL could easily be confused with minimal tumor extension to the preepiglottic fat space. There is air in the right and left vallecula seen on each side of the hyoepiglottic ligament. (*SH*, superior horn of thyroid cartilage) (*A*, courtesy of A. W. P. van Nostrand, Toronto General Hospital, Ontario, Canada. *B*, redrawn from Sabotta drawings in Clemente CD: Anatomy: A Regional Atlas of the Human Body. Copyright © 1975, Urban & Schwarzenberg, Munich)

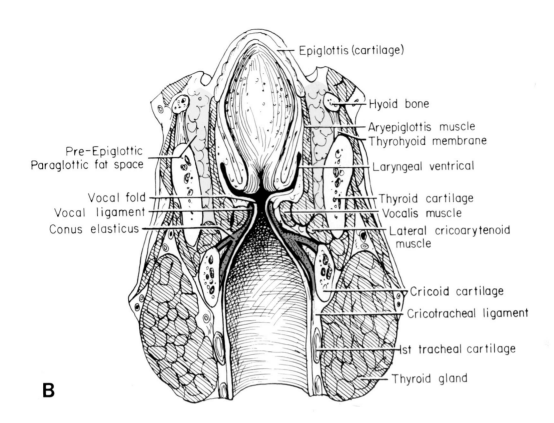

Epiglottis (cartilage)

Hyoid bone

Aryepiglottis muscle

Thyrohyoid membrane

Pre-Epiglottic
Paraglottic fat space

Laryngeal ventrical

Vocal fold

Thyroid cartilage

Vocal ligament

Vocalis muscle

Conus elasticus

Lateral cricoarytenoid
muscle

Cricoid cartilage

Cricotracheal ligament

1st tracheal cartilage

Thyroid gland

B

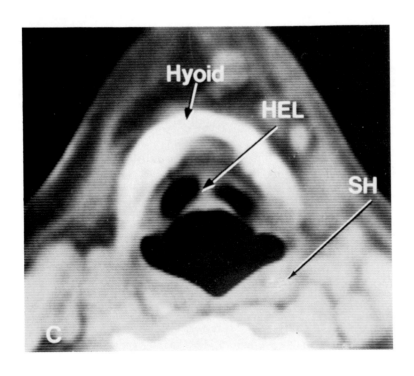

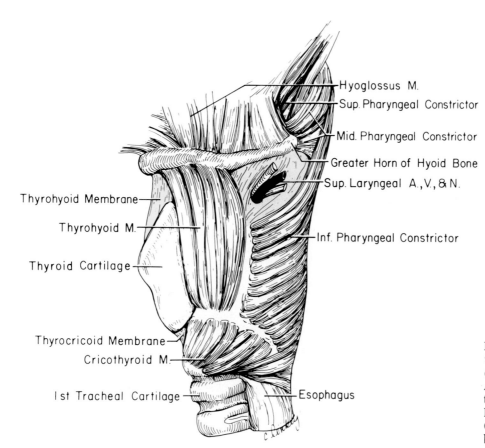

Hyoglossus M.
Sup. Pharyngeal Constrictor
Mid. Pharyngeal Constrictor
Greater Horn of Hyoid Bone
Sup. Laryngeal A., V., & N.
Thyrohyoid Membrane
Thyrohyoid M.
Thyroid Cartilage
Inf. Pharyngeal Constrictor
Thyrocricoid Membrane
Cricothyroid M.
1st Tracheal Cartilage
Esophagus

FIG. 19-3. External view of the larynx. (From Sabotta drawings in Clemente CD: Anatomy: A Regional Atlas of the Human Body. Philadelphia, Lea & Febiger, 1975. Copyright © 1975, Urban & Schwarzenberg, Munich)

surface of the cricoid, the vocal process of the arytenoid, and the lower thyroid cartilage; its free border is thickened into the vocal ligament.

Each arytenoid cartilage rests on top of the cricoid cartilage; the cricoarytenoid joint is lined by a synovial membrane (see Plate 11). The vocal ligaments and muscles attach to the vocal process of the arytenoid posteriorly and the thyroid cartilage anteriorly.

The two true vocal cords meet anteriorly to form the anterior commissure tendon, which inserts into the thyroid cartilage.

Muscles

The arrangement of the intrinsic muscles of the larynx, which primarily control the movement of the cords, is presented in Figure 19-2B and Plates 10 through 12. The extrinsic muscles are concerned primarily with swallowing, except for the cricothyroid muscle, which produces tension and elongation of the vocal cords and is innervated by the superior laryngeal nerve (Figs. 19-3 and 19-4).

Fat Spaces

The preepiglottic and paraglottic fat spaces are one continuous space lying between the external framework of the thyroid cartilage and hyoid bone and the inner framework of the epiglottis and intrinsic muscles (see Plates 10 through 12). This fatty areolar space is traversed by blood

and lymphatic vessels and nerves; there should be few, if any, capillary lymphatics arising in this area, and therefore invasion of the fat space should only indirectly be associated with lymph node metastases. The fat space is limited by the conus elasticus inferiorly; the thyroid ala, thyrohyoid membrane, and hyoid bone anterolaterally; the hyoepiglottic ligament superiorly; and the fascia of the intrinsic muscles on the medial side. Posteriorly it is in relationship to the anterior wall of the pyriform sinus. The fat space is thus semilunar or horseshoe-shaped on cross section and is easily seen on CT scan owing to the low contrast of fat (Fig. 19-2C).

Mucous Membrane

The laryngeal surface of the epiglottis and the free margin of the vocal cords are squamous epithelium, and the remainder is usually pseudostratified ciliated columnar epithelium. The stratified squamous epithelium of the vocal cord extends on the average 1.8 mm lateral and 2.3 mm inferior to the free edge of the vocal cord. Beneath the epithelium of the free edge of the vocal cord is the lamina propria, which can be divided into three layers.

The outer layer (0.3 mm thick) is loosely organized elastic and collagenous fibers with physical characteristics similar to soft gelatin; this layer is referred to as Reinke's space, the space where edema develops.

The intermediate and deep layers of the lamina propria (0.8 mm thick) are composed of densely organized elastic and collagenous fibers, and these two layers are referred

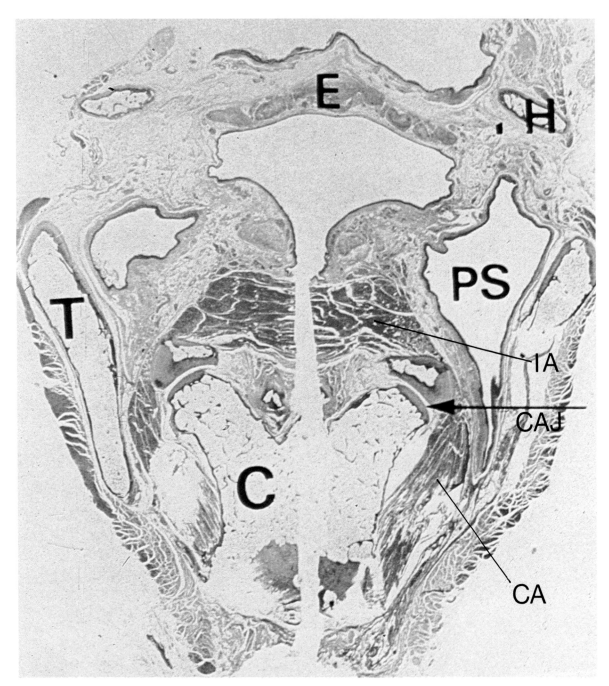

Plate 11. Whole-organ laryngeal coronal section of normal larynx through the posterior aspect of cricoid cartilage. The thyroid (*T*) and cricoid (*C*) cartilages are composed almost entirely of marrow-containing bone. The arrow points to the cricoarytenoid joint (*CAJ*); note proximity to the lower medial wall of the pyriform sinus (*PS*). The distance between the mucosa of the lateral wall of the pyriform sinus and the cartilage is narrow. The thyrohyoid and thyrocricoid membranes are indistinct. Fixation of the vocal cord may occur when tumor invades the cricoarytenoid joint, the cricoarytenoid muscle (*CA*), or the interarytenoid muscle (*IA*). (*E*, epiglottis; *H*, hyoid bone) (Courtesy of A. W. P. van Nostrand, Toronto General Hospital, Ontario, Canada)

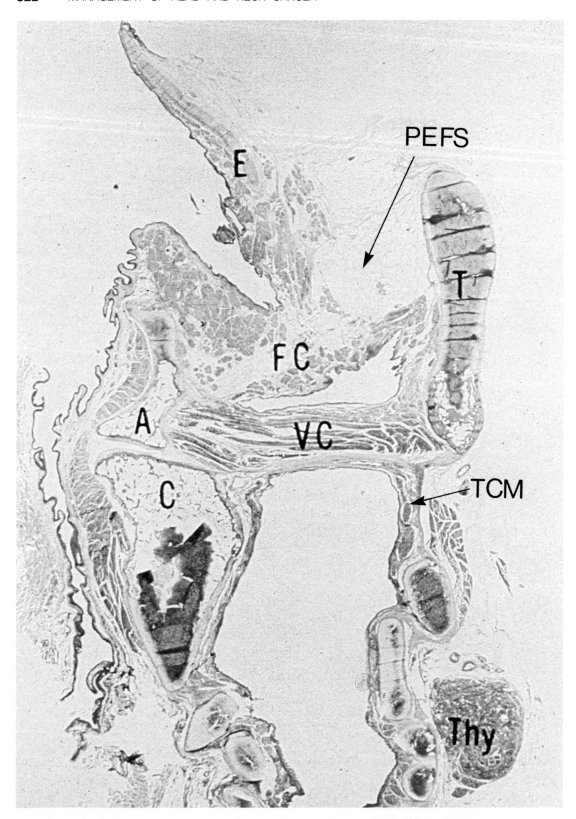

Plate 12.   Whole-organ sagittal section of normal larynx just to the left of the midline. The lower portion of the epiglottic (*E*) cartilage is perforated by the ducts of numerous minor salivary glands and appears discontinuous. The preepiglottic fat space (*PEFS*) is clearly seen. The ventricle lies between the false cord (*FC*) and the vocal cord (*VC*). The arytenoid (*A*) and cricoid cartilage (*C*) are ossified. The thyrocricoid membrane (*TCM*) can be identified. There is no obvious anatomical barrier to the spread of supraglottic lesions to the vocal cord or vice versa. (*Thy*, thyroid gland; *T*, thyroid cartilage) (Courtesy of A. W. P. van Nostrand, Toronto General Hospital, Ontario, Canada)

to as the vocal ligament. Fibers of the vocal ligament insert into the underlying vocalis muscle so that there is no sharp distinct border.

There is no true submucosal layer along the free margin of the vocal fold.[23]

Blood Supply

The laryngeal arteries are branches of the superior and inferior thyroid arteries.

Nerve Supply

The intrinsic muscles of the larynx are innervated by the recurrent laryngeal nerve. The cricothyroid muscle, an extrinsic muscle responsible for tensing the vocal cords, is supplied by a branch of the superior laryngeal nerve; isolated damage to this nerve causes a "bowing" of the true vocal cord (see Fig. 19-4). The vocal cord continues to be mobile, but the voice may become hoarse. Loss of the sensory function of one superior laryngeal nerve (the "watchdog of the larynx") does not usually produce problems.

Lymphatics

The supraglottic structures have a rich capillary lymphatic plexus. The lymphatic collecting trunks pass through the preepiglottic space and the thyrohyoid membrane and terminate mainly into the subdigastric lymph nodes; a few trunks drain directly to the middle internal jugular chain lymph nodes.

There are essentially no capillary lymphatics of the true vocal cords; as a result, lymphatic spread from glottic cancer occurs only when tumor extends to supraglottic or subglottic areas.

The subglottic area has relatively few capillary lymphatics. The lymphatic trunks pass through the cricothyroid membrane to the pretracheal (Delphian) lymph node(s) in the region of the thyroid isthmus, or the trunks may carry tumor to the lower internal jugular lymph nodes. The pretracheal nodes are midline in position and even when clinically positive are small (1 mm to 5 mm and rarely over 1 cm to 2 cm). The subglottic area also drains posteriorly through the cricotracheal membrane, with some trunks going to the paratracheal lymph nodes while others pass to the inferior jugular chain.

PATHOLOGY

The laryngeal surfaces of the epiglottis and vocal cords are lined with stratified squamous epithelium, and the remainder of the larynx is lined with pseudostratified ciliated columnar epithelium. Nearly all malignant tumors of the larynx arise from the surface epithelium and therefore are squamous cell carcinoma or one of its variants.

Carcinoma *in situ* occurs frequently on the vocal cords. Distinction between dysplasia, carcinoma *in situ*, squamous cell carcinoma with microinvasion, and true invasive carcinoma is a problem that the pathologist and the clinician frequently confront. Stripping of the entire cord in patients

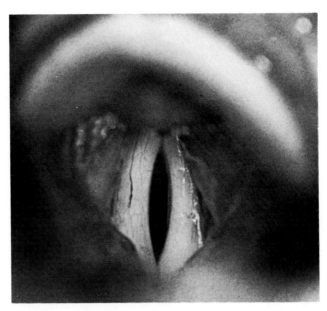

FIG. 19-4.   Bilateral superior laryngeal nerve paralysis results in "bowing" of the vocal cords.

with minimal lesions serves as the biopsy of the mucosa; the specimen tends to curl or fold, creating difficulty in orientation of the basement membrane.

Most of the vocal cord carcinomas are either well differentiated or moderately well differentiated. In a few cases there is an apparent carcinoma and sarcoma (i.e., carcinosarcoma) occurring together, but most of these are in reality a squamous carcinoma with pseudosarcomatous or spindle cell stromal reaction. It may be impossible for the pathologist to distinguish between a stromal reaction that mimics sarcoma in the presence of a carcinoma and a bona fide coexisting sarcoma and carcinoma. Only the course of the disease (i.e., metastasis) may settle the argument. Some of the carcinosarcomas present in the larynx and trachea as a polypoid or pedunculated tumor with a string-like umbilical cord.

Verrucous carcinoma occurs in 1% to 2% of patients with carcinoma of the vocal cord. The histologic diagnosis is difficult and must correlate with the gross appearance of the lesion.

Supraglottic carcinomas are less differentiated than those of the vocal cord, and verrucous lesions are rare. Carcinoma *in situ* is rarely diagnosed as a distinct entity in the supraglottic larynx, although a zone of carcinoma *in situ* is seen at the margin between invasive tumor and normal mucosa.

Small cell carcinoma ("oat cell") is rarely diagnosed in the supraglottic larynx and should be recognized as such because of its biologic potential for rapid growth, early dissemination, and responsiveness to chemotherapy.

Minor salivary gland tumors arise from the mucous glands in the supraglottic and subglottic larynx, but they are rare. Even more rare is the appearance of a chemodectoma, carcinoid, soft tissue sarcoma, malignant lymphoma, or plasmacytoma. (See the appropriate chapters for further discussion.) Benign chondromas and osteochondromas are reported, but their malignant counterparts are almost never seen.

PATTERNS OF SPREAD

Local Spread

The patterns of spread for squamous cell carcinoma are governed by the normal anatomical barriers and whether the lesion is infiltrative or develops with pushing borders. In explaining spread patterns, much has been made of the fact that the supraglottic larynx and the glottic/subglottic areas develop from different embryonic origins. While there is a tendency for supraglottic and glottic lesions to remain confined to their original compartments, there is no anatomical barrier to growth from one area to the next. Glottic lesions tend to be slow growing, but once they increase in size they quickly extend to the supraglottic and subglottic areas. Supraglottic lesions do not often start near the vocal cords, so that involvement of the cords on their external epithelial surface is a late phenomenon, but submucosal extension by way of the paraglottic area occurs earlier.

FIG. 19-5.   Horizontal section through supraglottic laryngectomy specimen. Early carcinoma of the tip of the epiglottis (*arrows*) with involvement of the lingual and laryngeal surfaces with minimal cartilage destruction. (*E*, epiglottis; *PES*, preepiglottic fat space; *H*, hyoid; *T*, thyroid cartilage) (Courtesy of A. W. P. van Nostrand, Toronto General Hospital, Ontario, Canada)

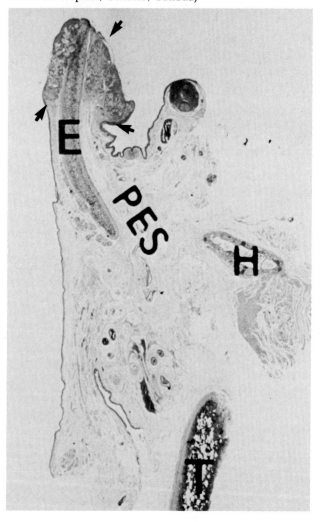

The fat space is an important avenue of submucosal tumor spread for infrahyoid epiglottis, false cord, and true vocal cord lesions (see Plates 10 through 12). As the false cord and true vocal cord lesions penetrate laterally, they quickly encounter the thyroid cartilage and then grow along the paraglottic fat space and even through the cricothyroid membrane before invading the perichondrium and cartilage. When thyroid cartilage invasion occurs, it usually occurs in the ossified section of the cartilage. In the thyroid and cricoid cartilages, the posterior portions are more commonly ossified.

Micheau and co-workers studied 120 cases of T2–T4 laryngeal cancer in patients without prior irradiation.[30] Partial or total ossification of the thyroid and cricoid cartilages occurred in 93%. Tumor invasion of cartilage was found in 70 patients, and in 66 the invasion occurred in the ossified portion. The most common site of thyroid cartilage invasion occurs at the anterior angle. They reported 3 unusual cases in which the internal portion of the cartilage was totally replaced by tumor, which expanded the cartilage, giving it a "blown-up" or expanded appearance. Isolated satellite nodules were reported in 18 of the 120 cases; in six instances, the satellites were distal.[30]

As the tumor grows down the paraglottic space, it is shunted at first by the conus elasticus toward and eventually through the cricothyroid membrane and into the tissues of the neck and the thyroid gland.

Fixation of the vocal cord is usually caused by invasion or destruction of the vocal muscle, invasion of the cricoarytenoid muscle/joint, or invasion of the recurrent laryngeal nerve. Other factors such as infection or mere bulk of tumor contribute to decreased mobility.

Perineural spread is uncommon in laryngeal malignancies.

SUPRAGLOTTIC LARYNX

The majority of lesions are epiglottic in origin. It is difficult to assign a site of origin for advanced lesions.

SUPRAHYOID EPIGLOTTIS

Lesions of the suprahyoid epiglottis may grow like a mushroom, producing a huge exophytic mass with little tendency to destruction of cartilage or spread to adjacent structures. Others may infiltrate the tip and produce destruction of cartilage and eventual amputation of the tip. The latter lesions tend to invade the vallecula and preepiglottic space, the lateral pharyngeal walls, and the remainder of the supraglottic larynx. A horizontal whole-organ section from a supraglottic laryngectomy for an early carcinoma of the tip of the epiglottis is shown in Figure 19-5.

INFRAHYOID EPIGLOTTIS

Lesions of the infrahyoid epiglottis tend to produce irregular outgrowths of tumor nodules with simultaneous invasion through the porous epiglottic cartilage and thyroepiglottic ligament into the preepiglottic fat space and toward the vallecula and base of the tongue (Plate 13). The hyoepiglottic ligament is fairly thick and represents an effective tumor barrier. However, the tumor may burrow through the epiglottic cartilage and preepiglottic fat space, penetrate the hyopiglottic ligament, and present in the vallecula and base of the tongue without involving the suprahyoid epiglottis.

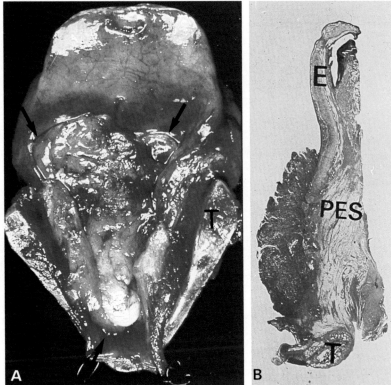

Plate 13. Carcinoma of the infrahyoid epiglottis. (*A*) Supraglottic laryngectomy specimen with large lesion (*arrows*) replacing the infrahyoid epiglottis. (*T*, thyroid cartilage) (*B*) Vertical section through specimen. The lesion is mostly exophytic. There is invasion of the thyroepiglottic ligament but minimal invasion of preepiglottic space. (*T*, thyroid cartilage; *E*, epiglottis; *PES*, preepiglottic space) (Courtesy of A. W. P. van Nostrand, Toronto General Hospital, Ontario, Canada)

Plate 14. (*A*) Total laryngectomy specimen showing an early carcinoma of the left false cord (*arrows*). The left true vocal cord appears grossly normal. (*B*) Coronal section through left false cord show submucosal extension of the tumor around the angle of the ventricle to the vocal cord. A conventional supraglottic laryngectomy would cut across the tumor. The dashed line shows the usual lower border for supraglottic laryngectomy; arrows point to the tumor margin. (Courtesy of A. W. P. van Nostrand, Toronto General Hospital, Ontario, Canada)

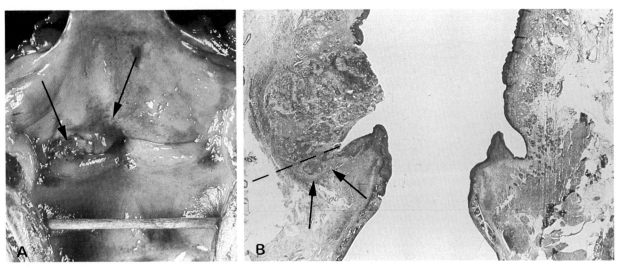

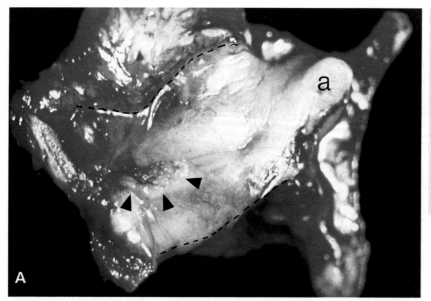

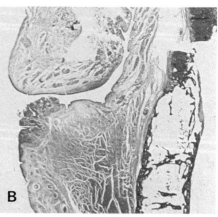

Plate 15. (A) Hemilaryngectomy specimen showing a carcinoma (*arrows*) confined to the anterior true vocal cord. Note the mucosal margins of resection (*dashed lines*). The inferior margin of resection corresponds to the top of the cricoid cartilage; the subglottic margin anteriorly is about 1.5 cm below the free margin of the vocal cord, gradually tapering to about 1.0 mm posteriorly. The superior mucosal cut corresponds to the superior border of the thyroid cartilage and would be 1.5 cm to 2.0 cm above the free margin of the vocal cord. The posterior border includes the arytenoid (*a*) in this specimen; the arytenoid is usually not removed unless necessary to obtain a margin. (B) Coronal section showing lesion confined to margin of cord with minimal invasion. (Olofsson J, van Nostrand AWP: Growth and spread of laryngeal and hypopharyngeal carcinoma with reflections on the effect of preoperative irradiation. Acta Oto-Laryngol [Suppl] 308:21, 1973)

Lesions of the infrahyoid epiglottis grow circumferentially to involve the false cords, aryepiglottic folds, and eventually the medial wall of the pyriform sinus and the pharyngoepiglottic fold. Invasion of the anterior commissure and cords is usually a late phenomenon, and subglottic extension occurs only in advanced lesions. Infrahyoid epiglottic lesions that extend onto or below the vocal cords are at high risk for cartilage invasion, even if the cords are mobile.[41]

FALSE CORD/VENTRICLE

False cord carcinomas are usually infiltrative and ulcerative with little exophytic component and are difficult to delineate accurately. They involve the paraglottic fat space early in their development and may spread a considerable distance beneath the mucosa without producing physical signs; they are therefore often understaged. These carcinomas extend to the perichondrium of the thyroid cartilage quite early, but cartilage invasion is a late phenomenon. Extension to the lower portion of the infrahyoid epiglottis with invasion of the preepiglottic space is common. Submucosal extension occurs to involve the vocal cord (Plate 14). Vocal cord invasion is often associated with thyroid cartilage invasion. Submucosal extension to the medial wall of the pyriform sinus occurs early. Subglottic extension is uncommon until the lesion is advanced.

ARYEPIGLOTTIC FOLD/ARYTENOID

Early lesions are usually exophytic growths. As the lesions enlarge, they extend to adjacent sites and eventually cause fixation of the larynx. The fixation may be secondary to mere bulk of tumor in some instances, but it is usually due to involvement of the cricoarytenoid muscle or joint or to invasion of the recurrent laryngeal nerve. It is usually impossible to distinguish the cause of fixation at the time therapeutic decisions are made. Advanced lesions invade the thyroid, epiglottic, and cricoid cartilages and eventually invade the base of the tongue and pharyngeal wall. It may be difficult to decide whether the lesion started on the medial wall of the pyriform sinus or on the aryepiglottic fold.

VOCAL CORD

The majority of lesions begin on the free margin and upper surface of the vocal cord (Plate 15). When diagnosed, about two thirds are confined to the cords, usually one cord. The anterior portion of the cord is the most common site, and extension to the anterior commissure is frequent. Anterior commissure involvement is said to occur when no tumor-free cord can be seen anteriorly; when the lesion crosses over to the opposite cord, anterior commissure invasion is certain. Small lesions isolated to the anterior commissure account for only 1% to 2% of all cases.

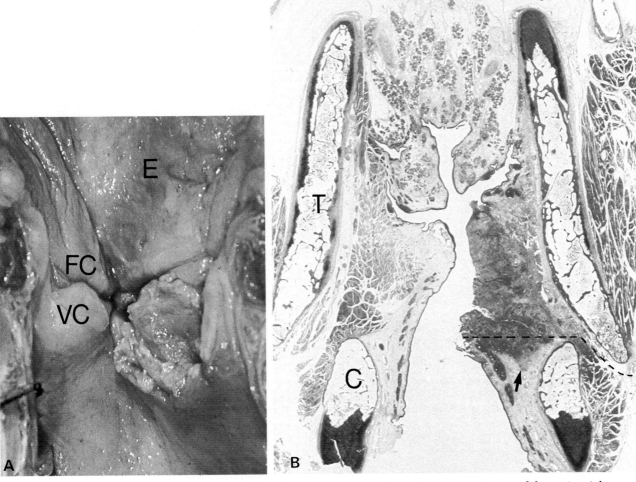

Plate 16. (*A*) Total laryngectomy specimen shows a carcinoma of the entire right vocal cord with obvious subglottic extension and invasion of the anterior commissure (T2). (*FC*, left false cord; *VC*, left true vocal cord; *E*, epiglottis) (*B*) Whole-organ coronal section at midcord level. The right vocal muscle is largely destroyed, and the tumor has penetrated the conus elasticus to involve the subglottic area. There is early involvement of the paraglottic fat space; note slight narrowing of space on the right compared with the left. There is no extension to the thyroid (*T*) or cricoid (*C*) cartilages. Dashed line shows the limits of conventional hemilaryngectomy. Arrow points to tumor margin. A portion of the cricoid would have to be removed to obtain a margin. (Olofsson J, van Nostrand AWP: Growth and spread of laryngeal and hypopharyngeal carcinoma with reflections on the effect of preoperative irradiation. Acta Oto-Laryngol [Suppl] 308:22, 1973)

Early lesions are frequently associated with zones of carcinoma *in situ* and atypism at the periphery of the lesion, and noncontiguous areas of carcinoma *in situ* or even early invasive tumor are seen in adjacent sites.

Tumors at the anterior commissure may extend anteriorly the short distance along the anterior commissure tendon (Broyles' ligament), which inserts directly into the thyroid cartilage and thus allows tumor access to the cartilage without the necessity of penetrating either a muscle or the perichondrium.[5] Early subglottic extension is also associated with involvement of the anterior commissure, and tumor may then grow through the cricothyroid membrane.

Lesions that arise on the posterior half of the vocal cord tend to extend along the submucosa toward the medial side of the vocal process to invade the cricoarytenoid joint and interarytenoid area. This extension is difficult to appreciate by clinical examination and results in understaging of the posterior vocal cord lesions. It probably accounts for the poorer local control rates by radiation therapy or hemilaryngectomy, compared with early lesions of the anterior half of the vocal cord.

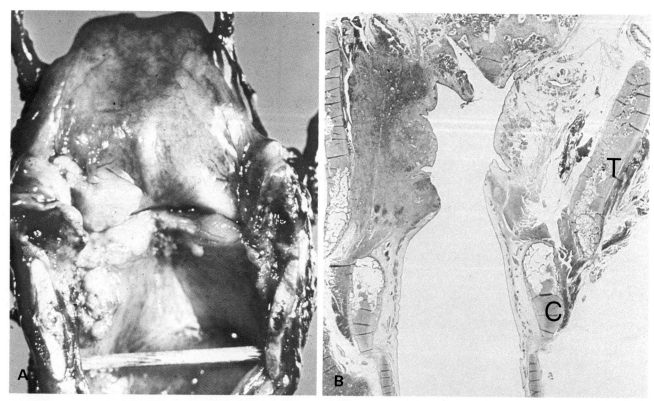

Plate 17. (*A*) Total laryngectomy specimen of an extensive vocal cord carcinoma with fixed left vocal cord (T3). There is obvious extension to the supraglottic and subglottic areas on the left with involvement of the anterior commissure and anterior half of the right vocal cord. (*B*) Coronal section at midcord level. There is extensive invasion of the left false cord. The paraglottic space is replaced by the tumor. Involvement of the subglottic area on this section is minimal. There is no invasion of cartilage. (*C*, cricoid cartilage; *T*, thyroid cartilage) (Courtesy of A. W. P. van Nostrand, Toronto General Hospital, Ontario, Canada)

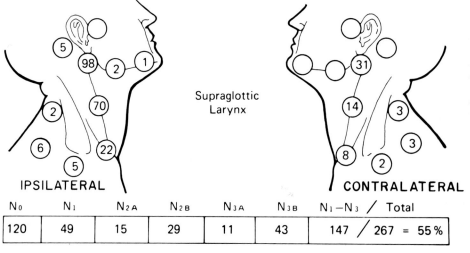

FIG. 19-6. Nodal distribution on admission, M. D. Anderson Hospital, 1948–1965. (Lindberg RD: Distribution of cervical lymph node metastases from squamous cell carcinoma of the upper respiratory and digestive tracts. Cancer 29: 1446–1450, 1972)

Supraglottic Larynx

IPSILATERAL   CONTRALATERAL

N_0	N_1	N_{2A}	N_{2B}	N_{3A}	N_{3B}	N_1-N_3 / Total
120	49	15	29	11	43	147 / 267 = 55%

Subglottic extension may occur by simple mucosal surface growth, but it more commonly occurs by submucosal penetration through the conus elasticus (Plate 16). One centimeter of subglottic extension anteriorly or 4 mm to 5 mm of subglottic extension posteriorly brings the border of the tumor to the upper margin of the cricoid, the limits of performing a conventional hemilaryngectomy. Lesions may spread beneath the epithelium along the length of the vocal cord within Reinke's space.[38]

As vocal cord lesions enlarge, they extend to the ventricle/false cord, vocal process of the arytenoid, and subglottic region (Plate 17). Infiltrative lesions invade the vocal ligament and muscle and eventually reach the paraglottic space and then the perichondrium of the thyroid cartilage. Once cancer reaches the perichondrium, it tends at first to grow up or down along the face of the cartilage in the paraglottic space rather than invading the cartilage. The conus elasticus acts only as a temporary barrier to subglottic penetration. The conus elasticus may direct tumor growth toward the thyrocricoid membrane. Advanced glottic lesions eventually penetrate through the thyroid cartilage or thyrocricoid membrane to enter the neck, where they may invade the thyroid gland. Lesions involving the anterior commissure often extend through the cricothyroid membrane after they extend subglottically.[38] Extension through the cricothyroid membrane is almost always associated with invasion of the adjacent edges of the thyroid or cricoid cartilage.

A fixed cord with less than 1 cm of subglottic extension and no false cord involvement does not ordinarily indicate invasion of the thyroid cartilage.[25] If the false cord is also involved, cartilage invasion is likely.

Jesse reported 48 patients whose disease was clinically staged T4.[24] In 47 the cancer was pathologically staged T4 due to cartilage invasion (54%), cricothyroid perforation (54%), extension to the pharyngeal wall (38%), or extension to or below the first tracheal ring (60%).

SUBGLOTTIC LARYNX

Subglottic cancers are rare. Most of them involve the vocal cords by the time they are diagnosed, so it is difficult to know whether the tumor started on the undersurface of the vocal cord or in the true subglottic larynx. The lesions are bilateral or circumferential in most instances since early diagnosis is uncommon. They involve the cricoid cartilage early, since there is no intervening muscle layer. Partial or complete fixation of one or both cords is the rule.

Lymphatic Spread

SUPRAGLOTTIC LARYNX

The distribution and N staging on admission prior to treatment for previously untreated patients with squamous cell carcinoma of the supraglottic larynx are given in Figure 19-6.[28] The spread pattern is mainly to the subdigastric area and internal jugular vein chain. The submaxillary area is rarely involved, and there is only a small risk for spinal accessory lymph node involvement.

The incidence of clinically positive nodes is 55% at the time of diagnosis; 16% are bilateral.[28] Elective neck dissection will show pathologically positive nodes in 16% of cases; observation of the neck will be followed by the ap-

pearance of positive nodes in 33% of cases.[11,34] Extralaryngeal spread to the pyriform sinus and vallecula/base of the tongue increases the risk of node metastases. The risk of late-appearing contralateral lymph node metastasis is 37% when the ipsilateral neck is pathologically positive. The risk is unrelated to whether the nodes in the ipsilateral neck were palpable before neck dissection.

VOCAL CORD

The incidence of clinically positive lymph nodes at diagnosis approaches zero for lesions confined to the cords (T1) and is 2% to 5% for T2 lesions and early, small-volume T3 lesions. The incidence of neck metastases increases to 20% to 30% for large T3 and T4 lesions.

Ogura and co-workers reported a 3% incidence of occult lymph nodes in 32 elective neck dissections for fixed cord lesions.[34] In six patients the risk for developing a contralateral lymph node when the ipsilateral neck was pathologically positive was zero. Supraglottic spread is associated with metastasis to the jugulodigastric nodes. Anterior commissure and anterior subglottic invasion is associated with midline pretracheal lymph node involvement (Delphian node).

Sessions and associates reviewed 132 glottic carcinomas with subglottic extension (>5 mm below the free margin of the vocal cord).[42] Only five patients had clinically positive lymph nodes on admission, in spite of the fact that 61% had greater than 1 cm of subglottic extension and 20% had greater than 2 cm of subglottic extension. Only four patients died due only to uncontrolled neck disease.

SUBGLOTTIC LARYNX

Lederman reported a 10% incidence of positive lymph nodes in 73 patients with subglottic carcinoma.[26]

CLINICAL PICTURE

Presenting Symptoms

VOCAL CORD

Carcinoma arising on the true vocal cords produces hoarseness at a very early stage. Sore throat, ear pain, pain localized to the thyroid cartilage, and airway obstruction are features of advanced lesions.

SUPRAGLOTTIC LARYNX

Hoarseness is not a prominent symptom for cancer of the supraglottic larynx until the lesion becomes quite extensive. Changes in voice quality are often described as a "hot potato" quality, the voice quality associated with unexpectedly swallowing a bite of very hot food. Pain on swallowing, usually mild, is the most frequent initial symptom. The pain is often described as a mild, persistant irritation or sore throat, and often the patient can point to the area with one finger. Mild difficulty in swallowing is frequent, and some patients report a sensation of a "lump in the throat." Cancer of the epiglottis may be quite large before symptoms are produced. Pain is referred to the ear by way of the vagus nerve and auricular nerve of Arnold (see Fig. 17-12 in Chapter 17). A mass in the neck may be the first

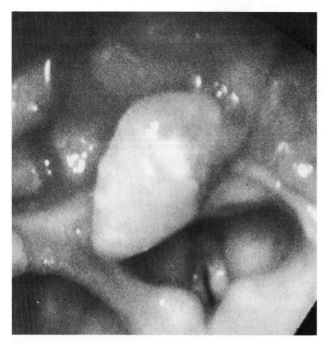

FIG. 19-7. Early squamous cell carcinoma of the vocal cord in a 60-year-old woman. The larynx was very small, and the tip of the epiglottis rested against the posterior pharyngeal wall and prohibited outpatient examination of the larynx. The right half of the tip was amputated with a biopsy forceps. This photograph was taken 1 year after radiation therapy. The patient was free of disease at 5 years. (For color photograph see Plate 1A in Chapter 3.)

sign of a supraglottic cancer. Late symptoms include weight loss, foul breath, dysphagia, and aspiration.

Physical Examination

Rigid and flexible fiberoptic illuminated endoscopes are now used routinely as a complement to the laryngeal mirror examination. The Hopkins rod with a right-angled lens gives excellent visualization of the infrahyoid epiglottis and anterior commissure, areas that may be difficult, if not impossible, to see with a laryngeal mirror. The mirror gives a larger image of the larynx/hypopharynx than that obtained by direct laryngoscopy or by fiberoptic endoscopes. The flexible fiberoptic laryngoscope is inserted through the nose and is useful in the more difficult cases (See Chapter 3, Examination with Fiberoptic Equipment.)

A horseshoe-shaped epiglottis or a posterior lying epiglottis may prohibit adequate laryngeal examination for even the most skilled examiner. The tip of the epiglottis may be amputated with a biopsy forceps in order to facilitate indirect examination of the larynx (Fig. 19-7). This is performed at the time of direct laryngoscopy. Loss of the tip of the epiglottis does not result in functional problems.

Determination of the mobility of the vocal cords frequently requires multiple examinations, since the subtle distinctions between mobile, partially fixed, and fixed cords are often difficult and in fact seem to change from examination to examination. A cord that appeared mobile to the surgeon prior to direct laryngoscopy may show sluggish motion or even fixation after biopsy.

Invasion of the preepiglottic space occurs more fre-

FIG. 19-8. Normal CT section at a level through the hyoid bone. The superior cornua of the thyroid cartilage (*SCT*) are seen posteriorly. Anterior to the airway, the epiglottis (*E*) and aryepiglottic folds (*AEF*) are seen. The epiglottis is composed of elastic cartilage and does not usually calcify. It is seen as a thin structure that is slightly more dense (*white*) than the airway and preepiglottic fat space. Also well seen are the hyoid bone (*HB*) and the low-density preepiglottic space (*PES*). The superior portions of the pyriform sinus (*PS*) contain air and are visible at this level lateral to the aryepiglottic folds. Lateral to the pyriform sinuses is the thyrohyoid membrane. The hyoepiglottic ligament (*HEL*) may be seen as an ill-defined midline density in the upper portion of the preepiglottic space; this normal structure can mimic early tumor invasion. The hyoepiglottic ligament is barely discernible on this reproduction. (*ICA*, internal carotid artery; *IJV*, internal jugular vein; *SCM*, sternocleidomastoid muscle)

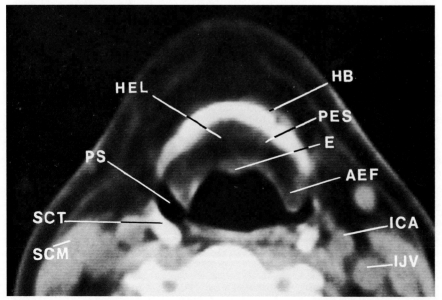

quently than can be diagnosed clinically. Ulceration of the infrahyoid epiglottis or fullness of the vallecula is an indirect sign of preepiglottic space invasion. Palpation of diffuse, firm fullness above the thyroid notch with widening of the space between the hyoid and thyroid cartilages signifies invasion of the preepiglottic space. Lateral soft tissue roentgenograms of the neck may show the presence of irregular air cavities inferior to the vallecula in patients with lesions of the suprahyoid epiglottis invading into the preepiglottic space by way of the vallecula. The preepiglottic space is a low-density area on the CT scan, and changes due to tumor invasion may be seen.

Postcricoid extension may be suspected when the laryngeal click disappears on physical examination. The thyroid carilage protrudes anteriorly, producing a picture of fullness of the neck. The diagnosis is confirmed by direct laryngoscopy, barium study of the hypopharynx, and laryngography.

Invasion of the thyroid cartilage remains a difficult clinical diagnosis. Localized pain or tenderness to palpation over one ala of the thyroid cartilage is suggestive. Tumor may actually penetrate through the thyroid ala and be felt as a small bulge.

METHOD OF DIAGNOSIS AND STAGING

Radiology*

In past years, larynx imaging was done by xeroradiography, plain film tomography, and contrast laryngography. These imaging techniques have largely been replaced in many centers by CT scans with contrast enhancement. *CT scan should be done prior to biopsy.* The normal CT anatomy of the larynx is shown in Figures 19-8 through 19-11. Contrast is helpful to outline the blood vessels and thyroid gland. Squamous cell carcinoma usually does not enhance, but enlarged metastatic lymph nodes may show irregular rim enhancement with low-density centers.

VOCAL CORD CARCINOMA

The CT scan does not show minimal mucosal lesions and is generally not indicated for well-defined, easily visualized vocal cord carcinomas. CT scanning finds its major use in diagnosis of moderately advanced to advanced lesions (Figs. 19-12 through 19-16). It is excellent for demonstrating subglottic extension and extension outside the larynx into the soft tissues of the neck. CT scan may show the cause of vocal cord fixation.

A potential area for CT diagnosis is determining thyroid or cricoid cartilage invasion. Early invasion of the thyroid and cricoid cartilages tends to occur at the edges of the cartilage rather than on the faces, and early involvement is difficult to detect with axial scans. The availability of direct coronal or sagittal scanning techniques may improve the detection of early cartilage invasion. Both the cricoid and the thyroid cartilage are unevenly ossified and normally have thick and thin areas that make interpretation of cartilage invasion difficult and, to our way of thinking, a bit unreliable. If the tumor mass extends through the cartilage to the soft tissues of the neck, then the diagnosis

* This section was written in conjunction with Derek J. Hamlin, MD.

(Text continues on p. 337.)

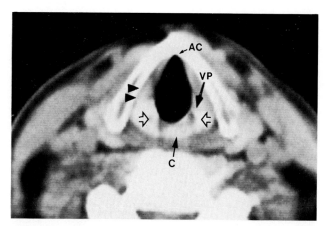

FIG. 19-9. Normal CT anatomy of the midplane of the true vocal cords. Open arrows indicate arytenoid cartilages. The top of the cricoid cartilage is partially visualized at this level (*C*). The vocal process (*VP*) of the left arytenoid cartilage is well demonstrated. A narrow low-density plane is seen between the right true vocal cord and the thyroid lamina (*arrowheads*); this is the inferior part of the paraglottic fat space. Note the complete lack of tissue at the anterior commissure (*AC*). Any tissue density here should be considered abnormal.

FIG. 19-10. Normal CT anatomy just below the midplane of the vocal cords. Arrows indicate low-density lower paraglottic fat space. The fibrofatty tissue in this space facilitates separation of the vocal vord and the adjacent thyroid lamina. If this clear space is maintained in the face of the thyroid lamina irregularity adjacent to the tumor, the lamina abnormality can be attributed to uneven calcification rather than tumor destruction. The posterior portion (*i.e.*, lamina) of the cricoid cartilage (*CC*) is seen. The outer and inner cortex of the cartilage is calcified; there is an intervening marrow space that is lower in density. The vertical height of the lamina is 2 cm to 3 cm. There is incomplete calcification of the thyroid cartilage anteriorly. (*IJV*, internal jugular vein; *ICA*, internal carotid artery; *T*, thyroid gland)

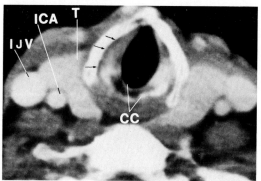

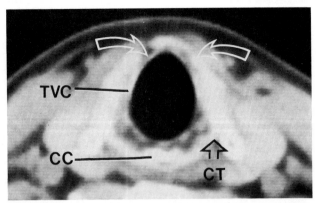

FIG. 19-11. Normal CT anatomy 5 mm below the free margin of the true vocal cord (*TVC*). The vocal cord appears thin due to abduction during scanning. There is bilateral paramedian incomplete calcification and thinning of the thyroid lamina (*arrows*). Note the normal lack of tissue density between the airway and the anterior arch of the thyroid cartilage. (*CC*, cricoid cartilage; *CT*, cricothyroid joint)

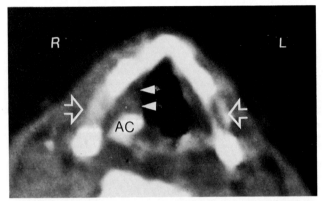

FIG. 19-12. Squamous cell carcinoma of the right true vocal cord (*arrowheads*). CT scan at the midplane of the true vocal cord. The tumor obliterates the right paralaryngeal space. The right arytenoid cartilage (*AC*) is well demonstrated. An important feature of this image is the incomplete calcification of the posterior third of the thyroid lamina just anterior to the takeoff of the inferior cornu (*open arrows*). This could easily be mistaken for tumor destruction of the thyroid cartilages.

FIG. 19-13. (*A*) Squamous cell carcinoma of the right vocal cord with subglottic extension. This section represents the transition from the true cord level to the infraglottis. Normally, there is no soft tissue density seen between the airway and the inner cortex of the cricoid cartilage. Subglottic tumor is seen on the right and extends from the anterior commissure to the posterior commissure; the left side is normal. Anatomical details determining this level include the cricoid lamina (*CL*) (which now only bounds the posterior aspect of the airway) and the inferior cornua (*IC*) of the thyroid cartilage; the arytenoids are no longer seen. (*B*) CT section 5 mm below *A*. This section is recognized anatomically by the cricoid lamina (*CL*) and cricoid arches (*CA*) surrounding the airway except anteriorly, where the airway is bounded by the thyrocricoid membrane (*white arrow*). Note faint ring of calcification of the cortex of the left cricoid arch (*crossed arrow*). Posteriorly, the cricothyroid joint (*open arrow*) is seen between the inferior cornu and the cricoid cartilage. On the right there is obvious subglottic extension (*arrowheads*).

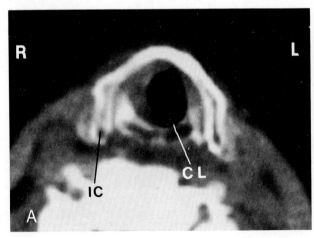

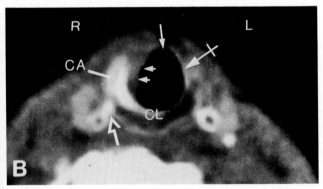

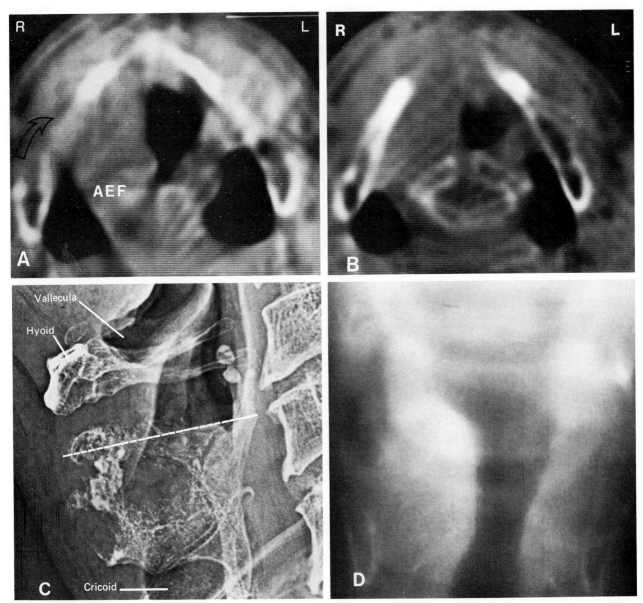

FIG. 19-14. A 70-year-old man presented with a 6-month history of progressive hoarseness. On physical examination, the right vocal cord was enlarged and fixed. There was extension to the right false cord, anterior commissure, and subglottic area. There was no palpable mass or tenderness over the thyroid cartilage. (*A*) CT section through the middle to low supraglottic level of the larynx. There was widening of the right aryepiglottic fold (*AEF*) and false cord on this side. The paraglottic space was preserved. There was irregularity of the posterior third of the thyroid lamina on the right side (*open arrow*). Note other areas of thyroid cartilage with irregular calcification. (*B*) CT scan at the level of the true vocal cords. The scan was taken during phonation. Both vocal processes rotated medially, even though the right vocal cord appeared fixed on indirect and direct laryngoscopy. The tumor crossed the anterior commissure to involve the anterior left vocal cord. There was incomplete calcification of the right anterior thyroid cartilage, suggesting tumor invasion. The paraglottic space was absent in this area. (*C*) Lateral xeroradiograph. There was patchy calcification of the thyroid cartilage. There was no evidence of a soft tissue mass extending through the cartilage. From this illustration it is easy to see why a CT scan is difficult to interpret accurately in regard to cartilage invasion. If the scanning gantry follows the dashed lines, a portion of the thyroid lamina will be partially out of the scan plane, resulting in the appearance of cartilage destruction. (*D*) Anteroposterior tomogram taken with patient in quiet respiration. The lamina of the right thyroid cartilage was absent. The tumor mass extended subglottically and supraglottically. The cord was fixed.

(continued)

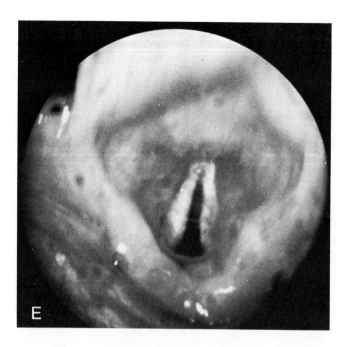

FIG. 19-14 (continued)

(*E*) Appearance at 7 months. The patient received 6750 rad/6 weeks, cobalt-60. He was free of disease at 2 years. There was complete return of motion in the right vocal cord. Should this lesion be classified T3 or T4?

FIG. 19-15.   A 45-year-old man presented with squamous cell carcinoma of the vocal cord. (*A*) Appearance following biopsy, prior to treatment. The entire right and left vocal cords were infiltrated with tumor. The right vocal cord was fixed, and the left vocal cord was partially fixed. There was extension into the left false cord and anterior commissure. There appeared to be tumor growing subglottically on the left. Direct laryngoscopy showed subglottic extension for at least 2 cm on both sides (T4N0). (*B*) CT section through midplane of the vocal cords taken during quiet respiration. Both vocal cords were enlarged. The anterior commissure was involved by tumor. The paraglottic space is not seen because of tumor invasion. (*A*, arytenoid cartilages) (*C*) CT scan at the transition from the true vocal cord to the infraglottic larynx. The mass extended across the midline, involved the anterior and left subglottic space. (*T*, thyroid cartilage; *IC*, inferior horn of thyroid cartilage; *CL*, cricoid lamina; *EA*, vertical ridge on posterior midline of cricoid lamina [site of attachment of the longitudinal fibers of the esophagus]) (*D*) CT section at midcricoid level, just below the undersurface of the true vocal cords. The mass involved the subglottic area in nearly a circumferential

(continued)

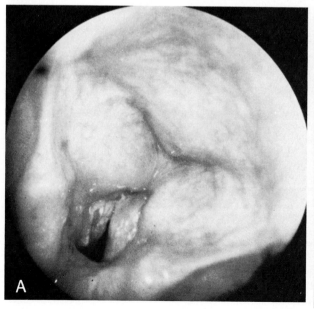

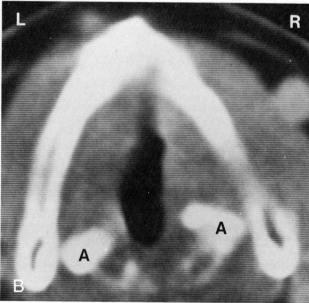

FIG. 19-15 (*continued*)

pattern. Only a few millimeters was spared posteriorly. Normally, no soft tissue density is present between the airway and the inner cortex of the cricoid cartilage. (*CL*, cricoid lamina; *CMS*, cricoid marrow space; *IC*, inferior cornu; *TC*, portion of the thyroid cartilage) (*E*) CT section 5 mm below *D*, through the cricoid and cricothyroid membrane. There was a circumferential tumor mass (*open arrows*). There was a soft tissue mass in front of the cricoid, continuous with the subglottic mass (*black arrows*). This extralaryngeal mass was not appreciated on clinical examination. Normally there is very little soft tissue anterior to the cricothyroid membrane. (*CA*, cricoid arches; *CL*, cricoid lamina) (*F*) Appearance of the larynx at 2 months. The patient was free of disease 1 year after receiving 7680 rad/6½ weeks, 120 rad twice a day.

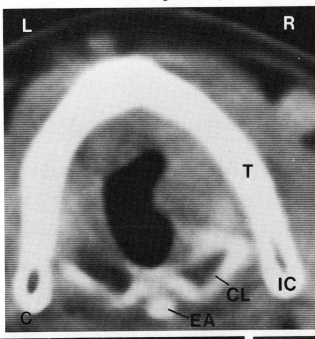

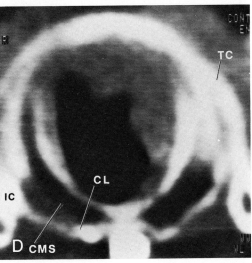

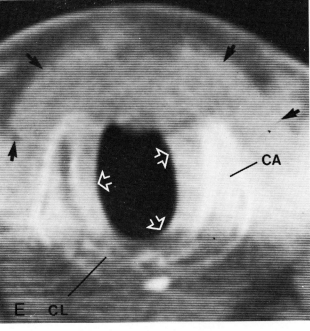

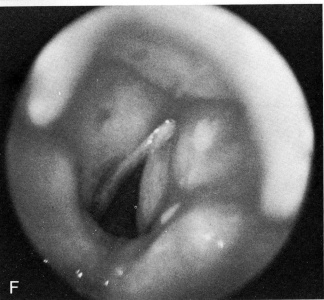

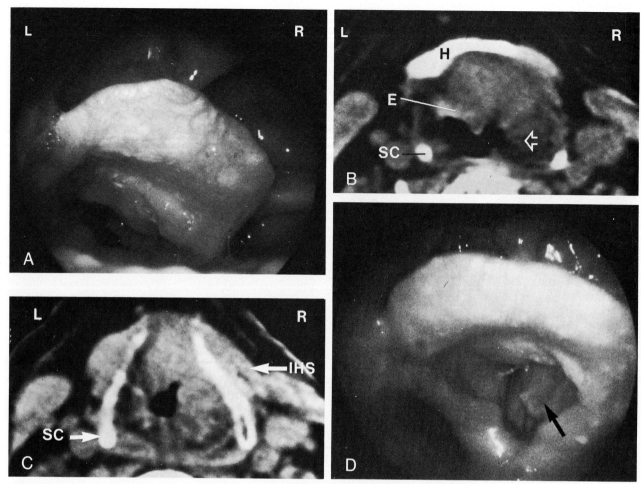

FIG. 19-16. A 70-year-old man presented with a 3-month history of sore throat and a 1-month history of hoarseness. (For color photographs see Plate 4C, D in Chapter 3.) (A) Direct and indirect laryngoscopy revealed a large lesion of the right infrahyoid epiglottis. The larynx was rotated clockwise. There was involvement of the right aryepiglottic fold, medial wall of the pyriform sinus, and right posterior false cord (not shown). Mobility of the right arytenoid was sluggish. The vocal cords were normal. (B) CT scan at the level of the hyoid bone. The epiglottis (E) was displaced to the left by a large mass in the preepiglottic space. The right pyriform sinus was obliterated. Only a portion of the hyoid bone (H) was visible. There was involvement of the aryepiglottic fold (open arrow). (SC, superior cornu of the thyroid cartilage) (C) Scan 5 mm below B at the midsupraglottis. The right paraglottic space was filled with tumor. The tumor extended toward the left preepiglottic space. The low-density fat space was preserved on the left. The thyroid notch marks the anatomical level. (IHS, infrahyoid strap muscle; SC, superior cornu) (D) Appearance at 2 months. The patient was treated with radiation therapy. There was a suspicion of persistence in the right false cord (arrow). Results of biopsies on three occasions were negative. The patient was free of disease at 2 years with marked supraglottic edema and hoarseness but no pain or airway obstruction. There was considerable fibrosis in the neck and persistent submental edema.

is reliable. However, in most of the cases there is merely some irregularity or low density of the cartilage next to an area of tumor, and it is very difficult to be sure about cartilage invasion. If the low-density plane of the paraglottic space is intact, cartilage invasion is probably not present.

SUPRAGLOTTIC CARCINOMA

The CT scan provides an excellent means for looking at the preepiglottic space and paraglottic fat spaces. Soft tissue extension into the neck or base of the tongue can also be seen.

The CT scan is also useful to determine extension to the subglottic areas.

The reader is referred to Mancuso and Hanafee's *Computed Tomography of the Head and Neck* for a full discussion of the normal and abnormal anatomy of this region.[29]

Differential Diagnosis

The differential diagnosis of laryngeal lesions includes hyperkeratosis (Fig. 19-17), papillomas, polyps, vocal nodules, fibromas, and granulomas. Papillomas can involve the epiglottis or false or true cords and can extend subglottically. They generally occur in children and young adults and may persist into adulthood. They may be confused with verrucous carcinoma in adults. However, four of our patients with vocal cord carcinoma were between the ages of 22 and 30 when they presented for diagnosis. There are 55 cases of laryngeal cancer reported in children 15 years of age or younger (aged 1 to 5 years in 7 cases). Carcinomas in children are often associated with papillomatosis, especially those in whom irradiation has been used.[17] Vocal polyps and vocal nodules occur at the junction of the middle and anterior thirds of the true vocal cords. There is usually a history of voice abuse followed by hoarseness.

Granulomas of the larynx usually occur as a result of intubation and are located on the posterior third of the vocal cords, near the posterior commissure. Endoscopic removal is the definitive treatment.

Contact ulcers occur over the vocal processes and are usually bilateral. They form granulation tissue around the ulcer and may be mistaken for carcinoma. Pain and hoarseness may be present.

Tuberculosis of the larynx, although rare, still occurs. Generally the lesion is destructive in nature and occurs at the posterior commissure of the glottis, the epiglottis, and the false cords. The appearance mimics cancer. Pulmonary tuberculosis is usually present.

Staging Procedures

Staging procedures for laryngeal cancer at the University of Florida include the following:

Indirect laryngoscopy (with photography)
CT scan with contrast enhancement (prior to biopsy)
Direct laryngoscopy with multiple biopsies
Chest roentgenogram

Direct laryngoscopy and biopsy with frozen section are usually performed with the patient under general anesthesia. A generous biopsy specimen is taken from the obvious lesion; additional biopsy specimens may be obtained

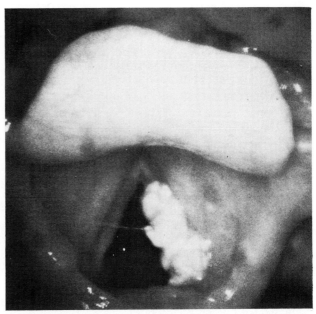

FIG. 19-17. A 61-year-old woman presented with a history of hoarseness for 2 years. There was an obvious lesion on the right vocal cord; mobility was normal. The entire lesion was removed in pieces with biopsy forceps. Microscopic diagnosis: hyperkeratosis with mild inflammatory atypia. This lesion grossly resembles either a verrucous carcinoma or an invasive squamous cell carcinoma.

from suspicious areas as well as from areas grossly involved, for purposes of staging. The mucosa of the margin of the cord may be stripped in order to provide adequate tissue when the lesion is distributed superficially along the cord and is not obviously a carcinoma. The ventricles, subglottic area, apex of the pyriform sinus, and postcricoid area must be carefully examined, since these areas are not consistently seen by any other method. Fiberoptic telescopes (0° and 30°) are introduced through the laryngoscope for inspection of these areas.

It may be nearly impossible to visualize the larynx by indirect laryngoscopy owing to the position of the tip of the epiglottis; the tip may be partially amputated with a biopsy forceps in order to facilitate examination (see Fig. 19-7). This procedure is rarely indicated since the availability of the flexible fiberoptic laryngoscope.

Staging

The American Joint Committee (AJCC) staging system for laryngeal primary cancer is listed below.[1] For lesions arising in the supraglottis, the sites of origin include false cords, aryepiglottic folds, suprahyoid (tip) epiglottis, infrahyoid epiglottis, and arytenoids. Only in the early T stages can one identify the specific site of origin with certainty. As the lesion enlarges, the site of origin is an educated guess based on the location of the greatest bulk of tumor.

Supraglottis

Tis Carcinoma *in situ*
T1 Tumor confined to region of origin with normal mobility
T2 Tumor involving adjacent supraglottic site(s) or glottis without fixation

T3   Tumor limited to the larynx with fixation or extension to involve the postcricoid area, medial wall of pyriform sinus, or preepiglottic space

T4   Massive tumor extending beyond the larynx to involve oropharynx, soft tissues of neck, or destruction of thyroid cartilage

Glottis

Tis   Carcinoma in situ

T1   Tumor confined to vocal cord(s) with normal mobility (includes involvement of anterior or posterior commissures)

T2   Supraglottic or subglottic extension of tumor with normal or impaired cord mobility, or both

T3   Tumor confined to the larynx with cord fixation

T4   Massive tumor with thyroid cartilage destruction or extension beyond the confines of the larynx, or both

The lower boundary of the vocal cord is considered to be the horizontal plane 1 cm below the apex of the ventricle according to the AJCC.[1] We prefer to consider the junction 5 mm below the free margin of the vocal cord.

More than 1.5 cm to 2.0 cm of subglottic extension would qualify for staging as T4 due to tracheal invasion. Caution is advised in overinterpretation of cartilage invasion by CT scan.

TREATMENT

Vocal Cord Carcinoma

SELECTION OF TREATMENT MODALITY

The goal is cure with the best functional result and the least risk of a serious complication. For purposes of treatment planning, patients may be considered to be in either an early group or a late group. The early group may be treated initially by irradiation or in selected cases by partial laryngectomy. The late group may be treated with radiation with laryngectomy reserved for failure or with total laryngectomy with or without radiation therapy.

DYSPLASIA, HYPERKERATOSIS, LEUKOPLAKIA

Complete stripping of the mucosa of the cord is often curative for lesions classified as leukoplakia, hyperkeratosis, or dysplasia. Careful observation is essential, since regrowth of the lesions often occurs. While repeated stripping with or without the use of a laser may seem a satisfactory plan of management, the cords may become thickened and the voice harsh, and it becomes increasingly difficult to tell whether or not invasive tumor is present. Irradiation may be recommended when there are repeated recurrences at short intervals.

CARCINOMA IN SITU

Lesions diagnosed as carcinoma in situ may sometimes be controlled by stripping the cord. However, it is difficult to exclude the possibility of microinvasion on these specimens. (See section on pathology.) Recurrence is frequent, and the cord may become thickened and the voice hoarse with repeated stripping.

We have come to recommend irradiation much earlier for carcinoma in situ, realizing that most cases would eventually come to this treatment and that earlier use of irradiation means a better chance of preserving a good voice.

Many of the cases treated as carcinoma in situ have obvious lesions that probably contain invasive carcinoma. We have often proceeded with radiation therapy rather than put the patient through a repeated biopsy procedure.

EARLY VOCAL CORD CARCINOMA

In most centers, irradiation is the initial treatment prescribed for early lesions, with operation reserved for salvage of irradiation failures. While hemilaryngectomy or cordectomy will produce comparable cure rates for selected T1–T2 vocal cord lesions, irradiation is generally the preferred initial therapy. The major advantages of irradiation compared with hemilaryngectomy or cordectomy are that the quality of the voice is likely to be better and that a major operation is avoided. The voice after hemilaryngectomy remains hoarse; we tell the patient that the voice will be "as hoarse as it is now or even worse." The voice after successful irradiation is usually better than before therapy, but occasional cases are seen in which there is no improvement or, uncommonly, a worsening. Hemilaryngectomy finds its major use as a salvage operation in suitable cases after irradiation failure. Even if the patient has a local recurrence after a salvage hemilaryngectomy, there is a third chance with total laryngectomy, which may still be successful.[3]

Verrucous lesions have the reputation of being unresponsive to irradiation and, in some instances, losing their verrucous nature to convert into invasive, often anaplastic, metastasizing lesions after unsuccessful irradiation. We recommend hemilaryngectomy for early verrucous carcinoma of the glottis, but we do not hesitate to recommend radiation therapy if the alternative is total laryngectomy. We have observed typical verrucous lesions that have disappeared with radiation therapy and not recurred. Burns and co-workers have also made this observation.[6] The patient must be advised of the risks when radiation therapy is used for verrucous carcinoma. Hemilaryngectomy is also used in patients who have had prior head and neck irradiation that prohibits further irradiation.

Fixed cord lesions may be subdivided into relatively early, favorable lesions and unfavorable lesions, the latter usually having extensive bilateral disease with a compromised airway. The patient with a favorable lesion is advised of the alternatives of radiation therapy with surgical salvage and immediate total laryngectomy. The local control rate with voice preservation with radiation therapy is 50% to 60% and 50% to 70% of failures are salvaged. The patient is advised that there is probably a slight reduction in the 5-year survival rate compared with immediate total laryngectomy. The patient must be willing to return for follow-up every month for the first 2 years and understand that total laryngectomy may be recommended purely on clinical grounds without biopsy-proven recurrence.

The major difficulty in the use of irradiation for the more advanced lesions is in distinguishing between radiation edema and local recurrence during follow-up examinations.

Extended hemilaryngectomy has been used with success by others in the treatment of well-lateralized fixed cord lesions. A permanent tracheostomy is required because a portion of the cricoid is resected, but a useful voice may be retained.[39]

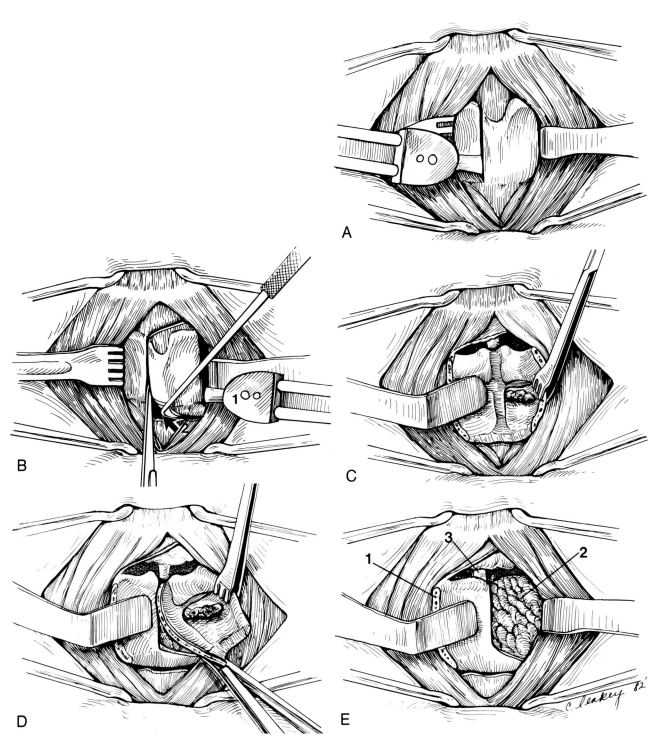

FIG. 19-18. Hemilaryngectomy for carcinoma of the left vocal cord with extension to the anterior commissure. (*A*) Strap muscles are retracted, exposing the thyroid cartilage. Perichondrium on the left is preserved. A saw cut is made just to the right of the midline. (*B*) A saw cut is made through the posterior edge of the thyroid cartilage, leaving 2 mm to 3 mm of cartilage posteriorly (*1*). The larynx is then entered anteriorly through the cricothyroid membrane (*2*). The lesion can then be viewed through a 1-cm exposure. A knife cut through the mucosa to the right of the midline is made under direct vision, and the incision is joined superiorly and inferiorly to the posterior cut. (*C*) The thyroid laminae are retracted, and the lesion is exposed. The posterior extent is now clearly visible. (*D*) The posterior mucosal cut is made along the line of the posterior cartilage cut. The final cut may include the arytenoid if it is involved. (*E*) Surgical defect after the specimen has been removed. Closure is completed by suturing the perichondrium from the left side to the perichondrium and thyroid cartilage on the right side (*1*). (*2*, mucosa of the pharyngeal wall; *3*, nasogastric tube)

ADVANCED VOCAL CORD CARCINOMA

The mainstay of treatment in most centers is total laryngectomy with or without postoperative irradiation. The most frequent sites of local failure after total laryngectomy are around the tracheal stoma, in the base of the tongue, and in the neck lymph nodes. If the neck is clinically negative prior to operation and if postoperative irradiation is planned, neck dissection is not done and irradiation is used to treat both sides of the neck. If the lymph nodes are clinically positive or if postoperative irradiation is not planned, a neck dissection is done. Postoperative irradiation may be used to control subclinical disease in the opposite neck as well as to help prevent recurrence in other areas.

Radical irradiation is prescribed for the patient who refuses total laryngectomy or is medically unsuitable for a major operation. Quite a few patients in this category will be cured and maintain a useful voice. Harwood and co-workers reported 50% local control by irradiation alone for unselected T3N0 glottic lesions.[21] Eighty-seven percent of the patients with treatment failure underwent laryngectomy, and 66% of those who had operations were cured. (See Table 19-13 in section on results of treatment.)

Harwood also reported the radiation therapy experience at the Princess Margaret Hospital for T4 glottic carcinomas.[22] Cartilage invasion was diagnosed by tomography and xerography. The 5-year actuarial local control was

FIG. 19-19. Treatment portal for early vocal cord carcinoma. The top border is adjusted according to the lesion. The bottom of the thyroid notch is the landmark for the very early lesions and the top of the notch for larger lesions or those with minimal supraglottic extension. The posterior border is the back edge of the thyroid cartilage if the lesion is confined to the anterior two thirds of the vocal cord; if the posterior one third of the vocal cord is involved, then the posterior border is placed 1.0 cm to 1.5 cm behind the cartilage. The inferior border is placed at the bottom of the cricoid cartilage when there is *no* subglottic extension.

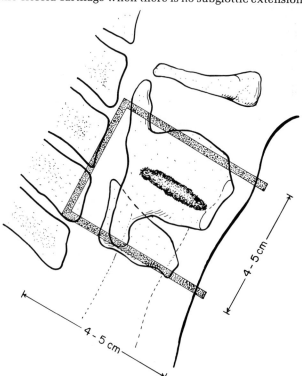

67% for 42 patients with involvement of cartilage, trachea, or base of the tongue and negative nodes, 19% for 14 patients with pyriform sinus involvement with or without cartilage invasion and negative lymph nodes, and 12% for 16 patients with clinically positive lymph nodes. The accuracy of clinical and radiologic assessment of cartilage involvement is admittedly imperfect, but there is a tendency to understage large lesions.[38,41]

SURGICAL TREATMENT

Stripping of the vocal cord implies transoral removal of the mucosa. The operating microscope is used by the surgeon in total stripping of the mucosa.

Thyrotomy with cordectomy is an excision of the vocal cord. Its use is usually confined to small lesions of the middle third of the cord. Cordectomy is generally reserved for that uncommon situation in which there is a postirradiation recurrence limited to the middle third of the cord with normal mobility. Following cordectomy, a pseudocord is formed and the patient has a useful, if somewhat harsh, voice. A portion of the adjacent thyroid cartilage may be removed with the cord.

Hemilaryngectomy is a partial, "vertical" laryngectomy that allows removal of limited cord lesions with preservation of voice (Fig. 19-18). There are definite restrictions in the use of this operation. One entire cord plus up to one third of the opposite cord is the maximum cordal involvement suitable for the operation in men; women have a smaller larynx, and usually only one vocal cord may be removed without compromising the airway. Partial fixation of one cord is not a contraindication to hemilaryngectomy, but only a few surgeons have attempted hemilaryngectomy for selected fixed cord lesions. The maximum subglottic extension allowable is 8 mm to 9 mm anteriorly and 5 mm posteriorly, in order to preserve the integrity of the cricoid. Tumor extension to the epiglottis, false cord, or both arytenoids is a contraindication to hemilaryngectomy. Less than 5% of hemilaryngectomies are converted to total laryngectomies at the time of operation in properly selected cases.

The last surgical alternative is total laryngectomy with or without neck dissection. Total laryngectomy is used as a salvage procedure for radiation failure in the early lesions that are not suited for conservative operations. It is the operation of choice for advanced lesions. The entire larynx is removed and the pharynx is reconstituted. A permanent tracheostomy is required. (See Chapter 20, Speech Rehabilitation After Total Laryngectomy.)

IRRADIATION TECHNIQUE

Irradiation for early vocal cord cancer (T1–T2) is delivered by small portals covering only the primary lesion. The incidence of lymph node involvement is so small (0 to 1%) that elective irradiation of lymph nodes is not recommended. Radiation portals extend from the thyroid notch superiorly to the inferior border of the cricoid; the posterior border depends on posterior extension of the tumor (Fig. 19-19). The field size ranges from 4 × 4 cm to 5 × 5 cm and is occasionally 6 × 6 cm for a large T2 lesion. Portals larger than this increase the risk of edema without increasing the cure rate. Since the portals are small and the skin of the neck is mobile, it is our practice to have the physician check the portal on the treatment table each

TABLE 19-1. Radiation Treatment Plan for Vocal Cord Cancer at the University of Florida (September 1980)

Stage	Description	External-Beam Irradiation (rad Tumor Dose)
T1	Early, no visible tumor	5625/25 fractions/5 weeks
T1	Moderate size	6300/28 fractions/5½ weeks
T1	Bulky	6525/29 fractions/6 weeks
T2	Early, normal motion	6300/28 fractions/5½ weeks
T2	Moderate size, reduced motion	6525/29 fractions/6 weeks
T3/T4	Fixed cord	See text

(Modified from Million RR, Cassisi NJ, Wittes RE: Cancer in the head and neck. In DeVita VT Jr, Hellman S, Rosenberg SA [eds]: Cancer: Principles and Practice of Oncology, pp. 301–395. Philadelphia, JB Lippincott, 1982)

FIG. 19-20. Comparison of portal arrangements (cobalt-60) for treatment of T1N0 squamous cell carcinoma of the anterior two thirds of the left vocal cord. (*A*) Ipsilateral portal, 4 × 4 cm. The maximum subcutaneous dose at 5 mm is 13% greater than the tumor dose (87%). (*B*) Normalized isodose distribution for parallel opposed portals, 4 × 4 cm, with wedges. Right to left = 1:1. The maximum subcutaneous dose occurs at 5 mm on both the right and left sides. The maximum subcutaneous dose is only 5% greater than the tumor dose. (*C*) Normalized isodose distribution for three-portal technique. The lateral wedged portals (4 × 4 cm) are each weighted 1.0 and the anterior portal (3.5 × 3.5 cm to 4 × 4 cm) is weighted 0.1 or 0.2. The maximum dose is shifted to the left side at a depth of 1 cm. The maximum dose is 5% greater than the tumor dose. This arrangement slightly reduces the high-dose volume and is the plan most often used in the past 5 years. The anterior portal is treated at the end of the treatment series after the lateral portals are completed.

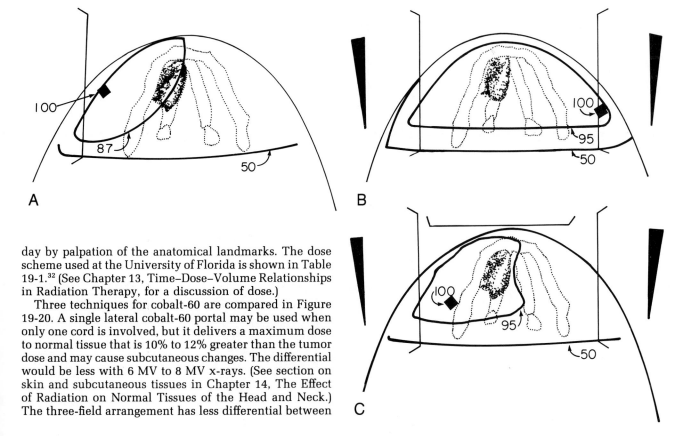

day by palpation of the anatomical landmarks. The dose scheme used at the University of Florida is shown in Table 19-1.[32] (See Chapter 13, Time–Dose–Volume Relationships in Radiation Therapy, for a discussion of dose.)

Three techniques for cobalt-60 are compared in Figure 19-20. A single lateral cobalt-60 portal may be used when only one cord is involved, but it delivers a maximum dose to normal tissue that is 10% to 12% greater than the tumor dose and may cause subcutaneous changes. The differential would be less with 6 MV to 8 MV x-rays. (See section on skin and subcutaneous tissues in Chapter 14, The Effect of Radiation on Normal Tissues of the Head and Neck.) The three-field arrangement has less differential between the maximum dose to normal tissue and the maximum dose to the tumor. The anterior portal is essentially a reduced portal and tends to center the high dose to the tumor. The weighting of the portals and the use of wedges or compensators are individualized to each case.

Irradiation of T3 and T4 lesions requires larger portals, which include the jugulodigastric and the middle jugular lymph nodes. The inferior jugular lymph nodes are included if there is greater than 1 cm of subglottic extension or for poorly differentiated carcinoma. The portals are reduced after 4600 rad (200 rad/fraction). The reduced portals cover only the primary lesion, and the dose per fraction is increased to 225 rad. The final dose is 6850 rad to 7075 rad/33 to 34 fractions. Twice-a-day fractionation (120 rad twice a day) to 7440 rad to 7680 rad/6½ weeks has been used successfully in a few large vocal cord lesions, and the functional result is excellent (Fig. 19-21).

MANAGEMENT OF RECURRENCE

Most recurrences appear within 18 months, but late recurrences may appear after 5 years.[14] The risk of metastatic disease in lymph nodes increases with local recurrence, and the lymph nodes should either be electively treated or watched very closely.

RECURRENCE AFTER RADIATION THERAPY

With careful follow-up, recurrence is sometimes detected before the patient notices return of hoarseness. There is often minimal lymphedema for 1 or 2 months after radiation therapy, which usually subsides or stabilizes. An increase in edema, particularly if associated with hoarseness or pain, is suggestive of recurrence, even if no obvious tumor is seen. Fixation of a previously mobile vocal cord usually implies local recurrence, but we have observed five patients who developed a fixed cord with an otherwise normal-appearing larynx and who have not shown evidence of recurrence. A paralyzed left vocal cord should also suggest the possibility of lung cancer.

It may be difficult to diagnose recurrence when the tumor is submucosal (Fig. 19-22). Generous, deep biopsies are required. If recurrence is strongly suggested, laryngectomy may rarely be advised without biopsy evidence of recurrence.

Irradiation failures may be salvaged by cordectomy, hemilaryngectomy, or total laryngectomy. An example of salvage of a radiation therapy failure by hemilaryngectomy is shown in Figure 19-23. Biller and co-workers reported a 78% salvage rate by hemilaryngectomy for 18 selected patients in whom irradiation failed.[3] Total laryngectomy

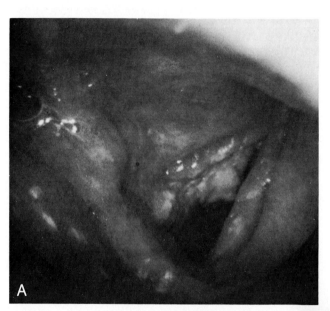

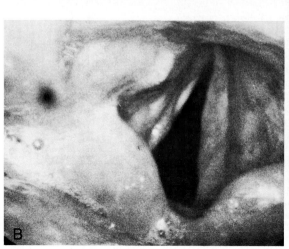

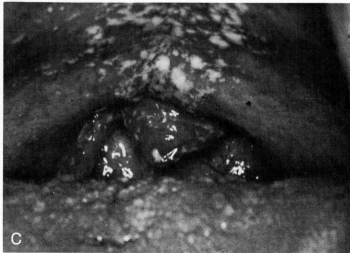

FIG. 19-21. Patient presented with a 3-year history of hoarseness and left-sided sore throat. (For color photographs see Plate 1B, C in Chapter 3.)(A) Squamous cell carcinoma of the left vocal cord with subglottic extension and involvement of the posterior left false cord and face of the arytenoid. The vocal cord was fixed (T3N0). Treatment was 7440 rad (120 rad twice a day) over 6 weeks, cobalt-60. The inferior treatment border was 2.5 cm below the cricoid cartilage. (B) Appearance 9 months after treatment. (C) The patient was asymptomatic until 3 years after treatment when he developed hoarseness, diffuse sore throat, and left ear pain. The midline soft palate and base of the tongue showed white patches consistent with candidiasis. The larynx was diffusely edematous and covered with patches of *Candida*. Further questioning disclosed the chronic use of a dexamethasone inhaler for chronic obstructive lung disease. He had failed to rinse his mouth following each application and developed candidiasis along the path of the drug due to local immune suppression. The condition was reversed with Mycostatin therapy and proper rinsing after inhalation therapy. The patient was free of disease at 3½ years.

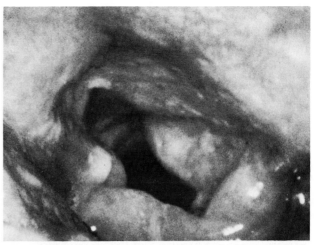

FIG. 19-23. A 57-year-old man presented with moderately well differentiated squamous cell carcinoma of the left vocal cord with minimal extension to the false cord (T2N0). The patient received 7000 rad/35 fractions (7 weeks), cobalt-60. Edema of the larynx and sore throat with ear pain developed at 6 months; results of biopsies were negative. Intermittent sore throat, hoarseness, and edema continued until recurrence became obvious on the left vocal cord at 15 months. A left vertical hemilaryngectomy was done; the arytenoid was spared. The tumor margins were free. This photograph was taken 6 years following left hemilaryngectomy. The patient's voice was hoarse. He was free of disease 8 years following hemilaryngectomy.

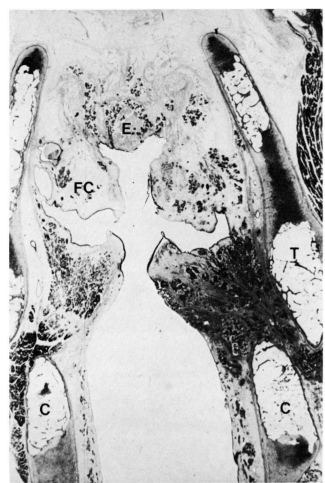

FIG. 19-22. Carcinoma of the vocal cord, recurring 3 years after radiation therapy (coronal section at the midcord level). The cord was fixed at the time of surgery. There was no gross evidence of disease in the specimen; the mucosa was smooth and intact. There was submucosal tumor replacing the vocal muscle and growing through the thyrocricoid space. There was subglottic extension to a level just below the top of the cricoid cartilage. (C, cricoid cartilage; T, thyroid cartilage; FC, false cord; E, epiglottis) (Courtesy of A. W. P. van Nostrand, Toronto General Hospital, Ontario, Canada)

was eventually required in 2 patients. Only 2 patients died of cancer. These investigators recommended the following four guidelines for the use of hemilaryngectomy: (1) contralateral vocal cord normal, (2) arytenoid not involved, (3) subglottic extension not exceeding 5 mm, and (4) vocal cord not fixed.

SURGICAL RECURRENCE

Salvage by radiation therapy for recurrences or new tumors that appear after hemilaryngectomy is about 50%. Lee and co-workers reported seven successes in 12 patients; one lesion was subsequently controlled by total laryngectomy.[27] Total laryngectomy will salvage almost all hemilaryngectomy failures not suitable for radiation therapy.

Radiation therapy will only occasionally cure a patient with recurrence in the neck or stoma after total laryngectomy.

Supraglottic Larynx Carcinoma

SELECTION OF TREATMENT MODALITY

For purposes of treatment planning, patients may be considered to be in either an early or favorable group suitable for radiation therapy or supraglottic laryngectomy or an unfavorable group often requiring total laryngectomy. Neck nodes are commonly involved and influence the overall treatment plan.

EARLY SUPRAGLOTTIC LESIONS

Treatment of the primary lesion for the early group is either by external-beam irradiation or supraglottic laryngectomy. Total laryngectomy would rarely be indicated as the initial treatment for this group of patients and is reserved for those who fail the initial treatment.

Irradiation and supraglottic laryngectomy are both highly successful modes of therapy for the early lesions, and for this reason it is seldom necessary to combine radiation therapy and surgery for initial management of the primary lesion; however, combined treatment may be indicated to control the neck disease.

The following paragraphs outline our guidelines for selection of supraglottic laryngectomy or radiation therapy. The patient and family are sometimes instrumental in making the decision, based on previous experience, good or bad, with surgery or radiation therapy.

Approximately one half of the patients seen in our clinic whose lesions are technically suitable for treatment by a

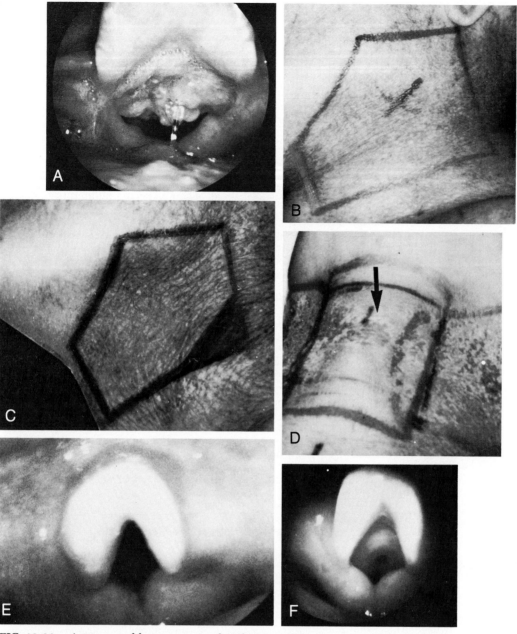

FIG. 19-24. A 64-year-old man presented with a 6-month history of dysphagia, hoarseness, and cough productive of mucus that was sometimes mixed with blood. His past history included coronary artery disease, hypertension, pulmonary emphysema, and adenocarcinoma of the prostate. (For color photographs see Plate 5A, B in Chapter 3.) (A) Exophytic, bulky squamous cell carcinoma of the infrahyoid epiglottis with minimal involvement of the false cords and aryepiglottic folds (T2N0). The anterior commissure and true vocal cords were free of disease. Irradiation was recommended since the patient was medically unsuitable for supraglottic laryngectomy and was a borderline risk for total laryngectomy. He received 7000 rad/7 weeks, cobalt-60. (B) Treatment plan was with parallel opposed lateral portals, cobalt-60, 4500 rad/5 weeks. (C) Parallel opposed reduced lateral portals, cobalt-60, 2000 rad/2 weeks. (D) Anteroposterior portal, cobalt-60, 500 rad/3 fractions. The lower neck was not treated. Note small area of skin change (*arrow*) in the anterior skin, even though an attempt was made to spare this strip of tissue. (E) Appearance 6 months after radiation therapy. The patient had a 2-week history of sore throat, hoarseness, and dysphagia. On indirect examination, there was 2+ lymphedema of the epiglottis and arytenoids but the vocal cords appeared normal. There was studding of the mucous membrane consistent with candidiasis. The edema gradually resolved over the next 6 months. (F) At 2 years there was persistent 1+ lymphedema but the airway was adequate. There was no evidence of disease at 5 years and minimal edema.

supraglottic laryngectomy are not suitable for medical reasons (e.g., inadequate pulmonary status or other major medical problems), and these patients are managed by radiation therapy (Fig. 19-24).

Analysis of local control by anatomical subsite within the supraglottic larynx shows no obvious differences in local control by radiation therapy when comparing similar stages. (See Table 19-17 in section on results of treatment.) Similarly, analysis of local control by anatomical subsite shows no obvious difference in local control by supraglottic laryngectomy when comparing similar stages. Transglottic lesions are not suitable for supraglottic laryngectomy, but they may be managed by radiation therapy in favorable cases (Fig. 19-25). Invasion of the preepiglottic space is not a contraindication to supraglottic laryngectomy or radiation therapy. The large, bulky infiltrative lesions are often selected for supraglottic laryngectomy.

The status of the neck often determines the selection of treatment of the primary lesion. Patients with clinically negative neck nodes and a high risk for occult bilateral neck disease may be treated by radiation therapy because of the ease of bilateral elective neck irradiation (e.g., poorly differentiated carcinoma of the suprahoid epiglottis with midline base of tongue involvement). Alternatively, supraglottic laryngectomy and bilateral conservation neck dissections may be done.

When a patient presents with an early-stage primary lesion but advanced neck disease (N2B or N3), combined treatment is frequently necessary to produce a high rate of control of the neck disease. In these cases the primary lesion is usually treated for cure by irradiation, with surgery added to the involved neck(s) (Fig. 19-26). If the patient has early, resectable neck disease (N1 or N2A) and surgery is elected for the primary site, postoperative irradiation is only added because of unexpected findings (e.g., positive margin or multiple positive nodes). We prefer to avoid routine high-dose preoperative or postoperative irradiation in conjunction with a supraglottic laryngectomy because the lymphedema of the remaining larynx may be considerable, although it will eventually subside.

ADVANCED SUPRAGLOTTIC LESIONS

The surgical alternative for these lesions is total laryngectomy. Selected advanced lesions, especially those that are mainly exophytic, may be treated by irradiation, since

FIG. 19-25. (*A*) Squamous cell carcinoma of the epiglottis (*arrow*) with extension to the left false cord. The right vocal cord appeared to be involved, but the biopsy result was negative. There was a 3-mm subglottic extension at the anterior commissure on direct laryngoscopy. The vocal cords were mobile (T2N0). Treatment was 6300 rad/28 fractions (5 weeks), cobalt-60. The lymph nodes were *not* electively irradiated. (*P*, petiole of epiglottis) (*B*) Appearance of larynx at 8 months. A 2.5-cm subdigastric lymph node appeared at 18 months. Radical neck dissection disclosed one lymph node that contained poorly differentiated carcinoma with extracapsular extension. Irradiation was added to the left upper neck (10-MeV electrons, 6000 rad/5 weeks). Patient was free of disease 37 months following irradiation of the larynx and 16 months after radical neck dissection.

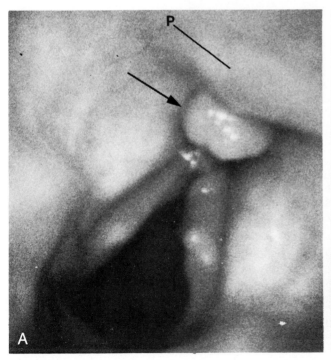
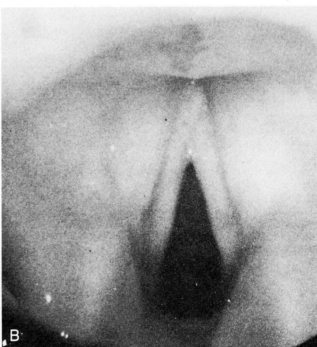

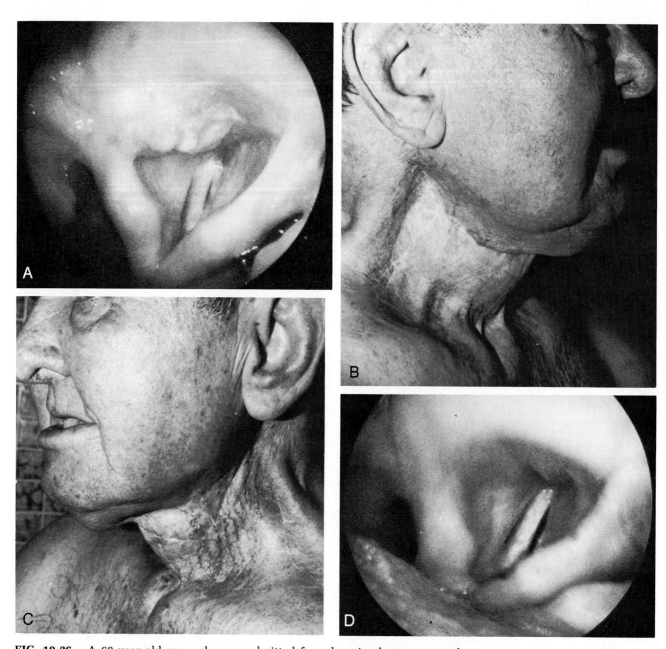

FIG. 19-26. A 68-year-old man who was admitted for a lens implant was noted to have a mass in the left upper neck. Examination revealed a squamous cell carcinoma of the infrahyoid epiglottis with multiple bilateral neck nodes (T2N3B). The largest lymph node on the left was 5 × 3 cm and the largest lymph node on the right was 3 × 2 cm. All of the lymph nodes were mobile. (For color photographs, see Plate 5C, D in Chapter 3.) (A) Lesion of the infrahyoid epiglottis with minimal extension to the aryepiglottic fold and pharyngoepiglottic fold. It was elected to treat the primary lesion with radiation therapy because of the desirability of combining radiation therapy and neck dissection for management of the neck. High-energy x-rays (17 MV) were selected in view of the planned bilateral neck dissection. The radiation treatment plan included 7000 rad/7 weeks, 17-MV x-rays, to the primary lesion and upper neck. The lower neck received 5000 rad/5 weeks, 8-MV x-rays. The posterior upper neck received 1000 rad, 10-MeV electrons. Staged neck dissection followed at 1 month and 2 months after radiation therapy. (B) Appearance of right side of neck after radical neck dissection; no tumor was found in 16 lymph nodes. (C) Appearance of left side of neck after radical neck dissection; no tumor was found in 44 lymph nodes. There were no postoperative wound complications. Moderate facial and submental lymphedema slowly subsided over the next 3 months. (D) At 20 months there was essentially no edema. The patient was free of disease at 24 months.

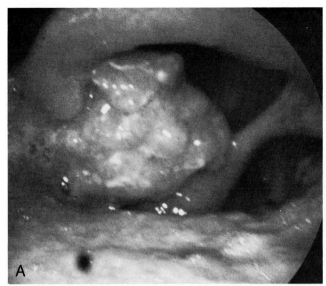

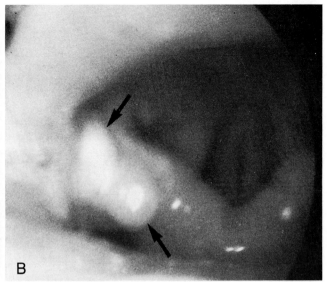

FIG. 19-27. A 74-year-old professor presented with a 3-month history of a loss of voice volume when lecturing and mild hoarseness. He was beginning to have difficulty swallowing certain foods. (*A*) Exophytic lesion of the left aryepiglottic fold with extension along the medial wall of the pyriform sinus to the apex. Mobility was normal. Biopsy revealed squamous cell carcinoma. The result of biopsy of the apex of the pyriform sinus was positive (T3N1). The treatment plan was 7000 rad/8½ weeks, cobalt-60, to the primary lesion and upper neck. The low neck received 4050 rad/3 weeks. (*B*) A small nodule persisted on the left aryepiglottic fold near the junction with the epiglottis (*arrows*). At 2 months it began to enlarge. Total laryngectomy was advised. (*C*) The patient was living, free of disease, at 4 years. He returned to lecturing using an electronic larynx with a microphone and an amplifier.

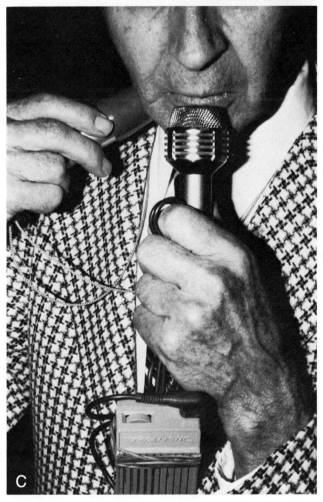

the control rate is fairly high, and total laryngectomy is reserved for failure (Fig. 19-27). (See section on results of treatment.) Borderline lesions are given a trial of irradiation to 4500 rad to 5000 rad, and if the response is good, irradiation is continued for cure (Fig. 19-28). If the response is unsatisfactory, irradiation is stopped and total laryngectomy is done 4 to 6 weeks later. There is no proof that one may select patients by this therapeutic trial, but many of the T3–T4 successes were culled out in this fashion.

Lesions unsuitable for irradiation are managed by total laryngectomy. If the neck disease is resectable, then operation is the initial treatment, and postoperative irradiation is added if needed. If the neck disease is unresectable, preoperative irradiation is used. (See section on management of the neck in Chapter 4.)

SURGICAL TREATMENT

SUPRAGLOTTIC LARYNGECTOMY

Supraglottic laryngectomy is a voice-sparing operation that can be used successfully for selected lesions involving the epiglottis, a single arytenoid, the aryepiglottic fold, and the false vocal cord. Extension of the tumor to the true vocal cord, the anterior commissure, or both arytenoids; fixation of the vocal cord; or thyroid or cricoid cartilage invasion excludes supraglottic laryngectomy. The supra-

glottic laryngectomy may be extended to include the base of the tongue as long as one lingual artery is preserved. In order to extend the procedure for involvement of the base of the tongue, the tongue extension must be lateralized to one side and should not extend beyond the circumvallate papillae. A neck dissection on one or both sides may be added as part of the supraglottic laryngectomy; 30% to 35%

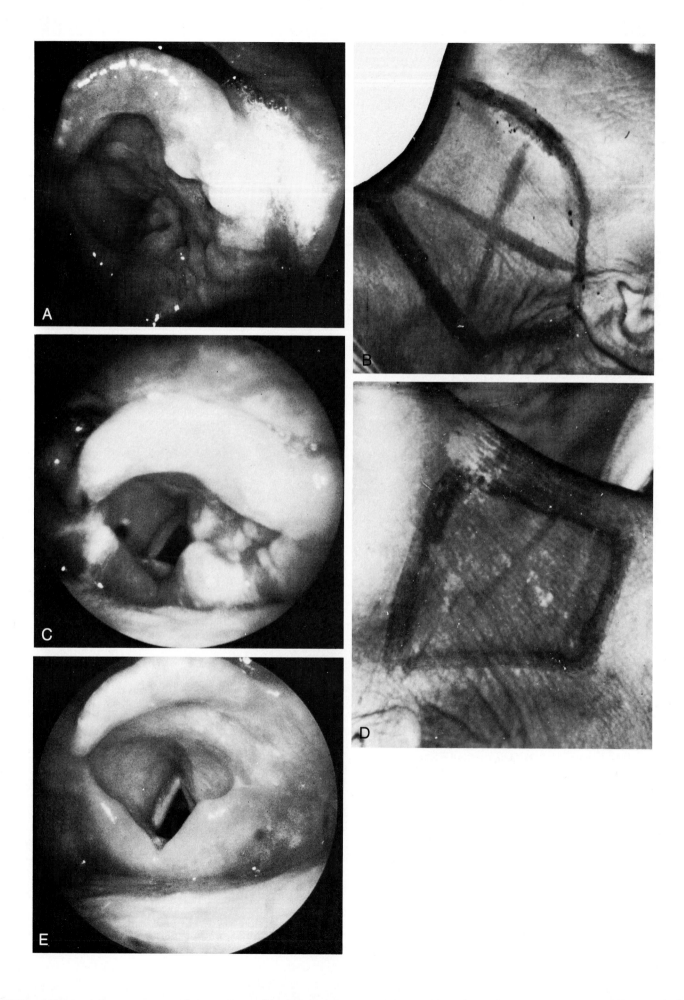

◄ **FIG. 19-28.** (*A*) Squamous cell carcinoma of the right aryepiglottic fold with extension to the false cord, pharyngoepiglottic fold, and vallecula and across the midline of the epiglottis (T3N0) in a 52-year-old woman. The surgical alternative was total laryngectomy. The treatment plan was 5000 rad and reevaluation. (*B*) External-beam portal (cobalt-60, 4600 rad/4 weeks, 120 rad twice a day). The lower border was located at the bottom of the cricoid cartilage. A small strip of skin was spared in the submental area. (*C*) There was an estimated 65% regression at 4500 rad, and it was recommended that full-dose radiation therapy be completed. (*D*) Reduced external-beam right lateral portal. The final dose was 7680 rad tumor dose (120 rad twice a day). (*E*) The patient was free of disease at 3 years, 8 months. (For color photograph see Plate 6A–C in Chapter 3.)

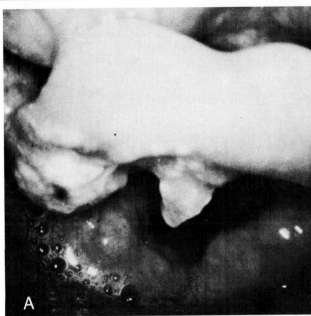

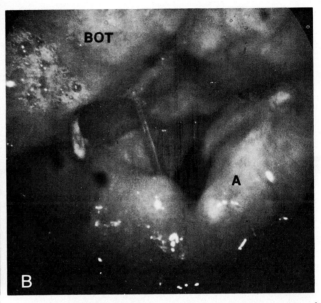

FIG. 19-29. (*A*) Squamous cell carcinoma of the infrahyoid epiglottis (T2N0). A trial of radiation therapy was recommended, but there was minimal regression after 4000 rad/4 weeks. Radiation therapy was discontinued and supraglottic laryngectomy was performed 1 month later. (*B*) Appearance 3 months following supraglottic laryngectomy. There was 2+ lymphedema, but the voice was normal and the patient swallowed without aspiration. He was free of disease at 3 years. (*BOT*, base of the tongue; *A*, right arytenoid)

of patients will have histologically positive nodes even when the neck is clinically negative. For small midline infrahyoid epiglottis lesions, which may spread to either side, neck dissection is usually reserved for the appearance of nodes, since the risk of subclinical disease is less for this site (11%) compared with the rest of the supraglottic larynx.[34]

All patients have difficulty swallowing with a tendency to aspirate in the immediate postoperative period, but almost all learn to swallow again in a short time; motivation and the amount of tissue removed are key factors in learning to swallow again. It is essential that adequate pulmonary reserve be present preoperatively, as evaluated by blood gas determinations, pulmonary function tests, chest roentgenography, and a work test (walking the patient up two flights of stairs to determine tolerance to pulmonary stress). The voice quality is generally normal following supraglottic laryngectomy.

Some centers use preoperative or postoperative irradiation as an adjunct to supraglottic laryngectomy. Routine use of preoperative irradiation is not indicated in carefully selected cases, since the cure with surgery alone is quite high, and radiation therapy increases the surgical complications and promotes lymphedema without substantially affecting the cure rate (Fig. 19-29). Postoperative radiation therapy may be advised for close or positive margins or when the risk of neck failure is substantial.

The structures removed include the entire epiglottis, both false vocal cords, the aryepiglottic folds, the preepiglottic space, a portion or all of the hyoid bone and thyroid cartilage, and, in some instances, one arytenoid. The neck incision is usually a modified Schobinger of half-H incision. If the likelihood of a total laryngectomy is high, then an apron flap is used. The neck dissection is completed and left attached to the thyrohyoid membrane. The supraglottic laryngectomy is outlined in Figure 19-30. The perichondrium of the larynx is elevated in continuity with the strap muscles and preserved in order to help close the surgical defect. Saw cuts are made through the thyroid cartilage and the hyoid bone so that the preepiglottic space is included in the specimen. Only the arytenoid(s) and true vocal cords remain after the specimen is removed. If one arytenoid must be sacrificed, the ipsilateral cord must be fixed in the midline to prevent aspiration. The defect is closed by suturing the previously saved perichondrium and muscle to the base of the tongue. Ten to 14 days later, the tracheostomy and nasogastric tubes are removed and

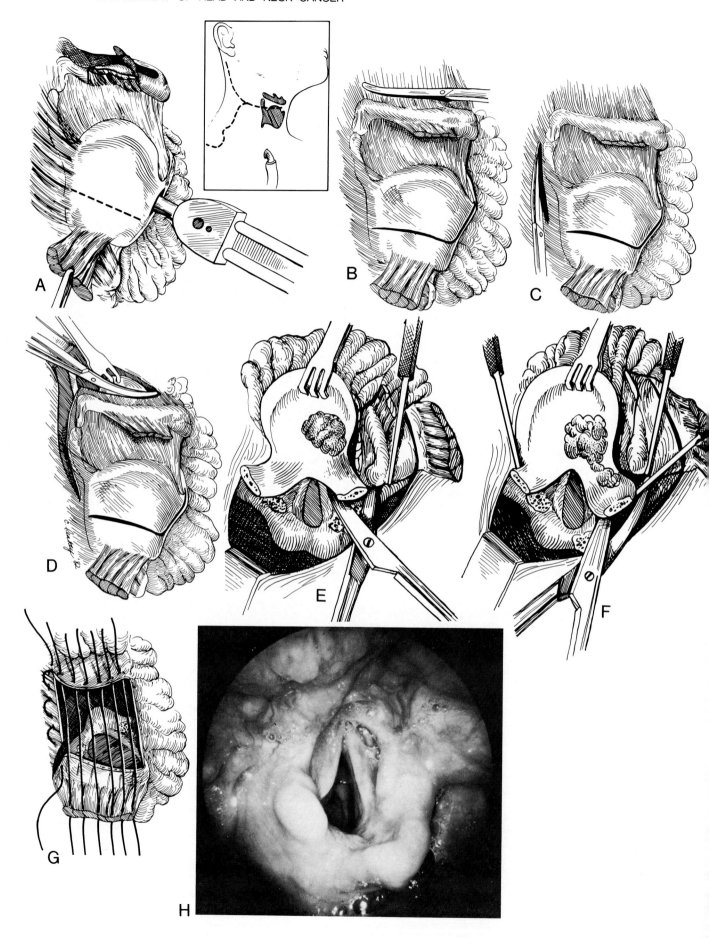

the patient is retrained in the act of swallowing. The patient is discharged when he can swallow 2000 ml or more without significant aspiration. A temporary gastrostomy may be required when the base of the tongue is resected, and it may remain as long as 3 months. Less than 5% of cases are converted to total laryngectomy at the time of operation with careful preoperative assessment.

WIDE-FIELD TOTAL LARYNGECTOMY

The entire larynx and preepiglottic space are resected en bloc and a permanent tracheostomy is fashioned. The strap muscles, the hyoid bone, and a portion of the thyroid gland are included with the specimen. The pharynx is reconstituted in most cases without a flap. Neck dissection is added as outlined in Chapter 4.

IRRADIATION TECHNIQUE

The primary lesion and both sides of the neck are included with opposed lateral portals; wedges are used to compensate for the contour of the neck. The anterior midline skin is shielded if possible. (See also section on irradiation technique in Chapter 21, Hypopharynx.) The dose for T1 lesions is 6000 rad to 6500 rad and for T2–T3 lesions, 7000 rad, occasionally 7500. (See also Chapter 13.) The early lesions that are encompassed by a small treatment volume receive 200 rad/fraction. The lesions requiring a large treatment volume receive 180 rad/fraction for the first 4500 rad to 5000 rad and either 180 or 200 rad/fraction for the remainder. The lower neck nodes are irradiated through a separate anterior portal. An anterior submental "boost" portal with photons or electrons may be used for the last 500 rad to 1000 rad for suprahyoid epiglottis lesions that invade the vallecula. (See section on base of tongue: irradiation technique in Chapter 18, Oropharynx.)

The addition of a neck dissection usually increases the risk of temporary lymphedema; however, neck dissection is preferable to the higher doses of radiation therapy required to control large neck nodes. (See section on management of the neck in Chapter 4.)

Patients develop a sore throat, loss of taste, and moderate dryness during irradiation. Edema of the arytenoids may occur and give a sensation of lump in the throat. Tracheostomy is seldom necessary even for bulky lesions; 180 rad/fraction treatment is favored for these lesions to avoid severe mucositis and edema.

Edema of the larynx may persist for several months to a year. Neck dissection increases the degree of lymphedema on the side of the operation. The lymphedema of the larynx and submental space resolves together. Patients who continue to smoke heighten the side-effects of dryness, dysphagia, and hoarseness.

COMBINED TREATMENT POLICIES

Either surgery alone or irradiation alone is recommended for management of the early primary lesions.

If total laryngectomy is required and the lesion is resectable, postoperative irradiation is preferred, since there is no evidence that preoperative irradiation produces any better local/regional control or improved survival. Radiation therapy is added for close or positive margins, invasion of soft tissues of the neck, subglottic extension, cartilage invasion, and N2B or N3 neck disease. The high-risk areas are usually the base of the tongue and the neck; the stomal area is mainly at risk when subglottic extension is present, but it usually may be shielded. Complications related to postoperative irradiation are relatively uncommon in this group if the pharyngeal wall is not resected.

Irradiation is used prior to total laryngectomy for patients with technically unresectable neck nodes and as a trial of radiation therapy prior to deciding on radiation therapy alone or total laryngectomy.

A number of patients either refuse laryngectomy or are unsuitable medically for the operation, and irradiation is the treatment by default. However, quite a few of these patients can be cured, and one should not take a hopeless attitude.[14]

MANAGEMENT OF RECURRENCE

Failures after supraglottic laryngectomy or irradiation can frequently be salvaged by further treatment, and recognition of recurrence should be vigorously pursued. Salvage of recurrence after combined total laryngectomy and radiation therapy is uncommon. Stomal recurrences are sometimes controlled by radiation therapy or surgery.

RESULTS OF TREATMENT

Vocal Cord Cancer

SURGICAL RESULTS

Neel and co-workers reported the results for 182 patients with early vocal cord carcinoma suitable for cordectomy; 177 had lesions that were confined to one cord.[33] The lesions

◀ **FIG. 19-30.** Supraglottic laryngectomy. Inset shows modified Schobinger skin incision. (A) Saw cuts on thyroid cartilage after the muscles and perichondrium have been reflected. The hyoid bone has been skeletonized. (B) Scissors cut through suprahyoid muscles to gain entrance into the pharynx by way of the vallecula for exposure of lesions of the false cord, pyriform sinus, or laryngeal surface of epiglottis. (C) Scissors cut through the pharyngeal constrictors to gain entrance into the pharynx by way of the pyriform sinus for lesions of the vallecula or lingual surface of the epiglottis. At this point the lesion can be seen, and the remainder of the incision (shown in D) is made under direct vision. (D) The incision into the pyriform sinus (in C) is extended superiorly through the suprahyoid muscles and the base of the tongue. (E) Removal of supraglottic lesion; both arytenoids are preserved. (F) Removal of supraglottic lesion including one arytenoid. (G) Closure of the defect, suturing muscle and perichondrium (inferiorly) to base of the tongue (superiorly). (H) Larynx after supraglottic laryngectomy (no irradiation). The base of the tongue extends to the anterior commissure of the glottis.

TABLE 19-2. Literature Results of Stage T4 Glottic Cancer

Author	Stage	No. Patients	Method of Treatment	Results (NED)
Jesse[24]	T4N0–N+	48	Laryngectomy	54% at 4 years
Ogura and co-workers[36]	T4N0	11	Laryngectomy	45% at 3 years
Skolnick and co-workers[46]	T4N0	7	Laryngectomy	30% at 5 years
Vermund[49]	T4N0	31	Laryngectomy	35% at 5 years
Stewart and Jackson[48]	T4N0	13	Irradiation with surgery for salvage	38% at 5 years
Harwood and co-workers[23]	T4N0	56	Irradiation with surgery for salvage	49% at 5 years*

* Actuarial survival, uncorrected for deaths due to intercurrent disease.
(NED, No evidence of disease)
(Modified with permission from Harwood AR, Beale FA, Cummings BJ, Keane TJ, Payne D, Rider WD: T4N0M0 glottic cancer: An analysis of dose-time volume factors. Int J Radiat Oncol Biol Phys 7:1507–1512, 1981. Copyright © 1981, Pergamon Press, Ltd.)

FIG. 19-31. (*A*) Invasive squamous cell carcinoma (2 mm) of the right vocal cord (T1N0). Treatment was 5625 rad/ 5 weeks, cobalt-60. (*B*) Appearance of larynx 17 months after treatment. The patient was free of disease at 5 years.

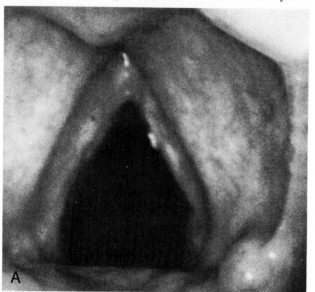

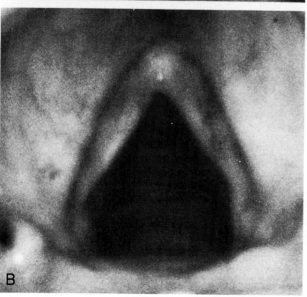

ranged from 2 mm to 25 mm in length. The follow-up was less than 3 years in 18% of cases. Four patients developed a laryngeal recurrence and 3 developed a neck recurrence. Only 3 patients (2%) died of their vocal cord cancer.

Ogura and associates reported a 3-year disease-free survival rate of 91% for 281 patients treated by hemilaryngectomy.[36] The local recurrence rate was 4% and the neck recurrence rate was 1.5%; 74% of treatment failures were salvaged.

A review of 61 patients with involvement of the anterior commissure treated by hemilaryngectomy resulted in an absolute survival of 74%.[43] There were three local recurrences (9%) and three neck recurrences (9%).

Som reported the results for hemilaryngectomy including the ipsilateral arytenoid for 130 cases of vocal cord carcinoma extending posteriorly to the vocal process and face of the arytenoid.[47] The cure rate for 104 patients with a T2 lesion was 74%, and for 26 patients with a T3 lesion it was 58%.

Bauer and co-workers analyzed the significance of the surgical margins in 111 hemilaryngectomy specimens.[2] Thirty-nine patients (35%) were found to have involved margins (usually the anterior margin). The local recurrence rate was 10% with a 5-year minimum follow-up. Seven recurrences were anterior. Only 7 (18%) of the 39 patients with an involved margin developed a recurrence, compared with 6% with uninvolved margins. Additionally, 5% had recurrence evident in the cervical lymph nodes. Four patients eventually died of cancer.

Ogura and co-workers reported that the 3-year determinate disease-free survival rate for patients treated by total laryngectomy with or without radical neck dissection was 80%.[36] The local and regional recurrence rate was 21%; approximately 46% of treatment failures were salvaged by surgery or radiation therapy, alone or combined.

The results of treatment of T4 vocal cord carcinoma from four surgical series and two irradiation series are summarized in Table 19-2.[22] The University of Florida results for total laryngectomy in T3 lesions are presented in Table 19-12 in the following section.

RADIATION THERAPY RESULTS

The appearance of a variety of lesions before and after radiation therapy is shown in Figures 19-31 through 19-34.

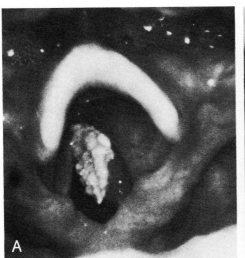
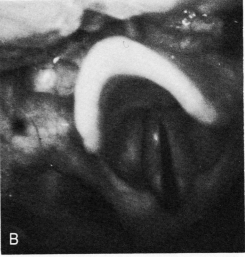

FIG. 19-32.   A 43-year-old man presented with a history of hoarseness for 1½ years prior to admission. Excisional biopsy of a right vocal cord lesion 1 year prior to admission revealed no cancer. He developed recurrent hoarseness, and rebiopsy 4 months prior to admission revealed verrucous carcinoma. Hoarseness did not improve, and lesion was growing. (A) Warty lesion of right vocal cord with extension to anterior commissure; mobility was normal. The right posterior cord was edematous and erythematous to the arytenoid. Rebiopsy revealed moderately well differentiated squamous cell carcinoma (T1N0). Treatment was 6300 rad/5½ weeks (28 fractions). (B) Appearance at 15 months. The patient was free of disease at 3 years.

FIG. 19-33.   (A) Squamous cell carcinoma of both vocal cords with 1.0-cm to 1.5-cm subglottic extension and early involvement of the right false cord. Both cords were mobile (T2N0). Treatment was 6300 rad/28 fractions (5 weeks), cobalt-60. (B) There was no evidence of disease at 3½ years. (For color photograph see Plate 2A, B in Chapter 3.)

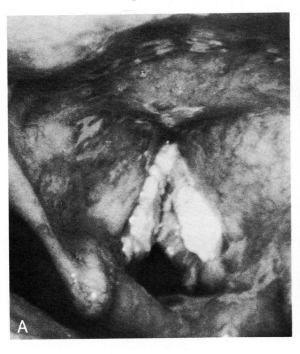
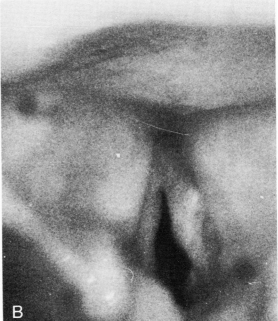

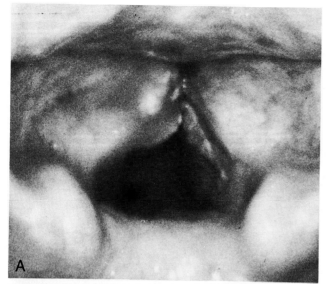

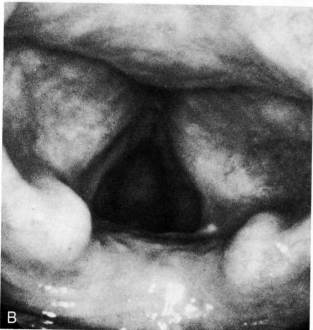

FIG. 19-34. (*A*) Squamous cell carcinoma of both vocal cords with involvement of the anterior commissure, left anterior false cord, and petiole of the epiglottis. There was reduced mobility of left vocal cord (T2N0). Treatment was 6750 rad/30 fractions (6 weeks), cobalt-60. (*B*) Appearance at 1 month after completion of therapy. The patient was free of disease at 5 years. (For color photographs see Plate 2C, D in Chapter 3.)

Harwood selectively treated 11 patients with hyperkeratosis; all were free of disease after 1 to 15 years.[20] Pêne and Fletcher reported the results for 79 patients with carcinoma in situ and 7 with dysplasia.[40] The local failure rate was 11% for lesions with a T1 anatomical distribution and 26% for lesions with a T2 anatomical distribution. Elman and co-workers reported similar results.[10]

The modern-day local control rates reported from several institutions for invasive squamous cell carcinoma are in the range of 90% for T1, 70% for T2, and 50% to 60% for T3–T4 disease. The surgical salvage rate for T1–T2 irradiation failures is 90% to 95%.

The local and regional control for 139 patients with squamous cell carcinoma of the vocal cord treated by irradiation is given in Table 19-3. One of the T1 and 4 of the T2 patients died of cancer. The five deaths were due to recurrence of vocal cord cancer in 2 patients who refused total laryngectomy, neck recurrence in 2 patients, and distant metastasis in 1 patient.

A few local failures appear after 5 years of follow-up. Some of these late failures occur on the opposite cord and undoubtedly represent new cancers. The same pattern of late recurrence is also seen after hemilaryngectomy.

Extension to the anterior commissure does not affect success with irradiation unless it is associated with bulky disease, especially in the subglottic area. Lesions confined to the posterior half of the cord have a slightly higher failure rate in the University of Florida series than lesions of a similar size in the anterior half; the reason is not known, but it is probably related to understaging.

The rate of local recurrence in relation to anatomical extent and volume of tumor is analyzed in Tables 19-4 through 19-8.[9] Within the T categories is a wide range of disease distribution and volume of tumor. The recurrence rate generally increases with a greater volume of tumor. For this reason, one cannot compare irradiation and surgical results by T stage only. Dickens and associates selected

TABLE 19-3. Local and Regional Control for Irradiation Plus Salvage for Vocal Cord Carcinoma—139 Patients

		Site of Failure		Salvage			Cause of Death		
Stage	No. Patients*	Primary Lesion	Neck	Hemilaryngectomy	Total Laryngectomy	Radiation Salvage	Larynx Cancer	Intercurrent Disease	Ultimate Control Above Clavicles
T1	90	7	0	1/3†	4/4	0	1	14	89/90 (99%)
T2	49	16‡	1	2/2	11/12	1/1§	4‡	6	46/49 (94%)

* Excluded from analysis of local control: 7 patients with stage T1 and 2 with stage T2 who died of intercurrent disease less than 2 years after treatment with primary lesion controlled at the time of death.

† Two patients with treatment failure had total laryngectomy; one died of neck node and distant metastasis, one died of intercurrent disease.

‡ Two patients refused total laryngectomy and died of larynx cancer.
§ Second failure salvaged by radiation therapy.
Note: University of Florida data; T1–T2 patients treated 10/64–12/77, analysis 3/80 by W. J. Dickens, MD.

TABLE 19-4. Local Failure Related to Involvement of One or Both Vocal Cords: Stages T1–T2 (139 patients)

Vocal Cord Involvement	Stage T1		Stage T2	
	No. Patients	Primary Recurrence	No. Patients	Primary Recurrence
One cord	74	4 (5%)	29	7 (25%)
Both cords	16	3 (19%)	20	9 (43%)
Total	90	7 (8%)	49	16 (33%)

(Dickens WJ, Cassisi NJ, Million RR, Bova FJ: Treatment of early vocal cord carcinoma: A comparison of apples and apples. Laryngoscope 93:216–219, 1983)

TABLE 19-5. Local Failure Related to Length of Vocal Cord Lesion: Stages T1–T2 (139 Patients)

Length of Lesion	One Cord Involved		Both Cords Involved	
	No. Patients	Primary Recurrence	No. Patients	Primary Recurrence
Less than 5 mm	16	0	4	2 (50%)*
5 mm–1.5 cm	51	2 (4%)	16	4 (25%)
Greater than 1.5 cm	35	9 (26%)	17	6 (35%)

* In 2 patients with extensive superficial carcinoma of both cords, the cords were stripped and there was no residual visible tumor prior to irradiation.

(Dickens WJ, Cassisi NJ, Million RR, Bova FJ: Treatment of eary vocal cord carcinoma: A comparison of apples and apples. Laryngoscope 93:216–219, 1983)

TABLE 19-6. Local Failure Related to Estimated Tumor Volume of Vocal Cord Lesion: Stages T1–T2 (139 Patients)

Tumor Volume	One Cord Involved		Both Cords Involved	
	No. Patients	Primary Recurrence	No. Patients	Primary Recurrence
Nonbulky	88	4 (5%)	33	8 (24%)
Bulky*	14	7 (50%)	4	4 (100%)

* *Bulky* refers to large exophytic and/or infiltrative lesion.

(Dickens WJ, Cassisi NJ, Million RR, Bova FJ: Treatment of early vocal cord carcinoma: A comparison of apples and apples. Laryngoscope 93:216–219, 1983).

TABLE 19-7. Local Failure Related to Subglottic Extension: Stage T2 (49 Patients)

Amount of Subglottic Extension	No. Patients	Primary Recurrence
None	27	7 (25%)
Less than 5 mm	16	6 (38%)
Greater than 5 mm	6	3 (50%)

(Dickens WJ, Cassisi NJ, Million RR, Bova FJ: Treatment of early vocal cord carcinoma: A comparison of apples and apples. Laryngoscope 93:216–219, 1983)

TABLE 19-8. Local Failure Related to Supraglottic Extension: Stage T2 (49 Patients)

Amount of Supraglottic Extension	No. Patients	Primary Recurrence
None	20	5 (25%)
Minimal extension to false cord	16	6 (38%)
Minimal extension to vocal process or arytenoid	9	3 (33%)
Moderate supraglottic extension	4	2 (50%)

(Dickens WJ, Cassisi NJ, Million RR, Bova FJ: Treatment of early vocal cord carcinoma: A comparison of apples and apples. Laryngoscope 93:216–219, 1983)

TABLE 19-9. Local Control and Voice Retention in Patients Managed by Irradiation and Surgical Salvage: 84 Patients Suitable for Hemilaryngectomy (Stages T1–T2)

Result	No. Controlled/ No. Treated	Comments
Control with irradiation alone	79/84 (94.0%)	
Surgical salvage		
Hemilaryngectomy	1/1	Alive and well over 5 years
Total laryngectomy	4/4*	Two alive and well over 8 years; two died of intercurrent disease at 3 and 8 years
Ultimate control of disease	84/84 (100%)	
Disease control with voice retained	80/84 (95.2%)	

* Hemilaryngectomy was not considered a treatment option at the University of Florida prior to 1973.
(Dickens WJ, Cassisi NJ, Million RR, Bova FJ: Treatment of early vocal cord carcinoma: A comparison of apples and apples. Laryngoscope 93:216–219, 1983)

TABLE 19-10. Local Control and Voice Retention in Patients Managed by Irradiation and Surgical Salvage: 70 Patients Suitable for Cordectomy (Stage T1)

Result	No. Controlled/ No. Treated	Comments
Control with irradiation alone	68/70 (97.1%)	
Surgical salvage		
Hemilaryngectomy	1/1	Alive and well over 5 years
Total laryngectomy	1/1	Died of intercurrent disease at 8 years
Ultimate control of disease	70/70 (100%)	
Disease control with voice retained	69/70 (98.6%)	

(Dickens WJ, Cassisi NJ, Million RR, Bova FJ: Treatment of early vocal cord carcinoma: A comparison of apples and apples. Laryngoscope 93:216–219, 1983)

84 patients (72 T1 and 12 T2) who were anatomically suitable for hemilaryngectomy.[9] The control rate by radiation therapy alone was 94%. In all 5 patients with recurrence, salvage was achieved by subsequent operations, in 4 by total laryngectomy, and in 1 by hemilaryngectomy (Table 19-9).

Dickens and associates also selected 70 patients with T1 lesions confined to one cord that would have been anatomically suitable for cordectomy.[9] The control rate by radiation therapy alone was 97.1% (Table 19-10). Salvage in 2 patients with recurrence was successful after total laryngectomy in 1 patient and hemilaryngectomy in the other.

The results for patients with T1–T2 disease who were anatomically suitable only for total laryngectomy are outlined in Table 19-11. There were three patients who were technically unsuitable for conventional hemilaryngectomy at presentation because of significant supraglottic exten-

TABLE 19-11. Local Control and Voice Retention in Patients Managed by Irradiation and Surgical Salvage: 55 Patients Not Suitable for Hemilaryngectomy (Stages T1–T2)

Result	No. Controlled/ No. Treated
Control with irradiation alone	36/55 (65.5%)
Surgical salvage	
Hemilaryngectomy	2/3* (66.7%)
Total laryngectomy	11/13† (84.6%)
Refused total laryngectomy: 2‡	
Total laryngectomy for treatment complication: 1§	
Ultimate control of disease	50/55 (90.9%)
Disease control with voice retained	38/55 (69.1%)

* Patient with recurrence after hemilaryngectomy who had total laryngectomy for salvage died of neck node and distant metastases.

† One died of neck node metastases only; one died of distant metastases only.

‡ Both died of disease; counted as uncontrolled.

§ Necrosis; no tumor found.

(Dickens WJ, Cassisi NJ, Million RR, Bova FJ: Treatment of early vocal cord carcinoma: A comparison of apples and apples. Laryngoscope 93:216–219, 1983)

TABLE 19-12. T3 Squamous Cell Carcinoma of the Vocal Cord—Survival and Control Above the Clavicles

Treatment	No. Patients	No. N+	Eligible for Control Analysis	Initial Control Above Clavicles	Salvage	Ultimate Control Above Clavicles	Survival Free of Disease			
							Absolute		Determinate	
							2-Yr	5-Yr	2-Yr	5-Yr
Irradiation	22	6	19	11/19 (58%)*	4/7	15/19 (79%)	77%	53%	89%	67%
Surgery	25	6	23	18/23 (78%)	3/5	21/23 (91%)	80%	65%	87%	87%
Surgery + irradiation	14	4	9	8/9 (89%)	0	8/9 (89%)	57%	17%	62%	29%
Irradiation + surgery	7	1	7	5/7 (71%)	0/1	5/7 (71%)	86%	66%	86%	66%

* Six failures at the primary site, one failure at the primary site and neck, and one neck failure.

Note: University of Florida data; patients treated 3/65–4/81; analysis 4/83 by W. M. Mendenhall, MD.

sion; however, they were thought to be suitable for hemilaryngectomy at the time of recurrence, since the recurrent disease was estimated to be confined to the vocal cord.

The survival and control rates of patients with fixed cord lesions (T3) treated at the University of Florida are presented in Table 19-12. Eleven patients in the radiation treatment group had preservation of their larynx. Two additional patients retained their larynx but died of other causes prior to 2 years of follow-up. The vocal quality varied from fair to near normal. There were two stomal recurrences in the 25 patients treated by surgery alone; in 1 patient salvage by radiation therapy was successful.

The 21 patients selected for combined treatment generally had more advanced local and regional disease.

The results of radical radiation therapy with surgery reserved for salvage for T3–T4 N0 and T1–T4 N1–N3 squamous cell carcinoma of the vocal cord treated at the Princess Margaret Hospital are detailed in Table 19-13.[20] Prior to 1970, the treatment plan was high-dose preoperative radiation therapy (5000 rad/4 to 5 weeks) followed 3 to 6 weeks later by total laryngectomy. A number of patients did not have immediate surgery and only had total laryngectomy if tumor was present. Approximately one third of patients with T3 lesions received only radiation therapy.

After 1970, nearly all patients have been treated with radical radiation therapy.[21] The patients staged T4N0 were separated into two prognostic groups: (1) invasion of cartilage, trachea, or base of the tongue and (2) pyriform sinus involvement. Almost all of the patients had a fixed cord; a few had anterior horseshoe-shaped lesions with cartilage invasion and mobile cords.* The pyriform sinus group did much worse than the cartilage group: 29% with voice spared versus 54%.[22]

The actuarial uncorrected 5-year survival rates for the T3 series and the T4 series are in the same range, approximately 50%.

Supraglottic Larynx Cancer

SURGICAL RESULTS

The 3-year determinate survival for 176 patients with supraglottic carcinoma managed by supraglottic laryngectomy is shown in Table 19-14; 109 patients received preoperative radiation therapy.[37] Only 11 patients (6%) developed a local recurrence; in 5 salvage by total laryngectomy or radiation therapy proved successful. Seventeen had treatment failures in the neck and salvage was achieved in 9. For patients with advanced lesions treated with preoperative radiation therapy followed by total laryngectomy and radical neck dissection, the 3- and 5-year survival rates were 70% and 67%, respectively.

Ogura and co-workers reported 59 patients with supraglottic carcinoma with extension to one arytenoid, treated by supraglottic laryngectomy; 56 of the patients had preoperative radiation therapy.[35] Five patients developed a local recurrence and 6 developed a neck recurrence. Salvage by total laryngectomy or radiation therapy was obtained in 4 of these patients.

Bocca reported 250 cases of supraglottic carcinoma (T1 and T2) managed by supraglottic laryngectomy and bilateral elective (or therapeutic) neck dissection.[4] The local recurrence rate was 11% and the neck recurrence rate was 5%; in nine patients salvage was achieved by further therapy. The 5-year survival rate was 79.7%.

RADIATION THERAPY RESULTS

An analysis of the results of treatment of the patients at the University of Florida who were managed by radiation therapy alone is outlined in Table 19-15. There is a very

* Harwood AJ: Personal communication, 1982.

high local control rate with doses of 6000 rad to 6500 rad for T1 lesions and 7000 rad for T2–T3 lesions.[14,44] (See Figures 13-6 and 13-7 in Chapter 13.)

Analysis of treatment failures by anatomical sites suggested that the infrahyoid epiglottis lesions were more difficult to cure compared with other sites. However, this was partly due to the unexplained use of lower doses. In recent years, control of infrahyoid epiglottis lesions parallels control of other supraglottic sites.

Fletcher and Goepfert reviewed the M. D. Anderson Hospital experience for radical radiation therapy for 181 supraglottic cancer cases. The results for two time periods are compared in Table 19-16.[13] There was an increase in dose of approximately 500 rad during the 1964–1972 era. The ultimate control rate after total laryngectomy for irradiation failures is shown in Table 19-17.[12] The percentage of patients with voice preservation and the number of patients with edema requiring either permanent or temporary tracheostomy are indicated in Table 19-18.[12]

COMBINED THERAPY RESULTS

The results of surgery alone (total laryngectomy in almost all cases) and total laryngectomy plus postoperative radiation therapy for resectable stage IV cases of squamous cell carcinoma of the supraglottic larynx are compared in Tables 19-19 and 19-20.[12,18]

FOLLOW-UP POLICY

Follow-up of patients with early lesions is planned for every 4 to 6 weeks for 2 years, every 3 months for the third year, and then every 6 months for life. Photographs are helpful for noting subtle changes. Follow-up by multiple examiners should be encouraged.

The follow-up of patients with vocal cord or supraglottic larynx lesions treated by irradiation or conservative surgery is almost more important than the treatment itself, since early detection of recurrence usually results in salvage and the salvage may include cure with preservation of voice. It is common to be suspicious of recurrence and yet obtain a negative result of biopsy at direct laryngoscopy, especially when edema is present; about one third of our patients with local recurrence have negative findings on the first biopsy. Persistent symptoms and abnormal physical findings are an indication to perform another biopsy.

TABLE 19-13.	**T3–T4 N0 and T1–T4 N1–N3 Squamous Cell Carcinoma of the Vocal Cord: Radiation Therapy Series (Princess Margaret Hospital)**			
Stage	**No. Patients**	**Local Control 5 Years With Larynx**	**Surgical Salvage**	**Uncorrected Actuarial Survival* at 5 Years**
T3 N0	131	50%	66%†	55%
T4 N0	68	56%	See note‡	49%
T1–T4 N1–N3	48	30%	See note‡	38%

* Uncorrected for death due to intercurrent disease.
† 66% salvaged of those attempted; approximately 13% had no attempt at salvage.
‡ Numbers not given, but percentage of treatment failures salvaged was small.
(Data from Harwood AR: Cancer of the larynx: The Toronto experience. J Otolaryngol 11 [suppl 11]: 3–21, 1982)

TABLE 19-14. Supraglottic Larynx Carcinoma: 3-Year Determinate Survival After Supraglottic Laryngectomy (176 Patients)

Primary Stage	N0		N1–N3	
	No. Surviving/ No. at Risk	Percentage	No. Surviving/ No. at Risk	Percentage
T1	64/78	82%	8/14	58%
T2	23/34	68%	8/12	67%
T3	7/10	70%	2/3	66%
T4	9/12	75%	8/13	62%
Totals	134		42	

(Ogura JH, Sessions DG, Spector GJ: Conservative surgery for epidermoid carcinoma of the supraglottic larynx. Laryngoscope 85:1808–1815, 1975)

TABLE 19-15. Carcinoma of the Supraglottic Larynx: Local Control by T Stage— Radiation Therapy Alone

Stage	Initial Radiation Therapy (No. Controlled/ No. Treated*)	Surgical Salvage (No. Salvaged/ No. Attempted)	Ultimate Control (No. Controlled/ No. Treated)
T1	11/12	1/1	12/12 (100%)
T2	20/26	3/6	23/26 (88%)
T3	9/14	2/4	11/14 (79%)
T4	2/11	3/4	5/11 (45%)
Total	42/63 (67%)	9/15 (60%)	51/63 (81%)

* 18 patients died less than 2 years after treatment with primary site controlled and are excluded from analysis of local control.

Note: University of Florida data; patients treated 10/64–5/81; analysis 5/83 by W. M. Mendenhall, MD.

TABLE 19-16. Squamous Cell Carcinoma of the Supraglottic Larynx: Control of Primary Lesion by Irradiation

Site	1954 Through 1963				1964 Through 1972*			
	T1	T2	T3	T4	T1	T2	T3	T4
Suprahyoid epiglottis	6/6	3/4	9/13	9/15	3/4	7/7	13/15	3/5
Infrahyoid epiglottis	3/5	5/8	0/0	1/4	5/5	11/12	3/4	1/1
Aryepiglottic folds	2/2	9/11	4/7	1/1	5/5	6/7	3/4	3/6
False cords	3/3	5/6	1/1	0/0	2/2	8/10	0/0	1/1
Arytenoids	0/0	2/3	0/1	0/0	2/2	1/1	0/0	0/0
Total	14/16	24/32†	14/22†	12/20	17/18	33/37†	19/23†	8/13

Approximately 500 rad higher dose in second period.

† T2 + T3, 1954–1963: 30% failure rate; T2 + T3, 1964–1972: 13% failure rate. $\chi^2 = 4.9386$; $p < 0.05$.

Note: M. D. Anderson Hospital data; analysis 8/76.

(Modified from Fletcher GH, Goepfert H: Larynx and pyriform sinus. In Fletcher GH: Textbook of Radiotherapy, 3rd ed, pp 330–363. Philadelphia, Lea & Febiger, 1980)

TABLE 19-17. Squamous Cell Carcinoma of the Supraglottic Larynx: Percentage of Ultimate Primary Control by Irradiation and Rescue Surgery*

Site	T1	T2	T3	T4
Suprahyoid epiglottis	90% (9/10)	100% (11/11)	85% (23/27)	62% (13/21)
Infrahyoid epiglottis	80% (8/10)	90% (19/21)	75% (3/4)	60% (3/5)
Aryepiglottic folds	100% (7/7)	94% (16/17)	75% (9/12)	71% (5/7)
False cords	100% (5/5)	94% (15/16)	(1/1)	(1/1)
Arytenoids	(2/2)	(4/4)	(0/1)	(0/0)

* Ultimate control after surgery for recurrence of primary irradiation failures (≧24 months after rescue surgery).
Note: M. D. Anderson Hospital data; patients treated 1954–1972; analysis 12/76.
(Fletcher GH, Goepfert H: Irradiation in the management of squamous cell carcinomas of the larynx. In English GM [ed]: Otolaryngology, vol 5, pp 1–45. Philadelphia, Harper & Row, 1981)

TABLE 19-18. Squamous Cell Carcinoma of the Supraglottic Larynx: Preservation of Normal Laryngeal Function

Stage	No. Patients	Failures	Severe Edema*	Laryngeal Voice Preserved
T1	18	1	0	94.5% (17/18)
T2	37	4	4	78.5% (29/37)
T3	23	4	2	74.0% (17/23)
T4	13	6	1†	54.0% (7/13)

* Necessitating either permanent or temporary tracheostomy.
† Tracheostomy for severe edema at 10 months and laryngectomy for recurrence at 33 months.
Note: M. D. Anderson Hospital data; patients treated 1964–1972; analysis 12/76.
(Fletcher GH, Goepfert H: Irradiation in management of squamous cell carcinomas of the larynx [1977]. In English GM [ed]: Otolaryngology, vol 5, pp 1–45. Philadelphia, Harper & Row, 1981)

TABLE 19-19. Squamous Cell Carcinoma of the Supraglottic Larynx: Active Disease Above the Clavicles After the Initial Surgery (Total Laryngectomy) in Resectable Stage IV Lesions*

Result	Surgery Only	Surgery + Postoperative Radiation Therapy
Definite failure above clavicles (2-year minimum follow-up after rescue surgery, if needed)	24% (28/116)	13% (7/53)

* Stage IV = T4 N0–N1, T1–T4 N2–N3.
(Adapted from Goepfert H, Jesse RH, Fletcher GH, Hamberger A: Optimal treatment for the technically resectable squamous cell carcinoma of the supraglottic larynx. Laryngoscope 85:14–32, 1975)

TABLE 19-20. Squamous Cell Carcinoma of the Supraglottic Larynx: Absolute Survival Rates* in Patients with Stage IV† Disease

Absolute Survival	Surgery Only‡	Surgery + Radiation Therapy
2 years	39.1% (34/87)§	68.5% (37/54)§
5 years	24.4% (19/78)ǁ	42.1% (16/38)ǁ

* Living, free of cancer.
† Stage IV: T4 N0–N1, T1–T4 N2–N3.
‡ All patients had a total laryngectomy.
§ $p < 0.005$.
ǁ $p < 0.08$.
Note: M. D. Anderson Hospital data; patients treated 1954–1972.
(Fletcher GH, Goepfert H: Larynx and pyriform sinus. In Fletcher GH: Textbook of Radiotherapy, 3rd ed, pp 330–363. Philadelphia, Lea & Febiger, 1980)

Five patients with early carcinoma of the vocal cord treated by radiation therapy developed a fixed cord but without edema, pain, or other findings to suggest recurrence. Follow-up for several years revealed no evidence of recurrence. Mobility returned after a few weeks to months in three cases.

When there is suspicion of recurrence and the biopsy result is negative, the patients are reexamined at 2-week intervals until the matter is settled.

Wagenfeld and co-workers studied 740 cases of glottic larynx cancer treated from 1965 to 1974 to determine the incidence of second respiratory tract malignancies.[51] There was a minimum follow-up of 5 years. There were 48 second respiratory tract malignancies, whereas only 14 were expected. Twenty-five were in the lung, and 23 were scattered among other head and neck sites (Table 19-21). Only 7 of the 23 second head and neck primary lesions resulted in death; these second lesions were frequently diagnosed in an early stage during routine follow-up for the glottic lesion.

Chest roentgenograms should be requested twice a year to look for asymptomatic lung cancer; several of our patients have been saved by early diagnosis.

COMPLICATIONS OF TREATMENT

Surgical Treatment

Repeated stripping of the cord for carcinoma in situ or dysplasia may result in a thickened cord and hoarse voice. A thickened cord with hoarseness is also suggestive of submucosal invasive carcinoma.

Neel and associates reported a 26% incidence of nonfatal complications for cordectomy.[33] Immediate postoperative complications included atelactasis and pneumonia, severe subcutaneous emphysema in the neck, bleeding from the tracheotomy site or larynx, wound complications, and airway obstruction requiring tracheotomy. Late complications included removal of granulation tissue by direct laryngoscopy to exclude recurrence, extrusion of cartilage, laryngeal stenosis, and obstructing laryngeal web.

The postoperative complications and sequelae of hemilaryngectomy include chondritis, wound slough, inadequate glottic closure, and anterior commisure webs. The rate of complications is given in Table 19-22 for 254 patients treated for hemilaryngectomy and for 171 patients treated by total laryngectomy for glottic carcinoma at Washington University School of Medicine, St. Louis.[16] The complications associated with subtotal (supraglottic) laryngectomy and total laryngectomy for supraglottic carcinomas are outlined in Table 19-23.[16] The risk of a complication increased when tumor margins were involved by tumor; there was no change in risk associated with age, sex, race, laryngeal site, stage of primary tumor, size of primary tumor, use of low-dose preoperative irradiation, or status of the positive nodes.

Radiation Therapy

GLOTTIC CARCINOMA

ACUTE COMPLICATIONS

The acute reactions from the treatment of early vocal cord cancer using 225 rad/day tumor dose to a total dose of 5625 rad to 6300 rad, 5 fractions/week, cobalt-60, and portals measuring 4 × 4 cm to 4 × 5 cm are relatively mild and almost never result in a treatment interruption. During the first 2 to 3 weeks, the voice may improve owing to regression of tumor. The voice then generally becomes hoarse again owing to the radiation-induced changes, even though the tumor continues to regress.

A mild sore throat develops beginning at the end of the second week, but it rarely requires medication. Approximately 50% of patients will develop the sensation of a lump in the throat; this sensation is probably related to some mild edema of the arytenoids and postcricoid area. The patient may associate this "lump" with cancer and should be forewarned of this expected event.

The voice begins to improve approximately 3 weeks after completion of treatment, reaching a plateau 2 to 3 months after radiation therapy. After irradiation, the quality and volume of the voice may tend to peter out at the end of the day, and many patients report temporary changes in voice with change in weather and with upper respiratory tract infections.

Patients with extensive lesions often recover a normal voice, and an occasional patient with an early lesion will not recover a normal voice, even though the vocal cords may appear normal.

LATE COMPLICATIONS

Edema of the larynx is the most common sequela following irradiation for glottic or supraglottic lesions. The rate of clearance of the edema is related to the dose of radiation, volume of tissue irradiated, addition of a neck dissection, continued use of alcohol and tobacco, and size and extent of the original lesion. For instance, glottic lesions involving the posterior cord(s) require a higher dose to the arytenoids and postcricoid structures than small anterior glottic lesions, and therefore the patients treated for posterior lesions have a higher incidence of edema. Edema may be accentuated by a radical neck dissection and may require 6 to 12 months to subside.

Soft tissue necrosis leading to chondritis occurs in less than 1% of patients, usually in those who continue to smoke. Soft tissue and cartilage necroses mimic recurrence, with hoarseness, pain, and edema; a laryngectomy may be recommended in desperation for fear of recurrent cancer, even though biopsy specimens show only necrosis.

Corticosteroids such as dexamethasone (Decadron) have been used to reduce edema secondary to radiation effect after recurrence has been ruled out by biopsy. If ulceration and pain occur, administration of an antibiotic such as tetracycline may be of help.

See Chapter 14, The Effect of Radiation on Normal Tissues of the Head and Neck, for a discussion of chondronecrosis.

SUPRAGLOTTIC CARCINOMA

ACUTE COMPLICATIONS

During the course of radiation therapy at 180 rad to 200 rad/day, the patient will develop a sore throat at the end of the first 2 weeks of treatment. This will persist until 3 to 4 weeks following completion of treatment. There will be an associated dry mouth from irradiation of the salivary and parotid glands, a loss of taste, and a sensation of a lump in the throat if the entire glottic area is also included.

It is unusual for the patient to require a tracheotomy prior to irradiation unless he develops severe lymphedema at the time of direct laryngoscopy and biopsy. However, in patients who have recovered from the direct laryngoscopy and biopsy without obstruction, we have never had to do a tracheotomy during the fractionated course of radiation therapy. Significant regression of the partially obstructing tumor usually occurs within the first 2 weeks, before the edema begins, and the tracheotomy is avoided.

Examples of acute chondritis requiring discontinuation of treatment have not been seen, even though almost all the epiglottic lesions, either suprahyoid or infrahyoid, have

TABLE 19-21. Site of Second Primary Respiratory Tract Tumors Among Patients With Glottic Cancer*

Site	No. Tumors	Dead From Second Primary Lesion
Lung	25	23 (92%)
Oral cavity	5	0
Oropharynx	9	1
Hypopharynx	2	2
Nasopharynx	1	1
Antrum	1	1
Esophagus	3	2
Larynx	2	0
Total	48	30

* Three patients had third respiratory tract primary lesions (1, hypopharynx; 2, lung).

(Wagenfeld SJH, Harwood AR, Bryce DP, van Nostrand AWP, DeBoer G: Second primary respiratory tract malignancies in glottic carcinoma. Cancer 46:1883–1886, 1980)

TABLE 19-22. Complications of Primary Treatment of Glottic Cancer With and Without Preoperative Irradiation

	Total Laryngectomy		Hemilaryngectomy	
	Without Preoperative Radiation Therapy	With Preoperative Radiation Therapy	Without Preoperative Radiation Therapy	With Preoperative Radiation Therapy
Total patients	118*	53*	237†	17†
No complications	85 (72%)‡	36 (68%)	199 (84%)	13 (76.5%)
Infection	1 (0.85%)	3 (5.7%)	1 (0.4%)	0
Wound slough	4 (3.4%)	1 (1.9%)	2 (0.8%)	0
Fistula	6 (5%)	1 (1.9%)	0	0
Hemorrhage	0	2 (3.8%)	2 (0.8%)	0
Carotid artery exposure and/or blowout	1 (0.85%)	0	9 (3.8%)	1 (5.9%)
Fatal complication	5 (4.2%)	0	2 (0.8%)	0
Other	16 (13.6%)	10 (18.9%)	22 (9.3%)	3 (17.6%)

* $\chi^2 = 15.934$; $v = 10.07$; $p > 0.10$.
† $\chi^2 = 0.712$; $v = 2.62$; $p > 0.50$.
‡ Number (percent incidence).
Note: Washington University Medical Center, St. Louis, data, 1955–1972.

(Gall AM, Sessions DG, Ogura JH: Complications following surgery for cancer of the larynx and hypopharynx. Cancer 39:624–631, 1977)

TABLE 19-23. Complications of Primary Treatment of Supraglottic Cancer With and Without Preoperative Irradiation

	Total Laryngectomy		Supraglottic Laryngectomy	
	Without Preoperative Radiation Therapy	With Preoperative Radiation Therapy	Without Preoperative Radiation Therapy	With Preoperative Radiation Therapy
Total patients	37*	25*	39†	94†
No complications	25 (67.6%)‡	22 (88%)	23 (59%)	67 (71.3%)
Infection	1 (2.7%)	0	0	0
Wound slough	0	1 (4%)	1 (2.5%)	7 (7.4%)
Fistula	3 (8.1%)	0	3 (7.7%)	3 (3.2%)
Hemorrhage	0	0	1 (2.5%)	2 (2.1%)
Carotid artery exposure and/or blowout	1 (2.7%)	0	2 (5%)	0
Operative death	0	0	1 (2.5%)	2 (2.1%)
Fatal complication	0	1 (4%)	1 (2.5%)	0
Other	7 (18.9%)	1 (4%)	7 (18%)	13 (13.8%)

* $\chi^2 = 30.307$; $v = 18.99$; $p < 0.05$.

† $\chi^2 = 7.769$; $v = 5.20$; $p > 0.10$.

‡ Number (percentage incidence).

Note: Washington University Medical Center, St. Louis, data, 1955–1972.

(Gall AM, Sessions DG, Ogura JH: Complications following surgery for cancer of the larynx and hypopharynx. Cancer 39:624–631, 1977)

cartilage invasion. The radiation reaction normally subsides 3 to 4 weeks after completion of treatment, and simultaneously the sore throat disappears. The patient recovers over the next weeks or months. The dryness is rarely severe, since there is protection of some of the minor salivary glands.

LATE COMPLICATIONS

The most common sequela of radiation therapy is temporary lymphedema.

The epiglottis, both suprahyoid and infrahyoid portions, will remain thicker than normal for long periods of time, but this thickening is not often associated with difficulty in swallowing, respiratory obstruction, or aspiration. Lesions of the suprahyoid epiglottis frequently destroy the tip of the epiglottis, and this may require some time for the exposed cartilage to heal (see Plate 7 in Chapter 3).

Successful irradiation of infrahyoid epiglottic tumors is not associated with a high rate of necrosis, even though almost all of these lesions penetrate through the porous epiglottic cartilage and certainly invade it. Examination of the epiglottis after radiation therapy is sometimes difficult because of the edema, but the fiberoptic laryngoscope has made a major improvement in our ability to examine this area.

There is frequently edema of the false cords prior to treatment. It may be very difficult to estimate the presence or absence of tumor in these cases. Lesions involving the aryepiglottic folds or arytenoids frequently disappear and leave a fairly normal-appearing larynx.

Shukovsky analyzed the risk of severe complications for 114 patients with squamous cell carcinoma of the supraglottic larynx.[44] There were 5 patients who developed a necrosis and 7 patients who developed severe edema. All but one of these complications appeared with doses in excess of 7000 rad/7 weeks or with a larger treatment volume.

Combined Treatment

Most surgeons agree that preoperative irradiation is generally associated with an increased risk of an operative complication and slightly prolonged hospitalization. If the same goal can be accomplished by postoperative irradiation, the overall complication rates are lower.

REFERENCES

1. American Joint Committee on Cancer: Manual for Staging of Cancer, 2nd ed, p 38. Philadelphia, JB Lippincott, 1983
2. Bauer WC, Lesinski SG, Ogura JH: The significance of positive margins in hemilaryngectomy specimens. Laryngoscope 85:1–13, 1975
3. Biller HF, Barnhill FR Jr, Ogura JH, Perez CA: Hemilaryngectomy following radiation failure for carcinoma of the vocal cords. Laryngoscope 80:249–253, 1970
4. Bocca E: Supraglottic cancer. Laryngoscope 85:1318–1326, 1975
5. Broyles EN: The anterior commissure tendon. Ann Otol Rhinol Laryngol 52:342–345, 1943
6. Burns HP, van Nostrand AWP, Bryce DP: Verrucous carcinoma of the larynx: Management by radiotherapy and surgery. Ann Otol Rhinol Laryngol 85:538–543, 1976
7. Clemente CD: Anatomy: A Regional Atlas of the Human Body. Philadelphia, Lea & Febiger, 1975
8. Devesa SS, Silverman DT: Cancer incidence and mortality trends in the United States: 1935–1974. J Natl Cancer Inst 60:545–571, 1978
9. Dickens WJ, Cassisi NJ, Million RR, Bova FJ: Treatment of early vocal cord carcinoma: A comparison of apples and apples. Laryngoscope 93:216–219, 1983
10. Elman AJ, Goodman M, Wang CC, Pilch B, Busse J: In situ carcinoma of the vocal cords. Cancer 43:2422–2428, 1979
11. Fletcher GH: Elective irradiation of subclinical disease in cancers of the head and neck. Cancer 29:1450–1454, 1972
12. Fletcher GH, Goepfert H: Irradiation in the management of squamous cell carcinomas of the larynx (1977). In English GM (ed): Otolaryngology, vol 5, pp 1–45. Philadelphia, Harper & Row, 1981

13. Fletcher GH, Goepfert H: Larynx and pyriform sinus. In Fletcher GH (ed): Textbook of Radiotherapy, 3rd ed, pp 330–363. Philadelphia, Lea & Febiger, 1980

14. Fletcher GH, Lindberg RD, Hamberger A, Horiot J-C: Reasons for irradiation failure in squamous cell carcinoma of the larynx. Laryngoscope 85:987–1003, 1975

15. Fraumeni JF Jr: Geographic distribution of head and neck cancers in the United States. Laryngoscope 88 (suppl 8):40–44, 1978

16. Gall AM, Sessions DG, Ogura JH: Complications following surgery for cancer of the larynx and hypopharynx. Cancer 39:624–631, 1977

17. Gindhart TD, Johnston WH, Chism SE, Dedo HH: Carcinomma of the larynx in childhood. Cancer 46:1683–1687, 1980

18. Goepfert H, Jesse RH, Fletcher GH, Hamberger A: Optimal treatment for the technically resectable squamous cell carcinomma of the supraglottic larynx. Laryngoscope 85:14–32, 1975

19. Hammond EC, Garfinkel L, Seidman H, Lew EA: "Tar" and nicotine content of cigarette smoke in relation to death rate. Environ Res 12:263–274, 1976

20. Harwood AR: Cancer of the larynx: The Toronto experience. J Otolaryngol 11 (suppl 11):3–21, 1982

21. Harwood AR, Beale FA, Cummings BJ, Hawkins NV, Keane TJ, Rider WD: T3 glottic cancer: An analysis of dose time-volume factors. Int J Radiat Oncol Biol Phys 6:675–680, 1980

22. Harwood AR, Beale FA, Cummings BJ, Keane TJ, Payne D, Rider WD: T4N0M0 glottic cancer: An analysis of dose-time volume factors. Int J Radiat Oncol Biol Phys 7:1507–1512, 1981

23. Hirano M: Structure and vibratory behavior of the vocal folds. In Sawashima M, Cooper FS (eds): Dynamic Aspects of Speech Production, pp 13–27. Tokyo, University of Tokyo Press, 1977

24. Jesse RH: The evaluation of treatment of patients with extensive squamous cancer of the vocal cords. Laryngoscope 85:1424–1429, 1975

25. Kirchner JA: Staging as seen in serial sections. Laryngoscope 85:1816–1821, 1975

26. Lederman M: Place de la radiothérapie dans le traitement du cancer du larynx (The place of radiotherapy in the treatment of cancer of the larynx). Ann Radiol 4:433–454, 1961

27. Lee F, Perlmutter S, Ogura JH: Laryngeal radiation after hemilaryngectomy. Laryngoscope 90:1534–1539, 1980

28. Lindberg RD: Distribution of cervical lymph node metastases from squamous cell carcinoma of the upper respiratory and digestive tracts. Cancer 29:1446–1449, 1972

29. Mancuso AA, Hanafee WN: Computed Tomography of the Head and Neck, pp 1–65. Baltimore, Williams & Wilkins, 1982

30. Micheau C, Luboinski B, Sancho H, Cachin Y: Modes of invasion of cancer of the larynx: A statistical, histological, and radioclinical analysis of 120 cases. Cancer 38:346–360, 1976

31. Million RR, Cassisi NJ: The management of local and regional laryngeal cancer. In Carter SK, Glatstein E, Livingston RB (eds): Principles of Cancer Treatment, pp 633–643. New York, McGraw-Hill, 1982

32. Million RR, Cassisi NJ, Wittes RE: Cancer in the head and neck. In DeVita VT Jr, Hellman S, Rosenberg SA (eds): Cancer: Principles and Practice of Oncology, pp 301–395. Philadelphia, JB Lippincott, 1982

33. Neel HB III, Devine KD, Desanto LW: Laryngofissure and cordectomy for early cordal carcinoma: Outcome in 182 patients. Otolaryngol Head Neck Surg 88:79–84, 1980

34. Ogura JH, Biller HF, Wette R: Elective neck dissection for pharyngeal and laryngeal cancers: An evaluation. Ann Otol Rhinol Laryngol 80:646–651, 1971

35. Ogura JH, Sessions DG, Ciralsky RH: Supraglottic carcinoma with extension to the arytenoid. Laryngoscope 85:1327–1331, 1975

36. Ogura JH, Sessions DG, Spector GJ: Analysis of surgical therapy for epidermoid carcinoma of the laryngeal glottis. Laryngoscope 85:1522–1530, 1975

37. Ogura JH, Sessions DG, Spector GJ: Conservation surgery for epidermoid carcinoma of the supraglottic larynx. Laryngoscope 85:1808–1815, 1975

38. Olofsson J, van Nostrand AWP: Growth and spread of laryngeal and hypopharyngeal carcinoma with reflections on the effect of preoperative irradiation: 139 cases studied by whole organ serial sectioning. Acta Oto-Laryngol (Suppl) 308:1–84, 1973

39. Pearson BW, Woods RD, Hartman DE: Extended hemilaryngectomy for T3 glottic carcinoma with preservation of speech and swallowing. Laryngoscope 90:1950–1961, 1980

40. Pêne F, Fletcher GH: Results in irradiation of the in situ carcinomas of the vocal cords. Cancer 37:2586–2590, 1976

41. Pillsbury HRC, Kirchner JA: Clinical vs histopathologic staging in laryngeal cancer. Arch Otolaryngol 105:157–159, 1979

42. Sessions DG, Ogura JH, Fried MP: Carcinoma of the subglottic area. Laryngoscope 85:1417–1423, 1975

43. Sessions DG, Ogura JH, Fried MP: The anterior commissure in glottic carcinoma. Laryngoscope 85:1624–1632, 1975

44. Shukovsky LJ: Dose, time, volume, relationships in squamous cell carcinoma of the supraglottic larynx. Am J Roentgenol Radium Ther Nucl Med 108:27–29, 1970

45. Silverberg E: Cancer statistics, 1982. CA 32:15–31, 1982

46. Skolnick EM, Yee KF, Wheatley MA, Martin LO: Carcinoma of the laryngeal glottis: Therapy and results. Laryngoscope 85:1453–1466, 1975

47. Som ML: Cordal cancer with extension to vocal process. Laryngoscope 85:1298–1307, 1975

48. Stewart JH, Jackson AW: The steepness of the dose response curve both for tumor curve and normal tissue injury. Laryngoscope 85:1107–1111, 1975

49. Vermund H: Role of radiotherapy in cancer of the larynx as related to the TNM system of staging. Cancer 25:485–504, 1970

50. Vincent RG, Marchetta F: The relationship of the use of tobacco and alcohol to cancer of the oral cavity, pharynx or larynx. Am J Surg 106:501–505, 1963

51. Wagenfeld DJH, Harwood AR, Bryce DP, van Nostrand AWP, DeBoer G: Secondary primary respiratory tract malignancies in glottic carcinoma. Cancer 46:1883–1886, 1980

52. Wynder EL: The epidemiology of cancers of the upper alimentary and upper respiratory tracts. Laryngoscope 88 (suppl 8):50–51, 1978

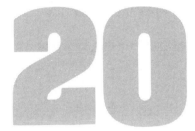

Speech Rehabilitation After Total Laryngectomy

GERALD E. MERWIN
LEWIS P. GOLDSTEIN

The diagnosis of laryngeal carcinoma need not always mean the loss of speech, owing to advances in radiation therapy and conservation surgery that preserve laryngeal tissue and function. Those patients whose disease dictates complete laryngectomy will be left voiceless, but they certainly need not be speechless. Overcoming cancer and restoring communication skills requires early interaction and team planning among the patient, family, physicians, and speech pathologists.

The purpose of alaryngeal rehabilitation is to supply the laryngectomee with a sound source, or voice, for use in speech production. There are four methods by which alaryngeal voice is produced: (1) intrinsic (buccal, pharyngeal, and esophageal); (2) prosthetic (artificial larynx); (3) surgical (tracheoesophageal fistula, "neoglottis"); and (4) surgical-prosthetic (pharyngotomy with prosthesis, tracheoesophageal fistula with valve). Each of these methods has specific applications with attendant advantages and disadvantages.

In choosing the best method for voice rehabilitation, one must consider that any given laryngectomee may be capable of using one or more methods. There is no proof to support the once widely held view that learning or using one method of speaking is detrimental to learning or using another method. At this medical center we offer an electronic artificial larynx to all laryngectomees when they have sufficiently recovered from surgery, usually within 10 days. In patients who have not had voicing procedures done at the time of primary surgery, esophageal speech training begins approximately 3 weeks following surgery. After no more than 3 months, patients are evaluated and consideration is given to potential surgical-prosthetic approaches to voice restoration. It is not unusual for patients to speak mainly with a tracheoesophageal puncture and valve, using esophageal speech for short utterances but still relying on an electronic artificial larynx when fatigued or experiencing respiratory difficulties.

Decisions regarding which method or methods are appropriate for a given patient are made jointly by the team after considerable teaching and counseling are provided for the family and patient by the speech pathologist and physician. The extent of surgery and the skills and communication needs of the patient should be considered.

INTRINSIC SPEECH DEVELOPMENT

The laryngectomee is capable of producing sound without the need for surgery and without a prosthetic device, using only the anatomy he possesses intrinsically. The three intrinsic methods are buccal, pharyngeal, and esophageal. Buccal speech consists of moving the air between the cheeks, tongue, and palate to produce sound. This results in a "Donald Duck" form of speech. Pharyngeal speech is produced by trapping air in the back of the throat. Vibration of the pharyngeal tissue produces a high-frequency, squeaky sound. Both of these methods yield poorly intelligible speech and are considered undesirable methods of communication.

Esophageal speech has been a major intrinsic form of oral communication for the laryngectomee. Production of an esophageal voice consists of using the esophagus as a pseudolung and the pharyngoesophageal segment as the vibrating source. The esophageal speaker must produce a pressure decrease across the pharyngoesophageal segment to achieve insufflation of air into the esophagus. The speaker must also develop a pressure differential across the pseudoglottis to drive it into oscillation.

One problem in developing esophageal speech is getting the air through the closed pharyngoesophageal segment and into the esophagus. The normal physiology of the pharyngoesophageal fibers prevents air from entering the esophagus. Diedrich reports two methods of air intake, based on cinefluorographic studies.[7] In the inhalation method the patient maintains an open airway either between the esophagus and the lips or between the esophagus and the nose. During inhalation of pulmonary air there is a decrease in the negative pressure into the esophagus if the pharyngoesophageal fibers are relaxed. In the injection method, oropharyngeal air is compressed by movements of the tongue into the hypopharynx. Contact between the tip of the tongue and the alveolar ridge prevents air from being expelled out of the mouth, and velopharyngeal closure prevents air from being expelled out of the nasal passages. Once again, pharyngoesophageal segment fibers must be relaxed to allow the compressed air to be pushed into the esophagus. As the esophageal speaker exhales pulmonary air, there is an increase of positive pressure within the esophagus. This change of pressure forces the air in the esophagus upward through the pharyngoesophageal segment, resulting in phonation.

Snidecor and Curry describe various characteristics of esophageal speech.[30,31] The results of evaluating the speech of six *superior* esophageal speakers reveal the following:

1. The mean fundamental frequency of male esophageal speakers was 65 Hz, approximately one full octave below that of normal male speakers.
2. Pitch variability was comparable to that produced in normal speech.
3. Superior esophageal speakers averaged between 85 and 129 words per minute.
4. Superior esophageal speakers averaged 5 words per air charge, while normal speakers average 12.5 words per breath.

Although esophageal speech is widely attempted, only a limited percentage of laryngectomees achieve a level of acceptable speech. There are many reasons why the laryngectomee may not acquire functional esophageal speech, and Diedrich and Youngstrom list some conditions that may contribute to this failure:[8]

Physical Conditions

Cicatrix
Recurring fistulas
Innervation disorder
Postirradiation fibrosis
Stenosis of the esophagus
Recurrence of the carcinoma
Strictures of the hypopharyngeal space
Extensive surgery, especially excision of the pharynx, base of the tongue, and floor of the mouth
Hearing loss
Edema and secretions in the hypopharynx
Pulmonary disease (e.g., tuberculosis, asthma, emphysema)
Either too much tonicity (spasm) or inadequate approximation of the pharyngoesophageal segment tissues

Psychological Considerations

Living alone
Emotional problems
Inability to accept the new voice
Inability to learn a new motor function
Lack of speech instruction
Lack of practice
Poor motivation

Prosthetic Artificial Larynx Speech Development

Although there are many artificial larynges on the market, they all fall into two broad categories determined by their source of power. They can be either pneumatic or electronic. A pneumatic artificial larynx can be either external or internal. The electronic artificial larynx can be either intraoral or transcervical.

Historically, the first internal pneumatic artificial larynx was developed by Joseph Lieter in conjunction with the first successful laryngectomy. Theodor Billroth in 1873 removed the larynx, but left a passage between the windpipe and the pharynx.[13] The prosthesis was inserted between the trachea and the pharynx and comprised three cannulae: laryngeal, tracheal, and phonatory, the last with a metal reed. The upper end of the laryngeal cannula had a lid held on by a spring acting as an epiglottis. Numerous modifications were made until the early 1900s, when surgeons no longer routinely left a passageway between the pharynx and trachea. This led to the use of externally applied prostheses. The Tokyo external pneumatic prostheses consist of a steel, plastic, or soft rubber cuff that fits over the stoma; pulmonary air is then directed through a chamber, which contains a vibrating source, either a rubber membrane or a reed (Fig. 20-1).[4] The device terminates with a plastic or rubber mouth tube that delivers the sound directly into the oral cavity. The pitch, tone, and loudness can be altered by adjusting the vibratory source and by varying the breathing pressure.

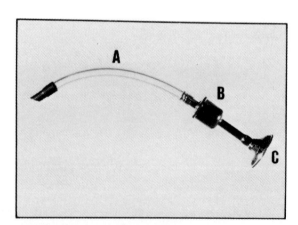

FIG. 20-1. Tokyo artificial larynx. (*A*, mouth tube; *B*, vibrator chamber; *C*, stoma cover) (Blom ED: The artificial larynx: Past and present. In Salmon SJ, Goldstein LP [eds]: The Artificial Larynx Handbook, pp 57–86. New York, by permission of Grune & Stratton, 1978)

The electronic artificial larynx was developed following the introduction of the transistor. The intraoral device consists of a battery-powered tone generator that places the sound directly into the oral cavity through an air-filled tube (Fig. 20-2).[4] Modifications have attempted to conceal the device within a pipe or to place it within a dental appliance. A transcervical device consists of a battery-powered vibrating head that, when coupled with neck tissue, transfers the sound into the pharynx and then oral cavity for articulation (Fig. 20-3).[4] Devices vary primarily in the manner used to produce sound.

The quality of sound, ease of use, and other physical characteristics vary greatly from device to device. The electronic hand-held artificial larynx requires inclusion in the speech circuitry of the arm, hand, and thumb in properly positioning the device and coordinating voicing (pressing the "on" button) and articulation. The person's ability to use a device, the extent of surgery, and the amount of training, as well as many other variables, will make the output of the same device different from patient to patient. These factors determine which device, if any, will be best suited to the individual patient. There have been numerous studies pertaining to listeners' judgments of artificial larynx speech as compared with other forms of speech. In all studies that compared normal speech with alaryngeal speech, normal laryngeal speech was always found to be easily differentiated and superior (Table 20-1). In comparing these and other studies, it is evident that no matter which parameter is being judged (intelligibility, preference, acceptability, or proficiency), the results are conflicting and more dependent on the speaking ability of the alaryngeal speaker than on the sound source.

In an attempt to determine which variables are important for good artificial larynx speech production, Goldstein and Rothman compared and analyzed the speech of five poor artificial larynx speakers and five good artificial larynx speakers.[11] Rate of speaking, intensity range, and frequency range were the three factors that differentiated significantly between the two groups. The good speakers spoke at a faster rate and achieved a wider range of intensity and frequency changes while speaking.

Salmon and Goldstein, in discussing the artificial larynx, make the following general points:[10,23]

1. Artificial larynx devices should be introduced early in the laryngectomee's speech rehabilitation program.
2. Artificial larynx devices should be selected for individual use based on the patient's needs, skills, preferences, and limitations.
3. Artificial larynx speech should be used initially and continued in conjunction with esophageal speech training.
4. Artificial larynx speech is acceptable, and the laryngectomee has the right to choose how he will incorporate its use with other forms of alaryngeal communication.
5. Artificial larynx speech is intelligible if properly taught and used.

Surgical Speech Development

Restoration of voice in the laryngectomee by surgically creating a fistula from the pulmonary power source by way of the trachea to a potential vibratory source, the pharyngoesophageal segment, dates back to the first lar-

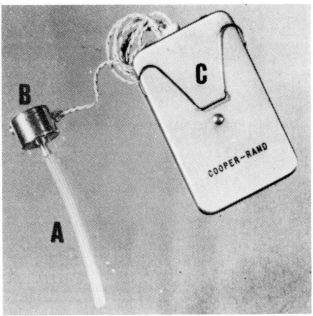

FIG. 20-2. Cooper-Rand electronic larynx. (*A*, mouth tube; *B*, hand-held tone generator; *C*, pulse generator and battery case) (Blom ED: The artificial larynx: Past and present. In Salmon S, Goldstein L [eds]: The Artificial Larynx Handbook, pp 57–86. New York, by permission of Grune & Stratton, 1978)

FIG. 20-3. Servox electronic larynx. (*A*, vibrator mechanism; *B*, pitch control; *C*, volume control; *D*, on-off switch; *E*, battery charger) (Blom ED: The artificial larynx: Past and present. In Salmon SJ, Goldstein LP [eds]: The Artificial Larynx Handbook, pp 57–86. New York, by permission of Grune & Stratton, 1978)

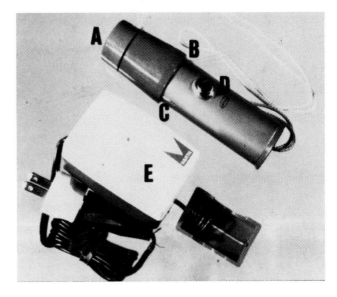

TABLE 20-1.   Listener Judgments of Alaryngeal Speech

Study	Subjects	Listeners	Stimuli	Parameters	Results
Hyman[14]	8 normal 8 esophageal 8 artificial larynx	120 students	(A) Standard passage (B) Words	Preference Intelligibility	Artificial larynx preferred
McCroskey and Mulligan[18]	5 esophageal 5 artificial larynx	10 professional 10 students 10 naive	Words	Intelligibility	Esophageal more intelligible by professional; artificial larynx more intelligible by naive
Bennett and Weinberg[3]	9 normal 5 esophageal 4 artificial larynx	37 naive	Standard passage	Acceptability	Tokyo artificial larynx most acceptable; esophageal more acceptable than other devices
Goldstein[9]	15 esophageal 15 artificial larynx	6 professional	Sentences	Proficiency	Equal proficiency

(Adapted from Goldstein LP: Listener judgments of artificial larynx speech. In Salmon SJ, Goldstein LP: The Artificial Larynx Handbook, pp 27–33. New York, by permission of Grune & Stratton, 1978)

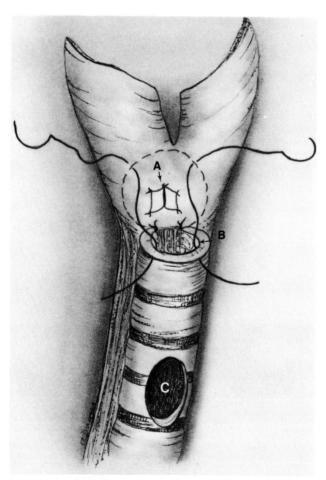

FIG. 20-4.   Staffieri surgical technique. Anterior hypopharyngeal wall with slit (A) is to be sewn over end of trachea (B). A tracheostomy (C) is created lower in the trachea.

yngectomy.[13] Throughout the history of surgical restoration of voice, the advantages of lung-powered speech have come at the cost of aspiration. In most early attempts, a passageway was created from the pharynx to the trachea. Various techniques and tissues have been used for this passageway, including anterior esophageal mucosa, vein, skin tube, and tracheal tube and side-to-side anastomosis.[1,2,5,6,16,19] While unacceptable aspiration has been the primary problem, recurrent stenosis of the tract has also occurred. If this type of fistula fails, the patient must undergo corrective surgery. Due to these problems, techniques of this type have not enjoyed continued use.

Tracheohypopharyngeal fistula voice with control of aspiration has been reported by Staffieri.[32] This surgical technique is employed at the time of primary surgery and requires a high tracheal resection at a point from the cricoid cartilage to the second tracheal ring. In some sense, this may represent less than a wide-field laryngectomy, and one must not consider this adequate for laryngeal tumors with subglottic or pharyngeal involvement. Breathing occurs through a tracheostomy created lower in the trachea. A 0.5-cm slit is created in the anterior esophageal mucosa; this mucosa is brought through the hypopharyngeal musculature and is then sutured over the open, truncated end of the trachea lying in the hypopharynx (Fig. 20-4). This slit is intended to allow tracheoesophageal airflow, yet prevent aspiration. The tracheostomy must, of course, be occluded, usually by a thumb or finger, in order to shunt airflow from the trachea through the fistula. Success, defined as good speech without clinically significant aspiration or swallowing difficulty, is reported in the range of 60% to 70% by those experienced in the technique.[28,32] Revision by endoscopic surgery for stenosis or leakage through the esophageal slit is required with some frequency. Preoperative radiation therapy, while not a contraindication, does impose restrictions. Staffieri recommends waiting 6 to 12 months after radiation therapy before beginning phonatory neoglottis surgery.[33] Griffiths suggests that a string be left through the esophageal slit during postoperative radiation therapy for dilatation of the slit and notes that spontaneous complete closure of the slit–fistula has occurred with radiation therapy.[12]

Some gratifying success has been achieved using this technique, with pulmonary-powered speech and successful protection of the lower airway, without the use of a prosthetic device. The limitations of the extent of tumors that can be safely resected while leaving sufficient tissue for creation of the fistula, coupled with restrictions regarding radiation therapy, limit the number of cancer patients for whom this technique may be useful. In addition, one must consider that secondary surgery occurs with some regularity in those with success; failure, which occurs in 30% to 40%, requires major surgery to close the fistula. With this technique, the patient must still occupy one of his hands in occluding the stoma in order to speak. It is too soon to determine the role that "neoglottis" procedures will play in the restoration of verbal communication, but at present they have limited application.

SURGICAL-PROSTHETIC SPEECH DEVELOPMENT

Surgical-prosthetic approaches have been designed to produce speech using a pulmonary air power source; either an external or internal prosthesis has been employed to connect the air source to the vocal tract. Three methods using an external prosthesis have been used but have had limited application. Two methods using internal prostheses have been introduced and would appear to offer simple and efficient options. The surgeon must attend to reconstructive techniques at the time of the laryngectomy to provide future options for voice restoration.

External Prosthesis

Taub and Bergner overcame the problem of aspiration by moving the pharyngeal fistula away from the trachea and interposing an air bypass valve.[34] A cervical esophagostomy is created in the lower lateral third of the neck. An external valved device connects the tracheostoma to the fistula. In addition to preventing aspiration, the air bypass valve responds differentially to pulmonary airflow pressure, allowing normal respiration (7 cm to 15 cm H_2O pressure) while shunting air for speech (22 cm to 40 cm H_2O pressure) to the vibrating pharyngoesophageal segment by way of its connection to the esophagostomy (Fig. 20-5). This then allows for alaryngeal speech without involvement of either hand. The low placement of the fistula is cosmetically appealing but puts the major vessels of the neck at risk. This technique is not widely used due to the incidence of carotid rupture and the problems of an external valve.

A surgical-prosthetic approach using a high-neck pharyngeal fistula, away from the great vessels, has been used successfully in patients who have been heavily irradiated or have required a control fistula.[17,29] The lightweight prosthesis connecting the tracheostoma and pharyngeal fistula contains an adjustable, pressure-regulated "flapper" valve allowing quiet breathing, coughing, and shunting of air to the pharynx for speech (Fig. 20-6). The vibratory source may be the fistula tract or pharyngeal tissues near the base of the tongue. A "duck bill" type of one-way valve permits low-pressure airflow while preventing salivary flow. The resulting functional speech in 65% of patients was reported as "well understood" and more closely approached the

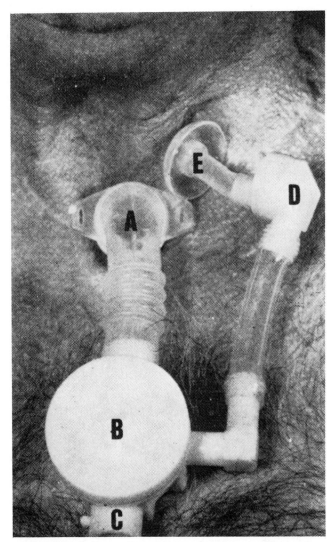

FIG. 20-5. LaBarge VoiceBak prosthesis. (*A*, tracheal interconnector; *B*, air bypass valve; *C*, adjustable breathing port; *D*, one-way fistula valve; *E*, flanged fistula tube) (Blom ED: The artificial larynx: Past and present. In Salmon SJ, Goldstein LP [eds]: The Artificial Larynx Handbook, pp 57–86. New York, by permission of Grune & Stratton, 1978)

acoustic characteristics of normal speech when compared with esophageal speech.[17] Unfortunately, problems relating to care and maintenance of the fistula and poor acceptance on a cosmetic basis have led to only limited application of this technique.

A third external prosthesis used with a high pharyngeal fistula employs a reed as a vibratory source for patients who lack an intrinsic vibrating segment (Fig. 20-7).[24,35] This technique is undesirable because it is attended by a fistula and a bulky external device; it is used in only a small percentage of patients, particularly those who have had complete laryngopharyngectomy with a control fistula.

Internal Prosthesis

Singer and Blom introduced a surgical-prosthetic approach to alaryngeal communication that combines a low-mor-

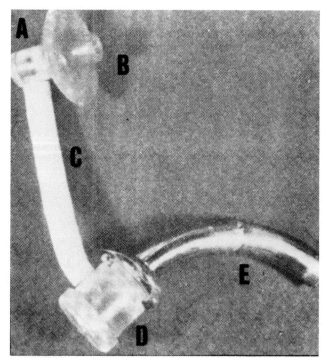

FIG. 20-6. Northwestern voice prosthesis. (*A,* one-way saliva valve; *B,* fistula fitting; *C,* conduit; *D,* pressure-sensitive respiratory valve; *E,* tracheal connector) (Sisson GA, McConnel FMS, Logemann JA, Yeh S: Voice rehabilitation after laryngectomy: Results with the use of a hypopharyngeal prosthesis. Arch Otolaryngol 101:178–181, 1975. Copyright © 1975, American Medical Association)

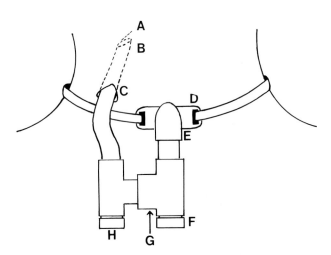

FIG. 20-7. Reed-fistula speech appliance. (*A,* inner valve; *B,* fistula tube in pharynx; *C,* fistula opening; *D,* tracheostomy tube; *E,* tracheal connector; *F,* inspiratory valve; *G,* reed housing; *H,* saliva trap) (Redrawn from Shedd D, Bakamjian V, Sako K, Mann M, Barba S, Schaaf N: Reed-fistula method of speech rehabilitation after laryngectomy. Am J Surg 124:510–514, 1972)

bidity endoscopic procedure with an internal "duck bill" type of valve.[25] A tracheoesophageal fistula, similar to the side-to-side fistula of Amatsu and co-workers,[1] is created by a simple puncture technique using a modified esophagoscope. Once a fistula has been created, a silicone-rubber prosthesis is placed in the fistula tract. Similar in shape to the end segment of a rubber catheter, the prosthesis has a slit in the esophageal end to allow air flow while preventing aspiration. The tracheostoma must be covered to divert air to the esophagus and pharyngoesophageal segment for voice production. Aspiration and stenosis are entirely prevented while the prosthesis is in place. The prosthesis must be cleaned regularly and replaced at intervals of 2 to 4 months. Functional speech in properly evaluated patients is achieved in 70% to 85% of laryngectomees.[15,27,36,37]

Few limitations are placed on the selection of patients for whom this technique may be used. The stoma must be no less than 1.5 cm in diameter, and the back wall of the trachea must be accessible for placement of the prosthesis 3 mm to 4 mm below the mucocutaneous junction. Hypopharyngeal constrictor muscle spasm can prevent passage of air through the pharyngoesophageal segment in some patients. This may be corrected with myotomy.[26] Speech using the Blom-Singer prosthesis closely resembles superior esophageal speech acoustically and normal speech in rate; such speech is preferred over artificial larynx speech.[20] Research continues in developing an optimum size and design for a prosthesis that will present the lowest resistance to air flow while preventing aspiration. In addition, an external valve worn over the stoma is being investigated that will function to allow normal respiration, yet differentially shunt air to the internal prosthesis for speech, thereby liberating the hands while the patient is speaking.*

A second internal valve has been developed by Panje.[21,22] A local anesthetic is administered in an outpatient setting and the fistula is placed lower in the trachea (Fig. 20-8). At this level the wall between the trachea and esophagus tends to be of relatively constant thickness. The "voice button" has a flange at each end to help maintain it in position. In most other respects, this surgical-prosthetic technique results in speech similar to that found in users of the Blom-Singer prosthesis. Satisfactory voice, without aspiration, and good patient acceptance have led to continued use of this technique and prosthesis. Stomal size must be adequate to place the prosthesis. There is less concern regarding parastomal configuration using this prosthesis, since it resides within the trachea and does not require external taping as does the Blom-Singer prosthesis. When selecting patients for use of either of these prostheses, one must ensure that they have sufficient visual and manual skill to deal with changing and cleaning the prosthesis.

Surgical Considerations

Planning for alaryngeal speech rehabilitation should be included when consideration is given to plans for treatment of the primary disease. Reconstruction of the hypopharynx must be accomplished without undue constriction or scarring to allow unrestricted swallowing and flow of tracheoesophageal air for voice production. Particular care and attention must be devoted to creating the tracheostoma.

* Blom ED: Personal communication, 1982.

The stoma should be of sufficient size to allow proper ventilation and to allow for possible future insertion of a button-type prosthesis. The tracheal stump should be properly beveled so that the cut end of the posterior tracheal wall lies in the plane of skin of the anterior neck, and the parastomal contour wall should be flat and flush with the beveled end of the trachea. This will allow the option of future placement of an internal valve and proper fitting for a stomal cover or valve.

APPROACH TO COUNSELING

For the patient and family, the diagnosis of "cancer of the voice box" engenders a multitude of fears. In addition to the fear of cancer, and all the emotions that mention of that word might elicit, there is the fear of major, life-threatening surgery, the fear of loss of speech and the ability to communicate, and the fear of becoming a social and psychological burden. These fears are real and must be dealt with by the health-care team, all of whom contribute their expertise and rehabilitation abilities.

The physician who makes the diagnosis of laryngeal cancer is often the surgeon who will perform needed surgery. His role should be that of coordinator for subsequent care. Consultation with a radiation therapist and speech pathologist must be obtained early. Planning for alaryngeal speech rehabilitation should be included when consideration is given to plans for treatment of the primary disease. The physician must provide support for the family and patient and know when to request help from those in counseling professions. Physicians take the primary role in educating about indications for and risks of the various approaches to treatment. Education about surgical approaches to alaryngeal speech rehabilitation also falls to the surgeon as well as to the speech pathologist. Following primary therapy for the disease, the physician provides continued surveillance for evidence of disease and remains alert for social, psychological, and communication problems so that early referral can be accomplished.

The objective of preparative counseling by a speech pathologist is to assure the patient that although he will be voiceless as a result of the removal of the larynx, he need not be speechless. As the speech pathologist outlines the rehabilitative program, each of the alaryngeal speech methods should be described and demonstrated. It is also beneficial to have the patient visited by an experienced alaryngeal speaker. The patient should be given reading material aimed at answering questions about this condition (available from the American Cancer Society). The patient's present speech pattern is recorded and analyzed so that the rate of speech, phrasing, and articulation can be integrated into alaryngeal speech rehabilitation.

REFERENCES

1. Amatsu M, Matsui T, Maki T, Kanagawa K: Vocal reconstruction after total laryngectomy: A new one-stage technique. Nippon Jibbiinkoka Gakkai Kaiho 80:779–785, 1977 (Japanese with English abstract)
2. Asai R: Laryngoplasty after total laryngectomy. Arch Otolaryngol 95:114–119, 1972
3. Bennett S, Weinberg B: Acceptability ratings of normal esophageal and artificial larynx speech. J Speech Hear Res 16:608–615, 1973
4. Blom ED: The artificial larynx: Past and present. In Salmon

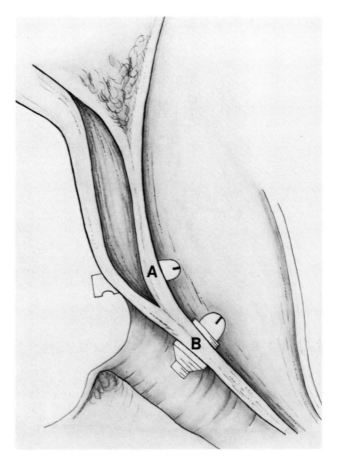

FIG. 20-8. Sagittal section showing position of Blom-Singer valve (*A*) and Panje button (*B*).

SJ, Goldstein LP (eds): The Artificial Larynx Handbook, pp 57–86. New York, Grune & Stratton, 1978
5. Calcaterra TC, Jafek BW: Tracheo-esophageal shunt for speech rehabilitation after total laryngectomy. Arch Otolaryngol 94:124–128, 1971
6. Conley JJ, DeAmesti F, Pierce MK: A new surgical technique for the vocal rehabilitation of the laryngectomized patient. Ann Otol Rhinol Laryngol 67:655–664, 1958
7. Diedrich WM: The mechanism of esophageal speech. Ann NY Acad Sci 155:303–317, 1968
8. Diedrich WM, Youngstrom KA: Alaryngeal Speech, p 130. Springfield, IL, Charles C Thomas, 1966
9. Goldstein LP: A Study of the Relationship Between Adience-Abience Scale Scores and Judgments of Verbal Communication Proficiency of a Group of Esophageal Speakers and a Group of Artificial Larynx Speakers, dissertation. University of Kansas, Lawrence, 1975 (Ann Arbor, MI: Xerox University Microfilming, Order No. 75-30,035)
10. Goldstein LP: Listener judgments of artificial larynx speech. In Salmon SJ, Goldstein LP (eds): The Artificial Larynx Handbook, pp 27–33. New York, Grune & Stratton, 1978
11. Goldstein L, Rothman H: Analysis of speech produced with an artificial larynx. Paper presented at the American Speech and Hearing Association Convention, Houston, Texas, 1976
12. Griffiths CM: Reconstruction of the glottis after total laryngectomy. Ear Nose Throat J 60:259–264, 1981
13. Gussenbauer C: Ueber die erste durch Th. Billroth am Menschen ausgeführte Kehlkopf-Exstirpation und die Anwendung eines künstlichen Kehlkopfes. Arch Klin Chir 17:343–356, 1874

14. Hyman M: An experimental study of artificial-larynx and esophageal speech. J Speech Hear Disord 20:291–299, 1955

15. Johns ME, Cantrell RW: Voice restoration of the total laryngectomy patient: The Singer-Blom technique. Otolaryngol Head Neck Surg 89:82–86, 1981

16. Komorn RM, Weycer JS, Sessions RB, Malone PE: Vocal rehabilitation with a tracheo-esophageal shunt. Arch Otolaryngol 97:303–305, 1973

17. McConnel FMS, Sisson GA, Logemann JA: Three years experience with a hypopharyngeal pseudoglottis for vocal rehabilitation after total laryngectomy. Trans Am Acad Ophthalmol Otolaryngol 84:63–67, 1977

18. McCroskey R, Mulligan M: The relative intelligibility of esophageal speech and artificial-larynx speech. J Speech Hear Disord 28:37–41, 1963

19. Miller AH: First experience with the Asai technique for vocal rehabilitation after total laryngectomy. Ann Otol Rhinol Laryngol 76:829–833, 1967

20. Merwin GE, Goldstein LP, Rothman HB: A comparison of speech using artificial larynx and tracheo-esophageal puncture with valve in the same speakers. Accepted for presentation at the meeting of the Association for Research in Otolaryngology, New Orleans, October 1982

21. Panje WR: Prosthetic vocal rehabilitation following laryngectomy. The voice button. Ann Otol Rhinol Laryngol 90:116–120, 1981

22. Panje WR, VanDemark D, McCabe BF: Voice button prosthesis rehabilitation of the laryngectomee: Additional notes. Ann Otol Rhinol Laryngol 90:503–505, 1981

23. Salmon SJ: Looking ahead. In Salmon SJ, Goldstein LP (eds): The Artificial Larynx Handbook, pp 145–147. New York, Grune & Stratton, 1978

24. Shedd D, Bakamjian V, Sako K, Mann M, Barba S, Schaaf N: Reed-fistula method of speech rehabilitation after laryngectomy. Am J Surg 124:510–514, 1972

25. Singer MI, Blom ED: An endoscopic technique for restoration of voice after laryngectomy. Ann Otol Rhinol Laryngol 89:529–533, 1980

26. Singer MI, Blom ED: Selective myotomy for voice restoration after total laryngectomy. Arch Otolaryngol 107:670–673, 1981

27. Singer MI, Blom ED, Hamaker RC: Further experience with voice restoration after total laryngectomy. Ann Otol Rhinol Laryngol 90:498–502, 1981

28. Sisson GA, Bytell DE, Becker SP, McConnel FMS, Singer MI: Total laryngectomy and reconstruction of a pseudoglottis: Problems and complications. Laryngoscope 88:639–650, 1978

29. Sisson GA, McConnel FMS, Logemann JA, Yeh S: Voice rehabilitation after laryngectomy: Results with the use of a hypopharyngeal prosthesis. Arch Otolaryngol 101:178–181, 1975

30. Snidecor JC, Curry ET: Temporal and pitch aspects of superior esophageal speech. Ann Otol Rhinol Laryngol 68:623–636, 1959

31. Snidecor JC, Curry ET: How effectively can the laryngectomee expect to speak? Norms for effective esophageal speech. Laryngoscope 70:62–67, 1960

32. Staffieri M: Laringectomia totale con ricostruzione di "glottide fonataria." Nuovo Arch Ital Otol 1:181–198, 1973

33. Staffieri M: Phonatory neoglottis surgery: Ear Nose Throat J 60:254–258, 1981

34. Taub S, Bergner LH: Air bypass voice prosthesis for vocal rehabilitation of laryngectomees. Am J Surg 125:748–756, 1973

35. Weinberg B, Shedd DP, Horii Y: Reed-fistula speech following pharyngolaryngectomy. J Speech Hear Disord 43:401–413, 1978

36. Wetmore SJ, Johns ME, Baker SR: The Singer-Blom voice restoration procedure. Arch Otolaryngol 107:674–676, 1981

37. Wood BG, Tucker HM, Rusnov MG, Levine HL: Tracheoesophageal puncture for alaryngeal voice restoration. Ann Otol Rhinol Laryngol 90:492–494, 1981

Hypopharynx: Pharyngeal Walls, Pyriform Sinus, and Postcricoid Pharynx

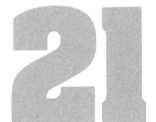

RODNEY R. MILLION

NICHOLAS J. CASSISI

The term *hypopharynx* ("low pharynx") refers arbitrarily to that portion of the pharynx from the level of the hyoid bone to the beginning of the esophagus at the plane of the lower border of the cricoid cartilage. However, the oropharyngeal and hypopharyngeal walls are continuous and will be considered together, since there is no distinct difference in the presentation, treatment, or prognosis. In this chapter, the posterior pharyngeal wall includes the oropharyngeal and hypopharyngeal walls. The great majority of hypopharyngeal lesions originate in the pyriform sinus. Postcricoid carcinomas are fortunately quite uncommon in the United States.

ANATOMY

The epithelium of the pharyngeal mucous membrane is squamous. It is continuous above with the mucous membrane of the nasopharynx; there is no visible point or line of transition. The dividing point between the nasopharynx and posterior pharyngeal wall is actually Passavant's ridge, a muscular ring that contracts to close the nasopharynx during swallowing. Beneath the mucous membrane of the posterior and lateral walls are the thin constrictor muscles. Between the constrictor muscle and the prevertebral fascia that covers the longitudinal spine muscles (longus colli and longus capitis) is a thin layer of loose areolar tissue, the retropharyngeal space. The entire thickness of the posterior pharyngeal wall from the surface of the mucous membrane to the vertebral body is no more than 1 cm in the midline. Lateral to the pharyngeal wall are the vessels, nerves, and muscles of the parapharyngeal space (see Fig. 18-2 in Chapter 18). The constrictor muscles are relatively thin, especially the superior constrictor, and do not present much of an obstacle to tumor penetration. There is a variable weak spot in the lateral pharyngeal wall just below the hyoid where the middle and inferior constrictor muscles fail to overlap. The lateral wall in this area is composed of the thin, fibrous thyrohyoid membrane, which is penetrated by the vessels, nerves, and lymphatics of the laryngopharynx (Fig. 21-1).[4]

The pharyngeal walls are continuous with the cervical esophagus below. The hypopharyngeal walls are visible by indirect mirror examination; the transition to cervical esophagus is below the arytenoids and invisible to mirror examination. The transition zone, 3 cm to 4 cm in length, is referred to as the postcricoid pharynx and will be dealt with separately, since tumors of this area present a special clinical picture.

The lateral pharyngeal wall is a narrow, ill-defined strip of mucosa. It lies behind the posterior tonsillar pillar in the oropharynx; it is partially interrupted by the pharyngoepiglottic fold, and then continues into the hypopharynx, where it becomes the lateral wall of the pyriform sinus. The lateral pharyngeal wall has a maximum width of 2 cm at any point. The superior horn of the thyroid cartilage may protrude into the lateral pharyngeal wall on one or both sides, producing a submucosal bulge.

The posterior pharyngeal wall is 4 cm to 5 cm wide and 6 cm to 7 cm in height. Submucosal bulges may be seen due to osteophytes on the anterior lips of the cervical vertebrae and may be mistaken for a submucosal tumor.

The pyriform ("pear-shaped") sinus is created by the intrusion of the larynx into the anterior aspect of the pharynx. This creates pharyngeal

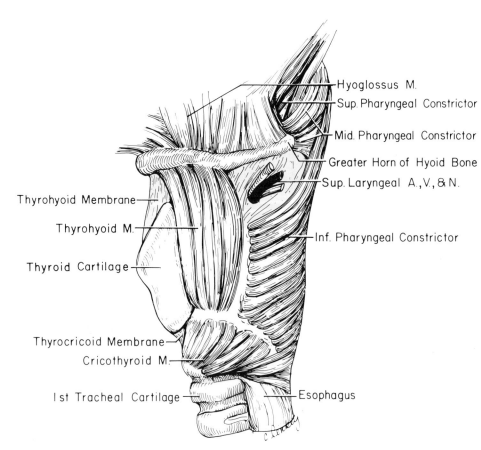

Hyoglossus M.

Sup. Pharyngeal Constrictor

Mid. Pharyngeal Constrictor

Greater Horn of Hyoid Bone

Sup. Laryngeal A., V., & N.

Thyrohyoid Membrane

Thyrohyoid M.

Thyroid Cartilage

Inf. Pharyngeal Constrictor

Thyrocricoid Membrane

Cricothyroid M.

1st Tracheal Cartilage

Esophagus

FIG. 21-1. Arrangement of the muscles and membranes that surround the hyoid bone and thyroid, cricoid, and tracheal cartilages. The lateral portion of the thyrohyoid membrane lies opposite to the upper lateral wall of the pyriform sinus. The thyrohyoid membrane presents a meager barrier to tumor spread. (Redrawn from Sabotta drawings. In Clemente CD [ed]: Anatomy: A Regional Atlas of the Human Body. Philadelphia, Lea & Febiger, 1975. Copyright © 1975, Urban & Schwarzenberg, Munich)

grooves lateral to the larynx. The superior margin of the pyriform sinus is the pharyngoepiglottic fold and the free margin of the aryepiglottic fold. The superolateral margin of the pyriform sinus is considered to be an oblique line along the lateral pharyngeal wall just opposite the aryepiglottic fold. The pyriform sinus therefore is made up of three walls, the anterior, lateral, and medial; posteriorly, the pyriform sinus is continuous with the pharyngeal cavity. The pyriform sinus tapers inferiorly to the apex and usually terminates at the level of the cricoid cartilage. The superior limit of the pyriform sinus is opposite the hyoid. The thyrohyoid membrane is lateral to the upper portion of the pyriform sinus (membranous pyriform sinus) and the thyroid cartilage is lateral to the lower portion (cartilaginous pyriform sinus). The cricoid lamina and the cricoarytenoid joint and muscles lie medial to the pyriform sinus. The internal branch of the superior laryngeal nerve lies in the anterior wall of the pyriform sinus and is said to produce a mucosal fold, but we have been unable to detect this often-described normal anatomy. The pathway for referred pain to the external auditory canal by way of the auricular branch of the vagus nerve is shown in Figure 17-12 in Chapter 17. The auricular branch is sensory to the skin of the back of the pinna and the posterior wall of the external auditory canal. Patients with referred pain from the larynx or hypopharynx will often point behind the ear and generally are vague about the location of the earache. (See the section on anatomy in Chapter 19, Larynx, for further details about the regional anatomy of the pyriform sinus.)

The postcricoid pharynx is funnel shaped to direct food into the gullet. There is no discrete superior margin, but it may be considered to begin just below the arytenoids.

The anterior wall lies behind the cricoid cartilage and is the posterior wall of the lower larynx; this wall is often referred to as the "party wall." The posterior wall is merely a continuation of the hypopharyngeal walls and is formed by the inferior constrictor muscle (see Fig. 21-1). The recurrent laryngeal nerve lies between the lateral wall and the deep surface of the thyroid gland. At the junction of the pharynx with the cervical esophagus, the muscular wall is incomplete posteriorly; this represents the site of herniation to form an esophageal diverticulum.

PATHOLOGY

Over 95% of malignant tumors are squamous cell carcinoma or one of its variants. Carcinoma *in situ* is commonly seen in surgical specimens at the edge of neoplasms of the pharyngeal wall, and multifocal skip areas of carcinoma *in situ* may make it difficult to obtain clear margins if excision is done. Minor salivary gland tumors are quite rare.

PATTERNS OF SPREAD

Posterior Pharyngeal Wall

Carcinomas of the posterior pharyngeal wall have a natural tendency to remain on the posterior wall, grow up or down the wall, and infiltrate posteriorly; they seldom spread circumferentially to the lateral walls even when quite advanced. Early lesions are red and sometimes have white patches sprinkled over the involved area. The uncommon early lesion (1 cm to 2 cm) may be exophytic. As the lesion progresses, the tumor enlarges submucosally and bulges into the pharyngeal cavity and a ragged, midline, linear ulceration appears. The posterior tonsillar pillars may become involved, with spread up the pillars eventually reaching the palate. Advanced lesions have a tendency to terminate inferiorly at the level of the arytenoids without growing into the postcricoid region. Superiorly they may extend into the nasopharynx. Direct invasion of the cervical vertebrae or base of the skull is uncommon.

Lateral Pharyngeal Wall

The lateral pharyngeal wall (including both the lateral oropharyngeal and the lateral hypopharyngeal wall) is a rather limited, ill-defined area, and only a few early lesions can be specifically designated to this site. Early tumors may be well-defined exophytic lesions. As they advance, they have a tendency to lateral penetration through the constrictor muscle and thyrohyoid membrane, thus entering the lateral pharyngeal space or the soft tissues of the neck to involve the neurovascular bundle. The direct expansion may form a mass and be palpable in the neck just below the hyoid and be confused with a lymph node.

The muscles of the pharynx originate from the base of the skull, eustachian tube, styloid process, pterygomandibular raphe, and hyoid bone, and tumor may spread along muscle and fascial planes to all muscular points of origin.[2] Tumor also courses along the glossopharyngeal and vagus nerves and the sympathetic chain. The thyroid gland is adjacent to the lower walls and is often invaded. Tumor secondarily invades the pharyngoepiglottic fold, the vallecula, and the anterior and lateral walls of the pyriform sinus.

Pyriform Sinus

Early lesions usually appear as nodular mucosal irregularities. Submucosal spread is a characteristic feature, with tumor often found more than 1 cm beyond the obvious tumor edge.

Medial wall lesions may extend superficially to involve the mucosa of the aryepiglottic fold and arytenoids or may invade directly into the false cord and aryepiglottic fold. They also grow posteriorly to the postcricoid region and extend to the opposite pyriform sinus. The vocal cord becomes fixed due to infiltration of the cricoarytenoid muscles, the crycoarytenoid joint, the thyroarytenoid muscles (vocalis muscle), or, less commonly, the recurrent laryngeal nerve. They penetrate toward the paraglottic and preepiglottic fat spaces (see section on anatomy in Chapter 19, Larynx) and then grow inferiorly along the inner face of the thyroid cartilage toward the thyrocricoid membrane. Spread into the cervical esophagus is a late event.

Lesions arising on the lateral wall tend toward early invasion of the posterior thyroid cartilage and the posterior-superior cricoid cartilage. The ipsilateral superior lobe of the thyroid gland may be invaded after tumor penetrates the cartilage, but thyroid invasion occurs without cartilage invasion when tumor penetrates behind the thyroid cartilage or through the cricothyroid membrane. Kirchner reports that thyroid cartilage invasion is associated with involvement of the apex of the pyriform sinus and the extent of invasion cannot be predicted on the basis of visible

disease.[8] Lesions of the lateral walls tend to spread submucosally onto the posterior pharyngeal wall. It is often difficult to estimate the extent of postcricoid invasion except at direct laryngoscopy, since these areas are impossible to visualize indirectly. Even with direct endoscopy, invasion is probably often underestimated.

Advanced lesions of the pyriform sinus invade all three walls, fix the larynx, involve the ipsilateral posterior pharyngeal wall, invade the thyroid cartilage and thyroid gland, affect the base of the tongue, and often escape into the soft tissues of the neck. The preepiglottic space is often involved. Perineural invasion of the recurrent laryngeal nerve may be seen in whole-organ sections.

Postcricoid Pharynx

Early lesions of the postcricoid area are rarely diagnosed. Lesions arising from the posterior wall tend to remain on the posterior wall. Lesions arising from the anterior wall tend to invade the posterior cricoarytenoid muscle and the cricoid and arytenoid cartilages. Advanced tumors eventually encircle the lumen. Since the apex of the pyriform sinus terminates in the postcricoid area, some lesions secondarily invade the apex of the pyriform sinus very early.

Lymphatics

PHARYNGEAL WALLS

The distribution and N staging on admission prior to treatment for 149 previously untreated patients with squamous cell carcinoma arising from the oropharyngeal walls is shown in Figure 21-2A; the majority of these lesions occur on the posterior pharyngeal wall.

The lymphatics of the pharyngeal walls terminate primarily in the jugular chain with a secondary avenue by way of the spinal accessory chain. The jugulodigastric node is the most commonly involved lymph node.

Lindberg reported 59% clinically positive nodes on admission; 17% were bilateral.[10] Ballantyne reported a 44% incidence of positive retropharyngeal lymph nodes in moderately advanced carcinoma of the pharyngeal walls and pyriform sinus treated by surgery.[2] Ogura reported a 66% incidence of subclinical disease for pharyngeal wall carcinomas.[15]

HYPOPHARYNX

The distribution and N staging on admission prior to treatment for 267 previously untreated patients with squamous cell carcinoma of the hypopharynx is shown in Figure 21-2B.[10]

The capillary lymphatics of the hypopharynx, especially the pyriform sinus, are profuse. The distribution of lymph node metastases is mainly to the jugular chain with a secondary pattern to the junctional and spinal accessory lymph nodes. The subdigastric lymph node is the most commonly involved, but midjugular involvement may occur without subdigastric involvement.

Seventy-five percent of patients have clinically positive lymph nodes on admission and at least 10% are bilateral. There is essentially no difference in the risk of lymph node metastases by T stage (see Table 2-2 in Chapter 2). Ogura and co-workers reported a 62% incidence of subclinical

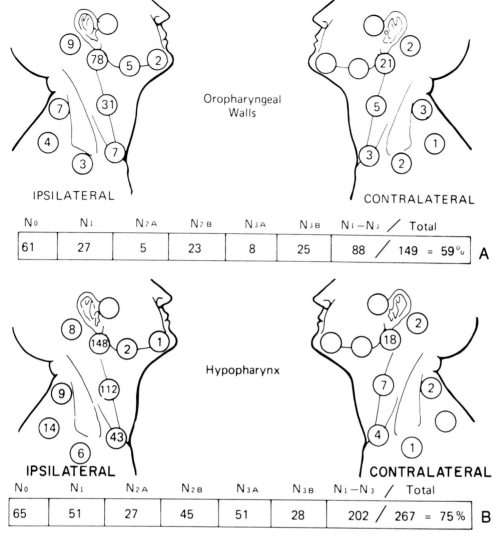

N_0	N_1	N_{2A}	N_{2B}	N_{3A}	N_{3B}	$N_1 - N_3$ / Total	
61	27	5	23	8	25	88 / 149 = 59%	A

N_0	N_1	N_{2A}	N_{2B}	N_{3A}	N_{3B}	$N_1 - N_3$ / Total	
65	51	27	45	51	28	202 / 267 = 75%	B

FIG. 21-2. Nodal distribution on admission, M. D. Anderson Hospital, 1948–1965. (*A*) Oropharyngeal walls. (*B*) Hypopharynx. (Lindberg RD: Distribution of cervical lymph node metastases from squamous cell carcinoma of the upper respiratory and digestive tracts. Cancer 29:1446–1450, 1972)

disease; some of the patients had 1500 rad to 3000 rad preoperative irradiation.[15] Biller and associates reported a 9% incidence of delayed-appearing contralateral nodes after an ipsilateral pathologically positive neck dissection.[3] The risk for late-appearing contralateral lymph nodes was independent of whether the positive ipsilateral lymph nodes were palpable.

CLINICAL PICTURE

The hallmark of pharyngeal wall and pyriform sinus cancers is sore throat. Tumors confined to the lateral pharyngeal wall or pyriform sinus produce a unilateral sore throat, a symptom rather specific for cancer since infectious sore throat is bilateral. The patient with cancer can point to the painful site with one finger, while the patient with inflammatory sore throat cannot. Dysphagia, sensation of foreign body, ear pain, blood-streaked saliva, aspiration,

and voice change occur later. Weight loss occurs in patients with advanced lesions. A neck mass may be the only presenting complaint.

Physical Examination

Lesions of the posterior pharyngeal wall may be overlooked even by competent physicians because of failure to look at the posterior pharyngeal wall routinely during indirect laryngoscopy.

Small lesions of the pyriform sinus are easily missed unless very careful examinations are done. Many of these patients have active gag reflexes, and complete topical anesthesia coupled with patience is required by the examiner. It may be difficult to differentiate between a lesion arising from the medial wall of the pyriform sinus and one arising from the aryepiglottic fold (Fig. 21-3).

Lesions of the apex of the pyriform sinus or postcricoid

area produce indirect findings that are clues to tumor not visible by indirect laryngoscopy. Pooling of secretions in the pyriform sinus and arytenoid area indicates obstruction of the upper gullet. Edema of the arytenoids and inability to see into the apex of the pyriform sinus are clues to postcricoid or low-lying pyriform sinus tumors. Invasion of the palatopharyngeus at its insertion into the inferior constrictor may cause shortening of the muscle and asymmetry of the posterior tonsillar pillars. (Most asymmetry of the posterior tonsillar pillars is due to scarring following tonsillectomy or chronic infection.) As postcricoid tumor enlarges it pushes the larynx anteriorly. This produces a full, expanded neck appearance. The thyroid click, which is produced by the superior thyroid horns hitting against the spine while the thyroid cartilage is rocked back and forth, is lost when the larynx and thyroid cartilage are forced anteriorly by the tumor mass.

METHODS OF DIAGNOSIS AND STAGING

Biopsy Technique

Biopsy of a lesion of the oropharyngeal wall can often be done in the outpatient clinic with the use of topical anesthesia. Biopsy of hypopharyngeal lesions is done under direct visualization and requires general anesthesia.

Staging Procedures

The most important staging tools are indirect and direct laryngoscopy, esophagoscopy, anteroposterior tomography, and computed tomographic (CT) scanning. Lateral soft tissue roentgenography, xerography, and laryngography contribute little and have been discontinued as routine studies. The findings on CT scan are not used to make major changes in treatment decisions at present until further experience is accumulated.

Staging

The American Joint Committee (AJCC) staging for the hypopharynx is satisfactory for disease of the pyriform sinus but unsatisfactory for that involving the pharyngeal wall:[1]

TX Minimum requirements to assess the primary tumor cannot be met.
T0 No evidence of primary tumor
Tis Carcinoma *in situ*
T1 Tumor confined to one site
T2 Extension of tumor to adjacent region or site without fixation of hemilarynx
T3 Extension of tumor to adjacent region or site with fixation of hemilarynx
T4 Massive tumor invading bone or soft tissues of neck

If there is definite decrease in mobility of the larynx, the lesion should be assigned to stage T3.

Lesions of the posterior pharyngeal wall tend to stay on the posterior pharyngeal wall rather than invade the larynx or lateral walls, and therefore fixation does not enter into staging. Posterior hypopharyngeal wall lesions are more appropriately staged by diameter of the tumor, as is done for lesions of the oropharyngeal wall. A posterior pharyngeal wall lesion could be 5 × 4 cm but confined to the posterior pharyngeal wall and could still be a T1 lesion, when in fact it would have a prognosis similar to a T3 lesion.

TREATMENT

Selection of Treatment Modality

POSTERIOR PHARYNGEAL WALL

The majority of lesions on the posterior pharyngeal wall are treated by radiation therapy, although the results are

FIG. 21-3. (A) Exophytic lesion on the left medial wall of the pyriform sinus. It is difficult to determine whether the carcinoma arises from the aryepiglottic fold or the medial wall of the pyriform sinus. (B) Photograph after 3000 rad shows 50% tumor regression. The mass has retracted to the medial wall of the pyriform sinus. The aryepiglottic fold is easily seen.

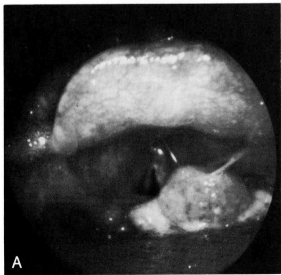
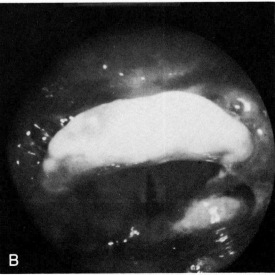

far from outstanding. Attempts have been made to combine surgery and radiation therapy for selected moderately advanced lesions with limited success.

All aspects considered, high-dose radiation therapy will produce cure rates similar to those produced by either surgery alone or combined surgery plus radiation therapy and with lesser morbidity. Salvage may be achieved by pharyngectomy in a few selected patients whose disease persists or recurs following irradiation.

LATERAL PHARYNGEAL WALL

There is very little information specifically related to the lateral walls. Small (T1–T2) lesions are usually exophytic and respond readily to irradiation. Larger lesions tend to be deeply infiltrative; control by irradiation or surgery is only modest at best, and combined therapy is often selected. An operation for a large lesion usually implies a laryngectomy in combination with pharyngectomy.

PYRIFORM SINUS

Lesions confined to the pyriform sinus with normal mobility (T1) are locally controlled in approximately 80% of cases by irradiation or partial laryngopharyngectomy.[12,14] Irradiation is our choice, since it leaves the patient with nearly normal swallowing and speech while permitting wider coverage of the regional lymphatics. Irradiation is more generally applicable, while there are certain restraints to the use of partial laryngopharyngectomy.

Lesions that extend outside the pyriform sinus with normal or reduced mobility (T2–T3) represent the group of cases where selection of treatment is more complex.

Invasion of the pyriform sinus apex is a contraindication to partial laryngopharyngectomy, but these same patients do poorly with radiation therapy also. These patients are usually selected for total laryngopharyngectomy plus postoperative radiation therapy, but they may be treated for cure by radiation therapy if apex involvement is minimal.

Fixation is a relative indication for total laryngopharyngectomy and postoperative radiation therapy. If the lesion is mainly exophytic and in the upper pyriform sinus, a trial of radiation therapy is offered as an alternative to total laryngopharyngectomy. If the disease shows a good response ($\geq$80% response) at 4500 rad to 5000 rad, radical irradiation is a reasonable choice, with total laryngopharyngectomy reserved for failure (Fig. 21-4). Partial laryngopharyngectomy is generally not attempted after 4500 rad to 5000 rad because of complications, so if the patient was suitable for partial laryngopharyngectomy at the initiation of radiation treatment, that option may be lost with a trial of radiation therapy. A select group of T2 lesions with minimal extension beyond the pyriform sinus and a normal apex are also suitable for partial laryngopharyngectomy. However, these are the very patients that do well with radiation therapy only. The local control rate by radiation therapy for T2–T3 lesions is 60% at the University of Florida. Some radiation therapy failures may be salvaged by total laryngopharyngectomy, although the mortality and morbidity are considerable after high-dose irradiation.

The more advanced, infiltrative lesions are best treated with immediate total laryngopharyngectomy, radical neck dissection, and postoperative radiation therapy. Preoperative irradiation is advised if the neck nodes are fixed.

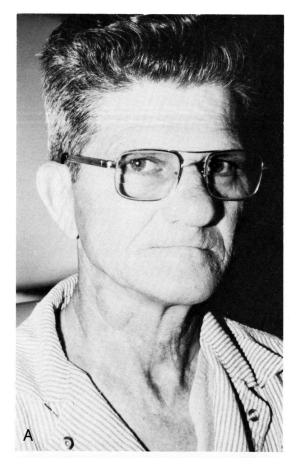

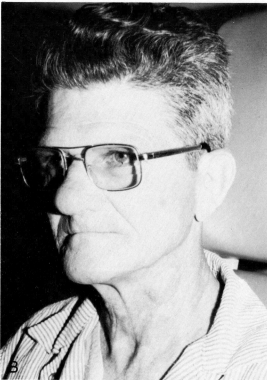

FIG. 21-4 (continued)

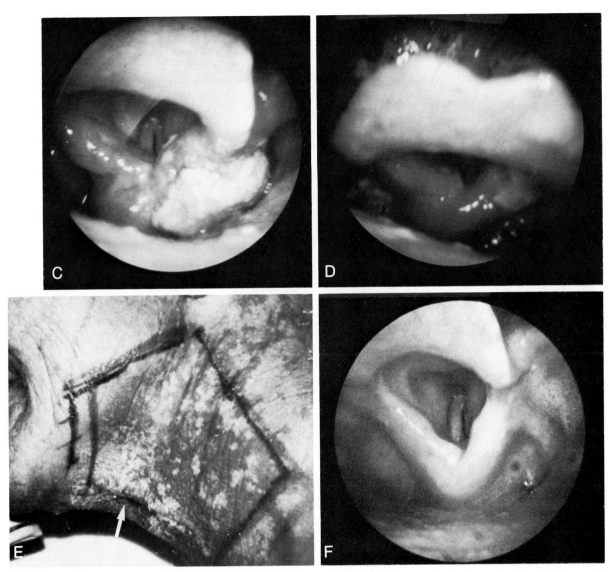

FIG. 21-4. A 54-year-old man presented with poorly differentiated squamous cell carcinoma of the left pyriform sinus. There was a 4 × 3-cm midjugular node in the right side (A) and left side (B) of the neck. (C) There was an exophytic lesion on the medial wall of the right pyriform sinus extending to the aryepiglottic fold and just onto the laryngeal surface of the epiglottis. The left postcricoid area was invaded submucosally. The right vocal cord was immobile, probably due to invasion of the cricoarytenoid muscle and/or joint (T3N3B—stage IV). (D) At 3000 rad, 80% tumor regression was noted. (E) Reduced portal at 4600 rad. The lower border of the original portal was 2 cm below the cricoid; the lower border of the reduced portal is the inferior border of the cricoid cartilage. A strip of midline neck skin is shielded on the reduced portal (arrow). (F) The final dose to the pyriform sinus and the lymph nodes was 7400 rad/ 6 weeks (120 rad twice a day). The enlarged lymph nodes disappeared after 4000 rad, and it was elected to observe the neck. The vocal cord regained full mobility 2 months after treatment. The patient had a normal voice and swallowing at 4 years. (For color photographs see Plate 8A, B in Chapter 3.)

Surgical Treatment

POSTERIOR PHARYNGEAL WALL

If the lesion is located high on the posterior wall, then a transoral approach can be used; however, for lower lesions the midline mandibulolabial glossotomy approach may be used. Alternatives are the transhyoid or a lateral pharyngotomy approach. The lesion is removed down to the prevertebral fascia, and a skin graft is used to cover the defect; postoperative irradiation is usually recommended.

PYRIFORM SINUS

PARTIAL LARYNGOPHARYNGECTOMY

A partial laryngopharyngectomy removes the false cords, epiglottis, and pyriform sinus; one arytenoid may be removed when necessary. The vocal cords are preserved.

Partial laryngopharyngectomy can be successfully used for early lesions confined to the pyriform sinus (T1) and selected lesions with minimal extension beyond the pyriform sinus (T2). In our clinic its use is advised only when radiation therapy cannot be used. The operation could be considered for salvage of a radiation therapy failure or for poor response to an initial trial of radiation therapy; these latter two situations occur infrequently and require surgical expertise. The following findings contraindicate partial laryngopharyngectomy:

  Extension to apex of the pyriform sinus
  Fixed cord
  Extension to contralateral arytenoid
  Poor pulmonary function
  Large, fixed lymph nodes

The apex of the pyriform sinus lies opposite the cricoid cartilage, and since the cricoid is the only cartilage that forms a complete ring about the airway, it must remain intact to prevent collapse. There is a greater tendency to aspiration after partial laryngopharyngectomy compared with supraglottic laryngectomy, and the patient must have the motivation to relearn to swallow.

TOTAL LARYNGOPHARYNGECTOMY

Total laryngopharyngectomy removes the larynx and varying amounts of pharyngeal wall. Advanced lesions require excision of nearly the entire circumference. The pharynx is reestablished by primary closure after a partial pharyngectomy, but a flap is required after total pharyngectomy. Since almost all these patients receive postoperative radiation therapy, the operation should be planned for one-stage reconstruction in order to start radiation therapy within 6 weeks. A planned controlled fistula speeds the healing process and largely eliminates the occurrence of an uncontrolled fistula, which delays healing and the start of radiation therapy. If a myocutaneous flap is used, a controlled fistula is unnecessary.

POSTCRICOID PHARYNX

Postcricoid carcinoma generally requires a total laryngopharyngectomy with immediate reconstruction, generally using a pectoralis major myocutaneous flap. If the lesion extends into the cervical esophagus, then reconstruction becomes more difficult. (See Chapter 22, Carcinoma of the Cervical Esophagus.)

Irradiation Technique

POSTERIOR PHARYNGEAL WALL

The irradiation technique for lesions of the posterior pharyngeal wall is opposed lateral fields to include the primary lesion and the regional nodes. Since these lesions tend to have mucosal skip areas, the entire posterior pharyngeal wall is included initially. If the lesion extends near the level of the arytenoids, the postcricoid pharynx, pyriform sinus, and upper cervical esophagus are included. The junctional, spinal accessory, and retropharyngeal lymph nodes are included even if the neck nodes are negative. High-energy x-rays (17 MV to 22 MV) are preferred if the neck nodes are negative, since this places the 90% to 95% depth dose at the tumor, with sufficient dose to the lymph nodes for subclinical disease. If the nodes are positive, then cobalt-60 or 4 MV to 8 MV irradiation is used for the initial portion of the treatment.

The critical portion of the treatment occurs when the portals are reduced at 4500 rad to 5000 rad to avoid the spinal cord. The posterior border of the portal corresponds to the posterior edge of the cervical vertebral bodies, which places the tumor very near the edge of the portal. Daily portal and imaging films and precision setups are required.

Size for size, posterior pharyngeal wall lesions are the most difficult head and neck squamous cell carcinomas to cure with radiation therapy. A time–dose analysis for local control shows a dependence on fraction size and total dose for T2–T3 lesions (see Fig. 13-18 in Chapter 13 and Table 6-9 in Chapter 6). It is difficult to deliver greater than 190 rad to 200 rad/fraction (e.g., 215 rad to 225 rad/fraction) to the initial large volume without major side-effects. Many of these patients are debilitated to start with, and one may prescribe 180 rad/fraction to ensure completion of therapy. A small nasogastric feeding tube will frequently make the difference in maintaining nutrition. The dose per fraction is increased to 215 rad to 225 rad after the portal reduction at 4500 rad whenever possible. There is little likelihood of surgical salvage of a radiation therapy failure, so every effort should be made to assist the patient through the acute effects in order to gain a reasonable chance of cure.

External-beam irradiation may be supplemented by either radon or gold seed single-plane implants (Fig. 21-5). A Crow-Davis retractor or suspension laryngoscope is used to expose the posterior pharyngeal wall. The seeds are implanted on a 1-cm grid. The implant usually adds 1000 rad to 3000 rad at 0.5 cm from the plane. It is impossible to put seeds in an ulcer since there is inadequate tissue to hold the seeds, and only the periphery of the ulcer can be implanted. If implants are planned, it is probably wise to reduce the spinal cord dose from external beam to 4000 rad and complete the treatment of the lymph nodes with either electrons or neck dissection. Local control for external-beam irradiation alone versus external-beam irradiation plus implant is compared in Table 21-1.

PYRIFORM SINUS

RADICAL IRRADIATION

Parallel opposed lateral portals are used to encompass the primary lesion and regional nodes on both sides (Fig. 21-6). The superior border is placed 2 cm to 3 cm above the tip of the mastoid in order to cover junctional lymph nodes. The retropharyngeal lymph nodes lie in front of C1 and must be included. The posterior border encompasses

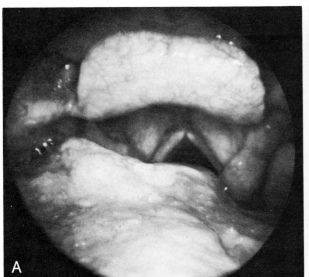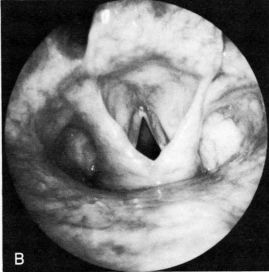

FIG. 21-5. (*A*) Squamous cell carcinoma of the posterior pharyngeal wall (T2N0). Treatment plan was external-beam irradiation, 6000 rad/6 weeks, and gold grain implant, 2000 rad to 2500 rad. (*B*) No evidence of disease at 3 years. (For color photographs see Plate 8*C, D* in Chapter 3.)

TABLE 21-1. Carcinoma of the Posterior Pharyngeal Wall: Control of Primary Site in 38 Patients*

T Stage	External-Beam Irradiation (No. Controlled/No. Treated)	External Beam Irradiation and Implant (No. Controlled/No. Treated)	No. Salvaged/ No. Attempted	Ultimate Control (No. Controlled/ No. Treated)
T1	No data	No data	No data	No data
T2	2/8	2/5	0/0	4/13 (31%)
T3	7/11	1/3	0/0	8/14 (57%)
T4	0/11	0/0	0/1	0/11 (0%)

* Excludes seven patients dead of intercurrent disease less than 2 years after treatment with primary site controlled.
Note: University of Florida data; patients treated 9/64–12/80; analysis 2/82 by C. M. Mendenhall, MD.

the spinal accessory lymph nodes. The spinal cord is shielded after 4500 to 5000 rad. Clinically positive nodes behind the plane of the spinal cord require the addition of a neck dissection or electron boosts. The anterior border is usually placed about 1 cm behind the anterior skin edge. When the anterior skin is shielded, the radiation therapist checks the setup daily because the margin for error is rather slim. Protection of the strip of anterior skin and subcutaneous tissue is thought to be important in providing an escape route for lymph through the dermal lymphatics, thereby reducing lymphedema of the larynx. A clothespin is sometimes used to isolate the tissues from the beam (Fig. 21-7). The inferior border is placed at least 2 cm below the inferior border of the cricoid for early lesions and lower for lesions with inferior extension. The inferior recess or apex of the pyriform sinus varies but generally terminates at the upper to middle cricoid.

There is usually a small area of unirradiated lower neck lymph nodes remaining when the inferior border is 2 cm to 3 cm below the cricoid. A small anterior low neck field is added to cover the lower jugular nodes, even for patients with a clinically negative neck. The tendency for pyriform sinus cancer to produce multiple nodes and frequent involvement of the inferior jugular or paratracheal nodes indicates generous use of elective neck irradiation.

Dosimetry is individualized using wedges, compensators, and unequal loadings as needed. Current dose recommendations are given in Table 21-2. (See Chapter 13, Time–Dose–Volume Relationships in Radiation Therapy, for dose analysis.) Twice-a-day fractionation schemes have given excellent results in several instances (see Figs. 21-4 and 21-6).

POSTOPERATIVE IRRADIATION

Opposed lateral portals are used for the upper neck portals and extend superiorly to include the junctional and lateral retropharyngeal lymph nodes, the base of the tongue, and the pharyngeal walls. The dose is 6000 rad/6 to 7 weeks with reduction off of the spinal cord at 5000 rad.

The lower neck is treated by an *en face* portal that includes the stoma. The minimum dose is 5000 rad given dose, but it may be higher in selected situations. Portals for preoperative irradiation are similar to those described in the section on radical irradiation.

Combined Treatment Policies

POSTERIOR PHARYNGEAL WALL

Operation should usually precede radiation therapy when a combination therapy is selected. There is a high incidence of operative mortality and complications with a preoperative dose of 2500 rad to 3000 rad.[11] When postoperative irradiation is used, a dose of 6000 rad to 6500 rad is usual.

PYRIFORM SINUS

A trial of irradiation may be given prior to deciding on total laryngopharyngectomy in selected T2–T3 lesions. They are reevaluated at 4500 rad. Irradiation is also used prior to operation for patients with a large fixed node in order to reduce the size of the mass and to help obtain surgical margins. The preoperative dose is usually limited to 5000 rad to the primary lesion, but the dose to the large lymph nodes may be 6000 rad or more depending on the response. (See Fig. 4-22 in Chapter 4.)

Following total laryngopharyngectomy with or without radical neck dissection, radiation therapy is recommended if there are close or positive margins, multiple or large positive nodes, extension of nodal disease through the capsule, or cartilage invasion. El-Badawi and co-workers showed a significant reduction in failure above the clavicle and an associated increased survival rate when comparing surgery alone to surgery plus postoperative radiotherapy.[7] In short, almost all patients receive postoperative radiation therapy. There is an increased risk of pharyngeal stenosis, especially if the pharyngeal closure is tight.

TABLE 21-2. Carcinoma of the Pyriform Sinus: Dose Recommendations for Radiation Therapy Alone to the Primary Lesion*

Stage	Dose/Time	Fraction Size†	No. Fractions
T1	6000 rad/6½ wk	180 rad	33
T2–T3	6500 rad/7 wk	190 rad	34
	7000 rad/8 wk	185 rad	38
T4	7500 rad/8½ wk	180 rad	42

* Selection of technique depends on portal size, general condition of patient, and willingness of patient to stop use of tobacco and alcohol.

† Increase daily fraction to 215 rad to 225 rad after field size reduction if no edema is present and a small field is used.

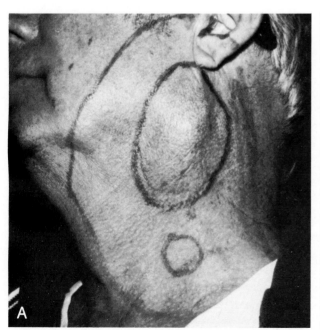

FIG. 21-6. A 64-year-old man with a history of mild sore throat for 1 year. One month prior to admission he felt a small, 1-inch knot in his neck. A biopsy of the neck showed squamous cell carcinoma; the mass enlarged rapidly after biopsy. (*A*) There was a 6 × 4-cm fixed mass in the upper neck with a well-healed biopsy scar. There was a 3 × 2-cm mobile low jugular lymph node. The lymph nodes are circled and the left lateral portal is outlined. The lower neck was irradiated through an anterior portal. (*B*) There was a small nodular lesion of the anterior wall of the left pyriform sinus with minimal extension to the medial and lateral wall. The apex was free of disease. There was early extension to the pharyngoepiglottic fold and vallecula. Mobility was normal (T2N3A). (*C*) Simulation film. The wire indicates the limits of the large lymph node. The initial treatment volume (*1*) received 4560 rad; the first reduced portal (*2*) was carried to 6000 rad and the final reduced portal (*3*) to 7680 rad (120 rad twice a day) over 6½ weeks. The posterior strips were boosted to 6500 rad with 10-MeV electrons. The right lower neck received 5000 rad given dose and the left lower neck received 6000 rad given dose in 6 weeks. (*D*) The large neck mass was reduced to 2 cm by the time of left neck dissection. Pathologic examination revealed pleomorphic squamous cell carcinoma in 2 of 16 lymph nodes. Photograph at 18 months shows 1+ edema of the epiglottis and aryepiglottic folds (patient was free of disease at 3 years).

(continued)

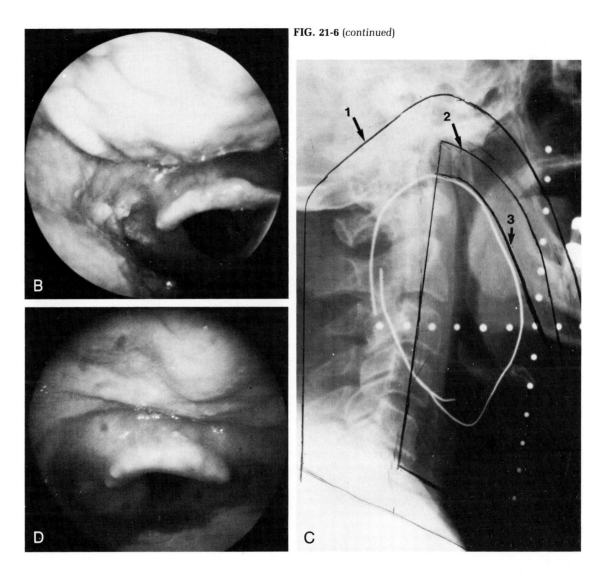

FIG. 21-6 (*continued*)

Management of Recurrence

POSTERIOR PHARYNGEAL WALL

Recurrence after radiation therapy may be limited to the posterior pharyngeal wall and may be suitable for surgical excision with occasional salvage. Meoz-Mendez and associates reported 11 of 68 local failures salvaged.[13] There has been no permanent salvage in 26 radiation therapy failures at the University of Florida (see Table 21-1). Irradiation salvage of a surgical failure would be unusual.

PYRIFORM SINUS

The hallmark of local recurrence after radical irradiation is persistent major edema, inability to visualize the pyriform sinus, pain on swallowing, and fixation of laryngeal structures. Direct laryngoscopy and biopsy are required, but biopsy may be negative and misleading. Eventually a decision may be made to recommend total laryngopharyngectomy for salvage without positive biopsy findings.

An irradiation failure may occasionally be salvaged by total laryngopharyngectomy with or without radical neck dissection. The risk of an operative mortality or major morbidity is high. The complications of total laryngopharyngectomy in seven radiation therapy failures are given in Table 21-3.[14] Four patients are living without recurrence 4, 5, 5, and 7 years after their operations.

Recurrence after total laryngopharyngectomy is usually in the soft tissues of the neck, the untreated opposite neck, the base of the tongue, or the stoma.

Surgical failures after total laryngopharyngectomy are occasionally salvaged by radiation therapy.[16] Surgical failures after partial laryngopharyngectomy for early lesions may be rescued by total laryngopharyngectomy.

RESULTS OF TREATMENT

Posterior Pharyngeal Wall

The treatment policy at the University of Florida has been primarily radical irradiation. The local control rate is shown in Table 21-1. The absolute and determinate survival rates are shown in Table 21-4.

Wang reported a 25% 3-year survival rate for 36 patients

TABLE 21-3. Summary of Surgical Complications From Carcinoma of the Pyriform Sinus Treated by Radiation Therapy ± Neck Dissection

Operation	No. Patients	Complications		Ultimate Control Above Clavicles	2-Year Disease-Free Survival
		Major	Fatal		
Immediate RND	13	2	1	6/11	6/13
Immediate PND	3	0	0	2/2	2/3
RND for recurrence	2	1	1	0/2	0/2
TLP for recurrence	2	1	1	1/2	1/2
TLP + RND for recurrence	5*	2	1	3/5	3/5

* 1—RND prior to TLP.
(RND, radical neck dissection, PND, partial neck dissection; TLP, total laryngectomy and partial pharyngectomy)
Note: University of Florida data; patients treated 10/64–12/80; 2-year to unlimited follow-up; analysis 2/83 by J. W. Devine, MD.

TABLE 21-4. Carcinoma of the Posterior Pharyngeal Wall: Survival

Stage	Absolute Survival		Determinate Survival*	
	2 Years	5 Years	2 Years	5 Years
I	No data	No data	No data	No data
II	4/8 (50%)	2/7 (29%)	4/8 (50%)	2/7 (29%)
III	3/13 (23%)	2/12 (17%)	3/11 (27%)	1/9 (11%)
IV	5/24 (21%)	2/24 (8%)	6/23 (26%)	2/21 (10%)
Total	12/45 (27%)	6/43 (14%)	13/42 (31%)	5/37 (14%)

* Excludes one patient dead of treatment complications at 22 months and two patients dead of intercurrent disease at less than 24 months.
Note: University of Florida data; patients treated 9/64–12/80; analysis 2/82 by C. M. Mendenhall, MD.

TABLE 21-5. Squamous Cell Carcinoma of the Pharyngeal Walls: Local Control

Stage	Local Control With Radiation Therapy Alone	Surgical Salvage	Ultimate Local Control
T1 (0–2 cm)	10/11 (91%)	1	11/11 (100%)
T2 (2–4 cm)	33/45 (73%)	2	35/45 (78%)
T3 (>4 cm)	38/62 (61%)	6	44/62 (71%)
T4 (massive)	15/46 (37%)	2	17/46 (41%)

Note: M. D. Anderson Hospital data; 164 patients treated 1954–1974.
(Adapted with permission from Meoz-Mendez RT, Fletcher GH, Guillamondegui OM, Peters LJ: Analysis of the results of irradiation in the treatment of squamous cell carcinomas of the pharyngeal walls. Int J Radiat Oncol Biol Phys 4:579–585, 1978. Copyright © 1978, Pergamon Press, Ltd.)

TABLE 21-6. Carcinoma of the Posterior Pharyngeal Wall: Local Control (Washington University, St. Louis)

Treatment	Local Control			
	T1	T2	T3	T4
Surgery*	6/8	7/12	4/12	0/1
Radiation therapy alone	1/1	3/6	0/5	1/1

* Twenty-nine patients had preoperative radiation therapy; two had postoperative radiation therapy; and two had surgery alone.
(Adapted with permission from Marks JE, Freeman RB, Lee F, Ogura JH: Pharyngeal wall cancer: An analysis of treatment results, complications, and patterns of failure. Int J Radiat Oncol Biol Phys 4:587–593, 1978. Copyright © 1978, Pergamon Press, Ltd.)

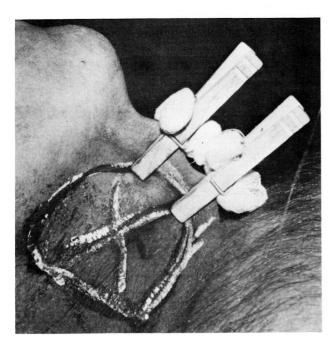

with carcinoma of the posterior pharyngeal wall treated by radiation therapy alone; the 3-year survival rate was 47% with clinically negative nodes.[17] Sixteen (66%) of 24 T1–T2 lesions and 3 of 13 T3 lesions were controlled.

Meoz-Mendez and co-workers reported the results of radiation therapy alone for 164 patients with lesions arising from the posterior and lateral pharyngeal walls.[13] The local control by T stage and the salvage of radiation therapy failures are shown in Table 21-5. The cause of death was local failure in 38%, neck recurrence in 6%, distant metastases in 10%, and second primary cancer in 16%.

Marks and co-workers compared low-dose preoperative radiation therapy (2500 rad to 3000 rad) followed by operation to radiation therapy alone (Table 21-6).[11] The local

FIG. 21-7. Clothespin applied to anterior midline strip of skin and subcutaneous tissues to increase the amount of tissue shielded. The portal is aligned with skin marks before the clamps are applied.

control was slightly better for the combined group, but the 3-year actuarial survival rate was 17% and the 3-year absolute survival rate was 14%. An operative mortality rate of 14% and a high risk of major surgical complications offset any gain in local control.

A group of 25 patients (5 stage T2, 20 stage T3–T4) were managed at M. D. Anderson Hospital by combined surgery and radiation therapy.[13] Nineteen received postoperative radiation therapy. Seven had positive margins, and 3 had close margins. Fifteen were dead at 5 years: 6 of local recurrence or neck recurrence, 5 of distant metastasis, 1 of intercurrent disease, and 3 of uncertain causes. The 5-year absolute survival rate was 4/19 (21%).

Pyriform Sinus

RADIATION THERAPY AND/OR NECK DISSECTION

Most reports paint a rather dismal outlook for pyriform sinus tumors treated by radiation therapy alone.[10,17] Kirchner and Owen reported only two 3-year survivors of 55 patients treated by radiation therapy alone; all but 4 patients had advanced disease.[9]

El-Badawi and co-workers reported results for 48 patients treated with cobalt-60.[7] Fifty-six percent were T1 and T2 lesions; 65% were staged N2 or N3. Eleven patients had a radical neck dissection after radiation therapy. Eleven (23%) developed a failure above the clavicle. Forty-eight percent were free of disease at 2 years. There was 1 patient who died of pharyngeal necrosis.

Million and Cassisi reported the results for radical irradiation for 42 patients with carcinoma of the pyriform sinus.[14] This study has recently been updated, and the new data are presented in Tables 21-7 through 21-10. T1 lesions

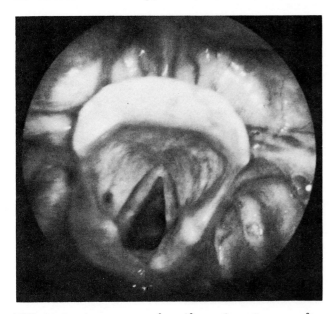

FIG. 21-8. Appearance of pyriform sinus 7 years after radiation therapy and right radical neck dissection for squamous cell carcinoma of the right pyriform sinus (T2 N3B [N2B–N1]).

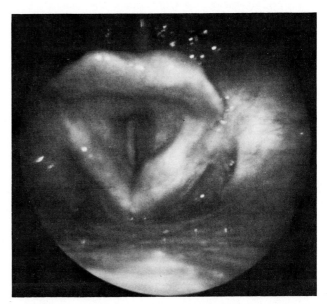

FIG. 21-9. Appearance of pyriform sinus 15 years after radiation therapy and right radical neck dissection for squamous cell carcinoma of the right pyriform sinus (T2N1).

TABLE 21-7. Carcinoma of the Pyriform Sinus: Local Control for 58 Patients Treated by Radiation Therapy ± Neck Dissection

Primary Stage	Excluded*	Local Control (No. Controlled/ No. Treated)	Surgical Salvage† (No. Salvaged/ No. Attempted)	Ultimate Control (No. Controlled/ No. Treated)
T1	1	12/15	0/1‡	12/15
T2	6	9/15	3/4	12/15
T3	5	5/8	1/1	6/8
T4	1	1/7	0/1	1/7

* Dead of intercurrent disease less than 2 years after treatment with primary lesion controlled.

† Successfully salvaged patients living 4, 5, 5, and 7 years.

‡ Patient refused operation for 1 year after recurrence was diagnosed.

Note: University of Florida data; patients treated 10/64–12/80; 2-year to unlimited followup; analysis 2/83 by J. W. Devine, MD.

TABLE 21-8. Carcinoma of the Pyriform Sinus: Control of Neck Disease in 58 Patients Treated by Radiation Therapy ± Neck Dissection

Neck Stage	Excluded*	Treatment	Neck Control (No. Controlled/ No. Treated)
N0	1	RT	10/10
N1	9	RT	4/4
	0	Excision + RT	1/1
	0	RT + RND	2/2
N2	3	RT	6/7†
	0	RT + PND	1/1
	1	RT + RND	2/2
N3	0	RT	1/5
	1	RT + PND	1/1
	2	RT + RND	4/8

* Seventeen patients excluded from analysis—dead of intercurrent disease or uncontrolled primary lesion in less than 2 years with neck disease controlled.

† One patient refused RND.

(RT, radiation therapy; PND, partial neck dissection; RND, radical neck dissection)

Note: University of Florida data, patients treated 10/64–12/80; 2-year to unlimited followup; analysis 2/83 by J. W. Devine, MD.

TABLE 21-9. Carcinoma of the Pyriform Sinus: Survival Free of Disease in Patients Treated by Radiation Therapy ± Neck Dissection

AJCC Stage	Absolute Survival		Determinate Survival	
	2 Years	5 Years	2 Years	5 Years
I, II	6/8	5/6	6/8	5/6
III	9/17 (53%)	3/12 (25%)	9/15 (60%)	3/8
IVA*	10/14 (71%)	4/10 (40%)	10/12 (83%)	4/6 (66%)
IVB	4/19 (21%)	1/13 (7%)	4/18 (22%)	1/13 (7%)
Total	29/58 (50%)	13/41 (32%)	29/53 (56%)	13/33 (41%)

* IVA—any combination of T1 or T2 and N2A, N2B, or N3A.

Note: University of Florida data; patients treated 10/64–12/80 (to 12/77 for 5-year figures); analysis 2/83 by J. W. Devine, MD.

TABLE 21-10. Carcinoma of the Pyriform Sinus: Cause of Death in Patients Treated by Radiation Therapy ± Neck Dissection

Stage	No. Patients	Living, NED	Cause of Death				
			P*	N	DM	ID	(Complication of Treatment†)
I, II	8	6	2	0	0	0	(1)
III	17	5	4	0	1	7	(2)
IVA	13	5	1	0	2	5	(0)
IVB	20	3	8	4	3	2	(2)
Total	58	19	15	4	6	14	(5)

* Five of 15 patients also had neck failure.

† Four patients died of a complication of surgical salvage attempt, and one died of laryngeal necrosis; they are also listed under another category.

(NED, no evidence of pyriform sinus cancer; P, primary recurrence; N, neck recurrence, primary controlled; DM, distant metastases only, primary and neck controlled; ID, intercurrent disease, no evidence of pyriform sinus cancer)

Note: University of Florida data; patients treated 10/64–12/80; 2-year to 5-year follow-up; analysis 2/83 by J. W. Devine, MD.

were selected for radiation therapy; T2 and T3 lesions were irradiated if they were exophytic and in the upper pyriform sinus, or if the patient refused operation. All T4 lesions were irradiated by default.

The local and regional control is shown in Tables 21-7 and 21-8. Neck dissection was added in 16 patients. Treatment failed in only four patients because of failure to control neck disease. Survivals at 2 and 5 years are presented in Table 21-9, and the cause of death is indicated in Table 21-10. The appearance of the larynx and pyriform sinus for two patients at 7 and 15 years after radiation therapy is shown in Figures 21-8 and 21-9.

Stage IV may be subdivided into a favorable group (IVA) with small primary lesions (T1–T2) and N2 or N3A neck disease, which can often be successfully managed by adding a neck dissection. In this group, the 2-year and 5-year determinate disease-free survival was similar to that for stages I through III (see Table 21-9).

PARTIAL LARYNGOPHARYNGECTOMY

The results of treatment are given in Table 21-11 for 80 patients with carcinoma of the pyriform sinus treated at Washington University, St. Louis, by 3000 rad of preoperative radiation followed by partial laryngopharyngectomy.[12] Seventy patients had the equivalent of AJCC T1 lesions, with disease limited to the pyriform sinus, and 10 patients had disease extending beyond the pyriform sinus. The cause of death was cancer in 26%, complications of treatment in 14%, and intercurrent disease in 20%. The 2-year absolute survival rate was 45/80 (56%), and the 5-year absolute survival rate was 25/66 (38%).*

TOTAL LARYNGOPHARYNGECTOMY

The results of treatment for 57 patients treated by preoperative radiation therapy followed by total laryngectomy

* Marks JE: Written communication, 1979.

and partial pharyngectomy are shown in Table 21-11. Thirty-five patients had lesions confined to the pyriform sinus (AJCC T1), and the remainder had extension beyond the pyriform sinus (AJCC T2–T4). The cause of death was cancer in 56%, complications of treatment in 11%, and intercurrent disease in 18%.

El-Badawi and co-workers compared results for 203 pa-

FIG. 21-10. Carcinoma of the pyriform sinus: actuarial survival comparing surgery only and surgery plus postoperative radiation therapy (M. D. Anderson Hospital data, 1949–1976, minimum follow-up 4 years). (Redrawn from El-Badawi SA, Goepfert H, Fletcher GH, Herson J, Oswald MJ: Squamous cell carcinoma of the pyriform sinus. Laryngoscope 92:357–364, 1982)

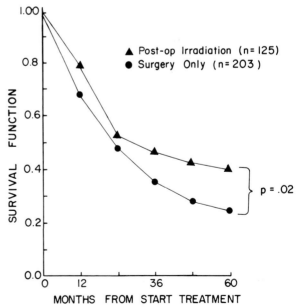

TABLE 21-11. **Carcinoma of the Pyriform Sinus: Results of Treatment by Preoperative Radiation Therapy Plus Partial Laryngopharyngectomy (PLP) or Preoperative Radiation Therapy Plus Total Laryngectomy and Partial Pharyngectomy (TLP)**

Result	PLP (80 Patients*)	TLP (57 Patients†)
Local recurrence ± neck recurrence	14%‡	14%
Neck recurrence ± distant metastases (primary lesion controlled)	9%	23%
Distant metastases alone	11%	21%
Five-year actuarial survival (no evidence of disease)	40%	22%

* T1, 70 patients, T2–T4, 10 patients (AJCC staging).
† T1, 35 patients; T2–T4, 22 patients (AJCC staging).
‡ Four patients had their treatment failure salvaged.
Note: Washington University, St. Louis, data, 1964–1974.

(Data from Marks JE, Kurnik B, Powers WE, Ogura JH: Carcinoma of the pyriform sinus: An analysis of treatment results and patterns of failure. Cancer 41:1008–1015, 1978)

TABLE 21-12. **Carcinoma of the Pyriform Sinus: Results of Treatment**

Treatment Modality	No. Patients	Failure Above Clavicles (%)	2-Year NED (%)	Cause of Death (>2 Year)
Surgery	203	39*	40†	DM—8 ID—23
Surgery and postoperative irradiation	125	11*	50†	N—1 DM—6 ID—7
Preoperative irradiation and surgery	17	29	47	DM—2 ID—2

* $p = <.001$.
† $p = .04$.
(NED, no evidence of pyriform sinus cancer; DM, distant metastasis; ID, intercurrent disease; N, neck nodes)
Note: M. D. Anderson Hospital data; patients treated 1949–1976; analysis 1/81.
(Adapted from El-Badawi SA, Goepfert H, Fletcher GH, Herson J, Oswald MJ: Squamous cell carcinoma of the pyriform sinus. Laryngoscope 92:357–364, 1982)

TABLE 21-13. **Carcinoma of the Pyriform Sinus: Ultimate Control Above the Clavicles (Including Salvage)—Surgery ± Radiation Therapy**

Stage	Preoperative Radiation Therapy	Postoperative Radiation Therapy	Surgery Alone
T1	0/1	0/0	0/0
T2	1/1	1/1	2/3
T3	8/15	10/15	3/6
T4	1/5	2/2	0/0

Note: University of Florida data; patients treated 10/64–12/80; 2-year to unlimited follow-up; analysis 2/83 by J. W. Devine, MD.

TABLE 21-14. Carcinoma of the Pyriform Sinus: Survival Free of Disease in Patients Treated by Surgery ± Radiation Therapy

AJCC Stage	Absolute Survival		Determinate Survival	
	2 Years	5 Years	2 Years	5 Years
I, II	0/2	0/2	0/2	0/2
III	9/14 (64%)	2/9	9/12 (75%)	2/7
IVA*	2/4	2/4	2/4	2/4
IVB	18/47 (38%)	7/41 (17%)	18/42 (43%)	7/35 (20%)
Total	29/67 (43%)	11/56 (20%)	29/60 (48%)	11/48 (23%)

* IVA—any combination of T1 or T2 and N2A, N2B, or N3A.
Note: University of Florida data; patients treated 10/64–12/80 (to 12/77 for 5-year figures); analysis 2/83 by J. W. Devine, MD.

tients treated by surgery alone and 125 patients treated by surgery (total laryngopharyngectomy) followed by 6000 rad of postoperative or 4500 rad to 5000 rad preoperative radiation.[7] The stages of the three groups were comparable. There was a minimum follow-up of 4 years (Table 21-12). The actuarial survival of the three groups is shown in Figure 21-10. The improvement in survival at 5 years is 15 percentage points. Note that the 22% actuarial 5-year survival rate for low-dose preoperative radiation therapy and total laryngopharyngectomy (see Table 21-11) is identical to the surgery alone (see Fig. 21-10). The rate of failure above the clavicle in the two groups is likewise almost identical (37% vs. 39%).

The ultimate control rates above the clavicles for 65 patients treated by total laryngopharyngectomy and 2 patients treated by partial laryngopharyngectomy at the University of Florida are present in Table 21-13. The patients with more advanced lesions in stage T2 and T3 were selected for an operation. Preoperative or postoperative radiation therapy was added in 54 of the patients. The ultimate control rate for T3 lesions treated by operation was 21 of 36 (58%) and for T4 lesions was 3 of 7. The survival figures are presented in Table 21-14.

Lateral Pharyngeal Wall

The lateral pharyngeal wall is seldom reported separately. The local control for eight evaluable lesions treated by radiation therapy, 1 fraction/day, at the University of Florida was poor: T2, 2/4; T3, 0/3; T4, 0/11. A good result for an advanced lesion treated with 2 fractions/day is shown in Figure 21-11.

FOLLOW-UP POLICY

Posterior Pharyngeal Wall

Ulceration is the hallmark of radiation failure, although two patients had ulceration that represented a soft tissue necrosis and that eventually healed. Radiation failures can only occasionally be salvaged by pharyngectomy.

Patients with pharyngeal wall lesions are at high risk for esophageal and lung cancers, and these areas should be monitored closely with biannual chest roentgenography and barium swallow.

Pyriform Sinus

Patients irradiated for cure must be followed monthly in order to permit early diagnosis of recurrence. The hallmark of persistence or recurrence is major edema of the arytenoids, pain, especially when swallowing, and development of hoarseness and a fixed cord. Patients who continue to smoke and drink make assessment more difficult. The addition of a radical neck dissection increases the edema. However, mild to moderate edema that is stable or slowly regressing without pain is usually safe to follow. Direct laryngoscopy should be considered if indirect examination is not satisfactory. We have been able to diagnose local recurrence by T1 and T2 lesions at a point when they could be cured by total laryngopharyngectomy, although salvage was not uniform due to other factors.

COMPLICATIONS OF TREATMENT

Posterior Pharyngeal Wall

SURGICAL COMPLICATIONS

Cunningham and Catlin reported an operative mortality rate of 9% and a complication rate of 57% for patients operated on during the period 1951 to 1961.[6] Mucocutaneous fistula was the most common problem.

Marks and co-workers reported a 14% operative mortality rate plus major complications including pharyngocutaneous fistula (31%) and carotid rupture (14%) for patients treated with preoperative radiation therapy, 2500 rad to 3000 rad.[11]

RADIATION THERAPY COMPLICATIONS

Meoz-Mendez and associates analyzed the complications for 164 patients with carcinoma of the pharyngeal wall treated by radiation therapy alone.[13] There was a 5% incidence of fatal complications. In 7 patients the fatality was secondary to carotid rupture, associated with attempts at surgical salvage. Only 2 patients developed severe la-

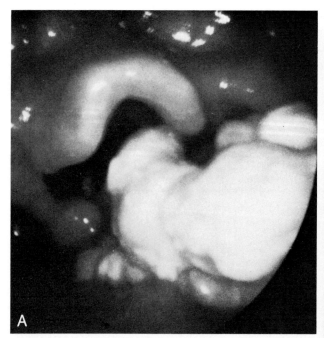

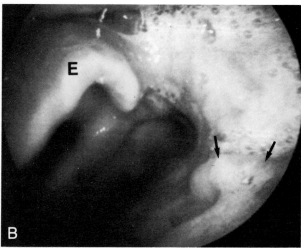

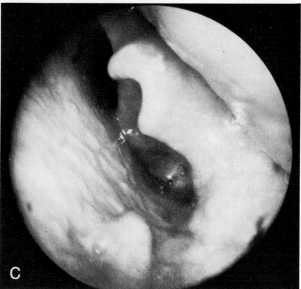

FIG. 21-11. (*A*) Extensive squamous cell carcinoma of the right lateral pharyngeal wall that extended from the level of the soft palate to the apex of the pyriform sinus. There was a single 2-cm subdigastric lymph node (T4N1). Treatment plan was 7720 rad total dose/6½ weeks (120 rad twice daily), parallel opposed portals (cobalt-60) with reductions at 4600 and 6000 rad. The right posterior tonsillar pillar remained enlarged and indurated 5 weeks after treatment. There was a 2 × 1-cm ulcer with rolled margins on the right pharyngeal wall at 2 months. Right radical neck dissection at 2½ months showed one positive midjugular lymph node. (*B*) Appearance at 4 months. Note submucosal bulge (*arrows*). Periodic examinations revealed persistent thickening along the palatoglossus (posterior tonsillar pillar), but patient remained asymptomatic. *E,* epiglottis. (*C*) Appearance at 40 months. Neck tissues soft and pliable. The submucosal bulge on the posterior pharyngeal wall is due to an osteophyte on the cervical vertebra.

ryngeal edema. Radiation myelitis was documented in 2 patients. The overall incidence of radiation therapy–related complications was 12% and increased in patients with advanced lesions.

Pyriform Sinus

SURGICAL COMPLICATIONS

The complications of partial laryngopharyngectomy include a 12% operative mortality rate, pharyngocutaneous fistula, carotid rupture, aspiration, and dysphagia.[12] The morbidity is significantly higher after preoperative radiation therapy.

The complications of total laryngopharyngectomy include a treatment-released mortality rate of 11%, fistula, carotid rupture, and pharyngeal stenosis.[12]

The complication rate is increased by the addition of radiation therapy. (See John Conley's *Complications of*

Head and Neck Surgery for a discussion of management of complications.[5])

Attempted surgical salvage of radiation therapy failures has a significant operative morbidity and mortality in the best of hands, but a few cures are produced (see Table 21-3). Pharyngocutaneous fistula and exposure of the carotid vessels are life-threatening complications.

COMPLICATIONS OF RADIATION THERAPY

Lymphedema of the larynx occurs temporarily in most cases and is increased by radical neck dissection. The edema gradually resolves in 2 to 6 months in successfully treated cases and may last for a year if bilateral neck dissection is added.

The major complication of radiation therapy is laryngeal necrosis. There have been two instances of laryngeal necrosis in the University of Florida series after radical irradiation. One patient had a total laryngectomy and is living free of disease at 5 years; the other patient died at home after tracheostomy. A third patient (stage T2N0) has developed fibrosis in the neck, which has produced bilateral hypoglossal nerve palsies and dysphagia that requires a gastrostomy. All three complications occurred after 7000 rad/7 weeks. Because of these three complications we advise that pyriform sinus lesions to be treated at the rate of 180 rad/fraction if one fraction per day is used or 120 rad/fraction if twice-a-day treatment is given.

REFERENCES

1. American Joint Committee on Cancer: Manual for Staging of Cancer, 2nd ed, p 33. Philadelphia, JB Lippincott, 1983
2. Ballantyne AJ: Principles of surgical management of cancer of the pharyngeal walls. Cancer 20:663–667, 1967
3. Biller HF, Davis WH, Ogura JH: Delayed contralateral cervical metastases with laryngeal and laryngopharyngeal cancers. Laryngoscope 81:1499–1502, 1971
4. Clemente CD (ed): Anatomy, A Regional Atlas of the Human Body. Philadelphia, Lea & Febiger, 1975
5. Conley JJ (ed): Complications of Head and Neck Surgery. Philadelphia, WB Saunders, 1979
6. Cunningham MP, Catlin D: Cancer of the pharyngeal wall. Cancer 20:1859–1866, 1967
7. El-Badawi SA, Goepfert H, Fletcher GH, Herson J, Oswald MJ: Squamous cell carcinoma of the pyriform sinus. Laryngoscope 92:357–364, 1982
8. Kirchner JA: Pyriform sinus cancer: A clinical and laboratory study. Ann Otol Rhinol Laryngol 84:793–803, 1975
9. Kirchner JA, Owen JR: Five hundred cancers of the larynx and pyriform sinus. Results of treatment by radiation and surgery. Laryngoscope 87:1288–1303, 1977
10. Lindberg RD: Distribution of cervical lymph node metastases from squamous cell carcinoma of the upper respiratory and digestive tracts. Cancer 29:1446–1449, 1972
11. Marks JE, Freeman RB, Lee F, Ogura JH: Pharyngeal wall cancer: An analysis of treatment results, complications, and patterns of failure. Int J Radiat Oncol Biol Phys 4:587–593, 1978
12. Marks JE, Kurnik B, Powers WE, Ogura JH: Carcinoma of the pyriform sinus: An analysis of treatment results and patterns of failure. Cancer 41:1008–1015, 1978
13. Meoz-Mendez RT, Fletcher GH, Guillamondegui OM, Peters LJ: Analysis of the results of irradiation in the treatment of squamous cell carcinomas of the pharyngeal walls. Int J Radiat Oncol Biol Phys 4:579–585, 1978
14. Million RR, Cassisi NJ: Radical irradiation for carcinoma of the pyriform sinus. Laryngoscope 91:439–450, 1981
15. Ogura JH, Biller HF, Wette R: Elective neck dissection for pharyngeal and laryngeal cancers: An evaluation. Ann Otol Rhinol Laryngol 80:646–653, 1971
16. Razack MS, Sako K, Marchetta FC, Calamel P, Bakamjian V, Shedd DP: Carcinoma of the hypopharynx: Success and failure. Am J Surg 134:489–491, 1977
17. Wang CC: Radiotherapeutic management of carcinoma of the posterior pharyngeal wall. Cancer 27:894–896, 1971

Carcinoma of the Cervical Esophagus

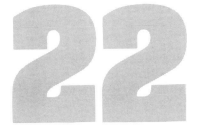

WILLIAM M. MENDENHALL

Cancer of the esophagus was described by Jurgani, a Persian medical writer, as early as 1100. Its incidence varies geographically, ranging from 130.8 per 100,000 people in Iran to 0.5 per 100,000 people in Nigeria. The incidence of cancer of the esophagus in the United States, according to the Third National Cancer Survey (1969–1971), is 4.7 and 1.3 for white males and females and 16.7 and 3.7 for black males and females, respectively. It is particularly common in black males in the coastal regions of North and South Carolina, Georgia, and northeast Florida. In addition, inhabitants of Puerto Rico have a high incidence of esophageal carcinoma. Cancer of the cervical portion of the esophagus is relatively rare, comprising 10% to 33% of all esophageal cancer. In contradistinction to cancers of the thoracic esophagus and other head and neck sites, malignancies of the cervical esophagus are more common in women, with a female-to-male ratio varying from 5:1 to 1:1. Patients are usually in the older age-group, with most presenting in their 50s and 60s. The disease occurs more frequently in patients with a history of excessive alcohol ingestion, cigarette smoking, a previous head and neck cancer (up to 20%), or the Plummer-Vinson syndrome (long-standing dysphagia, anemia, atrophy of mucous membranes, and brittle nails). The Plummer-Vinson syndrome is thought to be secondary to a nutritional deficiency and is seen with an increased frequency in Scandinavian and British women.

ANATOMY

The cervical esophagus is simply a narrow inferior extension of the pharynx. It begins at the cricopharyngeus at the level of C6 (approximately 16 cm from the incisors) and arbitrarily ends at the thoracic inlet (approximately 23 cm from the incisors), where it is continuous with the thoracic esophagus. The point at which the cervical esophagus becomes the thoracic esophagus is opposite the upper border of the manubrium (T4). There is no anatomical change in the esophagus *per se* at this transition. The cervical esophagus is 6 cm to 8 cm in length. As it descends in the neck, it deviates slightly to the left beyond the border of the overlying trachea. It is related to the trachea and recurrent laryngeal nerve on its anterior aspect, to the thyroid gland and carotid sheath laterally, and to the retroesophageal space and prevertebral fascia posteriorly. It is composed of squamous epithelium and two muscle layers: (1) an inner circular layer and (2) an outer longitudinal layer. There is no serosa.

The cervical esophagus receives its blood supply from the inferior thyroid artery and vein. The lymphatics of the cervical esophagus are moderately abundant and drain primarily to the peritracheal, periesophageal, lower internal jugular chain, and supraclavicular nodes. They communicate with the lymphatics of the pyriform sinus and postcricoid area, and thus tumor may spread to the upper internal jugular chain lymph nodes. The peritracheal and periesophageal chains provide an avenue of spread to the upper mediastinal lymph nodes.

PATHOLOGY

Cancer of the cervical esophagus is squamous cell carcinoma in over 90% of cases and is usually of moderate to poor differentiation. Less frequently, adenocarcinoma, carcinosarcoma, sarcoma, or tumors of minor salivary gland origin may be encountered. Carcinoma in situ is frequently seen adjacent to an area of frank carcinoma. Invasion of blood vessels, lymphatics, and perineural spaces is common.

PATTERNS OF SPREAD

Primary

Submucosal spread of the tumor beyond its gross extent is the rule in cancer of the esophagus. It has been reported to occur up to 8 cm from the edge of the obvious primary lesion.[18] As the tumor enlarges, it may extend to contiguous structures such as the hypopharynx, larynx, trachea, thyroid, recurrent laryngeal nerve, and great vessels. Large blood vessels, usually arteries, may be perforated by tumor; veins are more often compressed.

Lymphatics

The incidence of lymph node metastasis reported for the entire esophagus is related to the length of the primary lesion, with 50% of lesions less than 5 cm in length having lymph node metastases as compared with 90% when the primary lesion is longer than 5 cm.[39] The distribution of lymph node metastases in an autopsy series for carcinoma of the upper third of the esophagus was supraclavicular and infraclavicular, 5%; peritracheal and periesophageal, 69%; mediastinal, 23%; and abdominal, 9%. The incidence of clinically positive lymph nodes in the neck at the University of Florida is 12% (2 of 16) for carcinoma of the cervical esophagus. The lymph node metastases may be located at any level in the neck, but are most commonly found in the lower jugular chain. A deep medial mass in the low neck may be direct extension from the primary lesion. Computed tomographic (CT) scanning may help differentiate extension of the primary lesion from lymph node metastasis. Once the tumor has extended to the postcricoid area and pyriform sinus, it may spread through the lymphatic pathways in a manner similar to primary cancer in those locations and therefore reach the jugulodigastric lymph nodes without necessarily involving lymph nodes in the low jugular chain. I have observed two cases in which there was lymph node failure in the upper neck just above the irradiation portal.

Distant Metastasis

Distant metastasis is frequent, involving primarily the liver and the lung.[34] The approximate frequencies, based on an autopsy series, are liver, 16%; lung or pleura, 31%; bone, 9%; kidney, 4%; and adrenals, 2%.[11]

CLINICAL PICTURE

Symptoms

Dysphagia and weight loss, the two most common symptoms, are present in almost all patients at the time of diagnosis. These symptoms occur earlier than with lesions of the hypopharynx because the lumen of the cervical esophagus is smaller. Less frequently, patients may present with dyspnea, malaise, hoarseness (secondary to direct extension to the larynx or the recurrent laryngeal nerve), pain, cough, excess secretions, vomiting, and hematemesis. Patients with cancer of the cervical esophagus present with relatively early lesions compared with those with cancer of the thoracic esophagus.

Physical Findings

In addition to weight loss, the physical findings secondary to the lesion in the cervical esophagus include pooling of saliva in the pyriform sinus, visible tumor extending into the hypopharynx, direct extension into the soft tissues of the neck, loss of the thyroid click, anterior bowing of the trachea, fullness in the midline of the lower neck, and fixation of a vocal cord. Paratracheal masses may be felt on deep palpation of the lower neck and sternal notch. It may be difficult to distinguish between a metastatic lymph node and direct extension of tumor into the neck.

DIAGNOSIS AND STAGING

The differential diagnosis of carcinoma of the cervical esophagus includes any lesion arising in the lower neck and superior mediastinum that could invade and obstruct the esophagus. This would include thyroid cancer, lung cancer, thymoma, mediastinal lymphomas, soft tissue sarcomas, and metastatic disease to the regional lymph nodes. The diagnosis is usually made by contrast radiologic examination of the esophagus. Small lesions may be missed with conventional fluoroscopy and spot filming because of the rapid flow of barium through the cervical esophagus. Rapid filming devices are essential for detecting small lesions and for determining the extent of larger tumors.

Biopsy Procedures

Esophagoscopy and biopsy establish the diagnosis of cancer of the cervical esophagus. It is sometimes very difficult to establish the diagnosis by esophagoscopy because nondiagnostic tissue is obtained; constriction of the lumen above the lesion prevents access to tumor, and there is a reluctance to take deep biopsies because of the fear of perforation. Biopsy of a suspicious neck node or mass may be done when indicated. A specimen for cytology may be obtained using a Levin tube that is passed to the esophagogastric junction; as the tube is withdrawn, the esophagus is washed with saline. This technique was first described by Beale in 1853 and is reported to have an accuracy approaching 95%, with a false-negative rate of 10% and a false-positive rate of 2%.[5,36] I have no experience with this method. Occasionally, a decision must be made as to surgical exploration for diagnosis. If the lesion is to be treated by radiation therapy, the patient may be presented with the alternatives and will usually opt for treatment without a definitive diagnosis. This situation usually occurs with advanced, incurable lesions when the roentgenographic appearance and the clinical story are sufficient for diagnosis with almost no likelihood of error.

Staging Procedures

Esophagoscopy is used to establish the histologic diagnosis of cancer, as well as to define the location, extent, and mobility of the lesion. Barium swallow is also used to determine the location and extent of the cancer. Bronchoscopy will determine whether the lesion has invaded the trachea, and CT scan of the neck and upper thorax will help define the extent of the primary lesion and location of lymph node metastases (Fig. 22-1). Lateral soft tissue roentgenograms of the neck will determine if there is extraesophageal extension, as indicated by widening of the retrotracheal space. Chest roentgenograms and tomograms will show direct extension of the cancer to the superior mediastinum as well as distant metastasis in the lung. Bone scan, liver–spleen scan, and blood chemistry studies (e.g., liver function tests, alkaline phosphatase determination) will help determine if distant metastases are present at the time of diagnosis.

The American Joint Committee (AJCC) staging system for esophageal cancer is listed below.[2]

Primary Tumor

T0 No demonstrable tumor in the esophagus

Tis Carcinoma in situ

T1 A tumor that involves 5 cm or less of esophageal length, that produces no obstruction,* and that has no circumferential involvement and no extraesophageal spread†

T2 A tumor that involves more than 5 cm of esophageal length without extraesophageal spread† or a tumor of any size that produces obstruction* or that involves the entire circumference but without extraesophageal spread

T3 Any tumor with evidence of extraesophageal spread†

Regional Lymph Nodes

N0 No clinically palpable nodes

N1 Movable, unilateral, palpable nodes

N2 Movable, bilateral, palpable nodes

N3 Fixed nodes

The AJCC staging of the primary lesion seems overly complicated, difficult to apply, and impossible to remember. A system based only on the length of the lesion would simplify staging and make comparisons between institutions more reliable. Lesions as large as 2 cm are often curable, 2-cm to 5-cm lesions are only occasionally curable, and those greater than 5 cm are almost never curable.

TREATMENT

Factors in Selection of Treatment Modality

The choice of treatment is between surgical resection, radiation therapy, or a combination of the two.

* Roentgenographic evidence of significant impediment to the passage of liquid contrast material past the tumor or endoscopic evidence of esophageal obstruction.

† Extension of cancer outside the esophagus is seen by clinical, roentgenographic, and endoscopic evidence of (1) recurrent laryngeal, phrenic, or sympathetic nerve involvement; (2) fistula

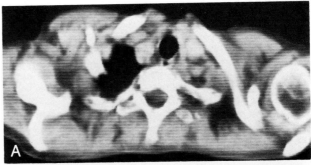

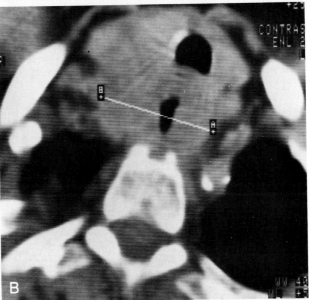

FIG. 22-1. (A) Normal anatomy on CT scan. (B) Carcinoma of the cervical esophagus extending to and surrounding the trachea.

Cure rates in unselected series are essentially the same for surgery, radiation therapy, or the combined approach. Radiation therapy is usually recommended as the initial treatment of these patients because the initial morbidity and mortality are less than when surgery is employed.

Surgical management is further complicated by the fact that a standard neck dissection does not remove the paratracheal and upper mediastinal lymph nodes. In the patient with a clinically negative neck, the risk for lymph node metastasis is bilateral, and there is no way to gauge which side of the neck is at risk.

Surgery

For the surgeon the pharynx combines three of the most formidable obstacles to the exercise of his art: it is inaccessible in a high degree, it is the seat of delicate and concentrated function, and it contains septic material to which the surrounding tissues are in no way immune.[47]

Wilfred Trotter, 1932

formation; (3) involvement of the tracheal or bronchial tree; (4) vena cava or azygous vein obstruction; and (5) malignant effusion. Mediastinal widening itself is not evidence of extraesophageal spread.

HISTORICAL PERSPECTIVE

Czerny is credited with the first resection of carcinoma of the cervical esophagus, performed in 1877 without reconstruction on a 51-year-old woman. Her postoperative course was relatively uncomplicated. She subsequently died with a local recurrence 15 months after her surgery.[24]

Mikulicz resected a carcinoma of the cervical esophagus in 1884 and reconstructed the defect with skin flaps.[24] Trotter, in his Hunterian lecture of 1913, described reconstruction of the gullet with skin flaps, a procedure that was further simplified and popularized by Wookey.[46,52,53] Roux proposed the use of a segment of jejunum in 1907, and Kelling and Vulliet independently reported the use of colon in 1911.[7] Torek described the first successful thoracic esophagectomy for carcinoma in 1913.[45] Eggers was the first to describe resection of cancer of the cervical esophagus in the United States in 1924.[13] Since that time, numerous methods to reconstruct the gullet have been devised, none of which has been entirely satisfactory.

CURATIVE RESECTION

The surgical treatment of cancer of the cervical esophagus may be divided into three groups of operations: curative resection, reconstruction, and palliative procedures. Obviously, the extent of the curative resection will depend on location and extent of the tumor. It will include a cervical esophagectomy with or without an en bloc laryngopharyngectomy.[7,9,15,52] Generally, at least an ipsilateral thyroid lobectomy is included, although some advocate total thyroidectomy because of the high likelihood that the thyroid is involved with tumor. A unilateral or bilateral radical neck dissection is included if the tumor clinically has metastasized to one or both sides of the neck.[6] Areas of controversy include the use of bilateral prophylactic neck dissection, total as opposed to partial esophagectomy, and routine dissection of the anterior superior mediastinal nodes, which usually entails splitting of the manubrium.[4] The rationale for these more extensive procedures is that cancer of the esophagus exhibits a propensity for lymph node metastasis and submucosal skip lesions.

FIG. 22-2. Bakamjian deltopectoral flap.

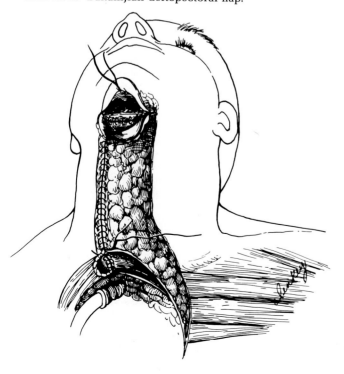

RECONSTRUCTIVE SURGERY

Some of the operations for excision of the esophagus which have been recommended and which are freely illustrated in books must be looked upon as largely armchair exploits and doomed to failure in practice.[48]

C. Grey Turner, 1936

There have been many advances over the past 56 years since Turner's observation, but a simple, safe method of reconstruction producing normal swallowing does not yet exist.

There are varied procedures that have been proposed to reconstruct the gullet after resection of the cervical esophagus. This attests to the lack of any one procedure that will consistently restore continuity to the gullet with an acceptable level of morbidity and mortality. Basically, reconstruction involves one of the following: primary closure or closure with pedicled skin flaps, free skin grafts, laryngotracheal allografts, free gut grafts, pedicled gut grafts, or, more recently, myocutaneous grafts.[44] These methods of reconstruction will be discussed with regard to technique, advantages, and disadvantages.

PRIMARY CLOSURE

One third of the circumference of the wall of the esophagus is required to attempt primary closure.[41] Should the defect be larger or the tissues devitalized by prior irradiation, primary closure is not possible. The diameter of the cervical esophagus is relatively small, and very few lesions would be suitable for this form of management.

PEDICLED SKIN GRAFTS

Wookey Procedure

Wookey described cervical esophagectomy with or without laryngectomy and reconstruction with cervical skin flaps in 1941.[52,53] This technique is, for the most part, considered to be outdated.

Bakamjian Deltopectoral Flap

The use of a medially based deltopectoral flap was described by Bakamjian in 1965.[3] The technique involves mobilization of the flap with a blood supply from the internal mammary artery. The flap is formed into a tube and anastomosed to the pharynx superiorly. The esophageal stump is then anastomosed to the side of the skin tube, and a nasogastric tube is placed through the nose, across the graft, and into the stomach. The inferior aspect of the tube is allowed to remain open (Fig. 22-2). A split-thickness skin graft may be used to cover any remaining raw areas. The inferior portion of the tube is closed, the nasogastric tube removed, and the inferior part of the flap transected 3 to 5 weeks postoperatively.

This is a well-vascularized, full-thickness flap that is available in sufficient length to bridge the defect. In addition, the flap originates on the chest and is therefore not included in the field of irradiation if preoperative treatment is given. A further advantage is that the temporary inferior opening of the tube is below the tracheostomy so that the chance of aspiration is less.

The disadvantages of the use of this flap are that it is bulky and nonperistaltic, a total esophagectomy is not performed, it is a multiple-stage reconstruction, and stenosis and fistula are common complications.[3]

FREE SKIN GRAFTS

The use of a free fascia lata graft sutured around a stent was initially described by Rob and Bateman in 1949.[38] A similar technique using a split-thickness skin graft instead of fascia lata was also described by Edgerton in 1952, Negus in 1952, and Conley in 1953.[10,12,31] The procedure is rarely used.

LARYNGOTRACHEAL AUTOGRAFT

The use of the laryngotracheal autograft was first described by Som in 1956.[42,43] The technique involves retention of the anterior half of the larynx, cricoid, and trachea to form the anterior and lateral walls of the gullet, and a split-thickness skin graft is used to reconstruct the posterior wall (Fig. 22-3).[21] The skin graft is sutured to the pharynx superiorly and to the cervical esophagus inferiorly, and the lateral margins are sutured together over a Som–Negus mold. A nasogastric tube is placed from the nose through the graft and into the stomach. The neck flaps are closed and the nasogastric tube is removed 10 to 12 days postoperatively; the stent is left in place for an additional 4 to 5 weeks.

The advantages of this procedure are that it is a one-stage procedure, it is relatively simple, and part of the gullet is restored using local tissues.

This innovative procedure is rarely applicable since it is suitable only for a relatively small lesion high in the cervical esophagus, with minimal involvement of the larynx.[21] Fistula and stricture may occur but are probably less common than with the Negus mold technique.

FREE GUT GRAFTS

The use of revascularized grafts of either jejunum (McKee and co-workers,[25] Som,[42] Jurkiewicz,[19] Seidenburg and co-workers[40]) or sigmoid colon (Nakayama[30]) has been reported. The technique using the jejunum will be described here. A 10-cm to 14-cm section of bowel is selected, and the direction of peristalsis is noted. The segment is then resected along with its vascular arcade. The mesenteric vessels selected for anastomosis have a luminal diameter of 3 mm to 4 mm. The graft may be perfused with heparinized Ringer's solution, and the vessels are then anastomosed to the superior thyroid artery and internal jugular or common facial vein. The graft is sutured, in an isoperistaltic direction, to the pharynx above and the esophagus below. McKee has used this graft with or without prior perfusion with heparinized Ringer's solution and notes no difference in the results.[25]

The advantages of this method of reconstruction are that the lumen of the graft is roughly the same caliber as the esophagus, the length may be tailored to fit the defect, the resection and reconstruction are completed in a single stage, and fistula and stricture are less likely than when skin flaps are used to reconstruct the defect.

It has been stated that when this method of reconstruction is successful, it is very successful, and when it fails, it is a disaster. The disadvantages of this procedure are that a graft necrosis or an anastomotic leak may result in fatal mediastinitis, the entire esophagus is not resected, revascularization is difficult and time consuming, obstruction of the graft may occur,[7] and bowel is said to be not particularly tolerant of postoperative radiation therapy.[4] However, high-dose irradiation (6500 rad) has been given to a jejunal graft used to reconstruct the pharynx and it

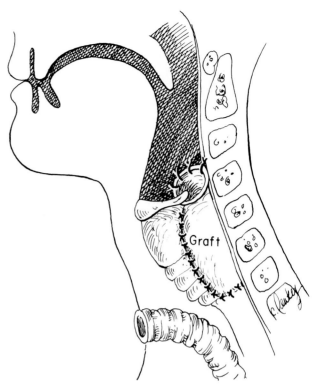

FIG. 22-3. Laryngotracheal autograft.

was observed to function well for several years with preservation of peristaltic activity.

PEDICLED GUT GRAFTS

There are essentially three forms of reconstruction using pedicled gut grafts: (1) transposition of the stomach, (2) reversed gastric tube, and (3) interposition of the colon with or without the terminal ileum. These techniques will be described in turn. The location of the graft may be either antethoracic, retrosternal, or posterior mediastinal. The pros and cons of each of these routes will be discussed later in the text.

Reversed Gastric Tube

Reconstruction using a reversed gastric tube was described by Heimlich.[18] The procedure involves constructing a pedicle tube about 12 inches in length from the greater curvature of the stomach such that the end of the tube is adjacent to the distal portion of the stomach (Fig. 22-4). The tube is then reversed and passed up to the neck, using an antethoracic, retrosternal, or posterior mediastinal route, and anastomosed to the pharynx.

The advantages of this procedure are that the graft has a good blood supply; a long segment of esophagus can be resected; the stomach remains in the abdomen; there is essentially only one anastomosis; the graft may be used in the antethoracic, retrosternal, or posterior mediastinal position; and the operation is completed in one stage.[18]

The disadvantages of this procedure are that necrosis of part of the graft or an anastomotic leak may result in mediastinitis; if the distance to be traversed is too long, the stomach must be moved into the mediastinum; and fistula and stricture may develop at the anastomotic site.[18,35]

Gastric Transposition

Gastric transposition was described by Ong and Lee in 1960[32] and later by LeQuesne and Ranger[23] and by Harrison.[16] The technique entails mobilization of the stomach with preservation of the right gastric and gastroepiploic vessels. The stomach is then transposed superiorly, usually through the posterior mediastinum, and the fundus is anastomosed to the pharynx (Fig. 22-5).[16]

The advantages of this technique are that it is completed in one stage, it has only one anastomosis and that is in the neck, the entire esophagus is usually resected, and the stomach has an excellent blood supply.[32] This is one of the more commonly employed techniques.

The disadvantages of this procedure are that there is regurgitation; the gastric juices tend to ulcerate adjacent pharyngeal mucosa; the stomach is dislocated from its normal location, so that nutrition may be impaired;[7] the bowel is not very tolerant of postoperative radiation therapy;[4] and postoperative mortality is approximately 10%.[23]

Colon Interposition

The use of colon to replace the esophagus was initially described independently by Kelling and by Vulliet in 1911.[20,49] Various parts of the colon and/or small bowel have been used; the technique that employs the right colon will be described here.[6,14] A laparotomy is performed after it is apparent that resection of the tumor is possible. The ascending colon is mobilized and its vascular pedicle preserved. The gut is transected at the cecum and the transverse colon. The cecum is then passed superiorly, by way of the antethoracic, retrosternal, or posterior mediastinal route, and is anastomosed to the pharynx and stomach. The transverse colon is anastomosed to the ileum, and a pyloroplasty is performed if the vagus nerves have been transected (Fig. 22-6).

The advantages of this technique are that it is completed in one stage, the colon is available in sufficient length that there should be no tension on the anastomosis, the caliber of the colon is sufficient for adequate swallowing, the colon is able to withstand regurgitation of the gastric juices, and the stomach is retained in its normal position.[6]

The disadvantages of this operation are that the blood supply of the graft is less dependable than that of the stomach; there are multiple anastomoses, and an anastomotic leak may result in fatal peritonitis or mediastinitis; the graft has a tendency to dilate; the chances of infection are higher than with use of the stomach; the grafted colon is a passive conduit;[6,7] the bowel does not tolerate postoperative radiation therapy well;[4] the entire esophagus is not always resected;[22] and the postoperative mortality is approximately 20%.

CHOICE OF LOCATION OF GUT GRAFT

The location of gut graft will be either antethoracic, retrosternal, or posterior mediastinal. The advantages and disadvantages of each of these routes will be discussed in turn.

Antethoracic

The major advantage of the antethoracic route is that

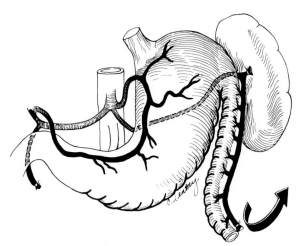

FIG. 22-4. Reversed gastric tube.

FIG. 22-5. Gastric transposition (*A*, mobilization; *B*, pyloroplasty; *C*, transection at esophagogastric junction; *D*, anastomosis to pharynx)

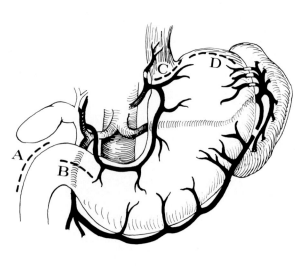

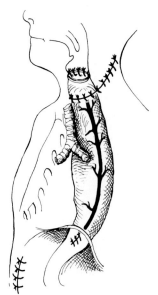

it is the safest location available. It is not necessary to enter the thorax, and a breakdown in anastomosis is readily accessible and should not result in mediastinitis.[6,14] Disadvantages are that it is longer, it results in a bulge on the chest wall, food must be milked through the graft, and the blood supply may be impaired by angulation over the costal margin.[7]

Retrosternal

The advantages of the retrosternal procedure are that it is cosmetically more appealing than the antethoracic route, it is more convenient to anastomose inferiorly, and incision of the pleura is not required.[6,7] The disadvantages of this location are that the bowel still emerges somewhat anteriorly and the blood supply may be embarrassed as the gut passes out of the thoracic inlet (which may require resection of the manubrium and medial clavicle[s]).[6,7]

Posterior Mediastinal

The advantages of the posterior mediastinal route are that it is the shortest route, it allows resection of the entire esophagus, and the vascular pedicle is more easily advanced.[7] The disadvantages are that it requires thoracotomy and is associated with the highest mortality and morbidity.[7]

PALLIATIVE PROCEDURES

The goal of palliation is to allow the patient to swallow his secretions and enough liquids to maintain adequate nutrition. The simplest way to achieve this palliative result is with a short course of palliative radiation therapy (e.g., 3000 rad/2 weeks). Radiation therapy fails to achieve the desired result in approximately 50% of cases, and some form of palliative operation must be considered. The use of Celestin stents in lesions of the cervical esophagus is rarely successful with regard to obtaining meaningful palliation.[7] Gastrostomy is useful in providing a means of internal alimentation but does nothing to treat the obstruction, which may result in aspiration of salivary secretions. Pyriformostomy may be used to reduce aspiration, but tracheostomy is frequently necessary. The use of any or all of these techniques is indicated in the patient who does not respond to a short course of palliative radiation therapy.

Radiation Therapy

Radiation therapy has been used in carcinoma of the cervical esophagus since the 1920s with results similar to those of surgery.[24] The introduction of megavoltage equipment in the 1950s allowed higher doses to be given with fewer complications and with a modest improvement in treatment results.[33]

TREATMENT PLANNING

The treatment planning for carcinoma of the upper esophagus represents one of the greatest technical challenges to the radiation therapist. The esophagus lies only 2 cm to 3 cm anterior to the spinal cord. Treatment planning includes the lower neck and upper thorax, which have dissimilar shapes and thicknesses, and the esophagus does not pursue a constant course in relation to the skin surfaces. In ad-

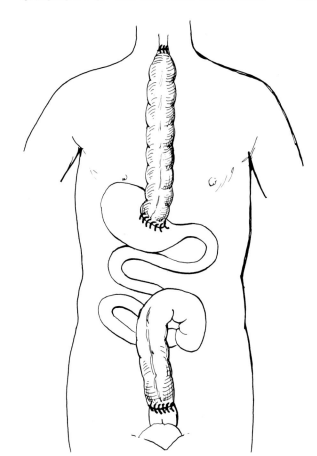

FIG. 22-6. Colon interposition.

dition, the lymph nodes at risk must be incorporated into the irregular treatment volume.

FIELD ARRANGEMENT

Parallel opposed lateral portals are suitable for a small lesion high in the cervical esophagus, but since most lesions are advanced, it is necessary to use some other arrangement because of the long diameter through the shoulders.

Paired anterior wedged fields and the three-field technique (anterior field and two posterior oblique fields) have the disadvantage of requiring complex angles and complex compensators on the oblique fields because the axis of the esophagus is not parallel to the axis of the body. In addition, it is difficult to interpret oblique port films. This is particularly problematic when reducing off the spinal cord.

A four-field box technique has been adopted at the University of Florida that consists of an anterior, a posterior, and parallel opposed lateral portals (Fig. 22-7).[27] Beeswax is used to fill the gap created by the deficit of tissues above the shoulder; it thus serves as a compensator (Fig. 22-8).[27] The advantages of this arrangement are that the dose to the spinal cord can be accurately calculated; the likelihood of hot or cold spots is minimized; port films may be more easily interpreted since the beams are not angled; the calculation of tumor doses is more precise; the field reductions are relatively simple; and contoured Cerrobend blocks may be designed so that the neck and mediastinal nodes may be included without a major increase in treatment volume. The disadvantage of this technique is that one must treat

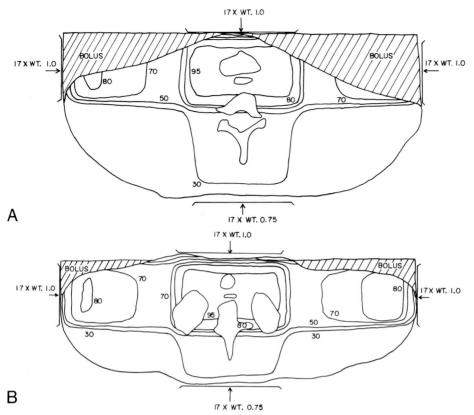

FIG. 22-7. Isodose curves for four-field box technique using 17-MV x-ray beam. (*A*) Section at level of C6 vertebra. (*B*) Section at level of T2 vertebra. (Reprinted with permission from Mendenhall WM, Million RR, Bova FJ: Carcinoma of the cervical esophagus treated with radiation therapy using a four-field box technique. Int J Radiat Oncol Biol Phys 8:1435–1439, 1982. Copyright © 1982, Pergamon Press, Ltd.)

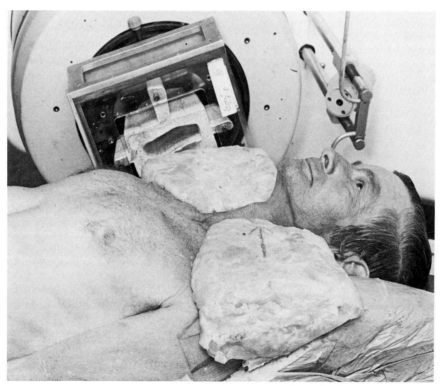

FIG. 22-8. Patient in position for treatment of right lateral portal. Note beeswax bolus, Cerrobend blocks, and foam body mold. The portal is set up by an isocentric method. The beeswax bolus is placed in position after the portal is aligned. The lateral portal should be checked frequently by imaging films. A strip of neck skin anterior to the thyroid cartilage can sometimes be spared and is shielded to reduce tangential irradiation of the skin and subcutaneous tissue and to decrease the likelihood of lymphedema. (Reprinted with permission from Mendenhall WM, Million RR, Bova FJ: Carcinoma of the cervical esophagus treated with radiation therapy using a four-field box technique. Int J Radiat Oncol Biol Phys 8:1435–1439, 1982. Copyright © 1982, Pergamon Press, Ltd.)

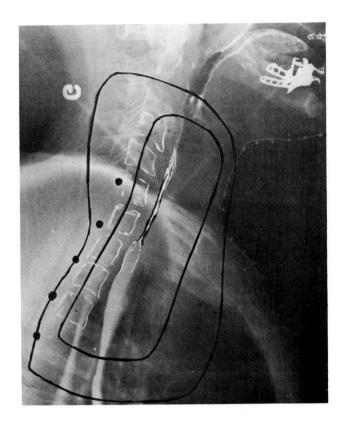

FIG. 22-9. Lateral and reduced lateral portals for a cancer of the cervical esophagus located at the inlet. A second and final reduction would just cover the gross lesion. The initial border is generous due to inability to evaluate the mediastinal nodes by palpation. The initial lateral portal bows posteriorly on its superior aspect to cover the posterior cervical nodes and bows anteriorly on its inferior aspect to cover the anterior mediastinal nodes. Note the proximity of the spinal cord to the esophagus. For this patient, it is 2.0 cm to 2.5 cm from the posterior wall of the esophagus to the anterior portion of the cervical spinal cord and about 3.0 cm to the thoracic spinal cord. Black dots mark the posterior aspect of the vertebral bodies. Solder wire with lead shot spaced at 1-cm intervals outlines the midline anterior skin surface. (Reprinted with permission from Mendenhall WM, Million RR, Bova FJ: Carcinoma of the cervical esophagus treated with radiation therapy using a four-field box technique. Int J Radiat Oncol Biol Phys 8:1435–1439, 1982. Copyright © 1982, Pergamon Press, Ltd.)

through the shoulders and apex of the lung so that the availability of high-energy x-rays, while not mandatory, is advantageous. (The lateral dimensions through the shoulder are similar to those through the pelvis, and there is extensive experience with the four-field box technique to irradiate pelvic lesions.) The margin of error on the lateral portals after reduction from the spinal cord is quite a fine line and requires careful attention to detail but so does any alternative method.

As an example, a typical course of radiation therapy for a carcinoma of the cervical esophagus would consist of 4500 rad/5 weeks using a four-field box technique to include the primary lesion and the regional lymph nodes. The anterior and posterior portals are discontinued, the lateral portals are redesigned to exclude the spinal cord, and the treatment is continued using parallel opposed lateral fields for an additional 2500 rad to 3000 rad (Fig. 22-9).[27]

LYMPH NODE TREATMENT

Lymph nodes at risk include the paraesophageal; paratracheal; upper, middle, and lower internal jugular chain; supraclavicular; spinal accessory; and upper mediastinal. I have observed two patients who developed lymph nodes in the upper neck above the irradiation portal. The entire neck on both sides is now included. The upper neck is at special risk when the pyriform sinus or postcricoid area is involved, or when there are clinically positive lymph nodes in the lower neck. It is possible to treat the upper neck lymph nodes through a separate en *face* portal with a midline shield in order to reduce mucosal and spinal cord irradiation.

If the patient has no clinically apparent adenopathy, the lymph nodes are treated electively with a dose of 4500 rad to 5000 rad/5 weeks. Small positive lymph nodes, 2.0 cm in diameter, may be treated by radiation therapy alone. Larger lymph nodes are best managed by a combined approach consisting of radiation therapy directed to the primary tumor and regional lymphatics followed by a neck dissection on the side involved. The conventional radical neck dissection does not resect all the nodes at risk and should not be relied on as a single mode of treatment.

SIMULATION

The patient is placed in the supine position with head and thorax in a customized foam mold to maximize setup reproducibility. A bite block may be used to assist in immobilizing the head. Simulation films are obtained with addition of a contrast medium to ascertain the exact location of the lesion, and the anterior aspect of the neck is outlined with wire (see Fig. 22-9).[27] Treatment portals are outlined and Cerrobend blocks are constructed. The superior and inferior borders of the field are arranged so that there is a 5-cm margin on the tumor, the extent of which is defined by barium swallow, indirect laryngoscopy, and esophagoscopy. The superior border may be somewhat more generous in the unlikely event that there are clinically positive lymph nodes in the upper neck. The cervical portion of the spinal cord is included in the initial fields to gain an adequate posterior margin beyond the tumor and to treat the lymph nodes in the neck. The thoracic portion of the spinal cord is included in the field primarily to gain an adequate margin beyond the esophageal lesion. Tattoos are used to mark the anterior source-to-skin dis-

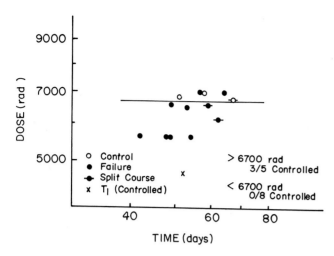

FIG. 22-10. Analysis of time-dose factors. Fourteen patients were evaluable for local control. Excluding the T1 lesion that was cured with 4750 rad, there were no controls below 6700 rad. (Two patients died of intercurrent disease less than 2 years after treatment without recurrence and were not evaluable.) (Reprinted with permission from Mendenhall WM, Million RR, Bova FJ: Carcinoma of the cervical esophagus treated with radiation therapy using a four-field box technique. Int J Radiat Oncol Biol Phys 8:1435–1439, 1982. Copyright © 1982, Pergamon Press, Ltd.)

tance and the field corners to ensure reproducibility in the event that the lines are inadvertently removed by the patient. All portals are set up daily from the anterior tattoo, and the treatment technique is isocentric. One cannot rely entirely on ink lines or tattoos to ensure daily reproducibility of the reduced lateral portals. *Imaging films are obtained daily in the lateral fields to ensure accurate treatment setup, particularly when the fields are reduced off of the spinal cord.*

DOSE

The large size of the initial treatment portals and the patient's poor nutritional status predict acute morbidity. Treatment is usually initiated at 180 rad/fraction and, if possible, the daily dose is increased to 200 rad/fraction once the portals are reduced in size, but only if the patient is tolerating the treatment and maintaining nutrition. The final tumor dose is 7000 rad to 7500 rad over 8 to 9 weeks. Field reductions are usually made at 4500 rad to 5000 rad and again at 6000 and 7000 rad. A time-dose analysis of 14 patients treated at the University of Florida with radiation therapy is shown in Fig. 22-10.[27] Twelve patients were treated primarily by irradiation (T1, 1 patient; T2, 3 patients; T3, 8 patients), and 2 patients underwent attempted resection but had gross residual tumor remaining after the operation and subsequently received postoperative irradiation. All patients had a minimum 2-year follow-up. There were no cures with less than 6700 rad except for the single T1 lesion.

PALLIATIVE RADIATION THERAPY

Patients with esophageal cancer almost always present with dysphagia, so that even if treatment is not expected to be curative, some sort of palliative treatment is indicated. Radiation therapy is the simplest noninvasive treatment and is usually the initial palliative step. The dose most often selected is 3000 rad/2 weeks or 2000 rad/2 fractions given 1 week apart using parallel opposed anterior and posterior portals. Tumor regression may appear within a few days, allowing the patient to swallow secretions and maintain nutrition. Approximately 50% of patients with advanced obstructive lesions will get useful palliation. Gastrostomy and pyriformostomy can usually be held in reserve for 2 to 3 weeks to observe the results of radiation therapy.

ACUTE AND LATE RADIATION SEQUELAE AND COMPLICATIONS

ACUTE

The major acute side-effect of radiation therapy is radiation esophagitis, which usually appears after 2 weeks of treatment, then plateaus or improves slightly during therapy, and finally resolves 3 to 4 weeks after the completion of treatment. It may be managed symptomatically with acetaminophen (Tylenol) elixir or Aspergum. Split-course irradiation will result in decreased severity of esophagitis, but it has been shown to also result in a lower cure rate in other head and neck cancers and is used only if necessary.

The patient will note erythema of the skin, which may progress to dry desquamation toward the end of treatment. Patches of moist desquamation are unusual.

Moderate xerostomia and loss of taste may be noted in the patient whose upper neck is irradiated. Taste generally begins to improve 1 to 2 months after treatment is completed and eventually reverts to near normal. Permanent xerostomia is usually absent or mild with this treatment since the parotid glands are not irradiated.

A mild, roentgenographic radiation pneumonitis may develop if the apex of the lung is included in the treatment volume. However, the apex is relatively resistant to developing symptomatic radiation pneumonitis. The course is usually self-limited and rarely requires treatment. The patient may notice a mild, dry cough 2 to 3 months after completion of treatment. The most serious acute treatment complication occurs when the tumor has invaded the trachea or a major blood vessel and, as it regresses, opens a fistula. This results in aspiration or hemorrhage, either of which may be fatal. If this complication is anticipated, slow fractionation and split course may help avoid the catastrophe. Tracheoesophageal fistula could occur if the tumor invades through the tracheal wall.

LATE

One of the late sequelae of radiation therapy is fibrosis, which may occur in any tissue included in the irradiated volume, specifically the skin, lung, and esophagus. Fibrosis of the lung, when it occurs, fortunately involves the lung apices, which contribute least to pulmonary function, and rarely results in symptoms. Fibrosis of the esophagus, usually at the site of the tumor, may result in a stricture, which could require periodic bougienage. Almost all successfully irradiated patients have a persistent narrowing on roentgenographic examination. These patients usually must alter their eating habits, but they can maintain adequate nutrition.

Another sequela of radiation therapy is Lhermitte's syndrome (see Chapter 14, The Effect of Radiation on Normal

Tissues of the Head and Neck), which usually becomes manifest 2 to 3 months after treatment and may last from several weeks to several months. The most severe late complication of radiation therapy is radiation myelitis. Hypothyroidism may occur since the entire gland is irradiated.

Chemotherapy

Cancer of the esophagus has been noted to respond, at times impressively, to some of the drugs commonly used for squamous cell carcinomas of the head and neck. There is no evidence at present, however, that indicates that chemotherapy, alone or in combination with other treatment modalities, improves the cure rate of patients with esophageal cancer.

Combined Treatment Policies

Combined radiation therapy and surgery is sometimes employed for carcinoma of the cervical esophagus.[15,21,29] After surgery there is usually a prolonged period of time before postoperative irradiation may be initiated. Preoperative irradiation plus surgery is associated with a high incidence of complications.

Management of Recurrence

Recurrence of tumor after definitive treatment is the rule rather than the exception in cancer of the cervical esophagus. Recurrence is usually at the primary site or in the regional lymph nodes and rarely will occur in distant sites alone. The consideration of radical treatment for recurrence at the primary site is usually out of the question, and palliative procedures, such as those previously described, are indicated. Ipsilateral recurrence in the lymph nodes of the neck, a rare occurrence, could be treated by a radical neck dissection with some hope of salvage.

RESULTS OF TREATMENT

Sixteen patients have been treated at the University of Florida with curative intent with irradiation. Local control of the disease was obtained in 4 of 16 patients, and survival analysis showed that these 4 patients were alive without evidence of cancer at 33, 47, 55, and 80 months. Two patients died of intercurrent disease at 4 and 15 months, and the remainder died of cancer.

The interpretation of treatment results in cancer of the cervical esophagus is hampered by several factors: the rar-

TABLE 22-1.   Results of Treatment by Surgery Alone

Study	No. Patients	Treatment	Results
Burdette and Jesse, M. D. Anderson Hospital, 1972[7]	10	Visceral subsitution	4/10 alive at 9 to 46 months
	12	Staged with skin flaps	2/12 alive at 22 months and 46 months
Goodner, Sloan-Kettering Institute, 1928–1968[15]	14	Surgery—various techniques	2/14 alive at 16 years and 20 years
Ballantyne, M. D. Anderson Hospital, 1971[4]	12	Flaps or skin grafts	5/12 alive at more than 5 years
Negus,* London, 1952[31]	5	Skin grafts	3/5 alive at 27 to 42 months*
Rob and Bateman, St. Thomas Hospital, 1949[38]	3	Skin grafts	0/3 alive
Harrison,† London, 1964–1970[17]	35	Gastric transposition	4/18 alive at 2 years and 2/13 alive at 3 years
Brain and Reading, Guy's Hospital, 1959–1965[6]	3	Colon interposition	0/3 alive
Postlethwait, Duke University Hospital, 1979[35]	4	Reversed gastric tube	4/4 alive at 5 to 39 months
Mustard,‡ Toronto, 1934–1959[28]	15	Wookey procedure	3/15 alive at 5 years
Pearson, Edinburgh, 1931–1967[34]	14	Various surgical procedures	3/14 alive at 5 years

* Selected series.
† Combined postcricoid and cervical esophagus; excludes six patients as having unresectable disease.
‡ Patients with small lesions; selected series.

TABLE 22-2.   Results of Treatment With Radiation Therapy Alone

Study	No. Patients	Technique	Dose	Results
Burdette and Jesse, M. D. Anderson Hospital, 1972[7]	9	Not specified	3000 rad/3 weeks to 6000 rad/7 weeks	1/9 alive at 14 months
Goodner, Sloan-Kettering Institute, 1928–1968[15]	36	175 to 250 kV or radium pack	Not specified	2/36 alive at more than 5 years
Pearson, Edinburgh, 1931–1967[34]	31	Supervoltage: anterior oblique wedged fields	5000 rad/4 weeks	7/31 alive at 5 years
Lederman,* London, 1967[21]	244	200 kV Supervoltage	4500–5500 rad/6 to 8 weeks 6000–7000 rad/6 to 8 weeks	19/244 alive at 5 years
Wara and co-workers, San Francisco, 1950–1973[51]	40	Not specified	5000–6000 rad/6 to 8 weeks	3/40 alive at more than 2 years
Rider and Mendoza, Toronto, 1950–1964[37]	5 3 39	200–400 kV Cobalt-60 + radium bougie Cobalt-60	6000 rad/35 days 7000 rad/28 days 6500 rad/42 days	0/5 alive at 3 years 0/3 alive at 3 years 4/39 alive at 3 years
Walker, Seattle, 1957–1963[50]	9	Cobalt-60	6000–6500 rad/6 weeks	3/9 alive at 2 and 5 years (one patient not specified)
Buschke and Cantril, Seattle, 1940–1952[8]	4	Supervoltage	6000–6500 rad/5 to 7 weeks	1/4 alive at 12 years
Marcial and co-workers,† Puerto Rico, 1966[26]	10	Supervoltage	6500–7000 rad/7 to 8 weeks	2/10 alive at 5 years
Mendenhall and co-workers, University of Florida, 1982[27]	16	Supervoltage	See text	4/16 alive at 33, 48, 55, and 80 months‡

* Report combines postcricoid and cervical esophagus tumors.
† Includes only those who completed treatment.
‡ Two dead of intercurrent disease at 4 and 15 months.

ity of the disease, the tendency to lump results with those of other sites such as the hypopharynx or the remainder of the esophagus, the failure to stage the lesions, and the tendency to report primarily on treatment technique in patients with inadequate follow-up (less than 2 years). Treatment results are presented from series treated by surgery, by radiation therapy, and by a combination of the two in Tables 22-1 through 22-3. A cure rate of 10% to 20% with adequate follow-up is consistent with most reported series, regardless of whether the patient is treated surgically, with irradiation, or with a combination of modalities.

STANDARD FOLLOW-UP POLICY

The main purpose of follow-up for cancer of the cervical esophagus is primarily to deal with treatment complications and to pick up second primary cancers in the head and neck area; salvage of radiation therapy or surgical failures is not likely except for the very early lesion. Follow-up examination includes a barium swallow, especially for those patients in whom salvage treatment is a possibility. Obstructive symptoms after radiation therapy may be due to tumor or fibrosis. Serial studies help differentiate the two. Esophagoscopy may be required to distinguish the cause. Careful dilatation may improve a stricture.

TABLE 22-3.   Results of Combined Surgery and Radiation Therapy

Study	No. Patients	Technique	Results
Burdette and Jesse, M. D. Anderson Hospital, 1972[7]	3	Surgery plus postoperative irradiation	1/3 alive at 29 months
Negus,* London, 1952[31]	5	Surgery plus postoperative irradiation	2/5 alive at 1 year
Goodner, Sloan-Kettering Institute, 1928–1968[15]	28	Surgery and irradiation (preoperative and postoperative)	4/28 alive at more than 5 years
Lederman, London, 1967[21]	24	Preoperative irradiation plus surgery	1/24 alive at 5 years
Adams and Smedal, Lahey Clinic, 1955[1]	2	6000 rad/35 days (supervoltage) plus resection	1/2 alive at 8 months

* Selected series.

REFERENCES

1. Adams HD, Smedal MI: Symposium on surgery of digestive tract: Treatment of carcinoma of the esophagus by resection and postoperative supervoltage roentgen therapy. Surg Clin North Am 35:647–652, 1955
2. American Joint Committee on Cancer: Manual for Staging of Cancer, 2nd ed, p 62. Philadelphia, JB Lippincott, 1983
3. Bakamjian VY: A two-stage method for pharyngoesophageal reconstruction with a primary pectoral skin flap. Plast Reconstr Surg 36:173–184, 1965
4. Ballantyne AJ: Methods of repair after surgery for cancer of the pharyngeal wall, postcricoid area, and cervical esophagus. Am J Surg 122:482–486, 1971
5. Beale LS: The Microscope in Medicine, 2nd ed. London, JA Churchill, 1858
6. Brain RHF, Reading PV: Colon transplantation into the pharynx and cervical esophagus. Br J Surg 53:933–942, 1966
7. Burdette WJ, Jesse R: Carcinoma of the cervical esophagus. J Thorac Cardiovasc Surg 63:41–53, 1972
8. Buschke F, Cantril ST: Results of supervoltage roentgenotherapy of esophageal carcinoma. J Thorac Surg 26:105–108, 1953
9. Colledge L: In discussion of C von Eicken: Malignant disease of the hypopharynx. J Laryngol Otol 47:261–263, 1932
10. Conley JJ: One-stage radical resection of cervical esophagus, larynx, pharynx, and lateral neck with immediate reconstruction. Arch Otolaryngol 58:645–654, 1953
11. Del Regato JA, Spjut JH: Ackerman and del Regato's Cancer: Diagnosis, Treatment, and Prognosis, 5th ed, p 450. St. Louis, CV Mosby, 1977
12. Edgerton MT: One stage reconstruction of the cervical esophagus or trachea. Surgery 31:239–250, 1952
13. Eggers C: Carcinoma of the upper esophagus and pharynx. Ann Surg 81:695–698, 1925
14. Goligher JC, Robin IG: Use of left colon for reconstruction of pharynx and oesophagus after pharyngectomy. Br J Surg 42:283–290, 1954
15. Goodner JT: Treatment and survival in cancer of the cervical esophagus. Am J Surg 118:673–675, 1969
16. Harrison DFN: Surgical management of cancer of the hypopharynx and cervical esophagus. Br J Surg 56:95–103, 1969
17. Harrison DFN: Role of surgery in the management of postcricoid and cervical esophageal neoplasms. Ann Otol Rhinol Laryngol 81:465–468, 1972

18. Heimlich HJ: Carcinoma of the cervical esophagus. J Thorac Cardiovasc Surg 59:309–318, 1970
19. Jurkiewicz MJ: Vascularized intestinal graft for reconstruction of the cervical esophagus and pharynx. Plast Reconstr Surg 36:509–517, 1965
20. Kelling G: Ösophagoplastik mit Hilfe des Querkolon. Zentralbl Chir 38:1209–1212, 1911
21. Lederman M: Role of irradiation in treatment of cancer of the hypopharynx, postcricoid and cervical esophagus. In Conley J (ed): Cancer of the Head and Neck, pp 347–356. Washington, DC, Butterworth, 1967
22. Leonard JR, Maran AGD: Reconstruction of the cervical esophagus via gastric anastomosis. Laryngoscope 80:849–862, 1970
23. LeQuesne LP, Ranger D: Pharyngolaryngectomy with immediate pharyngogastric anastomosis. Br J Surg 53:105–109, 1966
24. MacComb WS, Healey JE Jr, McGraw JP, Fletcher GH, Gallager HS, Paulus DD: Hypopharynx and cervical esophagus. In MacComb WS, Fletcher GH (eds): Cancer of the Head and Neck, pp 213–240. Baltimore, Williams & Wilkins, 1967
25. McKee DM, Peters CR: Reconstruction of the hypopharynx and cervical esophagus with microvascular jejunal transplant. Clin Plast Surg 5:305–312, 1978
26. Marcial VA, Tome JM, Ubinas J, Bosch A, Correa JN: The role of radiation therapy in esophageal cancer. Radiology 87:231–239, 1966
27. Mendenhall WM, Million RR, Bova FJ: Carcinoma of the cervical esophagus treated with radiation therapy using a four-field box technique. Int J Radiat Oncol Biol Phys 8:1435–1439, 1982
28. Mustard RA: The use of the Wookey operation for carcinoma of the hypopharynx and cervical esophagus. Surg Gynecol Obstet 111:577–592, 1960
29. Nakayama K: Preoperative irradiation in the treatment of patients with carcinoma of the oesophagus and of some other sites. Clin Radiol 15:232–241, 1964
30. Nakayama K, Yamamoto K, Tamiya T, Makino H: Vascular reconstruction in esophageal surgery, with special reference to autografting. J Int Coll Surg 38:358–371, 1962
31. Negus VE: Reconstruction of pharynx after pharyngoesophagolaryngectomy. Br J Plast Surg 6:99–101, 1952
32. Ong GB, Lee TC: Pharyngogastric anastomosis after oesopha-

gopharyngectomy for carcinoma of the hypopharynx and cervical oesophagus. Br J Surg 48:193–200, 1960

33. Pearson JG: The radiotherapy of carcinoma of the esophagus and postcricoid region in southeast Scotland. Clin Radiol 17:242–257, 1966

34. Pearson JG: The value of radiotherapy in the management of esophageal cancer. Am J Roentgenol Radium Ther Nucl Med 105:500–513, 1969

35. Postlethwait RW: Technique for isoperistaltic gastric tube for esophageal bypass. Ann Surg 189:673–676, 1979

36. Prolla JC, Taebel DW, Kirsner JB: Current studies of exfoliative cytology in diagnosis of malignant neoplasms of the esophagus. Surg Gynecol Obstet 121:743–752, 1965

37. Rider WD, Mendoza RD: Some opinions on treatment of cancer of the esophagus. Am J Roentgenol Radium Ther Nucl Med 105:514–517, 1969

38. Rob CG, Bateman GH: Reconstruction of the trachea and cervical esophagus: Preliminary report. Br J Surg 37:202–205, 1949

39. Rubin P: Cancer of the gastrointestinal tract: I. Esophagus: Detection and diagnosis. JAMA 226:1544–1546, 1973

40. Seidenberg B, Rosenak SS, Hurwitt ES, Som ML: Immediate reconstruction of the cervical esophagus by a revascularized isolated jejunal segment. Ann Surg 149:162–171, 1959

41. Shaw HJ: Repair of the laryngopharynx and cervical esophagus after irradiation. Br J Surg 59:524–532, 1972

42. Som ML: Laryngoesophagectomy: Primary closure with laryngotracheal autograft. Arch Otolaryngol 63:474–480, 1956

43. Som ML: Rehabilitation of the gullet after laryngoesophagectomy. In Conley J (ed): Cancer of the Head and Neck, pp 357–363. Washington, DC, Butterworth, 1967

44. Strawberry CW, de Fries HO, Deeb ZE: Reconstruction of the hypopharynx and cervical esophagus with bilateral pectoralis major myocutaneous flaps. Head Neck Surg 4:161–164, 1981

45. Torek F: The first successful resection of the thoracic portion of the esophagus for carcinoma. JAMA 60:1533–1534, 1913

46. Trotter W: Principles and technique of the operative treatment of malignant disease of the mouth and pharynx. (Hunterian lecture). Lancet 1:1075–1081, 1913

47. Trotter W: Treatment by excision. In discussion of C von Eicken: Malignant disease of the hypopharynx. J Laryngol Otol 47:252–258, 1932

48. Turner CG: Carcinoma of the oesophagus: The question of its treatment by surgery. Lancet 230:130–134, 1936

49. Vulliet H: De l'oesophageoplastic et des modifications. Sem Méd 31:529, 1911

50. Walker JH: Carcinoma of the esophagus: Cobalt-60 teletherapy: Experience and comparison with surgical results. Am J Roentgenol Radium Ther Nucl Med 92:67–76, 1964

51. Wara WM, Mauch PM, Thomas AN, Phillips TL: Palliation for carcinoma of the esophagus. Radiology 121:717–720, 1976

52. Wookey H: Surgical treatment of carcinoma of the pharynx and upper esophagus. Surg Gynecol Obstet 75:499–506, 1942

53. Wookey H: The surgical treatment of carcinoma of the hypopharynx and esophagus. Br J Surg 35:249–266, 1948

Nasal Vestibule, Nasal Cavity, and Paranasal Sinuses

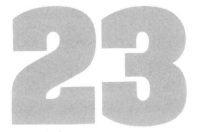

RODNEY R. MILLION

NICHOLAS J. CASSISI

DEREK J. HAMLIN

Tumors of the nasal vestibule, the anterior entrance to the nasal cavity, are considered separately from nasal cavity tumors because they are essentially skin cancers and have a different natural history.

Primary tumors arising from the nasal cavity and paranasal sinuses are considered together because the lesions are frequently rather advanced when first seen and it is not always possible to determine the site of origin with certainty. Primary lesions of the lower half of the maxillary sinus can usually be identified as such.

Cancer of the nasal cavity or paranasal sinuses is a relatively rare problem with a yearly risk factor estimated at approximately 1 case for every 100,000 people. These cancers occur more often in males (2:1) and usually appear after the age of 40 except for an occasional tumor of minor salivary gland origin or esthesioneuroblastoma that may appear before the age of 20.

Nasal cavity and ethmoid sinus adenocarcinomas have been linked to occupations associated with wood dust: the furniture industry, sawmill work, and carpentry.[2–4] Other dusty occupations such as bootmaking and shoemaking, baking, and the flour milling industry have also been implicated as a cause of adenocarcinoma.

Thorotrast is a known etiologic agent in maxillary sinus carcinomas. Thorotrast, containing the radioactive metal thorium, was used in past years as a contrast medium for roentgenographic study of the maxillary sinuses. The Thorotrast was retained in the sinus and was responsible for tumor induction.

Primary carcinomas of the sphenoid sinuses are rare. They mimic nasopharyngeal carcinoma and are most often diagnosed only after they penetrate to the nasopharynx.

Frontal sinus neoplasms are also rare.

ANATOMY

Nasal Vestibule

The nasal vestibule is the entrance to the nasal cavity. It is lined by skin in which there are numerous hair follicles and sebaceous glands. Each vestibule is a three-sided, pear-shaped cavity 1.5 cm to 2.0 cm in diameter that is surrounded by the lower lateral (alar) cartilage. The vestibule ends posteriorly at the limen nasi, the junction of the lower and upper lateral cartilages (Figs. 23-1 and 23-2). The medial wall is the mobile columella, formed by the medial wing of the alar cartilage and the anterior portion of the cartilagenous septum. The floor is less than 1 cm in length.

Nasal Cavity and Paranasal Sinuses

NASAL CAVITY

The nasal cavity begins at the limen nasi (the transition from skin to mucosa) and ends at the posterior nares, where it communicates directly with the nasopharynx. The composition of the midline septum and the bones and

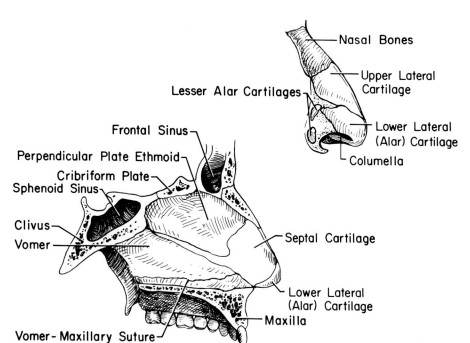

FIG. 23-1. Relationship of the bones and cartilages of the nose. (Million RR, Cassisi NJ: Cancer in the head and neck. In DeVita VT Jr, Hellman S, Rosenberg SA [eds]: Cancer: Principles and Practice of Oncology, p 370. Philadelphia, JB Lippincott, 1982)

FIG. 23-2. Coronal whole-organ section through the vestibule. The upper lateral alar cartilages fuse with the cartilaginous septum. The nasal bones overlap the cartilages. The limen vestibuli is the junction of the upper and lower lateral cartilages. (Bridger WM, van Nostrand P: The nose and paranasal sinuses—applied surgical anatomy. J Otolaryngol 7[suppl 6]:1–33, 1978)

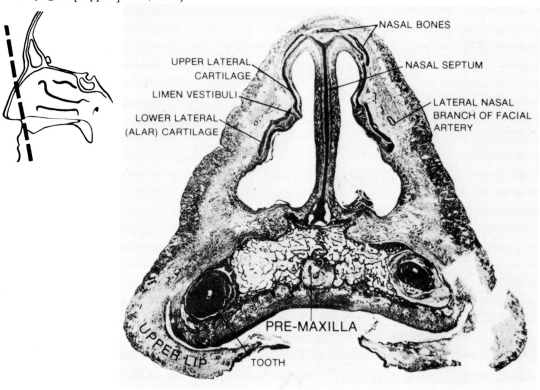

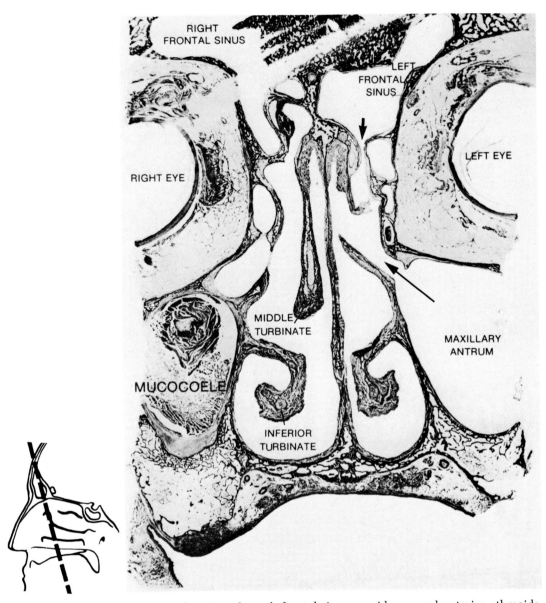

FIG. 23-3. Coronal section through frontal sinuses, midnose, and anterior ethmoids. Note left frontonasal duct and ostium of the left maxillary antrum, which open into the middle meatus. The middle turbinate appears to arise from the "roof" of the nasal cavity near the septum, which is the appearance during physical examination. (Bridger WM, van Nostrand P: The nose and paranasal sinuses—applied surgical anatomy. J Otolaryngol 7[suppl 6]:1–33, 1978)

cartilages that compose the roof and sides of the external nose are shown in Figure 23-1. Whole-organ sections of the nasal cavity and adjacent sinuses are shown in Figures 23-3 through 23-6. Each lateral wall is composed of thin bony folds that project into the nasal cavity. These are the inferior, middle, and superior nasal turbinates. The nasolacrimal duct enters the nasal cavity beneath the inferior turbinate. The frontal sinus and ethmoid bullae connect to the nasal cavity with openings into the middle meatus. The sphenoid sinus communicates with the nasal cavity by an opening on the anterior wall of the sphenoid sinus. (See Fig. 24-7 in Chapter 24, Nasopharynx.) The olfactory nerves enter the nasal cavity through the cribriform plate and distribute nerve fibers over the upper one third of the septum and superior nasal turbinate. Approximately 20 branches of the olfactory nerve penetrate the cribriform plate, and these perforations provide an avenue of tumor spread to the floor of the anterior cranial fossa (see Fig. 23-4). The olfactory epithelium is tall, pseudostratified, and columnar with highly specialized cilia. The lower half of the nasal cavity is the respiratory portion, and the epithelium is ciliated columnar. There are numerous collections of lymphoid tissue and mucous glands beneath the epithelium.

(Text continues on p. 412.)

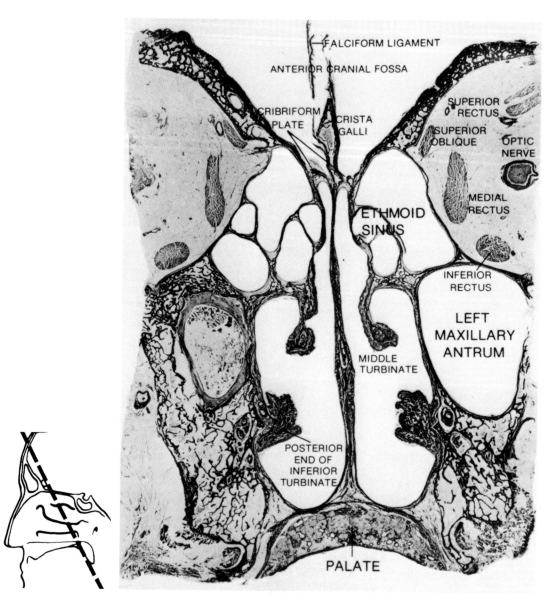

FIG. 23-4. Coronal section through the cribriform plate, middle ethmoid sinuses, and posterior inferior turbinates. Note the thinness of the walls separating sinuses from the orbits and nasal cavity. The right and left ethmoid sinuses are completely separated at all levels by the septum. The ethmoid cells may extend laterally above the orbits. (Bridger WM, van Nostrand P: The nose and paranasal sinuses—applied surgical anatomy. J Otolaryngol 7[suppl 6]:1–33, 1978)

FIG. 23-5. Coronal section just behind the maxillary antrum and just anterior to the ▶ sphenoid sinus and nasopharynx. Note relationships in the pterygopalatine fossa. (Bridger WM, van Nostrand P: The nose and paranasal sinuses—applied surgical anatomy. J Otolaryngol 7[suppl 6]:1–33, 1978)

FIG. 23-6. Horizontal section through lacrimal sac, orbit, and ethmoid and sphenoid ▶ sinuses. The posterior ethmoid cells lie farther laterally than those near the front. The sphenoid sinus is in close relationship to the optic nerve and orbital apex. Note the short distance between the anterior ethmoid sinuses and the inner canthus. (Bridger WM, van Nostrand P: The nose and paranasal sinuses—applied surgical anatomy. J Otolaryngol 7[suppl 6]:1–33, 1978)

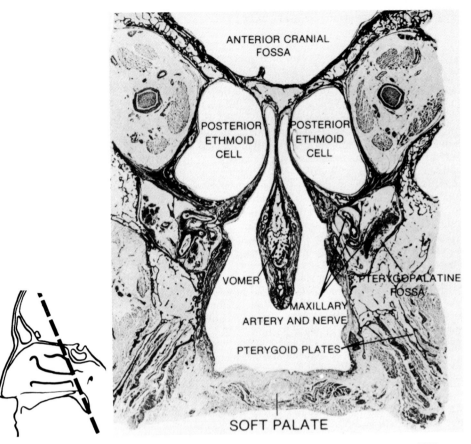

ANTERIOR CRANIAL
FOSSA

POSTERIOR
ETHMOID
CELL

POSTERIOR
ETHMOID
CELL

VOMER

PTERYGOPALATINE
FOSSA

MAXILLARY
ARTERY AND NERVE

PTERYGOID PLATES

SOFT PALATE

FIG. 23-5

FIG. 23-6

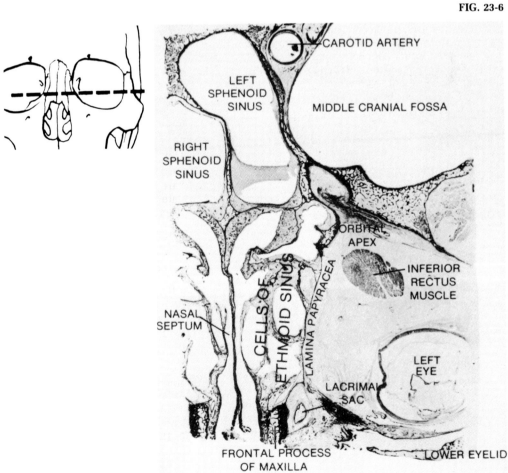

CAROTID ARTERY

LEFT
SPHENOID
SINUS

MIDDLE CRANIAL FOSSA

RIGHT
SPHENOID
SINUS

ORBITAL
APEX

INFERIOR
RECTUS
MUSCLE

NASAL
SEPTUM

CELLS OF ETHMOID SINUS

LAMINA PAPYRACEA

LEFT
EYE

LACRIMAL
SAC

FRONTAL PROCESS
OF MAXILLA

LOWER EYELID

ETHMOID SINUSES

The ethmoid sinuses consist of a labyrinth of air cells lying between the medial walls of the orbits and the lateral wall of the nasal cavity (see Figs. 23-3 through 23-6). The lateral border is the lamina papyracea, a very thin, incomplete porous bone easily penetrated by tumor. Medially the ethmoid air cells bulge into the lateral wall of the nasal cavity and form the superior and middle turbinates. The ethmoid cells communicate with the nasal cavity in the middle meatus. These bony walls are thin and easily traversed by tumor. The ethmoid air cells extend far anteriorly, and for this reason, anterior ethmoid lesions may present as a subcutaneous mass just in front of the inner canthus (see Fig. 23-6). The anterior cells are actually covered laterally by the lacrimal bone. The ethmoid bone is porous and presents little resistance to tumor spread. The right and left ethmoid cells are anatomically separated by the septum. To cross to the opposite nasal cavity and ethmoid sinuses, the tumor must first destroy the midline septum. The posterior nasal cavity and posterior ethmoid sinuses are slightly wider than the anterior portion.

SPHENOID SINUS

The sphenoid sinus is a midline structure in the body of the sphenoid bone. The pituitary lies above, the cavernous sinuses laterally, the nasal cavity and ethmoid sinuses in front, and the nasopharynx beneath. The clivus and brain stem are posterior. The pneumatization varies widely and can extend into all portions of the sphenoid bone. If the sphenoid sinus is extensively pneumatized, it may partially surround the optic nerve, carotid artery, and the maxillary and vidian nerves. The right and left sinuses may be separated by a septum but are considered as one in treatment planning, since the septum is often incomplete and thin. The sphenoid sinus connects anteriorly with the nasal cavity in the sphenoethmoidal recess. (See Fig. 24-7 in Chapter 24, Nasopharynx.)

MAXILLARY SINUS

Whole-organ sections through the maxillary antrum are shown in Figures 23-7 and 23-8. The maxillary sinuses are single pyramidal cavities with average measurements of approximately 3.7 cm in height by 2.5 cm in transverse diameter by 3 cm anteroposteriorly and a volume of approximately 15 cc in adults. The medial wall is the lateral wall of the nasal cavity and has one or several openings that communicate with the middle meatus under the me-

dial turbinate; an accessory ostium is usually present under the inferior turbinate (see Fig. 23-3).

The inferior wall or floor is the hard palate and superior alveolar ridge. The posterolateral wall is in relation to the infratemporal fossa and the pterygopalatine fossa. The complex anatomical relationships to the posterior wall of the antrum are shown in Figure 23-8; tumor extension through the posterior wall to invade the pterygoid area, the apex of the orbit, and the paranasopharyngeal area may imply inoperability for technical reasons. The superior wall or roof separates the maxillary sinus from the orbit. All walls may be invaded and destroyed by cancer. The medial wall is easily breached by tumor because it is thin, with one or several large natural perforations; the inferolateral wall is quite thin over the roots of the maxillary teeth.

FRONTAL SINUSES

The frontal sinuses are two irregular, asymmetrical air cavities separated by a thin bony septum. They connect to the middle meatus of the nasal cavity by the frontonasal duct (see Fig. 23-3). Frontal sinus cells may extend far laterally in the orbital process of the frontal bone. They are separated from the anterior ethmoid cells by thin bony walls. The posterior wall separating the frontal sinus from the anterior cranial fossa is thick in most patients.

Lymphatics

See also section on anatomy of the head and neck lymphatic system in Chapter 4.

NASAL VESTIBULE

The lymphatic trunks run mainly to the submaxillary nodes. There is a small risk for involvement of an intercalated facial node just behind the commissure of the lip along the course of the lymphatic trunk. Parotid area lymph nodes are occasionally involved, especially when tumor invades the lip or skin of the ala nasi.

NASAL CAVITY AND PARANASAL SINUSES

The lymphatics of the nasal cavity are separated into the olfactory group and the respiratory group. According to Rouvière, they do not communicate with each other.[36] There is a connection between the lymphatic network of

FIG. 23-7. Coronal section through the maxillary antrum. Note the thinness of all ▶ walls except the hard palate. Lateral to the antrum is the buccinator muscle and fat pad. (Bridger WM, van Nostrand P: The nose and paranasal sinuses—applied surgical anatomy. J Otolaryngol 7[suppl 6]:1–33, 1978)

FIG. 23-8. Sagittal section through antrum and apex of the orbit. The orbit apex ▶ communicates with the pterygopalatine fossa by way of the infraorbital fissure. Extension of the antral tumor through the posterior wall provides access to the middle cranial fossa along the cranial nerves and vascular foramina. (Bridger WM, van Nostrand P: The nose and paranasal sinuses—applied surgical anatomy. J Otolaryngol 7[suppl 6]:1–33, 1978)

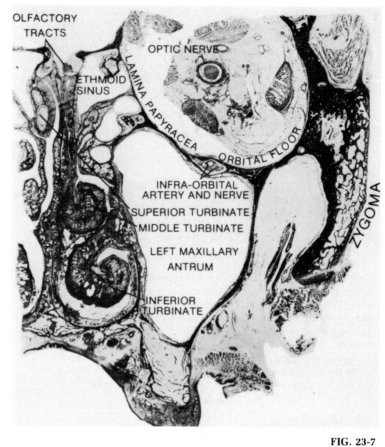

OLFACTORY
TRACTS

OPTIC NERVE

ETHMOID
SINUS

LAMINA PAPYRACEA

ORBITAL FLOOR

ZYGOMA

INFRA-ORBITAL
ARTERY AND NERVE

SUPERIOR TURBINATE

MIDDLE TURBINATE

LEFT MAXILLARY
ANTRUM

INFERIOR
TURBINATE

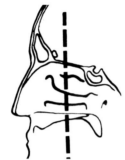

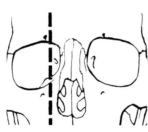

FIG. 23-7

FIG. 23-8

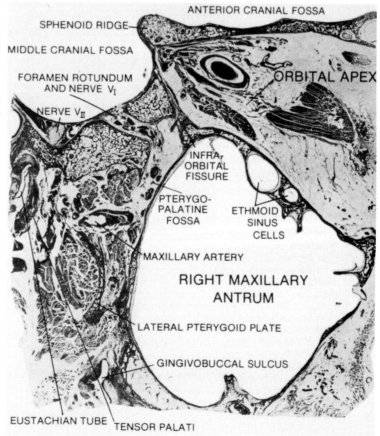

ANTERIOR CRANIAL FOSSA

SPHENOID RIDGE

MIDDLE CRANIAL FOSSA

ORBITAL APEX

FORAMEN ROTUNDUM
AND NERVE V_I

NERVE V_{II}

INFRA-
ORBITAL
FISSURE

PTERYGO-
PALATINE
FOSSA

ETHMOID
SINUS
CELLS

MAXILLARY ARTERY

RIGHT MAXILLARY
ANTRUM

LATERAL PTERYGOID PLATE

GINGIVOBUCCAL SULCUS

EUSTACHIAN TUBE   TENSOR PALATI

the olfactory region and the subarachnoid spaces, which allows some absorption of cerebrospinal fluid by the lymphatics.*

The lymphatics of the olfactory region of the nasal cavity run posteriorly to terminate in lymph nodes alongside the jugular vein at the base of skull in the lateral pharyngeal space. The lymphatics of the respiratory nasal cavity also run posteriorly to terminate a bit lower, either in a junctional lymph node or a subdigastric lymph node. The capillary lymphatic plexus of the nasal cavity is well developed over the middle and inferior turbinates, in the olfactory region, and around the choanae but is sparse over the lower septum.

Rouvière admits that knowledge of the lymphatics of the paranasal sinuses is imperfect.[36] He describes unusually delicate and sparse lymphatics of the frontal, ethmoid, and maxillary sinuses that connect with those of the nasal mucosa and thus have similar terminations. Metastases from carcinoma of the paranasal sinuses are uncommon, even though lesions are frequently quite advanced. It is literally unheard of for a paranasal sinus tumor to present with cervical lymphadenopathy and an asymptomatic primary lesion. Metastases probably only occur once tumor has extended beyond the paranasal sinuses to areas containing an abundant supply of capillary lymphatics, such as the nasopharynx, buccal mucosa, nasal cavity, and skin.

Enlarged lymph nodes associated with acute or chronic sinusitis are uncommon, which indirectly indicates a paucity or absence of capillary lymphatics in the sinuses.

PATHOLOGY

A wide variety of neoplasms, benign and malignant, affect this area.

Nasal Vestibule

Almost all of the vestibule lesions are squamous cell carcinomas; a few are basal cell carcinomas or adnexal carcinomas.

Nasal Cavity and Paranasal Sinuses

BENIGN TUMORS

Many so-called benign lesions destroy bone and soft tissues and, if uncorrected, cause death. The management of some of these problems is not unlike treatment of cancer.

Inflammatory polyps, giant cell reparative granuloma, benign mixed tumors of minor salivary gland origin, benign

---

* The importance of the lymphatic connections with the central nervous system is uncertain. In rabbits and cats, proteins and red blood cells can be partially removed from the cerebrospinal fluid and returned to the bloodstream by this route, although most absorption takes place through the arachnoid villi. An injection of Gerota substance into the subarachnoid space of humans near the cribriform plate is transmitted across the plate to the olfactory lymphatics of the nasal cavity. Földi has shown that complete obstruction of the cervical lymphatics in animals leads to a neurologic disorder that he termed "lymphogenic encephalopathy".[15] This syndrome was characterized by increased intracranial pressure with papilledema, cerebral edema, lymphedema of the head, listlessness, headache, and decreased mental ability.

odontogenic tumors, and necrotizing sialometaplasia are some of the benign lesions appearing in this area.[25]

MALIGNANT TUMORS

CARCINOMA

Squamous cell carcinoma or one of its variants is the most common neoplasm. Minor salivary gland tumors account for 10% to 15% of neoplasms in this region.

INVERTING PAPILLOMA

Inverting papilloma is a confusing condition often referred to as benign, but for practical reasons it is best classified as malignant, since it may have a rather aggressive clinical picture with multiple recurrences, extensive bone destruction, intracranial extension, and an association with squamous cell carcinoma. It is best approached as a "grade ½" neoplasm rather than as a benign polyp. At least one case with lymph node metastases has been reported.[37] The histologic picture is that of a papilloma that is growing into the stroma rather than growing outward. The lesion occurs predominantly in males 40 to 70 years of age. Any of the paranasal sinuses may be involved, as well as the nasal cavity. Squamous cell or transitional cell carcinoma is reported in association with inverting papilloma in 10% to 15% of cases. The squamous cell carcinoma is frequently present at the time of initial diagnosis and may be low grade or high grade.

LYMPHOMA

Malignant lymphoma, usually histiocytic, occurs in about 5% of cases. It is frequently a locally destructive lesion because it more often arises in bone than in soft tissue. (See Chapter 35, Lymphomas and Related Diseases Presenting in the Head and Neck.)

PLASMACYTOMA

See section on plasmacytoma in Chapter 35, Lymphomas and Related Diseases Presenting in the Head and Neck.

SARCOMA

A wide range of soft tissue and bone sarcomas is reported for the nasal cavity and paranasal sinus region, including chondrosarcoma, osteosarcoma, Ewing's sarcoma, and most of the soft tissue sarcomas. (See Chapter 33, Pediatric Tumors of the Head and Neck, and Chapter 34, Adult Mesenchymal Tumors Presenting in the Head and Neck.)

ESTHESIONEUROBLASTOMA (OLFACTORY NEUROBLASTOMA)

Esthesioneuroblastoma is a malignant tumor that originates from the olfactory nerves and has a histologic picture resembling adrenal neuroblastoma or retinoblastoma. Neurosecretory granules have been identified in ultrastructure examinations. Histologically, it may be confused with undifferentiated carcinoma or undifferentiated lymphoma. Esthesioneuroblastoma occurs at all ages, with cases commonly seen in the second and third decades. Kadish and co-workers report a 3-year-old boy with an advanced lesion, and we have treated a 12-year-old boy.[22]

MELANOMA

Malignant melanoma accounts for less than 1% of all neoplasms of the nasal cavity and paranasal sinuses. (See section on mucosal melanoma in Chapter 27, Melanoma of the Head and Neck.)

JUVENILE ANGIOFIBROMA

See Chapter 25, Juvenile Angiofibroma.

MIDLINE LETHAL NONHEALING GRANULOMA

Midline lethal granuloma is a nonspecific term that encompasses a variety of confusing histologic and clinical entities. Midline lethal nonhealing granuloma refers generally to a progressively destructive condition that involves the nose, paranasal sinuses, and hard palate and produces secondary erosion of contiguous structures. Unchecked, the disease is fatal, usually after an extended illness. Death results from extension to the central nervous system, hemorrhage, sepsis, or inanition. The etiology is debated. Midline lethal granuloma may be distinguished from Wegener's granulomatosis, which also produces inflammatory and destructive changes in the paranasal sinuses and nasal cavity. Wegener's granulomatosis also involves the lungs and kidneys with a necrotizing vasculitis. Kassel and associates subdivide midline lethal granuloma into three different histologic entities: (1) midline malignant (polymorphic) reticulosis, (2) malignant lymphoma (usually histiocytic lymphoma), and (3) Wegener's granulomatosis.[23] Regardless of the confusion in placing a proper name on the condition, most of these destructive lesions respond to radiation therapy with lymphomalike doses and many remain controlled for several years.

PATTERNS OF SPREAD

Nasal Vestibule

Lesions of the nasal vestibule invade the alar and septal cartilages and occasionally will grow through to the skin surface of the nose. The upper lip is frequently invaded. Posterior growth into the nasal cavity occurs late or after recurrence. Early lesions originating on the membranous septum or columella are often superficial lesions that ulcerate and produce a crust or scab. More advanced lesions often present with perforation of the membranous or cartilaginous septum.

Nasal vestibule carcinomas are quite deceptive to the novice since they are more extensive than one would imagine from the physical findings. This finding is confirmed by the numerous patients seen with positive margins or recurrences after attempted excision.

LYMPHATICS

Lymph node spread is usually to a solitary ipsilateral submaxillary node, but it may be bilateral. The facial nodes, preauricular nodes, and submental nodes are at small risk. Lymph node involvement is more likely in patients with extension to the floor of the vestibule, base of the columella, or upper lip and in patients with recurrent local disease.

Goepfert and co-workers report only 1 of 26 patients with clinically positive lymph nodes on admission, but 7 patients later developed positive lymph nodes, with 4 patients eventually showing bilateral disease.[17]

None of 11 patients seen at the University of Florida had clinically positive nodes when first seen, but 2 patients developed solitary submaxillary lymph node metastases with the primary lesion controlled.

Nasal Cavity and Paranasal Sinuses

NASAL CAVITY

The routes of spread are essentially the same for the various histologies with the exception that minor salivary gland tumors have a greater propensity for perineural spread, although squamous carcinomas and esthesioneuroblastomas may also follow nerve pathways.

Lesions arising in the olfactory region invade into the ethmoid sinuses, the orbit, and through the sievelike cribriform plate to the anterior cranial fossa. These lesions also tend to destroy the septum and may invade through nasal bone to the skin. Lesions arising on the lateral wall of the nasal cavity invade the medial wall of the maxillary sinus, the ethmoid sinuses, the pterygomaxillary fossa, and the orbit. The degree of orbital invasion is shown in Table 23-1.

The nasopharynx and the sphenoid sinus are secondarily invaded in advanced lesions. Tumor may follow the numerous nasal nerves posteriorly and then superiorly toward the sphenopalatine ganglion near the base of the skull

TABLE 23-1.   Degree of Orbital Invasion (37 Patients)

Primary Site	None	Minimal (Roentgenographic Changes)	Advanced*
Ethmoid sinus	2	4	6
Sphenoid sinus	4	0	0
Nasal cavity	13	4	4
Total	19	8	10

* Exophthalmos, blindness, palpable mass.

Note: University of Florida data; patients treated 10/64–1/79; analysis by J. T. Parsons, MD, 1981.

TABLE 23-2.   Inverted Papilloma: Findings at Lateral Rhinotomy (13 Patients)

Finding at Surgery	No. Patients
Papilloma in:	
Nasal fossa	13
Ethmoid sinus	10
Antrum	9
Frontal sinus	2
Sphenoid sinus	1
Orbit	1
Erosion of lamina papyracea	3

(Myers EN, Schramm VL, Barnes EL: Management of inverted papilloma of the nose and paranasal sinuses. Laryngoscope 91:2071–2084, 1981)

(pterygopalatine fossa) or along the maxillary branch of the trigeminal nerve (see Fig. 23-8).

Inverting papilloma almost always involves the lateral nasal wall. Extension to the adjacent paranasal sinuses, orbit, and anterior cranial fossa are frequent. The anatomical distribution of tumor at the time of lateral rhinotomy in 13 patients who had inverting papilloma with no squamous carcinoma is given in Table 23-2.

ETHMOID SINUSES

Lesions of the ethmoid sinuses have many options for local spread due to their location and the thin, porous bony walls, none of which offers particular resistance. Invasion through the lamina papyracea into the medial orbit is common and must be considered to have occurred even when physical examination and roentgenograms of the orbit are normal. The lamina papyracea is normally indistinct on roentgenographic examination, and this makes interpretation of early destruction nearly impossible. The lamina papyracea is the lateral wall for the middle and posterior ethmoid air cells; the anterior ethmoid cells are covered laterally by the small, thin lacrimal bone and the frontal process of the maxilla (see Fig. 23-6). Thus, the ethmoid air cells extend far anteriorly, within a centimeter of the inner canthus, and the tumor may present as a subcutaneous nodule. The medial surfaces of the ethmoid labyrinth are actually the middle and superior nasal turbinates, which are formed by a thin, convoluted bone, so that the tumor frequently presents in the nasal cavity.

The proximity of the maxillary antrum also provides ready access to tumor spread. Advanced lesions extend to the floor of the anterior cranial fossa, sphenoid sinus, nasopharynx, frontal sinus, skin, and pterygopalatine and infratemporal fossa.

SPHENOID SINUS

There is little information regarding spread patterns for tumors arising in the sphenoid sinus. The only early lesion we have seen (in a patient with a 1-year history of headache) was diagnosed just as it broke through the anterior wall of the sphenoid sinus; biopsy showed adenoid cystic carcinoma. It is probable that some of the advanced nasopharyngeal lesions are in reality primary sphenoid sinus lesions that are diagnosed when they erode into the na-

sopharynx. The fact that a disproportionate number of advanced nasopharynx lesions have no neck metastases is suggestive of their origin in the sphenoid sinus, a site with sparse, if any, capillary lymphatics, rather than from the nasopharynx with its copious lymphatics.

The sphenoid sinus is in close relationship with the cranial nerves in the cavernous sinus: the third, fourth, and sixth nerves and the ophthalmic and maxillary branches of the trigeminal nerve (see Fig. 24-10, in Chapter 24). Cranial nerve palsies and headache are frequently the first clinical evidence of a sphenoid sinus tumor. Diagnosis is usually made, however, when the tumor eventually grows through into the nasopharynx or nasal cavity, where it can be seen and biopsied.

The sphenoid sinus is closely related to the apex of the orbit and the optic nerve, depending on the degree of pneumatization (see Fig. 23-6). These structures are at risk for early tumor invasion. None of four patients seen at the University of Florida had evidence of orbit involvement (see Table 23-1).

MAXILLARY SINUS

The pattern of spread and bone destruction is largely dependent on the site of origin within the sinus. Lesions arising in the anterolateral infrastructure tend to invade through the lateral inferior wall and present in the oral cavity when tumor erodes through the maxillary gingiva or into the gingivobuccal sulcus. When the tumor erupts into the oral cavity, it is at first submucosal, causing elevation of the mucosa, loosening of teeth, or improper seating of a denture. Ulceration follows, with the development of an oral-antral fistula.

Lesions arising on the medial infrastructure readily develop extension to the nasal cavity due to the thin, porous nature of the medial wall.

Lesions of the posterior infrastructure erode through the posterolateral wall to the infratemporal fossa and pterygopalatine fossa. The diagnosis usually depends on sinus tomography and CT scan for definition. Recogition of this route of spread is important, since a tumor escaping posteriorly has immediate access to the base of the skull. Extension of lesions to the orbit occurs either directly through the roof of the maxillary sinus or by a circuitous route through the ethmoid sinuses and lamina papyracea or by way of the pterygopalatine fossa and infraorbital fissure.

Tumors arising in the upper half (suprastructure) of the antrum have two general patterns of development. One group develops laterally, invades the malar process of the maxilla and the zygomatic bone, and produces a mass just below the lateral floor of the orbit. The soft tissue mass may become quite large and eventually ulcerate through to the skin, producing an antrocutaneous fistula. The orbit is invaded laterally and displaces the eye inward and upward. The temporal fossa and zygomatic arch may become involved in very advanced lesions.

The suprastructure cancers that develop medially invade the nasal cavity, ethmoid sinuses and frontal sinus, the lacrimal apparatus, and the medial inferior orbit. It is usually impossible in these cases to determine whether the origin is the maxillary antrum, nasal cavity, or ethmoid sinus. These lesions are sometimes referred to as "crossroads" tumors because they develop at or near the junctions of the maxillary antrum, nasal cavity, and ethmoid sinuses.

LYMPHATICS

The incidence of lymphatic metastases on admission is 10% to 15% for nasal cavity, ethmoid sinus, and maxillary antrum. The risk of lymphatic metastases for primary sinus lesions is related to extension of the tumor outside the sinus to areas with capillary lymphatics. Maxillary sinus tumors that invade the oral cavity and involve the buccal mucosa or the maxillary gingiva/hard palate may spread to the submaxillary and jugulodigastric nodes. Lesions that invade the nasal cavity or nasopharynx spread posteriorly to the junctional (parapharyngeal) lymph nodes and then to the jugulodigastric area. Esthesioneuroblastoma, minor salivary gland tumors, melanoma, and sarcomas may all demonstrate lymph node metastases.

There is a case report of a garden-variety inverting papilloma managed by excision that developed three lymph node metastases 1 year later that showed characteristic inverting papilloma.[37]

CLINICAL PICTURE

Nasal Vestibule

Lesions of the nasal vestibule present with few symptoms other than a mass growing in the entrance to the nose with crusting, scabbing, and occasional minor bleeding. Pain, if it occurs, is usually modest, even with destruction of cartilage or involvement of the lip. Secondary infection may occur, in which case the nose is painful with manipulation. The lesion may be localized to one distinct area of the nasal vestibule, but it frequently fills the nasal vestibule so that the site of origin cannot be determined.

Nasal Cavity and Paranasal Sinuses

NASAL CAVITY

Patients with tumors in the nasal cavity often present with a history of chronic recurrent nasal obstruction and "sinus trouble," which has recently slowly begun to worsen. The symptoms are unilateral low-grade chronic infection with discharge, obstruction, and minor, intermittent bleeding. They mimic those associated with nasal polyps, and, since many of the patients with nasal neoplasms have a prior history of nasal operations for polyps, cancer is often missed in an early stage. The patient often complains of "sinus trouble" and intermittent anterior headache. Subsequent symptoms depend on the pattern of growth. Lesions arising in the olfactory region may cause unilateral or bilateral nasal expansion of the bridge of the nose, and a submucosal mass may appear near the inner canthus and eventually ulcerate. An obvious mass may protrude from the nose. Obstruction of the nasolacrimal system may cause epiphora and be a presenting complaint, with the patient treated by incision and drainage for dacryocystitis. Extension through the cribriform plate or into the ethmoid sinus is accompanied by frontal headache. Aberration or loss of smell is unusual but has been noted in one patient as an early symptom.

Invasion of the medial orbit produces proptosis and diplopia; a mass may be palpated in the orbit. Indirect examination of the nasopharynx may show early submucosal invasion through the posterior nares.

The symptoms and signs for inverting papilloma are similar to those for carcinoma.

Esthesioneuroblastoma has a bimodal age distribution with peaks at 11 through 20 and 51 through 60 years. The most common presenting complaints are nasal obstruction and epistaxis. Approximately 10% of patients develop cervical lymph node metastasis. Hypertension has been reported.[39]

MAXILLARY SINUS

Cancers of the maxillary sinus develop silently as long as they are confined to the sinus; they produce symptoms on extension outside the walls. If the tumor invades the oral cavity, the presenting symptoms relate to pain associated with the upper teeth; there may be loosening and eventually loss of teeth. The dentist is often the first one consulted, and the patient may have dental extractions without pain relief. Tumor may penetrate into the gingivobuccal sulcus or upper gum and eventually progress to an oral-antral fistula. If the patient wears upper dentures, the first symptom will be an ill-fitting denture. Palpation and observation of the face may show a mass. Early invasion of the floor of the orbit may be appreciated by feeling both orbits simultaneously with the tips of the index finger inserted between the bony rim and eyeball. Posterior invasion of the orbit will produce proptosis, diplopia, and edema of the conjunctiva. Invasion of the inferior orbital nerve or its branches in the floor of the orbit may cause paresthesias or anesthesia of the skin of the lower eyelid, upper lip, side of the nose, and the anterior premaxillary skin. Nasal obstruction and bleeding are common complaints, along with "sinus pain" or "fullness" over the involved antrum. Trismus and headache are associated with invasion posteriorly into the infratemporal fossa, with subsequent invasion of the pterygoid muscles and base of the skull.

Patients with cancer developing in the medial suprastructure of the antrum present with nasal obstruction, nasal discharge or bleeding, mild infraorbital pain, infected lacrimal sac, and displacement of the eye upward and laterally with proptosis, diplopia, and conjunctival edema.

Cancer developing in the lateral suprastructure produces a mass below the lateral canthus with associated pain. The eye may be deviated medially and upward when orbital invasion occurs. There is edema of the conjunctiva, narrowing of the palpebral opening, diplopia, and proptosis. Tumor may extend to the temporal fossa, producing a diffuse fullness.

ETHMOID SINUS

Mild to moderate sinus ache or pain referred to the frontal/nasal or retro-orbital area is an early symptom of tumors of the ethmoid sinus. A painless mass may present near the inner canthus. The mass may become infected and be interpreted by the patient as a boil. The physician may make the diagnosis of dacryocystitis, at which time an inappropriate incision and drainage procedure is done. Diplopia develops with invasion of the medial orbit. Proptosis is often present, and a mass can be felt by a deep digital palpation of the orbit. Nasal discharge, epistaxis, and obstruction are frequent presenting complaints. Paresthesias may occur over the distribution of sensory nerves.

Physical examination includes anterior and posterior rhinoscopy after thorough shrinking of the nasal mucosa.

A fiberoptic nasoscope is a great aid in visualizing the posterior and superior nasal cavity and the nasopharynx. Early invasion of the nasal cavity may produce only submucosal bulging into the superior or middle meatus, which is easily confused with allergic rhinitis, polyps, or inflammatory changes. Pus may be seen coming from beneath the turbinates.

Eye examination includes palpation of the orbit for masses. Palpation should be carried out simultaneously in both orbits, since the changes in the involved orbit are frequently subtle. Extraocular movements are examined, and proptosis is measured with a ruler; there may be only a 3-mm to 4-mm difference with early proptosis.

Invasion into the nasopharynx is usually submucosal and appears on the roof and lateral wall. Advanced lesions may obstruct the eustachian canal.

METHODS OF DIAGNOSIS AND STAGING

Biopsy Technique

Tumor in the nasal cavity is biopsied with a punch forceps. Examination and biopsy of tumor in the maxillary antrum is usually approached through a Caldwell–Luc procedure, which is an incision through the gingivobuccal sulcus and the canine fossa. This approach allows adequate visualization of the entire antrum.

Biopsy of ethmoid tumors is usually made of the tumor extending into the nasal cavity or inner canthus area. Tumor confined to the ethmoid sinuses may be found unexpectedly at the time of a lateral rhinotomy planned for diagnosis or treatment of benign disease. An orbital mass may occasionally be the site of biopsy.

Sphenoid sinus tumors are biopsied by way of the transseptal route for the rare localized disease, but biopsy is usually made of an extension to the nasopharynx or nasal cavity.

Frontal sinus tumors are approached by frontal sinus trephination.

Esthesioneuroblastomas are reported to produce catecholamines and vasopressin.[22,39]

Radiologic Evaluation

Modern radiologic procedures, including conventional and computed tomography (CT scanning), aid in the diagnosis and delineate the anatomical boundaries that are essential for treatment decisions and follow-up evaluations.

PLAIN FILM PARANASAL SINUS SERIES

The roentgenographic anatomy of the paranasal sinuses is particularly complex because the sinuses are projected over one another, thus obscuring anatomic detail, and there is a considerable spectrum of normal variation such as asymmetrical development and change in pneumatization with age.

The routine plain film sinus series consists of four views:[14,29]

1. Caldwell projection: useful in evaluating the frontal and ethmoid sinuses, lamina papyracea, nasal septum, medial antral walls, alveolar edge, and bony plate between the ethmoid cells and the maxillary sinus (Fig. 23-9A).

2. Waters' view: useful for evaluation of the maxillary antra, petrous ridges, and sphenoid sinus (Fig. 23-10A).
3. Lateral view: useful for evaluation of the anterior and posterior walls of the frontal and maxillary sinuses, floor of the anterior cranial fossa, ethmoid and sphenoid sinuses, base of the skull, and nasopharynx.
4. Submentovertex or base view: useful to show the posterolateral wall of the maxillary sinus, the posterior wall of the orbit, and the lesser and greater

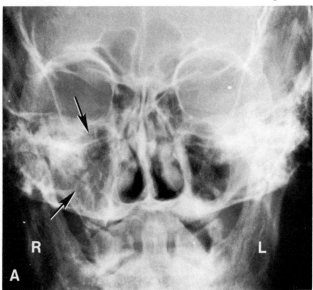

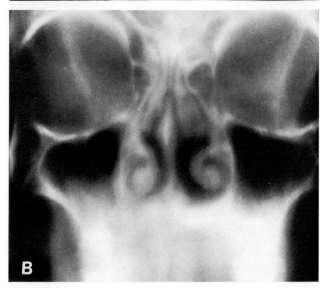

FIG. 23-9. (*A*) Caldwell projection plain film showing opacification of the right maxillary antrum (*arrows*). The floor of the antrum is not clearly shown. The relationship between the mass and hard palate destruction as demonstrated by tomography is not clear on this film. The mass appears to be confined within the antrum. (*B*) Anteroposterior tomogram clearly shows destruction of the medial aspect of the floor of the right maxillary antrum and adjacent hard palate. It is preferable to have air in the mouth (*i.e.,* mouth open, tongue depressed) to provide an air–mucosa interface to aid in the detection of early soft tissue changes.

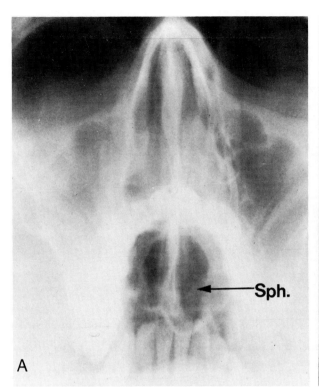
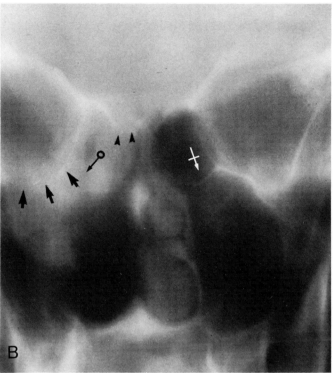

FIG. 23-10. (*A*) Waters' projection. The right maxillary antrum appears slightly opacified compared with the left. A mass lesion, orbital wall destruction, and extension into the ethmoid cells are not apparent but are easily seen with anteroposterior tomography. Petrous ridges are not identified due to the modified angulation to show the floor of the maxillary sinuses. (*Sph.*, sphenoid sinus) (*B*) Anteroposterior tomogram shows a right maxillary antral tumor mass with involvement of the right ethmoid sinus. The antral ethmoid septum is destroyed on the right (♂) compared with the left (↔). There is also destruction of the medial portion of the orbital floor (*arrows*). Turbinates on the right have been surgically removed. The tumor has also destroyed a portion of the cribriform plate on the right (*arrowheads*). Tumor extends slightly across the midline to involve also the left cribriform plate. A CT scan confirmed these findings. There was no frontal lobe involvement at this time.

wings of the sphenoid bone (Fig. 23-11). This view also shows the pterygoid plates, foramina (ovale, lacerum, spinosum), nasopharynx, and floor of the middle cranial fossa. This is the most useful of the plain films for evaluation of invasion of the base of the skull.

The plain film series is useful in providing a screening for paranasal sinus pathology, but usually it is inadequate for the diagnosis and delineation of anatomical extent.

CONVENTIONAL TOMOGRAPHY

Conventional plain film tomography (posteroanterior, lateral, and submentovertex projections) aids the demonstration of soft tissue masses and associated bone destruction. Linear or pluridirectional (stratomatic or polytome) tomography may be employed. Pluridirectional tomography is, however, best suited to this region because of the complex anatomy of the nasal and paranasal sinuses. The selection of appropriate projections is crucial in defining the nature and extent of sinus lesions.

The anatomical site of the tumor can frequently be judged from the routine plain film series. In general, frontal tomograms are appropriate for tumors involving the nasal cavity and ethmoid and sphenoid sinuses (Figs. 23-9*B* and 23-10*B*). Lateral tomography is indicated for abnormalities of the frontal sinus and posterior wall and roof of the maxillary sinus. The submentovertex projection demonstrates to best advantage tumors involving the posterolateral wall of the maxillary antrum and also lesions of the ethmoid sinuses.

It is important to assess whether the bone involvement is destructive, as with most malignant tumors, or expansile, which suggests a benign or slowly growing malignant lesion.[10,40]

COMPUTED TOMOGRAPHY

As the role of CT scanning expands, the emphasis previously placed on conventional pluridirectional tomography is decreasing. CT has proved to be a major advantage in the staging of paranasal sinus tumors, particularly in the demonstration of soft tissue tumor in the pterygoid region

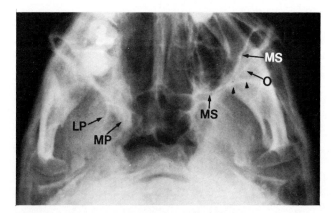

FIG. 23-11. The base view of the skull shows the S-shaped posterolateral wall of the maxillary sinus (*MS*). The posterior orbital wall is a straight line and is well seen (*O*). The anterior wall of the middle cranial fossa is formed by the lesser and greater wings of the sphenoid, represented by the curved line (*arrowheads*). The absence of teeth on the left improves the image. On the right, a rhabdomyosarcoma fills the maxillary antrum. Destruction of the antral walls was essentially superiorly and into the right ethmoid region. The lateral (*LP*) and medial (*MP*) pterygoid plates are intact. The patient has had previous surgery in the region of the right nasal turbinates and ethmoid sinuses. The foramina (ovale, spinosum, and lacerum) are not demarcated on this particular film.

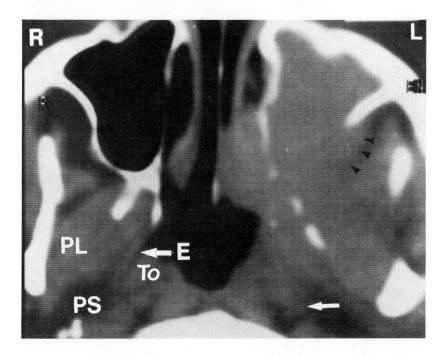

FIG. 23-12. Large tumor mass destroying the posterior wall of the left maxillary antrum and the pterygoid plates. The lesion extends into the infratemporal fossa (*arrowheads*), the parapharyngeal space (*white arrow*), and the nasal cavity. The left eustachian tube is also involved. (*PL*, lateral pterygoid muscle; *E* (*arrow*), right eustachian tube (normal); *To*, torus tubarius; *PS*, parapharyngeal space)

and orbit.[43] Early evaluation with the second-generation CT scanners already documented significantly greater sinus tumor demonstration with CT scans than with conventional roentgenograms.[34] Conventional radiologic techniques and clinical examination together frequently reveal bone destruction and gross soft tissue tumor extent, but the degree of involvement of surrounding structures may be missed or only determined later, at the time of surgery. Of particular importance to the surgeon in determining resectability is spread to the pterygopalatine fossa, pterygoid fossa, base of the skull, infratemporal fossa, orbit, cribriform plate, and nasopharynx. The parapharyngeal space is usually spared. Differentiation of the "clouded" sinus into tumor filled or fluid filled may be achieved using contrast-enhanced CT scanning to assess air–fluid levels, which change with positioning of the patient.[21]

Both axial and coronal CT scans are valuable in the evaluation of paranasal sinus disease. Contrast enhancement may not be helpful because both tumor and soft tissue may enhance equally.[19] Enhanced CT scanning is usually able to detect the hypervascularity of juvenile angiofibromas and other vascular lesions.

Thin (6 mm or less) section CT scanning is performed in the axial plane (Fig. 23-12) or coronal plane (Fig. 23-13) of the paranasal sinuses. Most sinus tumors are hypovascular; that is, enhancement is roughly the same as adjacent muscular planes. Contrast does opacify and aid recognition of blood vessels.

A major problem associated with the CT evaluation of bone destruction is that *small portions of bony structures may be "averaged" with adjacent soft tissue structures, making them appear destroyed when they are, in fact, uninvolved by tumor.* This is particularly misleading when thick sections are used. Also, bony septa that run parallel to the CT scan axis may appear as soft tissue densities rather than true bony margins (see Fig. 23-13). Therefore, when evaluating bone destruction, particularly in complex anatomical areas such as the paranasal sinuses and also

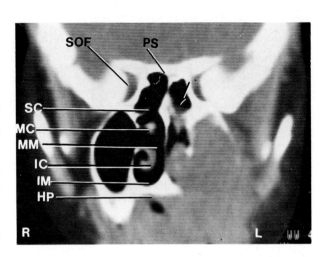

FIG. 23-13. Coronal CT scan through posterior portion of the maxillary sinuses shows tumor mass destroying medial wall, lateral wall, and floor of the left antrum. There is a soft tissue density in the floor of the left sphenoid sinus that may represent early extension into sphenoid sinus (*arrow*); the nasal cavity and infratemporal region are invaded. Hard palate destruction is also shown. Note that the medial wall of the right maxillary antrum appears to be "destroyed" due to the artifact of tissue averaging. (*SOF*, superior orbital fissure; *PS*, planum sphenoidale; *SC*, superior concha; *MC*, middle concha; *MM*, middle meatus; *IC*, inferior concha; *IM*, inferior meatus; *HP*, hard palate)

when the bone involved is a slender structure, thin (3-mm) CT sections are desirable (Fig. 23-14). Axial and direct coronal CT scans are frequently complementary studies.[35,42] Imaging in the additional plane results in more complete depiction of tumor extent and also improves the anatomical display of involved structures. Sagittal views are also frequently useful, particularly direct sagittal scans[32] as opposed to "reconstructed" or "reformatted" images.

PATTERNS OF SPREAD OF MALIGNANCIES OF THE MAXILLARY ANTRUM

Infrastructure Involvement

Anterolateral infrastructure lesions tend to invade the alveolar ridge, causing loosening of teeth and presenting in the oral cavity (Figs. 23-13 and 23-15). Tumors of the floor and anterior wall of the antrum may extend to invade the soft tissue of the overlying cheek (Fig. 23-16). Thickening of the skin of the cheek can be readily appreciated on the CT image. If more laterally placed, extension may be by way of the buccogingival groove or through the posterolateral wall into the infratemporal fossa (see Fig. 23-16).

Lesions arising on the medial infrastructure commonly extend into the nasal cavity. Invasion into the nasal cavity or hard palate is frequently shown to best advantage using conventional anteroposterior tomography (see Fig. 23-9) or with coronal CT scanning (see Fig. 23-13). CT scanning is superior to conventional films and tomography because of its ability to show air cleavage planes between the turbinates and tumor and between the nasal septum and tumor.[26] It is useful in assessing whether the tumor mass has crossed the midline (see Figs. 23-14 and 23-15) and spread to the nasopharynx.

Tumors of the posterior infrastructure may extend to the base of the skull and pterygoid plates, thus rendering the patient's disease inoperable. Posterior antral tumors

may extend into the region of the pterygopalatine fossa and infratemporal space (Fig. 23-17). The pterygoid fossa may also be involved once tumor destruction of the base of the pterygoid plates has occurred. Infratemporal fossa involvement is usually clearly depicted by a good CT study, even when early disease is present in this area. The normal low-density fat plane behind the antrum and around the lateral pterygoid muscle is maintained, even in the presence of chronic sinusitis. Inflammatory disease may thicken the bony walls of the antrum and cause indistinct margins of the fat plane anteriorly, but the lucency or low-density area around the lateral pterygoid muscle will remain intact.[26] CT evidence of invasion of the pterygoid muscle indicates tumor spread to the infratemporal fossa.[27] This is well shown in Figures 23-12 and 23-17.

Suprastructure Involvement

The antral roof may be directly involved by superiorly placed antral lesions or by central extension of tumor along the infraorbital canal. Invasion of the orbit from antral neoplasms that have spread to the ethmoid sinuses and then to the medial wall of the orbit is clearly depicted by both axial (Fig. 23-18) and coronal (Fig. 23-19) CT scans. Coronal and axial scans demonstrate invasion of the orbit. Lesions involving the "central surgical space" around the optic nerve and posterior apex of the orbit are in proximity to the sphenoid sinus and cavernous sinus.

Anterior cranial fossa spread may occur from antrum to anterior ethmoid air cells and from here to the anterior cranial fossa, or the tumor may spread by way of the nasal mucosa and then through the cribriform plate (see Fig. 23-19).

Caldwell views of the sinuses or conventional tomograms are frequently helpful in evaluating the possibility of intracranial extension. Intracranial spread is virtually ruled out if these views show the ethmoid sinuses to be normally aerated. However, if the ethmoid air cells are opacified, it

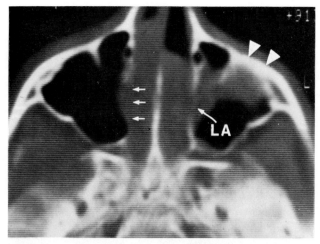

FIG. 23-14. A large tumor mass extended from the nasopharynx to involve the nasal cavity bilaterally. The medial maxillary antral wall on the right (*arrows*) is bowed laterally and partially destroyed. There is also transgression of the medial antral wall on the left (*LA*), and tumor extends into the middle and anterior regions of the antrum. Note that the anterior antral wall on this side is intact (*arrowheads*). Thin (3 mm) CT sections are essential when evaluating destructive lesions involving relatively thin bony structures. This technique minimizes problems of partial volume averaging whereby CT densities are averaged over the given recorded slice and small areas of intact bone look less dense (*i.e.,* partially or totally destroyed). This problem can also be avoided by using an additional CT plane, such as a direct coronal image.

is frequently difficult, if not impossible, to differentiate tumor from obstructed or infected sinuses. This problem also arises after radiation therapy, when a chronic sinusitis may be confused with recurrent tumor. (See section on radiation-induced sinusitis in Chapter 14, The Effect of Radiation on Normal Tissues of the Head and Neck.) To make this important differentiation, coronal CT scans with contrast enhancement are used to see if the lateral wall of the olfactory fossa is intact (*i.e.,* the bony plate forming the medial ethmoidal wall[33]) and to evaluate for tumor invasion into adjacent brain tissue.

PATTERNS OF SPREAD OF MALIGNANCIES OF THE ETHMOID SINUSES

Invasion through the lamina papyracea into the medial orbit is a common feature of spread from ethmoid sinus malignancy, and this extension may occur in patients with no abnormality on physical examination and with apparently normal plain roentgenograms of the orbit. Hence,

high-quality, thin-section axial or coronal CT examinations are of major importance in assessing patients with early (not advanced) ethmoid sinus disease (Figs. 23-18 through 23-21).

Advanced lesions may extend to the sphenoid sinus and even to the frontal sinuses (Fig. 23-22).

Esthesioneuroblastoma originates in the upper portions of the nasal cavity where olfactory epithelium is found. The roentgenographic findings are not specific for this histology. Frequently there is involvement of the cribriform plate, the paranasal sinuses, and the orbit. Invasion through the dura and into the frontal lobe is best demonstrated by enhanced CT scanning.

Staging Classification

NASAL VESTIBULE

The American Joint Committee (AJCC) skin cancer staging is appropriate, since nasal vestibule lesions arise from skin. (See section on staging in Chapter 26, Carcinoma of the Skin.) Many reports of nasal cavity carcinoma include the favorable vestibule cases.

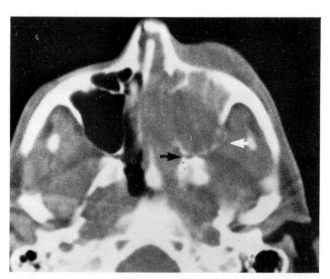

FIG. 23-15. Poorly differentiated lymphocytic lymphoma producing left maxillary antral destruction. There is spread to the entire left nasal cavity (*black arrowheads*). The left pterygopalatine fossa can still be recognized (*black arrow*). Note the normal pterygopalatine fossa on the right side. The pterygoid plates are intact. The mass does, however, extend posterolaterally toward the left infratemporal fossa (*white arrow*). There is also marked anterior destruction of the antrum with spread to the soft tissues of the cheek. CT demonstration of the pterygoid plates and the pterygopalatine fossa is important in the evaluation of tumor spread. The medial and lateral pterygoid plates unite to form a separation between the pterygopalatine fossa anteriorly and the pterygoid fossa posteriorly (*white arrowhead*).

FIG. 23-16. Adenocarcinoma of the right maxillary antrum extending through the anterior wall into the soft tissues of the cheek. The medial portion of the posterior antral wall and pterygopalatine fossa (*white arrows*) are normal. There is no extension of tumor into the nasal cavity. The medial wall of the antrum is also intact. There is lateral extension through the posterolateral antral wall, and early spread to the infratemporal space is suggested by the loss of the normal low-density region adjacent to the posterolateral antral wall (*black arrows*). Note the normal left side for comparison. White arrow indicates location of the pterygopalatine fossa, which is just beginning to appear on this section. (*E,* eustachian tube; *PL,* lateral pterygoid muscle; *M,* masseter muscle; *To,* torus tubarius; *L,* longus colli; *Ph,* lateral pharyngeal recess; *MH,* head of the mandible; *C,* carotid sheath; *S,* styloid process)

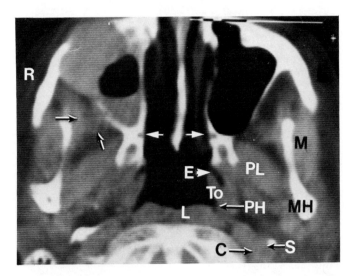

FIG. 23-17. The posterior wall of the right maxillary antrum is completely destroyed, and there is tumor extending into the infratemporal fossa (*arrowheads*). The pterygoid plates are also destroyed, and the pterygopalatine fossa is involved. The lateral pterygoid muscle is inseparable from the tumor mass. The CT scan clearly delineates the degree of tumor involvement of the infratemporal fossa. Massive destruction of the pterygoid plates is almost invariably present when the tumor has grown beyond the pterygopalatine fossa into the pterygoid fossa. The sphenopalatine ganglion lies in the pterygopalatine fossa but is not visible on CT. (*MC,* coronoid process of mandible; *MPP,* medial pterygoid plate; *LPP,* lateral pterygoid plate; *PL,* lateral pterygoid muscle) ▼

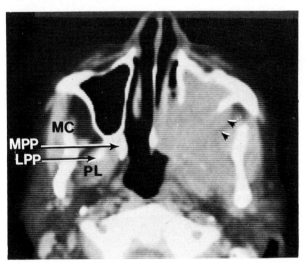

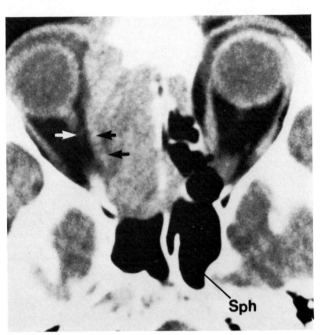

FIG. 23-18. Midorbit axial CT scan showing antral tumor ▲ spread to the right ethmoid sinus. The tumor mass has destroyed the lamina papyracea and is bulging into the right orbit. The medial rectus muscle is displaced laterally by the mass (*black arrows*). There is no mass effect in the region of the "central surgical space" around the optic nerve (*white arrow*). (*Sph,* sphenoid sinus)

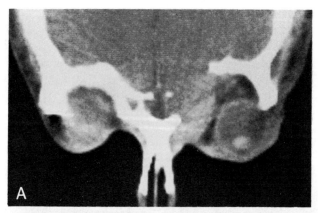

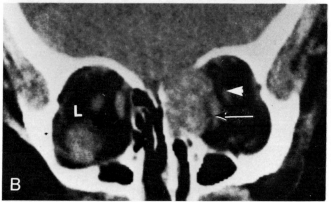

FIG. 23-19. (A) This coronal section shows anterior and lateral displacement of the globe by a lymphoma arising from the maxillary antrum. Cribriform plate and orbital roof destruction is well demonstrated, and there is tumor extension into the anterior cranial fossa. (B) Midorbit, behind globe. Bone destruction includes the planum sphenoidale, the cribriform plate, and the medial orbital roof. The medial rectus muscle is displaced laterally (white arrow). The optic nerve is not displaced (arrowhead). There is no extension across the midline at this level.

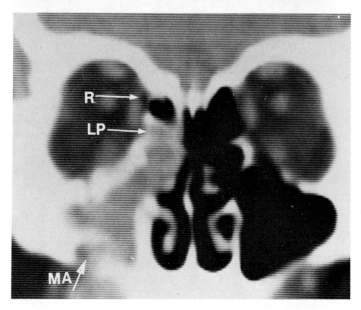

FIG. 23-20. Tumor involving the right ethmoid sinuses and right maxillary antrum, the floor of which is destroyed (MA). There is thickening of the lamina papyracea (LP), but no extension into the right orbit has occurred. The medial rectus muscle is in normal position (R). The cribriform plate is intact, and there is also no spread across the midline.

MAXILLARY SINUS

The AJCC staging system applies only to maxillary sinus tumors. Ohngren's line, a theoretic plane joining the medial canthus of the eye with the angle of the mandible, is used to divide the maxillary antrum into the anteroinferior portion (the infrastructure) and the superoposterior portion (the suprastructure). The primary tumor is staged as follows:[1]

TX Minimum requirements to assess the tumor cannot be met

T0 No evidence of primary tumor

T1 Tumor confined to the antral mucosa of the infrastructure with no bone erosion or destruction

T2 Tumor confined to the suprastructure mucosa without bone destruction, or to the infrastructure with destruction of medial or inferior bony walls only

T3 More extensive tumor invading skin of cheek, orbit, anterior ethmoid sinuses, or pterygoid muscle

T4 Massive tumor with invasion of cribriform plate, posterior ethmoid, sphenoid, nasopharynx, pterygoid plates, or base of the skull

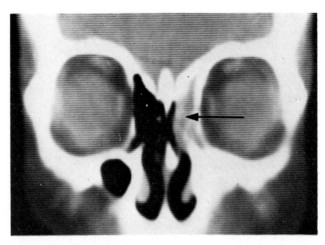

FIG. 23-21. Localized tumor in the left anterior ethmoid area (*arrow*). Cribriform plate is intact; the lamina papyracea is intact and appears thicker than the normal on the opposite side.

NASAL CAVITY AND ETHMOID SINUS

The staging system developed in 1981 at the University of Florida for tumors of the nasal cavity and ethmoid/sphenoid sinus is as follows:

I Tumor limited to nasal cavity and sinuses with or without skin infiltration

II Extension to orbit and/or nasopharynx

III Base of skull or pterygoid destruction; intracranial extension

TREATMENT

Nasal Vestibule

SELECTION OF TREATMENT MODALITY

Both surgical resection and radiation therapy produce a high degree of success when performed by experienced physicians.[9,17,18] Radiation therapy is the preferred treatment in our clinic since excision will almost always produce a deformity. Excision may be used for very small lesions, the removal of which will not produce cosmetic deformity nor require extensive reconstruction. However, few lesions fit this description since these tumors are frequently much more extensive than they appear (iceberg effect). Surgery is reserved for radiation failure. Radiation therapy has been successful in salvaging surgical failures, but the nasal deformity has already been produced and the value of irradiation lost. The local control rate with radiation therapy is shown in Table 23-3. Cases have been followed for 2 to 16 years.

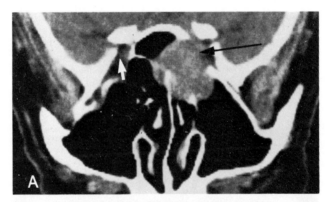
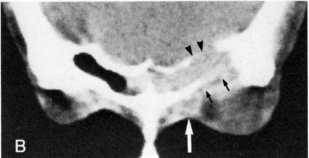

FIG. 23-22. (*A*) Coronal scan through the anterior clinoids and planum sphenoidale showing a posterior ethmoid histiocytic lymphoma extending into the left sphenoid sinus with destruction of the lateral wall of the sphenoid sinus and involvement of the superior orbital fissure (*black arrow*). Tumor extent is well shown because of surrounding air and bone. Normal superior orbital fissure (*white arrow*) contains the oculomotor, trochlear, trigeminal and abducens nerves, arteries, and veins. (*B*) The tumor mass also involves the frontal sinus on the left. Both the anterior wall (*black arrows*) and the posterior wall (*arrowheads*) are partially destroyed. There is bulging of the soft tissues (*white arrow*).

SURGICAL TREATMENT

Excision of lesions in the nasal vestibule usually involves removal of cartilage as well as skin. Depending on the site of the lesion, either the columella or the alar cartilages will be removed and may be difficult to reconstruct, particularly if the surgery is for radiation therapy failure. If the alar cartilage has been sacrificed, either a composite graft consisting of skin and cartilage from the ear or a nasolabial flap can be used to repair the defect. If the entire external nose is resected, a prosthesis is usually used to cover the defect, since examination for recurrent disease is easier and total nasal reconstruction is cosmetically unacceptable.

IRRADIATION TECHNIQUE

Irradiation techniques are not standardized, but success is good with several methods. Selection of technique will depend on the extent of the disease and the experience of the radiation therapist (Table 23-4).

EXTERNAL BEAM

Supervoltage beams are theoretically preferable to orthovoltage in order to reduce the dose in cartilage and adjacent bone. Orthovoltage therapy fractionated over 4 to 6 weeks, however, produces good results; shorter courses with higher daily fractions will cure the cancer, but the cosmetic result after a couple of years is poor, and the risk of a necrosis is increased.

There are two basic supervoltage external-beam treatment plans: (1) opposed lateral nasal portals and (2) an anterior portal with or without lateral portals. When the tumor volume can be encompassed by lateral portals, there is an advantage in avoiding unnecessary exit irradiation to the nasal cavity, nasopharynx, and central nervous system. This technique confines irradiation to the anterior nasal area but has the disadvantage of full skin reaction, since a wax bolus nose block is needed to ensure homogeneous irradiation. The portals may be angled posteriorly to ensure sufficient posterior coverage; wedges are added to compensate for the angle (Fig. 23-23). Fractionation schemes are those used for orthovoltage, since the bolus produces skin reactions comparable to orthovoltage therapy. (See Chapter 26, Carcinoma of the Skin.)

If the lesion extends posteriorly into the nasal cavity or is well localized to one side of the nose, either implantation or an anterior portal technique is used. Lesions that grossly involve the floor of the nasal vestibule or junction of the septum and nasal floor may be difficult to implant because of the underlying bone; these lesions are best treated with external-beam irradiation. A single anterior portal may be tailored to reduce irradiation of normal tissue as much as possible. Wax plugs are placed in the nares to fill the air cavities. A wax bolus is placed over the nose to obtain full dose at the skin surface and also to convert the irregular nasal surface to a boxlike contour to provide a better scattering medium to underlying tissues (Fig. 23-24). Either electrons or photons plus electrons may be used for tumor volumes extending from the anterior nasal vestibule to 4 cm to 5 cm posteriorly (Fig. 23-25). Extensive lesions are frequently managed by external-beam therapy, 5000 rad/ 5 weeks, followed by an interstitial implant.

Anterior and lateral portals with wedges may be used when sinus involvement is present (Fig. 23-26). The ip-

TABLE 23-3. Nasal Vestibule Carcinoma: Local Control by Radiation Therapy (No. Controlled/No. Treated)

Stage	No Prior Treatment	Recurrent After Surgery	No. Salvaged/No. Attempted	Ultimate Control
T1	3/3	2/2	0/0	5/5
T2	1/1	1/2	1/1*	3/3
T3	1/1	1/1	0/0	2/2
T4	1/1	0/0	0/0	1/1
Total	6/6	4/5	1/1	11/11

* Patient underwent partial rhinectomy for salvage 3 years afrer radiation therapy and then died of intercurrent disease 4 months later.

Note: University of Florida data; patients treated 2/66–4/80; analysis 4/82 by N.P. Mendenhall, MD.

TABLE 23-4. Nasal Vestibule Carcinoma: Local Control According to Radiation Treatment Technique (No. Controlled/No. Treated)

Status of Primary Lesion	External-Beam Radiation Therapy	External-Beam Radiation Therapy Plus Radium	Radium Alone
No prior treatment	5/5	0/0	1/1
Recurrent after surgery	0/0	2/3	2/2

Note: University of Florida data; patients treated 1/66–4/80; analysis 4/82 by N.P. Mendenhall, MD.

silateral lymph nodes may be electively irradiated when there is skin involvement or recurrent disease.

INTERSTITIAL IMPLANT

Interstitial implants of the nasal vestibule and nasal cavity are highly individualized. The basic implant is usually composed of two, three, or four planes of needles inserted through the skin surface of the external nose. The basic arrangement to cover the entire nasal vestibule and upper lip is presented in Figure 23-27. Needles may be subtracted for smaller lesions or added for superior coverage toward the nasal cavity.

The implant is done with the patient under general anesthesia. Postoperative pain and bleeding have been minimal. Computer-generated isodose distributions are essential since the implant does not comply with basic Paterson–Parker implant patterns. The dose has varied from 5500 rad to 7500 rad, depending on the size of the lesion (Figs. 23-28 and 23-29).

NASAL MOLDS

A nasal vestibule mold may be fashioned for treatment of a small ipsilateral lesion. A single radium or cesium source is inserted in the mold. Treatment is given on an outpatient basis with applications of 1 to 2 hours daily over a period of 7 to 9 days. Few lesions are suitable for this method.

COMBINED TREATMENT POLICIES

Locally advanced lesions may be considered for resection followed by radiation therapy. However, the cosmetic loss is severe, and the approach has generally been to use radical radiation therapy and reserve resection for failures.

TREATMENT OF LYMPHATICS

The results of management of the neck disease are shown in Table 23-5. The neck is usually observed when clinically negative because of the low risk (~15%) for subclinical disease. Elective neck irradiation is used for advanced, recurrent, or poorly differentiated lesions. Patients treated after multiple surgical recurrences may develop in-transit lymph vessel disease; electrons may be used to electively irradiate the transit lymph vessels at risk between the nose and submaxillary nodes (Fu Manchu technique).[44]

MANAGEMENT OF RECURRENCE

Lesions recurrent after radiation therapy are excised and surgical failures are usually treated by radiation therapy. Management of recurrence is often successful, but the associated cosmetic deformity may be quite severe. The risk of regional lymph node metastasis increases with recurrence.

Nasal Cavity

SELECTION OF TREATMENT MODALITY

The histology, extent, and location of the malignant tumor of the nasal cavity are all considered in making treatment decisions.

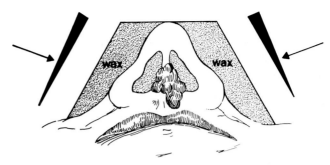

FIG. 23-23. Treatment plan for external-beam irradiation of a nasal vestibule carcinoma. (Million RR, Cassisi NJ, Wittes RE: Cancer in the head and neck. In DeVita VT Jr, Hellman S, Rosenberg SA [eds]: Cancer: Principles and Practice of Oncology, pp 301–395. Philadelphia, JB Lippincott, 1982)

Inverting papilloma (without carcinoma) is treated initially by surgical excision. Intranasal excisions, Caldwell-Luc procedures, and ethmoidectomies result in a high recurrence rate and possibly an increased risk to develop a carcinoma. Lateral rhinotomy and en *bloc* removal of the lateral nasal wall plus resection of involved mucosa in adjacent sinuses produces a low rate of recurrence.[31] Inverting papilloma associated with carcinoma is treated in the same fashion as other nasal carcinomas. When inverting papilloma begins to act aggressively with rapid recurrences and invasion of the sinuses, orbit, and cribriform plate, it should be considered a low-grade cancer and treated appropriately by more radical en *bloc* removal or irradiation. Experience with irradiation is limited, but it is definitely of value. One patient has been free of disease 8 years following irradiation for rapidly recurring inverting papilloma that had extended to the anterior cranial fossa and adjacent paranasal sinus. A recent case received preoperative radiation therapy (6000 rad) for an extensive recurrent inverting papilloma with a focus of squamous cell carcinoma involving the infratemporal fossa and orbit; the specimen was negative for tumor.

Squamous cell carcinoma and adenocarcinoma of the nasal cavity may be treated either with surgery, irradiation, or both. Most analyses of nasal cavity carcinomas are included with paranasal sinus cancer series. Since standardized staging is not applied, it is difficult to compare the results of various therapies. Since regional and distant metastases are relatively uncommon, local control is tantamount to cure.

Either surgery or radiation therapy is used for discrete early lesions. Operative management is usually indicated for early discrete lesions of the septum, where good surgical margins may be expected without cosmetic or functional loss. Radiation therapy is usually recommended for the remaining sites.

When carcinoma extends to the bone or cartilage of the external nose, adjoining sinuses, orbit, anterior cranial fossa, or nasopharynx, radical irradiation has been our treatment, with disease controlled locally in six of seven patients. The alternative in suitable cases would be a craniofacial procedure with postoperative irradiation.

Early stages of esthesioneuroblastoma may be treated by either radiation therapy or surgery with comparable results. Advanced lesions are managed by surgery and

(Text continues on p. 433.)

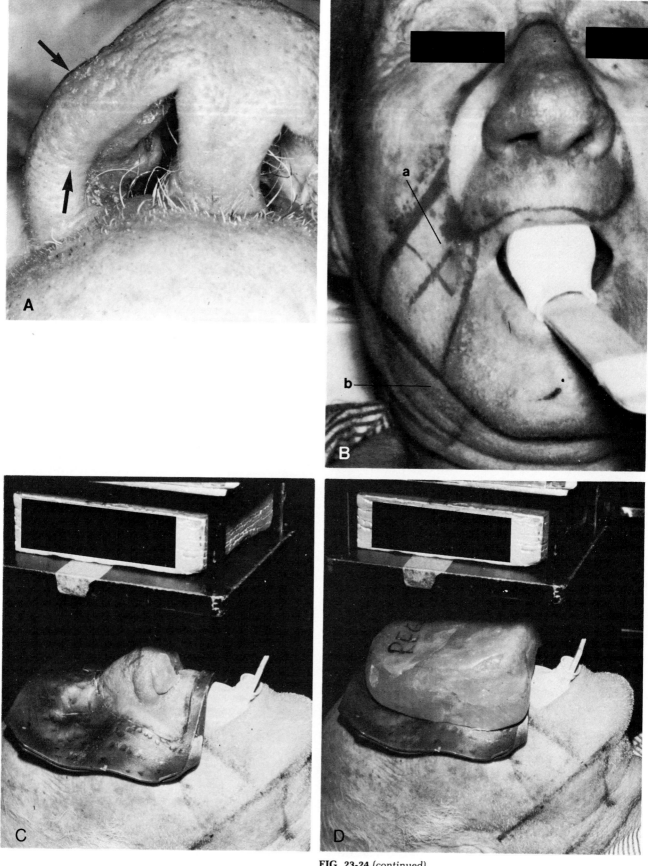

FIG. 23-24 (continued)

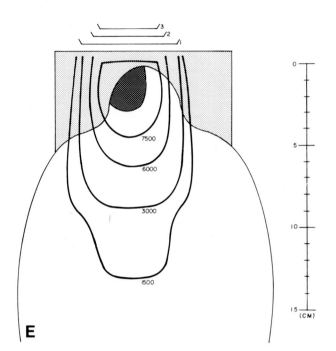

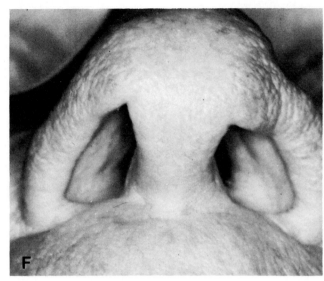

FIG. 23-24. An 84-year-old man presented with 3-month history of repeated episodes of nosebleeds. There was a 1.5-cm tumor on right lateral nasal vestibule with erythema and induration extending to the overlying skin of the tip and ala of the nose and just into the lip. There was probable invasion of the lateral alar cartilage. He also had a squamous cell carcinoma of the vocal cord (T1N0). (A) Squamous cell carcinoma of the right lateral wall of the nasal vestibule (arrows indicate skin invasion). (B) Outline of treatment portals. The transit lymphatics and facial lymph nodes were treated with electrons (a), and the submaxillary lymph nodes (b) were electively treated because of the significant dermal extension and the undesirability of doing a neck dissection if needed in this 84-year-old patient. (C) Treatment setup with lead shield, wax plugs in nose, and tongue depressor. (D) Wax bolus in place. Electron beam collimated by Cerrobend block on tray. Treatment plan was 7500 rad/8 weeks using a combination of photons and electrons. (E) Isodose distribution. Stippled area represents beeswax bolus/compensator.

Portal	Energy	Field Size (cm)	Given Dose (rad)
1	20 MeV	6 × 6	3720
1	17 MV	6 × 6	1830
2	20 MeV	4.5 × 4.5	1705
2	8 MV	4.5 × 4.5	440
3	17 MeV	3.5 × 3.5	550

(F) There was no evidence of disease at 2 years.

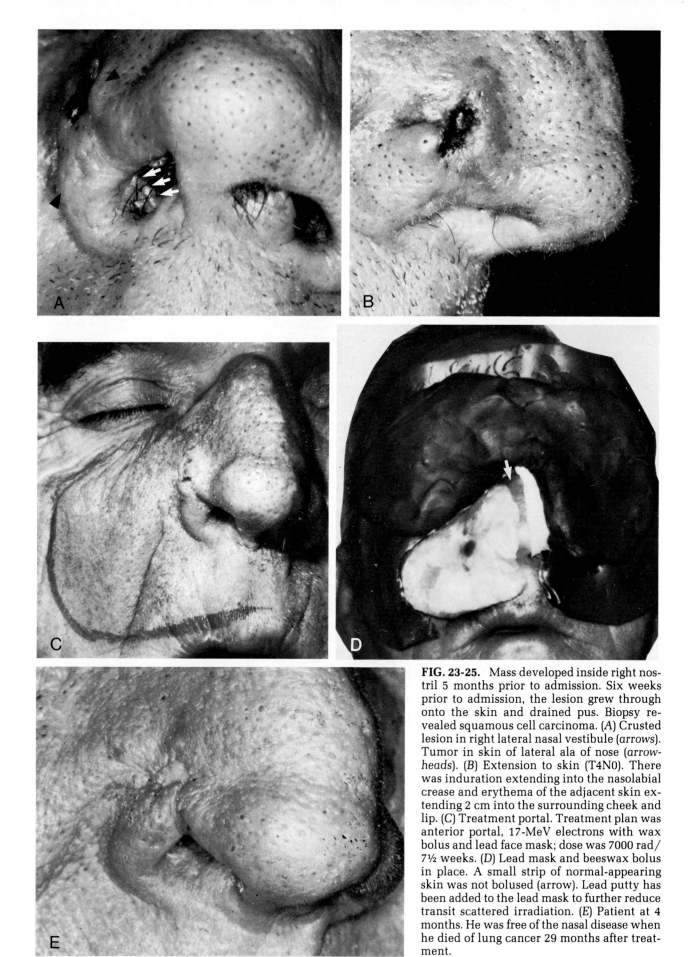

FIG. 23-25. Mass developed inside right nostril 5 months prior to admission. Six weeks prior to admission, the lesion grew through onto the skin and drained pus. Biopsy revealed squamous cell carcinoma. (*A*) Crusted lesion in right lateral nasal vestibule (*arrows*). Tumor in skin of lateral ala of nose (*arrowheads*). (*B*) Extension to skin (T4N0). There was induration extending into the nasolabial crease and erythema of the adjacent skin extending 2 cm into the surrounding cheek and lip. (*C*) Treatment portal. Treatment plan was anterior portal, 17-MeV electrons with wax bolus and lead face mask; dose was 7000 rad/ 7½ weeks. (*D*) Lead mask and beeswax bolus in place. A small strip of normal-appearing skin was not bolused (arrow). Lead putty has been added to the lead mask to further reduce transit scattered irradiation. (*E*) Patient at 4 months. He was free of the nasal disease when he died of lung cancer 29 months after treatment.

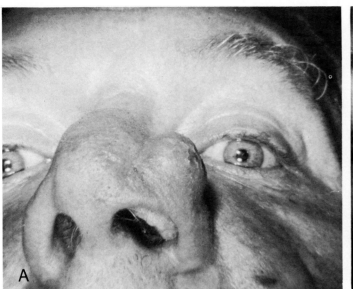
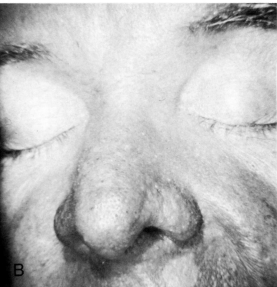

FIG. 23-26. (A) Squamous cell carcinoma of the left nasal vestibule with direct extension to the skin. Tomograms were reported to show possible erosion of the anterior ethmoid and medial wall of the maxillary sinus. Exploration of the maxillary sinus was negative. When the patient returned 10 days later, there was significant increase in size of the lesion. Treatment consisted of 7000 rad/8 weeks, cobalt-60, with anterior and left lateral portals with wedges. The adjacent sinuses were included and the skin of the nose was bolused. The regional lymph nodes were electively irradiated because of the history of rapid growth and skin infiltration. There was 90% regression after 3000 rad. (B) Appearance 3 months after end of treatment. The patient was free of disease at 5 years.

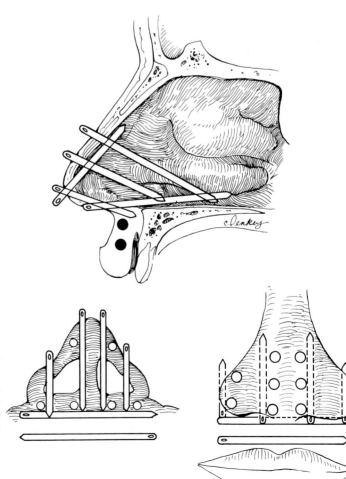

FIG. 23-27. Diagram of interstitial implant for carcinoma of the nasal vestibule. (Million RR, Cassisi NJ, Wittes RE: Cancer in the head and neck. In DeVita VT Jr, Hellman S, Rosenberg SA [eds]: Cancer: Principles and Practice of Oncology, pp 301–395. Philadelphia, JB Lippincott, 1982)

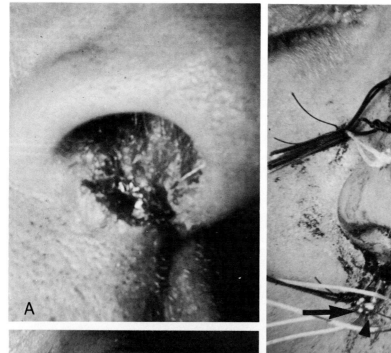

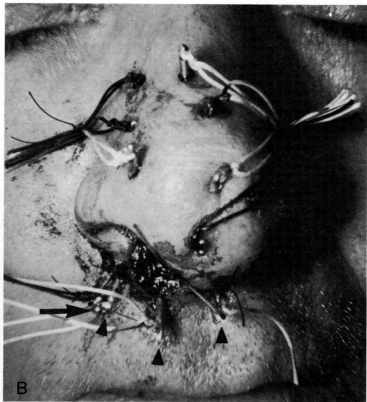

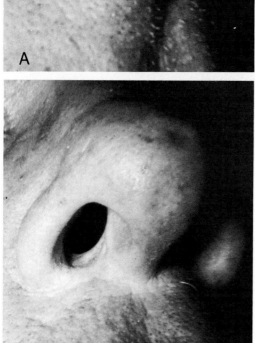

FIG. 23-28. (*A*) Squamous cell carcinoma of the nasal vestibule. The lesion was 2.5 cm in diameter. There was extension along the septum and floor of the nose and early involvement of the lip (*B*) Modified 2-plane implant. There are three needles in the floor of the nose (*arrowheads*) and a needle in the lip (*arrow*). Note that the needles in the floor of the nose protrude a few millimeters to enlarge the radiation field around the lesion. (*C*) Six months after treatment.

FIG. 23-29. Squamous cell carcinoma of the columella, 1.5 × 1.5 cm, treated with a modified three-plane implant in the nasal vestibule plus two needles in the lip and two needles in the floor of the nose (6500 rad/6 days). (*B*) Appearance 1 year after treatment.

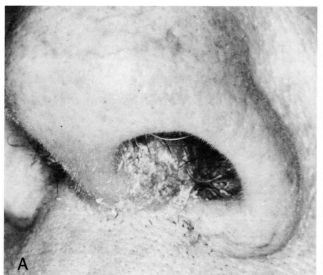

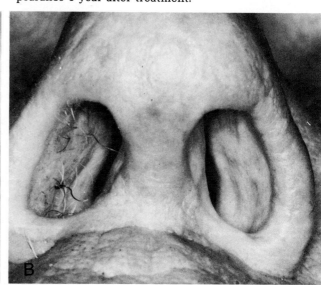

TABLE 23-5.   Nasal Vestibule Carcinoma: Neck Control—All Clinically Negative on Admission (No. With Neck Disease Controlled/No. Treated)

Result of Treatment of the Primary Lesion	No ENI	ENI	Salvage	Ultimate Control
Primary controlled	6/8	2/2*	2/2	10/10
Primary failure	1/1	0/0	0/0	1/1

*T3 lesions.
(ENI, elective neck irradiation)
Note: University of Florida data; patients treated 2/66–4/80; analysis 4/82 by N.P. Mendenhall, MD.

postoperative irradiation or radiation therapy alone. Elective neck treatment is generally not prescribed. However, recurrent lesions, lesions that extend to the nasopharynx, and poorly differentiated tumors have a higher risk of metastasis and selectively are given elective neck irradiation.

Midline lethal granuloma is treated by radiation therapy to the nasal cavity and all of the paranasal sinuses.

Surgical excision is usually the treatment of choice for sarcomas; preoperative or postoperative irradiation is added on an individual basis (see Chapter 34, Adult Mesenchymal Tumors Presenting in the Head and Neck).

For treatment of melanoma, see section on mucosal melanoma in Chapter 27, Melanoma of the Head and Neck.

SURGICAL TREATMENT

Excision of lesions of the lateral wall or septum is best carried out using a lateral rhinotomy approach. Generally, reconstruction is not necessary unless the entire cartilaginous septum has been removed, in which case there will be a saddle-nose deformity.

IRRADIATION TECHNIQUE

EXTERNAL BEAM

The majority of cases are treated by external beam irradiation that emphasizes an anterior portal with one or two lateral portals. Since satisfactory examination of the nasal cavity is difficult with cancer present, it is better to err on the side of a large treatment volume rather than rely too greatly on roentgenography and physical examination. This means that contiguous structures such as the medial portion of the maxillary sinus, ethmoid sinus, medial orbit, nasopharynx, base of the skull, and sphenoid sinus are generally included in the initial treatment volume, even though the lesion is thought to be rather localized. The treatment volume is reduced after 5000 rad to include the original gross disease with a margin.

Advanced lesions require inclusion of an entire orbit if tumor grossly invades the medial orbit; in these cases, loss of vision may occur, but an operation would require visual loss in any case. A two-field distribution for advanced nasal cavity lesions is shown in Figure 23-30.[30] (See section on the eye in Chapter 14, The Effect of Radiation on Normal Tissues of the Head and Neck, for further discussion.)

Treatment planning for midline lethal granuloma includes the nasal cavity and all of the paranasal sinuses. The dose is 4000 rad to normal areas and 5000 rad to areas of gross disease.

COMBINED TREATMENT POLICIES

If combined treatment is planned, we prefer to use the operation first to avoid obscuring the extent of tumor. Irradiation is started 4 to 6 weeks afterward. The dose is usually 6000 rad to 6500 rad/6½ to 7½ weeks.

MANAGEMENT OF RECURRENCE

Diagnosis of recurrent lesions is important since salvage may be possible. Once the patient has had an operation or irradiation it is difficult to determine the extent of recurrent disease by roentgenograms or CT scans because of changes from the previous therapy. The most common situation presenting for salvage treatment is a radiation or surgical failure that can be treated successfully by a craniofacial resection. Extension of tumor to the sphenopalatine fossa with definite destruction of a pterygoid plate may be a contraindication to a craniofacial procedure, as is cranial nerve involvement, invasion posteriorly near the optic chiasm, or sphenoid sinus invasion. It is often impossible to distinguish roentgenographically between tumor and inflammatory changes in the sphenoid sinus unless there is obvious bone destruction; surgical exploration may be necessary for final diagnosis. The anterior wall of the sinus may be removed, but the sinus itself cannot be resected.[24] Postoperative irradiation should be considered whether or not margins are positive. About 25% of patients may be cured by this approach. The limits of a craniofacial resection are shown in Figure 23-31.

Ethmoid Sinus

SELECTION OF TREATMENT MODALITY

Ethmoid sinus lesions are usually extensive when first diagnosed. Radiation therapy alone produces better results than surgery alone and is the preferred single treatment.[12] If resection is feasible with acceptable functional and cosmetic results, then the operation is carried out, followed by postoperative radiation therapy even if margins are clear.

SURGICAL TREATMENT

En bloc removal of an ethmoid sinus carcinoma requires a craniofacial resection. Lesser procedures are best described as piecemeal removal.

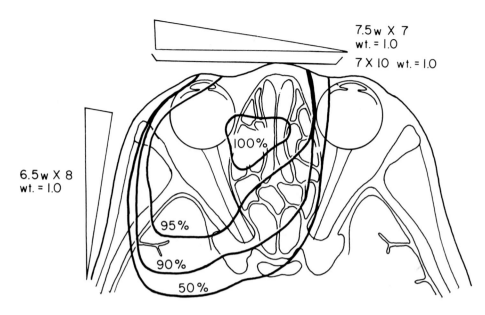

7.5w X 7
wt. = 1.0

7 X 10 wt. = 1.0

6.5w X 8
wt. = 1.0

100%

95%

90%

50%

FIG. 23-30. Isodose distribution for carcinoma of the ethmoid sinus with invasion of the orbit. The lateral portal is angled 5° posteriorly. (Million RR, Cassisi NJ, Wittes RE: Cancer in the head and neck. In DeVita VT Jr, Hellman S, Rosenberg SA [eds]: Cancer: Principles and Practice of Oncology, pp 301–395. Philadelphia, JB Lippincott, 1982)

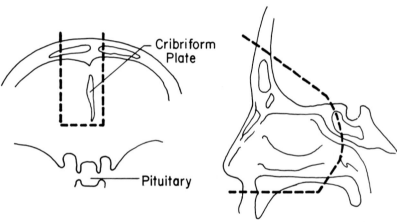

Cribriform Plate

Pituitary

FIG. 23-31. Lines of resection for craniofacial resection of advanced paranasal sinus tumor with intracranial extension. (Million RR, Cassisi NJ, Wittes RE: Cancer in the head and neck. In DeVita VT Jr, Hellman S, Rosenberg SA [eds]: Cancer: Principles and Practice of Oncology, pp 301–395. Philadelphia, JB Lippincott, 1982)

IRRADIATION TECHNIQUE

Radiation treatment is entirely by external beam, emphasizing treatment through an anterior field combined with one or two lateral fields (Fig. 23-32). A reduced anterior open field is often incorporated into the treatment plan to concentrate the dose to the major bulk of disease. This field arrangement, weighted 2:1 or 3:1 in favor of the anterior field, provides adequate treatment of the tumor volume while avoiding excessive irradiation of the contralateral eye. Wedges are added to achieve a satisfactory dose distribution.

If there is no evidence of extension of disease to the orbit (an uncommon situation), a rectangular or L-shaped anterior field is used that transects the ipsilateral eye just medial to the limbus. There is usually evidence of orbital invasion, and all or most of the orbit is included in the initial treatment field. The portal extends 1.5 cm to 2.0 cm across the midline to encompass the entire nasal cavity–ethmoid/sphenoid sinus complex and medial aspect of the contralateral orbit. The superior border encompasses the cribriform plate and includes all or part of the frontal sinus.

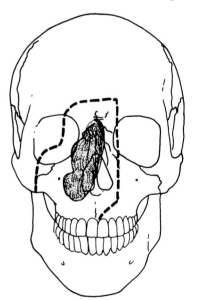

The inferior margin is low enough to cover the floor of the nose and all or part of the maxillary antrum as needed.

The anterior border of the lateral field is located at the lateral bony canthus. The posterior border is just anterior to the external auditory canal, ensuring adequate treatment of the pterygomaxillary space, sphenoid sinus, base of the skull, nasopharynx, and parapharyngeal nodes. The superior border of the lateral field is 1 cm above the base of the skull, unless there is evidence of extension to the cranial contents. With suspected intracranial extension, the superior borders are raised 2 cm to 3 cm. The lateral field is tilted 5° posteriorly to reduce contralateral eye irradiation.

Patients are instructed to gaze straight ahead and keep their eyes open during treatment. An eyelid retractor is used for patients who are unable to keep their lids open. A lacrimal gland shield is used, except in patients with extensive involvement of orbital tissues. (See section on the eye in Chapter 14, The Effect of Radiation on Normal Tissues of the Head and Neck, for further discussion of incidental eye irradiation.)

MANAGEMENT OF RECURRENCE

Recurrent disease is heralded by recurrent pain and cranial nerve palsies. Exploration of the sinuses is necessary for diagnosis.

Localized recurrence after surgery only may be managed by radiation therapy alone or craniofacial resection and postoperative radiation therapy. Radiation therapy failures may be treated by craniofacial resection.

Maxillary Sinus

SELECTION OF TREATMENT MODALITY

Surgical resection gives the best results. Early infrastructure lesions may be excised and cured by surgery alone, but for most other cases irradiation is given postoperatively even if the margins are negative. Extension of cancer to the base of the skull, the nasopharynx, or the sphenoid sinus contraindicates surgical excision. Many patients refuse the operation because of the defect imposed by maxillectomy and possible orbital exenteration. Radiation therapy alone produces a few cures even for advanced cases (Fig. 23-33).

SURGICAL TREATMENT

Surgery for carcinoma of the maxillary sinus depends on which walls are involved. If the roof of the sinus is free of disease, then the eye and the orbital rim may be left undisturbed and only the floor of the orbit removed. If, however, there is extension through the roof of the sinus into the orbit, then a maxillectomy and orbital exenteration must be performed. If the cancer extends through the posterior wall, the pterygoid muscle and ascending ramus of the mandible are usually removed. Lesions that spread medially and upward require removal of the ethmoid sinus and anterior wall of the sphenoid sinus. Lesions that grow anteriorly require excision of facial muscle and skin. A split-thickness skin graft is used to line the cavity, and a dental prosthesis is then used to fill the resulting deformity in the palate. It is preferable to construct the prosthesis prior to the surgery so it can be placed at the time of surgery and act as a stent. (See Chapter 10, Maxillofacial Prosthetics.)

IRRADIATION TECHNIQUE

Irradiation treatment planning includes the entire maxilla, adjacent nasal cavity, ethmoid sinus, nasopharynx, and pterygopalatine fossa, and at least a portion of the adjacent orbit. The entire orbit is included in patients with extension into the orbital fossa; failure to include the orbital contents is one of the most common causes of failure. The prescribed dose is 6500 rad to 7500 rad. An anterior portal combined with one or two lateral portals is the usual arrangement, designed to incorporate the tumor volume. (See section on the eye in Chapter 14, The Effect of Radiation on Normal Tissues of the Head and Neck.)

Drainage procedures are performed when needed, either before, during, or after radiation therapy.

COMBINED TREATMENT POLICIES

Except for the early infrastructure lesion, surgical resection is followed in 4 weeks by high-dose external beam radiation therapy. The dose should be 6000 rad to 6500 rad/6 to 7 weeks, since the recurrence rate at lower doses is substantial. Higher doses may be recommended for residual disease.

MANAGEMENT OF RECURRENCE

Recurrence following radiation therapy or surgery is sometimes suitable for craniofacial resection.

Sphenoid Sinus

The treatment planning for carcinoma of the sphenoid sinus is similar to that for advanced carcinoma of the nasopharynx.

RESULTS OF TREATMENT

Nasal Vestibule

The results for nasal vestibule carcinoma are often included under nasal cavity and may give a falsely high rate of success for nasal cavity.

Goepfert and co-workers reviewed the M. D. Anderson Hospital experience of 26 patients with squamous cell carcinoma of the nasal vestibule.[17] The absolute 5-year survival rate was 78%. Ten patients were treated initially by surgery; one developed a local recurrence and salvage was achieved by radiation therapy. Sixteen patients were treated by radiation therapy; of 3 who developed local recurrence, 2 had their disease controlled by an operation. Only 1 patient had a positive node on admission, but 7 patients later developed positive node(s); 4 patients developed bilateral nodes. All neck node metastases were successfully managed by surgery alone or by surgery and radiation therapy.

Mendenhall reviewed 11 patients treated by irradiation at the University of Florida for squamous cell carcinoma

(Text continues on p. 440.)

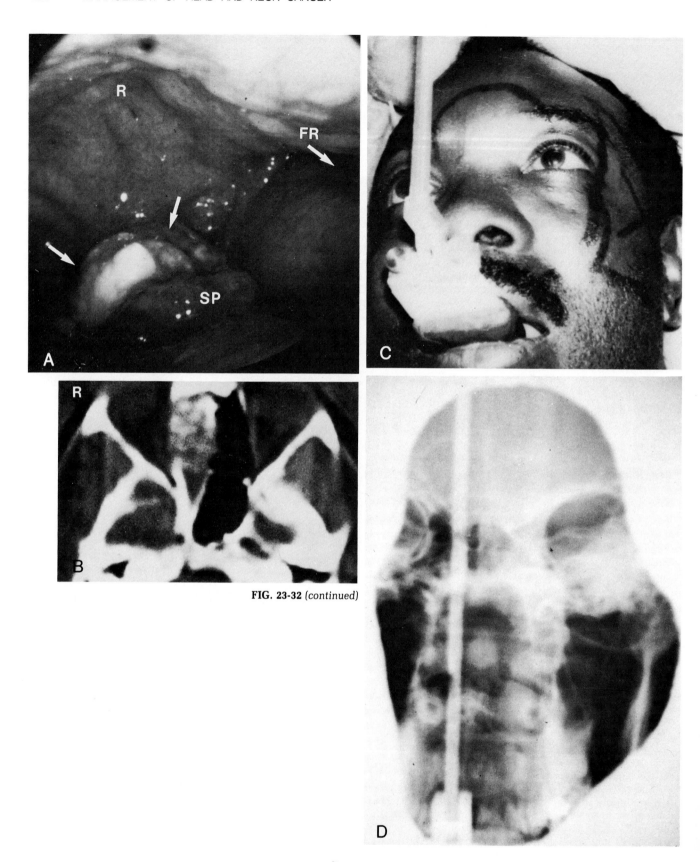

FIG. 23-32 (continued)

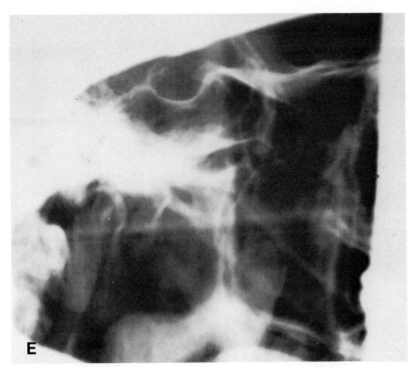

FIG. 23-32. A 33-year-old man presented with a 1-year history of left nasal congestion and frontal headaches, a 6-month history of epistaxis, and a 3-month history of tearing of the left eye. There was a granular lesion in the posterior nasal cavity and nasopharynx. Biopsy revealed squamous cell carcinoma of the ethmoid sinus. (A) Tumor mass extending into nasopharynx (*arrows*). (R, roof; SP, soft palate; FR, right fossa of Rosenmüller) (B) CT scan at level of orbit and ethmoid sinuses. There is opacification of the right ethmoid sinus and nasal cavity. The mass bulges into the medial aspect of the left orbit. Additional views showed opacification of the left sphenoid sinus and the left maxillary sinus, erosion of left pterygoid plates, and possible erosion of the cribriform plate. Diagnosis was squamous cell carcinoma of the ethmoid sinus with invasion of the maxillary sinus, sphenoid sinus, nasal cavity, and nasopharynx. The site of origin is actually an educated guess and could have been the nasal cavity or upper medial maxillary antrum. The tumor was thought to be inoperable because of involvement of the nasopharynx and possible sphenoid sinus invasion. (C) Radiation therapy treatment portals were anteroposterior and left and right laterals. The left upper lateral eyelid and the lacrimal gland were shielded since only the medial orbit was involved by tumor. (D) Simulation film of anteroposterior portal. Straight white line is the aluminum support for bite block. (E) Simulation film of lateral portal (5° posterior tilt). The treatment plan was 7000-rad minimum tumor dose in 7 weeks to 7700-rad maximum tumor dose in 7 weeks. The right and left upper necks received 4050 rad/3 weeks through an anterior portal with midline shielding. The visible tumor disappeared during therapy. The patient returned to full-time work as truck driver at 4 months. A cataract developed in the left eye at 36 months, but following extraction the patient was only able to count fingers at 2 feet, owing to radiation retinopathy. The patient was free of disease at 4½ years. (D and E from Ellingwood KE, Million RR: Cancer of the nasal cavity and ethmoid/sphenoid sinuses. Cancer 43:1517–1526, 1979)

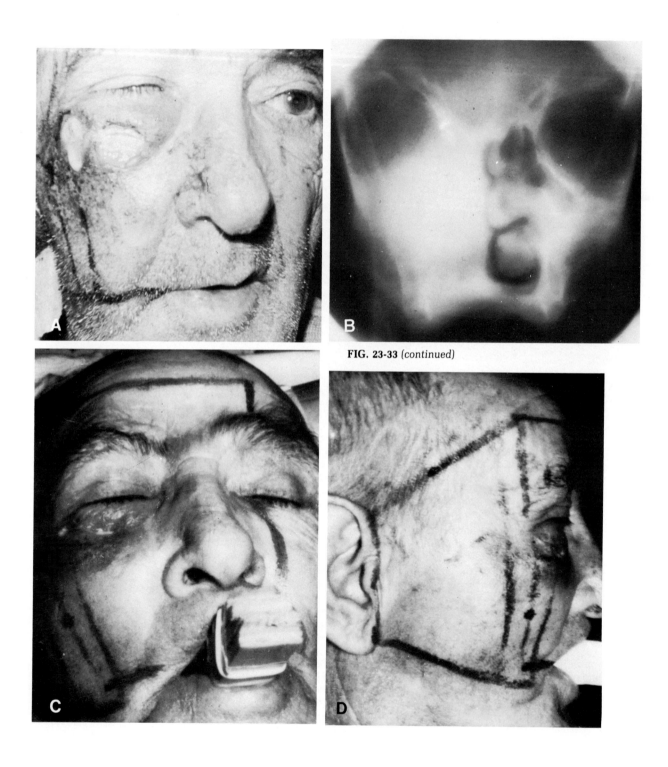

FIG. 23-33 (continued)

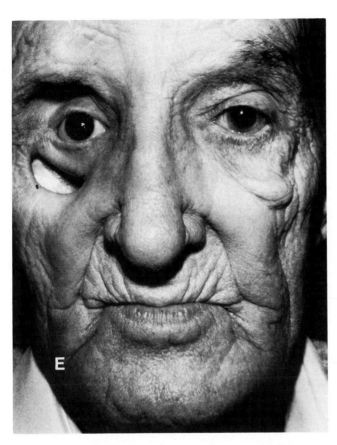

FIG. 23-33.   A 71-year-old man presented with a long history of sinusitis, including polypectomy and bilateral ethmoidectomies. Two months prior to admission he noticed pain in the right cheek and a mass below the right lateral eyelid. The mass spontaneously drained through the skin. There was recent onset of diplopia. (*A*) There was pus draining from the right cheek mass, the lids were red and edematous, and there was proptosis of the right eye. The orbit was filled with a rock-hard mass. The nasal cavity was occluded by tumor, but the nasopharynx was normal (T4N0). Biopsy revealed squamous cell carcinoma. (*B*) Tomography revealed an opacified right maxillary antrum, right ethmoid/sphenoid sinus, and right nasal cavity with destruction of the medial and inferior orbital walls. There was no intracranial extension. CT examination confirmed the above. The patient refused any form of operation. The radiation treatment plan was anterior (*C*) and right lateral (*D*) portals (cobalt-60). Tongue blades were used to depress the tongue out of the irradiation portal. The anterior and lateral portals overlapped approximately 2 cm. The minimum tumor dose was 7000 rad/8½ weeks to a maximum tumor dose of 8050 rad/8½ weeks. There was complete regression of obvious tumor at 5000 rad. The diplopia disappeared and vision returned to normal. Pneumatic equalization tubes were inserted for bilateral serous otitis media. Blurry vision developed at 14 months due to superficial keratitis secondary to dry eye and a cataract. The right cornea perforated spontaneously at 22 months and was repaired with a corneal transplant. The transplant failed, and the right eye was enucleated. (*E*) Appearance at 5 years. An artificial eye was inserted but caused intermittent discomfort. The antrocutaneous fistula persists but is asymptomatic and provides a porthole for antrum examination.

of the nasal vestibule; 5 had recurrent disease after 1 to 4 previous surgical excisions and 6 had had no prior treatment.* *Four patients had obvious cartilage invasion.* Radiation therapy was individualized. Ten of 11 lesions have been controlled for 2 to 16 years. Two patients developed a single submaxillary node that was treated and controlled by radical neck dissection; they are alive at 4 years and 9 years. Radiation therapy complications were minor. There was no example of persistent chondritis or soft tissue necrosis. Treatment of one patient failed 3 years after radiation therapy; he died of intercurrent disease 4 months after partial rhinectomy. The 2- and 5-year survival rates are shown in Table 23-6.

Nasal Cavity/Ethmoid Sinus

Frazell and Lewis reported a 56% 5-year cure rate for 68 nasal cavity neoplasms treated surgically.[16] The 5-year cure rate by radiation therapy was 18% for 28 patients treated. The selection and stage of patients for each modality was not analyzed. They reported 40% (4/10) of patients with ethmoid sinus carcinoma treated by radiation therapy were cured at 5 years, but only 4 of 21 patients treated by an operation were cured. They concluded, however, that the operation was the treatment of choice.

Bosch and co-workers reported their experience with 40 cases of cancer of the nasal cavity.[8] Eighty-five percent were treated by radiation therapy. The 5-year survival rate was 56% for the entire group and 50% for those treated by radiation therapy alone.

Boone and co-workers reported the M. D. Anderson Hospital experience for 28 patients with nasal cavity carcinoma.[7] The 5-year absolute cure rate was 63%; the local recurrence rate was 21%.

Parsons reviewed the results for 16 patients with squamous cell carcinoma of the nasal cavity or ethmoid sinus treated from October 1964 to January 1979 by radiation therapy.† The local control results by stage are shown in Table 23-7. Specification of the site of origin, except for stage I nasal cavity lesions, is an educated guess based on the bulk of disease, and therefore nasal cavity and ethmoid sinus lesions are combined for analysis. The 2- and 5-year local control results by histology for 37 patients treated with curative doses of radiation therapy are given in Table 23-8; 2 patients had surgical excision in conjunction with radiation therapy. Although the initial response and local control rates for adenoid cystic carcinoma were excellent, only 1 of 5 patients remained free of recurrence at 10 years; the other 4 patients developed recurrent disease at 3½, 4, 5, and 12 years after radiation therapy. There were no failures later than 2 years after treatment in the other histologies. The 5-year survival data for all histologies are given in Table 23-9.

Six patients had clinical and roentgenographic evidence of intracranial extension; 4 were free of disease at 3½, 4, 8, and 10 years. Elective neck irradiation was used in 16 patients, and no neck failures were observed. Two of 18 patients without elective neck irradiation developed a neck node, and salvage was achieved in both by radical neck dissection. Three patients presented with clinically positive lymph nodes; all were successfully managed by radiation therapy alone. Three patients died with distant metastases

* Mendenhall NP: Unpublished data, 1982.
† Parsons JT: Unpublished data, 1981.

TABLE 23-6. Nasal Vestibule Carcinoma: Survival—11 Patients

2 Years		5 Years	
Absolute	Determinate	Absolute	Determinate
11/11	11/11	5/7	5/5

Note: University of Florida data; patients treated 1/66–4/80; analysis 4/82 by N.P. Mendenhall, MD.

TABLE 23-7. Local Control by Stage in Squamous Cell Carcinoma of the Nasal Cavity and Ethmoid Sinuses: Primary Treatment by Radiation Therapy

Stage	Local Control (No. Controlled/No. Treated; Percentage)
I	4/4 (100%)
II	4/6 (66%)
III	2/6 (33%)

Note. University of Florida data; patients treated 10/64–1/79; analysis by J. T. Parsons, MD, 1981.

and the primary lesion controlled. Surgical salvage of local failure was unsuccessful in four attempts.

ESTHESIONEUROBLASTOMA

Elkon and associates reviewed the world literature on esthesioneuroblastoma and presented results for 78 patients.[11] The local control and salvage rates by treatment category are outlined in Table 23-10. All 24 stage A lesions were eventually controlled locally; 1 patient died with distant metastasis. Eighty-two percent of stage B lesions and 48% of stage C lesions were ultimately locally controlled. Eight patients developed regional lymph node metastases and 4 were cured. Only 1 patient with a spinal cord failure was listed.

The 5-year absolute survival rate for stage A was 75%; stage B, 60%; and stage C, 41%. The local recurrence rate after radiation therapy in this review is not explained by the doses prescribed. Local recurrence occurred at 6000 rad in five cases, but the disease was as often as not controlled with lower doses. This finding suggests inadequate treatment volume as a cause of failure.

INVERTING PAPILLOMA

Myers and co-workers reported no local recurrence in 13 cases of inverting papilloma excised through a lateral rhinotomy approach.[31] The follow-up was 1½ to 9½ years; three patients were followed for more than 9 years. Suh and associates reported recurrence in 4 of 34 inverting papillomas excised through a lateral rhinotomy.[41]

Myers and colleagues treated five patients for cure with mixed inverting papilloma and carcinoma; four had radiation therapy in addition to excision. Four patients had

TABLE 23-8. Local Control Following Radiation Therapy in Nasal Cavity and Ethmoid/Sphenoid Sinus Cancer (2-Year Minimum Follow-up)

Type of Tumor	Local Control*	
	2-Year	5-Year
Squamous cell carcinoma†	10/16 (63%)	5/9 (56%)
Esthesioneuroblastoma†	2/4 (50%)	1/3 (33%)
Minor salivary gland tumors† (excluding adenoid cystic)	5/6 (83%)	3/3 (100%)
Adenoid cystic‡	5/5 (100%)	2/5 (40%)
Miscellaneous (melanoma, sarcoma§)	2/3 (66%)	2/3 (66%)

* Six patients excluded from analysis of local control owing to death from intercurrent disease in less than 2 years with primary lesion controlled.
† Three patients were treated for postsurgical recurrences with advanced disease.
‡ One patient had resection of residual disease in nasal cavity 2 months following radiation therapy.
§ One patient had resection of fibrosarcoma with gross residual disease.
Note: University of Florida data; patients treated 10/64–1/79; analysis by J. T. Parsons, MD, 1981.

TABLE 23-9. Five-Year Results in Nasal Cavity and Ethmoid/Sphenoid Sinus Cancer (All Histologies)*

No. Patients at Risk	Absolute Survival	Absolute Survival Free of Disease	Death due to Intercurrent Disease	Determinate Survival
29	15/29 (52%)	13/29 (45%)	5	15/24 (63%)

* No. of patients in study (2-year minimum follow-up): stage I, 10; stage II, 10; stage III, 17.
Note: University of Florida data; patients treated 10/64–1/79; analysis by J. T. Parsons, MD, 1981.

TABLE 23-10. Esthesioneuroblastoma: Results of Treatment to Primary Tumor by Modality and Stage for 78 Patients With Follow-up of 6 Months to 32 Years (No. Controlled/No. Treated)

Modality	Stage A—Confined to Nasal Cavity		Stage B—Confined to Nasal Cavity and Paranasal Sinuses		Stage C—Beyond Nasal Cavity and Paranasal Sinuses	
	Initial Treatment	For Recurrent Disease at Primary Site	Initial Treatment	For Recurrent Disease at Primary Site	Initial Treatment	For Recurrent Disease at Primary Site
Radiation therapy alone	3/5	5/5	6/7	3/4	1/5	1/1
Surgery alone	5/9	2/2	3/6		1/1	0/0
Radiation therapy and surgery	9/10	0/0	15/20	0/1	7/15	0/0
Ultimate local control	24/24 (100%)		27/33 (82%)		10/21 (48%)	

(Modified from Elkon D, Hightower SI, Lim ML, Cantrell RW, Constable WC: Esthesioneuroblastoma. Cancer 44:1087–1094, 1979)

no evidence of disease at 3 to 6 years. One patient had a negative specimen after 6000 rad of preoperative irradiation.

MIDLINE LETHAL GRANULOMA

Fauci and co-workers reported results of ten patients with midline lethal granuloma treated by high-dose irradiation.[13] Long-term remissions (5 to 13 years) occurred in six patients. Four patients developed malignancies at other sites.

Maxillary Sinus

Jesse reviewed 87 patients with squamous cell carcinoma of the maxillary antrum.[20] The 3-year survival rate was about 30% for all cases, including 15 treated for palliation only and 9 that were too advanced for any treatment. Sixty-three were treated for cure, with a 3-year survival rate of 44%. Three-year survival after surgery alone for selected lesions was 9 of 20. Patients selected for combined treatment had either preoperative or postoperative irradiation, and the results were similar for both techniques. The local recurrence rate with combined treatment was 38%. Patients with infrastructure lesions and superolateral lesions had a 3-year survival rate of 68% (13/19), while those with superomedial or superoposterior lesions had a survival rate of only 29%.

Amendola and associates reported a 35% survival rate for 20 patients with squamous cell carcinoma of the maxillary antrum managed by radiation therapy alone; the 3-year local control rate was 66%.[5]

Bataini and Ennuyer reported Curie Foundation results for 31 patients with carcinoma of the maxillary antrum treated by supervoltage radiation therapy between 1959 and 1965.[6] Only three patients had limited primary disease; 30% had clinically positive lymph nodes. The 3- and 5-year survival rates were 39% and 32%, respectively.

FOLLOW-UP POLICY

Nasal Vestibule/Nasal Cavity

Careful follow-up is important since recurrences are often salvaged by second-line treatment.

Maxillary Sinus

If a maxillectomy has been done, follow-up is simplified by the ease of physical examination; it is much more difficult to appraise the patient who was treated only by radiation therapy, and Caldwell–Luc exploration is often necessary for suspicious symptoms. Baseline tomograms and CT scan are obtained about 6 months following treatment.

Ethmoid Sinus

Patients are followed by a routine physical examination. Roentgenograms and CT scans are requested for symptoms or signs suggesting local recurrence. Exploration of the ethmoid sinus is often required to substantiate recurrence. A few recurrences may be saved by a craniofacial procedure, radiation therapy, or both.

COMPLICATIONS OF TREATMENT

Maxillary Sinus

Complications of radiation therapy for maxillary sinus cancer include osteonecrosis, radiation-induced central nervous system disease, loss of vision, nasal obstruction, and otitis media. Complications of maxillectomy include failure of the split-thickness skin graft to heal, trismus, cerebrospinal fluid leak, and hemorrhage.

Ethmoid Sinus/Nasal Cavity

SURGERY

Complications of ethmoid sinus surgery include total blindness, loss of ocular motility, hemorrhage, meningitis, cerebrospinal fluid leak, cellulitis and pansinusitis, brain abscess, stroke, fistula between the cavernous sinus and internal carotid, and damage to the frontal lobe.[28] Complications of the craniofacial procedure are reported by Ketcham and co-workers.[24] About one third of the patients had a life-threatening complication requiring intensive care and prolonged hospitalization. The operative mortality rate was 4%. Complications included meningitis, subdural abscess, cerebrospinal fluid leak, diplopia, and hemorrhage. Most of these patients had recurrent or far-advanced disease prior to surgery.

IRRADIATION

The complications following radiation therapy for 37 patients are listed in Table 23-11. Eye complications are the most frequent and devastating of the complications of radiation therapy.[38] The majority of the 15 cases without complications died of cancer with a short follow-up. When

TABLE 23-11. Complications of Treatment of Tumors of the Nasal Cavity and Ethmoid/Sphenoid Sinuses (37 Patients)

Complication	No. Patients
Lhermitte's syndrome	2
Transitory central nervous system syndrome	3
Aseptic meningitis	1
Myelitis	0
Seizure disorders	0
Bone necrosis (mild)	1
Bone necrosis (severe)	1
Soft tissue necrosis	0
Sinusitis (symptomatic)	5
Nasal synechiae	5
Nasal septal perforation	2
Serous otitis requiring myringotomy	4
Blind in one eye	14
Blind in both eyes	1
None	15

Note: University of Florida data; patients treated 10/64–1/79; analysis by J. T. Parsons, MD, 1981.

only a portion of the ipsilateral eyeball is irradiated (medial one third) and the tears are preserved, it is possible to preserve vision in the majority of patients. However, when there is gross disease in the orbit, the entire eyeball is irradiated to a high dose with almost certain loss of vision; however, these same patients would require orbital exenteration if treated by surgery. (See Chapter 14, The Effect of Radiation on Normal Tissues of the Head and Neck.)

An estimated 10% of patients will develop a transitory central nervous system syndrome, which includes vertigo, headaches, decreased cerebration, and lethargy. This syndrome usually appears 2 to 3 months after completion of treatment but has been seen as late as 12 to 15 months. The early-appearing central nervous system syndromes usually last 1 to 2 months, but the late-appearing syndromes last 6 to 12 months before slowly resolving. Meningitis occurred 4½ years after treatment as a sequela to chronic sinusitis and was treated with antibiotics; the patient was alive and free of disease at 10 years.

Chronic, symptomatic sinusitis occurred in five patients. Exploration of the sinus was required in two patients to exclude recurrent disease and provide drainage. High-dose irradiation of the nasal cavity may cause narrowing and synechiae of the nasal cavity. Douching with salt water and daily self-dilations with petrolatum-coated cotton swabs will reduce this problem.

Septal perforations occur when tumor has destroyed part of the septum. These do not usually require treatment and some have closed spontaneously.

Destruction of the nasal bone and septum by tumor may result in cosmetic deformity. Two patients had successful reconstructive rhinoplasties after irradiation with doses of 7000 rad.

Maxillary necrosis may develop if dental extraction is undertaken, but this can usually be successfully managed because the blood supply is better in the maxilla than in the mandible.

Transient serous otitis is a frequent occurrence during or immediately after the course of therapy. Most cases resolve, but four patients required myringotomy and placement of pressure equalization tubes 2 to 13 months after treatment.

REFERENCES

1. American Joint Committee on Cancer: Manual for Staging of Cancer, 2nd ed, pp 43–48. Philadelphia, JB Lippincott, 1983
2. Acheson ED, Cowdell RH, Hadfield EH, Macbeth RG: Nasal cancer in woodworkers in the furniture industry. Br Med J 2:587–596, 1968
3. Acheson ED, Cowdell RH, Jolles B: Nasal cancer in the Northamptonshire boot and shoe industry. Br Med J 1:385–393, 1970
4. Acheson ED, Hadfield EH, Macbeth RG: Carcinoma of the nasal cavity and accessory sinuses in woodworkers. Lancet 1:311–312, 1967
5. Amendola BE, Eisert D, Hazra TA, King ER: Carcinoma of the maxillary antrum: Surgery or radiation therapy? Int J Radiat Oncol Biol Phys 7:743–746, 1981
6. Bataini J-P, Ennuyer A: Advanced carcinoma of the maxillary antrum treated by cobalt teletherapy and electron beam irradiation. Br J Radiol 44:590–598, 1971
7. Boone ML, Harle TS, Highott HW, Fletcher GH: Malignant disease of the paranasal sinuses and nasal cavity: Importance of precise localization of extent of disease. Am J Roentgenol Radium Ther Nucl Med 102:627–637, 1968
8. Bosch A, Vallecillo L, Frias Z: Cancer of the nasal cavity. Cancer 37:1458–1463, 1976
9. Bridger WM, van Nostrand P: The nose and paranasal sinuses: Applied surgical anatomy. J Otolaryngol 7(suppl 6):1–33, 1978
10. Dubois PJ, Schultz JC, Perrin RL, Dastur KJ: Tomography in expansile lesions of the nasal and paranasal sinuses. Radiology 125:149–158, 1977
11. Elkon D, Hightower SI, Lim ML, Cantrell RW, Constable WC: Esthesioneuroblastoma. Cancer 44:1087–1094, 1979
12. Ellingwood KE, Million RR: Cancer of the nasal cavity and ethmoid/sphenoid sinuses. Cancer 43:1517–1526, 1979
13. Fauci AS, Johnson RE, Wolff SM: Radiation therapy of midline granuloma. Ann Intern Med 84:140–147, 1976
14. Fletcher GH, Jing BS: The Head and Neck, pp 241–313. Chicago, Year Book Medical Publishers, 1968
15. Földi M: Lymphogenous encephalopathy. In Mayerson HS (ed): Lymph and the Lymphatic System, pp 169–198. Springfield, IL, Charles C Thomas, 1968
16. Frazell EL, Lewis JS: Cancer of the nasal cavity and accessory sinuses: A report of the management of 416 patients. Cancer 16:1293–1301, 1963
17. Goepfert H, Guillamondegui OM, Jesse RH, Lindberg RD: Squamous cell carcinoma of the nasal vestibule. Arch Otolaryngol 100:8–10, 1974
18. Haynes WD, Tapley ND: Radiation treatment of carcinoma of the nasal vestibule. Am J Roentgenol Radium Ther Nucl Med 120:595–602, 1974
19. Hesselink JR, New PF, Davis KR, Weber AL, Roberson GH, Taveras JM: Computed tomography of the paranasal sinuses and face: II. Pathological anatomy. J Comput Assist Tomogr 2:568–576, 1978
20. Jesse RH: Preoperative versus postoperative radiation in the treatment of squamous carcinoma of the paranasal sinuses. Am J Surg 110:552–556, 1965
21. Jing B-S, Goepfert H, Close LG: Computerized tomography of paranasal sinus neoplasms. Laryngoscope 88:1485–1503, 1978
22. Kadish S, Goodman M, Wang CC: Olfactory neuroblastoma: A clinical analysis of 17 cases. Cancer 37:1571–1576, 1976
23. Kassel SH, Echevarria RA, Guzzo FP: Midline malignant reticulosis (so-called lethal midline granuloma). Cancer 23:920–935, 1969
24. Ketcham AS, Chretien PB, VanBuren JM, Hoye RC, Bezley RM, Herdt JR: The ethmoid sinuses: A re-evaluation of surgical resection. Am J Surg 126:469–476, 1973
25. Maisel RH, Johnston WH, Anderson HA, Cantrell RW: Necrotizing sialometaplasia involving the nasal cavity. Laryngoscope 87:429–434, 1977
26. Mancuso AA, Hanafee WN: Computed Tomography of the Head and Neck, pp 203–243. Baltimore, Williams & Wilkins, 1981
27. Mancuso AA, Hanafee WN, Winter J, Ward P: Extensions of paranasal sinus tumors and inflammatory disease as evaluated by CT and pluridirectional tomography. Neuroradiology 16:449–453, 1978
28. Maniglia AJ, Chandler JR, Goodwin WJ, Jr, Flynn J: Rare complications following ethmoidectomies: A report of eleven cases. Laryngoscope 91:1234–1244, 1981
29. Meschan I: An Atlas of Anatomy Basic to Radiology, vol I, pp 297–300. Philadelphia, WB Saunders, 1975
30. Million RR, Cassisi NJ, Wittes RE: Cancer in the head and neck. In DeVita VT Jr, Hellman S, Rosenberg SA (eds): Cancer: Principles and Practice of Oncology, pp 301–395. Philadelphia, JB Lippincott, 1982
31. Myers EN, Schramm VL, Barnes EL: Management of inverted papilloma of the nose and paranasal sinuses. Laryngoscope 91:2071–2084, 1981
32. Osborn AG, Anderson RE: Direct sagittal computed tomographic scans of the face and paranasal sinuses. Radiology 129:81–87, 1978
33. Pagani JJ, Thompson J, Mancuso A, Hanafee W: Lateral wall of the olfactory fossa in determining intracranial extension of sinus carcinomas. AJR 133:497–501, 1979
34. Parsons C, Hodson N: Computed tomography of paranasal sinus tumors. Radiology 132:641–645, 1979
35. Rothman SLG, Allen WE, Simeone JF: Direct coronal computerized tomography. Comput Tomogr 1:157–165, 1977

36. Rouvière H: Anatomy of the Human Lymphatic System, pp 66–70. Michigan, Edwards Brothers, 1938

37. Schoub L, Timme AH, Uys CJ: A well-differentiated inverted papilloma of the nasal space associated with lymph node metastases. S Afr Med J 47:1663–1665, 1973

38. Shukovsky LJ, Fletcher GH: Retinal and optic nerve complications in a high dose irradiation technique of ethmoid sinus and nasal cavity. Radiology 104:629–634, 1972

39. Singh W, Ramage C, Best P, Argus B: Nasal neuroblastoma secreting vasopressin: A case report. Cancer 45:961–966, 1980

40. Som PM, Shugar JMA: The significance of bone expansion associated with the diagnosis of malignant tumors of the paranasal sinuses. Radiology 136:97–100, 1980

41. Suh KW, Facer GW, Devine KD, Weiland LH, Zujko RD: Inverting papilloma of the nose and paranasal sinuses. Laryngoscope 87:35–46, 1977

42. Tadmor R, Davis KR, Weber AL, New PFJ, Momose KJ: Computed tomography of skull and facial structures: Preliminary evaluation of direct coronal sections. Comput Tomogr 1:211–215, 1977

43. Takahashi M, Tamakawa Y, Shindo M, Konno A: Computed tomography of paranasal sinuses and their adjacent structures. Comput Tomogr 1:295–311, 1977

44. Tapley ND (ed): Clinical Applications of the Electron Beam, pp 104 and 111. New York, John Wiley & Sons, 1976

Nasopharynx

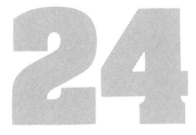

RODNEY R. MILLION
NICHOLAS J. CASSISI

Malignant tumors of the nasopharynx are uncommon in the United States, accounting for only a small percentage of all head and neck malignancies. The high incidence reported in Chinese is actually centered in the southeastern seabord among the Cantonese population of Kwangtung Province, including Hong Kong and Macao. The remainder of China has an intermediate to normal incidence. US statistics show that immigrant Chinese have a greater risk of developing a malignancy of the nasopharynx than those born in the United States, but the excess risk is maintained to a certain extent in subsequent generations. The risk is not associated with Asians in general, since the rate is low in Japanese. A number of possible factors have been suggested, such as inhalation of incense smoke containing nitrosamines, genetic susceptibility, and herpes-type viruses. Ho has suggested that the high incidence of carcinoma of the nasopharnyx in the boat people of Hong Kong may be related to a diet of salted fish fed to young children.[12] The salted fish contains nitrites, which are converted to nitrosamines in the absence of vitamin C. Nitrosamines are known to produce nasal carcinomas in WA albino rats and Syrian golden hamsters. Nasopharynx cancer has an association with elevated titers of the ubiquitous Epstein–Barr virus, and this finding is independent of geography.[12]

There is a 3:1 predominance of the disease in males. The age distribution is much younger than for cancer of other head and neck sites. Fifteen to 20% of patients are under 30 years of age; a 5-year-old patient has been reported.

ANATOMY

The anatomical features and relationships of the nasopharynx in a midsagittal section are shown in Figure 24-1.[8] The nasopharynx is roughly cuboidal with two lateral walls and a sloping roof, which is continuous with the posterior wall. The pharyngeal surface of the soft palate forms a mobile floor of the nasopharynx. The nasopharynx is in direct continuity with the nasal cavity, the oropharynx, and the middle ears by way of the eustachian tubes. The transverse diameter is about 3 cm anteriorly and 4 cm to 5 cm posteriorly at the level of Rosenmüller's fossa. The nasopharynx has an anteroposterior diameter of 2 cm to 4 cm. The distance from the skin of the upper lip to the posterior wall of the nasopharynx as measured through the nasal cavity is usually 7 cm to 8 cm in adults. The mucosa of the roof and posterior wall is often irregular due to the presence of the pharyngeal bursa, tonsil (adenoids), and hypophysis. A variety of views of the normal nasopharynx is given in Figure 24-2. The mucosa tends to become smooth and atrophied with age, but many folds may remain in the later years of life to add to the examiner's confusion as to whether a tumor is present. Submucosal lymphoid tissue may persist well past puberty and may even be present in elderly people. Following successful radiation therapy, the mucosa changes to a smooth, atrophic appearance.

The lateral walls include the eustachian tube openings, marked by the prominent and rounded posterior lips (torus tubarius) created by the underlying cartilaginous portion of the tube (Fig. 24-3). In the resting state, the torus appears prominent and rounded, but if the patient is gagging or swallowing, constriction of the muscles causes elongation and flattening of

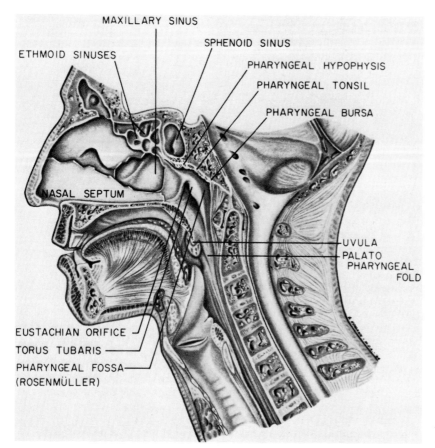

FIG. 24-1. Midsagittal section of the head, showing the nasopharynx and related structures. (Fletcher GH, Healey JE Jr, McGraw JP, Million RR: Nasopharynx. In MacComb WS, Fletcher GH [eds]: Cancer of the Head and Neck, pp 152–178. Copyright © 1967, the Williams & Wilkins Co., Baltimore)

the appearance of the lateral wall. The "tubal tonsil" as such does not exist.[5] Lymphoid tissue is present nearby in the submucosa of the fossa of Rosenmüller. Just behind the adenoids on the posterior wall is an inconstant blind sac or depression, the pharyngeal bursa, but this is not often identified. Anterior to the adenoids is the pharyngeal hypophysis landmark, which is also not easily identified. The pharyngeal hypophysis may consist of remnants of hypophyseal tissue derived from the craniopharyngeal canal (Rathke's pouch) and may be the rare site of origin of a craniopharyngioma.

Deep to the mucous membrane is the well-defined pharyngeal aponeurosis, which attaches to the bones of the base of skull and cervical spine. The line of attachment is outlined in Figure 24-4. Deep to the aponeurosis is the muscular wall, made up primarily of the superior constrictor muscle. The muscular wall is incomplete near the base of the skull, leaving a small muscular defect, the sinus of Morgagni (Fig. 24-5), through which the eustachian tube enters the nasopharynx. Therefore, tumor has only to penetrate the mucosa and the aponeurosis in this area to gain access to the parapharyngeal space and the lateral base of the skull.

The foramen lacerum is directly related to the roof of the nasopharynx (Fig. 24-6). The lower part of the foramen lacerum is filled with fibrocartilage, while the upper portion contains the internal carotid artery and, above this, the cavernous sinus. A whole-organ section of the nasopharynx, the sphenoid sinus, and posterior ethmoid sinuses is shown in Figure 24-7.

The blood supply to the nasopharynx is mainly through the ascending pharyngeal branch of the external carotid artery, the artery of the pterygoid canal (the vidian artery), and the sphenopalatine artery. Perfusion therapy would be accomplished by a catheter in the external carotid artery. Venous drainage is to a plexus of pharyngeal veins on the outer surface of the muscular wall. This plexus then drains to the pterygoid plexus and the internal jugular vein. Alternatively, the pharyngeal plexus may communicate with the orbital cavity by way of the inferior orbital vein.

The sensory nerves are the glossopharyngeal and the maxillary division of the trigeminal nerve, the latter supplying the anterior portion of the nasopharynx. Motor supply is from the vagus nerve except for the tensoris veli palatini and stylopharyngeus.

Lymphatics

There is an extensive submucosal capillary lymphatic plexus, attested to by the high incidence of neck metastases. The tumor spreads initially to the retropharyngeal, junctional, and jugulodigastric lymph nodes and then along the internal jugular and spinal accessory chain.

Although the majority of lymphatic channels empty into either the retropharyngeal, junctional, or jugulodigastric lymph nodes, inconstant lymphatic vessels are described as passing directly to the nodes below the bifurcation of the carotid (midjugular nodes) and to the spinal accessory nodes.[17]

(Text continues on p. 450.)

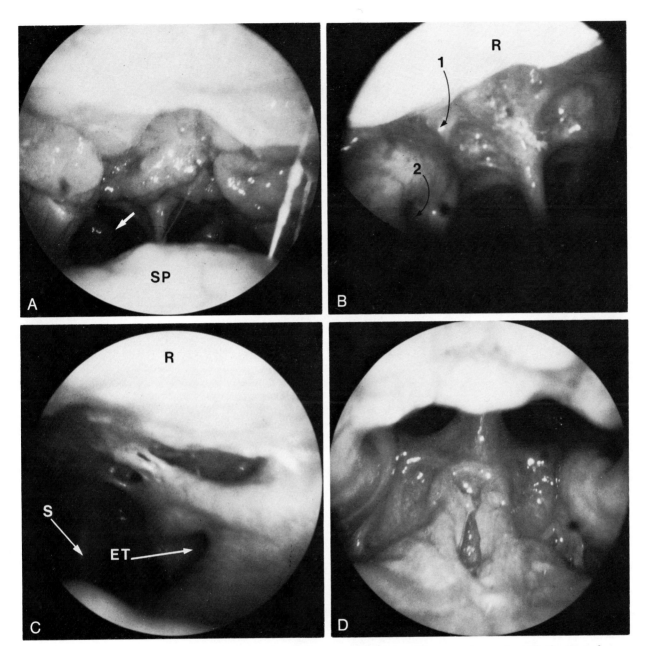

FIG. 24-2. Photographs of the nasopharynx. (Photographs made with the Storz laryngoscope. Photographs are oriented with the soft palate below and the roof to the top of the image. See Chapter 3, Examination with Fiberoptic Equipment.) (A) Normal nasopharynx in a 76-year-old man. Note prominent lymphoid tissue in anterior roof and filling both fossae of Rosenmüller. Arrow points to inferior nasal turbinate. (SP, soft palate) (B) Normal nasopharynx in an 80-year-old man. Arrow 1 points to left fossa of Rosenmüller. Arrow 2 points to eustachian tube opening. (R, roof of nasopharynx) (C) Synechiae between torus tubarius and roof of nasopharynx. (R, roof; ET, entrance to eustachian tube; S, nasal septum) (D) Normal nasopharynx in a 50-year-old man.

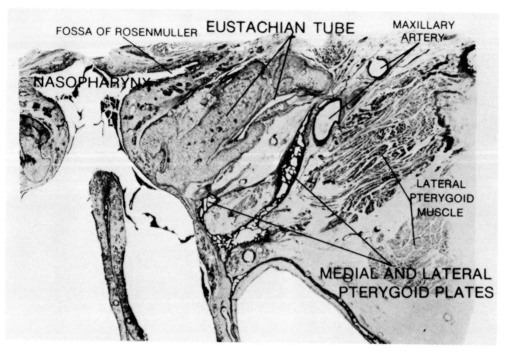

FOSSA OF ROSENMULLER EUSTACHIAN TUBE MAXILLARY ARTERY

NASOPHARYNX

LATERAL PTERYGOID MUSCLE

MEDIAL AND LATERAL PTERYGOID PLATES

FIG. 24-3. Horizontal section through the nasopharynx. Fossa of Rosenmüller created by protrusion of tube cartilage into lateral wall. (Bridger MWM, van Nostrand AWP: The nose and paranasal sinuses—applied surgical anatomy. J Otolaryngol 7 [suppl 6]:3–12, 1978)

FIG. 24-4. Basal view of skull to show the bony attachments of the nasopharyngeal wall. The bony foramina of the base of the skull are shown on the right, and structures occupying these foramina, on the left. (Fletcher GH, Healey JE Jr, McGraw JP, Million RR: Nasopharynx. In MacComb WS, Fletcher GH [eds]: Cancer of the Head and Neck, pp 152–178. Copyright © 1967, the Williams & Wilkins Co., Baltimore)

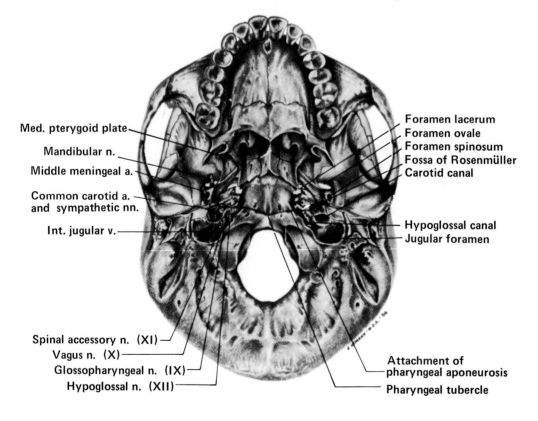

Med. pterygoid plate

Mandibular n.

Middle meningeal a.

Common carotid a. and sympathetic nn.

Int. jugular v.

Spinal accessory n. (XI)
Vagus n. (X)
Glossopharyngeal n. (IX)
Hypoglossal n. (XII)

Foramen lacerum
Foramen ovale
Foramen spinosum
Fossa of Rosenmüller
Carotid canal

Hypoglossal canal
Jugular foramen

Attachment of pharyngeal aponeurosis
Pharyngeal tubercle

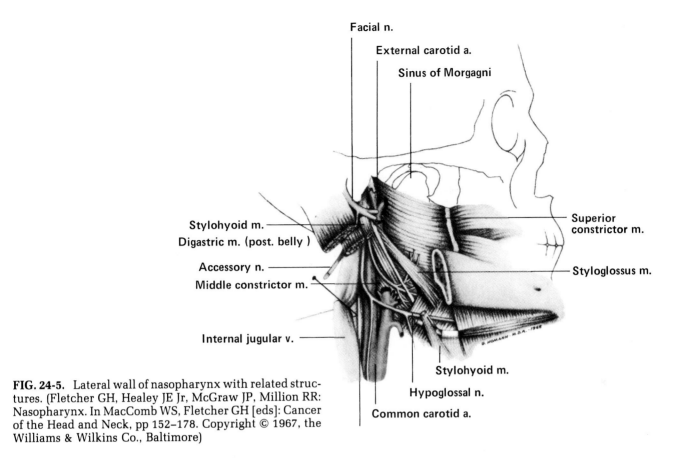

FIG. 24-5. Lateral wall of nasopharynx with related structures. (Fletcher GH, Healey JE Jr, McGraw JP, Million RR: Nasopharynx. In MacComb WS, Fletcher GH [eds]: Cancer of the Head and Neck, pp 152–178. Copyright © 1967, the Williams & Wilkins Co., Baltimore)

FIG. 24-6. Sagittal section through cavernous sinus, foramen lacerum, and nasopharynx, showing the interrelationships of these three structures. (Fletcher GH, Healey JE Jr, McGraw JP, Million RR: Nasopharynx. In MacComb WS, Fletcher GH [eds]: Cancer of the Head and Neck, pp 152–178. Copyright © 1967, the Williams & Wilkins Co., Baltimore)

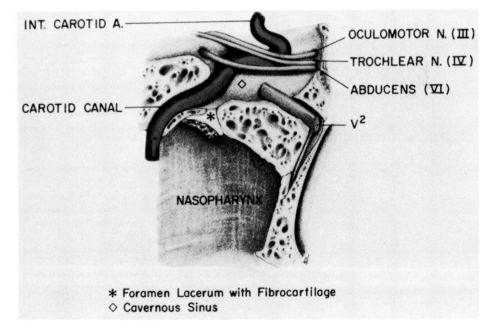

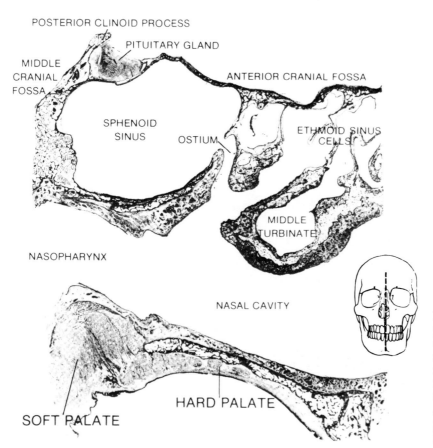

POSTERIOR CLINOID PROCESS

PITUITARY GLAND

MIDDLE CRANIAL FOSSA

ANTERIOR CRANIAL FOSSA

SPHENOID SINUS

OSTIUM

ETHMOID SINUS CELLS

MIDDLE TURBINATE

NASOPHARYNX

NASAL CAVITY

SOFT PALATE

HARD PALATE

FIG. 24-7. Sagittal section through nasopharynx and sphenoid sinus just to the left of midline. Note relationship of sphenoid sinus ostium to nasopharynx and posterior nasal cavity. The anterior wall of the sphenoid sinus and the floor of the pituitary are thin bone. (Bridger MWM, van Nostrand AWP: The nose and paranasal sinuses—applied surgical anatomy. J Otolaryngol 7 [suppl 6]:3–12, 1978)

The retropharyngeal nodes are an important route of spread. The lateral retropharyngeal nodes (node[s] of Rouvière) lie in the retropharyngeal space near the lateral border of the posterior pharyngeal wall and medial to the carotid artery (Fig. 24-8). Directly behind the nodes are the lateral masses of the atlas (C1). According to Rouvière, there is usually one node on each side, but occasionally two and rarely three nodes are found. These nodes are said to atrophy with age and may be absent on one side but are rarely absent entirely.[17]

A rare patient may present with a clinically involved parotid area lymph node. This route of spread is possible from the lymphatics of the eustachian tube, which may drain by way of the lymph vessels of the tympanic membrane and external auditory canal to the parotid area lymph nodes.[17]

PATHOLOGY

Carcinomas comprise about 85% and lymphomas about 10% of the malignant lesions of the nasopharynx. Lymphoepithelioma and transitional cell carcinoma are considered variants within the epithelial group. The incidence of lymphoepithelioma varies from 30% to 50%; the differences probably relate to variation in pathologists rather than geography. A miscellaneous group of malignant tumors that arise from the nasopharynx or adjacent tissues includes melanoma, plasmacytoma, adenocarcinoma, juvenile angiofibroma, chemodectoma, sarcoma, chordoma, nonchromaffin paragangliomas, craniopharyngioma, and unclassified malignancies.

PATTERNS OF SPREAD

Primary

The recognized spread to contiguous structures on admission prior to treatment in 99 patients with epithelial lesions is shown in Table 24-1.[9] These data were compiled prior to availability of computed tomographic (CT) scanning.

INFERIOR EXTENSION

Inferior extension along the lateral pharyngeal walls and tonsillar pillars is recognized in almost one third of the patients. When a submucosal mass is felt at the junction of the posterior and lateral pharyngeal walls, it is a moot question whether one is dealing with an extension of the primary lesion or an enlarged retropharyngeal node. Infiltration down the posterior pharyngeal wall is usually submucosal and may result in invasion of the prevertebral muscles and eventually the clivus or rarely the first cervical vertebra.

ANTERIOR EXTENSION

Extension into the posterior nasal cavity is common. Thorough shrinking of the nasal mucosa and examination with a small-diameter fiberoptic nasoscope is the best clinical method for detecting nasal extension (Fig. 24-9). The nasopharyngeal mass frequently occludes the view from the other direction, and it is difficult to adequately examine

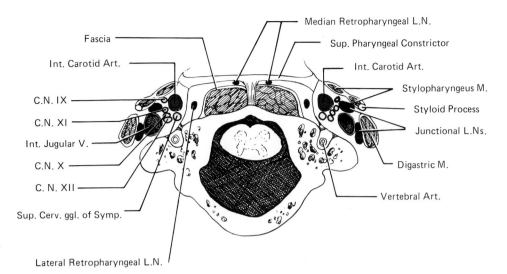

FIG. 24-8. Retropharyngeal lymph nodes.

the posterior nares with a nasal speculum. Tomography and CT scan are helpful to determine soft tissue extension into the nasal cavity, but inflammatory exudates or coagulated blood may give a false impression.

Invasion of the posterior ethmoids, the maxillary antrum, and the orbit occurs fairly often but must usually be diagnosed by tomograms and CT scan. These extensions are important to recognize since they dictate modification of standard treatment techniques.

SUPERIOR EXTENSION

Invasion into or through the base of the skull including the sphenoid sinus is recognized roentgenographically or clinically in at least 25% of patients prior to treatment.[6,9] Early, unrecognized invasion presumably occurs in a far greater number of patients, since the base of the skull, brain, and cranial nerves are frequent sites of local recurrence. Entry of tumor into the sphenoid sinus may occur through the nasosphenoid ostium or through direct penetration. Obstruction of the ostium produces inflammatory changes in the sphenoid sinus that are indistinguishable roentgenographically from tumor invasion until bone destruction can be recognized. Tumor may also erode through the foramen ovale, the foramen lacerum, and the foramen spinosum and eventually destroy large portions of the floor of the middle cranial fossa and the petrous portion of the temporal bone. The tumor eventually reaches the cavernous venous sinus and has access to the oculomotor, trochlear, trigeminal, and abducens nerves. The ophthalmic division and part of the maxillary division of the trigeminal nerve lie within the dural wall of the cavernous sinus and are frequently involved. The optic nerve is invaded by tumor only in very advanced cases, usually in cases with destruction of the sella turcica. The relationship of the nasopharynx to the sphenoid sinus, cavernous venous sinus, and cranial nerves is shown in Figure 24-10.

FIG. 24-9. Carcinoma of the nasopharynx protruding about 1 cm into the right posterior naris. Photograph taken through fiberoptic nasoscope. Arrow points to tumor. (*S*, septum; *T*, turbinate)

TABLE 24-1. Malignant Tumors of the Nasopharynx: Incidence of Spread to Contiguous Structures on Admission

Site of Spread	No. Cases*
Oropharyngeal wall	29
Base of skull (sphenoid sinus—11)	25
Tonsillar bed	15
Cranial nerves	12
Pterygoid fossa	9
Nasal cavity	5
Maxillary antrum	4
Orbit	3
Soft palate	3
Hard palate	2
Ethmoid sinuses	2
Hypopharynx	1

* In several patients, more than one structure was involved.
Note: M. D. Anderson Hospital data; patients treated 8/48–12/60.
(Fletcher GH, Million RR: Malignant tumors of the nasopharynx. Am J Roentgenol Radium Ther Nucl Med 93:44–55, 1965. Copyright © 1965, the Williams & Wilkins Co., Baltimore)

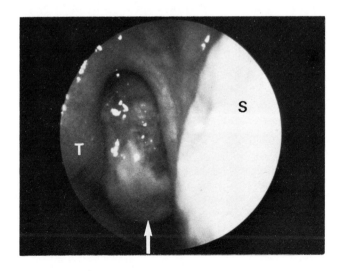

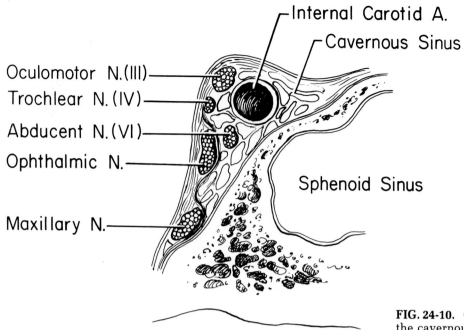

Oculomotor N.(III)
Trochlear N. (IV)
Abducent N.(VI)
Ophthalmic N.
Maxillary N.
Internal Carotid A.
Cavernous Sinus
Sphenoid Sinus

FIG. 24-10. Coronal section of the cavernous sinus.

LATERAL SPREAD

The lateral muscular wall of the nasopharynx is incomplete superiorly. This defect, referred to as the sinus of Morgagni, is traversed by the cartilaginous portion of the eustachian tube and the levator palatine muscle and provides an avenue of egress for the nasopharynx cancer to the lateral pharyngeal space and base of skull. Spread laterally and anteriorly to the pterygoid and infratemporal fossa occurs in advanced tumors with destruction of the pterygoid plates. Structures related to the lateral wall of the nasopharynx are shown in Figures 24-3 through 24-5 and 24-8. The nerves, major vessels, and lymph nodes are in the poststyloid portion of the lateral pharyngeal space. All of the nerves are vulnerable to lateral tumor extension or to enlarged lymph nodes; the spinal accessory nerve is least often affected because of its posterolateral position.

Lymphatics

The diffuse distribution of clinically positive nodes on admission is shown in Figure 24-11. There is an 85% to 90% incidence of metastatic neck node disease on presentation and approximately 50% have bilateral metastases.[9] The incidence of neck nodes does not correlate with T stage (see Table 2-2 in Chapter 2). There is actually a lower percentage of positive lymph nodes in T4 lesions than in T1–T3 lesions. Low-grade squamous cell carcinomas produce fewer metastases (73%) compared with high-grade carcinomas (92%). The incidence of subclinical disease in the neck is unknown because the high-risk areas are normally treated by irradiation, but the risk would be substantial, at least 70%, based on the known incidence and distribution of palpable disease. The actual incidence of spread to the lateral retropharyngeal lymph nodes is unknown; involvement is probably common but rarely diagnosed. Fortunately, these nodes are automatically included in the irradiated volume covering the primary lesion.

Much has been written about the normal lateral retropharyngeal lymph nodes, but there is little information about the true risk for their involvement in nasopharyngeal cancer. Ballantyne described finding positive lateral retropharyngeal lymph nodes in 44% of 34 patients operated on for advanced pharyngeal wall and 11 other miscellaneous head and neck tumors.[2] He reports that the nodes were often "minute or seemingly absent, whereas in others metastatic nodes measured up to 2.5 cm in diameter." He also notes that nodes up to 2 cm in size were reported not to contain carcinoma. In some patients it took as long as 2 years after initial treatment for recurrent nodes to reach a size where they produced symptoms or could be clinically identified. Ballentyne's observations suggest that the clinically positive lymph nodes do not usually produce masses large enough to be detected by clinical examination.[2]

Metastases to submental and occipital nodes appear only when there is blockage of the common lymphatic pathways either by massive neck disease or by an untimely neck dissection.

CLINICAL PICTURE

The most common presenting complaint is a painless upper neck mass or masses, which may be quite large when first discovered. The neck mass may enlarge quite rapidly due to necrosis or hemorrhage. A rare patient will report exquisite tenderness and will be unable to tolerate palpation of the masses.

Nasal obstruction and epistaxis are common. Decreased hearing and tinnitus due to otitis media are caused by obstruction of the eustachian tube. Otitis media is an uncommon diagnosis in adults and should always lead to a thorough examination for tumor.

Sore throat occurs in about 15% of patients and is related to spread along the oropharyngeal wall. Facial pain may be referred from any of the three divisions of the trigeminal nerve. Occipital or temporal headache is frequently seen. Pain in the scalp over the mastoid area may be related to

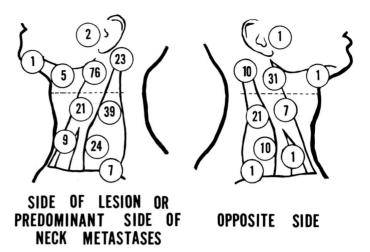

FIG. 24-11. Distribution of metastases to lymph node areas in epithelial tumors of the nasopharynx. The circled numbers indicate the number of times the particular lymph node is involved. Note the high incidence of involvement of the lymph nodes of the spinal accessory chain. Total cases = 99. No lymph nodes were involved in 10 patients (10%); lymph nodes were involved in 89 patients (89%). There was unilateral involvement in 38 patients (39%) and bilateral involvement in 51 patients (51%). (Fletcher GH, Million RR: Malignant tumors of the nasopharynx. Am J Roentgenol Radium Ther Nucl Med 93:44–55, 1965. Copyright © 1965, American Roentgen Ray Society)

SIDE OF LESION OR PREDOMINANT SIDE OF NECK METASTASES

OPPOSITE SIDE

involvement of a high jugular lymph node that has become fixed to the skull and spine.

Pain initiated by lifting the head and extending the neck is related to posterior infiltration of the prevertebral muscles or retropharyngeal lymph nodes.

Ballantyne reported that lateral retropharyngeal lymph nodes involved by carcinoma produced a syndrome of pain, often severe and difficult to pinpoint.[2] The pain is usually referred to the ipsilateral neck and ear, head, forehead, and orbit; it may be associated with a stiff neck or pain on extension of the neck.

Proptosis occurs with posterior orbital invasion and usually displaces the eyeball straight forward. Trismus is related to the invasion of the pterygoid region.

Neurologic symptoms and signs occur in about 25% of patients. Involvement of cranial nerves II–VI indicates intracranial extension into the cavernous sinus and pituitary region. Cranial nerves IX–XII and the sympathetic chain are involved in the lateral pharyngeal space.

Physical Examination

Fiberoptic nasoscopes and laryngoscopes are a great aid in examination of the nasopharynx. Early lesions occur on the lateral wall or roof; the nasopharyngeal surface of the soft palate is almost never the site of origin and not often invaded secondarily even by advanced lesions. In early lesions the findings may be quite subtle—only slight fullness in the fossa of Rosenmüller or a small submucosal bulge or asymmetry in the roof. Lymphomas and minor salivary gland tumors tend to remain submucosal until quite large.

Nasoscopy may show a tumor growing into the posterior and superior nasal cavity, or a tumor may be seen infiltrating submucosally along the posterior tonsillar pillars, and occasionally down the posterior pharyngeal wall.

The cranial nerves should be carefully evaluated; the sixth cranial nerve is the one most commonly involved. The eyes should be measured for proptosis. Ear examination may show findings of otitis media and decreased hearing.

The clinical appreciation of enlarged retropharyngeal nodes requires both visualization and palpation of the high

posterolateral pharyngeal wall, but the diagnosis is rarely made. Marked retropharyngeal lymph node enlargement, such as occurs in lymphoma, distorts the posterior tonsillar pillar, shifting it medially and anteriorly. Such a mass may be misdiagnosed as a peritonsillar abscess, followed by an inappropriate "incision and drainage" procedure.

The enlarged lymph node(s) said to be "classic" for nasopharyngeal carcinoma refers to several high internal jugular vein nodes, the junctional lymph nodes. When enlarged, these nodes bulge the sternocleidomastoid muscle just below the tip of the mastoid and may distort the earlobe. These lymph nodes are a technical problem for the surgeon because they lie in juxtaposition to the base of the skull and the internal jugular vein as it exits from the jugular foramen; they are not always removed in the "standard" radical neck dissection, as shown by postoperative cervical lymphangiograms.[7] (See Chapter 4, General Principles for Treatment of Cancers in the Head and Neck: Selection of Treatment for the Primary Site and for the Neck.)

METHODS OF DIAGNOSIS AND STAGING

Adults with large, easily visible masses may have a biopsy performed in the outpatient clinic. After the administration of a local anesthetic, a straight biopsy forceps is placed through the nose and the procedure is visualized indirectly from the nasopharynx, or a curved biopsy forceps may be inserted behind the retracted soft palate and biopsy is directed by nasoscopic visualization. Biopsy of a small lesion or random biopsies require administration of a general anesthetic; the palate is retracted with a Yankauer speculum, providing direct visualization of the nasopharynx. Since some of these lesions tend to grow submucosally, random biopsies must be deep in order to detect an invisible lesion. A mucosal sample is taken and then the biopsy forceps is placed back into the biopsy site and a deeper sample is obtained. If a juvenile angiofibroma is suspected, workup including an angiogram should precede the diagnosis and treatment. When a carcinoma of the nasopharynx is suspected, but not found on outpatient examination, a CT scan may be of assistance in locating a tumor mass *prior* to examination under anesthesia and biopsy.

Staging

The American Joint Committee (AJCC) staging system for nasopharyngeal primary tumors is listed below:[1]

Tis   Carcinoma *in situ*
T1   Tumor confined to one site of nasopharynx or no tumor visible (positive biopsy only)
T2   Tumor involving two sites (both posterosuperior and lateral walls)
T3   Extension of tumor into nasal cavity or oropharynx
T4   Tumor invasion of skull, cranial nerve involvement, or both

Staging requires tomography of the nasopharynx, nasal cavity, paranasal sinuses, and base of the skull. Coronal, sagittal, and submental vertical views are all useful. CT scans are usually obtained in axial and coronal planes. (It is not always possible to obtain coronal sections due to interference of metal in the teeth or to inability of the patient to flex the neck to enter the scanner.) The CT scan is particularly helpful in determining tumor extension to the orbit and parapharyngeal space. (See Chapter 23, Nasal Vestibule, Nasal Cavity, and Paranasal Sinuses, for normal CT anatomy of the nasopharynx.)

Chest roentgenogram, liver function studies, and occasionally bone scan are used for detecting distant metastases. Lymphoepitheliomas metastatic to bone may produce major bone pain for several weeks before the bone scan or roentgenograms become positive.

Baseline eye evaluation is recommended when the orbits are partially irradiated.

TREATMENT

Factors in the Selection of Treatment

The treatment of almost all malignancies of the nasopharynx is radiation therapy by default, since surgical resection is usually not appropriate. Occasionally a small adenocarcinoma or sarcoma may be locally excised. (See Chapter 25, Juvenile Angiofibroma.) Neck dissection is used less often in the management of neck disease in nasopharyngeal cancer compared with other sites because of the good success rate with radiation therapy alone, the high incidence of bilateral nodes, the frequent involvement of the junctional and retropharyngeal lymph nodes, which are not entirely removed by neck dissection, and the multiplicity of nodes, which usually predicts a higher failure rate with surgery. However, we have tended to add neck dissection more often in recent years, particularly in the patient with one or perhaps two large masses. While these large masses can often be controlled by radiation therapy alone, the large doses produce significant persistent fibrosis. The addition of a neck dissection in place of an extra 1500 rad to 2000 rad will produce less fibrosis in later years and improve neck control. Neck dissection should also be recommended for persistence or recurrence after irradiation.

Irradiation Technique

The anatomical planning is the same for the various grades of squamous cell carcinoma, the transitional cell carcinoma, and the lymphoepithelioma. Recommended doses by T stage and histology are summarized in Table 24-2.

Because of the large mucosal surface irradiated, the mucositis is severe with 1000 rad/week. The treatment is better tolerated at 850 rad to 900 rad/week.

TREATMENT PLANNING FOR T1, T2, AND EARLY T3 LESIONS

There is no place for small-volume irradiation even for an early epithelial tumor of the nasopharynx. If, after complete clinical and roentgenographic workup, the tumor is thought to be limited to the nasopharynx (T1 or T2) or to have minimal soft tissue extension (early T3), the following areas are included in the initial treatment volume:

1. Nasopharynx proper
2. Posterior 2 cm of the nasal cavity
3. Posterior ethmoid sinuses
4. Entire sphenoid sinus and basioccipital bone
5. Cavernous venous sinus
6. Base of skull (7 cm to 8 cm width encompassing the foramen ovale, carotid canal, and foramen spinosum)
7. Pterygoid fossae
8. Posterior one fourth of the orbit

TABLE 24-2.   Guide to Dosage for Primary Nasopharynx Tumors*

Stage	Squamous Cell Carcinoma (rad)	Lympho-epithelioma (rad)	Lymphocytic Lymphoma† (rad)	Histiocytic Lymphoma† (rad)
T1, T2, early T3	6500	6000	3000	5000
Late T3, T4	7000	6500	3500	6000

* 850 rad to 900 rad/week. A boost to the base of skull and nasopharynx is added to the basic dose. See the text for details.

† See Chapter 35, Lymphomas and Related Diseases Presenting in the Head and Neck, for additional information.

(Adapted from Fletcher GH, Million RR: Nasopharynx. In Fletcher GH [ed]: Textbook of Radiotherapy, 3rd ed, pp. 364–383. Philadelphia, Lea & Febiger, 1980)

9. Posterior one third of the maxillary sinus
10. Lateral and posterior oropharyngeal wall to the level of the midtonsillar fossa
11. Retropharyngeal nodes.

The high-dose volume, which is roughly cuboidal, is about 230 cc (5.5 cm anteroposterior, 7.0 cm wide, and 6.0 cm superoinferior).

A four-field arrangement (Fig. 24-12) with cobalt-60 or 3 MeV to 6 MeV is used to cover this central volume. The lateral fields deliver about two thirds and the facial fields about one third of the tumor dose.[10] Opposed lateral fields for the entire treatment course is not usually recommended, because a 5% to 10% higher dose is delivered to the temporomandibular joints, ears, and subcutaneous tissues as compared with the midline tumor.

The lateral fields are angled 5° to 10° posteriorly to ensure adequate posterior margins while avoiding direct ipsilateral irradiation of the external and middle ear and to reduce irradiation to the contralateral eye. A 5° posterior tilt shifts the field edge 8 mm backward at the midline and a 10° tilt moves it 15 mm at the midline (Fig. 24-13).

The anterior facial fields are angled 20° to 30°. Some radiation therapists object to the anterior angled fields as being difficult to set up and reproduce. However, by using the collimator lights as shown in Fig. 24-14, one can visualize the direction of the beam to determine the superior tilt and accurately reproduce the setup each day. The anterior facial fields with their inferior border at the level of the anterior commissure of the lip provide adequate inferior coverage to about the level of the midtonsillar fossa (angle of the mandible). When this technique becomes inadequate to cover low oropharyngeal extensions, by necessity one treats entirely with lateral fields. When only opposing lateral fields are used, a 6-MeV to 20-MeV beam improves the distribution and may be used for all or part of the treatment course depending on the presence or absence of clinically positive lymph nodes. Such an example for a patient with an enlarged lymph node is shown in Figure 24-15.

Six examples of volume distributions are given in Figure 24-16. The point of dose specification for the T1, T2, and early T3 lesions is the 4 × 4-cm volume that encompasses the nasopharynx.

Local failures may be partly related to less dose than planned in the posterior and superior aspect of the nasopharynx and base of skull for the following reasons:

1. Field edge effect: the posterior and superior aspect of the nasopharynx, the base of the skull, and the cavernous sinuses are on the edge or in the corner of the fields, and thus the dose is less than the dose at the central axis.
2. Bone: there is an almost continuous slab of dense bone at the level of the base of the skull, and even with high energies there is differential absorption (for cobalt-60, 3.5% per centimeter of bone).
3. Contour correction: the contour is usually taken at a level through the upper lip and the external auditory meatus; however, most patients are about 1 cm thicker at the level of the zygomatic arch, which causes an underdosage of about 5% from the lateral fields.
4. Field angulation: the anterior fields are angled superiorly, which is not allowed for in the contour; this adds about another centimeter that is not taken into consideration in the volume distribution of the an-

terior fields. Air in the sinuses and nasal cavity may partially compensate for this error.

A supplement of 500 rad is added to the base of the skull and nasopharynx through 5 × 4-cm opposed lateral fields to make up for the underdosage (Fig. 24-17). Corrections for homogeneity with CT treatment planning and off-axis treatment plans through the base of the skull will assist in treatment planning in the immediate future.

TREATMENT PLANNING FOR LATE T3 AND T4 LESIONS

BASE OF SKULL AND/OR INTRACRANIAL NERVE INVOLVEMENT

Extension to the base of the skull and/or involvement of cranial nerves II–VI requires that the superior border be raised to include all of the pituitary, the base of the brain in the suprasellar area, the adjacent middle cranial fossa, and the posterior portion of the anterior cranial fossa. A minimum dosage of 7000 rad is planned in patients with T3 and T4 squamous cell carcinoma and 6500 rad is the minimum in those with lymphoepithelioma. The point of dose specification encompasses a volume that is 7 cm to 8 cm wide and 4 cm to 5 cm anteroposteriorly. At the completion of the basic treatment with four fields, 500 rad is added to the nasopharynx and the base of skull/brain with a reduced field to compensate for underdosage (see Fig. 24-17). A weekly dose of 850 rad to 900 rad is preferred because of the severe mucosal reactions encountered at 1000 rad/week. With doses higher than 7000 rad, severe central nervous system and optic nerve complications can happen. Extreme care in treatment planning must be used.

ANTERIOR EXTENSION

In patients with anterior invasion of the orbit, ethmoids, or maxillary sinuses, the paired anterior fields may be discarded in favor of a single anterior field. A three-field arrangement requires the use of wedges on the lateral fields and partial use of wedges on the anterior field in order to produce a satisfactory volume distribution (see Fig. 24-16). The lacrimal gland should be shielded, if possible, to retain tears and help prevent development of a painful eye. When wedge fields are used on the lateral portals, it is not feasible to include the upper neck in the primary fields. The neck is then irradiated through anterior and posterior portals with photons or with lateral electron-beam portals to avoid overdose to the spinal cord. One such patient with an extensive destructive lesion of the base of skull and unilateral orbital involvement is living 7½ years following treatment, free of disease.

NECK NODES

A comprehensive en bloc plan must be developed to irradiate the neck to the level of the clavicles for both the epithelial lesions and the lymphomas (Fig. 24-18). Patients with no palpable disease in the neck should have full neck irradiation.[3]

UPPER NECK

The retropharyngeal nodes are included in the treatment of the primary lesion. The upper neck nodes are included in the lateral primary fields to the level of the thyroid notch. The posterior margin is placed 2 cm or more behind

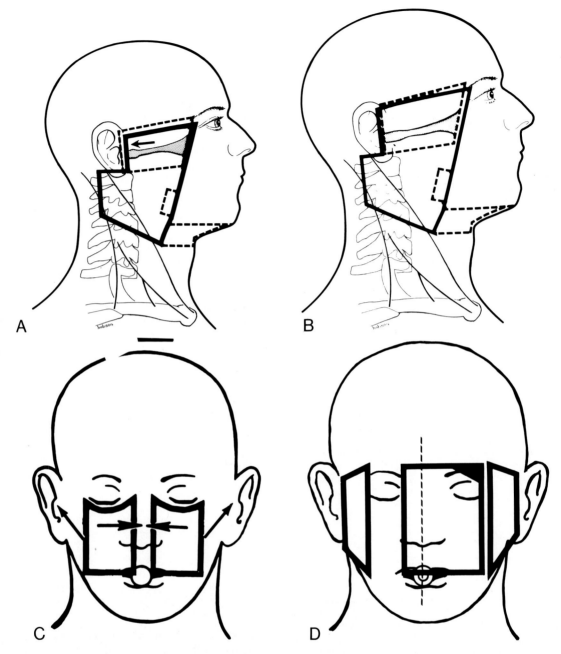

the upper border of the sternocleidomastoid in order to encompass the junctional and high spinal accessory nodes. The superior margin is 2 cm to 3 cm above the tip of the mastoid. The portals are extended anteriorly into the submental area only if there is disease in the submaxillary triangle or if the patient has had an untimely neck dissection prior to irradiation.

When the treatment of the primary lesion is shifted to the anterior facial fields, the upper neck nodes have usually received 4000 rad to 5000 rad. If there was no palpable neck disease prior to treatment, further neck irradiation is not required. Portions of the neck that are clinically involved must have the dose raised to appropriate levels. If only photons are available, anterior and posterior neck fields are designed to shield the midline and protect the spinal cord. Wedges are used to improve the distribution (see Fig. 16-1D in Chapter 16, The Unknown Primary). If electrons are available, they may be used to complete the neck treatment in suitable situations. An appropriate neck dissection should be considered.

LOWER NECK

The lower neck is treated through an anterior portal with a shield over the larynx. The midjugular nodes lie immediately adjacent to the lateral wings of the thyroid cartilage, so the lateral margin of the larynx block should be located 1 cm medial to the lateral border of the cartilage. The lower border of the tapered larynx shield is drawn 1 cm to 2 cm below the inferior border of the cricoid cartilage. The inferior jugular nodes move to a medial position in relation to the jugular vein in the low neck, and since the vein also assumes a paratracheal position in the lower neck, it is not advisable to block the midline more than 2 cm below the cricoid cartilage.

◀ **FIG. 24-12.** Portals for irradiation of the primary tumor. (*A*) Lateral portal for T1, T2, and early T3. The upper margin of the portal is drawn from the outer canthus to the upper margin of the tragus, usually 1 cm to 2 cm above the zygomatic arch. The portal film will show half of the pituitary fossa included in the treatment field. The posterior margin usually curves around the external ear canal and the posterior limb is placed 2 cm to 3 cm above the mastoid tip to ensure adequate treatment of jugular fossa. The posterior margin is then drawn behind the sternocleidomastoid muscle unless enlarged nodes are located farther posteriorly. The inferior margin of the portal is at the level of the thyroid notch. The anterior margin slopes from the external canthus inferiorly until it reaches the neck near the submaxillary gland. A small mandible block may be introduced to protect the third molar area. The submandibular and submental areas are included (*dashed lines*) when they contain clinically positive nodes or there is massive upper neck disease. The beam is angled 5° to 10° posteriorly, as determined by verification films. The reduced portal for the boost to the base of the skull is indicated by dashed lines and is not angled posteriorly. The posterior and superior borders of the boost portal may be outside the original margins to ensure adequate compensation for the low dosage at the base of skull. (*B*) Lateral portal used for late T3 and T4 lesions. The upper margin of the lateral portal is 1 cm to 2 cm higher than in *A* and on the verification film usually extends a centimeter above the pituitary fossa. The posterior margin of the portal is either the same as in *A* with tilt or may be located just behind the external auditory canal, in which case no tilt of the beam is necessary. The base of the skull "boost" portal (*dashed lines*) is located according to individual requirements. (*C*) Anterior portals. A cork and tongue blade are placed in the mouth to depress the tongue as far as possible out of the treatment fields. The beam is tilted medially on an average of 20° to 30°. The beam is aimed superiorly with the aid of the collimator light, as seen in Figure 24-14. The superior margins glance the eyeballs. The medial margins are usually 1 cm from the midline. The inferior borders are normally at the commissure of the lip, and the fields are usually about 6 cm wide. (*D*) Example of a three-field arrangement for lateralized anterior spread into the left orbit, ethmoid sinus, and posterior nose. The anterior field projects 2 cm across the midline and thus spares one eye. A lacrimal gland shield is used when possible. Wedges are used as necessary to produce the required volume distribution. If neck treatment is added, careful planning is necessary to avoid overdose to the spinal cord. The neck is best treated with anteroposterior arrangements with midline shielding; lateral neck portals with electrons may be incorporated into the treatment plan. (Fletcher GH, Million RR: Nasopharynx. In Fletcher GH [ed]: Textbook of Radiotherapy, 3rd ed, pp 364–383. Philadelphia, Lea & Febiger, 1980)

The junction of the upper and lower neck fields is a single line. By convention, the line is included when the upper portals are irradiated and excluded when the lower portals are treated. Occasionally one sees a small strip of moist desquamation at this junction. The junction may occasionally divide a large node, but this is not serious since there is a slight overdosage at the junction site. Occasionally one will feel a small strip of induration in the neck at the junction area during follow-up, but this has not created a symptomatic problem. Slight overdosage is more acceptable than attempting to calculate the field separation and risking underdosage.

DOSAGE TO NODES

Guidelines for selecting the dosage, depending on the histology and size of nodes, are presented in Table 24-3. Large neck nodes from a lymphoepithelioma may be just barely palpable on a Monday after 400 rad to 500 rad given the week before; conversely, they may on occasion still be palpable after 5000 rad/5 weeks. Squamous cell carcinomas have a slower, more predictable regression rate.

ACUTE SEQUELAE

The large volume of mucosa that is irradiated produces unpleasant side-effects during treatment. A sore throat begins at the end of the second week of therapy and persists for 3 to 4 weeks after the completion of treatment. Dryness is always present and may be quite severe. Loss of taste and appetite is often quite profound, but both return 1 to 6 months following completion of treatment.

The auditory tube is in the high-dose area, and obstruction may occur, resulting in secondary otitis media and hearing loss. This condition can be corrected by polyethylene tubes inserted through the eardrums to drain the middle ears. The obstruction often improves or clears completely following mucosal healing of the nasopharynx. Politzerization of the eustachian tubes may reopen the canal.

Although mild nausea may occur, severe nausea and vomiting are uncommon. The overall effect of the treatment is quite wearing on the patient, and a period of several months may be required for successfully irradiated patients to regain their sense of well-being.

(*Text continues on p. 460.*)

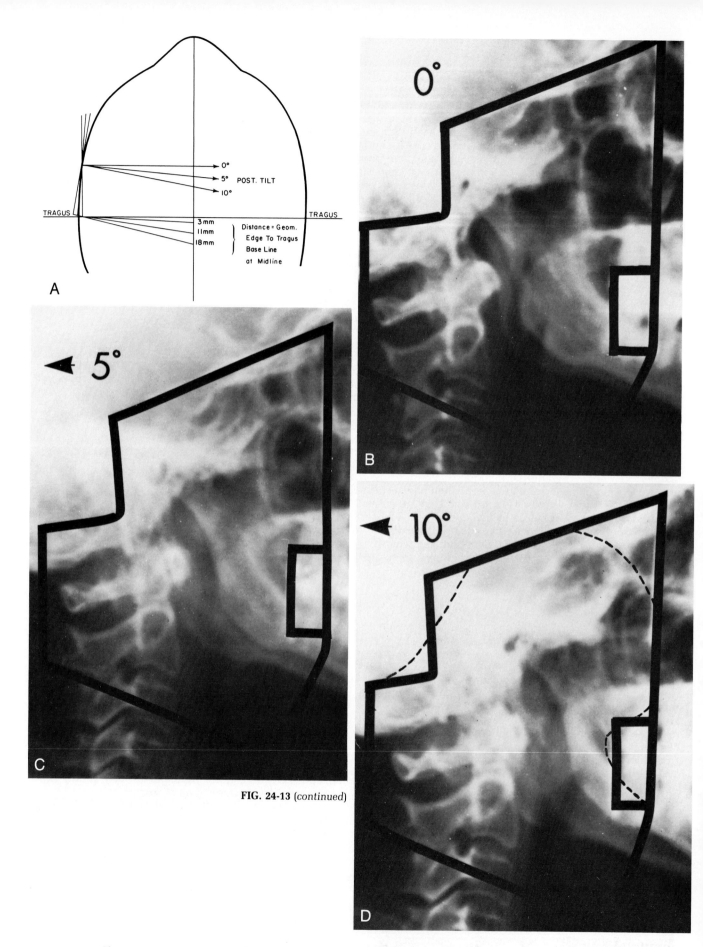

FIG. 24-13 (continued)

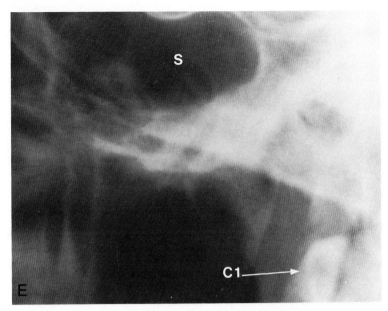

FIG. 24-13. (A) Change in the beam edge at a depth of 7 cm (corresponding to the midline skull) resulting from both 5° and 10° posterior tilt. The 5° tilt results in only 0.8-cm displacement, and the 10° tilt causes a 1.5-cm displacement at the midline (80 cm SSD). (B) A simulator film using lateral portals as described, without tilt, shows marginal coverage of the posterior wall of the nasopharynx. (C) A 5° tilt increases posterior coverage with the entire basiocciput enclosed in the field. Note the protection of the third molar area when the small mandible block is used with the lateral portals. (D) A 10° posterior tilt produces less coverage in the posterior nares, posterior ethmoid sinuses, and orbit with slight additional posterior coverage to about 1 cm behind the basiocciput. The dashed line shows portal modification adopted for Cerrobend blocking technique. (E) Verification film of the small portal used to compensate for underdosage. The roof of the nasopharynx is in the center of the portal; 500–1000 rad midline dose is added. (S, sphenoid sinus) (A through D from Fletcher GH, Million RR: Nasopharynx. In Fletcher GH [ed]: Textbook of Radiotherapy, 3rd ed, pp 364–383. Philadelphia, Lea and Febiger, 1980)

FIG. 24-14. Tilted anterior treatment fields. (A) Use of collimator lights for setup. (B) Schematic of A. (Fletcher GH, Million RR: Nasopharynx. In Fletcher GH [ed]: Textbook of Radiotherapy, 3rd ed, pp 364–383. Philadelphia, Lea & Febiger, 1980)

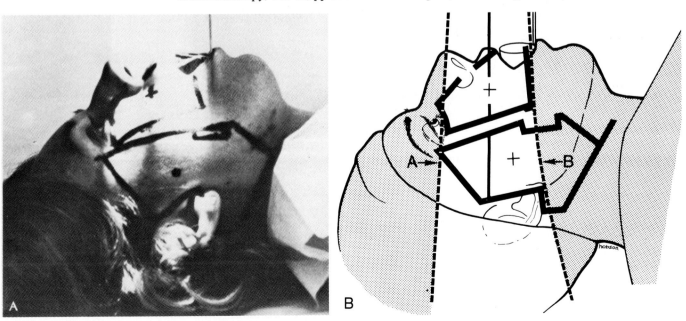

Management of Recurrence

The majority of recurrent squamous cell carcinomas are diagnosed within 2 years, but the lymphoepithelioma may reappear many years after initial therapy. Recurrence in the base of skull or middle cranial fossa may be difficult to diagnose even with CT scan. Headache and cranial nerve palsies usually indicate recurrence.

Re-treatment for recurrence may be rewarding, particularly for the lymphoepitheliomas.[6,14] Patients have been kept free of local disease for various lengths of time by irradiation through a limited portal with a high-energy beam or with brachytherapy sources inserted into the nasopharynx by mold technique. Fu and co-workers report a 41% 5-year survival rate and 25% 10-year survival rate for those patients with localized recurrence selected for re-treatment.[11] The longer the interval to recurrence, the better is the prognosis. There were six examples of soft tissue necrosis and three of osteonecrosis of the sphenoid sinus. No central nervous system necroses were reported.

RESULTS OF TREATMENT

The 5-year survival rate has improved considerably over the past 30 years. Survival rates of 10% to 30% were reported prior to the use of supervoltage techniques. More recent reports give an encouraging 44% to 59% 5-year survival (Table 24-4). The gains have not come from earlier diagnosis but from better staging of the primary lesion with tomography, use of a larger treatment volume and higher doses, and comprehensive irradiation of the neck. The local and regional control rates for patients treated at the University of Florida are given in Tables 24-5 and 24-6.

The 5-year survival rate for lymphoepithelioma is usually 20% to 30% higher than for squamous cell carcinoma. The high rate of local and regional control for lymphoepithelioma is partially offset by a 30% rate of distant metastasis.

FOLLOW-UP POLICY

Follow-up includes careful observation and laboratory testing for possible endocrine hypofunction of the thyroid and pituitary. Dental care must be closely monitored because of the severe xerostomia.

The neck should be carefully followed because a patient with isolated neck recurrence may be salvaged by neck dissection. Documentation of local recurrence is important, but salvage is rarely possible if high-dose, large-volume treatment has been given initially.

COMPLICATIONS OF TREATMENT

The unavoidable irradiation of part of the brain including the hypothalamus, temporal lobes, and pituitary to doses between 6000 and 7000 rad has not produced a single example of brain necrosis. Primary or secondary hypopituitarism due to a hypothalamic lesion has been reported. Hypothyroidism may result from either the direct irradiation of the thyroid gland or an indirect effect on the pituitary.[18] Delayed bone age and growth failure may be seen in young patients. A transitory central nervous system syndrome may appear 2 to 3 months after irradiation.[4] The greater the volume of central nervous system that is irradiated, the longer it takes the patient to recover his sense of well-being; some patients require 6 months to a year to regain their general strength. General weakness and extreme fatigue may be symptoms of low serum cortisol levels. Radiation myelitis of the cervical cord or brain stem is the most severe central nervous system complication.

Trismus occurs to varying degrees due to fibrosis and contracture of the pterygoid muscles rather than to temporomandibular joint fibrosis. This complication is more likely in those patients who are treated with two opposing portals for the entire course.

Palsy of cranial nerves IX–XII, especially the hypoglossal, may occur several years following treatment. This is a problem related to entrapment in the lateral pharyngeal space and is usually seen in patients who received a high dose of radiation therapy to a large upper neck node.

Eye complications such as retrobulbar optic neuritis may develop owing to irradiation of the optic nerve. Irradiation of the posterior eyeball to high doses may produce a radiation retinopathy with decreased vision or even total loss of one eye (see Chapter 14, The Effect of Radiation on Normal Tissues of the Head and Neck).

TABLE 24-3. Guide to Dose for Neck Nodes*

	Squamous Cell Carcinoma		Lymphoepithelioma		Lymphosarcoma, Reticulum Sarcoma	
	Minimum Tumor Dose	Boost to Residual†	Minimum Tumor Dose	Boost to Residual†	Minimum Tumor Dose	Boost to Residual†
No palpable nodes	5000		4500		4000	
Small nodes (1–2 cm)	6000	500–1000	6000	500–1000	4000	
Nodes (3–5 cm)	6000	1500–2000	6000	1000–1500	4000	500
Massive fixed nodes	6000	2000–3000	6000	1500–2000	4000	1000–1500

* Doses in rads, usually 850 rad to 1000 rad/week.

† Boost to residual: Boost dose added through portal just covering palpable residual disease. Neck dissection may be substituted for boost in selected cases (*e.g.*, grade II squamous, solitary 5-cm subdigastric node).

(Fletcher GH, Million RR: Nasopharynx. In Fletcher GH [ed]: Textbook of Radiotherapy, 3rd ed, pp 364–383. Philadelphia, Lea & Febiger, 1980)

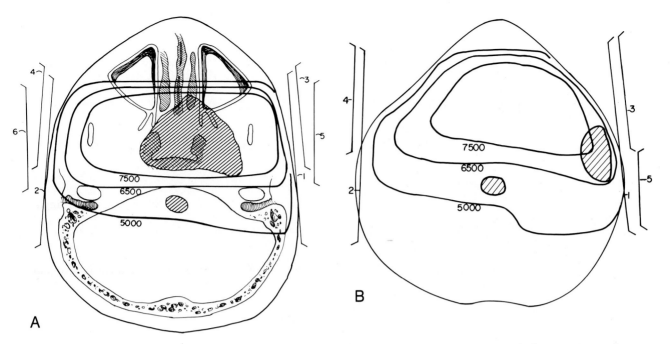

FIG. 24-15. (A) Isodose distribution using only lateral portals for treatment of a carcinoma of the nasopharynx (*hatched lines*) with one right subdigastric lymph node. The initial 5000 rad uses a right lateral cobalt-60 beam (portal 1) and a left lateral 17-MV beam (portal 2). The spinal cord is shielded, and treatment is continued with 17-MV photons (portals 3 and 4) weighted 2:1 in favor of the right. Portals 1 through 4 are angled 5° posteriorly. A boost to the base of the skull of 500 rad is added with 17-MV photons to reduced portals (5 and 6). The uncorrected high-dose volume (7500 rad) could be reduced by giving a small portion of the treatment from the anterior. The actual dose to the base of the skull in this instance is closer to 7000 rad.

Portal	Energy	Field Size (cm)	Given Dose (rad)
1	C-60	10 × 14	3220
2	17 MV	10 × 14	3220
3	17 MV	6 × 12	1934
4	17 MV	6 × 12	967
5	17 MV	6 × 4	456
6	17 MV	6 × 4	228

(B) Isodose distribution in the neck. The planned dose to the left neck is 4500 rad to 5000 rad for subclinical disease. The right neck lymph node is partially excluded from the reduced photon portals (portals 3 and 4) after approximately 5000 rad. A 12-MeV electron portal is added on the right (portal 5). The final minimum dose to the right upper neck lymph node is 6500 rad. The dose to the lymph node would be increased to 7000 rad with an appositional electron beam portal or with parallel opposed anteroposterior and posteroanterior portals with wedges.

Portal	Energy	Field Size (cm)	Given Dose (rad)
1	Co-60	10 × 14	3220
2	17 MV	10 × 14	3220
3	17 MV	6 × 12	1935
4	17 MV	6 × 12	970
5	12 MeV	6 × 12	1100

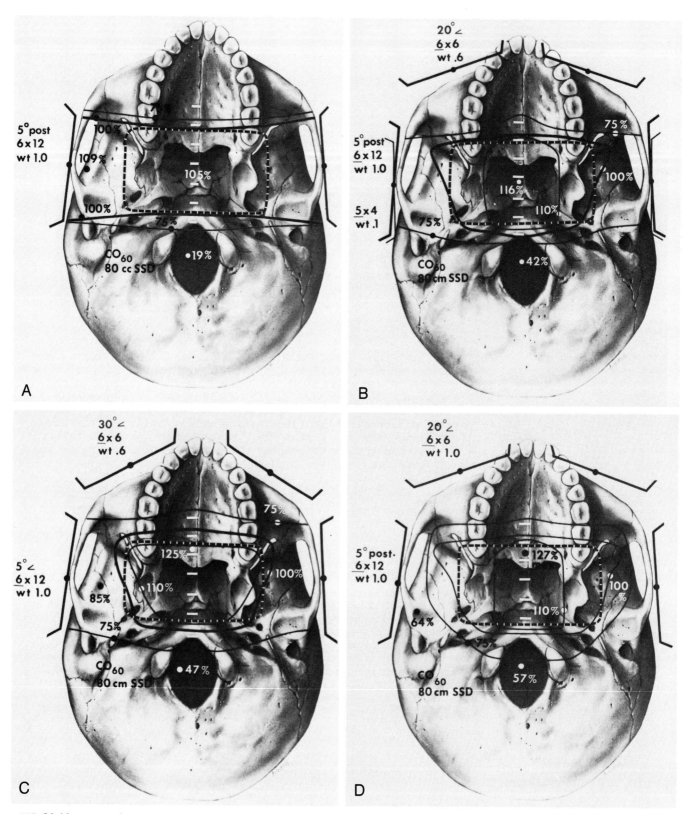

FIG. 24-16 (continued)

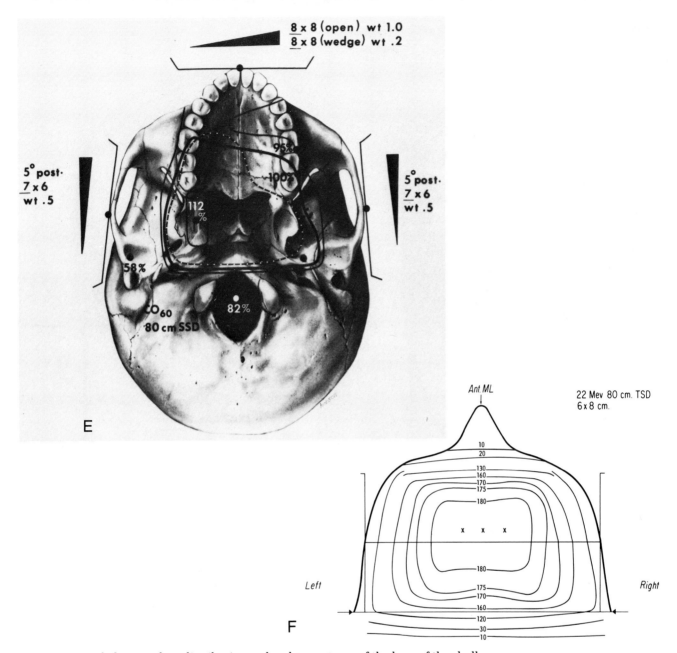

FIG. 24-16. Cobalt-60 isodose distributions related to anatomy of the base of the skull. The dashed line encompasses the usual treatment volume. Weights (wt) refer to the relative given dose to each field. (*A*) Opposed lateral portals result in 5% to 9% greater dose to the subcutaneous tissues, parotid, and temporomandibular joints. Posterior and anterior coverage is marginal. (*B*) The isodose for the four-field technique using 20° angle of anterior facial fields. The boost field (wt 0.1) is added to the volume distribution. The volume distribution from four fields produces a maximum dose in the anterior midline of the nasopharynx. For the T1, T2, and early T3 lesions the point of dose specification is the volume that roughly encompasses the nasopharynx (4 × 4 cm) and would correspond to the 110% normalized isodose on the illustrations. For late T3 and T4 lesions the point of dose specification encompasses the larger volume outlined by the dashed line and would correspond to the 100% normalized isodose; this area usually measures 7 cm to 8 cm wide and 4 cm to 5 cm anteroposterior. In this case, the nasopharynx proper would receive doses 10% higher than the specified dose, and the maximum dose would be 16% more than the specified dose. (*C*) A volume distribution using a 30° angle for the anterior fields; the boost field has not been added to this example. (*D*) Equal weighting of lateral and anterior portals produces about the same distribution in the central area compared with *B* and *C*. However, the dose to the brain stem and central nervous system is slightly greater. (*E*) A three-field technique devised for a patient with anterior extension into one nasal cavity. (*F*) Parallel opposed portals with a 22-MV photon beam produce maximum irradiation to the central volume with reduced dosage to the peripheral structures. (Fletcher GH, Million RR: Nasopharynx. In Fletcher GH [ed]: Textbook of Radiotherapy, 3rd ed, pp 364–383. Philadelphia, Lea & Febiger, 1980)

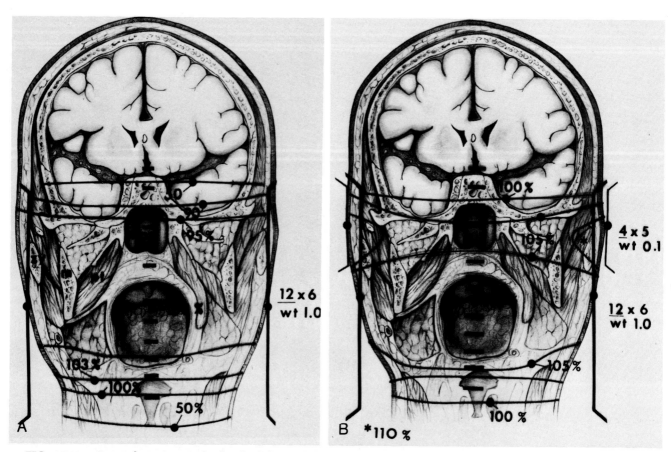

FIG. 24-17. Coronal section at the level of the midnasopharynx with superimposed volume distribution. (*A*) The treatment volume at the base of the skull receives less dose from the opposed lateral fields due to field edge effect, increased thickness of the head at this level, and bone absorption. (*npx*, nasopharynx; *zy*, zygomatic arch; *m*, mandible; *pt*, pterygoid muscle and lateral pteryoid plate) (*B*) A supplement or boost is added at the end of treatment to the base of the skull to compensate for the low dose. (Fletcher GH, Million RR: Nasopharynx. In Fletcher GH [ed]: Textbook of Radiotherapy, 3rd ed, pp 364–383. Philadelphia, Lea & Febiger, 1980)

FIG. 24-18. Portals for irradiation of the neck. (*A*) *En face* field used to irradiate the lower neck in conjunction with the lateral nasopharynx fields. The larynx, cricoid, and 2 cm of the trachea are blocked. It is not necessary to include the entire posterior cervical triangle in cases with minimal or no disease in the upper neck. The trapezius muscle may be blocked where possible. (*B*) Posterior split field may be used to supplement treatment to upper neck nodes. (*C*) Examples of reduced fields for boosting residual disease are shown. If there has been biopsy of a node, the scar is a potential site of recurrence and should receive additional irradiation. (Fletcher GH, Million RR: Nasopharynx. In Fletcher GH [ed]: Textbook of Radiotherapy, 3rd ed, pp 364–383. Philadelphia, Lea & Febiger, 1980)

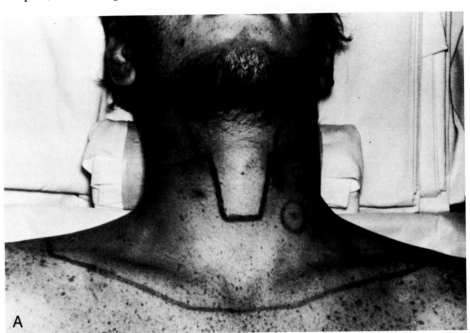

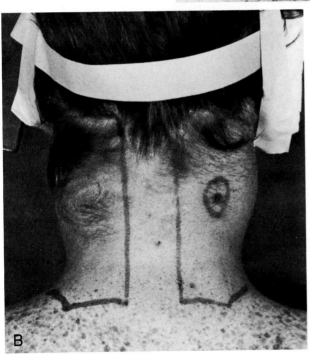

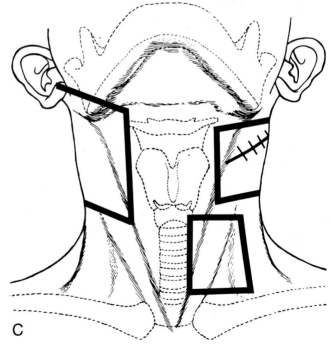

TABLE 24-4.   Nasopharynx Cancer—Results of Radiation Therapy

Insitition (Dates of Treatment)	No. Patients	5-Year Survival	Percentage of T4 Lesions	Percentage of Lymphoepithelioma
M. D. Anderson Hospital[15] (1954–1977)	251	52% (actuarial)	30%	45%
University of Florida* (1964–1978)	47	44% (absolute)	53%	24%
Stanford University[13] (1956–1973)	74	59% (absolute)	11%	36%
University of California[16] (1940–1968)	146	37% (absolute)	Not available	25%

* University of Florida data; patients treated 10/64–4/78; analysis 4/80 by J. W. Gefter, MD.

TABLE 24-5.   Local Control—Primary Lesion

Stage	No. Patients	
T1	4/4	(100%)
T2	4/5	(90%)
T3	9/10	(90%)
T4	10/20	(50%)
All stages*	27/39	(69%)

* Excludes eight patients dead of other causes less than 1 year after treatment or if cause of death was uncertain.

Note: University of Florida data; patients treated 10/64–4/78; analysis 4/80 by J. W. Gefter, MD.

TABLE 24-6.   Neck Control

Stage	No. Patients	
N0–N3A	21/21	(100%)
N3B	11/18	(61%)
All stages*	32/39	(82%)

* Excludes eight patients dead of other causes less than 1 year after treatment or if cause of death was uncertain.

Note: University of Florida data; patients treated 10/64–4/78, analysis 4/80 by J. W. Gefter, MD.

REFERENCES

1. American Joint Committee on Cancer: Manual for Staging of Cancer, 2nd ed, pp 31–36. Philadelphia, JB Lippincott, 1983
2. Ballantyne AJ: Significance of retropharyngeal nodes in cancer of the head and neck. Am J Surg 108:500–504, 1964
3. Berger DS, Fletcher GH, Lindberg RD, Jesse RH Jr: Elective irradiation of the neck lymphatics for squamous cell carcinomas of the nasopharynx and oropharynx. Am J Roentgenol Radium Ther Nucl Med 111:66–72, 1971
4. Boldrey E, Sheline G: Delayed transitory clinical manifestations after radiation treatment of intracranial tumors. Acta Radiol Ther 5:5–10, 1966
5. Bridger MWM, van Nostrand AWP: The nose and paranasal sinuses—applied surgical anatomy: A histologic study of whole organ sections in three planes. J Otolaryngol 7(suppl 6):1–33, 1978
6. Chen KY, Fletcher GH: Malignant tumors of the nasopharynx. Radiology 99:165–171, 1971
7. Fisch U: Lymphography of the Cervical Lymphatic System. Philadelphia, WB Saunders, 1968
8. Fletcher GH, Healey JE Jr, McGraw JP, Million RR: Nasopharynx. In MacComb WS, Fletcher GH: Cancer of the Head and Neck, pp 152–178. Baltimore, Williams & Wilkins, 1967
9. Fletcher GH, Million RR: Malignant tumors of the nasopharynx. Am J Roentgenol Radium Ther Nucl Med 93:44–55, 1965
10. Fletcher GH, Million RR: Nasopharynx. In Fletcher GH (ed): Textbook of Radiotherapy, 3rd ed, pp 364–383. Philadelphia, Lea & Febiger, 1980
11. Fu KK, Newman H, Phillips TL: Treatment of locally recurrent carcinoma of the nasopharynx. Radiology 117:425–431, 1975
12. Ho JHC: An epidemiologic and clinical study of nasopharyngeal carcinoma. Int J Radiat Oncol Biol Phys 4:183–198, 1978
13. Hoppe RT, Goffinet DR, Bagshaw MA: Carcinoma of the nasopharynx: Eighteen years' experience with megavoltage radiation therapy. Cancer 37:2605–2612, 1976
14. McNeese MD, Fletcher GH: Re-treatment of recurrent nasopharyngeal carcinoma. Radiology 138:191–193, 1981
15. Mesic JB, Fletcher GH, Goepfert H: Megavoltage irradiation of epithelial tumors of the nasopharynx. Int J Radiat Oncol Biol Phys 7:447–453, 1981
16. Moench HC, Phillips TL: Carcinoma of the nasopharynx: Review of 146 patients with emphasis on radiation dose and time factors. Am J Surg 124:515–518, 1972
17. Rouvière H: Anatomy of the Human Lymphatic System, p 10. Tobias MJ, trans. Ann Arbor, MI, Edwards Brothers, 1938
18. Samaan NA, Bakdash MM, Caderao JB, Cangir A, Jesse RH Jr, Ballantyne AJ: Hypopituitarism after external irradiation: Evidence for both hypothalamic and pituitary origin. Ann Intern Med 83:771–777, 1975

Juvenile Angiofibroma

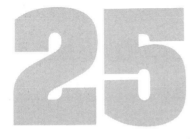

RODNEY R. MILLION
NICHOLAS J. CASSISI

Juvenile angiofibroma (JAF) is an uncommon, histologically benign vascular tumor with the potential to kill or cause serious morbidity due either to uncontrolled growth or complications of the treatment. The tumor occurs almost exclusively in males; a rare case in females has been documented in which female sex chromosomes were confirmed. Most tumors appear around the age of 12 to 15, but an occasional diagnosis is made before the age of 10 and after the age of 25. There is a case report of diagnosis at age 62.[10] Spontaneous regression has been reported but does not occur very often. There is no known etiology. Six tumors were studied for estrogen receptors and none were found.[6]

ANATOMY

The nasopharynx has often been regarded as the site of origin. Neel and co-workers determined the site of origin based on the patterns of spread, the clinical picture of early lesions, and the findings at surgery to be the posterolateral wall of the nose near the sphenopalatine foramen.[9] Sessions noted that irradiated lesions tended to regress toward the sphenopalatine area.[11] However, Hanafee reports cases without any involvement of the posterior nares.* It seems likely that there is more than one specific site of origin.

PATHOLOGY

JAF consists of large, dilated blood vessels with varying amounts of fibrosis, the fibrous stroma increasing in longstanding or recurrent tumors. There is no true capsule present. Because the tumor grows by expansion, there may be nerve, bone, and focal calcification within the tumor, but mucous glands and lymphoid aggregates are not normally present. Histologically, the lesion should be differentiated from nasal polyps, sclerosing hemangiomas, hemangioendotheliomas, and fibrosarcomas.

PATTERNS OF SPREAD

The early tumors are localized to the posterior nares, nasal cavity, or nasopharynx with or without early extension to a paranasal sinus. There are two case reports of lesions presenting as a cheek mass that, when dissected, involved the pterygopalatine fossa without a nasal component.[11] As the tumor enlarges it tends to extend along the roof of the nose and anteriorly into the nasal cavity, but it is usually confined to the ipsilateral nasal cavity. The hard palate may be eroded, producing a submucosal mass in the palate. Posterior growth occurs into the nasopharynx and often fills the entire nasopharynx, producing an obvious bulge in the soft palate. The tumor commonly extends laterally through the pterygopalatine fossa to the infratemporal fossa, where it grows anteriorly, pushing the posterior wall of the maxillary sinus forward and eventually destroying it by pressure. Less often, the tumor may enter the maxillary sinus through the medial wall of the

---

* Hanafee W: Personal communication, 1982.

467

antrum. The infratemporal fossa is often filled with tumor, producing enlargement of the cheek. Very large masses extend above the zygoma. Tumor in the pterygopalatine fossa has ready access to the orbit through the inferior orbital fissure. Superior extension may occur through the floor of the middle cranial fossa with eventual intracranial extension just lateral to the cavernous sinus, somewhat similar to that of nasopharyngeal carcinomas. Direct superior extension from the nasal cavity occurs into the sphenoid sinus with eventual expansion into the sella turcica with displacement of the pituitary gland and eventual pressure on the optic chiasm that may result in blindness. One instance of simultaneously occurring double JAFs has been reported.[11] Lymphatic and vascular metastases have not been reported.

CLINICAL PICTURE

The signs and symptoms are not always representative of the size of the lesion. Patients with minimal findings may turn out to have extensive lesions, while small lesions may produce alarming nosebleeds.

Nasal obstruction and epistaxis are the most common presenting symptoms. Early cases of nasal obstruction occur on only one side. Patients may present with moderate swelling of the cheek and, less commonly, proptosis. Other symptoms include nasal speech, sneezing, and nasal discharge. Conductive hearing loss occurs secondary to obstruction of the eustachian tubes. Cranial nerve palsies occur (e.g., trigeminal nerve) but are uncommon. Superior extension of the tumor may involve the optic nerve and produce partial blindness.

Physical Examination

The characteristic gross appearance of a JAF is a dark red to pale blue submucosal, smooth, nodular neoplasm, sometimes with evidence of recent hemorrhage. The lesions become more fibrous with time, which explains the variation in color; they are easily confused with a nasal polyp.

There may be obstruction of one or both nasal cavities with an obvious mass. The tumor may be seen extending through the posterior nares into the nasopharynx, completely filling the nasopharynx, and may cause bulging of the soft palate forward. There may be a submucosal bulge into the hard palate and gingivobuccal sulcus. Proptosis and an obvious, diffuse, soft swelling over the maxillary antral area and cheek may be evident. A larger, more extensive tumor may occasionally extend into the upper neck or temporal fossa. Cranial nerve palsies may occur in the more advanced lesions, expecially those with intracranial extension. Sexual maturation may be retarded or absent.

METHODS OF DIAGNOSIS AND STAGING

The diagnosis of JAF is usually established by computed tomographic (CT) scanning and, if necessary, arteriography. Biopsy may produce serious hemorrhage. If only a small sample is removed from the periphery of a JAF, it may not be representative and a mistaken diagnosis may occur.[12] If the patient has a characteristic JAF, we do not insist on a biopsy prior to radiation therapy.

Radiology

CT scan with contrast enhancement is usually the first diagnostic examination when JAF is suspected. The pattern of spread coupled with intense staining and contrast is usually diagnostic of JAF. If an operation is planned, arteriography is delayed until the day of operation in order to perform embolization of the tumor vessels after identifying the tumor vessels. If radiation therapy is planned, angiography is not essential if a good quality CT scan is available.

Bilateral selective internal and external carotid injections may be needed, since the tumor may be fed from multiple vessels and part of the arterial supply may come from the opposite side. Vertebral artery injections may be added, especially for recurrent lesions, when one external carotid has already been ligated. Subtraction techniques (which erase the overlying bone) aid in outlining the total extent of the tumor vessel. The typical findings at arteriography include dense contrast staining (tumor blush) during capillary phase and anterior displacement of the internal maxillary artery due to a mass in the pterygopalatine fossa.

The areas of tumor involvement as outlined by arteriography are shown in Table 25-1.[14] Intracranial tumor may be supplied from branches of the dural arteries and not demonstrated on carotid injections.

Axial CT scan with contrast enhancement characteristically shows a unilateral nasal mass with extension through the pterygopalatine fossa to involve the infratemporal fossa. The posterior wall of the maxillary sinus is bowed forward by the slowly expanding mass. The tumor may enter the orbit through the inferior or superior orbital fissure. Intracranial extension can usually (but not always) be diagnosed by contrast enhancement, but angiography may be necessary. JAF usually does not extend posterior to the styloid process and therefore does not involve the carotid area.[8]

The sinuses are often opacified and CT scan with contrast will help distinguish JAF from inflammatory exudates or blood.

Differential Diagnosis

Differential diagnosis in this age-group includes nasal polyps, nasal cavity and nasopharyngeal carcinomas, esthesioneuroblastoma, lymphomas, sarcomas (including rhab-

TABLE 25-1. Extension of Juvenile Angiofibroma in 16 Patients as Outlined on Angiography

Direction of Extension	No. Cases
Pterygopalatine fossa	15
Posterior ethmoid cells	4
Body of sphenoid and sphenoid sinuses	11
Posterior orbit	5
Maxillary sinus	10
Intracranial extension (extradural in the middle fossa)	6

(Wilson GH, Hanafee WN: Angiographic findings in 16 patients with juvenile nasopharyngeal angiofibroma. Radiology 92:279–284, 1969)

domyosarcoma, hemangioendothelioma), large adenoids, parapharyngeal tumors, foreign body, parotid gland tumor, and other rare tumors such as chordoma, meningioma, and plasmacytoma. A hemangiopericytomalike intranasal tumor may occur rarely in this age group.

TREATMENT

Although JAF is a histologically benign tumor, death may occur if the lesion is not treated. There is no evidence to support spontaneous remission by a certain age, and a policy of observation without treatment is seldom recommended. Death or serious morbidity may occur from the biopsy, arteriography, or the treatment; reasonable judgment is required in the selection of treatment, since both surgery and radiation therapy are curative.

If the lesion is resectable with little danger to the patient, then this is the treatment of choice. For the more extensive lesions in which resection will surely be incomplete and the patient faces a risk of major morbidity or even death, then radiation therapy is the preferred treatment. Cummings compared the lifelong risk factors of surgery and radiation therapy and concluded that they are comparable, but the surgical risks are immediate and the radiation risks are delayed (Table 25-2).[4] The doses now specified for JAF, 3000 rad to 3500 rad/4 to 5 weeks with supervoltage beams, produce minimal acute and chronic tissue changes even with years of follow-up.

There is considerable long-term follow-up experience in young patients treated with similar doses for lymphoma, although only orthovoltage beams were available at that time. The risk of a lethal radiation-induced neoplasm for a single course of supervoltage therapy is estimated to be 1 in 150 for someone 10 to 20 years of age and 1 in 400 for those older than 20 years of age.

The mortality risks associated with surgery include those of general anesthesia, blood transfusion, and the surgical procedure itself. The surgical risk varies, of course, with the extent of tumor to be resected, previous treatment of the tumor, and the experience of the surgical team.

The risks associated with radiation therapy in young people are real and should not be ignored, but it is irrational to recommend surgery and the possibility of immediate death or serious morbidity because of the tiny risk of a radiation-induced tumor that has a latent period of at least 7 years and usually more than 20 years.

It has been suggested that partial removal will reduce radiation portals and ensure a better result. However, the entire potential area of recurrence still must be irradiated, so this would not modify the radiation therapy portals. Whenever possible, a single treatment, either surgery or radiation therapy, should be chosen to minimize the total risk.

Surgical Treatment

Arteriography is planned just prior to surgery so that embolization with polyvinyl alcohol foam (Ivalon) will have a maximum effect. Embolization on the day prior to operation allows time for collaterals to compensate.

During the operative procedure, an attempt is made to tease tumor extensions by careful blunt dissection. Often, the dumbbell extensions through foramina or fissures are larger than the space through which they must be removed, and very careful dissection and adequate exposure are needed both to prevent major hemorrhage and to remove all tumor.

EARLY LESIONS

Tumors limited to the posterior nasal cavity and nasopharynx with minimal extension through the pterygopalatine foramen are approached through a transpalatal incision. The lesions are usually adherent to the anterior portion of the nasopharynx and the posterolateral wall of the nose. The extensions are teased from their adherent areas and are removed through the nasopharynx. If there is significant extension anteriorly and superiorly into the nasal cavity, lateral rhinotomy may be combined with a transpalatal approach. Minimal extension through the pterygopalatine foramen may be removed, particularly in a previously untreated case.[1]

LESIONS WITH MAJOR LATERAL EXTENSION

Large tumors or recurrent tumors that extend laterally toward the infratemporal fossa may require a midline mandibulotomy combined with transpalatine exposure in

TABLE 25-2. Estimated Risk for *Fatal* Complication Associated With Therapy for Juvenile Angiofibroma

Risks of Operation		Risks of Radiation Therapy	
General anesthesia	1:300	Radiation-induced cancer of the thyroid	1:400 to 1:1250
Arteriography	1:1700	Bone/soft tissue sarcoma	1:300
Blood transfusion		Arteriography	1:1700
Hemolytic treatment	1:3500	Benign neoplasm	Risk unknown
Anti-IgA anaphylaxis	1:1000	Late radiation therapy complications	See text
Hepatits	1:200		
Operation	1:500	Total estimated death risk (age 15):	
Total estimated death risk	1:100	Without blood transfusion	1:350
		With blood transfusion	1:100

Note: The exact estimated risks for operation in any single patient will vary with the extent of the neoplasm and whether there has been prior operation or radiation therapy. The risk data for radiation-induced neoplasia are not well established because few patients have been treated to 3000 rad to 3500 rad with supervoltage radiation to the head and neck area and then followed for more than 20 years. There is no doubt, however, that the radiation-induced neoplasms have a long latent period, at least 7 years and more often greater than 20 years.

(Data from Cummings BJ: Relative risk factors in the treatment of juvenile angiofibroma. Head Neck Surg 3:21–26, 1980)

order to gain access for dissection. The anterior, lateral, and posterior walls of the antrum and portions of the lateral pterygoid plate may need to be removed for best exposure. Recurrent lesions especially tend to be adherent, and exposure needs to be maximal. A sublabial or Caldwell-Luc exposure may assist removal of certain lesions.[1]

LESIONS WITH INTRACRANIAL EXTENSION

Although there are reports of successful removal of intracranial extension, the risks are substantial, and radiation therapy should be the initial treatment.[7,13] Should operation be required, an experienced team composed of a neurosurgeon and a head and neck surgeon is essential.

Radiation Therapy

The dose required for a high rate of local control is 3000 rad to 3500 rad/4 to 5 weeks. Most of the reported failures are due to inadequate treatment volume rather than to inadequate dosage, and one should err on the side of too large a volume, since the risks (except to the eye) are not changed. Since radiation therapy is generally reserved for patients with large or recurrent lesions, the treatment volume is generous. It is unwise to rely entirely on angiographic findings because all of the supplying vessels may not be perfused. The CT scan enhanced with contrast medium and the physical examination give valuable information about the extent of the tumor.

The treatment plan and response for a large lesion are shown in Figure 25-1. The initial response to radiation therapy is variable. Most patients show 30% to 50% regression during the course of radiation therapy, but complete regression usually does not occur until weeks or months later. A persistent shadow may be seen on follow-up CT examination and should not be cause for alarm as long as it remains stable.

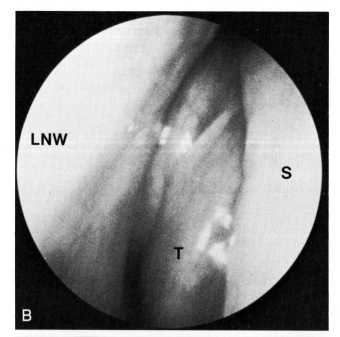

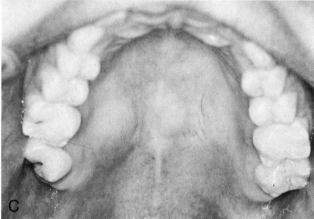

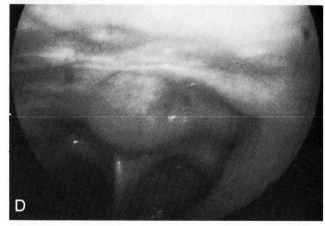

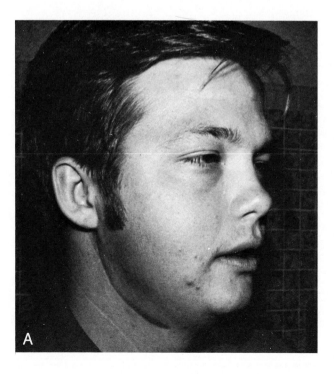

FIG. 25-1 (continued)

◀ **FIG. 25-1.** A 19-year-old man presented with 3-year history of fullness of the right cheek. Exploration of the right parotid revealed a "lipoma." Four months later he developed nosebleeds and right nasal obstruction. (A) Diffuse enlargement of the right cheek. There was 3-mm to 4-mm exophthalmos on the right. (B) Tumor mass at 5 cm in right nasal cavity. (S, septum; T, tumor; LNW, lateral nasal wall) (Photograph was taken through fiberoptic nasoscope.) (C) Submucosal bulge of right hard palate. There was also fullness in the right gingivobuccal sulcus (not shown). (D) Adenoids or tumor in the midline roof of the nasopharynx. Tumor could be seen filling the right posterior choana (not well seen). The left posterior choana is open. (E) CT scan with contrast. The mass fills the entire infratemporal fossa, extends posteriorly to the styloid process, and produces widening of the pterygopalatine fossa (arrow). The mass surrounds but does not destroy the pterygoid plates (arrowheads). There is characteristic anterior displacement of the posterior wall of the right maxillary antrum and mass in the right posterior nares. The scan was performed without intravenous contrast enhancement. Postinfusion scans reveal a densely staining mass which, coupled with the characteristic growth pattern, is highly diagnostic for JAF. (F) CT scan through orbits. There is early extension (arrow) through the inferior orbital fissure to the posterior orbit. There was 4 mm to 5 mm of proptosis on clinical examination. (G) Internal carotid angiogram. The anterior portion of the large angiofibroma is clearly demonstrated as a hypervascular mass with blood supply from the internal carotid system. The entire JAF is not outlined.

(continued)

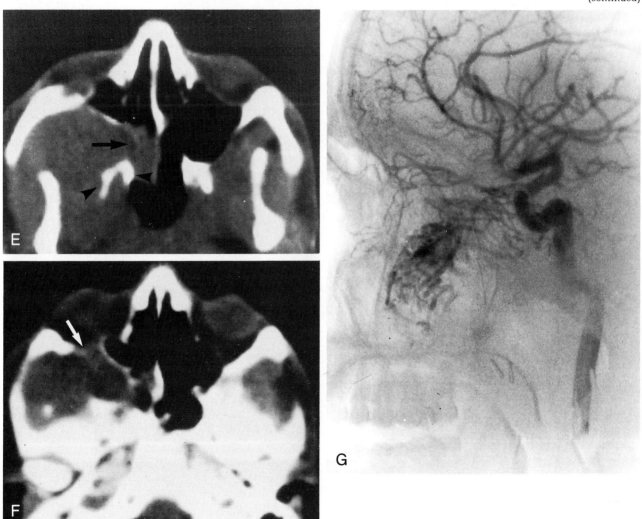

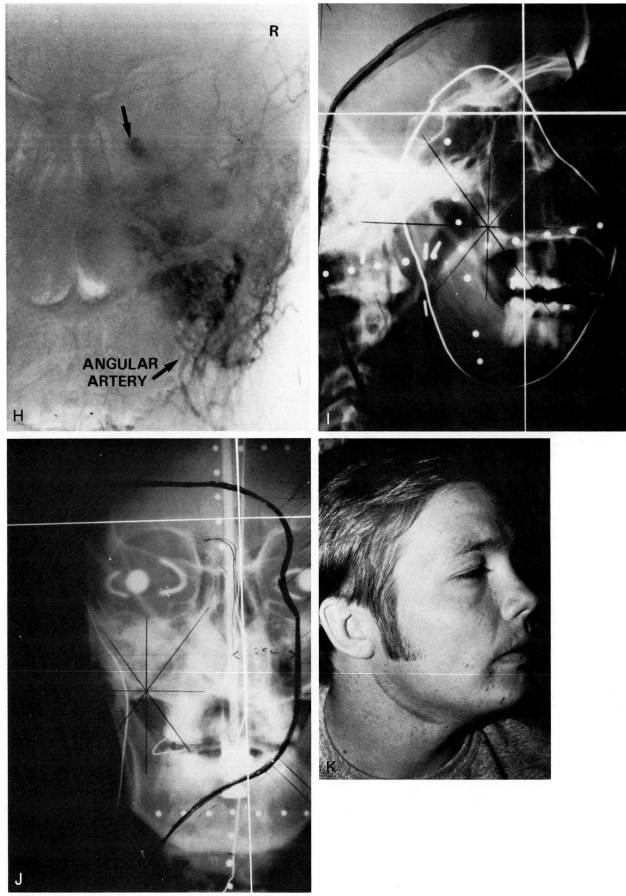

R

ANGULAR
ARTERY

H

I

J

K

FIG. 25-1 (continued)

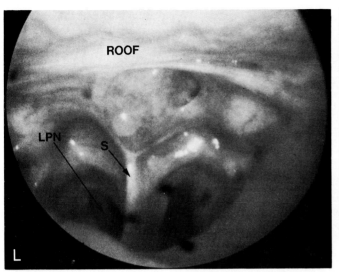

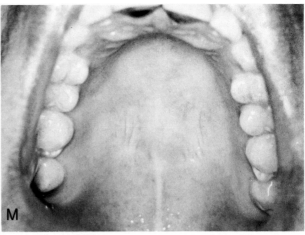

FIG. 25-1 (*continued*)

(*H*) Subtracted external carotid artery angiogram. A hypervascular mass (*arrow*) consistent with a large JAF is well demonstrated. Treatment plan: Radiation therapy was recommended because of the extension of the tumor to the orbit and the numerous feeding vessels. (*I*) Simulator film of lateral radiation therapy portal. Wire outlines palpable disease in the right cheek. The thick black line outlines portal. Note the generous portal size. (*J*) Simulator film of anterior radiation therapy portal. It was not possible to shield the eyeball due to tumor invasion of the orbit. Patient received 3500 rad/4½ weeks, 8-MV x-ray. (*K*) Appearance at 14 months. There was minimal regression at completion of therapy, 75% regression at 6 weeks, and complete clinical regression at 6 months. (*L*) Nasopharynx at 14 months. The submucosal nodule in the roof of the nasopharynx and the tumor in the right posterior nares have disappeared. (*S*, nasal septum; *LPN*, left posterior nares) (*M*) Appearance of hard palate at 14 months. There was no evidence of disease at 24 months.

Management of Recurrence

Recurrence of JAF following the course of radiation therapy may be treated by surgical removal or with repeat irradiation if the initial doses were on the order of 3000 rad to 3500 rad. Briant and co-workers report successful management of ten surgical failures by radiation therapy.[2] The same series details seven patients who had a second course of radiation therapy (3500 rad/3 weeks) with control of the lesion after the first series had failed. The most common cause for failure of radiation therapy is inadequate volume rather than inadequate dosage.

RESULTS OF TREATMENT

Operative Results

Neel and associates reported the surgical results from the Mayo Clinic, 1945–1971, for 56 patients with JAF.[9] The majority of these patients had had some prior form of irradiation or surgery. Fifteen required two or more secondary procedures. Five deaths from tumor occurred in patients with extensive sinus disease who had had prior treatment. Forty-five were alive and free of disease.

Biller and co-workers reported results of 43 male patients with JAF seen over a period of 34 years at the Barnes Hospital in St. Louis.[1] Prior to 1965, 26 patients were treated surgically with a variety of surgical approaches. Tumor persisted in 16 of 26 patients (61%). Sixteen patients were

operated on after 1965 and 6 patients had evidence of persistent tumor (37%). Five of the 6 patients with persistent tumor are now free of disease with secondary treatment with either radiation therapy or reexcision. Sequelae and complications are not reported.

Ward and colleagues reported 35 cases; 20% had evidence of intracranial extension.[13] They concluded that the operative risk was too great for the patient with intracranial extension and recommended the use of radiation therapy.

Operative results for JAF have improved in recent years with the use of arteriography to localize the tumor extent and preoperative arterial occlusion to reduce intraoperative blood loss. CT scans will further improve preoperative assessment of disease extent.

Radiation Therapy Results

Jereb and co-workers reported the results for 69 patients with JAF treated between 1919 and 1966 at the Radiumhemmet in Stockholm.[5] Three patients were treated by surgery alone, 16 by surgery plus radiation therapy, and the remaining 50 by radiation therapy alone. The doses varied from 2000 rad to 6000 rad. Of the 63 evaluable patients with at least a 5-year follow-up, 47 have been free of disease from 10 years to longer than 40 years, 10 patients have been free of disease for more than 5 years, and 6 for more than 1 year. No evidence of malignant disease occurred in any of the patients. Two patients died of treatment complications: one at the time of operation and the second of chronic osteitis and meningitis at the age of 51 after multiple courses of radiation therapy. Cataracts were noted in 2 patients.

Briant and co-workers reported the results for irradiation of 45 patients with JAF treated at the Princess Margaret Hospital.[2] The disease was eventually controlled in all patients. Thirty-five (78%) of 45 lesions were controlled by the initial treatment of 3000 rad to 3500 rad; seven failures were thought to be due to inadequate treatment volume. Seven patients had their tumors controlled by a second course of radiation therapy and three by operation. No radiation-induced neoplasms have been observed with a follow-up of 2 to 20 years.

The University of Florida experience with radiation therapy, 3000 rad/4½ weeks, has been limited to four patients with extensive disease. Two had intracranial extension and two had recurrent lesions after multiple excisions. None of the lesions has recurred with follow-up of 2, 4, 6, and 7 years; there is no evidence of persistent disease by physical examination or CT scan.

FOLLOW-UP POLICY

Patients are seen at frequent intervals for 2 years after surgery or radiation therapy. CT scan with contrast and physical examination are sufficient for follow-up in most cases. Arteriography is requested only if recurrence is suggested, since there is a potential risk of complications.

COMPLICATIONS OF TREATMENT

Radiation Therapy

At a dose level of 3000 rad to 3500 rad/4 weeks, one would expect temporary xerostomia, but most patients will have full return of their saliva. If the orbital contents are included, the possibility of cataract exists. However, usually only the posterior orbit need be included in the treatment field, and the risk of eye complications is small (see Chapter 14, The Effect of Radiation on Normal Tissues of the Head and Neck).

The risk of radiation-induced neoplasms is estimated at 1 in 150 patients irradiated between the ages of 10 and 18 years, and 1 in 400 for those older than 18 years.[4]

Repeat treatment to total doses of 5000 rad to 6000 rad will produce complications similar to those seen for carcinoma of the nasopharynx (see Chapter 24, Nasopharynx).

Sixty-nine patients with JAF were treated between the years 1919 and 1966 at the Radiumhemmet, Stockholm, with follow-up from 1 to more than 40 years. In the earlier years, rather large doses of radiation were used; in more recent years, doses in the range of 2000 rad to 3000 rad have been used. With the higher doses of radiation and long-term follow-up, the side-effects were similar to those seen for treatment of carcinoma of the nasopharynx.

Conley reported two cases of serious radiation complications: osteoradionecrosis of the maxilla in one case and extensive radiation-induced squamous cell carcinoma of the skin developing 18 years after 12,000 R (orthovoltage).[3]

Surgery

Operative death has been reported; the risk is increased with intracranial extension and recurrent disease.[3,13]

Conley reported the surgical complications for 55 operative procedures on 34 patients with JAF; 13 of the patients had recurrent disease when first seen. Complications included severe bleeding after biopsy, persistent palatal fistula, temporary cardiac arrest, meningismus, dacryocystitis, hepatitis, and nephritis. Many of the complications occurred in the years 1940 through 1960 and have decreased in frequency and severity.

Complications of lateral rhinotomy reported by Neel include nasal sequestra, neurologic changes consisting of diplopia or conductive deafness, serous otitis, perforation of the nasal septum, oral-antral fistula, and cerebrospinal fluid leak.[9]

REFERENCES

1. Biller HF, Sessions DG, Ogura JH: Angiofibroma: A treatment approach. Laryngoscope 84:695–706, 1974
2. Briant TDR, Fitzpatrick PJ, Berman J: Nasopharyngeal angiofibroma: A twenty-year study. Laryngoscope 88:1247–1251, 1978
3. Conley J, Healey WV, Blaugrund SM, Perzin KH: Nasopharyngeal angiofibroma in the juvenile. Surg Gynecol Obstet 126:825–837, 1968
4. Cummings BJ: Relative risk factors in the treatment of juvenile nasopharyngeal angiofibroma. Head Neck Surg 3:21–26, 1980
5. Jereb B, Änggård A, Båryds I: Juvenile nasopharyngeal angiofibroma: A clinical study of 69 cases. Acta Radiol Ther 9:302–310, 1970
6. Johns ME, MacLeod RM, Cantrell RW: Estrogen receptors in nasopharyngeal angiofibromas. Laryngoscope 90:628–634, 1980
7. Krekorian EA, Kato RH: Surgical management of nasopharyngeal angiofibroma with intracranial extension. Laryngoscope 87:154–164, 1977
8. Mancuso AA, Hanafee WN: Computed Tomography of the Head and Neck, pp 136–142. Baltimore, Williams & Wilkins, 1982
9. Neel HB, Whicker JH, Devine KD, Weiland LH: Juvenile angiofibroma: Review of 120 cases. Am J Surg 126:547–556, 1973
10. Pradillo JA, Rodriguez HA, Arroyo JF: Nasopharyngeal angiofibroma in the elderly: Report of a case. Laryngoscope 85:1063–1065, 1975
11. Sessions RB, Bryan N, Naclerio RM, Alford BR: Radiographic staging of juvenile angiofibroma. Head Neck Surg 3:279–283, 1981
12. Sessions RB, Wills PI, Alford BR, Harrell JE, Evans RA: Juvenile nasopharyngeal angiofibroma: Radiographic aspects. Laryngoscope 86:2–18, 1976
13. Ward PH, Thompson R, Calcaterra T, Kadin MR: Juvenile angiofibroma: A more rational therapeutic approach based upon clinical and experimental evidence. Laryngoscope 84:2181–2194, 1974
14. Wilson GH, Hanafee WN: Angiographic findings in 16 patients with juvenile nasopharyngeal angiofibroma. Radiology 92:279–284, 1969

Carcinoma of the Skin

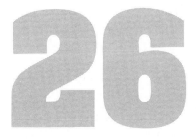

RODNEY R. MILLION
NICHOLAS J. CASSISI

Approximately 90% of skin carcinoma occurs in the head and neck area. The incidence in the United States is estimated to be 400,000 cases per year.[30] The risk increases in sunny climates. There is a low incidence in dark-skinned people; there is a corresponding increase in those with a fair, ruddy, "Scotch-Irish" complexion. Seventy-five percent of basal cell carcinomas in blacks occur in sun-exposed skin as contrasted to approximately a 90% rate in whites.[23] The mortality rate is approximately 1800/year or 0.45%.

Some of the conditions associated with carcinoma of the skin are listed below:

Actinic exposure
Ionizing radiation
Scar (e.g., burn scar)[33]
Chronic draining of sinus or fistulous tract (e.g., pilonidal sinus)
Immune disorders
  Chronic lymphocytic leukemia
  Transplant patients[14]
  Discoid lupus erythematosus[16]
Chemicals
  Arsenicals—herbicides, pesticides
  Psoralens and ultraviolet light (PUVA) treatment for psoriasis[32]
  Nitrates
  Tars, oils, and paraffins
Hereditary disorders
  Xeroderma pigmentosum
  Basal cell nevus syndrome
  Albinism
  Congenital epidermolysis bullosa[7]

ANATOMY

The epidermis is thinner in the face than in most portions of the body, measuring approximately 0.04 mm. There is no consistent change in the thickness of the epidermis with increasing age and no difference between that of men and women.

The dermis, which contains the blood and lymphatic vessels, adnexa, hair follicles, sweat glands, and sebaceous glands, is 1 mm to 2 mm thick; the dermis of the eyelid is thinner, 0.6 mm or less. Beneath the dermis lies the subcutaneous tissues containing the fat and the superficial fascia. There is no distinct transition from the dermis to the subcutaneous layer.

Lymphatics

There are no lymphatics in the epidermis. A superficial capillary lymphatic plexus lies in the dermis and is without valves.[37] The deep lymphatic trunks in the dermis and subcutaneous tissues have valves. The density of the capillary lymphatics has been noted to be approximately the same in all

475

areas except the sole of the foot and palm of the hand, where it is denser. Observation suggests that squamous cell carcinomas and malignant melanomas occurring on the skin of the temple are particularly prone to develop lymphatic metastasis.[5]

During the healing of wounds such as incisions or burns, there is a regeneration of lymphatic capillaries across the scar similar to the regrowth of small blood vessels.[37]

The first-echelon lymph nodes for carcinomas of the face and scalp are the superficial network of lymph nodes that form a ring around the top of the neck: submental, submaxillary, parotid area, postauricular (mastoid), and occipital lymph nodes, as well as inconstant intercalated lymph nodes.

See section on anatomy of the head and neck lymphatic system in Chapter 4, General Principles for Treatment of Cancers in the Head and Neck: Selection of Treatment for the Primary Site and for the Neck, and also Chapter 28, Major Salivary Gland Tumors, for additional discussion regarding lymphatics.

PATHOLOGY

Malignant carcinomas of the skin are basal cell carcinoma (65%), squamous cell carcinoma (30%), or one of their variants, and the remainder are adnexal carcinomas. Verrucous carcinoma of skin occurs most often on the foot and is rare in the head and neck area. Carcinoma in situ occurs frequently in the head and neck. Any of the carcinomas may show perineural invasion, particularly with recurrent disease.

Carcinomas (e.g., renal cell carcinoma) originating outside the head and neck area may metastasize to the skin, especially the scalp.

Basal Cell Carcinoma

The common basal cell carcinoma, which arises from the basal layer of the epithelium, may have a variety of growth patterns and gross appearances. Many of the different growth patterns merge into one another in the same tumor, and the different names applied to the gross and microscopic appearances have limited clinical meaning. The morphea type (sclerosing basal cell carcinoma) shows little surface disease and a marked infiltrative picture; it is an important subtype because of the higher risk for recurrence. Some lesions will have mixed basal cell and squamous cell carcinoma (basosquamous cell carcinoma).

Melanin pigment may be seen on both gross and microscopic examination of basal cell carcinoma.

Squamous Cell Carcinoma

Squamous cell carcinoma and its variants (i.e., verrucous carcinoma, spindle cell squamous carcinoma) are similar histologically to squamous cell carcinomas occurring in other sites. Most are well differentiated, but a small number are poorly differentiated. Evans and Smith identified two categories of spindle cell tumors of skin; one group was composed of obvious squamous cell carcinoma mixed with a spindle cell component, and the other group had only the spindle cell component present.[8] The spindle cell component was similar in both groups; mitoses, giant cells, and epithelioid cells were seen in some cases.

Keratoacanthoma

Keratoacanthoma is a benign tumor of the skin that grossly resembles a cystic basal cell carcinoma and microscopically resembles squamous cell carcinoma or squamous papilloma. Part of the difficulty in histologic diagnosis is due to an inadequate biopsy specimen. Ackerman concluded that "the diagnosis of keratoacanthoma can only be made with absolute certainty by biologic behavior in the form of eventual involution."[2]

Adnexal Carcinoma

Carcinomas may arise from the epithelium of the sweat glands or sebaceous glands and microscopically resemble the tissue of origin. Sweat gland carcinoma can arise from either the eccrine or apocrine glands, but there are no reliable histologic criteria to differentiate the origin. It is difficult to distinguish between benign and malignant sweat gland carcinoma in the absence of metastases. The differential diagnosis includes adenocarcinoma metastatic to skin and basal cell and squamous cell carcinomas with an adenoid cystic growth pattern. They are frequently misdiagnosed at the time of the first biopsy. Malignant tricholemmoma arising from hair follicles is extremely rare.

Dermatofibrosarcoma Protuberans

See Chapter 34, Adult Mesenchymal Tumors Presenting in the Head and Neck, for a discussion of dermatofibrosarcoma protuberans.

PATTERNS OF SPREAD

The patterns of spread for individual anatomical sites are outlined in the section on selection of treatment by anatomical site. Some lesions remain confined to the epidermis (carcinoma in situ) and may involve a large area of skin. Large in situ lesions occur more often on the trunk, but small areas of in situ disease are common on the head and neck skin.

Basal Cell/Squamous Cell Carcinoma

Both basal cell and squamous cell carcinomas are usually well differentiated and most have an indolent growth with distinct ("pushing") margins; a small proportion are poorly differentiated and grow rapidly. Basal cell carcinoma occurs more frequently around the central portion of the face, while squamous cell carcinoma occurs more often on the ears, preauricular and temporal area, scalp, and skin of the neck.

Most lesions remain superficial and invade the adjacent epidermis in a more or less circumferential (pagetoid) growth pattern. Invasion of the dermis is usually confined to the superficial (papillary) dermis. Eventually there is penetration to the reticular dermis, subcutaneous tissues, and other underlying structures. A few skin carcinomas tend to grow beneath the skin, and the surface lesion gives little indication of their extensive growth; this is more often seen in recurrent tumors. The great majority of early basal cell and squamous cell carcinomas show an orderly invasion of the superficial dermis, which allows successful local therapy. Both basal cell and squamous cell carcinomas will invade cartilage and bone, develop perineural spread, and eventually enter the lymphatics, although this is not common. Basal cell carcinoma in particular has a very low incidence of lymphatic involvement unless it is recurrent, while the incidence of lymph node spread for squamous cell carcinoma is 10% to 15%.

Scanlon and co-workers suggested the possibility that a small proportion of basal cell carcinomas spread along interstitial tissue planes and develop satellites.[28]

Squamous cell carcinomas may develop distant metastasis, whereas basal cell carcinomas rarely produce distant metastasis.

Basosquamous cell carcinoma is intermediate between basal cell carcinoma and squamous cell carcinoma as far as recurrence rates and risk of metastases.[29]

Spindle cell tumors of the skin have a gross appearance and growth pattern similar to squamous cell carcinomas.

Sweat Gland Carcinoma

Sweat gland carcinoma occurs with equal frequency in males and females. It predominantly affects elderly people, but it may occur even in early adulthood. The lesion is generally a subcutaneous nodular mass, which may be solitary or multiple, and the larger lesions may be ulcerated.

Sweat gland carcinoma occurs most often on the eyelid, face, and scalp. The growth rate varies from indolent to rapid. The tumor may be present for several years with little change and then suddenly begin to enlarge. Perineural invasion is frequent. Regional and distant metastases may develop. The scalp lesions are the ones most likely to develop regional lymph node metastases.

Recurrence following excision is said to be frequent, and often multiple recurrences are reported.[9] There is little information on the response to radiation therapy. In our limited experience, sweat gland carcinoma is sufficiently radioresponsive to justify irradiation, particularly in association with excision.

The mucin-producing adenocarcinoma of the sweat gland is a rare tumor; 47 cases have been reported to 1978. The eyelid is the primary site in approximately one half of the cases, and the face and scalp, another one fourth of the cases. The tumor presents most often in middle-aged men. Wright and Font reported 21 cases that originated on the eyelid.[36] Eight patients (40%) developed one or more local recurrences, one died with extensive persistent disease in the face after a 15-year interval, and only one patient had metastasis to the submandibular lymph nodes successfully treated by radical neck dissection. Regional or distant metastasis is a relatively infrequent event for lesions arising in the head and neck area.

Sebaceous Gland Carcinoma

Sebaceous gland carcinoma is rare. It occurs most often on the eyelids, predominantly on the upper lid in elderly women, but the lower lid and caruncle are also sites of origin; it may occur on other parts of the head and neck skin. It is often indolent in its growth, but it may be locally aggressive and develop regional and distant metastases. Local recurrence is common after excision because the lesions often have significant deep and lateral spread beyond the obvious lesion. Metastasis to regional lymph nodes is reported in approximately 20% of cases, and a small percentage of patients develop distant metastasis.[21] Inadequate treatment often occurs because of incorrect histologic diagnosis.

Keratoacanthoma

This benign lesion starts as a firm, round skin nodule and grows to 1 cm to 2 cm in a short time, usually a few weeks. As the lesion matures, the center becomes separate and can be removed, revealing a small crater. The lesion occurs most often in the exposed areas of the head and neck region. Keratoacanthoma is an unlikely diagnosis for a lesion of the lip vermilion. Typically, keratoacanthoma undergoes spontaneous regression. Conversion to squamous cell carcinoma is a controversial point because the lesions resemble squamous cell carcinoma in the beginning. Keratoacanthoma is twice as common in men than women. It occurs most often after the age of 40, but it may be seen as early as the second decade.

Basal Cell Nevus Syndrome

The basal cell nevus syndrome is an autosomal-dominant disorder with a high level of penetrance but a variable clinical picture. The clinical syndrome may be composed of any or all of the following:

Multiple basal cell carcinomas (differing only in their tendency to develop at an early age and on unexposed skin areas)
Jaw cysts (very common)
Palmar/plantar pits
Skeletal abnormalities (short fingers, hypertelorism)
Ectopic calcification
Eye muscle palsies
Hamartomas
Epidermal cysts (milia)

The age at onset is frequently in the second or third decade, and a family history is often positive for the disorder.[31]

Lymphatics

The overall risk of lymphatic metastases is 10% to 15% for squamous cell carcinoma of the skin. The risk increases with the size of the lesion, depth of penetration, histologic grade, and recurrence.

Jackson and Ballantyne reviewed the M. D. Anderson Hospital experience in the management of skin cancers metastatic to the parotid area lymph nodes.[15] The incidence of clinically positive lymph nodes in the ipsilateral neck was 24% for 149 nonbasal cell carcinomas, and 21% were pathologically positive. The incidence of disease in the clinically negative neck was 24% with elective neck dissection.

The skin site of origin for squamous cell carcinoma of the skin, metastatic to parotid area lymph nodes, is shown in Figure 26-1. The lymph nodes anterior to the ear (either the superficial preauricular or the parotid nodes) were involved in 28 cases, the tail of parotid lymph nodes in 6 cases, and both in 5 cases. The preauricular lymph nodes may be very small when first involved and easily missed unless a careful examination is carried out. Lesions arising

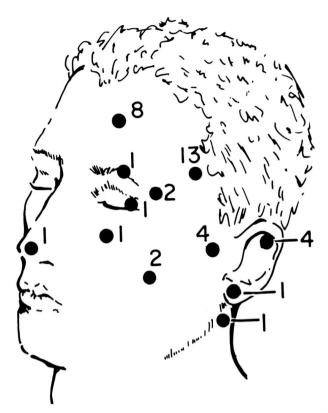

FIG. 26-1. Skin site of origin for 39 parotid area lymph node metastases. One preauricular lymph node was from an unknown primary site. (University of Florida data; patients treated 1/66–4/80; analysis 4/82 by N. P. Mendenhall, MD.)

from the temple area seem to have a high risk for lymph node metastases, but it is unknown whether this is related to a rich capillary lymphatic supply or to the size and depth of invasion. The risk for lymph node metastases from *de novo* basal cell carcinomas is less than 1% and is not related to size, depth of penetration, or histologic subtype; the risk increases for recurrent basal cell carcinomas, especially those with multiple recurrences occurring over several years. However, lymph node metastases are seen on rare occasions without a history of recurrence, and there may be an interval of several years between the treatment of the primary lesion and the appearance of the involved lymph node. Lymph node metastases, when they do occur, are often solitary.

Lesions of the posterior scalp spread to the occipital nodes; lesions of the parietal area spread to the postauricular nodes; lesions of the frontal scalp, temple, and eyelids spread to the preauricular lymph nodes; and lesions about the nose and lips spread to the submaxillary and parotid areas. The tiny buccal, facial, and mental foramen nodes and other inconstant intercalated lymph nodes near the nasolabial fold and external canthus are less common sites of lymph node metastasis and are often missed due to failure to look for them or recognize them when seen or palpated. Lesions that occur in overlapping lymphatic areas may spread in either or both directions.

When first involved, the superficial lymph nodes are frequently very small and easily missed unless thorough, gentle examination is carried out. This is particularly true

for the tail of parotid and superficial preauricular lymph nodes, which are probably the most commonly involved lymph nodes from skin cancer.

All of the first-echelon lymph nodes eventually drain to the internal jugular chain or spinal accessory chain lymph nodes.

CLINICAL PICTURE

It will never get well if you pick it.

American Proverb

Presenting Symptoms

The common history for basal cell carcinoma or squamous cell carcinoma is a slowly enlarging growth on or just beneath the skin surface. There is often a history of a sore that will not completely heal. Other symptoms such as bleeding or pain are unusual until the lesion becomes quite large, and even then the symptoms are relatively mild and infrequent. Patients with perineural spread may complain of paresthesias, especially the sensation of worms crawling under the skin. We have observed several cases that spread centrally along the facial nerve or branch of the trigeminal nerve (*i.e.*, infraorbital nerve), eventually producing multiple cranial nerve palsies and destruction of the apex of the temporal bone and floor of the middle cranial fossa. The diagnosis was delayed because the physicians did not associate the history of skin cancer and the possibility of tumor tracking along nerve sheaths to colonize a more central location. Advanced, neglected lesions with bone and cartilage destruction, orbit invasion, and regional metastases are still seen; these advanced lesions often produce few, if any, symptoms, and the patient simply "puts off" going to a physician.

Physical Examination

The regional lymph nodes must be carefully examined, even though they are not often involved. Because of the infrequent appearance of regional lymphatic metastases and because skin cancer patients are not often followed diligently, lymph node metastases are often missed. Although the lymphatic metastases may appear within a few months of the management of the primary lesion, in some cases many years intervene before the regional lymph nodes become apparent. It is not at all unusual for 5 years or more to intervene between the primary lesion and the appearance of metastasis. Patients with chronic lymphocytic leukemia and concomitant skin cancer often have enlarged lymph nodes from both processes and may have both squamous cell carcinoma and leukemia in the same lymph nodes.

When the lymph nodes in the preauricular area become involved, especially when there is a latent period of several years between treatment of the primary squamous cell carcinoma and the appearance of a metastatic node, they are frequently misdiagnosed as squamous cell carcinoma originating in the parotid gland. Failure to recognize their true origin results in inappropriate and unsuccessful treatment in most cases. *The squamous cell carcinoma (or adnexal carcinoma) arising from the temple area seems to have an especially high risk for lymphatic metastasis. These particular lesions should be watched very carefully.*

METHODS OF DIAGNOSIS AND STAGING

The majority of lesions should be biopsied prior to deciding on treatment. We do not always insist on biopsy for patients who are to be treated by radiation therapy, who have a typical skin carcinoma, and who have already had numerous lesions biopsied and treated; this is especially true for the elderly patient.

Small lesions occurring on the free skin areas (i.e., not involving the eyelid, ear, periorbital areas) can usually be biopsied and treated simultaneously with surgical excision. Larger lesions, or those involving areas where functional or cosmetic deficit might occur from excision, are first biopsied with a small incisional biopsy or with a skin punch. Biopsy with a skin punch should include the subcutaneous fat; punch biopsy is contraindicated when differentiating between keratoacanthoma and squamous cell carcinoma because of the small sample size.

The following is a partial list of conditions to be considered in the differential diagnosis of basal cell carcinoma and squamous cell carcinoma:

Senile keratosis
Keratoacanthoma
Nonpigmented nevi
Malignant melanoma
Cutaneous horn
Psoriasis
Lymphoma (mycosis fungoides)
Soft tissue sarcomas (dermatofibrosarcoma protuberans)
Hemangiosarcoma
Metastatic carcinoma
Adnexal carcinoma of skin

The American Joint Committee (AJCC) staging is based on the size, depth of penetration, and involvement of muscle, bone, or cartilage:[3]

TX   Minimum requirements to assess the primary tumor cannot be met.
Tis   Preinvasive caccrinoma (carcinoma *in situ*)
T0   No primary tumor present
T1   Tumor 2 cm or less in its largest dimension, strictly superficial or exophytic
T2   Tumor more than 2 cm but no more than 5 cm in its largest dimension or with minimal infiltration of the dermis, irrespective of size
T3   Tumor more than 5 cm in its largest dimension or with deep infiltration of the dermis, irrespective of size
T4   Tumor involving other structures such as cartilage, muscle, or bone

Neck node staging is the same as for other head and neck sites. (See Chapter 4, General Principles for Treatment of Cancers in the Head and Neck: Selection of Treatment for the Primary Site and for the Neck.) A computed tomographic (CT) scan may be helpful for a large parotid-area lymph node metastasis to determine the extent of tumor invasion to the deep lobe or parapharyngeal space.

The great majority of primary lesions can be staged by a simple physical examination and palpation. Larger lesions may require tomography or CT scanning to determine the extent of disease.

Patients suspected of having basal cell nevus syndrome should have appropriate radiographs to determine the extent of skeletal abnormalities.

TREATMENT TECHNIQUES

Treatment Modalities

A number of treatments are successful, including radiation therapy, a variety of surgical techniques, and topical chemotherapy; superficial basal cell carcinomas sometimes heal spontaneously.

TOPICAL CHEMOTHERAPY

Topical chemotherapy, usually with 5-fluorouracil, is successful for superficial lesions that are confined to the epidermis, such as precancerous keratosis, dysplastic skin, and carcinoma *in situ*. Topically applied 5-fluorouracil should not be used for invasive lesions since they appear to heal on the surface, allowing continued growth below the epidermis.[22] Invasive lesions treated with topical 5-fluorouracil have been observed to show temporary regression and then show an accelerated growth rate.

SURGICAL TECHNIQUES

Surgical techniques include scalpel excision, curettage and electrodesiccation, fulguration and curettage, cryotherapy, and chemosurgery. All of these techniques, when applied to appropriate lesions, are reported to produce excellent results in the hands of experienced clinicians.

CURETTAGE WITH ELECTROSURGERY

Curettage with electrosurgery is commonly used by the dermatologist and is very successful. It is usually reserved for relatively small, superficial, well-defined lesions. The area is anesthetized, and a sharp curet is used to scrape away the lesion until normal tissue is reached. The base of the wound is electrodesiccated to ensure destruction of remaining tumor cells and to obtain hemostasis. The physician depends on the feel of the curet to determine when normal tissue is reached. The process is repeated for larger lesions. Lesions of the tip and ala of the nose, lip vermilion, periorbital areas, auriculotemporal fold, or any large or deeply invasive lesions may be better treated by other means, since the cure rate, cosmetic result, and functional result may not be optimal.

Although successful for small lesions, this technique provides no specimen for checking the adequacy of the margins, which would be important in larger tumors. Healing occurs by second intention with a flat white scar. The healing time, usually 2 to 4 weeks, is longer than for a simple excision. The scar may be noticeable if adjacent to darker skin.

ELECTROFULGURATION AND CURETTAGE

The area is anesthetized, and a diathermy unit is used to coagulate the lesion and adjacent normal tissue. The initial coagulum is removed with a curet, after which repeated electrocoagulation is performed until normal-appearing tissue is reached. The wound heals in an average of 5 weeks. The cosmetic appearance is satisfactory when a small lesion is treated in this manner. Recurrence usually appears on the surface of the scar and is said to be easily detected, but recurrence may develop in the tissues deep to the scar and become extensive before appearing at the surface. There is no specimen available to determine adequacy of margins.

MICROSCOPICALLY CONTROLLED EXCISION

This technique was initially developed by Mohs and refers to a method in which the lesion is excised under microscopic control.[22] The tumor is either fixed in situ with an application of zinc chloride paste (fixed tissue technique), or the lesion is excised without prior fixation (fresh tissue technique).

Fixed Tissue Technique

The fixed tissue technique provides a more accurate microscopic control compared with the fresh tissue method and is therefore used for the more extensive and complicated cases. The usual procedure is to anesthetize the area and excise the obvious cancer mass, leaving a saucerized area. Hemostasis is achieved by application of dichloroacetic acid. The zinc chloride fixative is then applied and remains in place for a few minutes or as long as 2 days, depending on the depth of fixation desired and scheduling requirements. The depth of fixation is controlled by the thickness of the paste that is applied as well as the length of application. Local tissue factors may accelerate or retard the depth of fixation. The fixed tissue is then excised through the fixed area to avoid pain and bleeding. There may be considerable pain associated with the penetration of the fixative itself, and this may require analgesics ranging from aspirin to opiates. Successive horizontal layers are excised and frozen sections are prepared. A diagram is made of each layer and the layers are marked with dyes to orient anatomical landmarks. Successive areas are fixed but limited to the cancerous area, and successive excisions are performed until a cancer-free layer is reached (Fig. 26-2). The wound is usually allowed to heal by secondary intention; in certain cases, skin grafts may be applied.

This procedure is particularly useful for recurrent basal cell and squamous cell carcinomas. Physicians experienced in this technique are not available in all communities. Some patients complain of marked pain associated with the procedure due to the fixative, and some have flatly refused to undergo the procedure again.

Fresh Tissue Technique

The fresh tissue technique is usually indicated for cancers of small to moderate extent and has the advantage of being more rapid and less painful than the fixed tissue method. It can usually be accomplished in one procedure, whereas the fixed tissue technique may require several days. The major difference in the two techniques is that the in situ fixation is omitted. Hemostasis is accomplished by the application of a thin layer of Oxycel, superficial electrodesiccation, or the application of dichloracetic acid. Ligatures are occasionally required. The wound is usually allowed to heal by secondary intention, or in some cases it is covered with a split-thickness skin graft or a flap. This method adds an average of 2 hours to the surgical procedure but allows the entire excision to be finished in 1 day.

Advantages and Disadvantages

The major advantage of microscopically controlled excision is the selective removal of tumor ramifications, which may extend a considerable distance in a haphazard direction beyond the clinically visible or palpable borders of the neoplasm. The fixed tissue technique is especially

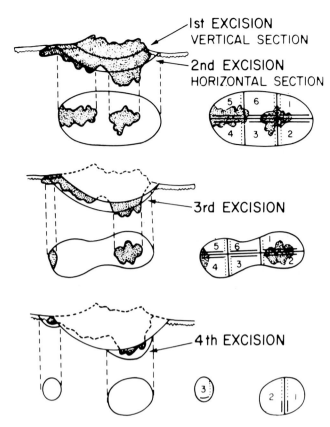

FIG. 26-2. Successive excisions in fixed tissue technique. (Reproduced with permission from Mohs FE: Chemosurgery for basal cell and squamous carcinomas of the skin. In M. D. Anderson Hospital and Tumor Institute, Houston: Neoplasms of the Skin and Malignant Melanoma, pp 173–188. Copyright © 1976 by Year Book Medical Publishers, Inc., Chicago)

applicable to large, complicated, often-recurrent lesions, for which it is very difficult for the surgeon and the radiation therapist to determine the margins. Involvement of the periosteum or nasal and orbital structures is not a contraindication. The procedure may be used for either basal cell or squamous cell carcinoma. The fresh tissue technique is preferred for lesions about the eyelid, inner canthus, and nasal ala, areas where it is difficult to obtain adequate margins when treated surgically. Cancers of the pinna are best removed by the fresh tissue technique because this permits salvage of the underlying cartilage, whereas with the fixed tissue technique the underlying cartilage must usually be removed even though it is not involved with cancer. The supporters of this technique report very high success rates at 5 years. The major advantage, compared with other surgical methods, is the ability to precisely determine whether all the tumor has been removed and, secondarily, to remove only as much normal tissue as is necessary, rather than guessing at the probable growth patterns.

The disadvantages of microscopically controlled excision include the appreciable pain from the fixative in the fixed tissue technique, the multiple injections of a local anesthetic required with either technique, and the increased operative time of about 2 hours with the fresh tissue method. An experienced dermatopathologist must be available. The cosmetic/functional losses may be considerable depending on the amount of tissue resected, the anatomical site affected, and whether healing is by secondary intention or reconstructive surgery.

CRYOTHERAPY

Cryotherapy produces excellent results for selected superficial basal cell carcinomas. A thermocouple is inserted into the base of the tumor to ensure a temperature of $-30°C$. A cryospray is used to freeze the lesion and a margin of normal tissue. The ice ball is allowed to thaw for 60 to 90 seconds and then the freezing is repeated. With properly selected lesions, the technique is successful with almost no risk of scarring, infection, or hemorrhage.

Liquid nitrogen may be applied topically to anesthetized lesions such as actinic keratosis, leukoplakia, carcinoma in situ, and multiple superficial basal cell carcinomas.

RADIATION THERAPY

The use of radiation therapy for treatment of skin cancer, while quite successful, has declined in recent years because of the greater availability of specialists to deal with the problems of skin cancer, the diminished use by dermatologists of x-ray therapy in their private offices, and the late morbidity observed after courses of radiation therapy given with a few high fractions. The radiation therapy skills available in the United States in the 1930s through the 1950s varied widely with correspondingly varied results. Radiation therapy, however, still plays a very important role in specific anatomical situations in which the functional or cosmetic result is better than for a surgical modality, for large lesions that are generally not suitable for surgical treatment, and for patients medically unable to undergo an operative procedure. Many of the skin cancers irradiated in past years were treated with a few high-dose fractions, which were often successful in curing the cancer but eventually produced a depressed, unsightly scar or worse. In addition, until recently, only orthovoltage radiation or implant techniques were available, so there was some constraint in treating large lesions involving cartilage or bone. With supervoltage radiations, the constraints have largely disappeared, so that radiation therapy may be applied in almost any anatomical and clinical situation.

Selection of Treatment Modality

Cancers of the facial skin
  were not a threat to Ann Boleyn.
Beheading's safe and comprehensive;
  we offer treatment less offensive. . . .

                    Jeffrey W. Gefter, MD

A comparison of the overall results of treatment of squamous cell carcinoma and basal cell carcinoma by radiation therapy and a variety of surgical techniques would suggest that the cure rates are similar. However, most comparisons are misleading since lesions are not staged, nor are results given by anatomical site. The large number of small, successfully treated lesions tends to obscure the less favorable results seen in the larger, more aggressive tumors. Cure rates are uncommonly reported for greater than 5 years (e.g., 10 to 15 years), and a significant number of cases recur late, which is in keeping with the indolent nature of the majority of lesions.

The selection of treatment generally follows this priority list:

1. Cure
2. Function
3. Cosmesis
4. Treatment time
5. Cost

The availability of specialists will often determine treatment selection. The following factors are considered in treatment decisions:

1. Anatomical location
2. Size
3. Invasion of contiguous structures
4. Histology (particularly grade)
5. Recurrent lesions
6. Medical condition
7. Mobility of the patient

Both basal cell and squamous cell carcinomas are equally treatable by surgery or radiation therapy; the histologic variants of basal cell carcinoma and squamous cell carcinoma, while perhaps suggesting a different prognosis and a minor adjustment in treatment technique, do not weigh heavily in the treatment decisions. Basal cell and squamous cell carcinomas are equally radiosensitive; the prescribed dose is based more on the size of the lesion, the extent of local invasion, and the contiguous normal tissues than on the histology. The grade of the tumor, particularly a squamous cell carcinoma that is poorly differentiated, may influence treatment decisions in one direction or another. Certainly, recurrent lesions require special planning, since their biology is often different from de novo lesions. A few of these recurrent lesions can never be controlled and eventually cause major morbidity after many years of unsuccessful treatment or the death of the patient. Keratoacanthoma, while generally managed by surgical modality, is reported to be as radiocurable as basal cell or squamous cell carcinoma.*

FAVORABLE AND UNFAVORABLE LESIONS

A favorable lesion is defined as a slow-growing lesion, with well-differentiated histology, discrete borders, and superficial penetration; not attached to contiguous structures nor involving the ear, periorbita, or nose; and less than 2 cm to 3 cm in diameter. The vast majority of favorable skin cancers can be managed successfully with either scalpel excision, curettage and electrodesiccation, or cryotherapy. These treatments work very well with little functional or cosmetic sequelae. Radiation therapy should be considered for favorable lesions if functional or cosmetic problems will result from the surgical procedure or if complex and costly repair will be needed.

Unfavorable characteristics include a history of rapid growth; poorly differentiated histology; infiltrative growth pattern (e.g., sclerosing basal cell carcinoma); fixation to underlying structures; involvement of the ear, periorbita, or nose; size larger than 2 cm to 3 cm; invasion of muscle, cartilage, bone, or nerve; and recurrent lesions.

A 1- to 3-cm lesion can be easily excised in many locations with adequate borders, but in some areas the re-

---

* Correa JN: Personal communication, 1982.

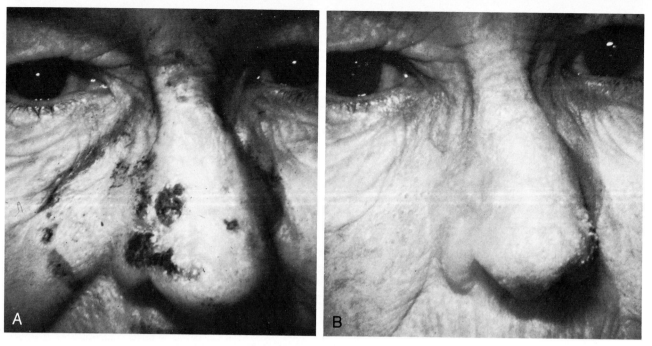

FIG. 26-3. (*A*) Multiple small superficial basal cell carcinomas of the nose and adjacent cheek with "normal" intervening skin. (*B*) Appearance at 1 month.

FIG. 26-4. (*A*) Squamous cell carcinoma invading the zygomatic arch, pinna, external auditory canal, temporal fossa, masseter, and parotid gland. Treatment plan was 6100 rad/5 weeks, cobalt-60, with wax bolus. (*B*) Appearance 1 month after treatment. (*C*) Appearance 2 months after treatment. (*D*) Appearance 6 months after treatment. Patient was alive with no evidence of disease at 6 years. (Courtesy of R. L. Lindberg, MD, Department of Radiation Therapy, M. D. Anderson Hospital and Tumor Institute, Houston)

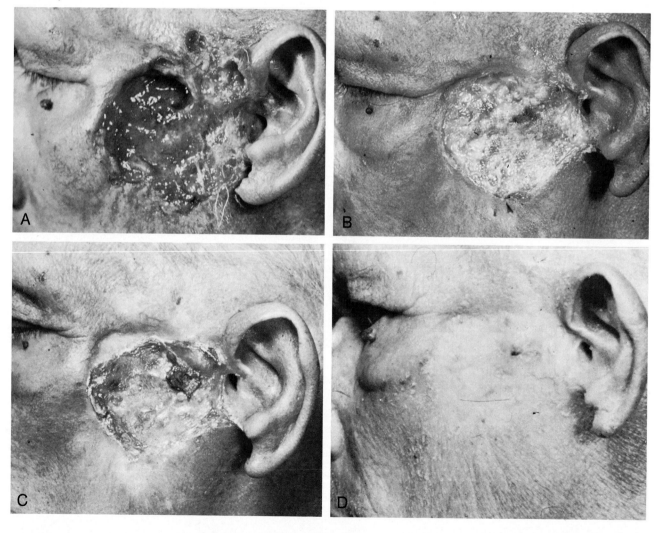

moval of 1 cm to 3 cm of tumor plus normal tissue implies functional and cosmetic loss as well as an increased likelihood of cut-through. Primary closure is not often possible and a graft or flap is required. For moderate-sized lesions, 1 cm to 3 cm, located in sites where excision may produce functional or cosmetic changes, consideration must be given to radiation therapy. Radiation therapy is often selected for larger lesions (i.e., >3 cm) that would require major resection and reconstruction and for small lesions (1 cm to 2 cm) of the eyelids, canthus, pinna, tip and alar areas of the nose, and the skin of the upper lip. Multiple small lesions in one general area (e.g., the nose) may be better treated with radiation therapy (Fig. 26-3). Large recurrent lesions may require combined treatment with surgery and irradiation.

There is an often repeated adage to the effect that lesions invading bone and cartilage should not be treated with radiation therapy. This simply is not true (Fig. 26-4). There is no doubt that the more advanced, neglected lesions invading cartilage or bone are more difficult to control by any means, but we have had a modest amount of success with radiation therapy for the treatment of lesions that involve bone and cartilage and do not consider this a contraindication to use of irradiation and, in fact, often prefer it. Certainly, the use of supervoltage irradiation in these situations has improved our ability to give larger doses to a large treatment volume and still obtain healing. There are numerous examples of cures by radiation therapy alone for lesions other than skin cancer that invade bone and cartilage (e.g., squamous cell carcinomas of the gingiva, paranasal sinuses, nasopharynx, nasal vestibule, and larynx). When tumor invades bone and cartilage, if the bone/cartilage is expendable and the loss acceptable to the patient, and if there is a good likelihood of obtaining adequate surgical margins, then surgical excision is selected; however, this set of circumstances is not often present with advanced lesions, and radiation therapy is often recommended as the sole modality or in combination with resection. Cartilage invasion may occur to a minimal degree in association with relatively small lesions of the ear, nasal vestibule, or nasal skin; there is no contraindication to radiation therapy in these cases, and the results are comparable to surgery.

Adult cartilage has no blood vessels and a large amount of interstitial substance with only a few cells of low mitotic activity. High-dose, properly fractionated radiation therapy (6000 rad to 7500 rad) incidentally delivered to normal adult cartilage (such as cartilage of the ears, larynx, nose, and ribs) essentially never produces a chondronecrosis (see section on cartilage necrosis in Chapter 14, The Effect of Radiation on Normal Tissues of the Head and Neck). When adult cartilage is invaded by tumor, the occurrence of radiation-induced chondronecrosis is still quite unusual, even with substantial doses. Cartilage destroyed by tumor is replaced by connective tissue rather than by cartilage.[31] A diagnosis of chondronecrosis should be viewed with suspicion, since the more likely diagnosis is recurrent cancer.

Another adage often repeated in surgical texts is that very large lesions might, in fact, be cured by irradiation, but the patient would be left with a large, unhealed defect. While this may happen, satisfactory healing by second intention does occur in most cases (Figs. 26-5 and 26-6). Healing of the large lesions is dependent on the redundancy and mobility of the adjacent tissues as well as on the protraction of treatment over several weeks. However, in the case shown in Figure 26-7 of a huge, destructive scalp lesion, although the lesion disappeared following radiation therapy, there was no way for the epithelium to cover the exposed bone and dura, and it was necessary to use local scalp flaps to cover the defect. We have successfully covered large defects with split-thickness skin grafts after therapy with 7500 rad (see section on the scalp).

SELECTION OF TREATMENT ACCORDING TO ANATOMICAL SITE

FREE SKIN

Free skin is a term used in some treatment centers to designate those areas of the cheek, temple, forehead, neck, and scalp that would not usually be associated with potential functional or cosmetic loss if a lesion were surgically excised. Small to moderate-sized lesions in these areas are preferably treated by a surgical modality, since the approach is successful, quick and simple, and less expensive compared with radiation therapy. Lesions that would require complicated and expensive reconstruction are often better treated with irradiation. Lesions that invade underlying bone, cartilage, or other adjacent structures (e.g., the facial nerve) are treated by radiation therapy alone or in combination with an operation. It is difficult to obtain a deep surgical margin in many of these cases, and radiation therapy often produces a more acceptable functional and cosmetic result; excision may be reserved for radiation therapy failure.

NOSE

Four nasal lesions prior to and after microscopically controlled excision of nonfixed tissues are shown in Figures 26-8 through 26-11.[24]

Nasal tip lesions tend to grow in a cephalocaudad direction and invade underlying cartilage (Fig. 26-8).

Lesions of the columella invade the upper lip and premaxilla (Fig. 26-9) (see Chapter 23, Nasal Vestibule, Nasal Cavity, and Paranasal Sinuses). The tooth roots may be invaded once tumor reaches the premaxilla.

Lesions arising on the lateral ala and/or the nasal labial crease tend to invade deeply ("iceberg" lesions) to involve the internal nose, inferior turbinate, and occasionally the nasolacrimal duct. Lateral spread occurs into the lip and cheek (Figs. 26-10 and 26-11).

Recurrence is observed more often for nasal skin cancer than for any other site, whether treated with radiation therapy or with surgery.[18]

Nasal carcinomas are often more extensive than expected. The problems with acceptable nasal reconstruction dictate removal of as little normal tissue as possible. Unless these lesions are very small and superficial, they are preferably treated with radiation therapy, which produces as good a local control rate and a better cosmetic result. Advanced lesions are often cured with radiation therapy, and although the cosmetic result is poor, it is usually more acceptable than total rhinectomy. Surgical excision, particularly of recurrent lesions, is more often successful using microscopically controlled excision.

EYELIDS/CANTHI

The inner canthus and lower lid are frequent sites of involvement for both basal cell carcinoma and squamous

(Text continues on p. 486.)

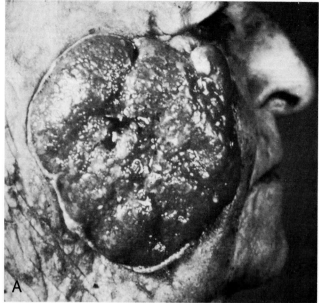

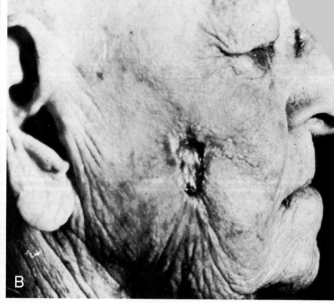

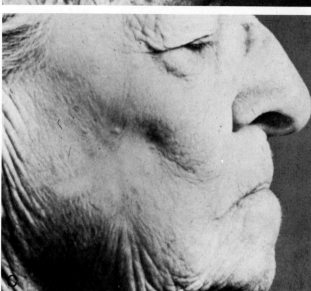

FIG. 26-5. (*A*) Squamous cell carcinoma of the right cheek. Note distinct borders. Treatment plan: 6500 rad/7 days, radium implant. (*B*) Partial healing at 3 months. (*C*) Complete healing at 1 year. There was no evidence of disease at 5 years. Healing of defect was aided by redundant skin. (Courtesy of R. L. Lindberg, MD, Department of Radiation Therapy, M. D. Anderson Hospital and Tumor Institute, Houston)

FIG. 26-6 (*continued*)

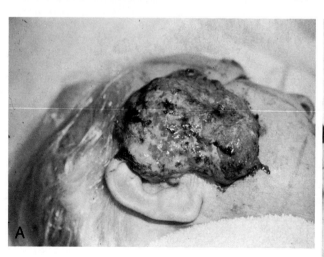

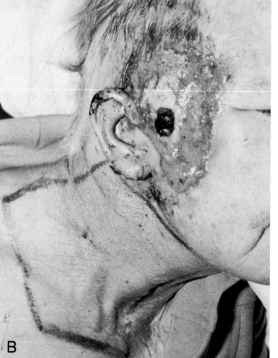

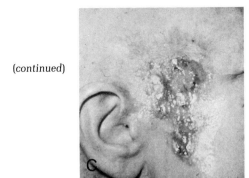

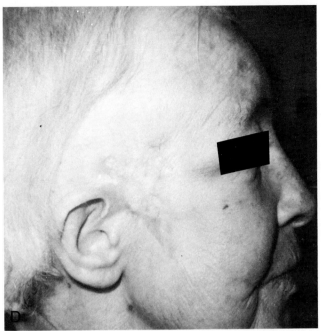

FIG. 26-6. Patient presented with a rapidly enlarging mass for 1 year. (*A*) A 12 × 16-cm squamous cell carcinoma was seen on the right cheek and temple with extension to the pinna. There was mild weakness of the frontal branch of the facial nerve and decreased sensation of the parietal scalp. Roentgenograms showed no bone destruction. Treatment plan: 6750-rad tumor dose/7 weeks, cobalt-60, with beeswax bolus, three fields. The neck received 5000 rad/5 weeks. (*B*) Fifty percent regression at 2500 rad. (*C*) Completion of treatment. (*D*) Appearance at 6 months. There was no evidence of disease at 5 years.

FIG. 26-7. (*A*) Extensive (18 × 14 cm) basal cell carcinoma involving 60% of the scalp. The patient's presenting complaint was shortness of breath due to anemia (Hbg = 9.6 g). There was obvious bone destruction with tumor extending to dura in one area. (*B*) Lytic changes in parietal bone. Treatment plan was 2500 rad (250 kV), and 4000 rad/cobalt-60/6½ weeks. Bolus was added during the cobalt-60 therapy. (*C*) Appearance 2 months after radiation therapy. There was extensive exposure of necrotic bone; dura could be seen in one area. The bone was debrided and a scalp flap was used to cover the defect. A helmet with attached wig was fashioned for protection. (*D*) Appearance of patient without helmet at 5 years with no evidence of disease.

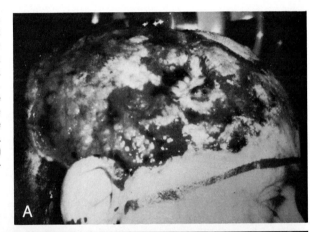

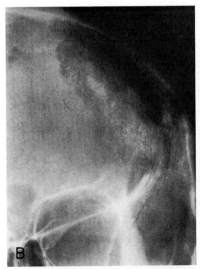

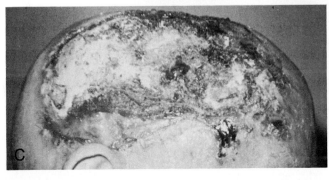

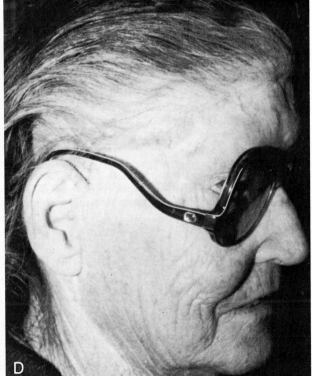

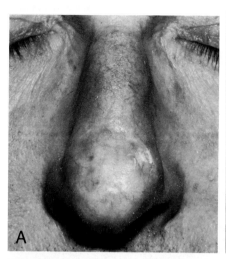
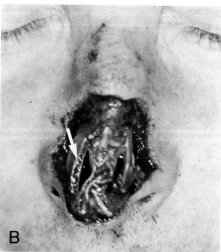

FIG. 26-8. (A) Preoperative photograph of carcinoma of the nasal tip. (B) Microscopically controlled excision. It was necessary to remove part of the underlying cartilage in order to obtain satisfactory margins (arrow). This defect is usually repaired with a skin graft. (Panje WR, Ceilley RI: The influence of embryology of the midface on the spread of epithelial malignancies. Laryngoscope 89:1914–1920, 1979)

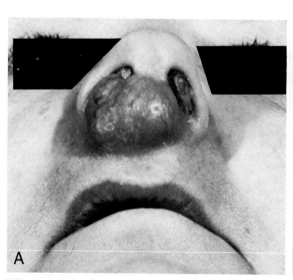
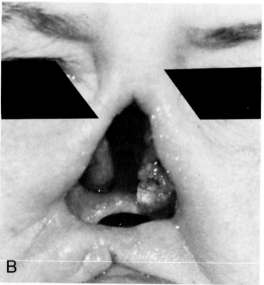

FIG. 26-9. (A) Skin cancer of the columella. (B) Postoperative appearance. (Panje WR, Ceilley RI: The influence of embryology of the midface on the spread of epithelial malignancies. Laryngoscope 89:1914–1920, 1979)

cell carcinoma.[10] Lesions arising in the medial canthus and root of the nose tend to invade deeply toward the medial orbit and lacrimal system and extend into the upper and lower lids. Lesions of the lateral canthus tend to invade the upper and lower lids, the lateral orbit, and the skin of the cheek and temple. Small lesions (0.1 mm to 0.5 mm) can often be treated by a surgical modality with a good functional and cosmetic result. However, the larger lesions

require excision of the underlying muscle (orbicularis oculi), the tarsal plate, or the lacrimal apparatus. Complicated repairs are required, the functional and cosmetic result may not be good, and the risk of local recurrence may be significant, even in experienced hands. Although the lids may look acceptable in a photograph, there are varying degrees of functional loss once a flap is inserted. It is our preference to treat most lesions that are greater

FIG. 26-10. (A) Lateral alar basal cell carcinoma. (B) Appearance after excision. (Panje WR, Ceilley RI: The influence of embryology of the midface on the spread of epithelial malignancies. Laryngoscope 89:1914–1920, 1979)

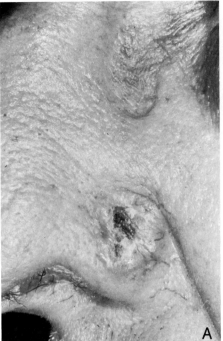
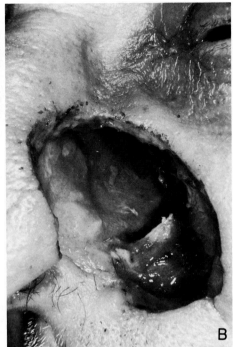

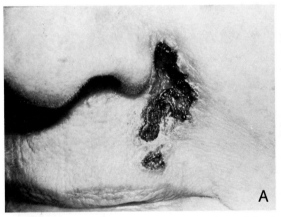
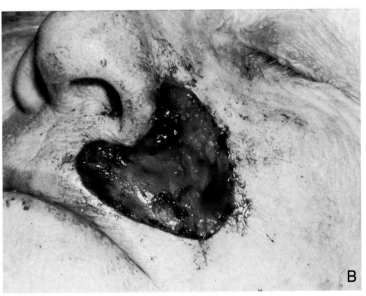

FIG. 26-11. (A) Basal cell carcinoma of nasolabial crease. (B) Appearance after excision. (Panje WR, Ceilley RI: The influence of embryology of the midface on the spread of epithelial malignancies. Laryngoscope 89:1914–1920, 1979)

than 0.5 cm and that involve the canthi and upper and lower lids with radiation therapy, assuming that the patient is willing to undergo at least a 3- to 4-week course of treatment. Short courses of irradiation produce satisfactory short-term results at 1 to 3 years, but the late side-effects may be undesirable, and only the more prolonged fractionated treatments give lasting cosmetic and functional results that compete favorably with excision.

Extensive lesions of the periorbital area that grossly invade the orbit may require a combination of radical surgery and radiation therapy, including evisceration of the eye. However, radiation therapy alone will cure some of these advanced lesions (Figs. 26-12 and 26-13). A craniofacial procedure may be required to obtain clear margins in ad-

vanced lesions that invade the paranasal sinuses (see Chapter 23, Nasal Vestibule, Nasal Cavity, and Paranasal Sinuses).

EAR

Basal or squamous cell carcinomas occurring on the external ear may be treated by either excision or radiation therapy. Surgical procedures for small lesions may result in a minor cosmetic loss, but if this loss is relatively unimportant to the patient, the results are satisfactory and the treatment expeditious. Radiation therapy produces equal results without the cosmetic loss, but requires a longer treatment course. The often-stated fear of producing

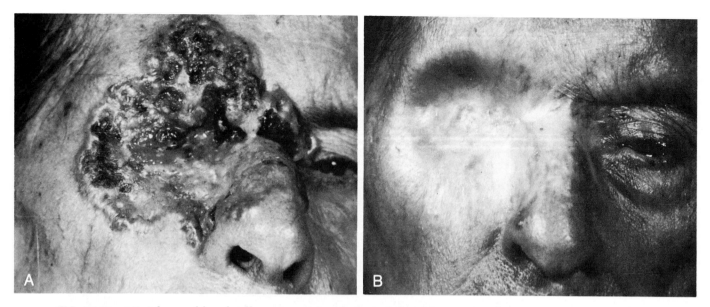

FIG. 26-12. (A) Advanced basal cell carcinoma has destroyed the right eye, involves most of the nose, and approaches the left eye. (B) Appearance 3 years following orthovoltage therapy. (Courtesy of R. L. Lindberg, MD, Department of Radiation Therapy, M. D. Anderson Hospital and Tumor Institute, Houston)

FIG. 26-13. (A) Squamous cell carcinoma of the right medial canthus that has destroyed the right eye and lids; cystic basal cell carcinoma of the left nasal alar skin. (B) Appearance 5 years following orthovoltage irradiation. (Courtesy of R. L. Lindberg, MD, Department of Radiation Therapy, M. D. Anderson Hospital and Tumor Institute, Houston)

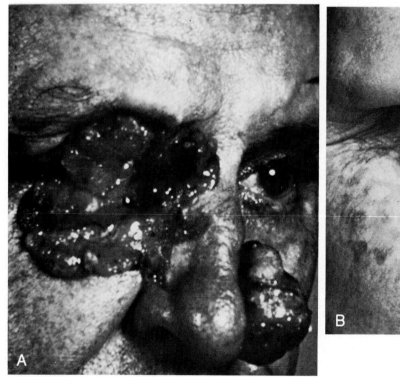

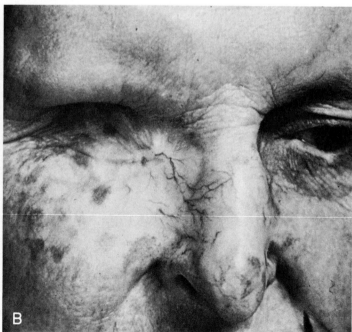

chondronecrosis with radiation therapy is unfounded if properly fractionated techniques are used.

Lesions in the concha frequently invade the external auditory canal and are less easy to cure by either surgery or radiation therapy. These lesions often have an infiltrative component that makes it difficult to define the extent of the lesion. If the cartilaginous canal is involved, then a sleeve resection or occasionally a temporal bone resection would be the surgical treatment (see Chapter 30, Temporal Bone). Radiation therapy is also used in these situations, probably with similar results.

SKIN OF THE UPPER LIP AND LIP COMMISSURE

Upper lip carcinomas tend to invade the lip vermilion, external nares, nasolabial crease, premaxilla, and lip commissure. Lesions less than 1 cm may be excised and closed primarily with an acceptable cosmetic result. Lesions involving more than 1 cm of the skin of the upper lip may require excision of part of the nose, the lip vermilion, and the commissure and then may need complicated reconstruction; for this reason, we favor radiation therapy for the majority of these lesions (Fig. 26-14). (See section on lip in Chapter 17, Oral Cavity.) Lesions involving the commissure are best treated with radiation therapy (Fig. 26-15).

ADVANCED LESIONS OF THE PREAURICULAR AREA/CHEEK

The large, deeply infiltrative lesions in the cheek often invade cartilage and bone, the parotid gland, the facial nerve, and the infratemporal fossa, and they may be dif-

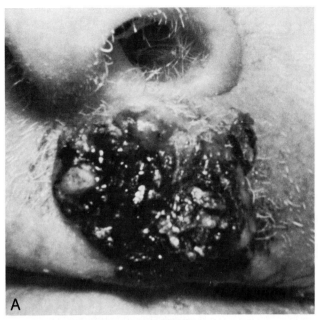

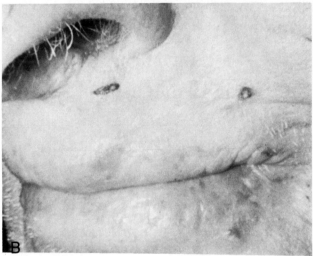

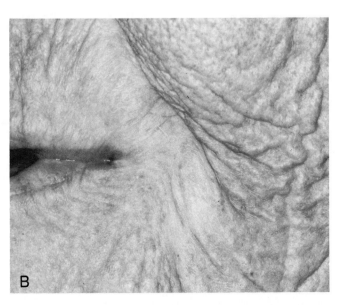

FIG. 26-14. (*A*) A 3.0-cm basal cell carcinoma of the upper lip. (*B*) Appearance 7 months after treatment with a single-plane radium needle implant (7000 rad at 0.5 cm). Patient died of intercurrent disease at 2 years.

FIG. 26-15. (*A*) Slowly enlarging superficial basal cell carcinoma of the cheek with involvement of the lip commissure. Treatment plan: 4750 rad/20 fractions/6 weeks; 250 kV (split-course). (*B*) There was no evidence of disease at 3 years. ▼

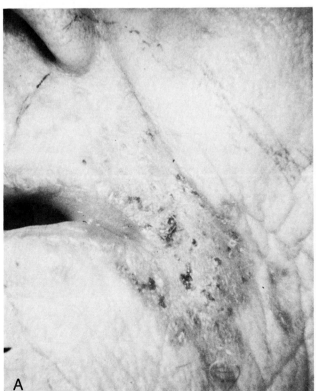

ficult to approach from the surgical standpoint. Radiation therapy is often recommended as the initial treatment. Examples of good results for these infrequent problems are shown in Figures 26-4 and 26-16.

SCALP

There is a preponderance of women in the small group of patients with large basal cell carcinomas of the scalp. These lesions tend to appear at an earlier age than most skin cancers.[4] Small, superficial lesions of the scalp are best approached with surgical excision. Larger, deeply infiltrating lesions require removal of the subjacent periosteum or even some calvarium; invasion of dura and spread to regional lymph nodes occurs in advanced lesions. Extensive lesions, either superficial or deeply invasive, may be treated with radiation therapy because of the large areas involved (see Fig. 26-7). Electrons may be of considerable advantage in these situations. Prior radiation therapy given for tinea capitis in childhood would be a relative contraindication to a curative course of radiation therapy. Microscopically controlled excision is also successful for the advanced lesions.[4]

REGIONAL LYMPH NODE METASTASIS

The management of lymphatic metastases is described in the section on management of the neck in Chapter 4, General Principles for Treatment of Cancers in the Head and Neck: Selection of Treatment for the Primary Site and for the Neck. However, metastases from skin cancers generally involve a different group of lymph nodes, and some comments are necessary.

Parotid Area Lymph Node Metastasis

Elective lymph node dissection in the parotid area is not generally recommended for squamous cell carcinoma of the skin, although some surgeons recommend it for malignant melanoma. However, if the primary lesion invades near or into the parotid gland, necessitating a parotidectomy, the lymph nodes would be removed at the same time.

If a patient is at high risk for lymphatic metastasis to the parotid area lymph nodes but none is palpable, a reasonable alternative would be elective irradiation to the parotid area and first-echelon neck lymph nodes.

When clinically positive parotid area lymph nodes are present, the philosophy of management is similar to that for a high-grade parotid neoplasm. Lateral lobectomy, total parotidectomy, or radical parotidectomy is the initial procedure if the lesion is resectable. The upper neck lymph nodes are removed. If the lymph nodes in the upper neck are clinically negative, then an elective neck dissection is not done if postoperative radiation therapy is planned to the parotid bed, since the ipsilateral neck is electively irradiated in all cases. If there are clinically positive lymph nodes in the neck, then a neck dissection is added to the parotidectomy. Postoperative radiation therapy is recommended in the majority of cases.

Jackson and Ballantyne reported 84% control above the clavicles in a select group of 43 patients treated by surgery alone and in whom the primary skin cancer was controlled.[15] Postoperative or preoperative radiation therapy was added in 26 patients selected for a high risk of recurrence. The control rate above the clavicles was 88% (23/26). Radiation therapy was used for salvage of surgical failures in 12 cases, and 5 (42%) were successfully controlled. If postoperative radiation therapy is not planned, a more extensive operation, at least a total parotidectomy, may be needed to ensure a high control rate. It is our prejudice to add irradiation in almost all cases rather than to increase the magnitude of the operative procedure.

If the parotid area metastasis is technically inoperable, then either preoperative irradiation or radiation therapy alone, including an interstitial implant, will cure a significant number of these patients (Fig. 26-17). Advanced preauricular metastases can produce a devastating situation since they may involve the tragus, a portion of the pinna, the external auditory canal, the facial nerve, the temporomandibular joint, the zygoma, the mandible, the temporal and infratemporal fossa, and the parapharyngeal space. Resection may produce a major functional and cosmetic loss, and therefore radiation therapy alone may be considered a viable alternative to radical excision. External-beam irradiation combined with an interstitial implant is the usual treatment plan.

Occipital Lymph Node Metastases

The regional metastases are removed by a posterolateral neck dissection; a supraomohyoid or standard neck dissection is added according to the situation. (See section on management of the neck in Chapter 4 and section on neck dissection in Chapter 5.)

FIG. 26-16. A 59-year-old woman presented with an 18-month history of an enlarging lesion on the right temple. There was decreased hearing and pain in the temporomandibular joint when chewing. An 11 × 10-cm lesion of the right preauricular area extended to within 2 cm of the lateral canthus. There was obvious destruction of the pinna, and the external auditory canal was filled with tumor. Paralysis of the orbital branch of the facial nerve was noted. Biopsy revealed basal cell carcinoma. Tomograms showed early erosion of the posterior zygoma, temporomandibular joint, and mastoid process. Treatment plan: ipsilateral cobalt-60 portal with a 5-mm layer of petrolatum gauze for bolus; 7000 rad at 0.5 cm/7 weeks. (A) Appearance prior to therapy. (B) Appearance after 2400 rad. (C) Appearance at end of treatment. (D) At 6 months there was 80% healing of the tumor bed; complete healing was evident at 8 months. The patient developed radiation caries. (E) Appearance at 3½ years. (F) At 3½ years there was persistent paralysis of the ophthalmic branch of facial nerve. The patient had no evidence of disease at 10 years.

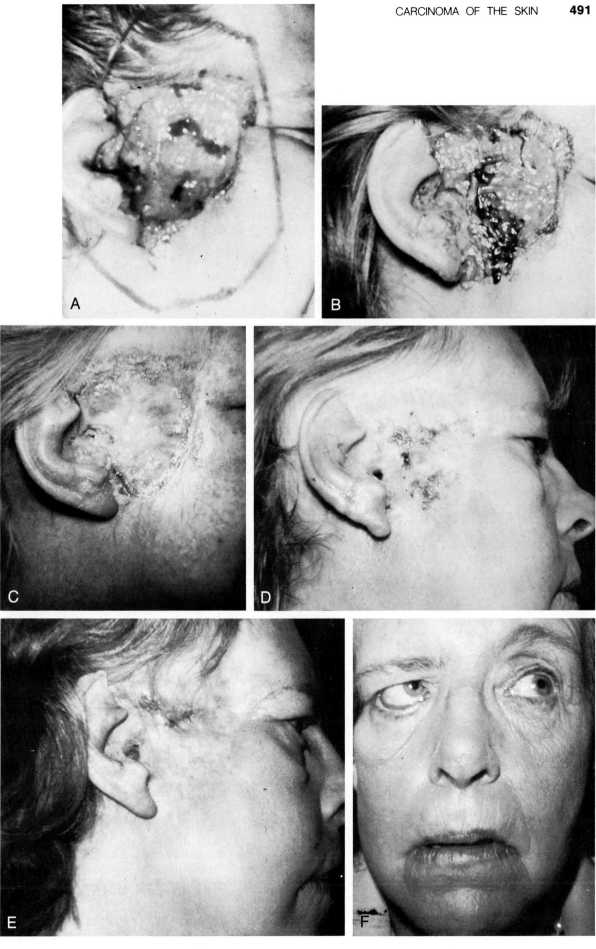

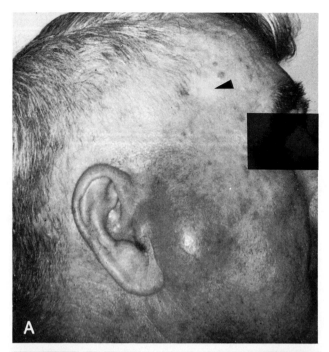

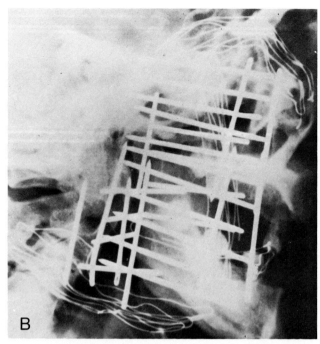

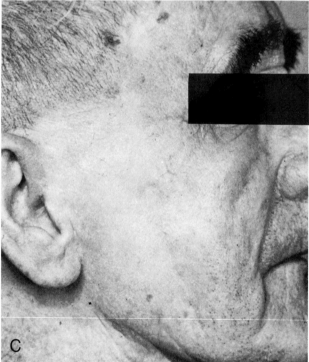

FIG. 26-17. (*A*) Squamous cell carcinoma metastatic to parotid lymph node. Squamous cell carcinoma of skin of temple treated 2 years prior to admission (*arrow*). Note that tragus is minimally involved, even when the parotid lymph node is 4 cm in diameter. If a superficial preauricular lymph node is involved, the tragus and pinna are involved early in the course. (*B*) Modified three-plane radium needle implant. One plane (four needles) is placed in the retromandibular deep lobe. (*C*) Lesion was completely healed at 1 year (no evidence of disease at 9 years). (Courtesy of R. L. Lindberg, MD, Department of Radiation Therapy, M. D. Anderson Hospital and Tumor Institute, Houston)

Postauricular/Mastoid Lymph Node Metastases

A regional lymph node dissection is done, and a supraomohyoid or standard neck dissection is added.

SELECTION OF TREATMENT FOR ADNEXAL CARCINOMAS

Surgical excision is the usual recommendation for the adnexal carcinomas. We have limited experience with radiation therapy for these histologies, and most of the experience is for postoperative radiation therapy or unfavorable recurrent lesions. However, gross lesions do respond to radiation therapy and a few of favorable size are probably cured (Fig. 26–18).

Surgical Excision

This section will deal primarily with scalpel excision. It is recognized that curettage and electrodesiccation, cryotherapy, fulguration, or microscopically controlled excision will produce good results when applied to suitable lesions. In-depth discussion of the technical aspects of these treatments is beyond the scope of this chapter, and the reader is referred to appropriate texts.

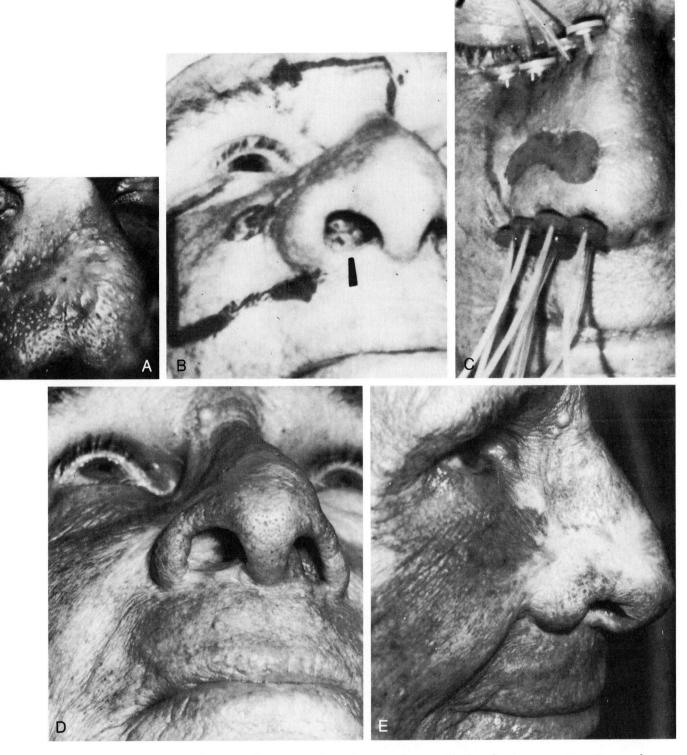

FIG. 26-18. A 69-year-old man presented with a slowly enlarging, asymptomatic growth on the right side of his nose beginning 10 years prior to admission. He underwent a reduction for rhinophyma 2½ years prior to admission. Microscopic diagnosis was sebaceous hyperplasia with rhinophyma. Shortly after the operation the nodularity reappeared and has grown slowly. He underwent repeat operation for rhinophyma and the tissue contained sebaceous carcinoma. (*A*) Appearance 1 month following surgery. There was a firm, white, slightly elevated scar overlying a 5 × 4-cm palpable mass of the right side of the nose and premaxilla with fullness in the nasolabial crease. (*B*) Tumor in lateral nasal vestibule. The mass extended approximately 3 cm into the nasal cavity. The patient refused operation and received 5000 rad/5 weeks, cobalt-60 (with bolus). There was 60% to 70% tumor regression. (*C*) Iridium implant. The dose was 3200 rad. (*D, E*) Appearance at 3 months. Patient was free of disease at 4 years. (Courtesy of T. Bloom, MD, and H. Kerman, MD, Department of Radiation Therapy, Halifax Hospital, Daytona Beach, Florida)

A margin of approximately 5 mm beyond the edge of the lesion is sufficient for small, discrete tumors; proportionately more is required for larger lesions. The most common site to cut across the tumor is not at the lateral edge but at the deep aspect, and this portion of the specimen should be checked by frozen section if there is any question about the adequacy of the resection. Lesions on the mobile skin are excised using an ellipse with a 4:1 ratio of length to width; the skin is mobilized and closed primarily. Lesions excised from an area of fixed skin such as the tip of the nose, or large lesions, may require either a split-thickness skin graft or a local flap closure. In the case of resection of very large or recurrent lesions, it is preferable not to cover the area with thick flaps, since it is difficult to observe for recurrence. In some cases, it is preferable to use a prosthetic device for the initial rehabilitation (e.g., following rhinectomy), allowing observation for 2 to 3 years before attempting reconstruction, unless the patient demands immediate repair.

SIGNIFICANCE OF POSITIVE MARGINS FOLLOWING EXCISION

It is not infrequent that a lesion is excised and the pathology report states that there is tumor close to the margins or that the margins are positive. The alternatives are reexcision, irradiation of the tumor bed, and observation.

Gooding and co-workers reported the results in 66 patients with positive margins following excision for squamous cell carcinoma.[11] These patients were treated from 1950 to 1960, and all patients had a 5-year minimum follow-up. This study includes nearly 1200 excisions, of which about 5% of the specimens had positive margins; the nose and nasolabial fold were the most common sites and accounted for 50% of positive margins. The incidence of recurrence for negative margins was not reported. Only 39% of patients with positive margins developed recurrence in the time frame of the study, and in all salvage was achieved by secondary treatment. However, clinical observation tells us otherwise. Because of the indolent nature of most skin cancers, many recurrences do not appear until 10 or 15 years after treatment, and certainly all recurrences are not permanently cured.

An individualized decision is made in each case when there is close or positive margins. One must weigh the factors of the anatomical site, the age of the patient, the histology, the previous therapy, and the history of the growth pattern in order to reach a decision to recommend additional treatment or just to observe the patient. For instance, the finding of a positive margin after excision of a basal cell carcinoma of the inner canthus or nasolabial fold is a potentially serious problem, since the recurrence may be difficult to detect and salvage might require major therapy. On the other hand, a small basal cell carcinoma excised from a free skin area with a close or positive margin might be safely watched, since recurrence is more easily diagnosed and treated. However, a small squamous cell carcinoma from a free skin site with a positive margin would dictate additional therapy, since the threat of lymph node metastasis, albeit low, would be an additional consideration.

Reexcision may be used in areas where there is ample tissue available to reexcise and not produce a functional or cosmetic problem. However, most cases with positive margins occur either in patients with large lesions who have already had a flap reconstruction, or in areas where resection of additional tissues may not be desirable.

Another difficulty with immediate reexcision is that there is usually a localized inflammatory reaction around the old surgical site, and since there is usually a minimal amount of tumor, the pathologist usually cannot assist the surgeon with margin checks. Radiation therapy has the advantage of being able to cover a fairly wide area, and this modality is often selected for patients with positive margins.

SURGICAL TREATMENT ACCORDING TO ANATOMICAL SITE

SCALP

Small lesions can be excised with primary closure. Larger lesions require full-thickness resection with perhaps a cuff of periosteum or even the outer table of the calvarium. A split-thickness skin graft or flap is required for coverage. A split-thickness skin graft can be applied over the bare skull and will usually take if the cortical bone is drilled down to bleeding bone. A scalp flap, posterior cervical flap, forehead flap, or free flap may be rotated to cover the defect. If the full thickness of the skull is removed, a protective helmet may be required.

FOREHEAD

Most lesions of the forehead may be excised with a primary closure along the natural skin lines. Larger lesions may require a split-thickness skin graft or local flap. Advanced lesions may invade the periosteum and require removal of adjacent bone (Fig. 26-19).[24]

EAR

Small, superficial lesions not invading cartilage can be excised with a cuff of perichondrium or cartilage. The skin is fixed to the underlying perichondrium, so other means of closure must be used. Through-and-through V excisions from the helix may be repaired with primary closure.

A retroauricular pedicle flap may be used to reconstruct small defects. Large lesions would require total or near-total removal of the external ear, often in connection with partial temporal bone resection; a prosthesis is required to reconstruct the external ear. It is advantageous to leave a small portion of the superior portion of the ear intact to help attach the prosthesis and to facilitate the wearing of glasses.

PERIORBITAL AREAS

Small lesions, 5 mm or less, on the eyelid may be excised and closed primarily without noticeable cosmetic or functional changes. Larger lesions that involve the edge of the eyelid are resected and repaired by either a rotation flap or a graft from the upper eyelid. Resection of one-third or more of the lid requires a more complex reconstruction. The lid may be reconstructed and have a decent appearance, but it has very little functional activity and the cosmetic appearance is not as good as it would appear in a still photograph. Lesions on the upper lid are often treated with radiation therapy, but up to about one fourth of the upper lid can be excised and directly approximated with acceptable results. Excision of greater portions of the upper lid requires a full-thickness pedicle flap. Large or recurrent lesions that invade the periorbital fat or muscles of the eyeball require an orbital evisceration or exenteration.

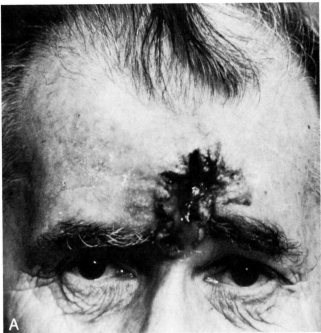

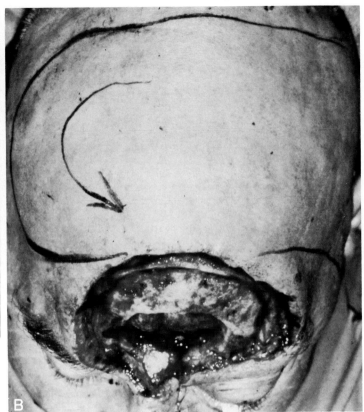

FIG. 26-19. (*A*) Basal cell carcinoma of the glabellar area. (*B*) Excision of lesion and underlying bone. (Panje WR, Ceilley RI: The influence of embryology of the midface on the spread of epithelial malignancies. Laryngoscope 89:1914–1920, 1979)

This defect is usually repaired with a split-thickness skin graft; postoperative irradiation is frequently advised in these cases.

NOSE

Small lesions on the bridge of the nose may be simply excised with primary closure, but larger lesions require a split-thickness skin graft or full-thickness rotation graft for coverage. Superficial lesions around the nasal alar areas or the tip of the nose are resected down to the perichondrium of the cartilages. The skin is immobile over these cartilages and must be repaired by a local flap or split-thickness graft. Lesions that are tethered to the cartilages require removal of underlying cartilage to obtain a tumor-free margin. These defects are usually repaired with a composite graft. The more deeply infiltrative lesions may extend through the crevices between cartilages and invade the submucosa of the nasal cavity. Microscopically controlled excision is desirable for these cases to avoid positive margins or excessive resection of normal tissue. Radiation therapy is usually preferable because of better cosmetic results.

Large lesions or recurrent lesions after irradiation may require partial or total nasal resection. This may be repaired either with a nasal prosthesis or by reconstruction with a forehead or tube-pedicle flap, with or without an autologous bone graft.

LYMPH NODE METASTASES

The operations for removal of parotid area lymph nodes are highly individualized because of the anatomy of the region and the close association of the lymphatic tissue with the facial nerve.

A contrast-enhanced CT scan may greatly assist in the planning of a surgical procedure in patients with larger clinically involved parotid area lymph nodes, particularly in regard to extension toward the parapharyngeal space.

Graham studied the distribution of the parotid lymph nodes in cadavers by serially sectioning either the entire parotid gland or the residual gland after a superficial parotidectomy in the plane of the facial nerve.[12] Study of the whole gland showed that the lymphatic tissue lay lateral to a plane passing through the main vascular bundle within the gland and that removal of that portion of the parotid lateral to the vascular bundle would be effective in removing parotid lymphatic tissue; dissection along the facial nerve would leave a substantial amount of lymphatic tissue in most instances.

In an elective parotid lymph node dissection, a lateral parotidectomy in the vascular plane rather than the facial nerve plane should encompass all the lymphatic tissue.

If there are clinically palpable nodes present at the time of the resection of the primary lesion, the primary lesion may be excised separately or through a single incision, as shown in Figure 26-20. In the majority of cases, the parotid area lymph node metastases appear at some point after successful treatment of the primary lesion. If the lymph nodes are small and mobile, then a lateral lobectomy in the plane of the vascular bundle in combination with an upper neck dissection is the treatment of choice. If the lymph nodes are large and there is a tumor growing through the capsule of the lymph nodes with fixation to skin, extension to the tragus or pinna, or gross invasion of the facial nerve, masseter muscle, mandible, or deep lobe of

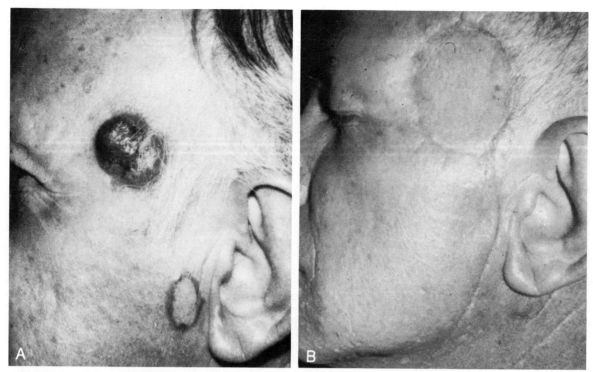

FIG. 26-20. A 55-year-old man presented with 6-year history of a dime-sized flat sore on the left temple and a 2- to 3-year history of a small subcutaneous lump in left preauricular area. He received a course of topical 5-fluorouracil to the temple lesion without a biopsy. The lesion suddenly began to grow after 6 weeks of treatment. (*A*) Elevated, red lesion on temple is 2.5 × 2 cm. There was a 2 × 1-cm mobile left parotid area lymph node. Recommendation was excision of primary lesion, parotidectomy, and postoperative radiation therapy. Findings were squamous cell carcinoma of skin with margins free and one positive parotid lymph node. (The gross appearance of the primary lesion was consistent with nodular melanoma.) (*B*) Appearance 6 weeks after surgery. The patient received postoperative radiation therapy to the tumor bed and left neck. The primary site and parotid bed received 6500 rad/7 weeks, mixed beam, 17-MV x-ray and 20-MeV electrons. The left lower neck received 5000 rad/5 weeks. Radiation therapy was recommended in spite of negative margins in view of the history of rapid growth, narrow margins, and small possibility of occult disease in the neck. There was no evidence of disease at 2 years.

the parotid gland, then an individualized major resection of the parotid and involved tissues is required. One should not rely on high-dose postoperative radiation therapy to sterilize the gross residual disease, and every attempt should be made to obtain a tumor-free margin.

If there are clinically or pathologically positive nodes in the neck, then an appropriate neck dissection is added to the parotid area lymph node dissection. If the upper neck lymph nodes are pathologically negative, no further neck dissection is done and the entire ipsilateral neck is included in the postoperative irradiation plan.

For a discussion of posterolateral neck dissection, see section on neck dissection in Chapter 5.

Radiation Therapy

With the increased availability of specialists dealing with the treatment of skin cancer by surgical modalities, the routine use of radiation therapy has greatly diminished

during the past 3 decades. Dermatologists generally have stopped giving radiation therapy in their offices in recent years, which further reduced its use as a treatment option.

The contraindications are prior high-dose irradiation within the area of the skin cancer, skin cancer developing on the site of a burn or chronic infection, and lesions of the palms and soles of the extremities. Relative contraindications include use in the young patient, especially those with complexions likely to develop a multiple number of skin cancers, prior use of low-dose irradiation (as in the treatment of acne), xeroderma pigmentosum, and lupus vulgaris. Involvement of bone or cartilage is not a contraindication, contrary to what is written in most surgical texts. There are numerous examples of cures by radiation therapy alone with bone and/or cartilage involvement. In fact, for large skin cancers we can find little difference in cure rate whether or not these tissues are involved. Certainly, the cure rates for advanced primary carcinomas of the nasal cavity, paranasal sinuses, nasopharynx, gingiva, and larynx with evidence of bone or cartilage invasion are not insignificant, and there is no reason to expect any difference with skin carcinoma. When tumor invades bone or cartilage, the treatment decision hinges more on whether the involved structure is expendable. For example, a portion of the ramus of the mandible or a portion of the maxilla might be resected with limited functional and cosmetic loss. However, resection of the lesions shown in Figures 26-4 and 26-16 would produce a major cosmetic defect with a low chance of obtaining adequate margins, and therefore radiation therapy is preferred. In fact, one of the indications for radiation therapy may be an advanced lesion invading bone or cartilage.

Radiation therapy is most commonly indicated for small lesions around the nose, eye, ear, upper lip, and commissure of the lip; for advanced lesions invading bone or cartilage; following an incomplete excision; for advanced lesions in general; for patients at poor medical risk for a surgical procedure; for multiple adjacent small lesions (e.g., on the nose); and for metastatic spread to regional lymph nodes.

A wide range of techniques is available for the treatment of skin cancer, including orthovoltage and supervoltage x-rays, electrons, and interstitial techniques. The selection of technique is highly individualized and depends on the tumor volume, normal tissues to be protected, available equipment, the experience of the radiation therapist, and the mobility of the patient.

The guidelines for selection of the external-beam dose, based on the size of the lesion, the functional or cosmetic result desired, and the patient's age and mobility, are given in Table 26-1. Short treatment schemes of one to five treatments are curative for small or medium-sized lesions, but eventually a depressed scar or other complications may result. The late effects of these short schemes have given radiation therapy a bad name in the management of skin cancer, and rightly so, since it usually falls on the surgeon to manage the late complications. These short, cauterizing treatments are particularly undesirable around the eye, nose, and ear. The short regimens are mostly used for the immobile, elderly patient who is able to make only a few visits to the radiation therapy department.

IRRADIATION TECHNIQUES ACCORDING TO ANATOMICAL SITE

EYELID

Almost all early lesions of the canthi and lids are treated with orthovoltage techniques. Low-energy electrons might seem advantageous compared with orthovoltage x-rays from a theoretical standpoint, but they have the same disadvantages of low doses at the beam edges, the production of high-energy x-rays in metal eye shields, scatter to the eyeball underneath the eye shields, and two to three times greater treatment expense. A set of eye shields is essential for treatment of these lesions and gives nearly complete protection of the eyeball. Radiation therapy should not be attempted without availability of these shields (Fig. 26-21).

A lead face mask is prepared in order to sharply limit the radiation field and to reproduce the exact treatment portal each day. (See Chapter 15, Treatment Planning for Irradiation of Head and Neck Cancer.) Since the treatment portals are irregular in outline, each one is calibrated separately. There is considerable reduction in percentage depth dose at the edge of small orthovoltage beams, which must be taken into account for treatment planning. These differences in depth dose give a built-in shrinking field technique, and therefore field reductions are seldom necessary. Additional layers of lead or lead putty must be added to the lead mask to further eliminate transit irradiation.

TABLE 26-1. Guidelines for Selection of External-Beam Dose

Orthovoltage Dose (rad)*	Examples
6500/7 weeks	Large untreated lesions with bone/cartilage invasion or large recurrent tumor†
6000/7 weeks	Large untreated lesion with minimal or suspected bone/cartilage invasion†
5500/6 weeks	Moderate to large inner canthus, eyelid, nasal, or pinna lesions (20–30 sq cm area)
5000/4 weeks	Small, thin lesion (less than 1.5 cm) around eye, nose, or ear (10 sq cm area)
4500/3 weeks	Moderate-sized lesion on "free" skin or postoperative cut-through of moderate size on "free" skin
4000/2 weeks or 3000/1 week	Small lesions (1 cm) on "free" skin

The following schemes are used when the late cosmetic result is not important and travel for the patient is difficult:

4000/10 fractions or 3000/5 fractions or 2000/1 fraction	Rapid fractionation schemes produce a high cure rate for small lesions, but the cosmetic result may be less than optimal after 5 years.

* Add 10% to dose for supervoltage therapy.
† All or a portion of the therapy given with supervoltage photons and/or electrons.
("Free," not involving ear, nose, eye, or lid)

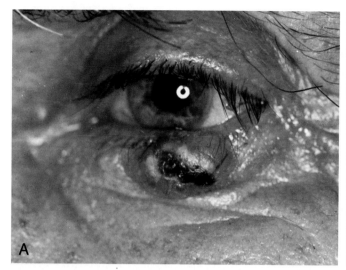

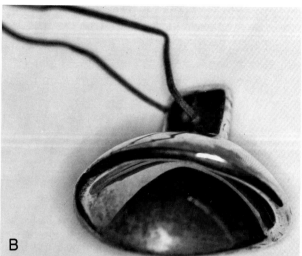

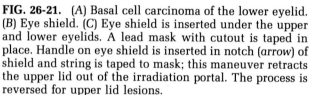

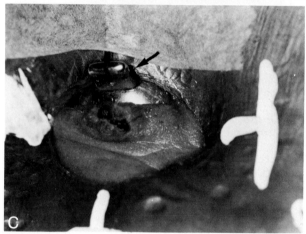

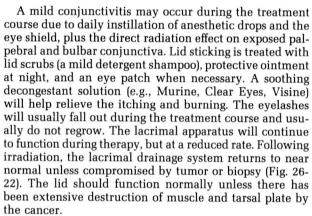

FIG. 26-21. (A) Basal cell carcinoma of the lower eyelid. (B) Eye shield. (C) Eye shield is inserted under the upper and lower eyelids. A lead mask with cutout is taped in place. Handle on eye shield is inserted in notch (*arrow*) of shield and string is taped to mask; this maneuver retracts the upper lid out of the irradiation portal. The process is reversed for upper lid lesions.

A mild conjunctivitis may occur during the treatment course due to daily instillation of anesthetic drops and the eye shield, plus the direct radiation effect on exposed palpebral and bulbar conjunctiva. Lid sticking is treated with lid scrubs (a mild detergent shampoo), protective ointment at night, and an eye patch when necessary. A soothing decongestant solution (*e.g.,* Murine, Clear Eyes, Visine) will help relieve the itching and burning. The eyelashes will usually fall out during the treatment course and usually do not regrow. The lacrimal apparatus will continue to function during therapy, but at a reduced rate. Following irradiation, the lacrimal drainage system returns to near normal unless compromised by tumor or biopsy (Fig. 26-22). The lid should function normally unless there has been extensive destruction of muscle and tarsal plate by the cancer.

Mild degrees of ectropion produced by the tumor may disappear after radiation therapy, but a more severe degree of ectropion will remain after successful treatment and may require reconstruction.

The permanent loss of eyelashes does not seem to produce any serious functional problems.

See Chapter 14, The Effect of Radiation on Normal Tissues of the Head and Neck, for a full discussion of the effects of radiation therapy on the eye and periorbita.

The skin of the eyelids is thin and delicate, and fractionation schedules of 3 to 5 weeks, which employ relatively small doses per fraction, should be adopted.

NOSE

Techniques for irradiation of nasal lesions vary from very simple to highly individualized and complex treatments. We prefer the preparation of a face mask for most *en face* portals for orthovoltage and electron-beam therapy. Lead strips covered with wax may be inserted into the nares to reduce the dose to normal tissues when orthovolt-age or electrons are used. A combination of photons and electrons may be used in certain situations to reduce depth dose. Supervoltage beams with bolus are useful when bone and/or cartilage are involved in order to gain a more homogeneous irradiation and avoid the increased dose in bone and cartilage associated with orthovoltage therapy. When supervoltage or low-energy electrons are used, a bolus is necessary to achieve full surface dose; uninvolved skin areas may not need a bolus. Lesions of the tip of the nose and nasal alar fold are frequently more extensive than judged by palpation, and treatment plans must be generous for these spread patterns.

There may be multiple small foci of cancer scattered over the nose and adjacent cheek with normal intervening skin. It is usually better to encompass all lesions in a single portal rather than to use multiple tiny adjacent portals.

Cartilage or bone necrosis should be a rare event with properly fractionated radiation therapy. Tumor that penetrates and destroys bone or cartilage may create a sinus between the skin and nasal cavity. This defect may contract and seal over after radiation therapy, or the sinus may remain open (Fig. 26-23). Surgical correction may be necessary if the defect is symptomatic (*e.g.,* whistling noises). Advanced nasal lesions may be successfully cured. The appearance is far from normal but may be more satisfactory than total rhinectomy.

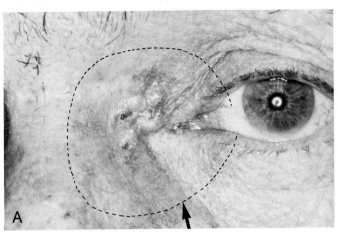

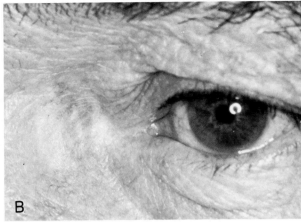

FIG. 26-22. (*A*) A 60-year-old man presented with basal cell carcinoma of the inner canthus. The lesion was tethered to the periosteum. Treatment plan was 5500 rad/6 weeks, 250 kV, 3.0 Cu HVL. Approximately 1.5 cm of each lid was included in the treatment. Dashed line indicates borders of portal. (*B*) Appearance 10 months after treatment. There is minimal tearing even though the proximal lacrimal system was included. There was no evidence of disease at 3 years.

FIG. 26-23. (*A*) Advanced basal cell carcinoma of the nose with extension to the cartilage and bone of nose, left lower lid and inner canthus, and right inner canthus. Patient refused rhinectomy. Treatment plan was 4500 rad, 250 kV and 1500 rad, cobalt-60, with a beeswax bolus, for a total of 6000 rad/7 weeks. (*B*) At 3 years there was no evidence of disease. There are two slitlike nasal-dermal sinuses that are asymptomatic.

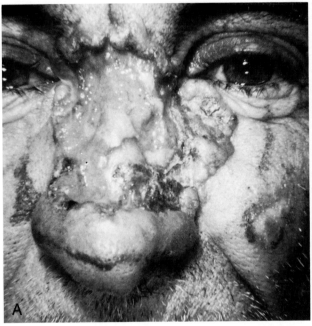

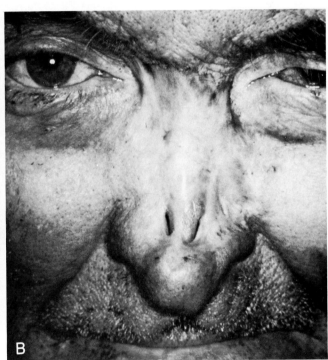

EAR

Small lesions of the pinna may be easily treated with single-portal orthovoltage irradiation. Large lesions, especially those invading cartilage and involving the postauricular sulcus, are frequently treated with supervoltage beam and a wax bolus to ensure homogeneous irradiation and reduce the differential absorption in bone and cartilage. Angled wedge fields, a three-field technique, or mixed beams will reduce irradiation to normal structures deep to the ear (Fig. 26-24). Lesions located in the concha and the external auditory canal are more difficult to control and have vague borders; surgical resection with postop-erative radiation therapy may be advantageous in the infiltrative, ulcerated lesions.

UPPER LIP

Lesions greater than 1 cm often involve the vermilion or the commissure of the lip or extend near the base of the columella or alar cartilages. They may be treated with external-beam irradiation, interstitial implant, or a

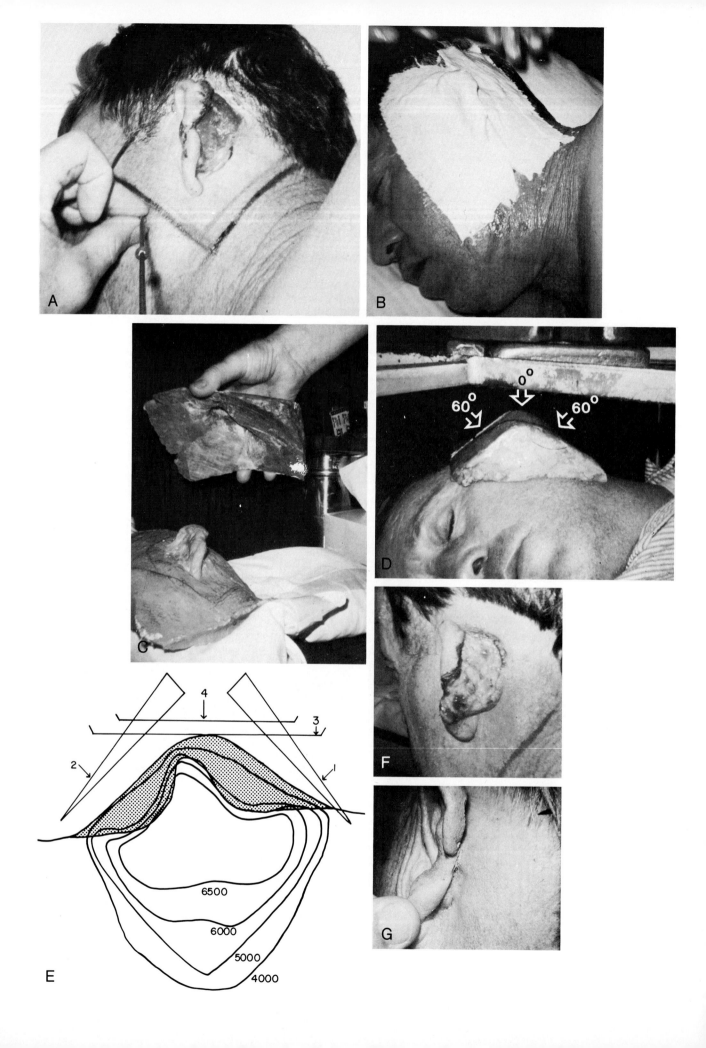

◀ **FIG. 26-24.** (*A*) Squamous cell carcinoma of the left ear with cartilage invasion (patient was blind in the right eye). Treatment plan is 6500 rad/7½ weeks, cobalt-60, with beeswax bolus, three-field technique. Superior and inferior portals angled 60° with wedges, and a straight lateral open field (0°). (*B*) Preparation of plaster mold. (*C*) Plaster cast. (*D*) Beeswax bolus in place. (*E*) Isodose distribution. Stippled area represents beeswax compensator. The dose to the midline was approximately 5000 rad/7½ weeks.

Portal	Energy	Field Size (cm)	Wedge Angle	Bolus	Given Dose (rad)
1	Co-60	8 × 8	60	yes	2940
2	Co-60	8 × 8	60	yes	2940
3	Co-60	10.5 × 10.5	open	yes	2730
4	Co-60	8 × 6	open	no	1540

(*F*) Appearance at 4000 rad. (*G*) There was no evidence of disease at 5½ years.

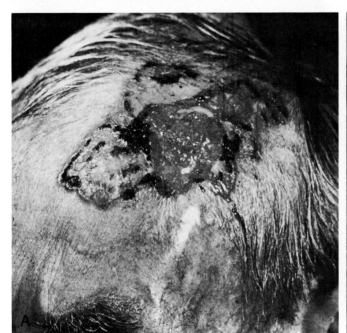

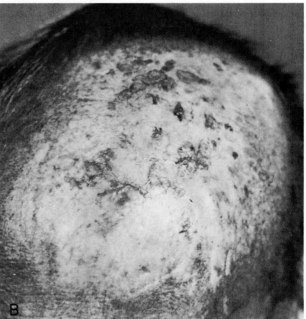

FIG. 26-25. (*A*) Squamous cell carcinoma of the scalp treated with radium mold. (*B*) At 4 years there was no evidence of disease. (Courtesy of R. L. Lindberg, MD, Department of Radiation Therapy, M. D. Anderson Hospital and Tumor Institute, Houston)

combination of both (see Fig. 26-14 and 26-28). A lead shield is inserted behind the upper lip to reduce transit irradiation when external-beam therapy is used; the shield is coated with wax. A gauze roll is inserted behind the upper lip at the time of the implant to reduce gingival irradiation. The dose to the lens from an upper lip implant is calculated to be 100 rad to 200 rad/6 days when the primary lesion receives 6000 rad at 0.5 cm from a 3 × 1.5-cm single plane implant.

SCALP

Small scalp lesions are usually managed by excision, but some lesions, although superficial, may involve an extensive area. The latter are usually managed by radiation therapy (Fig. 26-25). Advanced, destructive lesions or multiple invasive lesions have usually been treated by radiation therapy; the treatment plans are individualized and complex but often successful. Electrons are an advantage, but a variety of photon/electron beams can be mixed for the

desired effect (Figs. 26-7 and Fig. 26-26). A certain amount of brain irradiation is unavoidable in treatment of massive lesions.

TEMPLE

Small and moderate-sized lesions (2 cm to 3 cm) are usually managed by excision. Squamous cell carcinomas of the temple area are particularly prone to local and regional recurrence after surgical excision and should be watched closely. If the margins are close or positive, postoperative radiation therapy should be considered rather than reexcision. The larger carcinomas should be considered for radiation therapy (see Fig. 26-6). Electrons are advantageous to avoid unnecessary brain irradiation.

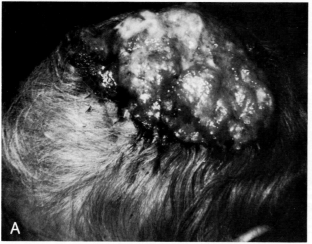

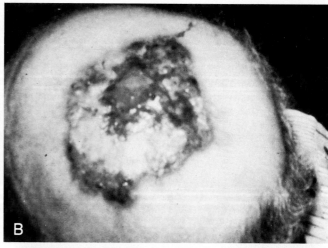

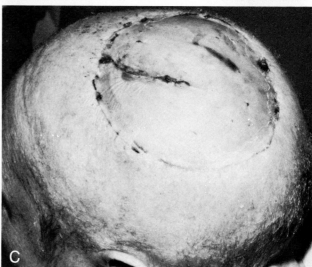

FIG. 26-26. A 70-year-old woman presented with 5-year history of an enlarging scalp mass. The patient entered the hospital because of anemia. The scalp lesion was obscured by a wig. Biopsy revealed squamous cell carcinoma. The cranium was intact, but the lesion was fixed to the periosteum. (*A*) Appearance prior to therapy. Treatment plan: radiation therapy with surgery reserved for persistence or recurrence: parallel opposed lateral portals, cobalt-60, with bolus, 4600 rad, 12-MeV electrons, 2900 rad; maximum dose, 7500 rad; minimum dose, 7000 rad/8½ weeks. (*B*) Appearance at 7 months. There was a persistent tumor that was 8 cm in diameter. (*C*) A wide local excision was performed. The periosteum was preserved, and a split-thickness skin graft was applied. There was no evidence of disease at 3 years.

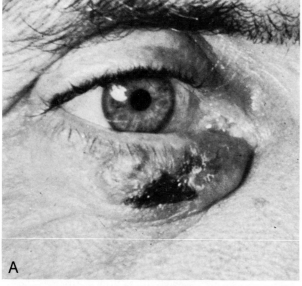

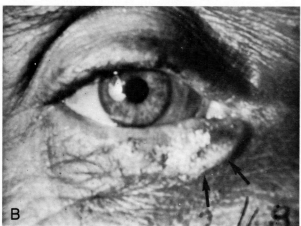

FIG. 26-27. (*A*) Basal cell carcinoma of the right lower lid (2.5 × 1 cm). The patient had a history of slow growth of the lesion for longer than 10 years. Treatment was with 250 kV, 5 mm copper filtration. The dose was 6500 rad/33 fractions/5½ weeks; the prescribed dose today would be 5000 rad/4 weeks. (*B*) Persistent abnormality 2 months after completion of treatment (*arrows*). The tumor regressed slowly and finally disappeared completely about 6 months after completion of treatment. (*C*). Appearance at 14 years. Patient has mild intermittent tearing.

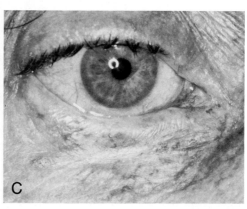

PREAURICULAR AREA (CHEEK)

The majority of the lesions in the preauricular area are early and can be successfully managed by a surgical modality. However, the advanced lesions require careful staging and treatment planning, since they frequently invade the parotid, the pinna, and the external and internal auditory canals; approximate or invade the facial nerve; and invade the zygoma or mandible. Some may be cured by radiation therapy alone in spite of cartilage and bone invasion (see Figs. 26-4 and 26-16). Surgical excision is either held in reserve for radiation therapy failure or combined with radiation therapy.

Radition therapy is usually a single lateral supervoltage external beam with a wax bolus to provide surface dose. A combination of photons and electrons or electrons alone produce the best distribution. The initial portals should be generous, and the depth-dose specification should be adequate.

LYMPH NODE METASTASES

In the early years, we had the opportunity to observe several patients with skin cancer metastatic to the parotid area lymph nodes that was initially managed by parotidectomy. Recurrence in the parotid area and the ipsilateral neck seemed to be the rule rather than the exception. Attempted salvage after recurrence was associated with a low rate of success and excessive morbidity. Parotidectomy followed routinely by postoperative radiation therapy became the standard management. The entire ipsilateral neck is electively treated for subclinical disease after two failures were observed in the low neck just below the treatment portals. Prior to the availability of electrons, the irradiation was delivered with superior and inferior, angled, cobalt-60 portals. A tailored ipsilateral portal is usually employed, and a combination of photons and electrons is selected to irradiate the anatomical areas at risk. (See Chapter 28, Major Salivary Gland Tumors.)

When the surgical margins are free of disease, the control rate is uniformly good with 6000 rad/6 to 7 weeks to the parotid area and 5000 rad to the undissected neck. However, when the treatment margins are close or positive, full radical doses, 6500 rad to 7000 rad, are advocated. Reducing fields are used when possible, and interstitial implants may be used in selected cases. When the tumor margins were negative, ten of ten cases were regionally controlled; when the margins were positive, four of six were controlled.

Metastasis to the parotid area lymph nodes may be managed by radiation therapy alone for a variety of reasons, with a significant success rate. The control rate related to the diameter of the lymph nodes is shown in Table 26-2. Two patients had cartilage involvement; the disease was controlled in one case. The disease was not controlled in three cases treated with less than 6500 rad, but it was controlled in all four cases treated with more than 6500 rad. An interstitial implant is desirable as part of the treatment unless tumor extends to the deep lobe and parapharyngeal space. The interstitial needles usually penetrate the tragal cartilage in order to obtain margins. High-dose preoperative radiation therapy, 6000 rad to 8000 rad, followed by parotidectomy is a reasonable approach for borderline operable cases.

TABLE 26-2. Parotid Area Lymph Node Metastases Treated With Radiation Therapy: Six Patients, Seven Lesions	
Size of Node	No. Controlled/No. Treated
1–3 cm	2/3
3–5 cm	1/2
5–7 cm	1/2

Note: University of Florida data; patients treated 1/66–4/80; analysis 4/82 by N. P. Mendenhall, MD.

Combined Treatment Policies

Combined treatment is recommended for some advanced skin lesions or difficult recurrent lesions, but there is precious little information on the success rate. The operation should be performed first to take advantage of frozen section control of the excision. Reconstruction should be as simple as possible to avoid delay in the start of radiation therapy. In particular, thick flaps should be avoided and split-thickness skin grafts used when possible. Local flaps add to the risk of regional implantation of tumor cells and may greatly increase the amount of tissue to be irradiated.

Follow-up

It is not practical to insist on frequent or long-term follow-up for the majority of small skin cancers. However, those patients with a significant risk for recurrence or complication should be followed every 1 to 3 months for 2 years and less often thereafter.

Irradiated lesions may not disappear for a few weeks to even months after completion of therapy; as long as they are regressing, biopsy is withheld (Fig. 26-27).

The diagnosis of recurrence is usually obvious, but some are heralded by paresthesias and difficult to target. Regional lymph node metastases may appear after 2 years and be confused with a parotid neoplasm or regarded as an unknown primary lesion.

PSEUDORECIDIVATION

Pseudorecidivation is a term used to describe an unusual process that is infrequently seen following irradiation of skin cancers. Usually occurring within 2 weeks of the completion of treatment, pseudorecidivation, or pseudorecurrence, consists of the appearance of a raised lesion on the previously irradiated skin. The new lesion may arise at the site of the original cancer or at the periphery of the field. The lesion may be skin colored, erythematous, yellow, or yellow brown; it may be smooth or verrucous in texture.[13] Biopsy reveals thickening of the prickle-cell (acanthosis) and horny (hyperkeratosis) layers and epidermal inclusion cyst formation. The lesions regress spontaneously, usually within 2 to 3 months. No treatment is indicated. Vaeth reported 5 cases of pseudorecidivation, all of which spontaneously disappeared within 12 weeks; tumor recurrence was not observed in any of the 5 patients.[34] It is important to recognize that the lesion is benign and self-healing so that unnecessary therapy is avoided (Fig. 26-28).

(Text continues on p. 506.)

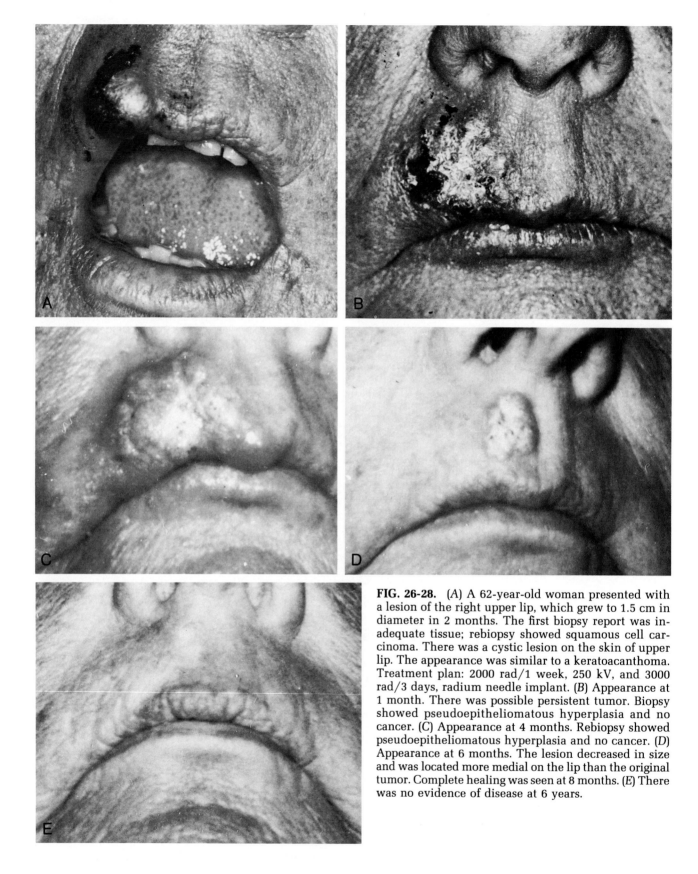

FIG. 26-28. (*A*) A 62-year-old woman presented with a lesion of the right upper lip, which grew to 1.5 cm in diameter in 2 months. The first biopsy report was inadequate tissue; rebiopsy showed squamous cell carcinoma. There was a cystic lesion on the skin of upper lip. The appearance was similar to a keratoacanthoma. Treatment plan: 2000 rad/1 week, 250 kV, and 3000 rad/3 days, radium needle implant. (*B*) Appearance at 1 month. There was possible persistent tumor. Biopsy showed pseudoepitheliomatous hyperplasia and no cancer. (*C*) Appearance at 4 months. Rebiopsy showed pseudoepitheliomatous hyperplasia and no cancer. (*D*) Appearance at 6 months. The lesion decreased in size and was located more medial on the lip than the original tumor. Complete healing was seen at 8 months. (*E*) There was no evidence of disease at 6 years.

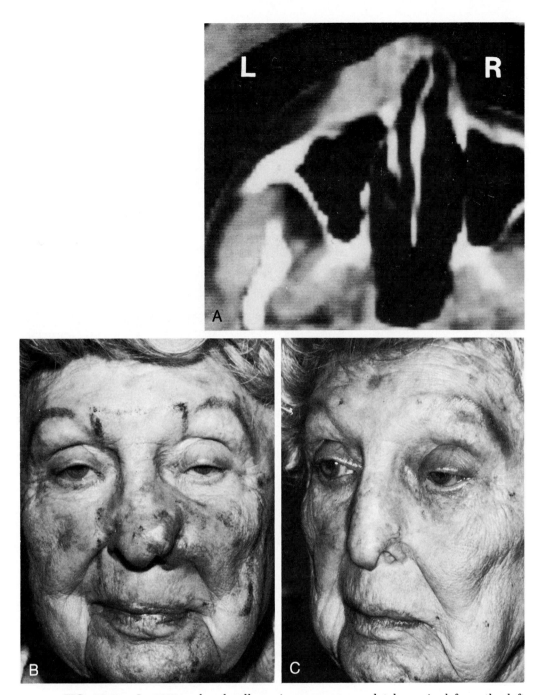

FIG. 26-29. In 1972, a basal cell carcinoma was completely excised from the left nasolabial crease of an 85-year-old woman. In 1979, a basal-squamous cell carcinoma was completely excised from the left alar rim, followed by reconstruction with a nasolabial flap. In 1980, there was regrowth of the mass in the left side of the nose accompanied by numbness of the upper lip. Biopsy revealed poorly differentiated squamous cell carcinoma. (*A*) CT scan shows soft tissue mass in the left nasal area. The anterior wall of the antrum is ill-defined adjacent to the mass, but there is no mass within the antrum. (*B*) There was a 4 × 3.5-cm indurated mass arising from the nasolabial fold and visible tumor in the nasal vestibule. The anterior portal is seen. The primary lesion received 7950 rad total dose/7½ weeks. Portal reductions were made after 5000 rad, 6000 rad, and 7125 rad; 20-MeV electrons were used for 6000 rad, 17-MeV electrons for 1000 rad, and 250 kV for the final 825 rad. The left upper neck and left parotid lymph nodes were electively irradiated to 5000 rad. (*C*) Appearance at 17 months. There was no evidence of disease at 3 years.

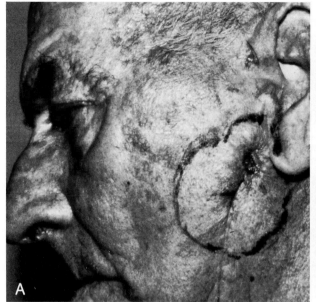
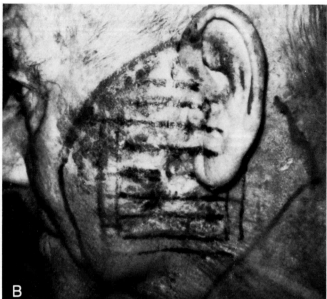
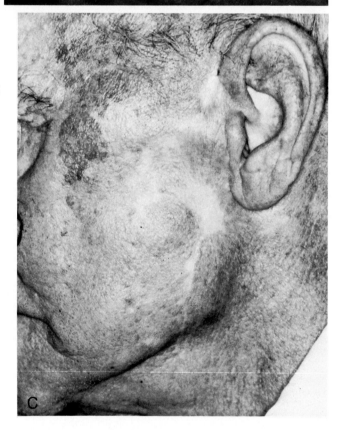

FIG. 26-30. A 69-year-old man presented with squamous cell carcinoma of the left cheek that had been excised; the margins were free of tumor. Nine months after excision the surgical site began to slowly enlarge. Biopsy 3 months later revealed poorly differentiated squamous cell carcinoma. (*A*) There was a 1-cm ulceration with surrounding induration measuring 4 × 5 cm. (*B*) Treatment plan to the primary site was electron-beam irradiation, 14 MeV, 5000 rad/5 weeks. The left lower neck received 8-MV x-rays, 5000 rad given dose/5 weeks. A single-plane radium needle implant added 3500 rad (58 hours). Photo at 5000 rad shows outline of electron beam portal and proposed radium needle implant. Note that needles penetrate ear cartilages. (*C*) There was no evidence of disease at 3 years.

Management of Recurrence

Although the overall risk of recurrence is reported to be small, the problem is not insignificant. Microscopically controlled excision is especially useful for the difficult cases. Radiation therapy may be used to advantage in certain cases because of the ability to cover rather generous potential areas of spread, both for horizontal and vertical spread (Figs. 26-29 and 26-30). The management of recurrent lesions is best placed in experienced hands, since a second recurrence often predicts eventual failure to obtain control.

Multiple sites of recurrence and/or new lesions are essentially incurable and test the imagination of the physicians to prescribe reasonable therapy. Frequent observation may be the only sensible approach, with palliative treatment added only when essential.

TREATMENT RESULTS

Results According to Histology

BASAL CELL AND SQUAMOUS CELL CARCINOMA

Treatment results for the various therapies are impossible to compare because of the selection for various treatments based on the size of the lesion, its location, and prior therapy

(whether untreated or recurrent). In addition, for patients with multiple lesions, it is often difficult to distinguish a treatment failure from a new cancer.

Most reports claim 95% or greater success rates for basal cell carcinomas and 90% or greater rates for squamous cell carcinomas. There is only a few percentage points' difference when comparing the various modalities. The success rate may be slightly inflated owing to the large number of early stage lesions, the lack of long-term follow-up, and the difficulty in discerning local recurrence versus a new skin cancer. Physicians who deal with a greater percentage of the more complicated, advanced stages, and often recurrent skin cancers, are somewhat less optimistic about the management of skin cancer.

Rigel and co-workers reviewed the results for 2960 basal cell carcinomas treated by microscopically controlled excision with a 5-year follow-up.[26] The overall recurrence rate was 2.6%. A group of lesions at high risk for recurrence (i.e., 10%) was identified: size (>4 cm in diameter); anatomical location (e.g., periauricular site); number of excisions to obtain tumor-free margins; and prior therapy.

Anderson reviewed the University of Florida experience of 55 patients who had lesions staged T2–T4 (AJCC) and treated by irradiation from 1964 to 1982.* There were 32 basal cell carcinomas and 23 squamous cell carcinomas. Follow-up ranged from 1 year to 19 years. The depth of dermal invasion was determined by the pathologist from the biopsy specimen. Bone and cartilage invasion was determined roentgenographically or clinically. Recurrent lesions were staged according to the findings at the time of recurrence when they presented for retreatment. The local control rates and the results of salvage therapy are presented in Tables 26-3 and 26-4, respectively. There will undoubtedly be additional failures in this series owing to the relatively short period of observation, but many of the patients with advanced lesions have had more than 5 years of follow-up and are probably cured. Photographs of some of these lesions appear throughout this chapter. The local control rate for the recurrent lesions was better than for the previously untreated lesions, which was an unexpected finding. A time-dose analysis for stages T3 and T4 failed to show a dividing line for success and failure. Survival data are shown in Table 26-5. There have been three deaths related to persistent skin cancer.

Levine reported the results for the surgical management of 60 patients with advanced skin cancer.[17] There were 40 basal cell carcinomas and 20 squamous cell carcinomas. All were recurrent after one or more previous therapies. All lesions were 3 cm or greater in maximum diameter; 39 involved cartilage, 28 involved bone, and 2 extended intracranially. All of these lesions were managed either by conventional surgery and total microscopic margin control (fresh tissue technique) or by Mohs' fixed tissue technique followed by the fresh tissue technique. With follow-up ranging from 1 to 4 years, 53 patients had no evidence of disease, 5 were alive with disease, and 2 were dead of disease.

SPINDLE CELL TUMORS

Evans and Smith reviewed 38 cases of spindle cell tumors of the skin.[8] The results of excision are related to the depth of invasion in Table 26-6 and to the margins of excision in Table 26-7. There was no difference in results regardless of whether the lesion was composed of spindle cells and squamous cells or contained only the spindle cell elements.

Judging from our limited experience, spindle cell/squamous cell carcinoma of the skin is curable with radiation therapy.

TABLE 26-3.   Skin Cancer Treated for Cure With Radiation Therapy: Local Control by T Stage (T2–T4)

Status of Primary Lesion	Local Control (No. Controlled/No. Treated)								
	T2			T3			T4		
	1 Yr	2 Yr	5 Yr	1 Yr	2 Yr	5 Yr	1 Yr	2 Yr	5 Yr
De novo	9/9	7/7	4/4	6/7	4/6	4/6	11/16	8/13	3/9
Recurrent	4/4	4/4	4/4	9/9	4/4	1/1	10/10	7/9	3/5
Total	13/13	11/11	8/8	15/16	8/10	5/7	21/26	15/22	6/14

Note: University of Florida data; patients treated 1/64–4/82; analysis 4/83 by N. H. Anderson, MD.

TABLE 26-4.   Advanced Skin Cancer Treated for Cure: Surgical Salvage of Radiation Therapy Failures

Stage	No. Patients	Status of Primary Lesion	No. Failed	No. Salvaged/No. Attempted		Ultimate Disease Control Rate
				First Recurrence	Second Recurrence	
T3	7	*De novo*	2	1/2	0/1	6/7
T4	16	*De novo*	6	3/5	0/1	13/16
T4	10	Recurrent	2	1/2	0/1	9/10

Note: University of Florida data; patients treated 1/64–4/82; analysis 4/83 by N. H. Anderson, MD.

---

* Anderson NH: Unpublished data, 1983.

TABLE 26-5. Advanced Skin Cancer Treated for Cure With Radiation Therapy: Survival by T Stage

Status of Primary Lesion	Survival					
	Absolute			Determinate		
	1 Year	2 Years	5 Years	1 Year	2 Years	5 Years
T2	13/13	11/12	8/10	13/13	11/11	8/8
T3	16/16	10/12	6/9	16/16	10/10	6/6
T4	25/26	19/20	6/9	25/26	19/20	6/8

Note: University of Florida data; patients treated 1/64–4/82; analysis 4/83 by N. H. Anderson, MD.

TABLE 26-6. Spindle Cell Tumors of the Skin: Results of Excision Related to Depth of Invasion

Depth of Invasion	No. Patients	Recurrence	Uncontrolled Recurrence	Metastases	Deaths
Dermis/subcutis	29	5	0	0	0
Muscle/bone	9	6	5	4	6

(Modified from Evans HL, Smith JL: Spindle cell squamous carcinomas and sarcoma-like tumors of the skin: A comparative study of 38 cases. Cancer 45:2687–2697, 1980)

TABLE 26-7. Spindle Cell Tumors of the Skin: Results of Excision Related to Margins of Excision

Margins of Excision	No. Patients	Recurrence	Uncontrolled Recurrence	Metastases	Deaths
Margins negative	31	5	1	2	2
Margins positive	7	6	4	2	4

(Modified from Evans HL, Smith JL: Spindle cell squamous carcinomas and sarcoma-like tumors of the skin: A comparative study of 38 cases. Cancer 45:2687–2697, 1980)

TABLE 26-8. Results of Radiation Therapy in Carcinoma of the Pinna

Stage	No. Patients	No. With Local Recurrence	Surgical Salvage
I	14	0	
II	10	2	1/2
III	14	2	0/2

Note: Follow-up 3 to 15 years.
(Data from Parker RG, Wildermuth O: Radiation therapy of lesions overlying cartilage: I. Carcinoma of the pinna. Cancer 15:57–65, 1962)

SEBACEOUS CELL CARCINOMA

Rulon and Helwig reviewed 59 cases of sebaceous cancer of the skin; 11 patients developed recurrence after excision and 8 developed metastasis to the parotid area lymph nodes.[27]

Results According to Anatomical Site

PINNA

Parker and Wildermuth reported the results for 38 carcinomas of the pinna treated with radiation therapy (Table 26-8) with a follow-up of 3 to 15 years.[25] There were ten patients with cartilage invasion prior to treatment. There were no instances of chondronecrosis. There were no local recurrences above an isoeffect line connecting 4250 rad/2 weeks (10 fractions), 4500 rad/3 weeks (15 fractions), and 5000 rad/4 weeks (20 fractions); these schemes are similar to those recommended in Table 26-1. The local recurrence rate was 4 of 38 (11%); in 1 patient salvage was achieved surgically. Two patients died of lymph node metastases.

Martin and Martin as well as del Regato and Vuksanovic reported similar results for the ear.[6,19]

EYELID

Fitzpatrick reported the results for 447 basal cell carcinomas and 30 squamous cell carcinomas of the eyelids treated by irradiation between 1958 and 1968.[10] The average diameter was 12 mm. The local recurrence rate was 5% for basal cell carcinoma and 3% for squamous cell carcinoma. Fifteen recurrences were in the center and ten at the edge of the lesion. There were no deaths due to eyelid cancer noted with follow-up of 3 to 13 years. The cosmetic and functional results were judged to be poor to fair in 6% of cases after 5 years' follow-up.

Abraham and co-workers reported a local recurrence rate of 7.4% for 68 patients with basal cell carcinoma of the medial canthal region treated by surgical methods.[1]

PAROTID AREA LYMPH NODES

The parotid area control rate for 39 patients with carcinoma of the skin metastatic to parotid area lymph nodes is outlined in Table 26-9, and the 2- and 5-year disease-free survival rates are shown in Table 26-10.*

* Mendenhall NP: Unpublished data, 1982.

Jackson and Ballantyne reported a 71% 2-year determinate survival rate for 123 non–basal cell carcinomas requiring a parotidectomy as part of their treatment; 18% of patients had postoperative or preoperative radiation therapy. Twenty-three patients died of local or regional failure and 11 of distant metastases.[15]

Wang reported the results for 28 patients who had parotid area lymph node metastases treated by radiation therapy alone (25 patients) or combined radiotherapy and parotidectomy (3 patients); two patients had recurrent disease after initial operation.[35] Radiation therapy usually combined a lateral wedge pair (cobalt-60) with boosts by interstitial implant and/or electron beam. The maximum dose in patients managed partly by implant was in the range of 8000 rad to 9000 rad. The parotid area and/or neck control rates are shown in Table 26-11. There were no reported complications of the facial nerve, temporomandibular joint, ear, bone, or muscles.

COMPLICATIONS

Surgery

True operative complications mostly involve problems with healing of flaps or split-thickness skin grafts. Reconstructive efforts may be unsatisfactory and require multiple revisions. Late complications are not likely.

Jackson and Ballantyne reported dysfunction of the facial

TABLE 26-9. Squamous Cell Carcinoma of the Skin Metastatic to Parotid Area Lymph Nodes: Parotid Area Control (39 Patients)

Initial Treatment (No. Patients)	Patients Excluded*	No. Evaluable for Parotid Area Control	Initial Parotid Area Control/No. Treated	No. Salvaged/No. of Salvage Attempts Evaluable†	Ultimate Control Rate
Surgery (14)	1	13	1/13	1/5	2/13
Radiation therapy (9)	3	6	3/6	0/0	3/6
Combined (16)	0	16	14/16	0/0	14/16

* Dead of intercurrent disease less than 2 years after treatment with no evidence of recurrence.

† Salvage attempts were considered evaluable if there was a minimum 2-year follow-up free of disease after the attempt.

Note: University of Florida data; patients treated 1/66–4/80; analysis 4/82 by N. P. Mendenhall, MD.

TABLE 26-10. Squamous Cell Carcinoma of the Skin Metastatic to Parotid Area Lymph Nodes: Survival Free of Disease

Initial Treatment (No. Patients)	2-Year Survival		5-Year Survival	
	Absolute	Determinate	Absolute	Determinate
Surgery (14)	1/14	1/14	1/9	1/9
Radiation therapy (9)	3/9	3/8	2/7	2/7
Combined (16)	13/16	13/16	6/10	6/8

Note: University of Florida data; patients treated 1/66–4/80; analysis 4/82 by N. P. Mendenhall, MD.

TABLE 26-11.	Parotid Area Lymph Node Metastases Treated by Radiation Therapy	
Stage*	Parotid and/or Neck Control	No. Patients NED
N1	7/8	6
N2A	3/4	3
N2B	5/8	3
N3A	3/4	1
Total	18/24 (75%)	13/24 (54%)

* See source article for details of staging system.[35]

Note: Follow-up 2 to 17 years, 11 patients died of disease; 6 died of parotid or neck recurrence, 5 died of distant metastases.

(NED, no evidence of disease)

(Adapted from Wang CC: The management of parotid lymph node metastases by irradiation. Cancer 50:223–225, 1982)

nerve in 7.3% of patients prior to operation for parotid area metastases.[15] The nerve was preserved in 57% of patients, partially preserved in 24%, and totally sacrificed in 19%.

Partial palsy of the facial nerve prior to operation for parotid area lymph node metastases was reported in 3 (21%) of 14 patients managed with combined treatment at the University of Florida.* Parotid area control is related to gross nerve involvement in Table 26-12. The uninvolved nerve was preserved in 7 of 14 patients, and the parotid area controlled in 6 of the 7.

Radiation Therapy

PRIMARY LESION

Acute complications vary with the anatomical site. The skin usually heals in 3 to 4 weeks after therapy for small lesions; two to four months may be required for large areas.

Late complications are site dependent. Skin damage is related to the fractionation scheme. Large defects heal by secondary intention and are often covered by a thin, atrophic, relatively avascular epithelium with spotty pigmentation and telangiectatic vessels; these areas do not have sweat glands, sebaceous glands, or hair. Needless to say, these areas do not tolerate trauma or infection very well. (See Chapter 14, The Effect of Radiation on Normal Tissues of the Head and Neck, for comments on cartilage and bone.)

Patients with cartilage invasion may report increased tenderness during the course of radiation therapy, but most report a decrease or no change in symptoms. Antibiotics may be used if infection is present.

Patients with obvious bone invasion and destruction are usually relatively asymptomatic and remain that way throughout therapy. Osteoradionecrosis of the calvarium occurred in past years when improper techniques were applied. Cerebral radionecrosis after radiation therapy for scalp cancer has been reported in 17 cases between 1930 and 1978.[20] The complications were related to single high-

* Mendenhall NP: Unpublished data, 1982.

TABLE 26-12.	Parotid Area Lymph Node Metastasis: 7th Nerve Injury (16 Patients—Combined Treatment)	
Status of Facial Nerve After Parotidectomy	No. With Parotid Area Controlled/No. Treated	
No injury	3/3	
Transient injury after operation	3/4	
Nerve preserved with gross tumor involvement	1/2	
Partial or complete sacrifice for gross tumor invasion*	6/7	

* Two patients had clinical deficits before surgery. Five patients had some transient or permanent injury to facial nerve branches other than those advertently sacrificed.

Note: University of Florida data; patients treated 1/66–4/80, analysis 4/82 by N. P. Mendenhall, MD.

dose treatment (2300 rad to 3000 rad), high daily fractions (i.e., >300 rad/fraction), high dose (7500 rad), or repeated courses of treatment. Ten of 12 patients operated on for brain necrosis were said to be cured.

Soft tissue necrosis may occur, particularly after successful treatment of large lesions, but it is an uncommon problem in our experience.

PAROTID AREA IRRADIATION

There has been no evidence of permanent damage to the normal facial nerve in patients treated with radiation therapy alone in spite of doses as high as 8000 rad to 9000 rad in some instances. One patient had a transient nerve palsy that recovered in 4 months. Other potential complications include trismus, hearing loss, serous otitis media, perforation of the tympanic membrane, and localized areas of necrosis.

REFERENCES

1. Abraham JC, Jabaley ME, Hoopes JE: Basal cell carcinoma of the medial canthal region. Am J Surg 126:492–495, 1973
2. Ackerman AB: Histopathology of keratoacanthoma. In Andrade R, Gumport SL, Popkin GL, Rees TD (eds): Cancer of the Skin: Biology, Diagnosis, and Management, p 795. Philadelphia, WB Saunders, 1976
3. American Joint Committee on Cancer: Manual for Staging of Cancer, 2nd ed, pp 123–126. Philadelphia, JB Lippincott, 1983
4. Binstock JH, Stegman SJ, Tromovitch TA: Large, aggressive basal cell carcinomas of the scalp. J Dermatol Surg 7:565–569, 1981
5. Cassisi NJ, Dickerson D, Million RR: Squamous cell carcinoma of the skin metastatic to parotid nodes. Arch Otolaryngol 104:336–339, 1978
6. Del Regato JA, Vuksanovic M: Radiotherapy of carcinoma of the skin overlying the cartilages of the nose and ear. Radiology 79:203–208, 1962
7. Didolkar MS, Gerner RE, Moore GE: Epidermolysis bullosa dystrophica and epithelioma of the skin: Review of published cases and report of an additional patient. Cancer 33:198–202, 1974

8. Evans HL, Smith JL: Spindle cell squamous carcinomas and sarcoma-like tumors of the skin: A comparative study of 38 cases. Cancer 45:2687–2697, 1980

9. Fierstein JT, Thawley SE, Druck NS, Ogura JH: Metastatic sweat gland carcinoma. Laryngoscope 88:1691–1696, 1978

10. Fitzpatrick PJ, Jamieson DM, Thompson GA, Allt WEC: Tumors of the eyelids and their treatment by radiotherapy. Radiology 104:661–665, 1972

11. Gooding CA, White G, Yatsuhashi M: Significance of marginal extension in excised basal cell carcinoma. N Engl J Med 273:923–924, 1965

12. Graham JW: Metastatic cancer in the parotid lymph nodes. Med J Aust 2:8–12, 1965

13. Herold SC, Nelson LM: Pseudoepitheliomatous reactions (pseudorecidive) following radiation therapy of epitheliomata. In Hellerström S, ed: Proceedings of the 11th International Congress of Dermatology, Vol. II, 426–432. Acta Derm Venereol (Stockholm), 1959

14. Hoxtell EO, Mandel JS, Murray SS, Schuman LM, Goltz RW: Incidence of skin carcinoma after renal transplantation. Arch Dermatol 113:436–438, 1977

15. Jackson GL, Ballantyne AJ: Role of parotidectomy for skin cancer of the head and neck. Am J Surg 142:464–469, 1981

16. Keith WD, Kelly AP, Sumrall AJ, Chhabra A: Squamous cell carcinoma arising in lesions of discoid lupus erythematosus in black persons. Arch Dermatol 116:315–317, 1980

17. Levine H: Cutaneous carcinoma of the head and neck: Management of massive and previously uncontrolled lesions. Laryngoscope 93:87–105, 1983

18. Levine HL, Bailin PL: Basal cell carcinoma of the head and neck: Identification of the high-risk patient. Laryngoscope 90:955–961, 1980

19. Martin CL, Martin JA: Long time studies of advanced cancer of the ear treated with electrosurgery plus radiation. Am J Roentgenol Radium Ther Nucl Med 117:584–594, 1973

20. Matsumura H, Ross ER: Delayed cerebral radionecrosis following treatment of carcinoma of the scalp: Clinicopathologic and ultrastructural study. Surg Neurol 12:193–204, 1979

21. Mellette JR, Amonette RA, Gardner JH, Chesney TM: Carcinoma of sebaceous glands on the head and neck: A report of four cases. J Dermatol Surg Oncol 7:404–407, 1981

22. Mohs FE: Chemosurgery for basal cell and squamous carcinomas of the skin. In M. D. Anderson Hospital and Tumor Institute, Houston: Neoplasms of the Skin and Malignant Melanoma, pp 173–188. Chicago, Year Book Medical Publishers, 1976

23. Mora RG, Burris R: Cancer of the skin in blacks: A review of 128 patients with basal-cell carcinoma. Cancer 47:1436–1438, 1981

24. Panje WR, Ceilley RI: The influence of embryology of the midface on the spread of epithelial malignancies. Laryngoscope 89:1914–1920, 1979

25. Parker RG, Wildermuth O: Radiation therapy of lesions overlying cartilage: I. Carcinoma of the pinna. Cancer 15:57–65, 1965

26. Rigel DS, Robins P, Friedman RJ: Predicting recurrence of basal-cell carcinomas treated by microscopically controlled excision: A recurrence index score. J Dermatol Surg Oncol 7:807–810, 1981

27. Rulon DB, Helwig EB: Cutaneous sebaceous neoplasms. Cancer 33:82–102, 1974

28. Scanlon EF, Volkmer DD, Oviedo MA, Khandekar JD, Victor TA: Metastatic basal cell carcinoma. J Surg Oncol 15:171–180, 1980

29. Schuller DE, Berg JW, Sherman G, Krause CJ: Cutaneous basosquamous carcinoma of the head and neck: Comparative analysis. Otolaryngol Head Neck Surg 87:420–427, 1979

30. Silverberg E: Cancer Statistics, 1982. CA 32:15–31, 1982

31. Southwick GJ, Schwartz RA: The basal cell nevus syndrome: Disasters occurring among a series of 36 patients. Cancer 44:2294–2305, 1979

32. Stern RS, Thibodeau LA, Kleinerman RA, Parrish JA, Fitzpatrick TB: Risk of cutaneous carcinoma in patients treated with oral methoxsalen photochemotherapy for psoriasis. N Engl J Med 300:809–813, 1979

33. Stromberg BV, Keiter JE, Wray RC, Weeks PM: Scar carcinoma: Prognosis and treatment. South Med J 70:821–822, 1977

34. Vaeth JW: Radiation-induced pseudorecidivation. Radiology 99:173–174, 1971

35. Wang CC: The management of parotid lymph node metastases by irradiation. Cancer 50:223–225, 1982

36. Wright JD, Font RL: Mucinous sweat gland adenocarcinoma of the eyelid: A clinicopathologic study of 21 cases with histochemical and electron microscopic observations. Cancer 44:1757–1768, 1977

37. Yoffey JM, Courtice FC: Lymphatics, Lymph Nodes, and Lymphoid Tissue. Cambridge, MA, Harvard University Press, 1956

Melanoma of the Head and Neck

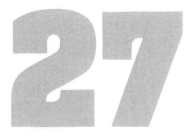

ANDREW R. HARWOOD

Melanoma primarily arising in the head and neck is a relatively uncommon problem, even for the physician dealing specifically with head and neck oncology. Particular emphasis will be given to the distinction of lentigo maligna and lentigo maligna melanoma from the other forms of melanoma and to the role of radiation therapy in the management of this disease. This is principally because these two areas have been sadly neglected in the literature concerning melanomas of the head and neck. The chapter is divided into two parts, the first dealing with cutaneous melanoma and the second with mucosal melanoma. Skin and mucosal melanomas are completely different in clinical appearance, treatment, and prognosis.

Ocular and conjunctival melanomas are usually considered specifically in ophthalmologic practice and will not be discussed here. However, they are frequently managed by radiation therapy with a good rate of success, which is in keeping with the observations on the response of skin and mucosal melanoma.

CUTANEOUS MELANOMA

Incidence, Epidemiology, and Etiology

Melanoma represents approximately 1% of all types of cancer in North America. The overall incidence is approximately four cases per 100,000 population per year in the United States and Canada.[40] Head and neck melanoma accounts for 20% to 35% of all cases of cutaneous melanoma. The incidence of melanoma seems to be slowly rising. It commonly occurs between the ages of 30 and 60 years, with the exception of lentigo maligna and lentigo maligna melanoma, which occur in the 60 to 80+ age-group.[18] It is extremely uncommon in children. Melanoma predominantly occurs in whites and is very uncommon in the head and neck region in blacks or orientals. There is strong evidence to implicate exposure to sunlight in the pathogenesis of the melanoma, since it is particularly common in people with white skin living close to the equator, where the duration of exposure to sunlight is more prolonged. Melanoma of the skin most commonly occurs in people who tolerate the sun poorly, particularly those who freckle, burn easily, and do not tan readily. The other known factor of importance in the etiology of melanoma is genetic. First-degree blood relatives of a patient with melanoma are 1.7 times more likely to develop cutaneous melanoma than members of the general population. It is estimated that approximately 11% of melanomas may be hereditary. In familial cases of melanoma, there is a greater tendency for multiple melanomas to occur (an average of approximately three tumors per person). Clark and co-workers have recently described an autosomal dominant B-K mole syndrome.[8] Patients with this syndrome have multiple pigmented moles on the skin and a high incidence of transformation of these moles into malignant melanomas.

TABLE 27-1. Summary of Clinical History, Appearance, Histology, Differential Diagnosis, Prognosis, and Treatment for Cutaneous Melanoma of the Head and Neck

	Lentigo Melanoma (LM)	Lentigo Maligna Melanoma (LMM)	Superficial Spreading Melanoma (SSM)	Nodular Melanoma (NM)
Clinical History	Slow growth of pigmented lesion, commonly on face of elderly person in sun-damaged skin	Development of nodule in preexisting LM that may have been present for many years; dermal invasion may occur prior to the development of a palpable nodule	More rapid growth than LM; does not grow as large as LM; palpable edge	Rapid growth of nodule, usually pigmented, in previously normal skin or preexisting nevus; there may be bleeding or discharge from a sore that will not heal; itching or other paresthesias may occur
Appearance	No palpable nodule; from a few millimeters up to 10 cm in size; varying degrees of pigmentation, black and brown; white areas of regression may be present; edge impalable, irregular, and serpiginous	The same as LM with the presence of a palpable nodule which may be ulcerated	Variety of color combinations (brown, black, blue, gray, even white); scaly, crusted surface; skin furrows lost; irregular outline; nodules may be present and ulcerated; surrounding red flare may be present	Nodular growth; variable colors from black to red to white; erythema of skin at periphery; satellites in surrounding skin
Differential Diagnosis	SSM; pigmented basal cell carcinoma; pigmented actinic or seborrheic keratosis; nevus	See LM; NM developing *de novo* or in a preexisting SSM	Same as LM and LMM	Pigmented basal cell carcinoma; squamous cell carcinoma
Prognosis	One third to one half ultimately develop dermal invasion (LMM)	Ten percent develop regional metastases; distant metastases uncommon	Twenty to 30% develop metastases to regional lymph nodes; distant metastases not uncommon; risk of metastases rises with increasing penetration of dermis (Clark level) and thickness of lesion (Breslow thickness)	Thirty to 50% develop metastases to regional lymph nodes and distant sites; risk of metastatic spread rises wtih increasing penetration of dermis (Clark level) and thickness of lesion (Breslow thickness)
Histology	Combination of severe solar degeneration of skin and linear proliferation of atypical melanocytes confined to epidermis	Similar to LM, but atypical melanocytes will have penetrated into the dermis	Proliferating melanocytes that invade the epidermis in a pagetoid fashion; dermal invasion nearly always present; invasive nodule may be composed of spindle or epithelioid cells	Downward growth of malignant melanocytes into dermis with minimal or no epidermal invasion
Treatment	Excision with 1–2 cm margins of normal skin; conventional fractionated irradiation	Excision of primary lesion alone; lymph node dissection not indicated unless nodes palpable; conventional fractionated irradiation	Excision of primary lesion is treatment of choice; conventional radiation therapy should be considered in certain cases	Wide excision of primary lesion; role of prophylactic lymph node dissection in selected cases controversial; local excision and irradiation indicated in selected cases

It is important for the clinician to recognize the hereditary form of malignant melanoma through careful follow-up of the patient for further primary melanomas and screening of blood relatives. This particularly applies to those patients with the B-K mole syndrome.

Pathology and Patterns of Spread

There are basically three types of cutaneous melanoma in the head and neck.[6,7] The treatment and prognosis are vitally dependent on an understanding of the differences between these three types: (1) lentigo maligna (LM); (2) superficial spreading melanoma (SSM); and (3) nodular melanoma, including those arising *de novo*, in a preexisting SSM, and in a preexisting LM (lentigo maligna melanoma [LMM]). Clinical appearance, pathology, prognosis, and treatment for each type are summarized in Table 27-1.

Nodular melanoma arising *de novo* has a 30% to 50% metastatic rate; arising in preexisting SSM, 30%; and arising in a preexisting LM, 10%. LM and SSM most commonly grow slowly by peripheral or centrifugal enlargement. This is called the "radial growth phase," and may last for many years in LM. Metastases rarely develop in a melanoma that is in the radial growth phase alone. The potential for metastases is markedly enhanced when the primary melanoma penetrates the deeper levels of the dermis. This is termed the *vertical growth phase*. The two methods of histologically staging melanoma recognize the importance of distinguishing these two growth patterns (see section on methods of diagnosis and staging).[5,6]

LENTIGO MALIGNA AND LENTIGO MALIGNA MELANOMA

Synonyms include Hutchinson's melanotic freckle,[33] circumscribed precancerous melanosis of Dubreilh,[19] benign melanoma, and senile freckle.[1] The clinical and pathologic features of this condition are summarized in Table 27-1. Since LM is confined to the epidermis, it is a precancerous lesion. Characteristically, it is a slowly growing, pigmented lesion on the skin of the head and neck of an elderly person (Fig. 27-1).[26] The most common sites are the cheek (60% to 70% of cases), ear, and nose. It rarely occurs in the hair-bearing scalp and is uncommon outside of the head and neck, although it does occur on the penis and extremities. Commonly, there is associated solar damage to the skin. It represents approximately 10% of all cutaneous melanomas of the head and neck. If left untreated, LM will slowly increase in size over a 5- to 10-year period and may reach up to 5 cm to 10 cm in diameter. Ultimately, approximately one third to one half will develop invasion of the dermis (LMM),[53] clinically manifested by a palpable nodule within the LM that may ulcerate and bleed. Microscopic dermal invasion in the larger LM (≥5 cm) can occur prior to the clinical development of a palpable nodule. Wayte and Helwig have suggested that the older and the larger the LM, the greater is the risk of the development of nodular melanoma.[53]

The clinical features of LMM are summarized in Table 27-1. These include the development of a palpable nodule, which may ulcerate and bleed, within or at the edge of a preexisting LM (Fig. 27-2). The biologic aggressiveness of a nodular melanoma arising in a preexisting LM is low, with a 10% or less chance of developing metastatic disease to the regional lymph nodes and distant sites. In our own experience with more than 30 patients with LMM, only one patient has developed regional lymph node metastases, one has developed distant metastases, and none has died of melanoma. This experience is similar to that of others.

The average time to onset of dermal invasion in an LM is 10 to 14 years.[1] Pathologically, LM and LMM are as distinctive microscopically as clinically. Frequently, severe solar damage is present in the affected skin. One observes linear proliferation of atypical melanocytes in the basal region of the epidermis, and this may extend into the external root sheaths of hair follicles. The presence of a dense lymphocytic infiltrate is also quite common. When dermal invasion by the atypical melanocytes is present, the lesion is classified as an LMM. It is relatively uncommon to observe advanced vertical growth phase (i.e., extension to Clark level 4 or 5) in a nodular melanoma arising in a preexisting LM.

FIG. 27-1. Lentigo maligna. (Reprinted with permission from Harwood AR: Conventional fractionated radiotherapy for 51 patients with lentigo maligna and lentigo maligna melanoma. Int J Radiat Oncol Biol Phys 9: 1019–1021, 1983. Copyright © 1983, Pergamon Press, Ltd.)

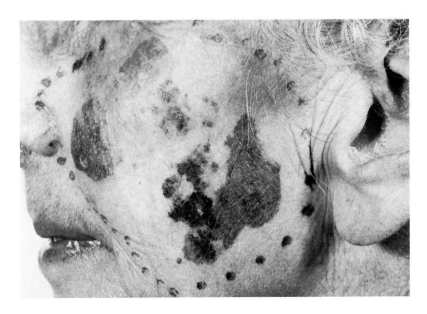

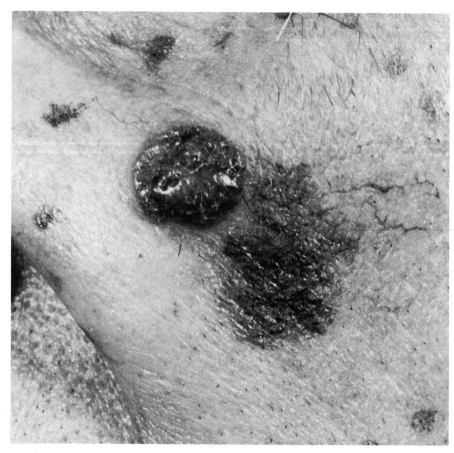

FIG. 27-2. Lentigo maligna melanoma.

SUPERFICIAL SPREADING MELANOMA

Superficial spreading melanoma accounts for 70% of all cutaneous melanomas and is intermediate in terms of biologic aggressiveness between LM and nodular melanoma arising *de novo* (see Table 27-1). Its peak incidence is in the fifth decade. As in LMM, there are both radial and vertical growth phases. The radial growth phase is shorter than in LM; the time to development of the vertical growth phase ranges from 1 to 2 years. The radial growth phase is associated with a metastatic potential of approximately 5% to 10%. Once the vertical growth phase develops, approximately 30% will develop metastases to regional lymph nodes or distant sites.

Clinically, SSM grows more rapidly than LM, and it rarely grows to the same size as LM. It has a palpable edge with an irregular outline, but it is more circumscribed than LM (Fig. 27-3). A variety of color combinations of brown, black, blue and frequently white areas of spontaneous regression may be present. It has a scaly, crusted surface, and the skin furrows may be lost. Nodules may be present and ulcerated. The vertical growth phase usually appears by the time the lesion is 1 cm to 2 cm in size. The radial growth phase is characterized histologically by proliferating melanocytes that invade the epidermis in a pagetoid fashion. Microscopic invasion of the papillary dermis is frequently observed. The vertical growth phase is characterized by deeper penetration of the dermis by malignant melanocytes associated with nodule formation.

NODULAR MELANOMA

Nodular melanoma arising *de novo* is the most malignant form of the three varieties of cutaneous melanoma (see Table 27-1). Metastatic potential is approximately 50%. Nodular melanoma arising *de novo* is composed exclusively of a vertical growth phase, with malignant melanocytes invading into the deeper levels of the dermis. The host cellular response (e.g., lymphocyte infiltration) is variable, but less than in LMM or SSM.[39]

Clinically, the lesion begins as a pigmented nodule in previously normal skin or in a preexisting nevus (Fig. 27-4). Growth is rapid, and ulceration and bleeding frequently occur. Occasionally, the nodular melanoma possesses no black or blue pigment and has the appearance of a reddish, nodular skin lesion; this amelanotic melanoma can resemble basal cell or squamous cell carcinoma and be difficult to diagnose both clinically and pathologically. The most common sites are the face (50%) and neck (20%), followed by the ear and scalp.[13] Pathologically, no radial growth phase is observed in nodular melanoma arising *de novo* and the lesion consists of malignant melanocytes in a nodule invading the dermis.

DISTANT METASTASES

LM does not produce distant metastases. LMM develops distant metastases only after regional metastases have appeared, and even then the risk is small. Distant metastasis occurs in less than 5% of SSM. Nodular melanoma commonly develops distant metastases, and they may occur without spread to the regional lymph nodes, although the incidence increases if lymph node metastases are present. The time to appearance of distant metastases is usually within 1 to 2 years of diagnosis, but they have been observed to appear capriciously up to 20 years or longer following primary therapy.

Methods of Diagnosis and Staging

The diagnosis is established by either incisional or excisional biopsy. It is frequently not possible to do an excisional biopsy in LM; the edge of the lesion should be biopsied, as well as any palpable nodule. The staging procedures for LM, LMM, and SSM in the radial growth phase are shown in Table 27-2. A full metastatic workup is not indicated in view of the very low incidence of distant metastasis. This should only be done in the case that is behaving locally in an aggressive manner or has metastasized to the regional lymph nodes. The biopsy of any palpable nodule is important, since it allows assessment of the presence or absence of invasion of the dermis and the level of penetration if the dermis is involved. Two parameters of pathologic microstaging of the primary lesion have been shown to be of importance in determining prognosis in melanoma: (1) Clark level of penetration of the dermis,[6] and (2) Breslow thickness.[5]

Clark levels of penetration of the dermis are as follows:[6]

Level 1   All tumor cells confined to the epidermis with no invasion of the basement membrane into the dermis (*i.e.*, melanoma *in situ*; *e.g.*, LM)
Level 2   Tumor cells penetrating the basement membrane into the papillary dermis, but not extending to the reticular dermis
Level 3   Tumor cells filling the papillary dermis and abutting, but not invading, the reticular dermis
Level 4   Tumor cells invading into the reticular dermis
Level 5   Invasion into the subcutaneous tissues

The Breslow thickness method involves measuring the maximal thickness of the vertical dimensions of microscopic sections of the primary melanoma using an ocular micrometer.[5] Both the Clark and the Breslow method of microstaging the primary melanoma are of prognostic importance (see section on prognosis). Correct assessment of

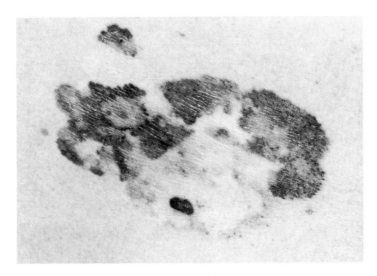

FIG. 27-3.   Superficial spreading melanoma.

FIG. 27-4.   Nodular melanoma.

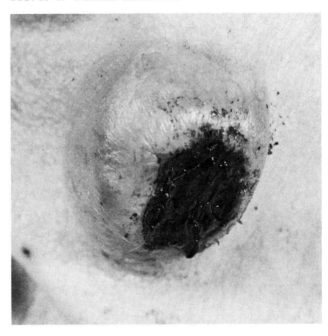

TABLE 27-2. Staging Procedures for LM, LMM, and SSM in Radial Growth Phase	
Procedure	**Rationale/Comment**
Physical examination	To assess extent of radial growth phase, presence of vertical growth phase (*i.e.*, nodule formation), and presence of regional lymph node metastases, in order to determine adequate treatment margins
Biopsy	
Edge of lesion	To establish diagnosis and assess whether dermal invasion is present and extent of radial growth phase, in order to determine adequate treatment margins
Any palpable nodule	To establish whether dermal invasion is present and, if it is, to assess Clark level of penetration and Breslow thickness
Metastatic workup*	Not indicated unless lymph node metastasis is present or unexpected finding of Clark ≧3 or Breslow >0.75

* See Table 27-3.

TABLE 27-3. Staging Procedures for Nodular Melanoma Arising *de Novo* or in an SSM

Procedure	Rationale/Comment
Physical examination	To assess extent of local disease (satellites), presence of lymph node metastases, and presence of distant metastases
Biopsy (excisional, if possible)	To assess Clark level of penetration of the dermis and Breslow thickness of the lesion
Metastatic workup: mandatory	
Peripheral blood hematology and biochemistry (alkaline phosphatase, serum glutamic oxaloacetic transaminase, lactic dehydrogenase	To assess presence of possible bone marrow, liver, or bone metastases
Chest roentgenogram and whole lung tomograms	To assess presence of lung metastases
Metastatic workup: optional	
Brain CT scan	Done only if central nervous system symptoms are present
Liver scan	Done if there is hepatomegaly or elevated alkaline phosphatase or serum glutamic oxaloacetic transaminase levels
Bone scan	Done if bone pain is present or bony alkaline phosphatase level is elevated

Clark level and Breslow thickness clearly requires careful attention to biopsy technique and proper pathologic sectioning of the specimen.

The staging procedures for a nodular melanoma arising *de novo* or in an SSM are shown in Table 27-3. Since distant metastasis is quite frequent in this form of melanoma, a limited metastatic workup is indicated. Chest roentgenography and whole lung tomography or computed tomographic (CT) scanning have the highest detection rate for occult metastatic disease. In view of the low detection rate, liver and bone scanning is not done routinely unless there is an indication on clinical assessment or biochemical investigation that bone or liver metastases may be present.[52] A brain CT scan should be done in all cases when *any* symptom indicative of brain metastases is present.[52]

A variety of clinical staging systems are used, distinguishing melanomas confined to the primary site, those with lymph node metastases, and those with distant metastases. The most commonly used staging system is shown in Table 27-4. When a lymph node dissection has been undertaken, a record of the number of nodes involved, size of nodal involvement, and presence or absence of penetration of the lymph node capsule is of prognostic importance, and these parameters should be determined by the examining pathologist.

Treatment

In view of the major and sometimes capricious differences in biologic behavior for LM/LMM, SSM, and nodular melanoma arising *de novo* or in a preexisting SSM, the treatment of these three entities is considered separately.

LENTIGO MALIGNA AND LENTIGO MALIGNA MELANOMA

In North America, the traditional method of treatment of LM and LMM has been by surgical removal,[4,10,14] although

TABLE 27-4. Clinical Staging System for Melanoma

Stage	Definition
I	Local
IA	Primary lesion alone
IB	Primary and satellites within a 5 cm radius of the primary lesion
IC	Local recurrence within a 5 cm radius of a resected primary lesion
ID	Metastases located more than 5 cm from the primary site but within the primary lymphatic drainage area
II	Regional nodal disease
III	Disseminated disease

in continental Europe radiation therapy has been frequently employed.[2,16,41] LM or LMM is predominantly a disease of the skin of the face of elderly people. Quite frequently, the lesion reaches a large size prior to diagnosis. Surgical excision of a large area of skin requires skin grafting to repair the defect; the cosmetic blemish created by the resection of a large LM, particularly on elderly, unfit patients, has led to other techniques of treatment being tried, including 5-fluorouracil cream, cryotherapy, and electrodesiccation and cautery.[38,48] These methods have met with varying degrees of success. In the experience at the Princess Margaret Hospital, with more than 40 cases, irradiation has proved to be a simple, well-tolerated, outpatient treatment that produces an excellent cosmetic result, superior to that produced by excision and full-thickness skin grafting (Table 27-5). This is illustrated in Figure 27-5 in which a patient with a large LM is shown before

TABLE 27-5.   Results of Radiation Therapy in the First 40 Cases of Lentigo Maligna and Lentigo Maligna Melanoma

Tumor Type	No. Patients	Controlled (Follow-up)	Comment
Lentigo maligna	17	15 (6 months–13 years)	Two local failures controlled by further irradiation and surgery
Lentigo maligna melanoma	23	21 (6 months–7 years)	Two local failures both controlled by further surgery; one regional failure controlled by surgery and adjuvant irradiation

FIG. 27-5. Large lentigo maligna just lateral to the eye. (*A*) Appearance prior to treatment. (*B*) Appearance after radiation therapy.

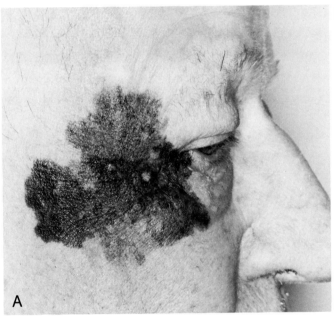
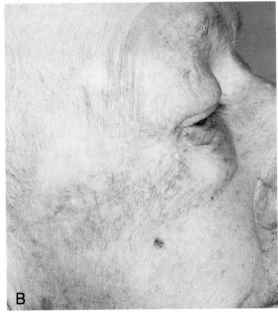

and after radiation therapy, and in Figure 27-6, which shows a similar patient before and after surgical treatment, including repair with a full-thickness skin graft.

Therefore, in view of the favorable experience with conventional irradiation at the Princess Margaret Hospital, the following management policy for LM and LMM is recommended:

1. Small LM/LMM on the free skin of the face should be primarily excised, provided this can be accomplished without a major resection requiring skin graft for reconstruction.
2. Small LM/LMM in sites where excision may produce cosmetic or functional deficits (*e.g.,* ear, eyelid, nose) should be treated primarily with fractionated irradiation, reserving surgery for the patients (less than 10%) who fail this management policy.

3. Large LM/LMM should be treated with conventional fractionated irradiation, reserving surgery for failure of irradiation to control the disease.

SURGERY

Surgery has been the traditional treatment for this disease, and the majority of patients have been cured. In view of the relatively benign nature of this type of melanoma, wide excision (i.e., 5 cm border of normal tissue) is not routinely required. It has generally been conceded that a margin of 1 cm to 2 cm of normal skin around the lesion constitutes an adequate margin of resection.[4,10] Skin grafting is not routinely required unless the defect created is too large for coverage by advancement of flaps. Lymph node dissection is not indicated unless there are clinically positive malignant nodes in the neck.

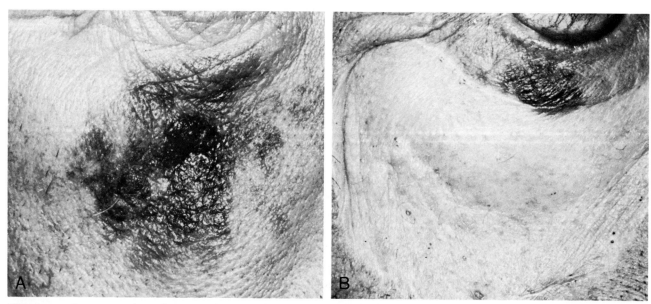

FIG. 27-6. Lentigo maligna beneath the right lower eyelid. (*A*) Appearance prior to treatment. (*B*) Appearance after surgical treatment. Repair was a full-thickness skin graft. Note persistent disease in lower lid.

TABLE 27-6. **Results of Radiation Therapy for SSM of the Head and Neck**

Site	Clark Level	Age/Sex	Previous Treatment	Radiation Treatment	Result
Ear	3	54/M	Biopsy	4500 rad/10 fractions/2 weeks	NED 3 years
Cheek	3	78/F	Biopsy	4500 rad/10 fractions/2 weeks	NED 3 years
Cheek	2	55/F	Local excision, margins involved	4500 rad/10 fractions/2 weeks	NED 3 years
Eyebrow	2	27/F	Local excision, margins involved	5000 rad/10 fractions/2 weeks	Dead at 1 year*
Scalp	3	46/M	Recurrent after surgery	5000 rad/10 fractions/2 weeks	NED 5 years

* Local control; patient died of distant metastases.

(NED, no evidence of disease)

RADIATION THERAPY

Irradiation using the Miescher technique has been used for many years in Europe.[2,16,41] This technique involves the use of very superficial irradiation using a contact therapy machine (10 KeV to 20 KeV, 50% depth dose 1 mm) and the application of extremely high doses of irradiation (2000 rad per treatment once weekly for five to six treatments).[41] The results achieved by several authors on more than 100 patients show a recurrence rate of less than 5%.[2,16,41] The major disadvantage with this technique is that the penetration of the x-ray beam is extremely limited and the fall-off of radiation dose is very rapid. If, therefore, the lesion is only slightly thicker than appreciated on clinical examination (e.g., with undetected but marked microscopic extension into the dermis), then the deeper portion of the tumor will be undertreated and subcutaneous recurrence will develop. This is probably the reason why

the experience of Kopf and co-workers with this technique was less favorable, with several recurrences consisting of invasive melanoma seen in the subcutaneous tissue.[36] It is well recognized, particularly in the larger LM, that unrecognized microscopic invasion of the dermis can occur in the absence of a palpable nodule.

In Toronto, my colleagues and I have for many years employed fractionated orthovoltage radiation therapy (100 KeV to 250 KeV).[12,25,26] The most commonly used fractionation regimens have been 3250 rad/5 fractions/1 week for LM smaller than 2 cm in size, 4500 rad/10 fractions/ 2 weeks for LM 2 cm to 5 cm in size, and 5000 rad/15 fractions/3 weeks for very large LM, such as illustrated in Figure 27-1. The method of irradiation that we have used avoids the problem of possible undertreatment of unappreciated deep extension, since the penetration of even the most superficial x-ray beam that we have used (100 KeV) results in a 50% depth dose at 6 mm. Generally, a margin of 1 cm to 2 cm of normal skin is treated around the clinically obvious LM (Fig. 27-1).[26] More penetrating irradiation (175 KeV to 250 KeV) has been used on thicker LMM (more than 0.7 mm thick). We have now treated more than 40 patients with fractionated irradiation; the results are summarized in Table 27-5.[25] Thirty-eight of the 40 patients had lesions of the head and neck. Two LM patients failed irradiation. One patient was 92 years of age when referred for treatment and refused fractionated irradiation. She was treated with a single exposure of 2000 rad. The lesion faded and then regrew; 2½ years following the irradiation, the recurrence was excised, and the patient is free of disease. The other patient was irradiated with an inadequate margin of normal tissue, developed an edge recurrence, was reirradiated, and is alive and well 13 years following treatment of the recurrence.

Two LMM patients developed local recurrence following irradiation, and salvage was achieved with subsequent surgery. There has recently been 1 regional lymph node recurrence in a patient with a level 5 nodular melanoma arising in an LMM on an ear. The primary lesion was controlled with conventional irradiation, but regional recurrence developed 18 months following primary treatment; neck dissection was carried out, followed by postoperative irradiation, since tumor was penetrating the lymph node capsule. The patient is free of local and regional disease. To date, there have been no deaths from melanoma in this group of patients. *Characteristically, the lesion may take up to 24 months (median 9 months) to completely regress following irradiation.* The cosmetic results of irradiation have, in general, been excellent. A representative example is given in Figure 27-5. There have been no major complications of irradiation in this group of patients; all patients developed an acute fibrinous irradiation reaction in the area of treatment that soon healed.

SUPERFICIAL SPREADING MELANOMA

Excision remains the treatment of choice for SSM of the head and neck; however, radiation therapy should be considered as primary treatment when there is a contraindication to surgery due to medical reasons or for locations where it is not feasible to do an adequate excision.

SURGERY

The principle of wide surgical excision for melanomas has been advocated for more than 70 years and was based on pathologic studies of the frequency of dermal lymphatic permeation into the surrounding skin.[40] Generally, surgeons have advocated full-thickness excision of the skin with margins of 3 cm to 4 cm in all directions around the lesion. However, such a philosophy presents problems in the head and neck region where, due to anatomical considerations, such wide excision is not always feasible. Recently, the necessity for such wide excisions has been questioned, particularly for SSM without the vertical growth phase or SSM with a vertical growth phase measuring less than 0.76 mm.[5] Breslow studied 62 melanomas less than 0.76 mm thick that were treated with a variety of resection margins varying from 0.1 to 5 cm. In these "thin" melanomas, no difference in local recurrence rates was found between those patients with margins less than 0.5 cm wide compared with those with margins greater than 3 cm. Although this was a retrospective analysis and no prospective study has been done on this point, it seems

reasonable to recommend for patients with SSM in the radial growth phase, particularly in the head and neck, that more limited resection with a margin of normal tissue both clinically and pathologically in the range of 0.5 cm to 1.5 cm is quite adequate.[15] In many cases, this will allow primary closure without the necessity for skin grafting. Where doubt exists as to the adequacy of the margins of the excision, postoperative irradiation can be applied as an alternative to further wide excision (see section on nodular melanoma).

The incidence of lymph node metastases in SSM in the radial growth phase is 5% to 10%. Prophylactic lymph node dissection is therefore not indicated.

RADIATION THERAPY

There is very little information in the English language literature on the use of primary radiation therapy for SSM.[27] Only five patients have been treated in Toronto for SSM of the head and neck by radical radiation therapy (Table 27-6). In all five patients, the disease was locally controlled by irradiation; one patient died of distant metastases without local recurrence. Consideration should be given to the use of conventional fractionated irradiation for patients with SSM of the head and neck when there are positive or close margins following excision or when conventional excision with an adequate margin cannot be carried out due to anatomical considerations, age, or medical condition.

NODULAR MELANOMA

Nodular melanoma arising *de novo* or in an SSM is the most virulent form of cutaneous melanoma of the head and neck and is the area in which controversy about management is most marked.

Surgery is recommended as the treatment of choice for nodular melanoma of the head and neck region. Two large surgical series report an overall survival rate of 25% at 5 years, with 50% to 60% of stage I patients and 12% to 30% of stage II patients alive at 5 years.[3,9] Little information exists in the literature specifically on the curative use of irradiation in nodular melanoma. The experience at the Princess Margaret Hospital suggests that local excision followed by high-dose irradiation is an option that deserves further study.[29] Generally, we recommend wide local excision of the primary lesion. Lymph node dissection is recommended only when palpable lymphadenopathy is present, for all levels of nodular melanoma. Local excision plus high-dose irradiation is applied when conventional surgical therapy is not felt to be appropriate because of the medical condition of the patient or because the location of the primary lesion makes wide excision impossible or too mutilating.[29] Irradiation is given for unresectable melanoma in lymph nodes (either primary or recurrent) and is given to patients following lymph node dissection who are thought to have a high risk of recurrence within the neck. (See section on radiation therapy.) Adjuvant chemotherapy or immunotherapy is not used unless the patient is participating in a clinical trial.

SURGERY

Surgical resection of the primary lesion and/or lymph nodes has been accepted and in the majority of reports represents the sole treatment for nodular melanoma of the head and neck for the past 70 years.[3,9,18,44,46,51] With respect to the primary lesion, wide excision with a 3-cm to 5-cm cuff of normal skin around the lesion has been recommended where feasible. Some centers have been recommending less aggressive surgical excisions for lesions thinner than 0.76 mm in maximum vertical height. In this situation, a number of centers have shown that local excision with a 0.5-cm to 1.0-cm margin of normal tissue around the lesion is quite adequate and associated with a very low local recurrence rate.

For the thicker lesions (Breslow thickness >0.75 mm or Clark level 4 or 5), wide excision is still recommended as standard treatment (minimum 2.5-cm to 5-cm margin where anatomically feasible in the neck and scalp).[51] Lesions of the ear and nose are frequently treated by amputation. With such radical excisions, the local recurrence rate is 4% to 15%, although the cosmetic defects produced may be substantial.[3,51] In a series by Storm and co-workers, all patients referred with local recurrences were found on assessment of the initial pathology report to have had an inadequate excision with a margin of less than 2.5 cm.[51] Whether the defect should be covered by primary closure, rotation of flaps, or split-thickness skin grafting depends more on local factors than on any feeling that a particular method of reconstruction results in a higher recurrence rate.[3] Generally, wide excisions on the nose, scalp, or forehead require split-thickness skin grafts for closure.[3]

When palpable lymph nodes are present, the generally accepted method of treatment is radical neck dissection. Frequently, in addition to dissecting the neck contents on the side involved, a superficial parotidectomy and dissection of the parotid area lymph nodes are carried out, particularly when the primary lesion is on the forehead, temple, cheek, or ear. (See Chapter 26, Carcinoma of the Skin, for management of parotid area lymph nodes.) A posterolateral lymph node dissection is frequently carried out for primary lesions on the posterior skin of the ear and the posterior scalp.[3] (See Chapter 5, General Principles for Treatment of Cancers in the Head and Neck: Surgery, for posterior lateral neck dissection.) We are currently studying the use of adjuvant irradiation following surgical dissection of lymph nodes for certain high-risk patients. The survival after radical neck dissection for patients with gross melanoma in regional neck nodes is poor, however, with 5% to 30% surviving 5 years.[3,9,46]

The most controversial area relates to the value of adjuvant elective or prophylactic lymph node dissection in patients with nodular melanoma. No randomized prospective studies have been carried out on melanomas of the head and neck to study the benefit of elective lymph node dissection. There is a general consensus in the literature that the following groups of patients should not have elective lymph node dissection in the absence of clinically palpable nodes: patients with nodular melanoma arising in a preexisting LM; those with thin nodular melanoma (<0.76 mm) arising *de novo* or in an SSM; and elderly patients or those in poor general condition.[3]

The controversy on elective lymph node dissection therefore revolves on the benefit of this procedure in patients with nodular melanoma, arising *de novo* or in an SSM, that is thick (level 3 lesions > 0.76 mm in size, level 4 and 5).

Ballantyne, in a retrospective series of stage IA patients (no palpable lymph nodes, disease confined to the primary site, not recurrent), analyzed 115 patients who did not have an elective lymph node dissection and 75 who did.[3] The reasons for selection of treatment were not given.

Twenty-seven (23%) of 115 patients who did not have an elective lymph node dissection subsequently required therapeutic neck dissection. The overall survival rate for this group was 60.8%. Of 73 patients who underwent elective lymph node dissection, 11 (15%) had positive nodes; the overall survival rate for this group was 77% at 5 years. The differences in survival were due to a lower incidence of distant metastases in the elective dissection group (22% vs. 31%) and a lower incidence of primary recurrence (5% vs. 9%). Olson and co-workers found no difference in survival between those patients receiving elective neck dissection and those who did not.[44] Of particular interest in the Olson study was that skip involvement of nodes was not encountered; if proximal nodes were negative, more distal nodes were also negative. The incidence of occult positive nodes in Olson's series was 23%. When three or more nodes were found in the operative specimen, prognosis was extremely poor (<20%). Others have found that once melanoma has metastasized to regional lymph nodes, this is strongly predictive of the presence of disseminated disease.[21,46]

In view of these findings, it is difficult to justify elective lymph node dissection in any form of nodular melanoma of the head and neck in the absence of a randomized study to test this form of treatment. We have not carried out elective lymph node dissections in the absence of clinically significant palpable lymphadenopathy, since there is little concrete evidence to support the thesis that it improves survival, even for selected patients.

RADIATION THERAPY

It has been repeatedly stated in the literature that nodular melanoma is a radioresistant tumor.[34] Rarely, however, are data provided to justify such an opinion. My colleagues and I have undertaken a detailed historical review on the radiosensitivity of nodular melanoma.[27] Generally, reports quoting radioresistance of melanoma are based on limited experience with orthovoltage irradiation used only when the disease was far advanced and unsuitable for surgery.[27] In Toronto, Richards treated nodular melanomas by local excision followed by high-dose postoperative irradiation (5000 R/10 fractions/2 weeks). The results of Richards' work were analyzed by Dickson in 1958.[17] Of 121 patients treated by local excision and irradiation, 41% were alive and well at 5 years, a result comparable to that achieved by wide local excision during the same time period. In contrast, 71 patients treated by local excision alone had a 20% 5-year survival rate. The reason for this success was probably twofold. First, he was treating a series of patients probably similar to those submitted to surgery rather than a highly selected, unfavorable group of recurrent or palliative cases. Second, by pure chance, Richards was using large doses of radiation per fraction. As a result of Dickson and Richards' work, a limited number of patients with nodular melanoma have been treated by the technique described by Dickson.[17]

There has been a substantial amount of work done on the radiobiology of melanoma in recent years to determine if it is indeed an intrinsically radioresistant tumor.[27] Studies on experimental melanoma lines in cell culture and on human melanoma cell lines grown *in vitro* indicate that the melanoma cell is not intrinsically radioresistant, but that melanoma cells have a large capacity to repair sublethal radiation damage. This would therefore indicate that in order to overcome this effect, large doses per fraction are necessary (270 rad or more). Our own clinical experience plus that of others would tend to support this contention.[23,27,31,45] It is quite apparent that there are major differences in radiosensitivity between different melanomas, since some response is even observed to 200-rad daily fractions.[11] There is also some evidence to suggest that hypoxia may be present in melanomas, and substantial evidence that in some cases melanoma may be slow to regress following irradiation, further contributing to the impression of radioresistance.[27]

There has been only one randomized prospective study carried out on 56 patients with pathologically positive lymph nodes to test whether postoperative irradiation of the neck improves survival for head and neck melanoma.[11] The dissected neck received 5000 rad/28 fractions with a 3- to 4-week split after 2500 rad. Three of 27 irradiated patients developed recurrence in the treatment field. There was only one recurrence in 29 patients treated with neck dissection alone. No survival benefit was seen in the adjuvant irradiation group.

As a result of the historical experience of Dickson and Richards, 16 patients with nodular melanoma of the head and neck were treated with a technique of incisional (14 patients) or excisional (2 patients) biopsy followed by high-dose postoperative irradiation as an alternative to wide excision.[27,29] The results are summarized in Table 27-7. Fourteen of the 16 patients had local control of disease, and 6 of the 14 are alive and well from 2 to 14 years following irradiation.

Another 16 patients were treated with irradiation for locally or regionally recurrent disease following unsuccessful surgery. In contrast to the primary cases, only 2 of the 16 patients with recurrence achieved local/regional control with irradiation, and in 3 additional patients salvage following irradiation failure was achieved with further surgery. Ten died of melanoma and 1 died of intercurrent disease with no melanoma.

Analysis of local control versus irradiation fraction size revealed that local control was 71% if a dose of greater than 400 rad/fraction was used, compared with 25% if less than 400 rad/fraction was used.

The data in the primary cases treated by the Dickson technique indicate that this method of treatment is worthy of further study in nodular melanoma of the head and neck. We continue to use the technique of local excision followed by high-dose postoperative irradiation in selected cases in which, due to the age or medical condition of the patient or the location of the primary lesion, the more traditional wide local excision is too hazardous or would result in a poorer cosmetic result.

The results of irradiation for recurrent head and neck melanoma were less favorable; however, surgical therapy is also relatively ineffective in this situation.[3] Only when there is recurrence of the primary lesion alone can salvage be achieved in a significant proportion of cases by surgery. In our patients with recurrent head and neck melanoma treated by irradiation, we only had three such patients, one of whom had salvage by irradiation.

The disadvantage of the Dickson technique is that it can only be applied to relatively small volumes of tissue (skin and subcutaneous tissue) and is therefore only suitable for treatment of primary disease.[27] *When disease occurs in lymph node–bearing areas, large volumes of tissue must be treated, and the Dickson fractionation regimen is greater than the radiation tolerance for normal tissue.* As a result of this and the belief that large dose-per-fraction irradiation

TABLE 27-7.   Results of Radiation Therapy for Nodular Melanoma of the Head and Neck

Result	No. Patients
No evidence of disease (2 to 14 years)	6
Local failure, dead of melanoma	2
Local control, dead of melanoma:	
Regional and distant	2
Distant only	3
Dead of intercurrent disease, no melanoma	3
Total patients with no local recurrence	14
Total patients treated	16

provided higher response rates in melanoma, a fractionation regimen employing an 800-rad tumor dose as a single dose given on three occasions on day 0, 7, and 21 was initiated in 1975.[35] This "day 0, 7, 21" regimen is useful for treatment of large volumes, such as the entire neck, but once again it is not applicable for systemic metastases in brain, lung, or liver where such radiation doses are above the limits of normal tissue tolerance, although limited volumes of these organs may occasionally be treated in this fashion. *Care also has to be taken with this regimen, since it is above spinal cord tolerance, and generally the dose to the spinal cord is limited to a maximum of 2 fractions of 800 rad.*

Three clinical subtypes of disease have been treated: (1) microscopic residual melanoma following surgery (generally after lymph node dissection); (2) gross residual melanoma (large volume) after surgery; and (3) recurrent melanoma.[35]

The first group consisted of 22 patients who were referred for treatment following complete surgical excision but who were considered to be at high risk for microscopic residual tumor and subsequent development of recurrence in the surgical field. This group included patients who on pathologic assessment of the specimen had a tumor penetrating through the lymph node capsule, multiple nodes involved in the specimen, or one node greater than 3 cm in size with complete destruction of the node by melanoma. Eighteen of the 22 patients so treated have had no recurrence in the irradiated volume to date (12 to 50 months following irradiation) and 10 are alive and well (12 to 50 months following irradiation). The four in-field recurrences all occurred within 15 months of irradiation, and 2 patients died less than 7 months following irradiation with an extremely aggressive form of melanoma that was unresponsive to therapy. The 8 patients who died despite local/regional control of their disease died of metastatic melanoma (6 in less than 15 months following irradiation). This illustrates the highly aggressive nature of some melanomas and emphasizes the need for effective systemic therapy in this group of patients. The results suggested that large dose-per-fraction irradiation reduced the recurrence rate in the surgical field, and randomized prospective studies to test this are indicated.

Thirty-two patients were treated with day 0, 7, 21 radiation therapy with gross residual or recurrent unresectable melanoma. Twelve (37%) had complete remission of frequently massive disease, and 7 are alive and well up to 56 months following irradiation. Only 2 patients had progression of disease within the treated volume within 3 months of irradiation. The response rate is higher than we have previously observed with conventional irradiation, although a randomized comparison has not been done.

Morbidity of the treatment has been low, provided that care is taken to limit the maximum given dose to 825 rad/fraction to avoid excessive fibrosis.[35] We continue to use this fractionation regimen in melanomas of the head and neck for gross residual or unresectable (principally nodal) recurrent melanoma when a large volume (>5 cm of skin and subcutaneous tissue) must be irradiated. It offers good palliation with a much higher complete response rate than achieved by any chemotherapeutic combination currently in use. It is well tolerated, and survival may be prolonged in some patients.

Irradiation is often useful for palliation of distant metastases to brain, bone, and other tissues.

CHEMOTHERAPY AND IMMUNOTHERAPY

A detailed review of chemotherapy for metastatic melanoma is outside the scope of this review and has been published elsewhere.[40] Dacarbazine is the most active single agent in melanoma with response rates of the order of 20% being observed. The complete response rate is 5% or less, significantly poorer than for day 0, 7, 21 irradiation applied to localized masses.

There is little specific information on the use of adjuvant immunotherapy for malignant melanomas of the head and neck with the exception of 1 report of 25 patients treated with adjuvant BCG in head and neck melanoma with lymph node metastases.[20] The results were compared with those of 17 nonrandomized, concurrent patients with neck node metastases. Survival benefit was shown in favor of the patients receiving adjuvant immunotherapy. This benefit has not yet been confirmed in other centers. There have been a number of major randomized studies carried out in both the United States and Canada testing the value of immunotherapy in cutaneous melanoma. Conclusive data supporting improved survival with adjuvant immunotherapy are lacking. At this time, therefore, adjuvant immunotherapy or chemotherapy cannot be recommended for use in head and neck melanoma unless carried out as part of a prospective randomized clinical trial.

Treatment Results

The type of melanoma is a factor of major prognostic importance: With LM, there is essentially a 100% cure rate; with LMM, 95% or better 5-year survival rate; and with SSM, 90% to 95% 5-year survival rate. However, there is an approximately 50% 5-year survival rate for nodular melanoma de novo and 75% 5-year survival rate for nodular melanoma arising in SSM.

Since the prognosis for LM and SSM is so favorable, the majority of series analyzing prognostic factors have limited further analysis to nodular melanoma arising de novo or in SSM.[9,18,21,40,54] In nodular melanoma, prognostic factors of importance include clinical stage and pathologic microstaging of the primary lesion. When the disease is confined to the primary lesion, there is a 50% to 75% 5-year survival rate; with metastases to regional lymph nodes, 5% to 30% 5-year survival rate; and with distant metastases, no 5-year survival. The results are shown by Clark level and Breslow thickness in Table 27-8. Women have a better prognosis than men (by 10% to 20% at 5 years).[21] Patients with scalp or ear melanomas have a poorer prognosis than patients with face melanomas.[21] The more intense the lymphocyte infiltration, the better is the prognosis.[21] Within clinical stage II (lymph node metastases), involvement of more than four nodes, penetration of the lymph node capsule, and node size greater than 5 cm are associated with a poor prognosis.[35,54]

MUCOSAL MELANOMA

Mucosal melanomas of the head and neck represent 0.5% to 2.0% of all malignant melanomas.[42] A review of the literature in 1969 indicated 195 reported cases of mucosal melanoma of the nose and paranasal sinuses.[32] The most common location within the head and neck is the nasal cavity, where melanomas represent 13% to 18% of all malignant tumors.[37,50] In contrast, Lederman reported only 10 melanomas (6%) in 172 ethmoid tumors and only 1 primary melanoma (0.3%) in 356 antral tumors. The Toronto experience is similar, with melanomas representing 14% of all malignant nasal cavity tumors and 2% of all malignant maxillary antral tumors. Melanomas arising in other sites within the head and neck region are rare, with only isolated cases being reported. There is a 2:1 male-to-female inci-

TABLE 27-8.   Results of Treatment According to Pathologic Microstaging (Clinical Stage I)

Pathologic Microstaging	Percentage 5-Yr Survival	Percentage With Lymph Node Metastases
Clark level		
1	100	0
2	94	6–10
3	76	29–33
4	69	32–43
5	57	33–63
Breslow thickness (mm)		
<0.7	95	ND
0.7–1.5	72	ND
≧1.5	53	ND

(ND, no data)

dence ratio, and the majority of cases occur in the sixth and seventh decades.[47]

It is a very rare disease in blacks, although pigmentation of the oral mucosa is very common in black Africans.[47] The reason why mucosal melanoma is predominantly a disease of white North Americans is unclear. Melanoma of the oral cavity is more common among the Japanese and is frequently associated with melanosis. An associated mucosal melanosis is seen less frequently in mucosal melanomas arising in whites.

Pathology

The gross appearance of the tumor is variable. It is commonly a solid, polypoid growth. The color may be white to pink, red, gray, brown, or black. The median diameter of the lesion at the time of diagnosis is 1.5 cm.[32] Microscopically, the lesions are also variable. They generally consist of solid growths of medium-sized cells with large nuclei. In contrast to cutaneous melanomas, lymphocyte infiltration is rarely seen. Melanoma pigment is readily identified with special staining (Fontana stain) in two thirds of specimens. In one third of cases, persistent searching for melanosomes is required, including the use of electron microscopy. Approximately one third of malignant melanomas arising in the nasal cavity are amelanotic. In view of the major differences in treatment and prognosis between mucosal melanoma and other anaplastic malignant tumors of the nasal cavity and paranasal sinuses, it is important for the pathologist to consider melanoma in the differential diagnosis. The correct diagnosis was missed initially in two cases in our series and inappropriate treatment was prescribed.

Patterns of Spread

Local extension is common and may be extensive, with bone destruction and extension from the nasal cavity into the other sinuses; the local patterns of spread are similar to the carcinomas of these regions. (See Chapter 23, Nasal Vestibule, Nasal Cavity, and Paranasal Sinuses, for a full discussion of the anatomy and patterns of spread.) Nodal disease is present in 10% to 23% of patients when first seen.[24,47] Subsequent development of regional lymph node metastases in the absence of local recurrence or disseminated disease is uncommon, occurring in less than 5%.[47] Nodal disease may appear at some time in the course of the disease in up to 25% of patients, although this is most common in association with local recurrence and distant metastases.[24,49] Hence, regional lymph node metastasis in most series has not presented a significant problem in management, and in very few patients did the lymph node metastases *per se* contribute to death.[49] Distant spread to liver, lungs, brain, and subcutaneous tissues is very common and is the major cause of death. Five to 10% of patients have distant metastases at presentation, and the vast majority of patients with this disease ultimately die of distant metastases.[47] There is a continual attrition rate from distant metastases more than 5 years following treatment, and there is little evidence to suggest that this disease can be cured.[22,32]

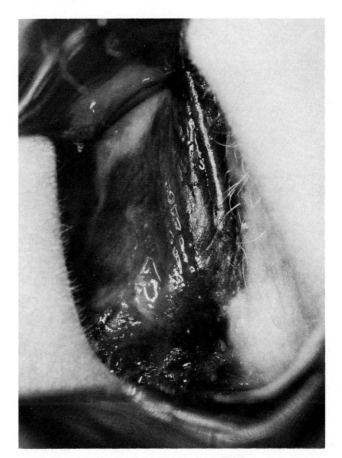

FIG. 27-7. Patient presented with nasal bleeding. Anterior rhinoscopy revealed an area of black melanosis on the nasal septum and a reddish, fleshy nodule at the base of the septum. Biopsy revealed nodular melanoma. The patient was treated with day 0, 7, 21 radiotherapy and went into complete remission for 1 year; a local recurrence developed, which was excised. She was alive and well 2 years later.

Clinical Picture

The clinical picture clearly depends on the site of origin of the melanoma within the head and neck. Nasal melanomas present with the same symptoms as other nasal tumors: bleeding, obstruction, and discharge.[32,49] A typical case is shown in Figure 27-7. Anterior rhinoscopy usually reveals a solid submucosal mass that may be polypoid and that bleeds easily. Approximately 50% of cases are obviously pigmented on clinical assessment. Extensive disease with extension into the sinuses with associated bone destruction is common. Lymph node and distant metastases may be present when the patient is first seen. It is extremely uncommon to see an associated nevus in a melanoma of the nasal cavity. Symptoms may have been present up to 2 years, and it is not uncommon for the patient to have had previous nasal polypectomies.[32]

In the oral cavity, the primary tumor is frequently associated with intraoral melanosis, and the lesion may be

TABLE 27-9. **Results of Radiation Therapy in Mucosal Melanoma of the Head and Neck (25 Patients)**

Result	No. Patients
Incomplete remission (7 patients)	
Dead of melanoma	6
Salvaged by surgery	1
Complete remission (18 patients)	
Alive and well (6 months–3½ years)	5
Local recurrence, dead of melanoma	7
Local control, regional/distant recurrence	2
Alive and well (1)	
Dead of melanoma (1)	
Dead of intercurrent disease, no melanoma	4

TABLE 27-10. **Local Control in Mucosal Melanoma Versus Irradiation Fraction Size**

Dose/Fraction (rad)	No. Controlled/ No. Treated	Duration (months)
0–399	5/18	9–54
≥400	6/7	6–42

quite large, covering an extensive portion of the oral cavity prior to diagnosis.[49] Ulceration and bleeding are the most common symptoms of oral cavity melanoma; significant pain is rarely seen.[49]

Methods of Diagnosis and Staging

The diagnosis of oral cavity melanoma is relatively easy, in view of its typical appearance and frequent association with melanosis. Nasal cavity melanoma can be difficult to diagnose in approximately one third to one half of cases due to clinical lack of pigmentation in one half of cases and absence of melanosomes under light microscopy in one third of cases pathologically.

A deep wedge scalpel biopsy should be made to permit accurate assessment of the degree of thickness and penetration of the primary lesion. When difficulty is encountered in trying to visualize melanosomes under light microscopy, electron microscopy is beneficial to establish the diagnosis. The deep biopsy also permits accurate assessment of the degree of thickness and penetration of the primary lesion.

A summary of staging procedures is essentially the same as shown for cutaneous melanoma (Table 27-3) with the exception of pathologic microstaging, which is of little known benefit in mucosal melanomas. The size of the lesion is also of limited benefit in terms of prognosis. Because the vast majority of patients with this disease die of it, irrespective of extent of disease, the need for an extensive staging system is not great. Most series confine themselves

to a simple clinical staging system in which stage I indicates disease confined to the primary site; stage II, primary lesion plus lymph node metastases; and stage III, distant metastases.

Treatment

We have undertaken a detailed review of the literature on the treatment of this form of melanoma with particular attention to the relative roles of surgery and irradiation.[28] A review of the literature to 1969 revealed an 11% 5-year survival rate and only one patient (0.5%) surviving 10 years.[32] Similarly, a large series of 56 patients from the Mayo Clinic failed to show any evidence of cure in patients with mucosal melanoma.[22] Quite clearly, these data must influence treatment decisions, since treatment for this condition is essentially palliative, although the palliation may be prolonged (5 to 10 years in some cases).

Generally, the tumor has been stated to be radioresistant, but these observations have generally been based on the results in advanced cases.[24, 28, 32, 43] My own experience plus that of others who have used irradiation in earlier stage disease quite clearly shows that the concept of radioresistance is incorrect. Since the most common site for mucosal melanomas of the head and neck is the nasal cavity and the results for primary radical surgery are equivalent to radical radiation therapy in equivalent-stage patients, radiation therapy (day 0, 7, 21) is used as the initial treatment and extensive *en bloc* excision is reserved for those who fail to respond to irradiation or who have recurrence following irradiation. It is difficult to justify major resections initially when the results are so poor; resection should be reserved for use only in those patients for whom irradiation fails.

SURGERY

Surgery has been the recommended primary method of management in most series.[22,24,32,43,49] Generally, wide *en bloc* excision has been recommended for the primary lesion in the absence of regional or distant metastases. Elective lymph node dissection is not indicated, in view of the low incidence of subsequent development of lymph node metastases in the absence of local or distant recurrence and the fact that the most common primary site is in the midline (nasal cavity). There is no evidence that extending the limits of excision has any influence on survival. The majority of long-term survivors with surgery also had irradiation.[28]

Therapeutic neck dissection is indicated for lymph node metastases in the neck in patients who have no evidence of distant metastatic disease.

RADIATION THERAPY

My colleagues and I have reviewed the literature on the irradiation of mucosal melanomas of the head and neck, together with our own experience in Toronto.[28] Only 24 cases reported in the literature (including 12 cases of our own: seven nasal cavity, three oral cavity/oropharynx, and two antral tumors) allow detailed review of the radiation parameters and outcome; these are individually reported in detail elsewhere.[28] The complete remission rate locally is 72% (18 of 25 areas treated, 1 patient being treated twice). Seven of the 18 patients who achieved complete local remission relapsed locally from 9 to 144 months following irradiation (median 36 months). Eleven patients remained in complete remission locally from 9 to 54 months (median follow-up, 20 months). Five are alive and well (6 months to 3½ years); 4 died of intercurrent disease without melanoma; 1 developed an isolated regional recurrence, was treated surgically, and is alive and well; and 1 died of distant metastases with no local/regional disease.

Of 7 patients who failed to completely respond to irradiation, 6 are dead of melanoma and 1 is alive and well following surgery (this patient had a partial response and the residuum was excised). All patients with local recurrence following a complete remission are dead of melanoma. The results are summarized in Table 27-9. In view of the risk of late relapse, none of the patients alive and well following irradiation can be considered cured. It is apparent that those patients who respond to irradiation have a substantially longer survival than those who do not. Local control versus irradiation fraction size in the 25 areas treated is analyzed in Table 27-10. Follow-up is somewhat shorter in the large dose-per-fraction group, since this method of treatment has only been used in recent years. Although patient numbers are small, large dose-per-fraction irradiation seems to produce a greater chance of local control, as in cutaneous melanoma of the head and neck. Our own policy is to use the day 0, 7, 21 regimen discussed in the section on cutaneous melanoma. We have now treated seven mucosal melanomas with this fractionation regimen; it is well tolerated, and we have experienced *no major morbidity, provided that the spinal cord and brain are shielded for the third fraction or the dose to the spinal cord and brain does not exceed 500 rad to 600 rad/fraction.* If the patient does not achieve complete clinical and radiologic remission within 3 months of irradiation, then surgical excision is undertaken, provided that there is no evidence of distant metastases. This approach allows optimization of treatment so that some patients may achieve prolonged palliation without a major resection. For those who fail irradiation and still have localized disease, the surgical option is still available.

The technique used for irradiation depends on the site (e.g., nasal cavity, oral cavity) and extent of the lesion. For small nasal cavity melanomas, frequently a direct anterior electron field or high-energy x-ray field (20 MV to 25 MV) with appropriate bolus is used. For more extensive nasal cavity or sinus tumors, multiple-field techniques are used, generally employing a direct high-energy x-ray beam (8×8 cm to 10×10 cm in size) with bolus and a cutout for the eye combined with two lateral wedged cobalt-60 fields ("bull's-eye technique").[30] The neck is not irradiated.

CHEMOTHERAPY

There is little information in the literature on chemotherapy in mucosal melanoma. Generally, mucosal melanomas respond more poorly to chemotherapy than cutaneous melanomas, and we have not seen a single complete remission with chemotherapy. Generally, dacarbazine or mephalan is tried.

Prognosis

As noted above, the prognosis for mucosal melanomas is extremely poor, and there is a constant attrition rate with time, so that it cannot be considered a curable disease, although prolonged palliation can be obtained in some patients. In a review of the literature until 1969, Holdcraft and Gallagher found an 11% 5-year survival rate and a 0.5% (1 patient) 10-year survival rate.[32] There has been a report of 26 well-documented cases with a 5-year survival rate of 38%.[49]

REFERENCES

1. Andrade R: Circumscribed precancerous melanosis (Dubreuilh). In Andrade R, Gumport SL, Popkin GL, Rees TD (eds): Cancer of the Skin: Biology, Diagnosis, Management, pp 679–702. Philadelphia, WB Saunders, 1976
2. Arma-Szlachcic M, Ott F, Storck H: Zur Strahlentherapie der melanotischen Präcancerosen (Studie anhand von 88 nachkontrollierten Fällen). Hautarzt 21:505–508, 1970
3. Ballantyne AJ: Malignant melanoma of the skin of the head and neck: An analysis of 405 cases. Am J Surg 120:425–431, 1970
4. Becker FF: Lentigo maligna and lentigo maligna melanoma: Recognition and treatment. Arch Otolaryngol 104:352–356, 1978
5. Breslow A, Macht SD: Optimal size of resection margin for thin cutaneous melanoma. Surg Gynecol Obstet 145:691–692, 1977
6. Clark WH Jr, From L, Bernardino EA, Mihm MC Jr: The histogenesis and biologic behavior of primary human malignant melanomas of the skin. Cancer Res 29:705–727, 1969
7. Clark WH Jr, Mihm MC Jr: Lentigo maligna and lentigo-maligna melanoma. Am J Pathol 55:39–67, 1969
8. Clark WH, Reimer RR, Green M, Ainsworth AM, Mastrangelo MJ: Origin of familial malignant melanomas from heritable melanocytic lesions: "The B-K mole syndrome." Arch Dermatol 114:732–738, 1978
9. Conley J, Hamaker RC: Melanoma of the head and neck. Laryngoscope 87:760–764, 1977
10. Costello MJ, Fisher SB, DeFeo CP: Melanotic freckle: Lentigo maligna. AMA Arch Dermatol 80:753–771, 1959
11. Creagan ET, Woods JE, Cupps RE, O'Fallon JR: Radiation therapy for malignant melanoma of the head and neck. Am J Surg 138:604–606, 1979
12. Dancuart F, Harwood AR, Fitzpatrick PJ: The radiotherapy of lentigo maligna and lentigo maligna melanoma of the head and neck. Cancer 45:2279–2283, 1980
13. Davis NC, Beardmore GL, Quinn RL: Primary cutaneous melanoma: A report from the Queensland melanoma project. CA 26:80–107, 1976
14. Davis J, Pack GT, Higgins GK: Melanotic freckle of Hutchinson. Am J Surg 113:457–463, 1967
15. Day CL, Mihm MC, Sober AJ, Fitzpatrick TB, Malt RA: Narrower margins for clinical stage I malignant melanoma. N Engl J Med 306:479–481, 1982
16. DeGroot WP: Provisional results of treatment of the mélanose précancéreuse circonscrite Dubreuilh by Bucky-rays. Dermatologica 136:429–431, 1968
17. Dickson RJ: Malignant melanoma: A combined surgical and radiotherapeutic approach. Am J Roentgenol Radium Ther Nucl Med 79:1063–1070, 1958
18. Donnellan MJ, Seemayer T, Huvos AG, Miké V, Strong EW: Clinicopathologic study of cutaneous melanoma of the head and neck. Am J Surg 124:450–455, 1972
19. Dubreuilh MW: Lentigo malin des vieillards. Bull Soc Fr Dermatol Syphiligr 5:460–467, 1894
20. Eilber FR, Townsend CM Jr, Morton DL: Results of BCG adjuvant immunotherapy for melanoma of the head and neck. Am J Surg 132:476–479, 1976
21. Fitzpatrick PJ, Brown TC, Reid J: Malignant melanoma of the head and neck: A clinicopathological study. Can J Surg 15:90–101, 1972

22. Freedman HM, DeSanto LW, Devine KD, Weiland LH: Malignant melanoma of the nasal cavity and paranasal sinuses. Arch Otolaryngol 97:322–325, 1973

23. Habermalz HJ, Fischer JJ: Radiation therapy of malignant melanoma: Experience with high individual treatment doses. Cancer 38:2258–2262, 1976

24. Harrison DFN: Malignant melanomata of the nasal cavity. Proc R Soc Med 61:13–18, 1968

25. Harwood AR: Conventional radiotherapy in the treatment of lentigo malignum and lentigo malignum melanoma. J Am Acad Dermatol 6:310–316, 1982

26. Harwood AR: Conventional fractionated radiotherapy for 51 patients with lentigo maligna and lentigo maligna melanoma. Int J Radiat Oncol Biol Phys 9:1019–1021, 1983

27. Harwood AR, Cummings BJ: Radiotherapy for malignant melanoma: A re-appraisal. Cancer Treat Rev 8:271–282, 1981

28. Harwood AR, Cummings BJ: Radiotherapy for mucosal melanomas. Int J Radiat Oncol Biol Phys 8:1121–1126, 1982

29. Harwood AR, Dancuart F, Fitzpatrick PJ, Brown TC: Radiotherapy in nonlentiginous melanoma of the head and neck. Cancer 48:2599–2605, 1981

30. Harwood AR, Keane TJ: General principles of irradiation therapy as applied to head and neck cancer. J Otolaryngol 11:69–76, 1982

31. Hellriegel W: Radiation therapy of primary and metastatic melanoma. Ann NY Acad Sci 100:131–141, 1963

32. Holdcraft J, Gallagher JC: Malignant melanomas of the nasal and paranasal sinus mucosa. Ann Otol Rhinol Laryngol 78:5–20, 1969

33. Hutchinson J: On tissue-dotage. Arch Surg (London) 3:315–317, 1892

34. Jansen GT, Westbrook KC: Cancer of the skin. In Suen JY, Myers EN (eds): Cancer of the Head and Neck, p 234. New York, Churchill Livingstone, 1981

35. Johanson C, Harwood AR, Cummings BJ, Quirt I: 0, 7, 21 radiotherapy in nodular melanoma. Cancer 51:226–232, 1983

36. Kopf AW, Bart RS, Gladstein AH: Treatment of melanotic freckle with x-rays. Arch Dermatol 112:801–807, 1976

37. Lederman M: Cancer of the upper jaw and nasal chambers. Proc R Soc Med 62:65–72, 1969

38. Litwin MS, Krementz ET, Mansell PW, Reed RJ: Topical chemotherapy of lentigo meligna with 5-fluorouracil. Cancer 35:721–733, 1975

39. McGovern VJ (ed): Malignant Melanoma. Clinical and Histological Diagnosis. New York, John Wiley & Sons, 1976

40. Mastrangelo MJ, Rosenberg SA, Baker AR, Katz HR: Cutaneous melanoma. In DeVita VT Jr, Hellman S, Rosenberg SA (eds): Cancer: Principles and Practice of Oncology, pp 1124–1170. Philadelphia, JB Lippincott, 1982

41. Miescher G: Über melanotische Präcancerose. Oncologia 7:92–94, 1954

42. Milton GW: Melanoma of the nose and mouth. In Hilton GW (ed): Malignant Melanoma of the Skin and Mucous Membrane, pp 157–163. Edinburgh, Churchill Livingstone, 1977

43. Moore ES, Martin H: Melanoma of the upper respiratory tract and oral cavity. Cancer 8:1167–1176, 1955

44. Olson RM, Woods JE, Soule EH: Regional lymph node management and outcome in 100 patients with head and neck melanoma. Am J Surg 142:470–473, 1981

45. Overgaard J: Radiation treatment of malignant melanoma. Int J Radiat Oncol Biol Phys 6:41–44, 1980

46. Roses DF, Harris MN, Grunberger I, Gumport SL: Selective surgical management of cutaneous melanoma of the head and neck. Ann Surg 192:629–632, 1980

47. Shah JP, Huvos AG, Strong EW: Mucosal melanomas of the head and neck. Am J Surg 134:531–535, 1977

48. Silvers DN: Focus on melanoma. J Dermatol Surg 2:108–110, 1976

49. Snow GB, VanDerEsch EP, VanSlooten EA: Mucosal melanomas of the head and neck. Head Neck Surg 1:24–30, 1978

50. Stewart TS: Nasal malignant melanoma. J Laryngol Otol 65:560–574, 1951

51. Storm FK III, Eilber FR, Morton DL, Clark WH Jr: Malignant melanoma of the head and neck. Head Neck Surg 1:123–128, 1978

52. Thomas JH, Panoussopoulous D, Liesmann GE, Jewell WR, Preston DF: Scintiscans in the evaluation of patients with malignant melanomas. Surg Gynecol Obstet 149:574–576, 1979

53. Wayte DM, Helwig EB: Melanotic freckle of Hutchinson. Cancer 21:893–911, 1968

54. Woods JE, Soule EH, Borkowski JJ: Experience with malignant melanoma of the head and neck. Plast Reconstr Surg 61:64–69, 1978

Major Salivary Gland Tumors

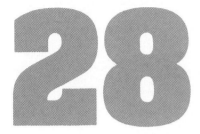

RODNEY R. MILLION
NICHOLAS J. CASSISI

Tumors of the parotid, submandibular, and sublingual glands account for 3% to 4% of all head and neck neoplasms. Radiation-induced neoplasms have been reported.[19] There may be an increased risk of major salivary gland tumors associated with female breast cancer. The average age of patients with malignant neoplasms is 55 years, and for benign tumors it is about 40 years. Approximately one fourth of parotid tumors and one half of submandibular tumors are malignant. About 80% of all major salivary gland tumors occur in the parotid gland.

ANATOMY

Parotid Gland

The parotid ("around the ear") gland, the largest of the major salivary glands, is a relatively simple structure with rather complex and important anatomical relationships (Figs. 28-1 through 28-4).[5] The gland is shaped by the surrounding muscles, bones, vessels, and nerves that come in contact with it. It is roughly L shaped, with its superior border at the zygomatic arch. The anterior border, although variable, does not extend beyond the orifice of the parotid duct, which is located in the buccal mucosa opposite the second maxillary molar tooth. The inferior border is the upper border of the posterior belly of the digastric muscle. Posteriorly and superiorly, the gland lies adjacent to the anterior and inferior portions of the external auditory canal and then extends to the tip of the mastoid. Deep to the anterior portion of the parotid gland is the masseter muscle and the horizontal ramus of the mandible. The retromandibular part of the gland extends between the horizontal ramus of the mandible and the mastoid tip. The deep portion is in relationship to the styloid process with its three attached muscles (the stylohyoid, styloglossus, and stylopharyngeus), the lateral process of C1, the internal pyterygoid muscle, and the contents of the parapharyngeal space. The small superior portion of the parotid gland is tucked between the external auditory canal and the condyle.

That portion of the superficial lobe that lies between the angle of the mandible and the mastoid tip is referred to as the "tail" of the parotid; the tail represents about 20% of the total mass of the gland and measures about 2 cm in diameter and is 1 cm to 2 cm thick. In older, obese patients, the gland becomes infiltrated with fat, enlarges, and becomes more distinct to palpation; the tail of the parotid may then be confused with a lymph node or parotid mass. The fatty parotid tails are usually similar on both sides, which helps in making the diagnosis.

A number of accessory lobes have been reported in a variety of locations, particularly along Stensen's duct.

529

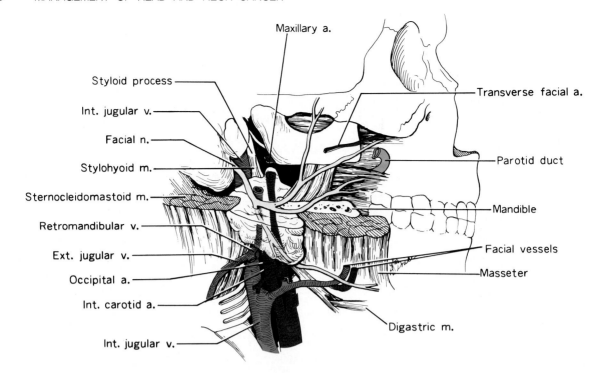

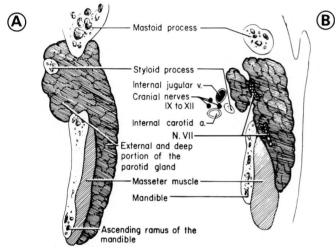

▲
FIG. 28-1.   Regional anatomy of the parotid. (Note: Posterior facial vein is cut away.) The main trunk of the facial nerve divides into the superior branch, which is made up of the temporal, zygomatic, and buccal branches, and the inferior branch, which is made up of the marginal and cervical branches. (Redrawn from Beahrs OH, Adson MA: The surgical anatomy and technic of parotidectomy. Am J Surg 95:885–896, 1958)

◀ **FIG. 28-2.**   Anatomical relationships of the parotid gland (transverse sections): just below ear canal (A), tip of the mastoid (B), and angle of mandible (C). (Modified from Rafla-Demetrious S: Mucous and Salivary Gland Tumours. Springfield, IL, Charles C Thomas, 1970)

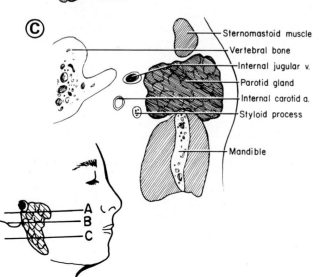

Embedded within the gland are the facial nerve, filaments from the auriculotemporal nerve, part of the external carotid artery and its two terminal branches, the maxillary and superficial temporal arteries, the posterior facial vein, and a number of lymph nodules and nodes (see Fig. 28-1).

The facial nerve courses through the parotid gland, and for this reason the surgeon artificially divides the parotid gland into a lateral (superficial) lobe and a medial (deep) lobe. There is no fascial plane separating the two lobes. The lateral lobe accounts for 70% to 80% of the parotid gland. There is little or no deep lobe lateral to the horizontal ramus of the mandible and masseter muscle, with most of the deep lobe occurring in the retromandibular portion of the gland (Fig. 28-4). Anterior to the ramus of the mandible, the nerve lies on the undersurface of the gland, essentially on the surface of the masseter muscle.[14]

The parotid gland is encompassed by fascia that is sufficiently dense to contain most parotid infections and benign and low-grade malignant tumors until they become massive. The superficial fascia overlying the gland is usually dense and connected by multiple fibrous septa that penetrate deeply into its stroma.[40] However, the fascia between the parotid gland and the conchal and tragal cartilages is quite thin; this is a weak spot through which tumor and infection may penetrate toward the ear canal. The fascia separating the deep lobe from the parapharyngeal space (stylomandibular fascial membrane) is thin, particularly in the upper and lower portion; therefore, tumors involving the deep lobe may produce a mass bulging into the posterolateral pharyngeal wall, tonsil, palate, and nasopharynx.

The facial nerve penetrates the parotid gland almost immediately (within 1 cm or less) on leaving the stylomastoid foramen. It forms extensive anastomoses between the five major branches, but in 13% of cases there are no anastomoses between the terminal nerve branches. Damage to these smaller anastomotic branches does not usually produce significant facial weakness. Anastomoses are frequent between terminal branches of the three temporofacial divisions and less frequent between the two branches of the cervicofacial division.

The auriculotemporal nerve, a branch of the trigeminal nerve, runs deep to the deep lobe of the gland and gives branches that contain parasympathetic fibers to the gland. This nerve provides one route of perineural spread to the base of the skull and the intracranial contents. Section of these branches may contribute to the development of Frey's syndrome (gustatory sweating).

The parotid gland is richly supplied from several arteries, which freely anastomose within the gland. The external carotid artery divides within the deep portion of the gland into the posterior auricular, superficial temporal, and internal maxillary arteries. Branches of the posterior auricular, external facial, transverse facial, and occipital arteries send branches to the gland.

The superficial temporal and internal maxillary veins combine within the gland to form the retromandibular vein (see Fig. 28-1). Both the retromandibular and posterior facial veins usually lie deep to the facial nerve. Branches of these veins may produce troublesome bleeding during

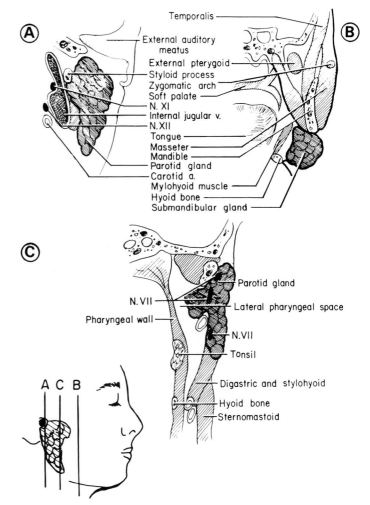

FIG. 28-3. Anatomical relationships of the parotid and submaxillary glands: coronal section behind the mandible (*A*), coronal section through the submaxillary gland (*B*), and coronal section showing relationship of the parotid gland to the parapharyngeal space (*C*). (Modified from Rafla-Demetrious S: Mucous and Salivary Gland Tumours. Springfield, IL, Charles C Thomas, 1970)

FIG. 28-4. Relationships of the facial nerve to the parotid gland, mastoid, and masseter muscle.

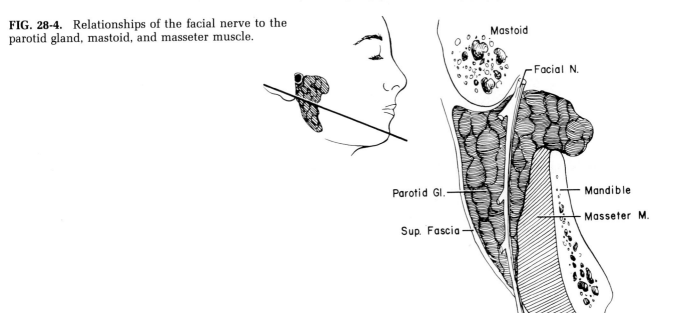

parotidectomy or during a radical neck dissection when the tail of the parotid is transected.

The sensory nerve supply to the parotid skin and part of the pinna is by way of the greater auricular nerve (C2–3). This nerve is usually severed during parotidectomy, causing a permanent loss of sensation in the earlobe, which may be disconcerting to the female (and occasional male) patient who wears earrings. A portion of the greater auricular nerve may be used as a nerve graft to repair the facial nerve.

LYMPHATICS

The parotid area lymph nodes are shown in Figure 28-5. The superficial preauricular nodes, usually one or two in number, lie outside the fascia of the parotid gland and immediately in front of the tragus and in close relationship to the superficial temporal vessels. These lymph nodes drain the skin of the ear, temple, and upper face, including the eye and the nose. They are most frequently involved by metastatic skin cancer (carcinoma and melanoma) and lymphoma but not usually by parotid neoplasms. The superficial preauricular lymph nodes are not true parotid nodes *per se*; secondary invasion of the gland and facial nerve may occur when they are involved by metastatic tumor. (See Chapter 26, Carcinoma of the Skin.)

The preauricular lymph nodes drain either to the superficial lymph nodes (inferior parotid lymph nodes) along the external jugular vein as it crosses the sternocleidomastoid muscle, or they may communicate directly with the internal jugular chain of lymph nodes.

The true parotid lymph nodes are represented by two groups within the fascia of the parotid gland. One group, lying within the substance of the parotid gland, is represented by numerous lymph follicles and four to ten small lymph nodes scattered along the retromandibular, posterior facial, and jugular veins. Thus, they may lie deep to the facial nerve and may not be removed by lateral lobectomy. A second group lies between the gland and the superficial fascia. One or two nodes lie in front of the ear, and one or two between the inferior aspect of the tail of the parotid and the anterior border of the sternocleidomastoid muscle, in association with the external jugular vein. These latter are referred to as the subparotid or tail of parotid lymph nodes. An enlarged subparotid node is difficult to distinguish from a mass originating in the tail of the parotid gland.

Submaxillary and Sublingual Glands

For the anatomy of the submaxillary and sublingual glands, see Chapter 17, Oral Cavity.

FIG. 28-5. Parotid area lymphatics. The superficial preauricular and inferior parotid lymph nodes lie outside the fascia of the parotid gland. The parotid lymph nodes lie between the fascia and the lateral surface of the parotid. There are multiple intraparotid lymph nodules. (Modified from Conley J: Salivary Glands and the Facial Nerve. New York, Grune & Stratton, 1975)

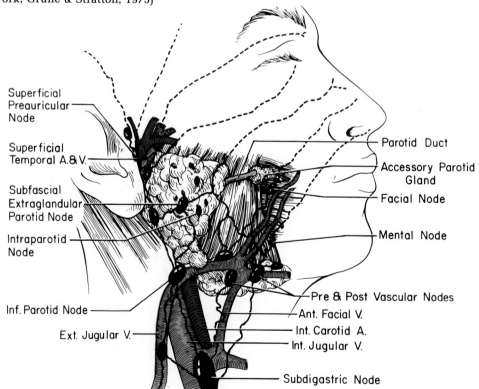

PATHOLOGY

There is a large variety of benign and malignant neoplasms that occur in the major salivary glands. The approximate incidence of the various neoplasms in the parotid gland is given in Table 28-1. The initial diagnosis for parotid masses is most often made by frozen section at the time of exploration. It may be difficult to distinguish between benign and malignant neoplasms on frozen section, and the patient must be advised of this possibility.[28]

Miller and co-workers analyzed the accuracy of frozen-section diagnosis for 132 parotid lesions.[28] The frozen-section diagnosis was the same as the final diagnosis in 110 cases (83%). Six cases (5%) were called benign on frozen section and changed to malignant on final diagnosis. In three instances, the malignant portion of the tumor was not included in the sample taken for frozen section. Fifteen tumors were called malignant on frozen section, and none was changed to benign. A definitive diagnosis could not be given on frozen section in ten cases; four turned out to be malignant and six were benign. There is variability and overlap in the microscopic appearance of this group of neoplasms. The clinical picture should be considered as well in determining the treatment plan.

Benign Tumors

BENIGN MIXED TUMORS

Benign mixed tumors are the most common salivary gland neoplasms. They first appear in patients in their early 20s, with a mean age at presentation of 40 years. Benign mixed tumors may grow to enormous size, but they are usually 2 cm to 7 cm in diameter. Consistency of the mass varies with the relative amount of connective tissue, cartilage, and cystic degeneration. They are discrete, slow-growing neoplasms surrounded by an imperfect pseudocapsule that is traversed by fingers of tumor. Enucleation or removal with a narrow cuff of normal tissue results in recurrence in at least 20%.

The histologic distinction between benign and malignant mixed tumor is only occasionally difficult. Lesions considered benign for many years may unexpectedly become clearly malignant and develop metastases. Some benign mixed tumors recur innumerable times and display a locally aggressive behavior in spite of a benign histologic appearance.

PAPILLARY CYSTADENOMA LYMPHOMATOSUM (WARTHIN'S TUMOR)

A benign tumor, usually 1 cm to 3 cm in diameter, papillary cystadenoma lymphomatosum probably arises from lymphoid elements. It accounts for 5% to 10% of all parotid neoplasms. The tumor is encased by a thin, but complete capsule. It occurs predominantly in the tail of the parotid in older men, is bilateral in approximately 10%, and may be multiple in one or both sides. Recurrences are rare following excision.

BENIGN LYMPHEPITHELIAL LESIONS (GODWIN'S TUMOR)

Benign lymphepithelial lesions account for about 5% of benign lesions. The tumor may be bilateral and is more common in women. Excision may be followed by recurrence.

ONCOCYTOMA

Oncocytoma (oxyphiladenoma) is usually a benign, slow-growing tumor found mostly in an older age-group. The well-circumscribed, encapsulated tumor has a dark appearance reminiscent of melanoma. There are case reports of low-grade malignant oncocytomas.

BASAL CELL ADENOMA

The basal cell adenoma is an uncommon benign lesion appearing in older people. It is histologically and clinically benign and is cured by simple excision. It must be distinguished from basal cell carcinoma of the skin metastatic to parotid lymph nodes.

Malignant Tumors

LOW-GRADE MALIGNANCY

ACINIC CELL CARCINOMA

Acinic cell tumors typically are classified as slow-growing, low-grade neoplasms. They appear in all age-groups and are more common in women. Grossly, they may appear encapsulated, but microscopically some lesions invade contiguous structures such as bone, nerve, skin, and blood vessels.[1,4] This neoplasm should not be considered benign. Batsakis and associates collated ten series reported between the years 1954 and 1979.[4] Ninety-four (37%) of 257 patients developed a local recurrence, and 15% developed metastasis. These tumors will recur (or a new acinic cell carcinoma will develop?) after inadequate removal, sometimes as long as 25 to 30 years after initial treatment. Metastases occur in a significant percentage of cases; histologic grading is unreliable for predicting metastases.

MUCOEPIDERMOID CARCINOMA, LOW GRADE

The majority of mucoepidermoid carcinomas are low-grade, solid or cystic, slow-growing lesions that appear in any age-group. There is little or no capsule, although they are well circumscribed and are readily cured by wide excision. A few tumors act aggressively and may widely infiltrate the normal gland or become fixed to the skin. The mucin produced by the neoplasm may incite inflammatory changes about the edge of the mass.

TABLE 28-1. Relative Frequency of Parotid Neoplasms	
Histology	**Incidence (%)**
Benign mixed tumors	65
Miscellaneous benign tumors	15
Malignant mixed tumors	4
Mucoepidermoid carcinoma	6
Adenoid cystic carcinoma	3
Acinic cell carcinoma	3
Adenocarcinoma	3
Miscellaneous malignant tumors	1

HIGH-GRADE MALIGNANCY

MUCOEPIDERMOID CARCINOMA, HIGH GRADE

A few of the mucoepidermoid carcinomas behave in a very agressive fashion and widely infiltrate the salivary gland and produce lymph node and distant metastases. They may be difficult to distinguish histologically from a high-grade epidermoid carcinoma. Perineural invasion is infrequent, and late recurrences are uncommon.

ADENOCARCINOMA; POORLY DIFFERENTIATED CARCINOMA; ANAPLASTIC CARCINOMA; SQUAMOUS CELL CARCINOMA

These histologies tend to appear late in life and have an aggressive behavior. True squamous cell carcinomas may arise from the salivary glands or their ducts in rare cases; almost all cases are either metastases to the preauricular or parotid lymph nodes from squamous cell carcinoma of the skin[10] or high-grade mucoepidermoid carcinomas that are producing scant amounts of mucin. (See Chapter 26, Carcinoma of the Skin.)

MALIGNANT MIXED TUMORS

Malignant mixed tumors account for 5% or less of all mixed tumors. Mixed tumors may be malignant when first diagnosed. A small percentage of benign mixed tumors probably progress to a frank malignancy and have a very aggressive behavior. The malignant portion may be epithelial only, or all the components may appear malignant. It may be small and discrete or may dominate the mass to the point that recognizable benign mixed tumor elements are difficult to identify. The malignant portion is usually the epithelial component and may appear as an adenocarcinoma, epidermoid carcinoma, or undifferentiated carcinoma, or all types may coexist.

ADENOID CYSTIC CARCINOMA

This neoplasm is uncommon in the major salivary glands. The growth rate varies from slow to rapid. Metastases to regional lymph nodes and distant sites occur. Perineural involvement is a characteristic finding, and facial nerve palsy may be present at the time of diagnosis. Recurrences may appear many years after initial treatment in the slow-growing lesions. The high-grade lesions have a greater proportion of solid epithelial pattern on histologic examination.

PATTERNS OF SPREAD

Parotid Gland

BENIGN MIXED TUMORS

Benign mixed tumors grow by expansion and local infiltration, and because of their slow growth rarely cause facial nerve palsy, although the nerve may be severely stretched by large masses. When incompletely excised, multiple nodules of tumor develop within the surgical bed. The skin may become involved in recurrent lesions by implantation. Bone invasion rarely occurs; a large mass may cause pressure defects of adjacent bone.[30] A sudden increase in the growth rate may indicate a malignant change, although a few benign mixed tumors may intermittently grow rapidly. Facial nerve palsy is an almost certain sign of malignant change.

MALIGNANT TUMORS

The malignant tumor tends to be smaller than the benign lesion. The malignant neoplasms infiltrate the parotid gland, invade the facial nerve or the auriculotemporal nerve, and spread along nerve sheaths. Tumor may invade the adjacent skin, muscles, and bone, depending on the site of origin. Adenoid cystic carcinoma, in particular, infiltrates widely all adjacent tissues without respect for anatomical planes. The external jugular vein may become thrombosed, and the external carotid may be narrowed by compression. Obstruction of the parotid duct is rarely seen. Deep lobe tumors invade the parapharyngeal space and base of the skull and compromise cranial nerves.

Lymph node metastases may occur from all of the malignant neoplasms. Approximately 20% of patients with malignant tumors will have clinically positive or occult metastases in lymph nodes at the time of diagnosis. Low-grade mucoepidermoid carcinoma and acinic cell adenocarcinoma have a low rate of lymph node metastasis. There is little difference in the rate of lymph node metastasis among the various high-grade lesions. The risk for lymph node metastasis increases with recurrent disease.

The risk for lymph node metastasis by anatomical site for 179 malignant major and minor salivary gland tumors is shown in Table 28-2.[32] Approximately one half of the metastases are present at the time of first diagnosis.

Submaxillary Gland

Malignant tumors that extend through the capsule of the submaxillary gland fix the tumor to the adjacent mandible, invade the mylohyoid muscle and eventually the tongue and the lingual and hypoglossal nerves, and extend to the oral cavity or oropharynx. Skin invasion occurs in advanced cases. Lymph node metastases are common. Obstruction of the submaxillary duct is not a feature of malignant or benign tumors.

CLINICAL PICTURE

Parotid Gland

The great majority of patients with either benign or malignant tumors present with a solitary, painless mass that is easily seen and felt just in front of or just below the earlobe. Mild, intermittent pain is associated with a few of the masses, but it does not reliably distinguish between benign and malignant lesions. A more pronounced pain is more often associated with malignant neoplasms or inflammatory conditions. Patients with benign mixed tumors and low-grade malignant tumors may have a history of the presence of a mass for many years with little or no observable growth, and then an increase in size is noticed that brings the patient to the physician. Facial nerve weakness is an infrequent presenting complaint (2% to 3%), but when present it indicates malignancy. Tumors involving the deep lobe may produce dysphagia, sore throat, ear symptoms, headache, and, rarely, cranial nerve palsy or trismus.

An occasional patient will present with a slowly pro-

TABLE 28-2. Incidence of Lymph Node Metastases in Malignant Salivary and Mucous Gland Tumors

Site	No. of Cases With Malignant Tumors	No. of Cases With Lymph Node Metastasis
Parotid gland	66	16 (24%)
Submandibular and sublingual glands	21	8 (38%)
Oral cavity	31	9 (29%)
Upper air passages*	40	4 (10%)
Larynx and trachea	8	1 (12.5%)
Pharynx	6	4 (66%)
Esophagus	1	0 (0%)
Lacrimal glands	6	1 (16.7%)
Totals	179	43

* Including nasopharynx.

(Rafla-Demetrious S: Significance and treatment of lymph node metastases of malignant mucous and salivary gland tumors. Am J Roentgenol Radium Ther Nucl Med 117:595–604, 1973)

gressive facial palsy, which is at first regional and often associated with temporary periods of improvement. The paralysis eventually becomes complete and may be accompanied by mild pain. A complete investigation or multiple investigations fail to disclose a mass or cause. Conley and Selfe reported 14 such cases in which a neoplasm was eventually discovered.[13] The usual culprit was a malignant tumor or neurilemoma adjacent to the nerve in the deep lobe or isthmus. The diagnosis was made by exploration of the extraosseous main trunk of the nerve. Bell's palsy was the most common erroneous diagnosis.

PHYSICAL EXAMINATION

The mobility of the mass depends on its size and location. Minimal to moderate fixation or reduced mobility may occur in both benign and malignant neoplasms and does not distinguish between the two. Tumors presenting in the deep lobe may bulge the palate and lateral pharyngeal wall. Deep lobe tumors may present as a retromandibular mass with little or no bulge into the oropharynx. Most lesions originating in the deep lobe are large at the time of diagnosis and present in both the oropharynx and the upper neck.

Salivary flow is not affected by either benign or malignant tumors.

Advanced malignant lesions may affect the facial nerve. The mandibular branch of the trigeminal nerve may be involved when tumor tracks along the auriculotemporal nerve to the base of the skull; pain is an associated finding. More rarely, the glossopharyngeal, vagus, spinal accessory, and hypoglossal nerves and the sympathetic chain are affected if the parapharyngeal space is invaded.

Tumor may become fixed to the skin or even ulcerate through to the surface.

Submandibular Gland

Both benign and malignant neoplasms present as a mass beneath the mandible. Mild pain is occasionally a feature but does not distinguish between benign and malignant lesions. Moderate to severe pain usually indicates malignancy. Nerve palsy is rarely seen.

PHYSICAL EXAMINATION

Bimanual examination is used to evaluate size, mobility, local extension of the mass, and the presence of stones in the duct. The tumor mass is usually tethered or fixed to the mandible unless quite small. Loss of mobility occurs with both benign and malignant lesions. It is often difficult to distinguish between an enlarged submandibular gland involved with cancer and an enlarged, fixed lymph node involved with cancer. The tumor may infiltrate the skin in malignant lesions.

METHODS OF DIAGNOSIS AND STAGING

Differential Diagnosis

PAROTID GLAND

It is often easy to distinguish nonneoplastic from neoplastic conditions by history, physical examination, and simple diagnostic tests. The distinction between benign and malignant neoplasms is more difficult unless there is obvious nerve palsy, pain, or metastatic cervical lymph nodes.

Gallia and Johnson reviewed 140 patients who eventually underwent parotidectomy for diagnosis.[16] Only 11% had malignant masses; the remainder had benign neoplasms (62%) or nonneoplastic conditions (27%).

Conditions that may be confused with a parotid tumor include the following:

Metastatic cancer, lymphoma, or leukemia involving parotid area lymph nodes
Fatty replacement, tail of parotid
Chronic parotitis
Boeck's sarcoid
Stone in duct
Cysts (branchial cleft, dermoid)
Hypertrophy associated with diabetes

Hypertrophy of masseter muscle, unilateral or bilateral
Neoplasms of the mandible
Prominent transverse process of C1 (atlas)
Penetrating foreign bodies
Hemangioma/lymphangioma
Lipoma

SUBMANDIBULAR GLAND

The differential diagnosis of a submandibular mass centers around inflammatory disease, squamous cell carcinoma metastatic to a lymph node, and a primary neoplasm of the submandibular gland.

Episodic pain and mass are the hallmark of inflammatory disease, but approximately one third of the lesions will be asymptomatic.[15]

Obstructive sialadenitis is a common cause of submandibular gland enlargement. It is caused by stricture of the duct or stone in the duct. There is pain and swelling associated with eating, which recedes after several hours. There may be erythema over the mass. A stone may be palpated in the duct, and occasionally pus can be stripped from the submandibular duct. A sialogram will show the site of the obstruction. Sialolithiasis may be found, however, in the presence of submandibular carcinoma.

A solitary squamous cell carcinoma metastatic to a submandibular lymph node in the absence of an obvious oral cavity primary lesion is uncommon. (See Chapter 16, The Unknown Primary.) A primary submandibular neoplasm, benign or malignant, is a relatively rare event, but failure to recognize the possibility may result in an inappropriate and sometimes disastrous initial step in management.

Gallia and Johnson reviewed 110 submandibular lesions in patients who underwent biopsy.[16] Ninety-three (85%) were nonneoplastic, usually inflamed glands, and 9 (8%) were benign tumors. Eight patients (7%) had malignant lesions, of which 3 were lymphoma, 3 were metastatic carcinoma, and 2 were primary submandibular gland carcinoma.

Radiology*

Since its inception in 1925, the use of sialography for the accurate delineation of salivary gland abnormalities has declined, since the information provided by this procedure, particularly with respect to determining the malignancy of a mass, is frequently distrusted.[9,27,38] To avoid the inaccuracies and diagnostic pitfalls of routine sialography, sialography followed by fluoroscopy and tomography has been tried and is reported to increase the accuracy of detecting and delineating mass lesions of the parotid gland.[21]

Computed tomographic (CT) scanning with intravenous administration of a contrast medium or after retrograde injection of Stensen's duct with a contrast medium has been introduced. The normal CT anatomy of the parotid gland is shown in Figures 28-6 and 28-7.

The parotid and submandibular glands can be outlined with intravenous contrast enhancement and modern rapid CT scanning techniques, or a retrograde parotid sialogram can be done to outline the parotid duct and the gland.

On CT scans *without* simultaneous sialography, the density of the parotid gland is less than that of adjacent muscles

---

* This section was written in conjunction with Derek J. Hamlin, MD.

FIG. 28-6. (*A*) Normal CT scan anatomy of the parotid gland after intravenous contrast injection. The gland (*arrows*) has been largely replaced by fat and appears radiolucent on this examination. On physical examination, a fatty gland feels firm and discrete and resembles an enlarged lymph node. (*IJV*, internal jugular vein; *SCM*, sternocleidomastoid muscle; *RMV*, retromandibular vein; *MAS*, masseter muscle) (*B*) Normal CT-assisted parotid sialogram. Stensen's duct is clearly outlined. The parotid is largely replaced by fat (compare to *A* and to Fig. 28-7). The arrowheads point to the low-density fascial planes that separate the deep lobe and the parapharyngeal space (*B* from Mancuso AA, Hanafee WN: Computed Tomography of the Head and Neck, pp 168–202. Baltimore, Williams & Wilkins, 1981)

---

and usually approaches the density of subcutaneous fat (see Fig. 28-6A). Unfortunately, no particular architectural changes of the fibrous septations within this fat are detectable by CT scanning, and the only structures commonly recognized within the substance of the gland are the branches of the facial vein and the external carotid artery.

CT scanning of the parotid gland finds its major use in determining the extent of deep lobe and parapharyngeal space invasion and in outlining primary deep lobe or parapharyngeal space masses (Figs. 28-8 and 28-9). It is not used routinely for discrete masses limited to the superficial portion of the gland. It may also be indicated to outline the relationships of a large metastatic lymph node in the upper neck.

CT scanning together with simultaneous contrast sialography (CT sialography) may aid in the differentiation between intrinsic and extrinsic lesions and may show the relationships of the tumor mass to the facial nerve.[8,26,35] CT scanning may also aid in the differentiation of benign from malignant neoplasms of the parotid gland. Malignant lesions may have an obvious, lobulated, irregular pattern, with extension into adjacent structures such as the sternocleidomastoid muscle, while benign tumors typically have a rounder, more sharply circumscribed appearance. Very slow growing malignant lesions may infiltrate ducts and glandular elements, causing the gland to fill poorly.[26]

Biopsy Technique

PAROTID GLAND

The biopsy and the definitive surgical treatment are often the same for parotid masses. Lesions lying in the superficial lobe are best biopsied by performing a superficial parotidectomy. Lesions involving both the superficial and deep lobe or just the deep lobe are "biopsied" by total parotidectomy. This approach avoids contamination of the tumor bed. Incisional or excisional biopsy increases the risk of tumor recurrence and facial nerve damage and increases the definitive surgical procedure by necessitating wide removal of the biopsy site.

There are several advocates of fine-needle aspiration for diagnosis; it is essential that the pathologist be familiar with this method. Needle biopsy can be used in the inoperable or recurrent lesion when radiation therapy is the initial treatment.

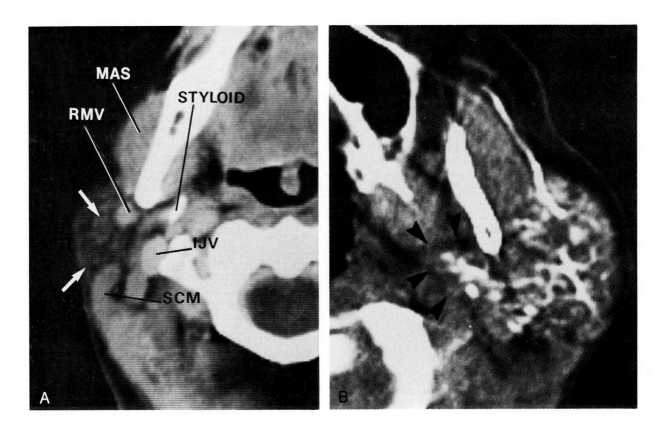

FIG. 28-7. (*A*) Normal CT parotid sialogram (axial section through mastoid tip and just below external ear canal). There is scant deep lobe (*DL*) at this level. Arrow points to stylomastoid foramen. (*S*, styloid process; *MPM*, medial pterygoid muscle) (*B*) Axial section just above the angle of mandible, below the tip of the mastoid. The facial nerve is not visualized on CT scans. There is a small deep lobe extending between the styloid process and the mandible. Stensen's duct is clearly outlined. (*Open arrow*, retromandibular vein [radiolucent area just behind the mandible]; *solid arrow*, sternocleidomastoid muscle indents the parotid gland; *white arrowheads*, fascial planes between deep lobe and parapharyngeal space) (Mancuso AA, Hanafee WN: Computed Tomography of the Head and Neck, pp 168–202. Baltimore, Williams & Wilkins, 1981)

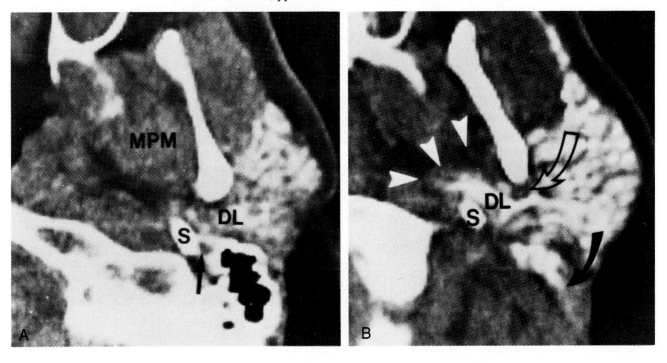

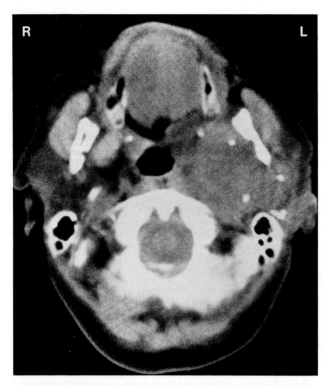

FIG. 28-8. CT scan (with contrast) at level of tip of mastoid and submandibular gland. There is a large adenocarcinoma of the left parotid gland that fills the parapharyngeal space, bulges the soft palate and lateral pharyngeal wall, and extends to tongue muscles.

SUBMANDIBULAR GLAND

Needle biopsy is often misleading and may delay diagnosis. If a careful search of the head and neck area fails to reveal a primary mucosal lesion, the submandibular triangle is dissected as the biopsy procedure. Incisional or excisional biopsy increases the risk of tumor recurrence, even when followed by appropriate treatment, and increases the surgical morbidity by requiring excision of the biopsy site.

Staging

The American Joint Committee (AJCC) staging for salivary gland tumors is listed below.[3]

TX Minimum requirements to assess the primary tumor cannot be met.

T0 No evidence of primary tumor

T1 Tumor 2 cm or less in greatest diameter without significant local extension*

T2 Tumor more than 2 cm but not more than 4 cm in greatest diameter without significant local extension

T3 Tumor more than 4 cm but not more than 6 cm in greatest diameter without local extension

T4A Tumor over 6 cm in greatest diameter without significant local extension

T4B Tumor of any size with significant local extension*

* Significant local extension is defined as evidence of tumor involvement of skin, soft tissues, bone, or the lingual or facial nerves.

The AJCC staging for neck nodes is also listed.

NX Minimum requirements to assess the regional nodes cannot be met.

N0 No evidence of regional lymph node involvement

N1 Evidence of regional lymph node involvement

STAGING PROCEDURES FOR PAROTID TUMORS

The majority of parotid neoplasms are small, benign, discrete lesions in the superficial lobe, and routine roentgenographic studies are not justified. Malignant tumors may invade the mandible, the parapharyngeal space, or

FIG. 28-9. CT scan below the tip of the mastoid of a 67-year-old man who presented with a 3-month history of rapidly enlarging right cheek mass and a 1-week history of sudden increase in size and onset of severe pain in the cheek, radiating to the scalp. There was an 8 × 8-cm fixed parotid mass with early partial facial nerve palsy and a 2-cm hard jugulodigastric lymph node. Diagnosis: Poorly differentiated adenocarcinoma of the parotid. Note that the low-density fascial planes of the right parapharyngeal area are intact. The findings from physical examination suggested that the mass involved the deep lobe and perhaps the parapharyngeal space. The arrow points to an area of subcutaneous change associated either with the incisional biopsy or with tumor extension. The right retromandibular vein (RMV) is displaced laterally by the tumor mass. (PG, normal left parotid gland; SCM, sternocleidomastoid muscle.) Treatment plan: A course of preoperative irradiation was recommended because of the large size, fixation, possible subcutaneous involvement, and poorly differentiated histology. There was 50% regression after 4500 rad/5 weeks, and radiation therapy was discontinued and operation planned. Total parotidectomy was done 6 weeks later. The specimen was negative for residual tumor. The patient died of pulmonary metastases 14 months after the start of treatment with no evidence of local recurrence.

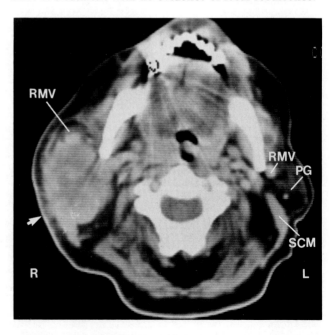

the adjacent areas of the skull such as the mastoid, styloid process, and base of the skull, and appropriate roentgenograms and CT scans are requested if invasion is suspected.[25,35] Occasionally the unsuspecting surgeon will encounter extensive tumor in the retromandibular deep lobe and parapharyngeal space and be unprepared for the management of the situation. A preoperative CT scan may help avoid this problem. Routine sialograms are not recommended to distinguish between malignant and benign neoplasms. Sialograms are only helpful when there is obstruction of the parotid duct, which usually indicates a nonneoplastic process such as a stone, a stricture, or sialectasis.

A Warthin's tumor will concentrate technetium-99m and show as a hot nodule on the scan.

TREATMENT

Selection of Treatment Modality

Surgical resection is the mainstay of treatment for major salivary gland tumors. The concept of adding radiation therapy to the surgical management of salivary gland tumors has been "rediscovered," but it is hardly a new one. Ahlbom concluded in 1935, on the basis of 254 cases managed at the Radiumhemmet, that a combination of surgery and irradiation produced a relatively greater frequency of local control than is customarily seen with surgery or radiation alone.[2] He also observed that the regional lymph nodes should be irradiated along with the primary site.

In 1940, Cade made the same observation from his records, namely that either preoperative or postoperative irradiation or both greatly added to the efficacy of the surgical treatment of this group of tumors.[8]

Rafla-Demetrious reviewed the experience of the Royal Marsden Hospital with major and minor salivary gland tumors in 1970.[33] There are several examples in his monograph of patients managed entirely by radiation therapy, thus demonstrating the radiocurability of both benign and malignant neoplasms.

Jesse and Fletcher of M. D. Anderson Hospital pioneered the concept of combining surgery and radiation therapy to conserve the facial nerve.

PAROTID GLAND

BENIGN TUMORS

Surgical removal with a cuff of normal tissue is the treatment of choice for benign tumors of the parotid gland. This margin can be accomplished by a superficial lobectomy in most cases. Postoperative radiation therapy is considered when there is recognized tumor spill[18] or suspicion of malignancy. The few recurrences after operation alone are usually successfully managed by further resection (see section on management of recurrence), but the risk of facial nerve damage is increased (see section on results of treatment). The routine use of postoperative radiation therapy is not advised, especially in younger patients, because of a slight risk of radiation-induced malignancy and other late complications; these factors must be balanced against the substantial risk of facial nerve loss that is associated with operation for recurrent disease.

LOW- TO MODERATE-GRADE MALIGNANCIES

The majority of low- to moderate-grade malignancies can be managed by a superficial lobectomy; a few require

total parotidectomy. Postoperative irradiation is usually not needed, but it may be used in the case of positive or close margins, rupture of the capsule, surgical dissection close on the facial nerve, or recurrent tumor.

ADENOID CYSTIC CARCINOMA

Microscopically, adenoid cystic carcinoma appears as a low-grade malignancy and often has a history of slow growth, but it is best approached as a *high-grade malignancy*. The management of this histologic type can be one of the most frustrating experiences in oncologic practice; it frequently demonstrates a capricious unpredictable behavior reminiscent of malignant melanoma. A seemingly slow-growing, localized lesion that is completely excised and given generous postoperative radiation therapy may develop late evidence of local/regional recurrence or distant metastasis. These tumors are radiosensitive, but the term *curative* must be applied with caution. The natural history of this tumor requires a treatment strategy that gains the maximum local/regional control and survival with acceptable morbidity. The usual approach is wide surgical resection followed by radiation therapy to a generous volume including the perineural pathways and ipsilateral neck. Wide surgical excision may be easier to recommend than to perform, and positive margins are frequent. Borderline resectable lesions should be considered for preoperative irradiation or even radiation therapy alone.

Asymptomatic, slowly evolving lung metastasis may be present at the time of initial diagnosis or at a time when the patient presents for management of a local or regional recurrence. Some of these patients live several years with distant metastasis, and the approach to management of the local/regional problem may not differ much from the patient without distant metastasis.

HIGH-GRADE TUMORS

High-grade neoplasms are usually managed by parotidectomy and postoperative radiation therapy. The risk for local recurrence is 35% to 55% with surgery alone, and the addition of postoperative irradiation can reduce the risk to about 10%. If the facial nerve is uninvolved by tumor, the mass can sometimes be removed, leaving the nerve intact. If the tumor extends through the isthmus to the deep portion of the gland, the nerve is gently retracted and the deep portion excised in continuity with the superficial lobe. If the tumor grossly invades the facial nerve, one or more branches may have to be sacrificed. If the tumor merely lies adjacent to the nerve, it may be carefully dissected from the nerve; postoperative irradiation is essential in this situation. *There should be no evidence of gross residual tumor around the nerve, however, since the risk of local recurrence in this situation is substantial even with postoperative irradiation.* The irradiation will not necessarily apologize for an incomplete gross resection.

The lymph nodes adjacent to the parotid gland are removed in continuity with the specimen. A neck dissection is added only if the neck lymph nodes are positive. Postoperative irradiation is added in almost all cases, regardless of the margins, and includes the entire ipsilateral neck.

Preoperative radiation therapy should be considered for patients with unresectable disease; the masses become smaller and more discrete and develop a tougher capsule, which aids dissection. Unresectable tumors are treated by radiation therapy alone, usually a combination of external-beam and interstitial implant therapy; a few cures are reported for these cases.

See Chapter 26, Carcinoma of the Skin, for management of squamous cell carcinoma that is metastatic to parotid area lymph nodes.

SUBMANDIBULAR GLAND

Submandibular triangle dissection is used to make the diagnosis. If frozen-section diagnosis shows a malignant lesion and there is no involvement of nerves, mandible, or soft tissues, the operation is concluded, and postoperative irradiation is given to the submandibular bed and ipsilateral neck.

If there is perineural invasion, bone invasion, a clinically positive lymph node, or extension to contiguous soft tissues, then the resection is enlarged to encompass the necessary areas. This resection may include the mandible, mylohyoid muscle, digastric muscle, adjacent floor of the mouth or tongue, and involved nerves and also a neck dissection. Postoperative radiation therapy is added.

Unresectable lesions are biopsied and given preoperative radiation therapy or radiation therapy alone.

Surgical Treatment

LATERAL LOBE PAROTIDECTOMY (SUPERFICIAL PAROTIDECTOMY)

The initial approach for resectable lesions confined to the lateral lobe is exploration and *en bloc* lateral lobectomy for both diagnosis and treatment. Lumpectomy, enucleation, or excisional biopsy should not be done because the recurrence rate, even for benign lesions, is high, the surgical field is violated, and damage to the facial nerve is likely.

An incision is made in the preauricular crease and is then curved under the earlobe posteriorly and then into the upper neck. An anterior cheek flap is developed to expose the fascia and underlying gland. The upper neck and inferior portion of the ear are then exposed. Singleton and Cassisi reported that thin flaps are more likely to produce gustatory sweating than thick flaps.[34] The facial nerve must be identified in all superficial parotidectomies; the nerve is in a more superficial position at the stylomastoid foramen in children. Once this is accomplished, sharp dissection is carried out between the mass and the facial nerve (Fig. 28-10). There is no cleavage plane between the nerve and the gland nor between the lateral lobe and the deep lobe.

The lateral lobectomy may be modified for different anatomical situations. Neoplasms involving the isthmus may attach to the fascia of the masseter, and a cuff of muscle must be included to satisfy the deep margin.

The large, bulky tumors require a modification in approach in order to identify the facial nerve. One method is an inferior dissection to first identify a lower branch and then trace this branch to the main trunk.

TOTAL PAROTIDECTOMY

The term *total parotidectomy* is a slight exaggeration since it is nearly impossible to remove all the glandular tissues. It is quite difficult at the operating table to distinguish

FIG. 28-10. Lateral lobectomy for a mass confined to the left lateral lobe. Sharp dissection proceeds along the course of the facial nerve.

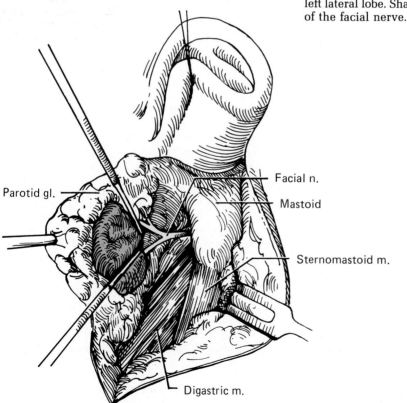

Parotid gl.

Facial n.

Mastoid

Sternomastoid m.

Digastric m.

between the borders of the gland and the adjacent fat; and if the facial nerve is preserved, the term *total* is even less appropriate.

Total parotidectomy includes the entire gland and a cuff of normal tissue, and it may be done with complete sparing of the facial nerve or with partial or complete facial nerve resection. The facial nerve can usually be spared for a benign tumor that extends toward the deep lobe and for some large low-grade or even small, discrete malignant tumors that invade the isthmus or deep lobe. Some normal parotid tissue remains, and the chance of residual tumor is more likely.

A radical parotidectomy may include the facial nerve, the skin, the superficial fascia and platysma muscle, a portion of the masseter, the posterior digastric muscle, a section of the internal pterygoid muscle, the stylohyoid muscle, the tip of the mastoid, a portion of the sternocleidomastoid muscle, and sometimes the external auditory canal. A partial mandibulectomy is required when the tumor is fixed to the periosteum or actually invades the mandible. When pain or paresthesias are present, the auriculotemporal nerve should be explored to the base of the skull.

Either elective neck dissection or elective neck irradiation is advised for high-grade lesions, since the risk of lymph node metastasis is approximately 30%. If the lymph nodes prove positive for disease, a neck dissection is added.

Benign tumors arising from the deep lobe and lateral pharyngeal space are approached by first doing a lateral lobectomy to gain exposure and preserve the facial nerve. The tumor mass is then removed by retracting the branches of the facial nerve. It may be necessary to divide the mandible behind the third molar to expose a large, deep lobe mass.

NERVE GRAFTS

See section on complications of surgical treatment for a discussion of nerve grafts.

Irradiation Technique

Tumors of the salivary glands have an undeserved reputation for being resistant to radiation therapy. There are instances of unresectable or recurrent tumors controlled by radiation therapy alone, and even examples of benign mixed tumors that disappear or remain under control with radiation therapy alone. There appears to be little difference in the response of the various malignant histologies except that the malignant mixed tumor may respond less often than the others.

PAROTID GLAND

Radiation therapy plays its major role as an adjunct to surgery and is usually given postoperatively, although preoperative treatment may be considered in special situations. Postoperative irradiation is indicated for most high-grade lesions, for close or positive margins, for tumors involving the deep lobe, for recurrent tumors, and for multiple regional lymph node metastases.

The minimum treatment volume includes the parotid bed and upper neck nodes. Perineural involvement indicates enlargement of the portals to cover the nerve pathways. The entire neck is electively irradiated for high-grade lesions or for clinically positive nodes in the radical neck dissection specimen. The tumor dose to the primary area is 5000 rad/5 weeks to 6000 rad/6 weeks if there is no gross residual; higher doses are used for gross disease or positive margins. There are no good data to show a difference in dose required for the various histologies, although the treatment failure rate for malignant mixed tumors may be greater.[19,20]

INTERSTITIAL IMPLANT

Interstitial implant may be used for postoperative irradiation if the primary tumor was located in the preauricular portion of the superficial lobe. A modified two-plane implant, the deep plane extended into the retromandibular area, for 6000 rad/6 to 7 days will cover the tumor bed, but it gives inadequate coverage of the perineural spread and borderline coverage of the retromandibular portion of the parotid bed. Alternatively, the interstitial implant may be added as a boost treatment after external beam therapy for a specific area that is at especially high risk due to a positive margin, to boost treatment along a scar, or to boost treatment of a residual mass when irradiating unresectable or locally recurrent disease. The implant is relatively simple to perform. In order to gain the margin along the external ear canal, the needles and sources usually penetrate the tragal cartilage. The implantation of the retromandibular deep lobe area is a blind procedure, but it may be done safely and with ease. (See Fig. 26-17 in Chapter 26).

EXTERNAL BEAM

The majority of patients with parotid gland tumors are managed by external-beam radiation therapy. Two basic techniques are used. One technique involves a wedge pair, with the direction of the portals being superior and inferior to direct the exit dose away from the orbits and oral cavity. Anterior- and posterior-directed wedge portals are often possible as long as the technique avoids exit irradiation to the contralateral orbit. The disadvantage of the angled wedge technique is the inability to shape the fields to avoid irradiation of some normal tissues in the high mastoid–retroauricular area.

A second basic technique uses simple ipsilateral portals that are shaped to fit the anatomy. The usual outline is an L-shaped field. A treatment scheme using a combination of high-energy photons and high-energy electrons produces a homogeneous dose distribution and delivers 3000 rad or less to the opposite salivary glands (see Chapter 15, Treatment Planning for Irradiation of Head and Neck Cancer). This technique is preferred over the wedge-pair portals because of the ability to shape the fields, to reduce them easily when desired, and to attach an ipsilateral antero-posterior neck field easily. In those patients with malignancies with a proclivity to perineural spread, one must include the intraosseous pathway of the facial nerve and the auriculotemporal nerve. Tumor may spread peripherally as well as proximally along the facial nerve so that adequate coverage along the peripheral distribution is also required. When tumor involves the deep lobe or otherwise extends near the midline, it is necessary to use parallel opposed photon portals weighted to the side of the lesion for the first portion of the therapy. Calculation of the brain stem-spinal cord dose must be precise in these plans.

The dose to the parotid bed depends on the level of risk for residual disease: 5000 rad/5 weeks to 6000 rad/6 weeks is prescribed, depending on the risk factors for recurrence;

higher doses are recommended for positive margins or gross residual disease.

An interstitial implant boost is recommended to boost treatment of gross disease whenever technically possible; the dose in these cases will often be 5000 rad to 6000 rad from external-beam therapy plus 2000 rad to 3500 rad from the implant. (See section on parotid area lymph node metastasis in Chapter 26, Carcinoma of the Skin.)

SUBMANDIBULAR GLAND

Ipsilateral external-beam portals are tailored to the extent of disease found in the surgical dissection. The possible sites of local recurrence include the submandibular triangle, adjacent oral cavity, pterygomaxillary fossa, base of the skull, parotid gland, and neck. The entire ipsilateral neck is always included; the opposite neck is not usually treated. The energy used depends on the depth at risk. An electron beam, photon beam, or a combination of both is selected, depending on the situation. The postoperative dose is 6000 rad to 6500 rad/6 to 6½ weeks if there is no gross residual disease. Higher doses are used if there is gross residual disease. An interstitial implant may be added to the tumor bed if residual disease is suspected.

Management of Recurrence

BENIGN MIXED TUMORS

Recurrent benign mixed tumors can usually be successfully reoperated, but the risk of damage or sacrifice of the facial nerve is higher due to the presence of scar tissue from previous operation(s). Postoperative radiation therapy is added on an individualized basis for recurrent or residual disease, especially when recurrence is multinodular. In patients with unresectable benign mixed tumors salvage may be achieved by radiation therapy alone. Observation alone is appropriate for some recurrences.

MALIGNANT TUMORS

Malignant tumors that recur after an operation are managed by reoperation and postoperative radiation therapy or, if unresectable, by radiation therapy alone.

RESULTS OF TREATMENT

Benign Mixed Tumors

Enucleation or excision with a narrow rim of normal tissue will eventually result in a local recurrence rate of approximately 20% after 10 to 15 years of follow-up. Rafla-Demetrious reported only a 2.7% recurrence rate when enucleation or excision was followed by postoperative radiation therapy.[31] Gleave and co-workers reported a 1.9% recurrence rate after capsular dissection in 257 patients and a 1.8% recurrence rate after nerve dissection in 112 patients.[17] Forty-nine patients received postoperative radiation therapy owing to tumor spill or question of malignancy; 1 patient in this group had tumor recurrence.

Piorkowski and Guillamondegui reported on the management of 45 patients who had recurrent benign mixed tumors and 13 patients who had had incomplete excision.[30] The operative procedure was individualized and varied from excision of a tumor nodule to total parotidectomy

with total resection of the facial nerve. Only 3 patients received postoperative radiation therapy. The recurrence rate was 14%. The facial nerve was partially resected in 24% of cases and completely in 16%.

Fee and associates reported 65% surgical success for the first recurrence, while 29% were controlled after the second and 25% after the third recurrence.[15] There was permanent facial nerve paralysis in 29% of cases, usually involving 20% or less of the nerve. Cleave and co-workers reported a 12.6% recurrence rate after operation for recurrent benign mixed tumors of the parotid gland; 41% had postoperative radiation therapy.[17] There was a 12.6% incidence of permanent facial nerve injury.

Death due to benign mixed tumor should be a rare event.

Malignant Tumors

PAROTID GLAND

Woods and co-workers from the Mayo Clinic reported the results for the treatment of 228 malignant parotid tumors for two time periods.[39] There was a minimum 5-year period of observation for all cases. In the period 1940 to 1954, local excision or biopsy followed by irradiation was used in 65% of cases, and all or a portion of the facial nerve was sacrificed in only 20% of cases. The local recurrence rate was 17% (3 of 18) for low-grade carcinomas (low-grade mucoepidermoid and acinic cell) and 58% (38 of 65) for high-grade carcinomas. In the second period (1955 to 1969), local excision or biopsy plus irradiation was used in only 8% of cases, and a total of 17% received postoperative irradiation. The initial operations were more radical, with 34% of patients having all or a portion of the facial nerve removed. The local recurrence rate was 6% (5 of 78) for low-grade carcinomas and 53% (35 of 66) for high-grade carcinomas.

Spiro and colleagues reported the Memorial Sloan-Kettering Hospital results for 288 previously untreated malignant tumors of the parotid gland treated between 1939 and 1968.[36] There were 89 low-grade tumors and 199 high-grade tumors. The incidence of clinically positive lymph nodes on admission in the patients with high-grade tumors was 19%; the incidence of occult disease revealed in neck dissection specimens was 8%. An additional 8% of the patients later developed metastatic disease in the neck. The overall risk for neck disease for patients with high-grade carcinomas was therefore 35%. Curative resection was attempted in 264 patients; only 12 patients received postoperative radiation therapy. The sites of recurrence by stage are shown in Table 28-3. Local recurrence was recorded in 27% of cases. All but two of the patients with neck failure also had recurrence at the primary site. The local recurrence rate for mobile, solitary lesions 1 cm to 3 cm in size (stage I) is only 7%. The recurrence rate increases to 21% for 3-cm to 6-cm masses (stage II), which may be mobile or partially fixed. The advanced lesions (stage III), which were almost all high-grade lesions, were larger than 6 cm, or had multiple tumor masses, ulceration, deep fixation, facial nerve palsy, or clinically positive lymph nodes, had a 58% rate of local failure. Thirty-four patients were treated for recurrent disease, and in fifteen the disease was controlled. Prognostic factors are listed in Table 28-4.[36] Low histologic grade and early stage promised a better prognosis, but the site of origin within the gland (i.e., body, tail, or deep lobe) was irrelevant to prognosis.

Guillamondegui and colleagues reported the M. D. An-

TABLE 28-3.   Treatment Failure According to Stage*

Disease	Stage I (104 Patients)	Stage II (83 Patients)	Stage III (99 Patients)	Total (286 Patients)†
Local recurrence	7 (7%)	17 (21%)	46 (58%)	70 (27%)
Uncontrolled neck disease	1 (1%)	8 (10%)	26 (33%)	35‡ (13%)
Distant metastasis	2 (2%)	8 (10%)	31 (39%)	41§ (16%)
No information or palliation only	1	3	20	24

* See reference cited in credit line for staging system.
† Excluded two unstaged cases.
‡ All but two had local recurrence also.
§ Local disease controlled in 13 patients.

(Spiro RH, Huvos AG, Strong EW: Cancer of the parotid gland: A clinicopathologic study of 288 primary cases. Am J Surg 130:452–459, 1975)

TABLE 28-4.   Malignant Tumors of the Parotid: Factors Affecting 5-Year Absolute Cure Rate (288 Patients)

Factor	No. Patients	No Evidence of Disease at 5 Years (%)
Facial nerve intact	212	66
Nerve palsy	43	14
Tumor spill	32	58
No tumor spill	256	50
Neck negative (N0)	157	74
Neck positive (N+) on admission	57	9
Neck positive (N+) delayed	18	17
No local recurrence	194	79
Local recurrence	71	21

Note: Memorial Sloan-Kettering data; patients treated 1939–1968.
(Modified from Spiro RH, Huvos AG, Strong EW: Cancer of the parotid gland: A clinicopathologic study of 288 primary cases. Am J Surg 130:452–459, 1975)

derson Hospital results for 120 previously untreated malignant parotid tumors that were treated between 1944 and 1965.[18] The period of observation ranged from 7 to 28 years. Surgery was the initial treatment in 104 patients, surgery and postoperative radiation therapy in 10 patients, and radiation therapy in 6 patients. The local recurrence rate after surgery alone was 8% for 38 low-grade tumors, and all 3 failures were controlled. The local recurrence rate after surgery alone was 35% for 66 high-grade carcinomas; 3 of the recurrences were controlled with subsequent treatment for an ultimate local failure rate of 30%. The absolute 5-year survival rate for each histology is shown in Table 28-5.

McNaney and co-workers reported the M. D. Anderson Hospital experience for 77 patients with malignant parotid tumors who received postoperative radiation therapy.[24] Parotidectomy was performed for a *de novo* tumor in 54 patients (70%) and for a recurrent tumor in 23 patients (30%). Patients with a history of more than two surgical procedures for parotid tumor were excluded. There was a minimum follow-up of 3 years; follow-up was greater than 5 years in 81% and greater than 10 years in 27% of the patients. Table 28-6 shows the sites of local–regional failures according to the estimated extent of residual dis-

ease after parotidectomy. The overall incidence of local failure was 8% (6 of 77), and the incidence of neck failure alone was 5% (4 of 77). There have been no failures after 4 years of observation. There were no local or regional failures in the 14 patients with low-grade lesions. Therefore, the local failure rate for high-grade tumors was 10% (6 of 63). Analysis of local recurrence according to the extent of facial nerve sacrifice showed 1 local failure in 35 cases in which the nerve was preserved, 1 local failure in 21 cases after partial facial nerve resection, and 3 local failures in 21 cases after total resection of the nerve. Distant metastases developed in 18 patients (23%).

Black and co-workers reviewed the results of 62 cases of adenoid cystic carcinoma managed at the Princess Margaret Hospital between 1957 and 1974.[6] Fifty cases were in major salivary glands and twelve were in minor salivary glands. Ten percent had clinically positive lymph nodes on admission, and another ten percent subsequently developed positive lymph nodes. The results by method of treatment are shown in Table 28-7.[6] The postoperative dose was 5000 rad/4 weeks. The actuarial 5- and 10-year survival rates were 78% and 57%, respectively. The 10-year survival rate with lesions less than 3 cm was 73% and for those greater than 3 cm it was 38%. The lesions

TABLE 28-5. Parotid Cancer: Absolute 5-Year Survival— 120 Patients

Histology	No. Patients	5-Year Survival (%)
Acinic cell	12	92
Mucoepidermoid (low grade)	28	76
Adenocarcinoma	12	66
Malignant mixed	27	50
Adenoid cystic	10	50
Squamous cell	6	50
Mucoepidermoid (high grade)	13	46
Undifferentiated	12	33

Note: M. D. Anderson Hospital data; patients treated 1944–1965.

(Guillamondegui OM, Byers RM, Luna MA, Chiminazzo H Jr, Jesse RH, Fletcher GH: Aggressive surgery in treatment for parotid cancer: The role of adjunctive postoperative radiotherapy. Am J Roentgenol Radium Ther Nucl Med 123:49–54, 1975. Copyright © 1975, American Roentgen Ray Society)

TABLE 28-6. Postoperative Radiation Therapy in Malignant Tumors of the Parotid Gland: Local–Regional Failures by Extent of Residual Disease

Residual Disease	No. Patients	Site of Failure		
		Primary Site	Neck	Primary Site and Neck
Gross (any grade)	14	1	1	0
Microscopic (any grade)	26	2	1	0
High grade (good margin)	16	1	2	0
Unknown grade (good margin)	17	1	0	1
Low grade (questionable margin)	4	0	0	0
Total	77	5	4	1

(Adapted with permission from McNaney D, McNeese MD, Guillamondegui OM, Fletcher GH, Oswald MJ: Postoperative irradiation in malignant epithelial tumors of the parotid. Int J Radiat Oncol Biol Phys, in press 1983. Copyright © 1983, Pergamon Press, Ltd.)

TABLE 28-7. Adenoid Cystic Carcinoma

Initial Therapy	No. Patients	Persistence After Therapy	Local Recurrence	Salvage (Surgery + Radiation Therapy)	Neck Recurrence With Primary Lesion Controlled	Distant Metastases	No Evidence of Disease (5–20 Years)
Surgery	19	2	11/17	5	0	0	6
Surgery + radiation therapy	35	0	6	0	2	4	23
Radiation therapy	8	3	4/5	0	1†		0

* Major salivary glands, 50 cases; minor salivary glands, 12 cases.
† Salvage by surgery and radiation therapy.
Note: Data from Princess Margaret Hospital, Toronto.

(Modified from Black KM, Fitzpatrick PJ, Palmer JA: Adenoid cystic carcinoma of the salivary glands. Can J Surg 23:32–35, 1980)

TABLE 28-8. Morbidity After Treatment of Benign Mixed Tumors (BMT) of the Parotid

Disorder	New BMT (369 Cases)	Recurrent BMT (103 Cases)
Facial nerve paresis		
Temporary	15%	21.4%
Permanent	1.3%	12.6%
Frey's syndrome	11.1%	28%
Amputation neuroma	5.7%	9.7%
Salivary fistula	0.2%	1.94%
Radiation-induced malignancy	0	0.97%

(Adapted from Gleave EN, Whittaker JS, Nicholson A: Salivary tumors: Experience over thirty years. Clin Otolaryngol 4:247–257, 1979)

in all six survivors treated by surgery alone were less than 3 cm. Twenty-three patients developed pulmonary metastasis. Eleven survived for 3 years, and one is asymptomatic after 7 years. Six patients were treated by chemotherapy without objective response.

Tapley reported the M. D. Anderson Hospital results for 13 unresectable malignant parotid tumors treated by radiation therapy.[37] Only 3 patients were observed to develop local recurrence, but 8 developed distant metastases. A single patient was alive, free of disease, at 5 years. Tapley also analyzed 38 patients treated by radiation therapy for recurrent disease after initial surgery. Twenty-four percent developed local recurrence. Eight patients (21%) were living, free of disease, for 3 to 20 years.

SUBMANDIBULAR GLAND

Byers and associates reported the results of treatment for 22 malignant tumors of the submandibular gland with no prior therapy.[7] Treatment was resection followed selectively by postoperative irradiation. The local control rate was 64%, and the survival rate was 50%.

FOLLOW-UP POLICY

Late recurrences develop in the benign mixed tumors, acinic cell carcinoma, and adenoid cystic carcinoma, requiring lifetime follow-up. Neurologic symptoms or signs in the absence of physical findings of recurrent disease are often the harbinger of perineural recurrence.

COMPLICATIONS OF TREATMENT

Surgical Treatment

BENIGN MIXED TUMORS

Gleave and co-workers reported the operative complications for 369 new and 103 recurrent benign mixed tumors of the parotid gland (Table 28-8).[17] Postoperative irradiation was used in 13% of new cases and 41% of recurrent cases.

Amputation neuromas occur in 5% to 10% of cases, but they seldom require excision unless constant irritation from clothing causes symptoms.

MALIGNANT TUMORS

Loss of sensation in the earlobe after surgical treatment of a malignant tumor is a minor annoyance, particularly to women.

Gustatory sweating (Frey's syndrome) occurs in 5% to 25% of patients after parotidectomy, but it can be reduced by cutting thicker skin flaps.[34] This problem uncommonly requires treatment, but it can sometimes be managed with a topical application of scopolamine. Symptoms usually decrease with time. Tympanic neurectomy is reasonably successful in controlling the syndrome when it is sufficiently annoying.

Temporary paresis of the facial nerve occurs in approximately 50% of uncomplicated lateral lobectomies due to intraoperative manipulation. Some degree of paresis may be expected in nearly all parotidectomies performed for more complicated problems. Recovery normally occurs in 1 to 6 months; it is unknown whether postoperative radiation therapy slows recovery, but we have observed gradual recovery of nerve function even during the course of irradiation.

If there is unexpected complete paralysis in the immediate postoperative period, it may be necessary to reexplore the nerve to exclude the possibility that the nerve was inadvertently severed or ligated, and if so, to repair the nerve immediately. If one or more branches or the main trunk has been resected, a decision must be made regarding immediate grafting. If postoperative radiation therapy is not to be added, then immediate nerve graft is usually preferred. However, if postoperative radiation therapy is to be added, there is mixed opinion as to the likelihood of success.[11,12,22,23,29]

Pillsbury and Fisch studied nine patients treated by facial nerve graft and postoperative radiation therapy.[29] Facial movements were reduced from an average of 70% of normal without radiation therapy to 25% of normal. They recommend the use of fascia lata slings and muscle transfer to restore facial symmetry as an alternative to nerve grafting when irradiation is recommended. If nerve grafting has been done, it would seem prudent to wait as long as is practical before starting the radiation therapy.

There is little reported experience with delayed nerve grafting after postoperative irradiation. Delayed nerve grafting is difficult in unirradiated patients owing to scarring in the surgical bed, and the additional fibrosis incurred by radiation therapy would make it nearly impossible.

A few cases have been reported of return of facial movement without grafting after complete resection of the trunk of the facial nerve.[12]

Radiation Therapy

Xerostomia is usually avoided by techniques that spare the contralateral salivary tissues, but it occurs to a moderate degree in some cases even with techniques that restrict the dose to the contralateral salivary tissues to 3000 rad or less.

There may be trismus due to fibrosis of the masseter and pterygoid muscles. The temporomandibular joint almost always receives a high dose but seldom develops symptomatic ankylosis.

Serous otitis media may occur, and a dry ear canal occurs in nearly all cases.

Localized hair loss may occur with some techniques.

Radiation damage to the facial nerve has not been observed even with doses in the range of 8000 rad to 9000 rad; however, other motor nerves have shown late-onset radiation-induced neuropathy, and presumably the facial nerve is not immune to this risk. Brain stem injuries have been reported.

Osteoradionecrosis of the mandible is infrequent.

REFERENCES

1. Abrams AM, Cornyn J, Scofield HH, Hansen LS: Acinic cell adenocarcinoma of the major salivary glands: A clinicopathologic study of 77 cases. Cancer 18:1145–1162, 1965
2. Ahlbom HE: Mucous and salivary gland tumors: A clinical study with special reference to radiotherapy, based on 254 cases treated at the Radiumhemmet, Stockholm. Stockholm, Acta Radiol [Suppl] 23:1–78, 1935
3. American Joint Committee on Cancer: Manual for Staging of Cancer, 2nd ed, pp 49–54. Philadelphia, JB Lippincott, 1983
4. Batsakis JG, Chinn EK, Weimert TA, Work WP, Krase CJ: Acinic cell carcinoma: A clinicopathologic study of thirty-five cases. J Laryngol Otol 93:325–340, 1979
5. Beahrs OH, Adson MA: The surgical anatomy and technic of parotidectomy. Am J Surg 95:885–896, 1958
6. Black KM, Fitzpatrick PJ, Palmer JA: Adenoid cystic carcinoma of the salivary glands. Can J Surg 23:32–35, 1980
7. Byers RM, Jesse RH, Guillamondegui OM, Luna MA: Malignant tumors of the submaxillary gland. Am J Surg 126:458–463, 1973
8. Cade S: Malignant Disease and its Treatment by Radium, ed 1, vol II, p 366. Baltimore, Williams & Wilkins, 1940
9. Calcaterra TC, Hemenway WG, Hansen GC, Hanafee WN: The value of sialography in the diagnosis of parotid tumors. Arch Otolaryngol 103:727–729, 1977
10. Cassisi NJ, Dickerson DR, Million RR: Squamous cell carcinoma of the skin metastatic to parotid nodes. Arch Otolaryngol 104:336–339, 1978
11. Conley JJ: Facial nerve grafting. Arch Otolaryngol 73:322–327, 1961
12. Conley JJ: Salivary Glands and the Facial Nerve, pp 12, 302, 349. New York, Grune & Stratton, 1975
13. Conley J, Selfe RW: Occult neoplasms in facial paralysis. Laryngoscope 91:205–210, 1981
14. Davis RA, Anson BJ, Budinger JM, Kurth LRE: Surgical anatomy of the facial nerve and parotid gland based upon a study of 350 cervicofacial halves. Surg Gynecol Obstet 102:385–412, 1956
15. Fee WE Jr, Goffinet DR, Calcaterra TC: Recurrent mixed tumors of the parotid gland: Results of surgical therapy. Laryngoscope 88:265–273, 1978
16. Gallia LJ, Johnson JT: The incidence of neoplastic versus inflammatory disease in major salivary-gland masses diagnosed by surgery. Laryngoscope 91:512–516, 1981
17. Gleave EN, Whittaker JS, Nicholson A: Salivary tumours: Experience over thirty years. Clin Otolaryngol 4:247–257, 1979
18. Guillamondegui OM, Byers RM, Luna MA, Chiminazzo H Jr, Jesse RH, Fletcher GH: Aggressive surgery in treatment for parotid cancer: The role of adjunctive postoperative radiotherapy. Am J Roentgenol Radium Ther Nucl Med 123:49–54, 1975
19. Katz AD: Unusual lesions of the parotid gland. J Surg Oncol 7:219–235, 1975
20. King JJ, Fletcher GH: Malignant tumors of the major salivary glands. Radiology 100:381–384, 1971
21. Kushner DC, Weber AL: Sialography of salivary gland tumors with fluoroscopy and tomography. AJR 130:941–944, 1978
22. Lathrop FD: Management of the facial nerve during operations on the parotid gland. Ann Otol Rhinol Laryngol 72:780–801, 1963
23. McGuirt WF, McCabe BF: Effect of radiation therapy on facial nerve cable autografts. Laryngoscope 87:415–428, 1977
24. McNaney D, McNeese MD, Guillamondegui OM, Fletcher GH, Oswald MJ: Postoperative irradiation in malignant epithelial tumors of the parotid. Int J Radiat Oncol Biol Phys (in press)
25. Mancuso AA, Hanafee WN: Computed Tomography of the Head and Neck, pp 168–202. Baltimore, Williams & Wilkins, 1981
26. Mancuso A, Rice D, Hanafee W: Computed tomography of the parotid gland during contrast sialography. Radiology 132:211–213, 1979
27. Meine FJ, Woloshen HJ: Radiologic diagnosis of salivary gland tumors. Radiol Clin North Am 8:475–485, 1970
28. Miller RH, Calcaterra TC, Paglia DE: Accuracy of frozen section diagnosis of parotid lesions. Ann Otol Rhinol Laryngol 88:573–576, 1979
29. Pillsbury HC, Fisch U: Extratemporal facial nerve grafting and radiotherapy. Arch Otolaryngol 105:441–446, 1979
30. Piorkowski RJ, Guillamondegui OM: Is aggressive surgical treatment indicated for recurrent benign mixed tumors of the parotid gland? Am J Surg 142:434–436, 1981
31. Rafla-Demetrious S: Submaxillary gland tumors. Cancer 26:821–826, 1970
32. Rafla-Demetrious S: Significance and treatment of lymph node metastases of malignant mucous and salivary gland tumors. Am J Roentgenol Radium Ther Nucl Med 117:595–604, 1973
33. Rafla-Demetrious S: Mucous and Salivary Gland Tumours, pp 26–32. Springfield, IL, Charles C Thomas, 1970
34. Singleton GT, Cassisi NJ: Frey's syndrome: Incidence related to skin flap thickness in parotidectomy. Laryngoscope 90:1636–1639, 1980
35. Som PM, Biller HF: The combined CT-sialogram. Radiology 135:387–390, 1980
36. Spiro RH, Huvos AG, Strong EW: Cancer of the parotid gland: A clinicopathologic study of 288 primary cases. Am J Surg 130:452–459, 1975
37. Tapley ND: Irradiation treatment of malignant tumors of the salivary glands. Ear Nose Throat J 56:110–114, 1977
38. White IL: Sialoangiography: X-ray visualization of major salivary glands. Laryngoscope 82:2032–2049, 1972
39. Woods JE, Chong GC, Beahrs OH: Experience with 1360 primary parotid tumors. Am J Surg 130:460–462, 1975
40. Work WP, Gates GA: Tumors of the parotid gland and parapharyngeal space. Otolaryngol Clin North Am, pp 497–514, October 1969

Minor Salivary Gland Tumors

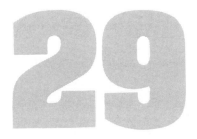

RODNEY R. MILLION
NICHOLAS J. CASSISI

Tumors of minor salivary gland origin are uncommon, accounting for 2% to 3% of all malignant neoplasms of the upper aerodigestive tract. They may appear at any age, but their presentation is uncommon before age 20 and rare under age 10. They occur most often in the oral cavity, nasal cavity, and paranasal sinuses. Thus, the site of origin is related more to the population density of the minor salivary glands in a particular tissue than to any environmental factor. The adenocarcinomas of the nasal cavity are reported to be associated with certain occupations (see Chapter 23, Nasal Vestibule, Nasal Cavity, and Paranasal Sinuses).

ANATOMY

Minor salivary glands are ubiquitous in the mucosa of the upper aerodigestive tract, with the exception of the gingivae and the anterior portion of the hard palate, in which they are absent. The glands are distributed on the undersurface of the anterior and lateral oral tongue and on the base of the tongue. Aberrant salivary tissue is sometimes seen in lymph nodes, in the body of the mandible just behind the third molar teeth, in the vestigial remnant of the nasopalatine canal that lies in the anterior maxilla, in the middle ear, in the lower neck, in the sternoclavicular joint, in the thyroglossal duct, and at other sites.

PATHOLOGY

Approximately one half of minor salivary gland tumors are malignant. The histologic varieties of malignant tumors include adenoid cystic carcinoma, mucoepidermoid carcinoma, adenocarcinoma, and malignant mixed, acinic cell, and oncocytic carcinomas. About two thirds of the malignant tumors are adenoid cystic. The mucoepidermoid carcinoma and adenocarcinoma arise predominantly in the oral cavity (Table 29-1).[10]

The great majority of benign tumors are benign mixed tumors (Fig. 29-1) with a sprinkling of intraductal papillomas, papillary cystadenomas, basal cell adenomas,[12] and benign oncocytomas.

PATTERNS OF SPREAD

The sites of origin for minor salivary gland tumors in 118 patients are listed in Table 29-1. Tongue lesions usually originate from the base of the tongue. There are no minor salivary glands in the anterior one half or the midline of the hard palate, so tumors arise on the posterolateral hard palate and all of the soft palate. The site of origin for salivary gland tumors of the floor

TABLE 29-1.   Site of Presentation and Histology for 118 Malignant Minor Salivary Gland Tumors

Site	No. Patients	Adenoid Cystic	Mucoepidermoid		Adeno-carcinoma	Malignant Mixed	Acinic Cell
			High Grade	Low Grade			
Lip	2	1	0	0	1	0	0
Buccal mucosa	16	9	1	3	3	0	0
Tongue	17	10	2	1	4	0	0
Floor of mouth	22	10	4	3	4	0	1
Gingivae	13	3	5	1	4	0	0
Palate	23	15	1	3	4	0	0
Paranasal sinuses and nasal cavity	20	16	1	1	2	0	0
Nasopharynx and pharynx	3	1	0	1	0	1	0
Trachea	1	1	0	0	0	0	0
Larynx	1	1	0	0	0	0	0
Total	118	67	14	13	22	1	1

Note: M.D. Anderson Hospital data; patients treated 1/70–2/78.
(Schell S, Barkley HT Jr, Chiminazzo H Jr: Treatment of malignant minor salivary gland tumors, in preparation, 1983)

FIG. 29-1. Benign mixed tumor of hard palate. The patient was elderly and elected no treatment.

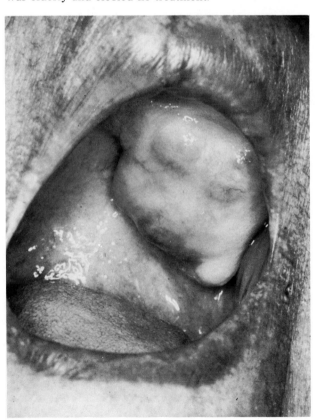

of the mouth is moot—either the sublingual gland or a minor salivary gland.

These tumors grow by extensive local infiltration with eventual invasion of muscle, bone, cartilage, nerves, and blood vessels. Perineural spread is a common feature, par-ticularly for adenoid cystic carcinoma. The tumor may track both centrally and peripherally along nerves, but the central spread is the more common event because most lesions arise near the terminations of the nerves. Extension along nerves eventually may traverse the base of the skull and present intracranially, although this spread pattern may not be recognized for several years after the original treatment. Tumor growth along a nerve may be characterized by skipped areas, so that a normal nerve segment is no assurance of free margins. Adenoid cystic carcinoma may grow along the haversian systems of bone without showing bone destruction.[8]

Lymphatic Spread

The risk for lymph node metastases is related to the site of origin and the grade of the tumor. Lymph node metas-tases are most likely from sites with a dense capillary lym-phatic network (*e.g.*, nasopharynx, tonsillar fossa, base of the tongue). The incidence of lymph node metastasis was 59% (10 of 17) in patients with oropharynx or nasopharynx primaries and predictably low for the hard palate, 7% (1 of 14) and paranasal sinuses, 6% (20 of 34).[7] The patterns of spread are similar to those for squamous cell carcinoma.

Adenoid cystic carcinoma, low-grade mucoepidermoid carcinoma, and acinic cell carcinoma are at low risk to spread to lymph nodes. Approximately 20% of adenoid cystic carcinomas spread to lymph nodes, but this low incidence is partly related to their frequent site of origin in the hard palate and paranasal sinuses, areas that infre-quently produce lymph node metastases. The high-grade tumors (high-grade mucoepidermoid carcinoma, adeno-carcinoma, and malignant mixed tumor) have approxi-mately a 30% incidence of lymph node involvement on admission, and eventually 51% showed lymph node me-tastases.[7] Schell and co-workers report a 17% incidence of positive nodes on admission for all histologies and grades and subsequent appearance in 11%.[10] Most were staged N1 or N2A and were usually associated with lesions of the tongue or floor of the mouth.

Distant Metastasis

At least 25% of patients will develop distant metastasis and the rate for adenoid cystic carcinoma is closer to 50%. The lung is the site first recognized, but no site is exempt.

CLINICAL PICTURE

The clinical picture obviously depends on the site of origin. The signs and symptoms differ somewhat from those of squamous cell carcinoma arising from the same anatomical area. Many of the lesions are indolent, and the history may go back many months or even years; about 25% will give a history of a mass being present over 10 years. Since the lesions develop under the epithelium, the initial lesion is a submucosal mass that is often painless until ulceration develops. Perineural involvement is expressed as pain, nerve palsies, or paresthesias; the neurologic syndromes may be perplexing and difficult to reconcile with the gross extent of disease as determined by physical examination and roentgenographic examination. There is often a delay of several months during which the symptoms remain unexplained in the face of normal tomograms, normal computed tomographic (CT) scans, and minimal neurologic findings. Persistent unexplained symptoms should be considered *prima facie* evidence of perineural spread beyond the site of origin. Otherwise, the clinical picture resembles that for squamous cell carcinomas for a given size and site. Lymph node metastases surface at predictable sites. The clinically positive nodes are usually small and mobile, but a neck dissection on such a patient may show numerous small, clinically undetectable positive nodes, particularly in the case of adenoid cystic carcinomas.

METHODS OF DIAGNOSIS AND STAGING

The differential diagnosis includes lesions that produce an enlarging submucosal mass, such as an abscess, a stone in a duct, a cyst of soft tissue or bone, a sarcoma, or a lymphoma.

Because of the infrequency of these lesions, faulty histologic interpretation is not unusual and often leads to inappropriate therapy.

The staging systems applied to squamous cell carcinomas may be used, although very few reported series bother to correlate size and extent of tumor with results by various treatment modalities. Roentgenographic studies are similar to those used for squamous cell carcinomas for a specific site. Studies to rule out metastases are usually limited to a chest roentgenogram.

TREATMENT

Selection of Treatment Modality

Surgery and irradiation are the only curative therapies available. There is little disagreement about the value of operation, but there remains considerable disagreement regarding the results of irradiation.

Most series reporting poor results from radiation therapy mention neither the selection of patients for irradiation nor the doses and volumes used. Since radiation therapy has often been used as a last-ditch effort for high-grade, advanced lesions after multiple surgical procedures, it is hardly surprising that results in some reports have been poor. Those series using radiation therapy alone for early lesions or as an immediate postoperative adjunct to surgical removal have had a favorable experience. After all, the histologies of the minor salivary gland tumors are the same as those of parotid gland tumors, and it is generally accepted that routine postoperative irradiation will decrease the local recurrence rate in high-grade parotid lesions and that irradiation alone will even control a few locally recurrent or inoperable tumors.[4] The response of malignant minor salivary gland tumors to irradiation is generally similar to that of a squamous cell carcinoma of the same size and same anatomical site, and the doses used are quite similar.

LOW-GRADE TUMORS

The low-grade lesions (*i.e.,* low-grade mucoepidermoid carcinoma, acinic cell carcinoma, and benign mixed tumors) are treated initially by an operation when feasible, but irradiation is sometimes used as the initial primary treatment for inaccessible lesions (e.g., nasopharynx, sphenoid sinus) or when the functional loss would be considerable (Fig. 29-2). If there is failure to respond to radiation therapy, the treatment is discontinued and operation is advised (Fig. 29-3). Postoperative irradiation is added for close margins or for those lesions that have recurred more than once. If the patient presents after excisional biopsy of a small lesion, irradiation is an alternative to reexcision, particularly if the procedure would produce significant cosmetic or functional loss.

The benign mixed tumors also respond to radiation therapy, although complete regression is unusual. Long-term cure by radiation therapy alone has been reported. Surgery, however, remains the treatment of choice, and the major use of radiation therapy has been an adjunct to operation in cases at significant risk for recurrence. The benign mixed tumors of minor salivary gland origin are reputed to be more radiosensitive than those arising in the parotid gland, but this may be a function of tumor volume rather than of inherent differences in radiosensitivity.

HIGH-GRADE TUMORS

The treatment of high-grade lesions (adenocarcinomas, high-grade mucoepidermoid and malignant mixed tumors) varies immensely, depending on the site of origin, stage of disease, and willingness of the patient to accept a major cosmetic or functional change subsequent to an operation. Except for malignant mixed tumors, our approach is to accept radiation therapy as a curative therapy, and we essentially approach most lesions as we would a squamous cell carcinoma of similar stage and similar anatomical site. We have no experience with radiation therapy alone for malignant mixed tumors and would select surgery as the main treatment option.

ADENOID CYSTIC CARCINOMA

The management of adenoid cystic carcinomas is a frustrating experience. Histologically, they are low grade, but biologically they are high grade in the sense that they are difficult to cure because of their insidious growth pattern.

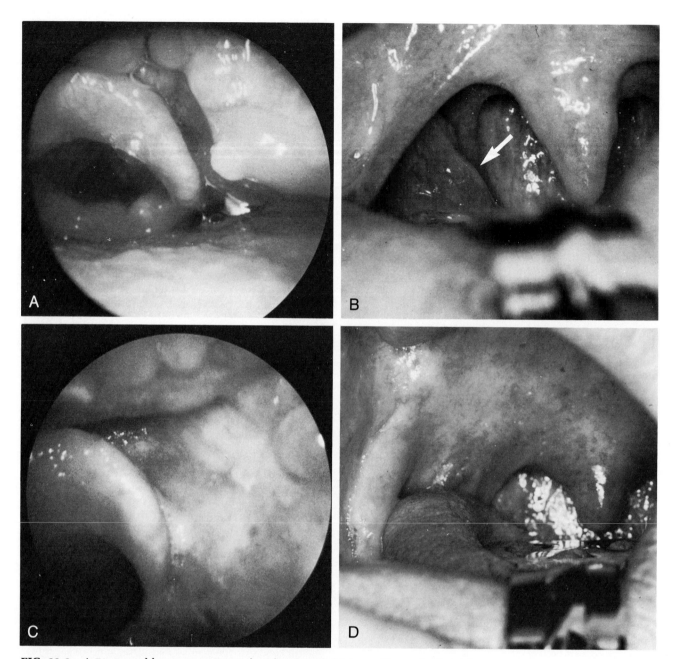

FIG. 29-2. A 71-year-old woman presented with 4-month history of lump in the right side of her throat. (For color photographs see Plate 9C, D in Chapter 3, Examination With Fiberoptic Equipment.) (*A*) There was a 4 × 5-cm submucosal lesion in the right base of the tongue extending to the vallecula. (*B*) Extension of submucosal tumor mass into right tonsillar fossa. Neck was negative. Biopsy showed mucoepidermoid carcinoma, low grade. Treatment plan was 7500 rad tumor dose/8½ weeks, cobalt-60. There was 70% regression at completion of treatment. (*C, D*) There was complete disappearance of tumor at 5 months (patient was free of disease at 30 months).

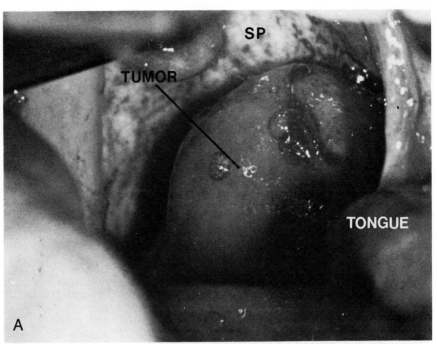

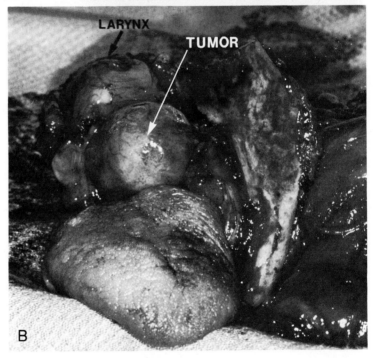

FIG. 29-3. A 52-year-old man presented with an 8-month history of hoarseness and dysphagia. There was a huge submucosal mass probably arising from the left vallecula. Biopsy showed mucoepidermoid carcinoma. The patient was started on radiation therapy, but there had been only 25% regression after 5000 rad and radiation therapy was discontinued. (A) Large submucosal mass occluded the oropharyngeal aperture. *SP,* soft palate. (B) Surgical specimen including the entire tongue, larynx, hemimandible, and neck specimen. The patient is free of disease 9 years after treatment.

Treatment is individualized based on anatomical site, tumor size, and age of the patient. Small to moderate-sized lesions may be resected, but the surgeon is always in a quandary regarding the amount of tissue to resect because of the proclivity to perineural spread; the tumor margins are frequently positive even after a generous resection. Adenoid cystic carcinomas are generally quite radiosensitive, and even large lesions disappear. A typical response for primary adenoid cystic carcinoma of the palate treated by radiation therapy alone is shown in Figures 29-4 through 29-6.[5] If the lesion fails to disappear, surgical excision follows immediately (Fig. 29-7). However, eventually most will recur after several years of apparent healing. Our approach has sometimes been to use radiation therapy as the initial treatment, reserving operation for radiation therapy failure. This gives the patient several years without the functional loss from the operation. The opposite tack may be chosen in which operation is used initially and radiation therapy is reserved for recurrence. There is no evidence that any one sequence of therapies is best, and therefore each case is individualized. In some cases, combined therapy may be used from the outset.

(*Text continues on p. 554.*)

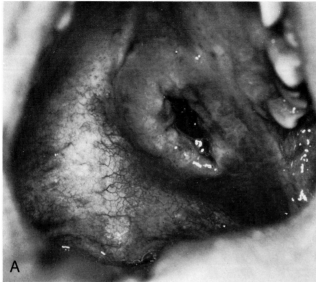

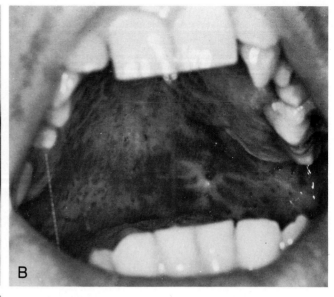

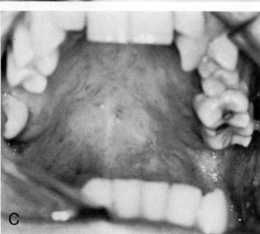

FIG. 29-4. A 34-year-old woman presented with an asymptomatic lesion that was discovered by her dentist on a routine visit for treatment of dental caries. On close questioning, she admitted to numbness over the left malar area for 2 months. (*A*) There was a 2 × 3-cm submucosal lesion with central ulceration on the left posterior hard palate. Roentgenograms showed intact bones and normal sinuses. Biopsy showed adenoid cystic carcinoma. Treatment plan was 1250 rad/5 fractions through intraoral cone, 6000 rad/6½ weeks through three-field external-beam technique, for a total of 7250 rad/8½ weeks. (*B*) Complete regression at completion of treatment. (*C*) Photograph at 3 years (living, free of disease, at 5 years). (Million RR, Cassisi NJ, Wittes RE: Cancer in the head and neck. In DeVita VT Jr, Hellman S, Rosenberg SA [eds]: Cancer: Principles and Practice of Oncology, pp 301–395. Philadelphia, J.B. Lippincott, 1982)

FIG. 29-5. (*A*) Adenoid cystic carcinoma of the right maxillary sinus with destruction of maxilla and tumor present submucosally in right hard palate (*arrows*). (*B*) Coronal tomogram shows mass in maxillary antrum (*arrowhead*) and bone destruction of floor of the sinus (*arrow*). The patient refused operation. Treatment plan was 7000 rad/7 weeks, cobalt-60, three fields (anteroposterior and right and left lateral). The eyes were shielded. There was complete disappearance of the submucosal mass at completion of therapy. (*C*) Appearance at 1 month. (*D*) There was no evidence of disease at 4 years.

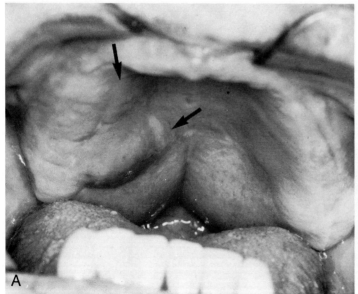

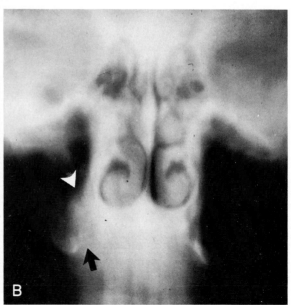

(continued)

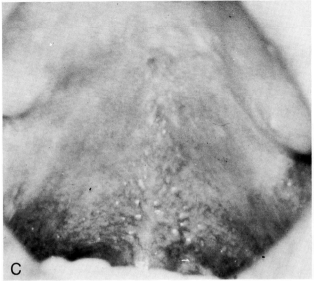

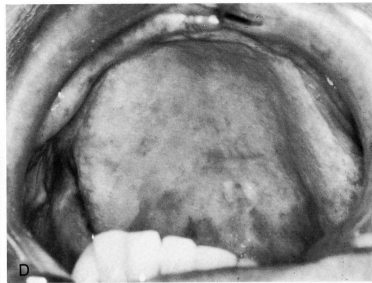

C

D

FIG. 29-5. (*continued*)

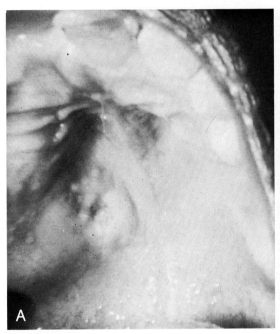

A

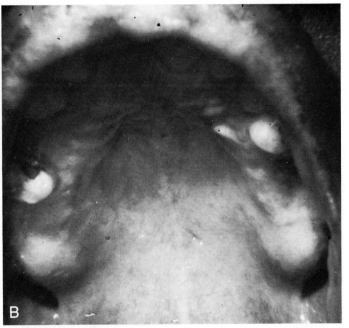

B

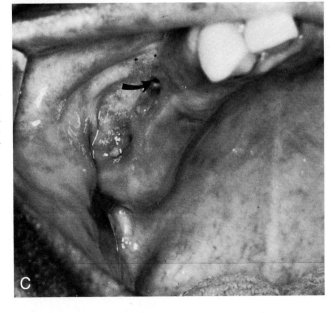

C

FIG. 29-6. A 42-year-old woman presented with a 1-year history of a lump on the hard palate. Biopsy showed adenoid cystic carcinoma. (*A*) Tomograms of paranasal sinuses showed a 2-cm well-defined mass in the floor of right maxillary antrum. Aspiration of right antrum was negative for tumor. Treatment plan was 7200 rad/8½ weeks, cobalt-60. The lesion disappeared completely prior to completion of therapy. (*B*) There was no evidence of disease at 7 years. (*C*) Appearance at 8 years. An oral-antral fistula developed spontaneously (*arrow*). Fullness was noted in the gingivobuccal sulcus. There was obvious recurrence a few months later, and a maxillectomy was performed.

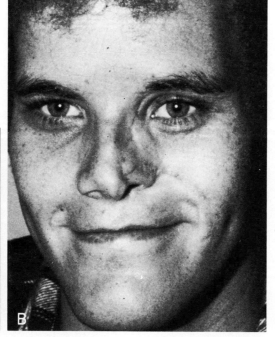

FIG. 29-7. A 14-year-old boy presented with epistaxis. There was a 2 × 2-cm bulge of the left side of the nose and a mass enlarging the left inferior turbinate that did not decongest. Biopsy revealed adenoid cystic carcinoma. Tomograms showed no sinus or orbital involvement. (*A*) Mass of left lateral nose. Treatment plan was to use anteroposterior and left lateral portals, cobalt-60, 6500-rad minimum tumor dose (7000 rad maximum)/9 weeks (split course). There was approximately 50% regression at completion of radiation therapy. (*B*) A persistent, well-encapsulated mass was resected 2 months later. Pathology showed adenoid cystic carcinoma. The patient was free of disease at 11 years.

When combined treatment is indicated, the operation should precede radiation therapy in order to facilitate healing and gain knowledge of tumor extent for radiation treatment planning.

Chemotherapy

Because of the rarity of these neoplasms, information about chemotherapy is almost entirely anecdotal. Some evidence of antitumor effects has been seen with 5-fluorouracil, hydroxyurea, methotrexate, and *cis*-platinum with bleomycin,[6,9,13,14] but the magnitudes of responses are often difficult to evaluate in the context of broad phase II studies or retrospective reviews of medical records. Using a combination of methyl-CCNU, doxorubicin (Adriamycin), and vincristine, Hayes and co-workers reported significant responses in adenoid cystic carcinoma.[3]

Surgical Treatment

Benign tumors are removed by wide local excision that includes a cuff of normal tissue. Local excision or enucleation is insufficient owing to the high recurrence rate associated with limited procedures.

For malignant lesions, the surgical approach is dictated by the histology and anatomical site. Small low-grade lesions may be treated with a wide local excision including a shell of normal tissue. Large low-grade lesions and high-grade lesions require a radical resection, which would be similar to that used for a squamous cell carcinoma of the same location and extent. Elective neck dissection is not often advised. Postoperative radiation therapy is often recommended. Resection of adenoid cystic carcinoma must allow for propensity for perineural and direct extension far beyond the gross lesion. It is not possible, of course, to

remove all the nerves potentially involved, but nerves that are involved should be sacrificed wherever reasonable to do so. As an alternative, postoperative irradiation may be used to cover the perineural routes of spread. Since unsuccessfully treated patients often live many years before they eventually die of their disease, careful planning must go into reconstruction and rehabilitation.

Irradiation Technique

The irradiation techniques are similar to those for squamous cell carcinomas of the same anatomical site and similar tumor size with the exception that nerve pathways must be covered, especially for high-grade lesions and adenoid cystic carcinomas. Recurrences are frequently manifested in and about the base of the skull at the origin of the cranial nerves.

Dose and fractionation schedules are similar to those used for squamous cell carcinomas.

The regression rate of adenoid cystic carcinoma during treatment is similar to that of squamous cell carcinoma. Successfully treated adenocarcinomas or low-grade mucoepidermoid carcinomas may require several weeks or months to disappear after completion of treatment. The regional lymphatics are electively irradiated depending on the site of origin and the grade of the lesion.

The response of benign mixed tumors is predictably slow and often incomplete.

Management of Recurrence

Minor salivary gland tumors have an honest reputation for late recurrence, but *70% of recurrences appear within 2 years.* Most of the late failures occur in the adenoid cystic carcinomas. Local recurrences in the tumor bed are usually easy to diagnose, but recurrences that develop from perineural spread are often difficult to diagnose. The symptoms and signs precede the changes in roentgenograms and CT scans by many months. Neurologic symptoms or signs should be considered evidence of recurrence until proved otherwise.

Patients with recurrent lesions are often "salvaged" by subsequent therapy. Most reported series have a high proportion of previously treated patients, and yet a considerable number of these patients with recurrences have a prolonged, useful life with further treatment. There are some patients (usually with adenoid cystic carcinoma) who have recurrent disease for whom there is no reasonable treatment available, and they are merely observed. Some of these observed patients lead a reasonably good life for several months or years with minimal symptoms and should not be harrassed by inappropriate therapy.

RESULTS OF TREATMENT

Spiro and co-workers reported the Memorial Sloan-Kettering results for 434 malignant minor salivary gland tumors, of which 90% were treated surgically.[11] The determinate 5-, 10-, and 15-year cure rates were 44%, 32%, and 21%, respectively; 51% died of the original cancer.

Patients with adenoid cystic carcinoma had the poorest prognosis, with about 20% surviving without recurrence. Those with adenocarcinoma had an intermediate outlook, about 35% surviving without recurrence. Mucoepidermoid carcinomas had the best control rate, with about 70% long-term cures. Local control differed considerably by site (Table 29-2), but this difference is partly explained by the higher incidence of advanced adenoid cystic carcinoma in the sinuses. Local control was also better for small lesions and those without bone or lymph node involvement. Previous treatment had little effect on cure rate.

Bardwil and co-workers report a similar series (87 cases) from M. D. Anderson Hospital with shorter follow-up (3 to 20 years) in which surgery was the sole treatment in 82% of cases (Table 29-3).[1] Local control was reported to be 75%, but 47% of the patients died of their original cancer, a percentage similar to that of the Memorial Sloan-Kettering series.

Schell and associates have reported a group of 118 malignant minor salivary gland tumors of which only 10% were treated by operation alone, 58% by surgery plus radiation therapy, and 32% by radiation therapy alone (Table 29-3).[10] The group treated by radiation therapy alone included 15 early and 23 advanced lesions. Follow-up was 2 to 10 years. The initial local control rate for the entire group was 79%, and 11 patients had their treatment salvaged by subsequent operation for an ultimate control of 88%. The risk of local recurrence by treatment category and histology is shown in Table 29-4. The low incidence of recurrence with radiation therapy alone for adenoid cystic carcinoma indicates that this histology responds consistently to radiation, which corresponds with our own observations. However, most cases eventually recur, if followed long enough. There are too few cases in the other categories to reach any conclusions except that surgery plus radiation therapy seems to provide better initial control than surgery alone for high-grade lesions; however, the eventual survival may be only slightly enhanced.

Byers and co-workers reported 14 patients with malignant minor salivary gland tumors of the lip.[2] This is a rare presentation, representing 1% of all malignant minor salivary gland tumors, and 1% of all lip cancers seen at the M. D. Anderson Hospital. Ten occurred on the lower lip, which is contrary to most reports. The free-of-disease sur-

TABLE 29-2. Results of Surgical Treatment of Minor Salivary Gland Tumors—267 Patients*

Site	No. Patients	Local Control (%)
Oral cavity/oropharynx	198	68
Sinus/nasal/nasopharynx	58	28
Larynx	11	55

* 60%, no prior treatment; 14%, clinically positive nodes on admission; 90%, treated surgically; follow-up 5 years.

Note: Memorial Sloan-Kettering Hospital data; patients treated 1939–1963.

(Data from Spiro RH, Koss LG, Hajdu SI, Strong EW: Tumors of minor salivary origin: A clinicopathologic study of 492 cases. Cancer 31:117–129, 1973)

TABLE 29-3. Results of Treatment of Malignant Minor Salivary Gland Tumors (M. D. Anderson Hospital)

Study	No. Patients	No Prior Treatment	Follow-up	Local Control	Distant Metastases	DOD or LWD	Method of Treatment	
Bardwil and co-workers[1] (1945–1962)	87	56%	3–20 yr	75%	30%	47%	S S + RT RT	(71) (10) (6)
Schell and co-workers[10] (1970–1978)	118	42%	2–10 yr	79%*	25%	36%	S S + RT RT	(11) (69) (38)

* Eleven patients had repeated operations, for an ultimate control rate of 88%.

(DOD or LWD, dead of disease or living with disease; S, surgery; RT, radiation therapy)

(Million RR, Cassisi NJ, Wittes RE: Cancer in the head and neck. In DeVita VT Jr, Hellman S, Rosenberg SA [eds]: Cancer: Principles and Practice of Oncology, pp 301–395. Philadelphia, JB Lippincott, 1982)

TABLE 29-4.   Malignant Minor Salivary Gland Tumors: Primary Recurrence Related to Treatment Modality (No. of Patients With Recurrence After Initial Treatment/Total Patients Treated)

Histology	Surgery Only	Surgery + Radiation Therapy	Radiation Therapy Alone	Total
High grade				
Adenoid cystic	3/4	9/40	0/23	12/67
Mucoepidermoid	0/1	0/6	4/7	4/14
Adenocarcinoma	3/4	3/14	1/4	7/22
Malignant mixed	0/0	0/1	0/0	0/1
Low grade				
Mucoepidermoid	1/2	0/7	1/4	2/13
Acinic cell	0/0	0/1	0/0	0/1
Total	*7/11	†12/69	6/38	25/118

* Five patients salvaged by repeated surgical resection.
† Six patients salvaged by surgery.
Note: M. D. Anderson Hospital data.
(Schell S, Barkley HT Jr, Chiminazzo H Jr: Treatment of malignant minor salivary gland tumors, in preparation)

TABLE 29-5.   Malignant Minor Salivary Gland Tumors (No. Locally Controlled/ No. Treated)

Method of Treatment	Local Control	Salvage	Ultimate Control
Surgery	3/6	1/3	4/6
Radiation therapy	4/8	2/2	6/8
Surgery + radiation therapy	6/8	0/1	6/8

Note: University of Florida data; patients treated 1/60–4/78; analysis 4/80 by J. R. Russell, MD.

TABLE 29-6.   Benign Minor Salivary Gland Tumors (No. Locally Controlled/ No. Treated)

Method of Treatment	Local Control	Salvage	Ultimate Control
Surgery	2/3	1/1	3/3
Surgery + radiation therapy	2/2	0	2/2

Note: University of Florida data; patients treated 1/60–4/78; analysis 4/80 by J. R. Russell, MD.

TABLE 29-7.   Incidence of Recurrence of Pleomorphic Adenoma of Minor Salivary Glands in the Royal Marsden Series: Distribution According to the Method of Treatment

Method of Treatment	No. Patients	No. With Recurrence	Length of Follow-up
Radiation alone	11	0	5 for 5+ years
Preoperative irradiation and surgery	14	2	9 for 5+ years
Surgery and postoperative irradiation	18	0	14 for 5+ years 9 for 10+ years
Surgery alone	1	0	1 for 5 years
Total	44	2	29 for 5+ years

(From Rafla-Demetrious SF: Mucous and Salivary Gland Tumours, p 118. Courtesy of Charles C Thomas, Publisher, Springfield, IL, 1970)

vival rate was approximately 20%. These researchers recommended that all but the smallest lesions be treated with a combination of surgery and radiation therapy. There was a substantial risk for regional node and perineural invasion.

Twenty-two patients with malignant minor salivary gland tumors were treated at the University of Florida from 1960 to April 1978.* The results of treatment are given in Table 29-5; 50% were dead of disease with a 2- to 20-year follow-up.

* Russell JR: Unpublished data, 1980.

Benign mixed tumors of minor salivary gland origin have a good prognosis. Enucleation, however, is followed by recurrence, and a cuff of normal tissue is required. Recurrence can usually be successfully managed by reexcision.

Bardwil and co-workers reported 13 patients with benign mixed tumors, all of whom were cured, 12 by operation and 1 by radiation therapy alone.[1]

Five patients with benign mixed tumors were treated at the University of Florida, and all five had control of disease (Table 29-6).

Rafla-Demetrious reported the Royal Marsden experience of 44 cases of benign mixed tumor (Table 29-7).[7] Eleven patients were treated by radiation therapy alone, and none of the tumors regrew, although not all had complete regression. Several photographs in Rafla's book demonstrate the response to radiation therapy. Local recurrence of benign mixed tumor may appear after many, many years, and an occasional patient may eventually die of uncontrolled disease.

FOLLOW-UP POLICY

The majority of local recurrences appear by 2 or 3 years, but the benign mixed tumors and adenoid cystic carcinomas may show a recurrence many years after initial treatment. Early recognition of recurrence may be important because in some patients salvage is achieved by further treatment.

COMPLICATIONS OF TREATMENT

The surgical and radiation complications are similar to those already outlined by anatomical site.

REFERENCES

1. Bardwil JM, Reynolds CT, Ibanez ML, Luna MA: Report of one hundred tumors of the minor salivary glands. Am J Surg 112:493–497, 1966
2. Byers RM, Boddie A, Luna MA: Malignant salivary gland neoplasms of the lip. Am J Surg 134:528–530, 1977
3. Hayes DM, Magill GB, Golbey RB, Krakoff IH: Methyl CCNU, Adriamycin, and vincristine (MAV) chemotherapy of adenoid cystic carcinoma. Proc Soc Surg Oncol, p 35, 1976
4. King JJ, Fletcher GH: Malignant tumors of the major salivary glands. Radiology 100:381–384, 1971
5. Million RR, Cassisi NJ, Wittes RE: Cancer in the head and neck. In DeVita VT Jr, Hellman S, Rosenberg SA: Cancer: Principles and Practice of Oncology, pp 301–395. Philadelphia, JB Lippincott, 1982
6. Moore GE, Bross IDJ, Ausman R, Nadler S, Jones R Jr, Slack N, Rimm AA: Effects of chlorambucil (NSC-3088) in 374 patients with advanced cancer. Eastern Clinical Drug Evaluation Program. Cancer Chemother Rep (Part I) 52:661–666, 1968
7. Rafla-Demetrious S: Mucous and Salivary Gland Tumors. Springfield, IL, Charles C Thomas, 1970
8. Ranger D, Thackray AC, Lucas RB: Mucous gland tumors. Br J Cancer 10:1–16, 1956
9. Rentschler R, Burgess MA, Byers R: Chemotherapy of malignant major salivary gland neoplasms. A 25-year review of M. D. Anderson Hospital experience. Cancer 40:619–624, 1977
10. Schell S, Barkley HT Jr, Chiminazzo H Jr: Malignant tumors of minor salivary glands, in preparation
11. Spiro RH, Koss LG, Hadju SI, Strong EW: Tumors of minor salivary origin: A clinicopathologic study of 492 cases. Cancer 31:117–129, 1973
12. Thawley SE, Ward SP, Ogura JH: Basel cell adenoma of the salivary glands. Laryngoscope 84:1756–1766, 1974
13. Vermeer RJ, Pinedo HM: Partial remission of advanced adenoid cystic carcinoma obtained with Adriamycin: A case report with a review of the literature. Cancer 43:1604–1606, 1979
14. Wittes RE, Brescia F, Young CW, Magill GB, Golbey RB, Krakoff IH: Combination chemotherapy with cis-diamminedichloroplatinum (II) and bleomycin in tumors of the head and neck. Oncology 32:202–207, 1975

Temporal Bone

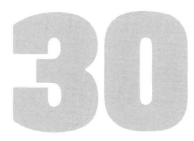

RODNEY R. MILLION
NICHOLAS J. CASSISI

Primary carcinomas of the external auditory canal and middle ear are uncommon. They are usually associated with a longstanding history of chronic infection, and with the availability of antibiotics, the problem of chronic infection has mostly disappeared. Metastatic lesions and secondary invasion of the temporal bone by tumors arising from contiguous areas are more common. Temporal bone tumors are often misdiagnosed until advanced, at which time the success of therapy is understandably poor. This section will deal mainly with the carcinomas (see Chapter 31, Chemodectomas [Glomus Body Tumors]).

ANATOMY

The temporal bone is a complex structure housing the organs of hearing and balance. It is traversed by the internal carotid artery, internal jugular vein, and the facial, vestibulocochlear, glossopharyngeal, vagus, and spinal accessory nerves and some of their branches (Fig. 30-1).

The cartilaginous portion of the external ear canal is covered by skin with numerous hair follicles and sebaceous and ceruminous glands. The skin of the bony portion of the canal is firmly adherent to the underlying periosteum. The canal, which is 2 cm to 4 cm in length, is formed by bone over the medial two thirds and fibrocartilage over the outer one third. The cartilage is incomplete, particularly superiorly and posteriorly; the intervals are filled with fibrous tissue. Immediately anterior to the external auditory canal are the temporomandibular joint and the parotid gland. Behind the canal is the mastoid bone and inferiorly the canal is in relation to the tail of the parotid and the facial nerve. Lymphatic drainage is to the preauricular, jugular chain, and mastoid lymph nodes. The tympanic membrane probably has significant capillary lymphatics on the external surface only.

The middle ear is subdivided into the tympanic cavity, mastoid, and eustachian tube. The tympanic cavity and mastoid antrum and air cells are lined by columnar epithelium, both ciliated and nonciliated. The epithelium is continuous along the eustachian (auditory) tube to the nasopharynx. The epithelium lining the cartilaginous portion of the eustachian tube is thick and vascular and contains numerous mucous glands; the epithelium is ciliated columnar.

The tympanic cavity and mastoid probably do not have significant capillary lymphatics[13] nor does the internal ear (labyrinth). Capillary lymphatics are described for the mucous membrane of the cartilaginous portion of the eustachian tube; the drainage is to the jugular chain and retropharyngeal lymph nodes. A potential pathway from the eustachian tube to the preauricular nodes is described by Arnould.[1]

The internal ear or labyrinth is lined by epithelium and presumably could be the site of a primary carcinoma, although no record of such has been found.

PATHOLOGY

A rare benign neoplasm is squamous cell papilloma, usually occurring in the external auditory canal and rarely in the middle ear.[12] These tumors are more frequent in southern China and are said to be sensitive to irradiation.

559

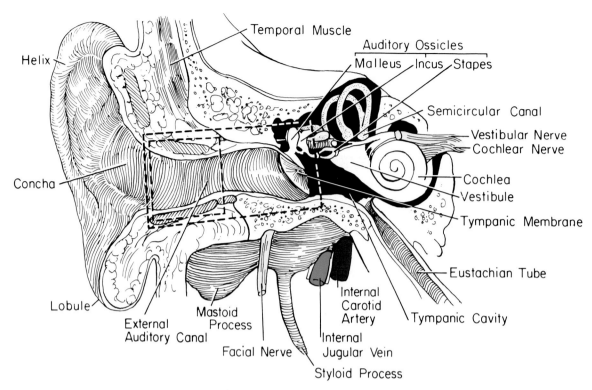

FIG. 30-1. Dashed lines outline the surgical margins of excision of the cartilaginous portion of the external auditory canal and for the entire canal, including the tympanic membrane, malleus, and incus.

Chemodectomas are the most common neoplasm seen in the temporal bone. They are best considered as a low-grade malignancy in the sense that they are locally aggressive tumors that rarely disseminate to regional lymph nodes or distant sites (see Chapter 31, Chemodectomas [Glomus Body Tumors]).

Carcinomas of the external auditory canal are essentially squamous cell or basal cell skin carcinomas; malignant melanoma may also arise in the canal. Ceruminous gland adenocarcinoma is a rare tumor developing from the modified sweat glands of the external auditory canal.[16] Tumors arising from the tympanic cavity, mastoid, or eustachian tube include squamous cell carcinoma and benign malignant and salivary gland tumors, particularly along the medial two thirds of the eustachian tube and the middle ear. Twenty-six cases of middle ear adenomas and adenocarcinomas have been reported.[10]

Embryonal cell rhabdomyosarcoma is a rare sarcoma of the middle ear occurring in children. The histiocytoses frequently involve the temporal bone. Ewing's sarcoma and osteosarcoma have been reported but are rare (see Chapter 33, Pediatric Tumors of the Head and Neck).

Metastases occur to the temporal bone and must be distinguished from lesions originating in the temporal bone. The breast is a common site for a primary lesion.[5]

PATTERNS OF SPREAD

External Auditory Canal

Basal cell carcinoma of the external auditory canal tends to begin in the entrance to the canal. As the lesion progresses, it quickly attaches to the perichondrium and eventually invades and destroys cartilage and extends to the concha, the tympanic membrane, and finally the middle ear and mastoid.

A squamous cell carcinoma of the external auditory canal may occur anywhere along the canal. It may appear as a red, polypoid mass, usually associated with chronic infection. Since growth is contained by the bony/cartilaginous walls and the tympanic membrane, the neoplasm tends to fill up the canal and attach to underlying perichondrium or periosteum. Eventually the tumor invades cartilage or bone or grows through the tympanic membrane to reach the middle ear, mastoid, and facial nerve.

Jesse and co-workers report a 21% incidence of lymph node metastases on admission.[6]

Middle Ear: Tympanic Cavity, Mastoid, and Eustachian Tube

Since the areas of the middle ear are not readily available for visual examination, the growth pattern of early lesions remains speculative. When first diagnosed, most lesions have destroyed bone and invaded cranial nerves and the sensory organs of hearing and balance. The neoplasm may then proceed along any of several routes. The temporal bone is literally riddled with numerous channels carrying nerves, muscles, the eustachian tube, and blood vessels; these tunnels allow early spread without destroying bone.

Posterior growth through the mastoid brings tumor to the sigmoid sinus and contents of the posterior cranial fossa.

Superior extension occurs through the thin roof of the tympanic cavity (tegmen tympani) to the middle cranial fossa.

Erosion through the thin floor of the hypotympanic recess brings the tumor into relationship with the tail of the parotid, facial nerve, jugular vein, internal carotid artery, and soft tissues of the upper neck.

The tumor may extend medially and anteriorly along the eustachian tube to the nasopharynx; this spread pattern is often accompanied by destruction of the petrous apex and possible extension into the carotid canal. Anterior growth eventually invades into the temporomandibular joint, parotid gland, and parapharyngeal space.

Access to the cranial cavity is through direct bony penetration or along the facial and vestibulocochlear nerves and the lesser superficial petrosal nerve.

Lymphatic spread is unusual, since significant capillary lymphatics occur only in the medial two thirds of the eustachian tube. Boland and Paterson report lymph node metastases on admission in 10 of 86 patients (12%).[2]

CLINICAL PICTURE

External Auditory Canal

The initial symptom is similar to that of any skin cancer—a painless lump or growth in the canal. As the lesion enlarges, the patient may notice minor bleeding, pain, itching, and intermittent serous drainage. Both the patient and the physician assume that the diagnosis is external otitis, and local treatment is prescribed over a period of several months. A loss of hearing occurs when the canal is occluded or when the tumor involves the tympanic membrane or middle ear. Pain may be severe in advanced cases.

Early lesions of the external canal appear as a nodule, possibly with crusts and dried blood from scratching. As the lesions enlarge, they tend to grow under the skin and produce narrowing of the canal with the appearance of a polypoid mass filling the canal. Examination of the tympanic membrane is aided by an operating microscope and suction since a large amount of debris is frequently present. A preauricular mass or fullness may be seen due to parotid invasion, and trismus may result with invasion of the temporomandibular joint. The tumor may be seen eroding into the posterior auricular sulcus. The concha is often involved

Middle Ear: Tympanic Cavity, Mastoid, and Eustachian Tube

Carcinomas of the middle ear are associated with chronic ear infection in the majority of patients, many of whom have had a mastoid operation. The onset of symptoms due to cancer is associated with increasing pain and discharge. The pain may be quite severe and is usually temporal. Facial nerve palsy is a common cause for seeking medical advice. Hearing loss is often present from the chronic otitis, but there may be further loss due to the neoplasm. Vertigo and tinnitus are infrequent. Cranial nerves II–XII may be invaded.

A rare lesion probably arises in the auditory tube and produces syndromes that mimic nasopharyngeal cancer. The patient has pain, otitis with hearing loss, and cranial nerve deficits due to involvement of the cavernous sinus and erosion of the petrous apex and adjacent base of the skull. The nasopharynx is negative to examination, which delays diagnosis. Lederman and co-workers describe four such cases, and we have observed two cases at the University of Florida.[7] Computed tomographic (CT) scans and tomograms should be helpful in these rare cases.

On physical examination, a small mass may be seen on the tympanic membrane, or, more often, the deep portion of the external auditory canal is blocked by a friable, bleeding tumor. There may be diffuse edema and erythema of the external auditory canal or of the skin around the concha. Tugging on the pinna may cause pain. Anterior growth may be associated with trismus. A submucosal mass may be seen in the nasopharynx. Cranial nerves should be evaluated.

METHODS OF DIAGNOSIS AND STAGING

The differential diagnosis of external auditory canal lesions includes the following:

> Extension of middle ear tumor to the external auditory canal
> Otitis externa
> Malignant external otitis (*Pseudomonas* infection occurring in diabetes mellitus)
> Squamous cell papilloma
> Foreign body
> Furuncle
> Osteoma

Diagnosis is established by incisional biopsy. The differential diagnosis of carcinomas of the middle ear, mastoid, or eustachian tube lesions includes the following disorders:

> Chronic otitis media
> Cholesterol granuloma[9]
> Cholesteatoma
> Mastoiditis
> Glomus tumors
> Metastatic cancer
> Carcinoma of the nasopharynx
> Acoustic neuroma
> Fibrous dysplasia
> Meningioma

If a mass is readily accessible in the external auditory canal or neck, biopsy may be performed immediately; if not, roentgenographic studies including tomography and CT scan should precede exploration and biopsy. If the diagnosis of chemodectoma is considered, angiography (digital vascular imaging) or CT scan enhanced with a contrast medium should precede exploration and biopsy (see Chapter 31, Chemodectomas [Glomus Body Tumors]).

There is no staging system for these rare tumors.

Pretreatment workup should include audiograms, tomograms of the temporal bone and base of the skull, including C1 vertebra, and CT scans. Preoperative evaluation for middle ear lesions includes carotid arteriography to determine the involvement or displacement of the internal carotid as it courses through the foramen lacerum. The sigmoid sinuses are evaluated to be sure the opposite one is patent, in case it should be necessary to obliterate the ipsilateral sinus at the time of operation.

TREATMENT

Selection of Treatment Modality

Radiation therapy and operation, either alone or combined, are the only curative options. The number of cases managed even in a large cancer hospital is so small that it is impossible to gauge the relative effectiveness of excision and radiation therapy. The selection of treatment modality is therefore based more on an educated hunch than on firm data. While the morbidity from excision of external auditory canal tumors is relatively minor, a major temporal bone resection poses the threat of immediate death and rather major morbidity, so that irradiation, even with the risk of late central nervous system damage, is a more tempting initial modality, with operation reserved for persistence.

Surgical Treatment

EXTERNAL AUDITORY CANAL

A tumor confined to the cartilaginous portion of the ear canal and adjacent concha without involvement of the bony canal or the tympanic membrane is treated by a sleeve resection of the canal (partial temporal bone resection) (see Fig. 30-1). This is similar to coring an apple: circumferential incisions are made around the external meatus, and a core of skin, cartilage, and possibly bone is resected. The defect is lined by a split-thickness skin graft. Tumor involving only the bony portion of the external auditory canal can be treated by sleeve resection with preservation of the facial nerve and removal of the tympanic membrane, including one or two ossicles (see Fig. 30-1). There is minor hearing loss (less than 10 dB). The defect is repaired by split-thickness skin graft. Minimal extension to the tympanic cavity or adjacent mastoid may be encompassed by extended sleeve resection.

Extensive tumor invading the middle ear and/or mastoid requires a subtotal temporal bone resection. Mastoidectomy is not sufficient treatment for the advanced lesions of the external auditory canal; it has been tried by Lewis[8] and at the M. D. Anderson Hospital,[6] and was successful in only 2 of 23 patients from both series.

Sleeve resection of tumors confined to the external auditory canal enlarges the canal to a 2-cm to 3-cm circular defect. Hearing is preserved and the pinna remains intact. Larger lesions may require removal of part of the pinna, parotid gland, temporomandibular joint, mastoid, or tympanic membrane. The cosmetic and functional losses are minimal unless the facial nerve is lost.

MIDDLE EAR

If there is more than minimal involvement of the middle ear, the application of the principle of *en bloc* cancer surgery requires a subtotal temporal bone resection. Prior to the description of subtotal temporal bone resection in 1954,[11] treatment consisted of either radical mastoidectomy (and thus incomplete removal of tumor) followed by postoperative radiation therapy, or piecemeal removal of tumor and temporal bone and postoperative radiation therapy. The subtotal temporal bone resection is a combination extracranial-intracranial procedure. Extension of tumor to the petrous apex, cavernous sinus, internal auditory canal, internal carotid artery, middle or posterior cranial fossa, C1, C2, or the basioccipital bone are contraindications to a surgical attempt. The patient is first explored through a temporal craniotomy, and the temporal lobe and dura are retracted to expose the petrous portion of the temporal bone. Minimal involvement of the dura can be excised with the specimen. The entire temporal bone except for the petrous apex is removed *en bloc* down to the dura of the middle and posterior cranial fossae. The sigmoid sinus is exposed and may be sacrificed if necessary, if the opposite sinus is patent. With the use of chisels, the petrosal segment is fractured at a level just lateral to the carotid canal and the specimen is removed. The internal carotid artery at the apex of the petrous bone is preserved and forms the medial margin of the resection. The defect is then covered by a flap. Extension of disease to the parotid, the mandible, or the neck may dictate an in-continuity parotidectomy,

FIG. 30-2. A 50-year-old man presented with a history of chronic right middle ear infection of long duration. There was recent increased pain. Exploration revealed squamous cell carcinoma in the middle ear. (A) Axial CT scan. There is destruction of the right petrous apex and floor of the middle cranial fossa. The foramen lacerum is enlarged. The temporal bone is sclerotic. (B) Coronal CT scan. Note destruction of the right petrous apex and floor of the middle cranial fossa. (C) Simulator planning film. The large portal corresponds to portals 1 and 2 in D. The smaller portal corresponds to portal 4. (EAC, external auditory canal) (D) Isodose distribution. The tumor extended within 1 cm of the brain stem near the foramen magnum. It was necessary to deliver approximately 2000 rad to the right eye in order to limit the dose to the brain stem (*black*). The minimum tumor dose was 6000 rad/8½ weeks, but the gross disease probably received 7000 rad.

Portal	Energy	Field Size (cm)	Wedge Angle	Given Dose (rad)
1	8 MV	12 × 9	open	4300
2	17 MV	12 × 9	open	2000
3	8 MV	9 × 9	open	500
4	17 MV	6 × 5	60	1200
5	17 MV	5 × 9	30	1300
6	17 MV	5 × 9	30	1300

(E). Positioning device. (See Chapter 15, Treatment Planning for Irradiation of Head and Neck Cancer, for details of preparation.) There was no evidence of disease at 24 months; the patient was asymptomatic and working full time.

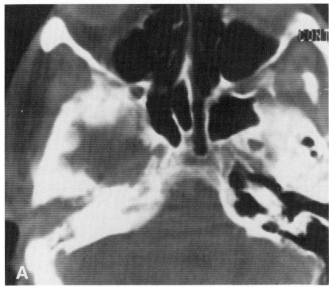

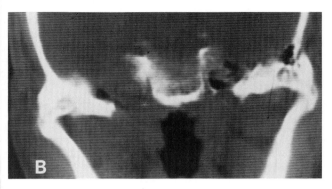

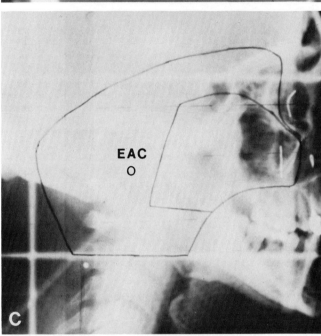

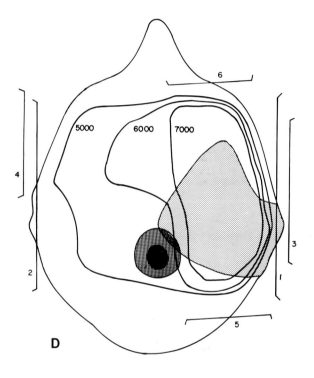

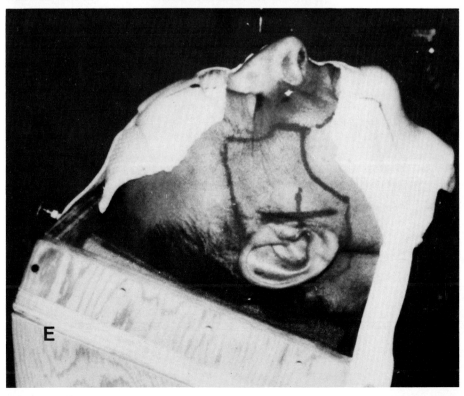

partial mandibulectomy, or radical neck dessection. It is possible to remove the entire temporal bone, but the dura is extremely adherent to the cavernous sinus and, should bleeding occur at this point, the results could easily be catastrophic; so, from a standpoint of safety, a small portion of the apex remains; hence, the "subtotal" temporal bone resection.

Temporal bone resection usually implies loss of hearing, temporary or permanent loss of balance due to loss of the semicircular canals, difficulty chewing due to loss of the horizontal ramus of the mandible, facial palsy due to sacrifice of the facial nerve, and loss of the pinna.

Irradiation Technique

EXTERNAL AUDITORY CANAL

Lesions confined to the external auditory canal and adjacent structures are usually treated with a pair of superior and inferior angled wedge portals, sometimes in conjunction with a single ipsilateral portal. Mixed-beam or electron techniques would also produce a satisfactory and simpler technique. The incidental doses delivered to the spinal cord, brain stem, and brain are well within the limits of tolerance. The treatment is fractionated at 180 rad/day due to underlying cartilage, bone, and the central nervous system. Small lesions would receive 6000 rad/7 weeks and larger lesions, 6500 rad to 7500 rad. Reducing field techniques are employed. The preauricular, postauricular, and subdigastric nodes would usually be encompassed by the irradiation plan.

MIDDLE EAR

There is no standard portal arrangement for irradiation of lesions of the middle ear. Angled wedge fields may be used for the smaller lesions (see Chapter 31, Chemodectomas [Glomus Body Tumors], for examples). Those lesions invading near the midline require highly individualized treatment planning. The radiation therapist faces the same technical problem as the surgeon, namely, the central nervous system. Since the apex of the temporal bone is within 2 cm of the brain stem, it is a technical nightmare to deliver the high dose required (7000 rad to 7500 rad) to have a chance at cure for an advanced lesion (Fig. 30-2). The dose to the brain stem will be at least 6000 rad and possibly more, and the patient must accept a small risk of myelitis in the face of a uniform fatality from the neoplasm. If only a small portion of the brain stem/spinal cord receives 6000 rad at 180 rad/day, the risk of transverse myelitis is estimated at 10%, and for a dose of 7000 rad the risk is considerable.

Combined Treatment Policies

Irradiation is added after operation for incomplete resection or for large lesions even when margins are considered to be free.

Management of Recurrence

A number of the surgical successes have occurred after an unsuccessful full dose of irradiation.[3]

RESULTS OF TREATMENT

Results from several series by treatment and site of origin are listed in Tables 30-1 through 30-5.[2,3,4,6,7,8,14,15] Comparison between institutions is full of hazards. Irradiation series often include lesions and patients not suitable for operation, surgical series often include irradiation failures, and there is no standard reporting method to separate external auditory canal from middle ear lesions.

Early carcinomas of the external auditory canal are equally well treated by irradiation or sleeve resection of the canal. Advanced carcinomas of the external auditory canal with minimal involvement of the tympanic cavity or mastoid may be managed by extended sleeve resection with postoperative irradiation added as needed or with irradiation alone in patients not suitable for operation.

For carcinomas of the middle ear there seems to be a small advantage to surgical resection and postoperative irradiation in patients with lesions suitable for the operation; this treatment should produce about a 50% cure rate. However, the cure rate for middle ear lesions by irradiation alone is approximately 33% and the hazards are far less, although not insignificant. Many patients treated curatively by irradiation would not be suitable for surgical resection due to extension to the middle cranial fossa or apex of the petrous bone, or cranial nerve involvement (other than the facial or vestibulocochlear nerve). If there is doubt about resectability, it seems prudent to proceed with a full course of radiation therapy and to reserve an operation for persistence.

FOLLOW-UP POLICY

Radiation failures may occasionally by salvaged by an operation. Biopsy should be performed when an ulcer fails to heal or if there is persistent mass or pain. Exploration of the middle ear and mastoid may be required for diagnosis. Baseline roentgenograms should be ob-

TABLE 30-1.   Carcinoma of the External Auditory Canal: Surgical Series (No. Controlled/No. Treated)

Type of Treatment	Conley and Novack[3] (5 Years)	Lewis[8] (3 Years)	M. D. Anderson Hospital[6] (3 Years)	University of Florida (2 Years)
Early—sleeve resection ± mastoidectomy	2/8	5/6	3/4	1/1
Late—temporal bone resection	0/2	11/13	3/4	1/1

tained and follow-up studies ordered periodically for comparison.

COMPLICATIONS OF TREATMENT

Surgical Treatment

The operative mortality should be very low for sleeve resection. Patients may complain of dizziness in cold weather due to the increased exposure of the semicircular canals created by the defect.

Conley and Novack report a 60-day operative mortality rate of 27% (3/11) for temporal bone resection; 8 of the 11 patients had had prior radiation therapy or surgery.[3] In experienced hands, the operative mortality has diminished, but it still remains a significant deterrent to the novice.

Hemorrhage is often considerable, and ample blood must be available for transfusion.

The carotid may be injured, resulting in hemiplegia.

Cerebrospinal leak may lead to meningitis and brain abscess. Removal of the semicircular canals results in vertigo and loss of equilibrium; the patient usually recovers in 2 to 4 weeks, although a degree of unsteadiness may persist for several months and is more severe in the dark. Loss of the facial nerve requires a tarsorrhaphy. The pinna is usually lost with resection of the larger lesions; a prosthesis may be constructed if desired.

Hearing loss occurs with temporal bone resection and is permanent.

TABLE 30-2. Carcinoma of the External Auditory Canal: Radiation Therapy Series

Study	Follow-up	No. Controlled/No. Treated
Boland and Paterson[2]	5 years	9/11
University of Florida	2 years	4/5*
Lederman and co-workers[7]	5 years	6/25

* One failure subsequently salvaged by subtotal temporal bone resection for ultimate control in 5/5.

TABLE 30-3. Carcinoma of the Middle Ear: Surgical Series

Study	Follow-up	No. Controlled/No. Treated
Conley and Novack[3]	5 years	2/11
Lewis[8]	3 years	3/12
Jesse and co-workers[6]	3 years	1/3

TABLE 30-4. Carcinoma of the Middle Ear: Radiation Therapy Series

Study	Follow-up	No. Controlled/No. Treated
Holmes[4]	5 years	28/78 (36%)
Lederman and co-workers[7]	5 years	12/39 (31%)

TABLE 30-5. Carcinoma of the External Auditory Canal and Middle Ear: Treatment by Surgery and Radiation Therapy (No. Controlled/No. Treated)

Location	M. D. Anderson Hospital[6] (3 Years)	Wang[15] (5 Years)	University of Florida (2 Years)	Sørenson[14] (5 Years)	Conley and Novack[3] (5 Years)
External auditory canal					
Early stage		4/4			1/1
Late stage	0/1	3/11			1/1
Middle ear	0/3	4/8	1/2	5/11	

Radiation Therapy

EXTERNAL AUDITORY CANAL

Serous otitis will develop in at least half of the patients, and some will require pressure-equalization tubes for relief. Soft tissue or bone necrosis may occur adjacent to the external auditory canal. Hearing should not be seriously affected unless a chronic otitis develops.

MIDDLE EAR

Holmes reports three cases of central nervous system damage (two fatal) and seven cases of bone necrosis in a group of 78 radically irradiated patients.[4] Treatment for bone necrosis was debridement and antibiotics. One patient at the University of Florida developed multiple cranial nerve palsies but lived for 5 years free of disease.

Combined Treatment

Wang reports five cases of osteonecrosis of the temporal bone in 20 patients treated by excision and postoperative radiation therapy; three of the patients survived more than 5 years.[15] A dose equivalent to 7000 rad/7 weeks or greater was correlated with complications.

REFERENCES

1. Arnould N: A propos des lymphatiques de la face interne du pavillon et du conduit audifit externe. Ann Anat Pathol Anat Normale Méd-Chir 4:224, 1927
2. Boland J, Paterson R: Cancer of the middle ear and external auditory meatus. J Laryngol Otol 69:468–478, 1955
3. Conley JJ, Novack AJ: The surgical treatment of malignant tumors of the ear and temporal bone: I. AMA Arch Otolaryngol 71:635–652, 1960
4. Holmes KS: Carcinoma of the middle ear. Clin Radiol 16:400–404, 1965
5. Jahn AF, Farkashidy J, Berman JM: Metastatic tumors in the temporal bone: A pathophysiologic study. J Otolaryngol 8:85–95, 1979
6. Jesse RH, Healey JE Jr, Wiley DB: External auditory canal, middle ear, and mastoid. In MacComb WS, Fletcher GH (eds): Cancer of the Head and Neck, pp 412–427. Baltimore, Williams & Wilkins, 1967
7. Lederman M, Jones CH, Mould RF: Cancer of the middle ear; technique of radiation treatment. Br J Radiol 38:895–905, 1965
8. Lewis JS: Cancer of the ear: A report of 150 cases. Laryngoscope 70:551–579, 1960
9. Miglets AW, Booth JB: Cholesterol granuloma presenting as an isolated middle ear tumor. Laryngoscope 91:410–415, 1981
10. Pallanch JF, McDonald TJ, Weiland LH, Facer GW, Harner SG: Adenocarcinoma and adenoma of the middle ear. Laryngoscope 92:47–52, 1982
11. Parsons H, Lewis JS: Subtotal resection of the temporal bone for cancer of the ear. Cancer 7:995–1001, 1954
12. Rogers KA Jr, Snow JB Jr: Squamous cell papilloma of the external auditory canal and middle ear treated with radiation therapy. Laryngoscope 78:2183–2187, 1968
13. Rouvière H: Anatomy of the Human Lymphatic System. Tobias MJ, trans. Ann Arbor, MI, Edwards Brothers, 1938
14. Sørenson H: Cancer of the middle ear and mastoid. Acta Radiol 54:460–468, 1960
15. Wang CC: Radiation therapy in the management of carcinoma of the external auditory canal, middle ear, or mastoid. Radiology 116:713–715, 1975
16. Wetli CV, Pardo V, Millard M, Gerston K: Tumors of ceruminous glands. Cancer 29:1169–1178, 1972

Chemodectomas (Glomus Body Tumors)

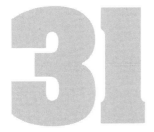

RODNEY R. MILLION
NICHOLAS J. CASSISI

Chemodectomas are a fascinating but uncommon group of neoplasms that may originate anywhere glomus bodies are found. The lesions are uncommon before the age of 20, and there is a female predominance in some series. They may occur in multiple sites in 10% to 20% of cases, especially in families with a history of this tumor.[26] Carotid body tumors are associated with conditions producing chronic hypoxia, such as living in areas of high altitude, and chronic hypoxemia, such as occurs in association with cyanotic heart disease. A few of the tumors demonstrate endocrine activity and produce symptoms similar to a pheochromocytoma or a carcinoid apudoma.

ANATOMY

The normal glomus bodies in the head and neck vary from 0.1 mm to 0.5 mm in diameter. An autopsy study showed a correlation between carotid body size and increased right ventricular weight secondary to emphysema.[4] Because of their small size, their total number and distribution in the head and neck remain speculative. Tumors arising from glomus bodies (i.e., chemodectomas or nonchromaffin paragangliomas) occur most often from the carotid and temporal bone glomus bodies, with rare reports of tumors arising from the orbit, nasopharynx, larynx, nasal cavity, paranasal sinuses, tongue, jaw, and trachea.

The glomus bodies of the temporal bone require special mention in regard to their distribution, since the site of tumor development explains the different clinical pictures.

Guild reports an average of 2.82 glomera per temporal bone with a range of 0 to 12.[10] Since the glomera are so tiny, this realistically represents a minimum number. The temporal bone glomus bodies are not consistently found in any location but vary from person to person. The distribution of the glomus bodies in the temporal bone and along the cranial nerves near the base of the skull is shown in Figure 31-1. At least one half of the glomus bodies are found in the general region of the jugular fossa and are located in the adventitia of the superior bulb of the internal jugular vein. The remainder are distributed along the course of the nerve of Jacobson (a branch of the glossopharyngeal nerve) and the nerve of Arnold (a branch of the vagus nerve). Approximately 20% of all temporal bone glomus bodies lie in the tympanic canaliculus and approximately 10% lie in relation to the cochlear promontory. A few glomus bodies are located in the descending part of the facial canal.

The carotid bodies are located in relation to the bifurcation of the common carotid; orbital glomus bodies are located in relation to the ciliary nerve.

The vagal bodies are found adjacent to the ganglion nodosum of the vagus nerve.

The superior laryngeal glomus bodies are situated in the false cord/aryepiglottic fold region, and the inferior laryngeal glomus bodies usually lie lateral to the cricoid cartilage. Their position is variable.[16]

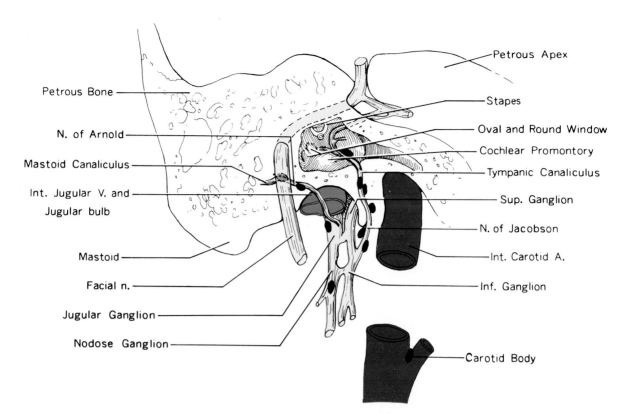

FIG. 31-1. Anatomical location of glomus bodies in the temporal bone. Approximately half of the glomus bodies are located in the region of the superior jugular bulb of the internal jugular vein.

PATHOLOGY

Chemodectomas are histologically benign tumors that resemble the parent tissue and consist of nests of epithelioid cells within stroma containing thin-walled blood vessels and nonmyelinated nerve fibers. The tumor mass is well circumscribed, but a true capsule is not seen. Dense fibrous bands occur in some tumors and account for the firmness of some masses. The histologic appearance varies, depending on the relative amounts of epithelioid and vascular tissue present. The criterion of malignancy is based on the clinical progress of the disease rather than on the histologic picture. Chemodectomas without cellular atypia may metastasize to regional nodes or to distant organs. Metastases are infrequent, probably occurring in less than 5% of cases.

Endocrine activity has been reported in a few head and neck chemodectomas.[5] Lawson concluded that the glomus cell is a modified neuroblast of neural crest origin with the ability to synthesize biogenic monoamines in tissue culture, and therefore is a true neurocrine cell.[15] Although the glomus bodies and glomus tumors are normally nonchromaffin, areas of positive staining cells may be seen, which suggests the presence of catecholamines. The presence of serotonin (5-hydroxytryptamine) has also been demonstrated by histochemical staining. The infrequency of clinically detectable endocrine activity is probably related to the sparseness of the secretory granules in these tumors.

PATTERNS OF SPREAD

Chemodectomas usually grow slowly, and it is usual to have a history of symptoms for a few years and occasionally for 20 years or longer.

Primary Spread

CAROTID BODY TUMORS

Carotid body tumors are located at the bifurcation of the common carotid and, as they expand, tend to displace and encircle the internal and external carotid vessels. The tumor begins in the adventitia of the artery and initially derives its blood supply from the vasa vasorum. An accessory blood supply may come from branches of the vertebral artery and the ascending pharyngeal artery.[27] The tumor is usually closely adherent to the wall of the carotid adjacent to its vascular pedicle, and there may be thinning of the arterial wall due to pressure by the mass. Large masses extend toward the cervical spine, the base of the skull, the angle of the mandible, and the lateral pharyngeal space and its contents.

TEMPORAL BONE TUMORS

Glomus tympanicum lesions tend to be small when diagnosed because they produce symptoms early in their course. Tumor may involve the ossicles, tympanic membrane, mastoid, external auditory canal, semicircular canal, and the facial, Jacobson's, and Arnold's nerves. Cranial nerve involvement is not common, however, for this site.

Glomus jugulare tumors invade the base of the skull, petrous apex, jugular vein, middle ear, and middle and posterior cranial fossae. Cranial nerves V–XII and the sympathetic chain are frequently involved. Spector and coworkers reported a 15% incidence of intracranial extension.[24]

The remaining temporal bone glomus tumors do not have a specific name affixed to them; their spread patterns and clinical pictures are predictable, based on the site of origin.

LARYNGEAL TUMORS

Sixteen glomus body tumors in the supraglottic larynx and one tumor along the lateral surface of the thyroid cartilage have been reported.[29] The tumors average 3 cm to 4 cm in size. Metastatic disease may be found in the lymph nodes.

The supraglottic lesions usually present as a smooth, submucosal, cystic-appearing mass in the aryepiglottic fold–false vocal cord area. Subglottic and tracheal cases are reported.[16]

Lymphatic Spread

Lymphatic metastases are uncommon but are reported for carotid body and laryngeal chemodectomas. An upper neck mass may be an inferior extension of a temporal bone tumor rather than a lymph node metastasis. Capillary lymphatics have been described that drain the dura around the jugular foramen and could be the site of origin for temporal bone lymph node metastasis.[7]

Distant Metastases

Distant metastases have been reported, usually to the lung. Considering the frequency of jugular vein invasion by temporal bone tumors, the risk of distant spread is quite small. The risk is greater for carotid body tumors than for temporal bone tumors.

CLINICAL PICTURE

Symptoms may be present from a few months to many years prior to diagnosis; the average is 3 to 4 years. Tumors usually present after the age of 20 but a few have been reported between the ages of 10 and 20.

Glomus tumors may be associated with an endocrine syndrome similar to that of a pheochromocytoma or, more rarely, a functioning carcinoid tumor.

Hypertension may by cyclical. Control of the tumor by surgery or radiation therapy may improve or eliminate the hypertension.[15]

Patients with carcinoid syndrome have a history of recurring bouts of explosive diarrhea, headaches, flushing, and hypertension.[5]

Carotid Body Tumors

PRESENTING SYMPTOMS

The most common presenting symptom is an asymptomatic, slow-growing mass in the upper neck near the bifurcation of the carotid. Large masses may encroach on the parapharyngeal space and produce dysphagia, pain, and cranial nerve palsies. A carotid sinus syndrome may occur owing to the pressure of the mass.

PHYSICAL EXAMINATION

On examination the mass usually lies deep to the sternocleidomastoid muscle and is tethered to surrounding structures. The borders of the mass are discrete. It is difficult to distinguish a small carotid body tumor from a normal carotid bulb. Fixation occurs only in large tumors that extend to the spine and base of the skull. A submucosal bulge may be seen in the tonsillar area. A bruit may be heard. Steady compression of the mass may reduce its size; it then rebounds when the pressure is released. This maneuver is discouraged, since it may initiate a syncopal attack due to pressure on the carotid sinus. Ipsilateral enlarged lymph nodes may represent regional spread.

Temporal Bone Tumors

PRESENTING SYMPTOMS

Since there is variation in the distribution of glomus bodies, the initial symptoms and signs depend on the site of origin.

Patients with tumors arising in or near the middle ear present with an insidious conductive hearing loss, pulsatile tinnitus, vertigo, and headache.

Patients with lesions developing in or around the jugular fossa develop headache that is often pulsatile and referred to the orbit or temple. Cranial nerves V–XII and the sympathetics become affected.

When lesions develop in the facial canal patients present with facial nerve symptoms. Otorrhea and hemorrhage may occur when tumor breaks through into the external auditory canal.

Intracranial extension is usually associated with multiple cranial nerve palsies, severe headache, and symptoms and signs of increased intracranial pressure. Invasion of the middle cranial fossa may result in paralysis of cranial nerves III–VI and retro-orbital pain. Proptosis occurs with posterior orbital invasion. Extension to the posterior cranial fossa may produce ataxia, pulsatile occipital headache, and paralysis of cranial nerves V–XII.

PHYSICAL EXAMINATION

A characteristic blue red mass may be seen bulging the tympanic membrane or actually occupying the external auditory canal. Brown has described a diagnostic test he terms the "pulsation sign."[1] An ear speculum fitted with an air bulb is inserted into the external auditory meatus. As the pressure is gradually increased, the mass at first shows increased pulsation, but then the pulsations cease and the tumor blanches; when the pressure is released, the color and pulsations return. A mass may be seen or felt in the upper neck between the mandible and mastoid and at times may be quite large. Lymph node metastases are rare.

Cranial nerves V–XII and the sympathetic nerves may show varying neurologic loss. Papilledema occurs with increased intracranial pressure. Proptosis and visual loss are reported for advanced lesions.[24]

Vagal Body Tumors

Vagal chemodectomas produce symptoms similar to glomus jugulare chemodectomas, but they are more likely to have an associated mass in the neck.

Laryngeal Chemodectomas

The symptoms are similar to carcinoma of the supraglottic larynx: hoarseness or voice change, dysphagia, sore throat, ear pain, stridor, and a mass in the neck.

Orbital Chemodectomas

Patients with these rare lesions present with exophthalmos, diplopia, and loss of vision.

METHODS OF DIAGNOSIS AND STAGING

Radiology*

CAROTID BODY TUMORS

Carotid body tumors arise between the internal and external carotid arteries at the level of the bifurcation. The distortion and separation of the carotid arteries by the encircling abnormal vessels are shown to best advantage with angiography (Fig. 31-2A, B).[6] In addition to its obvious role in the diagnosis, angiography accurately delineates the overall tumor extent and also demonstrates the adjacent vascular anatomy, thus facilitating a comprehensive presurgical evaluation.

Additional x-ray "imaging" is now available with computed tomographic (CT) scanners. Chemodectomas take up intravenous contrast agents, resulting in an intense contrast enhancement of the mass (Fig. 31-2C, D).[6] The tumor is then readily diagnosed and differentiated from other abnormalities that occur in this area, such as carotid artery aneurysm, cystic masses (e.g., branchial cleft cyst), and solid masses (benign tumors, e.g., neuroma, lipoma). CT scanning also demonstrates local extension of larger masses to bone (skull base, spine) and adjacent soft tissues of the lateral pharyngeal space.

Improved anatomical orientation may result from "reformatting" or direct CT images in coronal and sagittal planes. Until these newer CT techniques are further refined, the x-ray diagnosis and staging of carotid body tumors rests principally with the angiographer, whether by conventional arterial catheterization or the less invasive, simpler, and safer "digital vascular imaging," whereby venous injection of small amounts of contrast agent is followed by digital subtraction.

Temporal Bone Tumors

As with carotid body tumors, the temporal bone chemodectomas are usually clearly demonstrated by angiography (Fig. 31-3A, B). The main blood supply is usually from the ascending pharyngeal branch of the external carotid artery. A vertebral injection may demonstrate additional feeder vessels (Fig. 31-3B). Thus, angiography facilitates accurate

---

* This section written with the assistance of Derek J. Hamlin, MD.

diagnosis and staging and aids differentiation from other vascular anomalies and variants, other tumor masses, and the sequelae of infections of the temporal bone.

Retrograde jugular venography may at times be useful to demonstrate tumor in the jugular vein when the venous phase of the arteriogram does not adequately fill the vein.

CT scanning is perhaps of more use with temporal bone tumors than with carotid body tumors. Glomus jugulare tumors that have destroyed portions of the petrous apex will usually have a soft tissue component bulging into the posterior cranial fossa. This soft tissue component enhances during intravenous contrast administration and becomes clearly delineated during CT evaluation (Fig. 31-3C, D). Although conventional tomography usually demonstrates the bone involvement, the soft tissue component remains concealed.

Modern CT techniques, using thin scan "slices" to increase spatial resolution and special computer software to reduce beam hardening and artifacts off dense bony structures, have added greatly to the roentgenographic diagnosis and staging of glomus tumors but have not yet replaced angiography. If the patient is to be treated by radiation therapy, a CT scan enhanced with a contrast medium may be sufficient for diagnosis and treatment planning.

Differential Diagnosis

CAROTID BODY TUMORS

The differential diagnosis includes enlarged lymph nodes, aneurysm of the carotid artery, branchial cleft cyst, benign tumors (e.g., lipoma), and direct extension of a lateral pharyngeal wall or pyriform sinus cancer into the soft tissues of the neck.

Carotid angiography and CT scan with contrast provide the preoperative diagnosis. Biopsy usually produces serious hemorrhage and is not recommended.

TEMPORAL BONE TUMORS

The differential diagnosis includes the presentation of an internal carotid artery in the middle ear either as an aberrant vessel or as an aneurysm.[14] These patients also present with hearing loss, pulsatile tinnitus, and a pulsatile mass behind the eardrum. Needless to say, biopsy of the "carotid tumor" may have a rather disastrous result.

A high jugular bulb may present as a vascular mass in the middle ear and mimic a glomus tumor.[8]

Other diagnoses to be considered include the following:

Polyp of ear canal
Malignant tumor of the nasopharynx with extension to the temporal bone

---

FIG. 31-2. (A) Arterial phase of angiogram shows widening of limbs of the carotid ▶ artery bifurcation. (B) Subtraction view of capillary phase of angiogram shows a prominent vascular blush in an egg-shaped tumor between the proximal portions of the external and internal carotid arteries (*arrows*). (C) Precontrast CT section shows an oval mass outlined by arrows in the left side of the neck. (D) Postcontrast CT study shows prominent vascular blush of the periphery of the mass (*arrows*). The CT value (500 scale) of the enhanced periphery is 43 to 45. The CT value of the center of the mass is 33 to 36. (Ferris RA, Kirschner LP, Mero JH et al: Case report: Computed tomography of a carotid body tumor. J Comput Assist Tomogr 3:834–835, 1979)

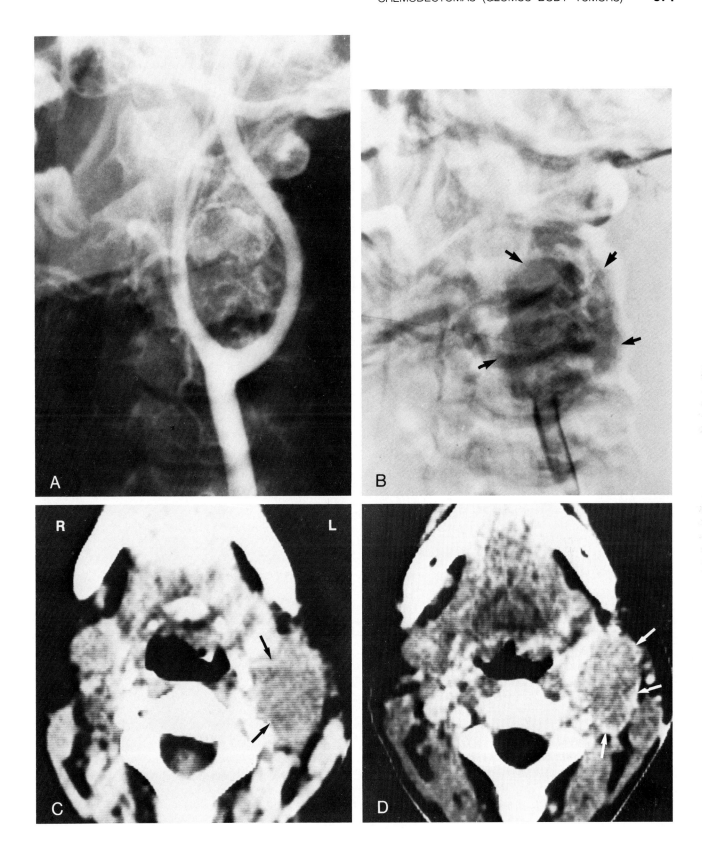

Acoustic neuroma
Carcinoma of the middle ear
Metastatic carcinoma (especially breast cancer)
Cholesteatoma
Histiocytosis
Chronic serous otitis and mastoiditis

The diagnosis of glomus tumor is established by arteriography and CT scan with enhancement. Biopsy may be associated with serious or even fatal hemorrhage and is avoided if possible. If an operation is planned for a localized lesion of the tympanic cavity, then excision of the lesion is the biopsy.

Staging

There is no accepted staging scheme for chemodectomas. Patients are considered to have an early lesion when there is little or no bone destruction and an advanced lesion when there is extensive bone destruction or cranial nerve deficits. Tumors recurring after prior treatment are usually advanced because of the delay in diagnosis.

A 24-hour urine sample may be examined for vanillylmandelic acid (VMA) and metanephrines if hypertension is present, and for 5-hydroxyindoleacetic acid (5-HIAA) if a carcinoid picture is present.

TREATMENT

Selection of Treatment Modality

Although chemodectomas have a low potential for metastatic spread and a slow growth pattern, if unchecked they may cause major disability and eventually death. It may be appropriate to recommend no active treatment in selected nonprogressive, stable cases, but the great majority should be treated.

TEMPORAL BONE TUMORS

Surgical excision is satisfactory for small lesions that can be removed without significant risk of major hemorrhage or damage to normal structures.

Early lesions of the tympanic cavity are successfully managed by excision without loss of hearing or vestibular function. The remainder of the temporal bone and vagal lesions are best managed by irradiation. Partial removal of the tumor prior to irradiation does not improve the results but only increases the overall morbidity and puts the patient at risk for a fatal complication.

There remains a great deal of confusion regarding the results of radiation treatment for chemodectomas. A review by Kim and co-workers of over 200 patients showed that the recurrence rate after adequate radiation therapy for temporal bone chemodectomas was 2% with doses of 4000 rad or greater.[13] Most of the failures noted in early radiation therapy series were most likely due to inadequate treatment volume (i.e., geographic miss). In some cases, examination of the temporal bone after radiation therapy has shown either no definable tumor or a few microscopic residuals. In the majority of patients the tumor mass regresses, but stable remnants may be seen for years. Success in these patients is equated with the lack of tumor regrowth and permanent improvement in signs and symptoms.

CAROTID BODY TUMORS

Small lesions (1 cm to 5 cm) may be successfully removed with little risk to the patient. However, if ligation or replacement of the carotid vessels is anticipated or if a large lesion is fixed or unresectable because of size, radiation therapy may be the preferred initial treatment. These lesions are identical histologically to temporal bone chemodectomas, and the response to radiation should be similar. There are scattered reports of patients with regression of the mass, while other reports declare little or no immediate response. There are anecdotal cases in which patients lived many years after radiation therapy with no recurrence or progression, even though there was a residual tumor mass. The doses in some cases were well below the currently accepted level of 4000 rad to 5000 rad, and the lack of immediate regression is not necessarily tantamount to a therapeutic failure.[28]

Surgical Treatment

TEMPORAL BONE TUMORS

Small glomus tympanicum lesions are approached through the eardrum or mastoid and are removed. Hearing loss

FIG. 31-3. (A) External carotid artery injection (anteroposterior projection, subtraction technique). Mass is supplied by the ascending pharyngeal artery. There is rapid venous filling ("vascular stain"), which outlines the lesion. The mass extends inferiorly through the jugular foramen (arrow). (ECA, external carotid artery; APA, ascending pharyngeal artery) (B) Right vertebral angiogram (anteroposterior projection, subtraction technique) shows a glomus jugulare tumor. There is a hypervascular mass with intense stain occupying most of the petrous and tympanic portions of the temporal bone. Angiography accurately identifies the widely diversified blood supply, including a supply from the lateral marginal artery to the cerebellum (arrow). This implies extension into the posterior cranial fossa. Also demonstrated is an enlarged anterior meningeal branch from the vertebral artery. This indicates that the lesion has parasitized the dura in the posterior fossa (arrowhead). The bone destruction is best shown on the CT scans. (C) Axial CT scan with contrast. There is destruction of the petrous and tympanic portions of the temporal bone. The extent of the enhancing mass is especially well depicted adjacent to the air in the external auditory canal. The extension of the mass into the posterior fossa (arrowheads) is not optimally seen due to the wide window settings used to better delineate the bone destruction (see D). (D) The mass (arrowheads) is more easily demonstrated with proper window settings (compare with C).

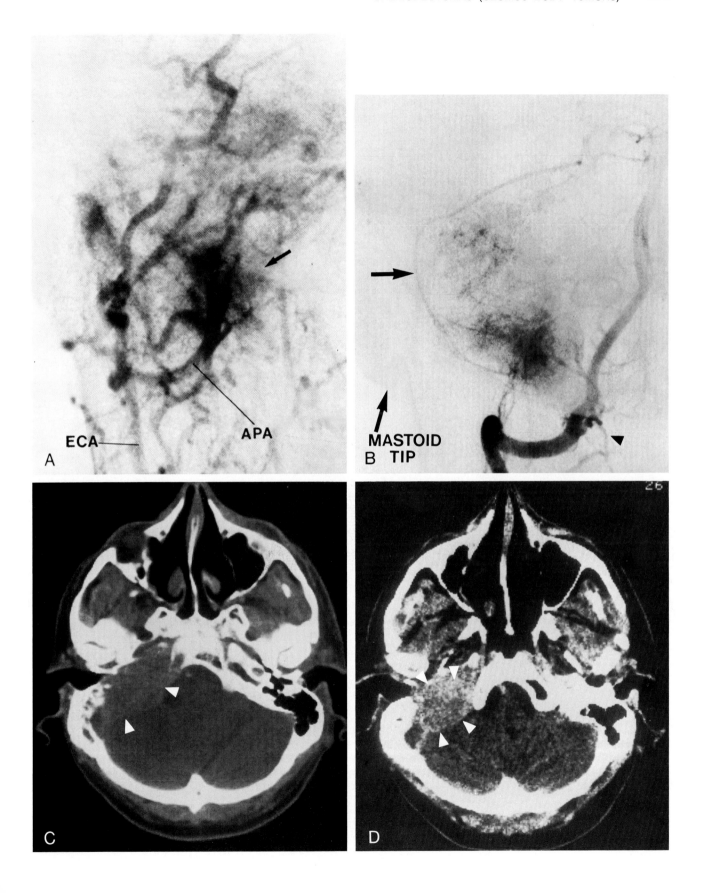

may occur from the operation, but if there is conductive hearing loss from the tumor, it may be correctable.

For the glomus jugulare tumors, operation is reserved for radiation failure, in which case a radical mastoidectomy or a subtotal temporal bone resection would be required. Some surgeons advocate a base of the skull approach.[18]

CAROTID BODY TUMORS

When an adequate workup indicates that the most likely diagnosis is a carotid body tumor, hypertension, if present, should be treated. A standard neck incision is made in a skin crease at the level of the carotid bulb, and the carotid sheath and its contents are identified. The tumor mass is usually lying at the crotch of the internal and external carotid arteries, often displacing these vessels. Marked drops in blood pressure and bradycardia can be avoided by injecting the bulb area with lidocaine (Xylocaine). Troublesome bleeding can be avoided by using the bipolar electrode prior to excising the mass. The mass is then removed, preserving the carotid arteries.

Irradiation Techniques

Treatment planning starts with collation of tumor extent from the arteriogram (Fig. 31-4) and CT scan (with contrast). An allowance should be made for tumor extensions that may not be visualized roentgenographically. Small to moderate-sized lesions are treated by superior and inferior angled wedged portals in order to reduce the dose to the midline and to avoid an exit dose to the eye (Fig. 31-5).[3,25] Large lesions, especially those that extend near the midline, usually require opposed lateral portals weighted 2:1 or 3:2 to the ipsilateral side.

Multiple series now show nearly 100% long-term control with doses greater than 4000 rad and an *adequate treatment volume*. The current treatment plan is 4500 rad/5 weeks, 180 rad/fraction, to a generous tumor volume. All portals should be treated each day. There is no evidence at present that larger lesions require higher doses, but we frequently use 5000 rad for the more advanced lesions. This dose is below the tolerance of the brain stem and spinal cord.

Tumor-related symptoms may begin to improve during the first week of treatment, and the tumor mass, if visible, may show a decrease in size. Frequently, however, the regression rate then slows, and a persistent mass is usually seen at the completion of treatment. In some cases, there is no measurable reduction in mass size during the course of radiation therapy. Some patients eventually show complete gross disappearance of visible or palpable tumor, but many have a persistent, stable gross lesion for many years.

Nausea and vomiting are uncommon side-effects at 180 rad/fraction. The patient will have temporary hair loss in the entrance and exit areas beginning about the third week. The hair should regrow over a period of 2 to 4 months but may show a slightly different texture or color.

Management of Recurrence

TEMPORAL BONE TUMORS

The diagnosis of recurrence is often delayed because of the inaccessibility to examination. A baseline CT scan should be obtained for reference.

Regrowth of tumor after proper irradiation is uncommon, and the diagnosis must be made only after complete re-evaluation and evidence of progression of symptoms or an enlarging mass. Pulsatile tinnitus may persist after irradiation because of incomplete regression of the vascular component of the tumor.[17,19]

Documented recurrence after operation is usually treated by irradiation; the complication rate in this group is higher than for those treated initially by irradiation. Recurrence after irradiation should be treated by operation if feasible; if operation is not possible, reirradiation may be considered. The potential for a complication would be significant, but in the face of advancing neoplasm the risk would probably be acceptable.

CAROTID BODY TUMORS

Recurrence of carotid body tumors after excision is related to the size of the initial lesion; in some series the recurrence rate is substantial. Management of recurrence is individualized, but radiation therapy should be considered in the treatment planning.

RESULTS OF TREATMENT

Chemodectomas in some, but not all, cases may show persistent evidence of tumor mass, presumably the vascular component, following irradiation. Reliable indications of successful treatment of a chemodectoma of the temporal bone structures include amelioration of symptoms, return of cranial nerve function, and absence of disease progression with long-term follow-up.

Temporal Bone Tumors

Between September 1964 and September 1976, 17 patients with chemodectomas arising in temporal bone structures were evaluated and treated at the University of Florida.[3] There was a minimum follow-up of 5 years, and 10 have been followed for more than 10 years. One patient died 22 months after treatment of intercurrent disease with no clinical evidence of chemodectoma.

All 3 of the patients treated by surgery alone had excision of early, localized glomus tympanicum tumors. The 14 patients treated by radiation therapy and the 3 patients treated by surgery alone have had control of disease for 5 to 15 years (Table 31-1).[3] Of the 8 patients with cranial nerve paralysis prior to radiation therapy, 5 had return of function of one or more cranial nerves. Four of 6 patients had return of function of the glossopharyngeal nerve and 4 of 7 patients had return of function of the vagus nerve. None of the 7 patients with facial nerve paralysis prior to radiation therapy regained function of that nerve.

The local control rates for five irradiation series of chemodectomas in which adequate doses (3500 rad or more) were prescribed and the treatment volumes were adequate are listed in Table 31-2.[2,3,12,22,25] No patient had documented evidence of disease progression in 71 patients treated. The local control reported in five surgical series is given in Table 31-3.[9,11,20,21,23] Most surgical reports do not distinguish between tympanicum and jugulare (nontympanicum) lesions. Spector and co-workers reported success in 10 (91%) of 11 glomus tympanicum tumors treated by transcanal tympanotomy (five patients) or radical mastoidectomy (six

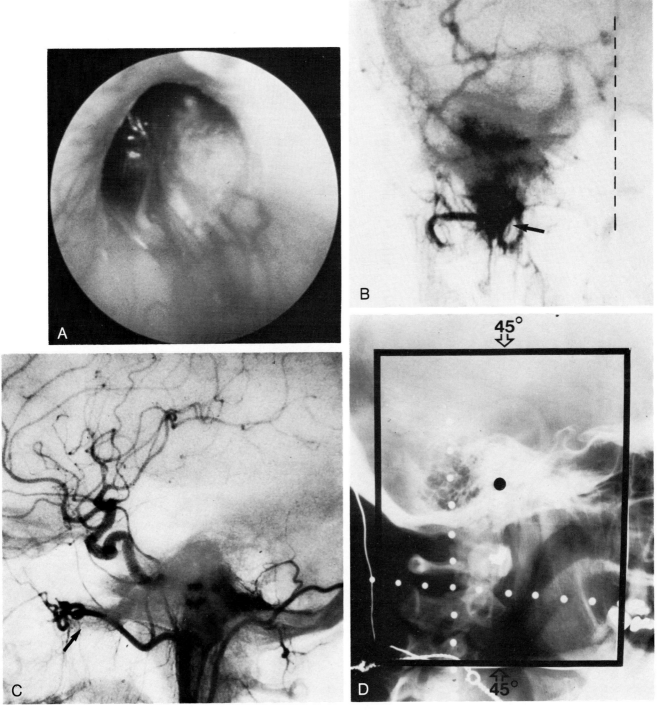

FIG. 31-4. Treatment planning for a moderately advanced chemodectoma of the temporal bone. The treatment volume should be generous in order to avoid missing tumor that may not show on arteriogram or CT scan. (A) Blue red mass bulging into external auditory canal (photograph taken through a fiberoptic nasoscope). (B) Anteroposterior arteriogram (subtraction technique). The mass extends to within 1 cm of the midline and 3 cm to 4 cm below the jugular fossa (*arrow*). (C) Arteriogram, lateral view. Note anterior extension of tumor (*arrow*). (D) Treatment planning film. Black dot locates the external auditory canal. Compare location of anterior and posterior borders to the arteriogram (*B* and *C*). Superoinferior angled portals were used. See Fig. 31-5*B* for representative isodose distribution.

patients).[23] Thirty-five (78%) of 45 glomus jugulare tumors were cured by radical mastoidectomy or hypotympanic resection (nine patients). Follow-up ranged from 2 to 27 years (average 9 years).

It is difficult to understand reports that persist in recommending that irradiation should only be used for palliation and that operation is the treatment of choice, even though the recurrence rate after operation is higher than

50% in some series and the operative risk for large lesions is immediate.

CAROTID BODY TUMORS

The rate of control is related to the tumor size and spread. The rate of control for complete surgical excision is very good. Incomplete removal is followed by local recurrence. Operative mortality is significant in some series.[28] Only anecdotal data are available for radiation therapy, but occasional successes are reported for advanced disease.

FOLLOW-UP POLICY

A baseline CT scan may be useful for following temporal bone tumors. Repeat angiograms are ordered only if recurrence is suggested. Although late recurrences are often predicted following treatment with modern irradiation techniques, they are seldom observed. It is not unusual to have a persistent blue red mass behind the eardrum after irradiation, even though the patient is clinically improved and there is no evidence of progression. Five to 10% of all patients will develop a second chemodectoma, often in the head and neck area; about one third to one half of the patients with a familial history may have multiple glomus tumors. CT scanning with enhancement is used for screening.

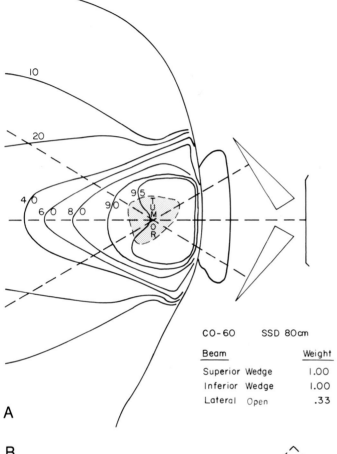

CO-60   SSD 80 cm

Beam		Weight
Superior Wedge		1.00
Inferior Wedge		1.00
Lateral	Open	.33

A

B

FIG. 31-5. (A) Three-field technique for relatively small temporal bone chemodectoma. The open lateral portal can be shaped to fit the tumor distribution. The dose to the brain stem is approximately one half the tumor dose. (B) Isodose distribution from superoinferior wedge portals with 45° angle. This distribution is used for large tumors extending near the midline. The 100% isodose is within 1 cm to 2 cm of the midline; the dose to the brain stem/spinal cord is 10% to 20% less. (A from Dickens WJ, Million RR, Cassisi NJ, Singleton GT: Chemodectomas arising in temporal bone structures. Laryngoscope 92:188–191, 1982; B from Tidwell TJ, Montague ED: Chemodectomas involving the temporal bone. Radiology 116:147–149, 1975)

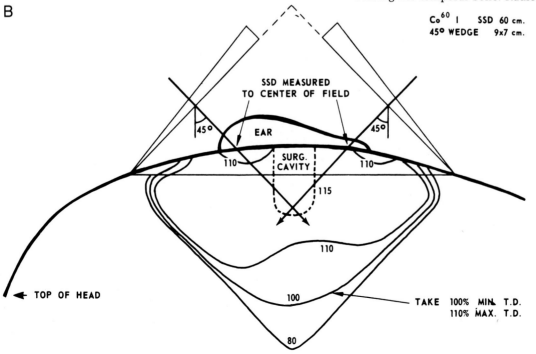

Co⁶⁰ I   SSD 60 cm.
45° WEDGE   9x7 cm.

TABLE 31-1. Chemodectoma: Results of Treatment at the University of Florida

Modality	Stage	Free of Recurrence	Years of Control
Radiation*	Early	6/6	5, 8, 10, 10, 11, 13
	Advanced	8/8	5, 6, 6, 7, 9, 10, 11, 12
Surgery	Early	3/3	13, 13, 15

* Includes five patients treated for recurrence after operation and three patients treated in the immediate postoperative period for residual disease. Average tumor dose was 4550 rad.

Note: University of Florida data; patients treated 10/64–10/77; analysis 10/79.

(Data from Dickens WJ, Million RR, Cassisi NJ, Singleton GT: Chemodectomas arising in temporal bone structures. Laryngoscope 92:188–191, 1982)

TABLE 31-2. Local Control of Chemodectomas with Irradiation

Institution	Tumor Dose* (rad)	Local Control†	Follow-up
M. D. Anderson Hospital[25]	4250–5000	17/17	4–18 years
University of Florida[3]	3750–5640	14/14	5–13 years
Baylor Medical Center[12]	4000–5000	9/9	1–7 years
Geisinger Hospital[2]	4000–5000	11/11	1–12 years
Princess Margaret Hospital[22]	3500/3 weeks	20/20	2–20 years

* The dose per fraction is 180 rad to 200 rad except for Princess Margaret Hospital.

† Local control = regression and absence of disease progression.

TABLE 31-3. Local Control of Chemodectomas With Operation

Study	Year	No. Patients	No. With Recurrence or Persistence
Newman and co-workers[20]	1973	14	11
Grubb and Lampe[9]	1965	9	5
Hatfield and co-workers[11]	1972	16	8
Rosenwasser[21]	1967	8	3
Spector and co-workers[23]	1976	11 (GT)	1
		45 (GJ)	10

(GT, glomus tympanicum; GJ = glomus jugulare)

(Adapted from Tidwell TJ, Montague ED: Chemodectomas involving the temporal bone. Radiology 116:147–149, 1975)

COMPLICATIONS OF TREATMENT

Surgical Treatment

Fatalities have been reported from biopsy and resection. The major risk during operation is for hemorrhage and injury to cranial nerves. Other complications include hemiparesis, cerebrospinal fluid leak, and hearing loss.[8]

Radiation Therapy

There have been isolated reports of brain necrosis; these cases were associated with high doses, high daily fractions, or repeat courses of irradiation. This complication should not occur at a dose of 4500 rad to 5000 rad or less given at 180 rad/day, 5 days/week. Other complications include cholesteatoma and sequestrum of the mastoid, and serous otitis. Detectable damage to the hearing mechanism and vestibular apparatus has not been reported to occur with 4500 rad to 5000 rad to the normal temporal bone. Cranial nerve palsy due to irradiation should not occur. The complication rate is greater when both operation and irradiation are used.[3]

REFERENCES

1. Brown LA: Glomus jugulare tumor of the middle ear: Clinical aspects. Laryngoscope 63:281–292, 1953
2. Cole JM: Glomus jugulare tumor. Laryngoscope 87:1244–1258, 1977

3. Dickens WJ, Million RR, Cassisi NJ, Singleton GT: Chemodectomas arising in temporal bone structures. Laryngoscope 92:188–191, 1982

4. Edwards C, Heath D, Harris P: The carotid body in emphysema and left ventricular hypertrophy. J Pathol 104:1–13, 1971

5. Farrior JB III, Hyams VJ, Benke RH, Farrior JB: Carcinoid apudoma arising in a glomus jugulare tumor: Review of endocrine activity in glomus jugulare tumors. Laryngoscope 90:110–118, 1980

6. Ferris RA, Kirschner LP, Mero JH, Fields RL, Fulcher TM: Case report: Computed tomography of a carotid body tumor. J Comput Assist Tomogr 3:834–835, 1979

7. Földi M: Lymphogenous encephalopathy. In Mayerson HS (ed): Lymph and the Lymphatic System, pp 169–198. Springfield, IL, Charles C Thomas, 1968

8. Glasscock ME III, Harris PF, Newsome G: Glomus tumors: Diagnosis and treatment. Laryngoscope 84:2006–2032, 1974

9. Grubb WB Jr, Lampe I: The role of radiation therapy in the treatment of chemodectomas of the glomus jugulare. Laryngoscope 75:1861–1871, 1965

10. Guild SR: The glomus jugulare, a nonchromaffin paraganglion, in man. Ann Otol Rhinol Laryngol 62:1045–1071, 1953

11. Hatfield PM, James AE, Schultz MD: Chemodectomas of the glomus jugulare. Cancer 30:1164–1168, 1972

12. Hudgins PT: Radiotherapy for extensive glomus jugulare tumors. Radiology 103:427–429, 1972

13. Kim J-A, Elkon D, Lim M-L, Constable WC: Optimum dose of radiotherapy for chemodectomas of the middle ear. Int J Radiat Oncol Biol Phys 6:815–819, 1980

14. Lapayowker MS, Liebman EP, Ronis ML, Safer JN: Presentation of the internal carotid artery as a tumor of the middle ear. Radiology 98:293–297, 1971

15. Lawson W: The neuroendocrine nature of the glomus cells: An experimental, ultrastructural, and histochemical tissue culture study. Laryngoscope 90:120–144, 1980

16. Lawson W, Zak FG: The glomus bodies ("paraganglia") of the human larynx. Laryngoscope 84:98–111, 1974

17. Maruyama Y, Gold LHA, Kieffer SA: Clinical and angiographic evaluation of radiotherapeutic response of glomus jugulare tumors. Radiology 101:397–399, 1971

18. Mischke RE, Balkany TJ: Skull base approach to glomus jugulare. Laryngoscope 90:89–94, 1980

19. Myers EN, Newman J, Kaseff L, Black FO: Glomus jugulare tumor: A radiographic-histologic correlation. Laryngoscope 81:1838–1851, 1971

20. Newman H, Rowe JF Jr, Phillips TL: Radiation therapy of the glomus jugulare tumor. Am J Roentgenol Radium Ther Nucl Med 118:663–669, 1973

21. Rosenwasser H: Current management: Glomus jugulare tumors. Ann Otol Rhinol Laryngol 76:603–610, 1967

22. Smith PE: Management of chemodectomas (glomus jugulare). Laryngoscope 80:207–216, 1970

23. Spector GJ, Fierstein J, Ogura JH: A comparison of therapeutic modalities of glomus tumors in the temporal bone. Laryngoscope 86:690–696, 1976

24. Spector GJ, Gado M, Ciralsky R, Ogura JH, Maisel RH: Neurologic implications of glomus tumors in the head and neck. Laryngoscope 85:1387–1395, 1975

25. Tidwell TJ, Montague ED: Chemodectomas involving the temporal bone. Radiology 116:147–149, 1975

26. Van Baars F, Van Den Broek P, Cremers C, Veldman J: Familial non-chromaffinic paragangliomas (glomus tumors): Clinical aspects. Laryngoscope 91:988–996, 1981

27. Ward PH, Jenkins HA, Hanafee WN: Diagnosis and treatment of carotid body tumors. Ann Otol Rhinol Laryngol 87:614–621, 1978

28. Warren KW: Symposium on surgical lesions of neck and upper mediastinum: Tumors of the carotid body: Recognition and treatment. Surg Clin North Am 53:677–693, 1953

29. Wetmore RF, Tronzo RD, Lane RJ, Lowry LD: Nonfunctional paraganglioma of the larynx: Clinical and pathological considerations. Cancer 48:2717–2723, 1981

Carcinoma of the Thyroid

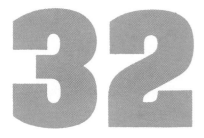

JAMES T. PARSONS
WILLIAM W. PFAFF

Thyroid carcinoma represents a spectrum of diseases with markedly different clinical behaviors. Opinions vary considerably regarding the means of establishing the diagnosis, the extent of initial surgery, and the role of various surgical adjuvant treatments. Because there are a number of factors that influence the course of disease, treatment must be individualized.

EPIDEMIOLOGY

Thyroid carcinoma is a relatively rare disease. In 1982, the National Cancer Institute predicted 10,100 new cases (7,200 women, 2,900 men) and 1,050 deaths (700 women, 350 men) in the United States.[91] The prevalence seems to be fairly uniform throughout the world wherever adequate statistics are available.[29] In the United States, there is a higher incidence of thyroid cancer in whites than blacks.[28]

The disease occurs primarily in young and middle-aged adults (Fig. 32-1).[111] Only about 5% of all cases occur before 15 to 20 years of age, and these are mostly papillary carcinomas in patients with a history of low-dose neck irradiation for benign disease.[43,80] The peak incidence of papillary carcinoma occurs 15 to 20 years earlier than that of follicular carcinoma, which is about 10 years before that of anaplastic carcinoma.[48,111] At the M. D. Anderson Hospital, only 8% of patients with anaplastic carcinoma were under 50 years of age.[1]

While most medullary carcinomas (approximately 80%) occur sporadically, they may also occur as a component of two complex endocrine syndromes, multiple endocrine neoplasia type IIA (MEN IIA) or type IIB (MEN IIB). The peak incidence of sporadic disease is in the sixth decade versus the second or third decade for familial disease.[16,107] All types of medullary carcinoma produce elevated plasma calcitonin levels.

MEN IIA is inherited as an autosomal dominant trait and is often associated with pheochromocytoma and parathyroid adenoma or hyperplasia. The variant syndrome, MEN IIB (medullary thyroid carcinoma, mucosal neuromas, and pheochromocytomas), is usually sporadic, but familial cases have also been reported.[74,107]

For both papillary and follicular carcinomas, the female-to-male ratio is 2.5 to 3.0:1.[19,111] The sex ratio for anaplastic and medullary carcinomas is approximately equal.[1,19,60,111]

ETIOLOGY

Low-dose radiation given for benign conditions during infancy and childhood has produced thyroid cancer in a small percentage of patients; the exact incidence is unknown. Most radiation-induced cancers are well differentiated. The usual latent interval is 10 to 30 years, but cases outside both time limits have been observed. (See Chapter 14, The Effect of Radiation on Normal Tissues of the Head and Neck.) In some series up to one third of the total thyroid cancer population gave a history of prior head and neck or chest irradiation.[80] Since for the past 20 years radiation has seldom been given to young patients with benign disease, the number of cases secondary to irradiation should decline in future years.

579

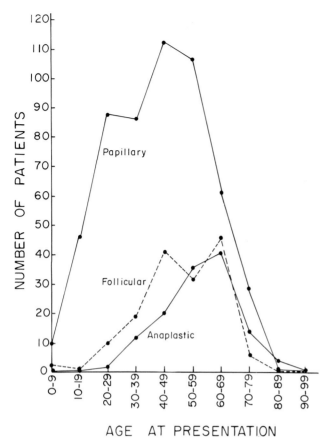

FIG. 32-1. Age distribution for 828 patients with differentiated or anaplastic thyroid carcinoma seen at the Mayo Clinic, 1926–1955. (Data from Woolner LB, Beahrs OH, Black BM, McConahey WM, Keating FR Jr: Classification and prognosis of thyroid carcinoma: A study of 885 cases observed in a thirty-year period. Am J Surg 102:354–387, 1961)

Although it has been suggested that some tumors are hormone dependent, there is no strong evidence to indicate that human thyroid cancer develops in response to elevated levels of thyrotropin (TSH), as has been shown in animals. Attempts to link the geographic distribution of nodular goiter to that of thyroid cancer have yielded inconclusive findings.

ANATOMY

Although the majority of anatomical variations in the region of the thyroid gland are rather minor, they occur frequently and are therefore of considerable importance to the surgeon. Too great reliance must not be placed on the "normal" anatomy if one is to avoid major surgical complications, primarily recurrent laryngeal nerve palsy and/or hypoparathyroidism.

The thyroid gland is situated anteriorly in the low neck in close proximity to the larynx, trachea, esophagus, parathyroid glands, recurrent laryngeal nerves, cervical sympathetic chain, and carotid sheath and its contents (Fig. 32-2).[33] The lateral lobes are approximately 5 cm in length and extend to the level of the mid-thyroid cartilage su-

periorly and to the sixth tracheal ring inferiorly; the lobes are connected in the midline by the isthmus at the level of the second to fourth tracheal rings (Fig. 32-3).[69] The isthmus is occasionally absent.[105] A pyramidal lobe is present in 40% to 50% of patients[31,50] and ascends for a variable distance toward the hyoid bone, usually slightly to the left of midline.

The functional unit of the thyroid gland is the follicle, which consists of a single layer of cuboidal epithelium surrounding a colloid-filled space. The follicles are separated from each other by a highly vascular connective tissue in which are situated the parafollicular cells, which secrete calcitonin. Connective tissue fibers from the capsule penetrate the gland, separating groups of follicles into lobules.

The capsule of the gland is formed rather late in fetal life from adjacent mesenchymal tissue; consequently, tissues foreign to the thyroid gland, such as the parathyroid glands, are often enclosed within it.[31] Although the recurrent laryngeal nerve is also said to occasionally pierce the capsule and enter the substance of the gland, such an occurrence must be quite rare and was never observed by Martin or his colleagues over a 30-year period at Memorial Sloan-Kettering Hospital in the performance of up to 225 thyroid operations per year.[63]

The right recurrent laryngeal nerve recurs around the right subclavian artery and the left recurs around the aortic arch. In the region of the thyroid gland, the nerves usually lie in a protected position in the tracheoesophageal grooves, although in some cases they may be lateral or, more rarely, anterolateral to the trachea.[50] Before it enters the larynx under cover of the inferior constrictor muscle (behind the articulation of the inferior cornu of the thyroid cartilage with the cricoid cartilage), the nerve is intimately related to the medial surface of the thyroid gland. The inferior thyroid artery is a useful guide to the location of the recurrent laryngeal nerve;[31] the nerve may pass in front of or behind the artery or through its branches. The recurrent laryngeal nerve may branch well below the larynx.[19,63,71] Simply visualizing the nerve in the tracheoesophageal groove is no insurance that it will not be injured higher up. The most frequent site of recurrent laryngeal nerve injury is under the upper pole of the gland,[63,71] where the nerve is frequently embedded in the fascial attachment (adherent zone, ligament of Berry) of the thyroid gland to the cricoid cartilage and upper tracheal rings and where more than one branch of the nerve may be present.[19,50,63,105] The nerve may also be injured during ligation of the inferior thyroid artery.

If the right recurrent laryngeal nerve cannot be located at operation, the possibility of a nonrecurrent nerve should be entertained. This variation, associated with an anomaly of the aortic arch and its branches, is probably present in less than 1% of patients, but it will be seen by any surgeon who performs a large number of thyroid operations.[31,50,63,71,75] Instead of looping under the subclavian artery, a nonrecurrent nerve may originate from the cervical trunk of the vagus at the level of the cricoid or thyroid cartilage and pass horizontally to the larynx, or it may first descend for several centimeters and then ascend in essentially the position of a normal recurrent laryngeal nerve.[75] Such a nerve may be injured by an unsuspecting surgeon. We have not seen reports of the anomaly on the left side.

The normal parathyroid glands vary in size, number, and position and are not easily identified at surgery.[19,63] Their color, texture, and relationship to the branches of

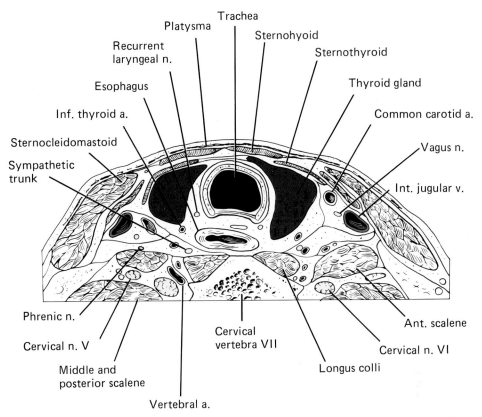

FIG. 32-2. Cross section of the neck through the C7 level. (Redrawn from Eycleshymer AC, Schoemaker DM: A Cross-Section Anatomy, p. 55. New York, D. Appleton-Century, 1938. Copyright © 1938, Mary Elizabeth Eycleshymer)

FIG. 32-3. Regional anatomy of the thyroid gland. © Copyright 1965, CIBA Pharmaceutical Company, Division of CIBA-GEIGY Corporation. Reprinted with permission from THE CIBA COLLECTION OF MEDICAL ILLUSTRATIONS, illustrated by Frank H. Netter, M.D. All rights reserved.

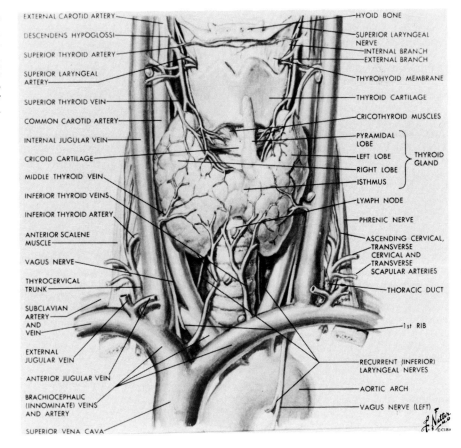

the inferior thyroid artery may help distinguish the glands from lymph nodes, fat, or thyroid tissue.[31] Typically, the glands are 6 mm long, 3 mm to 4 mm wide, and 1 mm to 2 mm thick; sometimes, in the region of the normal glands, there may only be many minute islands of parathyroid tissue scattered in the connective tissue and fat.[105]

Generally, there are two superior and two inferior glands. The upper glands are relatively constant in position; they are usually adherent to the capsule of the thyroid gland at the junction of its upper and middle thirds (at approximately the level of the upper portion of the cricoid cartilage). Embryologically, the lower parathyroid glands develop cephalad to the superior glands, in close association with the thymus; they are drawn below the superior glands when the thymus migrates caudad. The parathyroid glands normally descend only as far as the lower pole of each thyroid lobe. However, because of their "embryologic motility",[31] the inferior glands are more variable in position than the superior ones. They may be found within the substance of the thyroid gland, or they may migrate with the thymus into the chest; if they fail to migrate, they remain above the superior parathyroids, near the bifurcation of the common carotid artery.

The upper parathyroid glands are generally cephalad to the inferior thyroid artery and its uppermost branches, while the lower glands are caudad to the lowermost branches (Fig. 32-4). When the glands are hard to find, it may be of some help to trace the arterial branches.[31]

Lymphatic capillaries are arranged around the thyroid follicles and drain into a lymph network in the capsular region of the gland. From there, collecting trunks drain to a number of nodal sites, including those of the internal jugular chain, the Delphian node (one or two nodes overlying the cricothyroid membrane, present in about one-half of patients), and the pretracheal and paratracheal nodes in the lower neck.[85] Spread of thyroid cancer into the mediastinum is generally limited to lymph nodes in the anterosuperior segment, behind the manubrium and cephalad to the innominate veins. Lymphatics in the anterosuperior mediastinum can be considered as the lowest component of the cervical lymphatic system; spread of cancer to this region is almost always associated with spread to lateral cervical lymph nodes. Drainage to more inferiorly located mediastinal nodes is rarely seen in the absence of extensive anterosuperior mediastinal or pulmonary metastases.[10] McCormack and Sheline described seven thyroid cancer patients seen over a 20-year period at the University of California, San Francisco, in whom metastases occurred to parapharyngeal or retropharyngeal lymph nodes, as recognized by the occurrence of a submucosal mass in the pharynx.[59]

PATHOLOGY

Carcinomas of follicular cell origin are subdivided into papillary, follicular, and anaplastic carcinoma; those arising from parafollicular cells are called medullary (solid) carcinoma. The relative frequencies of thyroid carcinomas in 1181 patients treated at the Mayo Clinic over a 35-year period are shown in Table 32-1.[112] Papillary and follicular lesions (often referred to as the well-differentiated thyroid carcinomas) accounted for 80% of the total group. The percentage of patients with anaplastic carcinoma was higher at the Mayo Clinic than in some other large series; only 7% of 1174 thyroid carcinomas seen at the M. D. Anderson Hospital were true anaplastic lesions.[1]

The majority of papillary carcinomas contain both papillary and follicular elements in varying proportions; whether the lesion contains equal proportions of the two patterns or is mostly papillary or mostly follicular does not affect its biologic behavior. Microscopic diagnosis is not difficult in the majority of cases. The lesions are typically unencapsulated, have a high incidence of multifocality within the gland (whether these multifocal lesions represent true multicentric foci of origin or intrathyroidal lymphatic dissemination is not known),[19] and have almost no tendency toward vascular invasion. Psammoma bodies are frequently present.[111] Metastases generally contain both papillary and follicular elements.

Follicular carcinomas tend toward gross encapsulation. Papillary structure is, by definition, absent. Two morphologic subtypes are recognized, depending on invasiveness. The diagnosis of a carcinoma with slight or equivocal invasion is made on the basis of vascular invasion in the capsular region.[45] Often, the pathologist must examine multiple histologic sections from this region in order to distinguish a well-encapsulated follicular carcinoma from an adenoma. Follicular carcinomas with moderate to marked invasion are generally of a higher grade than less invasive lesions and often demonstrate obvious invasion of thyroid parenchyma.[45] The Hürthle cell carcinoma is a variant of follicular carcinoma.

"Anaplastic" has often been used as a wastebasket classification into which some investigators have placed spindle and giant cell carcinomas, squamous cell carcinomas, occasional sarcomas, small cell carcinomas, and perhaps some lymphomas. The task of distinguishing these various neoplasms may be difficult for the pathologist, but it should be attempted so that appropriate therapy may be planned. It is believed by some authors that many so-called small cell anaplastic carcinomas are, in reality, lymphomas.[1,109] Histopathology may not allow one to distinguish between the two, and electron microscopy and cell surface markers specific for lymphoid tissue are necessary. Our own feeling is that most of these lesions represent lymphoma, and a diagnosis of small cell carcinoma should be viewed with suspicion. Clinicopathologic correlation is important.

The M. D. Anderson Hospital group regards spindle and giant cell carcinoma as the only anaplastic neoplasm of thyroid epithelial origin and provides evidence that these lesions develop from preexisting differentiated carcinomas. Eighteen (21%) of 84 patients had a prior history of differentiated carcinoma; histologic sections from 66 patients (78%) revealed coexisting differentiated and anaplastic carcinoma, frequently with areas of transition from one pattern to the other.[1]

Medullary thyroid carcinoma is the only thyroid cancer that contains an amyloidlike substance. Although a frequent finding, this material need not be present to establish the diagnosis. Both the primary lesion and the metastases usually contain the substance.[45] Histologically, sporadic medullary thyroid carcinoma appears no different from that occurring in patients with the MEN II syndromes. However, in MEN IIA or MEN IIB, the cancer is virtually always bilateral within the gland. The sporadic form may be either unilateral or bilateral, more commonly the former.[47,108]

PATTERNS OF SPREAD

Each histologic type of thyroid carcinoma possesses its own distinctive natural history.

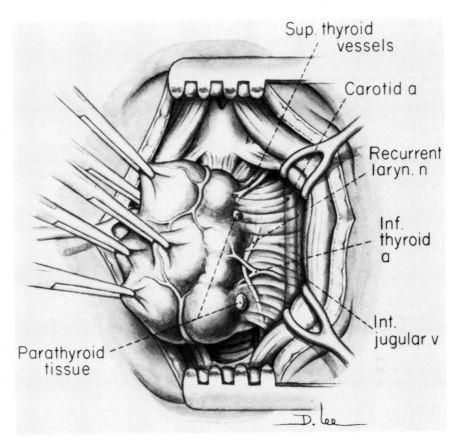

Sup. thyroid vessels

Carotid a

Recurrent laryn. n

Inf. thyroid a

Int. jugular v

Parathyroid tissue

D. lee

FIG. 32-4. Idealized diagram showing relationship of inferior thyroid artery to recurrent laryngeal nerves and parathyroid glands. (Dozois RR, Beahrs OH: Surgical anatomy and technique of thyroid and parathyroid surgery. Surg Clin North Am 57:647–661, 1977)

TABLE 32-1.	Classification of Thyroid Carcinoma		
Histology		**No. Patients**	**Percentage**
Papillary carcinoma		736	62.3
Follicular carcinoma		208	17.6
Slight or equivocal invasion		104	
Moderate to marked invasion		104	
Medullary (solid) carcinoma		77	6.5
Anaplastic carcinoma		160	13.6
Total		1181	100.0

Note: Data from Mayo Clinic, 1926–1960.

(With permission from Woolner LB, Beahrs OH, Black BM, McConahey WM, Keating FR Jr: Thyroid carcinoma: General considerations and follow-up data on 1181 cases. In Young S, Inman DR [eds]: Thyroid Neoplasia, pp 51–79. New York, Academic Press, 1968. Copyright ©: Academic Press Inc. [London] Ltd.)

Papillary carcinomas are characterized by slow growth. Extension of the primary tumor through the capsule of the gland into the soft tissues of the neck with invasion of surrounding viscera is unusual (5% to 10%) at presentation;[5,35,65] most of the patients in whom such extension occurred in the Mayo Clinic series were over 40 years of age at diagnosis.[111] Seven percent of previously untreated patients at Memorial Sloan-Kettering Hospital, New York City, had grossly unresectable disease secondary to invasion of the great vessels, larynx, trachea, or pharynx.[35]

Forty to 50% of patients with papillary carcinoma have gross evidence of regional lymph node metastases at operation;[45,65,111] in patients under 15 years of age, the incidence approaches 90%.[43] The true incidence of lymphatic metastases at presentation is higher than 50% because at least half of the patients with grossly normal lymph nodes are found to have metastases if they are systematically sampled.[35,63,65,72] The earliest metastases are generally to neck nodes ipsilateral to the primary lesion. Mediastinal metastases usually occur later; mediastinal metastases large enough to be detected on a chest roentgenogram were noted in 4 of 265 previously untreated patients at Memorial Sloan-Kettering Hospital.[35] Involved lymph nodes tend to remain discrete and mobile, without extension of tumor through the capsule.[43,95] Distant metastasis at presentation is quite unusual (3% of previously untreated patients at Memorial Sloan-Kettering Hospital)[15,35] and encountered mainly in patients with extracapsular extension;[78] less than

10% of patients developed distant metastases (usually to the lung) at some time during the course of their disease.[41,65,111]

Follicular carcinomas, like papillary lesions, are characterized by slow growth. As with papillary carcinoma, locally advanced, unresectable primary disease is unusual at presentation.[15,112] Lymph node metastases are seldom seen, except in the presence of extensive capsular invasion, recurrent tumor,[110] or extraglandular extension.[15] Twelve (7%) of 178 patients with follicular carcinomas had evidence of distant metastases, usually to the lung or bone, on referral to the Lahey Clinic;[15] if one assumes that virtually all of these metastases occurred in patients with moderate to marked capsular and vascular invasion, then one might expect metastases at presentation in 15% to 20% of this group.[5] Distant metastasis following treatment is a frequent problem in patients with highly invasive lesions.[111]

Anaplastic carcinomas are among the most aggressive of human tumors. In 84 cases seen at M. D. Anderson Hospital over a 28-year period, only three patients had limited disease confined to the gland without evidence of regional or distant metastases.[1] The primary lesions tend to be large and fixed, with invasion of adjacent structures. Skin invasion and fixation are not rare, giving rise to dermal lymphatic metastases on the chest and abdominal walls. Neck nodes are usually involved, although sometimes the primary tumor is so extensive that regional node status is difficult to assess. Axillary nodes are involved in some instances. In contradistinction to the mobile lymph nodes of differentiated lesions, those of anaplastic carcinoma are often fixed. Almost half (41 of 84) of the M. D. Anderson Hospital patients had distant metastases on admission.[1]

Medullary carcinoma is bilateral in virtually all familial cases, and it may be unilateral or bilateral in sporadic cases. At presentation, 25% of patients have palpable lymph nodes; 50% to 75% of all patients have positive lymph nodes at thyroidectomy. Involvement of mediastinal lymph nodes is frequent. Distant metastases occur most often in the liver, lungs, and bones.

CLINICAL PICTURE

Since the thyroid is an endocrine organ, one might expect to find malignant tumors that produce excessive quantities of thyroid hormone, but such a situation is exceedingly rare.

Differentiated carcinoma commonly presents as an asymptomatic unilateral mass that is either found incidentally on a routine examination or is noted by the patient. In many instances, some abnormality of the gland has been known to be present for several years prior to diagnosis.[29] While rapid enlargement may suggest malignancy, such enlargement may also occur secondary to hemorrhage into an adenoma or cyst. Pain and tenderness suggest thyroiditis.[5,19] Lymphadenopathy may occur in Hashimoto's thyroiditis as well as in malignant conditions.[19]

In 149 (21%) of 704 Mayo Clinic patients with papillary carcinoma, the primary was a clinically unsuspected, small ($\leq$1.5 cm) lesion that produced no lymph node metastases and was incidentally found when operation was performed for a goiter or some other benign problem.[103,112]

Another relatively common presentation (95 of 704 patients or 13% at the Mayo Clinic and approximately 15% at Memorial Sloan-Kettering Hospital) of papillary carci-

noma is with regional lymph node metastases (usually multiple nodes, sometimes massive) from a clinically inapparent, small primary cancer.[35,112] In the older medical literature, before the true nature of this presentation was recognized, these nodal metastases were thought to represent "lateral aberrant thyroid" tissue; true aberrant thyroid tissue of embryonic origin occurs in the midline, along the path of the thyroglossal duct. This "unknown primary" presentation is most commonly seen in young patients.[5] In cases of unilateral lymph node metastases, the primary lesion will generally be found in the ipsilateral lobe.[35,63]

Patients with follicular carcinoma rarely have lymph node metastases on admission. Occasionally, a pathologic fracture is the presenting symptom.[19,89]

Primary anaplastic carcinomas are typically large, hard, and fixed and grow rapidly. Local symptoms due to compression and/or invasion of the esophagus, airway, or recurrent laryngeal nerves are often marked and may overshadow symptoms of distant metastases, which also occur frequently. Symptoms include pain, a sensation of tightness, dysphagia, dyspnea, stridor, and hoarseness.

In the M. D. Anderson Hospital series, 18 of 84 patients with anaplastic carcinoma had a well-documented prior history of differentiated thyroid carcinoma, and 31 other patients had a history of longstanding, histologically undiagnosed goiter that suddenly grew rapidly. In only a handful of patients was the anaplastic lesion an incidental small focus within a larger, well-differentiated lesion.[1]

At initial presentation, most patients with medullary carcinoma are asymptomatic and are referred for evaluation of a painless thyroid mass.[16,47] Ten percent present with symptoms due to extensive local invasion (pain, dysphagia, or hoarseness) and their tumor is locally unresectable in a substantial number of cases.[47] Twenty to 30% of patients have significant diarrhea at presentation, most commonly when extensive regional or distant metastases are present.[47,96] The mechanism is unknown, but it is probably due to elaboration of a hormone by the tumor. Diarrhea frequently precedes the diagnosis of cancer by months to years, and occasionally is the only complaint at presentation.

Almost all patients with medullary thyroid carcinomas large enough to be palpated have elevated basal plasma thyrocalcitonin levels. Even in the presence of markedly elevated levels, hypocalcemia is almost never seen in medullary carcinoma; in fact, hypercalcemia is more common and occurs in patients with MEN IIA. The occurrence of parathyroid hyperplasia is probably not a reactive phenomenon that occurs in response to the hypocalcemic effect of thyrocalcitonin because it is not seen in patients with sporadic disease or MEN IIB, despite markedly elevated thyrocalcitonin levels. Hyperparathyroidism occurs in approximately 60% of MEN IIA patients and is detected by an elevated blood calcium concentration.[108]

In patients with MEN IIA or MEN IIB, it is essential to exclude the presence of, or treat, a pheochromocytoma prior to any neck operation in order to avoid a possible hypertensive crisis.[74,107] The pheochromocytomas associated with medullary carcinoma usually present in the second or third decade, are bilateral in approximately 70% of cases, and almost always are confined to the adrenal gland. They are present in 40% or more of patients with MEN II syndromes.[16,108] Elaboration of adrenocorticotropic hormone (ACTH), histaminase, prostaglandins, and serotonin have been reported in patients with medullary carcinoma and may produce a variety of symptoms.

MEN IIB patients are characterized by typical facies (*i.e.*, puffy lips, soft tissue prognathism, broad base of the nose, and everted eyelids), multiple mucosal neuromas, marfanoid habitus, and a variety of skeletal abnormalities.[74]

METHODS OF DIAGNOSIS

A thyroid nodule can be palpated in 3% to 4% of the US population at large;[2,52,78,97] the incidence increases with age and is higher in females than males.[2] The frequency with which nodules are found at autopsy is higher than the clinical incidence.[67] Since the prevalence of thyroid cancer is low compared with these figures, it is obvious that the majority of nodules are benign and, unless symptomatic, need not be resected. The problem for the thyroid surgeon is to separate out the small group of malignant lesions from the larger group of benign lesions.

At one extreme, the diagnosis of malignancy may be strongly suspected on clinical grounds alone, such as a young patient with a prior history of head and neck irradiation who presents with a steadily enlarging, firm, solitary thyroid mass with or without lymphadenopathy. Similarly, a thyroid nodule in a child is highly suspect.[5] A patient with a family history of thyroid cancer or a patient with marked symptomatology suggestive of anaplastic carcinoma likewise generally presents little diagnostic challenge. Such patients generally require open exploration regardless of the findings of various laboratory tests.

At the other extreme, the clinical picture may be near-diagnostic of a benign condition, such as an older patient with a relatively soft, multinodular goiter that has not changed for many years. Observation alone may suffice unless there is some other reason (cosmesis or pressure symptoms) to remove the mass.

Between these two extremes, one finds many patients in whom the history and clinical findings are not so conclusive. Often the mass is unilateral, asymptomatic, and thought to be of recent origin. Diagnosis in these cases is difficult, and the differential diagnosis includes cysts, cancer, adenomas, or some type of thyroiditis. Although there are some helpful clues (*e.g.*, the likelihood of malignancy in nodular goiter is greater in males than females and greater in solitary than multinodular glands), often the answer is unclear even after the patient has undergone a number of the laboratory tests discussed below.[5,21,53,55,76]

An ultrasound is usually ordered because, if the lesion is cystic (approximately 15% of cases),[23,83] it may be aspirated and thereby treated. The aspirated fluid is sent for cytologic examination, but only rarely is cancer present. If a mass persists after aspiration, further evaluation (generally open or needle biopsy) is necessary.[27] Large (>4 cm) cysts are probably best treated by surgery.[83]

Although a radioisotope thyroid scan is usually performed, in many cases it is not particularly helpful in establishing the diagnosis. The clinician is looking for a "cold" nodule, and that is just what he finds in the majority of cases since most nodules, whether benign or malignant, are cold.[76] Only 10% to 20% of biopsied solitary cold nodules are due to cancer.[53,76] The main usefulness of a scan would be in the detection of a "hot" nodule, which rarely contains malignancy,[76] or in the detection of multiple nodules within a gland clinically thought to harbor a solitary lesion, thus making likely the diagnosis of a multinodular goiter.

Tests of thyroid function are rarely helpful in establishing a diagnosis since the vast majority of patients with benign and malignant lesions are euthyroid. We do obtain the tests, however, since they are simple, cheap, and establish a baseline. Elevated serum thyroglobulin levels can be seen in patients with a variety of thyroid diseases and have no significant diagnostic value.[100] Measurement of antithyroid antibodies is not helpful.[54]

Computed tomographic (CT) scanning does not distinguish benign from malignant conditions, but it may be of some use in showing the local and regional extent of advanced or recurrent cancer prior to surgery. On the CT scan the thyroid gland usually shows significantly higher attenuation values than the surrounding soft tissues owing to its iodine content (see Fig. 19-10 in Chapter 19). Infusion of a contrast medium increases the difference.[62]

In most US centers, histologic examination of thyroid tissue obtained by large-bore needle biopsy or cytologic examination of smears from fine-needle aspirates are not considered substitutes for open biopsy. Although there are some exceptions,[27,34,104] most American physicians have not adopted needle techniques for routine clinical use, generally because they fear misdiagnosis. Few centers have a cytopathologist with experience in reading aspiration biopsies. Some have recommended needle biopsy only when the probability of malignancy is low.[5] The largest experience with aspiration biopsy cytology has been in the Scandinavian countries, where thousands of procedures have been performed over the past 30 years.[58] In a 50-year review of the literature concerning aspiration and large-bore needle techniques, Ashcraft could find only one instance of tumor seeding in the needle track.[3] If the clinical suspicion of malignancy is strong, one should not hesitate to perform open biopsy despite a negative needle biopsy finding.

Although a 3- to 6-month trial of thyroid suppression is used in some clinics in an attempt to distinguish between benign and malignant nodules, significant regression and/or complete disappearance occur in a rather low percentage of the total patient group with solitary thyroid nodules.[3,12] If the nodule fails to regress, as is rather common, one has only postponed the decision about what to do. If the nodule continues to grow, suggesting possible malignancy, definitive surgery has been delayed by several months. If thyroid suppression is attempted, it would seem reasonable to perform a needle biopsy beforehand: if the biopsy is positive, immediate surgery is undertaken; and if it is negative, one at least has some reassurance that more definitive therapy is not being unnecessarily delayed. Extreme caution should be exercised in prescribing thyroid hormone to old patients with thyroid nodules for fear of precipitating angina or myocardial infarction in a patient who probably has a benign lesion; suppression is contraindicated if underlying coronary disease is known to be present.

Although we have no "routine" workup for the patient who presents with a thyroid nodule, all University of Florida patients first undergo a careful head and neck examination, with special attention to indirect laryngoscopy. We obtain thyroid function tests and a chest roentgenographic examination. A radionuclide scan and ultrasound are performed to help establish a diagnosis. A CT scan is performed if mediastinal lymph node metastases are suspected, and a bone scan is done if symptoms suggest metastases. Results of liver function tests are generally obtained. Bronchoscopy is indicated if tracheal invasion is suggested.

If open biopsy of a thyroid nodule is indicated, the recommended procedure is lobectomy. Lesser procedures (e.g., "nodulectomy") are not advised since a diagnosis of cancer will necessitate reoperation, which is technically more difficult and increases the risk of recurrent laryngeal nerve injury. At the time of operation, the gland is fully exposed to allow inspection and palpation of both lobes and adjacent structures. Should an enlarged lymph node or nodes be found, immediate frozen section may aid in planning the appropriate surgical procedure. Previously unrecognized contralateral thyroid nodules also influence the scope of the operation.

Screening of High-Risk Populations

Calcitonin, a hormonal product of the cell of origin (the parafollicular or C cell) of medullary carcinomas, serves as a marker by which family members with C-cell hyperplasia (the presumed premalignant precursor of medullary carcinoma) or early, clinically inapparent medullary cancers can be identified.[107] Provocative testing is necessary since family members with early disease often have normal basal calcitonin levels but abnormal levels after stimulation.[93] Yearly screening following calcium and/or pentagastrin infusion has been recommended for family members over 5 years of age; a single screening is not sufficient since some who have a negative test initially are noted to convert to a positive test when followed for a period of time.[107] Although such screening is not yet proven to increase the cure rate, almost certainly this will be the case since thyroidectomies are now being performed in some very young, asymptomatic patients with very small primary lesions and no lymphatic metastases.[37,107]

Screening of the relatives of 36 Mayo Clinic patients presumed to have the sporadic form of medullary thyroid carcinoma (i.e., no family history of medullary carcinoma, pheochromocytoma, or hyperparathyroidism) resulted in detection of 57 new cases in seven families.[93] Thus, 19% of patients (7 of 36) presumed to have sporadic disease were actually index cases to kindreds with familial disease.

In addition to family members of patients with medullary carcinoma, another high-risk population that should be screened consists of patients known to have received low-dose irradiation during infancy and childhood. If the results of the baseline physical examination are normal, such patients should undergo careful reexamination every 1 to 2 years. We do not recommend routine thyroid scans in the absence of a palpable abnormality. Evaluation of thyroglobulin levels has little value as a screening procedure.[88]

TREATMENT

Well-Differentiated Carcinomas

SURGERY

There still exists a fair difference of opinion among surgeons as to how radical the thyroidectomy and node dissection should be. At the University of Florida, the operation is individualized according to the nature and extent of the disease, with a tendency toward a fairly conservative surgical approach in the majority of cases; external-beam irradiation or radioiodine is used for the occasional patient with a high likelihood of microscopic residual cancer. The minimum operation that is adequate would be a total lo-

bectomy, usually with resection of the isthmus. For patients with small intraglandular papillary carcinomas or low-grade encapsulated follicular carcinomas, this may be the only treatment necessary.[24] If a small, unsuspected cancer is found in a lobe resected for a benign condition, reoperation is usually not indicated. Similarly, if cancer was suspected but the frozen section was negative (e.g., follicular adenoma), reoperation is usually not necessary after lobectomy if the pathologist later returns a diagnosis of minimally invasive follicular carcinoma on permanent sections.[42,49] There is no reason to add radioiodine to ablate the residual gland[5] or to add external-beam irradiation for these cases.

If frozen section reveals follicular carcinoma with moderate to marked vascular invasion or if the tumor is larger, no matter what the histology, total or "near-total" (ipsilateral total and contralateral subtotal lobectomy) thyroidectomy is indicated. The bilateral presence of gross disease calls for a total thyroidectomy.[24] If distant metastases are present or suggested, a total thyroidectomy will facilitate the use of iodine-131 for both detection and treatment.[5] Because the local and distant failure rates are high and the survival rate is low following thyroidectomy for markedly invasive follicular carcinoma,[24,48,112] adjuvant radiation therapy is recommended.

More advanced presentations require more extensive individualized operations. The goal of surgical therapy is removal of all gross cancer with preservation of function whenever possible. The larynx, trachea, and recurrent laryngeal nerves are rarely sacrificed unless there is intraluminal tumor extension or extensive involvement. If the strap muscles are invaded, they are removed en bloc with the gland. Tumors adherent to the trachea, larynx, and esophageal wall are most often "shaved off," following which external-beam irradiation, radioiodine, or both are administered for microscopic residuum.[11,30,90] In some instances, partial resection of the trachea or removal of a thyroid ala is necessary. Total laryngectomy along with resection of a length of trachea is not frequently necessary for well-differentiated thyroid carcinoma.[11,30] If gross residual disease will definitely be left behind, operation is often best withheld; radioiodine, external-beam irradiation, or both are administered in such instances. If all of the tumor does not disappear, it is sometimes made resectable by the radiation.

Gross evaluation of lymph nodes in the tracheoesophageal grooves and anterosuperior mediastinum should be made at the time of operation.[9,10] Resection of limited disease in the anterosuperior mediastinum can generally be accomplished through the cervical incision; attempts to resect more advanced disease necessitate splitting the sternum. Elective lymph node dissections are not routinely performed for papillary or follicular carcinoma. If positive neck nodes are noted at surgery, they are usually adequately resected by way of modified neck operation with preservation of the internal jugular vein, sternocleidomastoid muscle, and spinal accessory nerve. Radical neck dissection is necessary in 10% or less of patients with papillary carcinoma,[5,111] usually only when tumor extends through the capsule of nodes. Although lymph node "plucking" or "berry picking" procedures are performed by some surgeons, we prefer to do a modified neck dissection in the presence of gross nodal metastases, since it is a more complete operation and can be accomplished without functional loss.

Local or regional recurrences are managed by completion thyroidectomy and/or neck dissection(s) as the need arises.

If recurrent tumor extends into the soft tissues of the neck or if it is unresectable, external-beam irradiation and radioiodine (if uptake is demonstrable) are added, since failure to achieve both distant[24] and local-regional control is frequent.

SUPPRESSION WITH THYROID HORMONE

Suppression of thyrotropin by administration of exogenous thyroid hormone has been reported to prevent recurrences after surgery and to result in temporary and occasionally permanent regression of metastatic well-differentiated thyroid cancer; the best results have been obtained in young patients.[24] In patients who have undergone total or near-total thyroidectomy or who have had their glands ablated with radioiodine, administration of thyroid hormone is necessary just to meet physiological needs. In patients who have remaining functional thyroid tissue, thyroid hormone is administered for its suppressive effect. We recommend that thyroid hormone, in amounts sufficient to suppress thyrotropin, be administered indefinitely with interruptions only for radioiodine studies or treatments.[17]

Just as there is controversy over the surgery and radiation therapy for these tumors, so the role of thyroid hormone as a therapeutic agent remains controversial. Jesse and Clark found no evidence for suppression of any type of thyroid cancer following administration of 3 grains of desiccated thyroid per day to over 700 patients who underwent total thyroidectomy at the M. D. Anderson Hospital.[18,51] Likewise, Block noted no apparent benefit from suppressive therapy after surgery for well-differentiated lesions.[8] At the Lahey Clinic, there was a 5% reduction in death rate due to papillary cancer in those who received thyroid hormone postoperatively but no difference for follicular carcinoma.[15] Several other investigators who have tried to suppress gross disease with thyroid hormone have noted partial, short-lived regression in only a small percentage of patients, most often to some, but not all, sites of involvement; eventual regrowth of tumor was noted in all cases.[38,92] The fact that some thyroid tumors are initially responsive to thyroid hormone, but later lose their responsiveness, is hardly surprising because this is what is routinely observed in other hormonally responsive cancers (e.g., breast and prostate). Whenever treatment is indicated for known or suspected residual differentiated cancer, thyroid hormone should be administered only as a supplement to other therapy.

RADIATION THERAPY

There are no precise guidelines for when to use external-beam irradiation or radioiodine either alone or in combination for well-differentiated carcinomas of the thyroid. Any claims for the superiority of one technique over another are difficult to substantiate. The indications for the use of these treatments vary from center to center and often vary considerably even within a single institution. Controlled trials have not been performed, but they would require a very large number of patients who could be carefully stratified according to a number of risk factors and followed for many years.

For the majority of patients, routine ablation of the remaining thyroid gland with radioiodine or external-beam irradiation is not indicated after adequate surgery since cure has usually already been achieved by the operation alone; this is particularly true of patients under 40 years of age. Although the risk of developing acute leukemia following treatment with iodine-131 is admittedly small (probably ≦1%), we feel that the risk does constitute a relative contraindication to its routine prophylactic use in patients who have little risk of tumor recurrence. For patients over 40 years of age the prognosis is worse, and some authors recommend prophylactic treatment even after apparently complete surgery;[99] radioiodine ablation of residual glandular tissue followed by diagnostic radioiodine total body scans is an approach that we commonly use, even though it is difficult to find solid evidence for the effectiveness of such treatment in this group of patients. When there is known gross or microscopic residual cancer, radioiodine is used in preference to external-beam irradiation in many US centers, unless the lesion does not concentrate radioiodine. The rationale of administering a systemic dose of radiation for a local problem has been questioned.[90] We believe that postoperative external-beam irradiation is rational treatment for the following: suspected residual disease when tumor has extended through the capsule of the gland or through the capsule of nodes into surrounding soft tissues, since the risk of local-regional failure in this circumstance is high;[40,64,112] markedly invasive follicular carcinoma, since the rates of local and distant failure are both high;[5,111] and known gross residual cancer in the neck after operation.[92,99] In a number of institutions, including the Institut Gustave-Roussy, the Princess Margaret Hospital, the Royal Marsden Hospital, and the Glasgow Institute of Radiotherapeutics, external-beam irradiation is frequently combined with radioiodine;[38,40,92,101] such a combination would seem particularly appropriate in patients with, or at high risk of developing, both local and distant failure. Radioiodine ablation of remaining normal thyroid tissue in patients who are at substantial risk of developing distant metastases has an additional advantage in that it helps in the detection of metastases by way of iodine-131 scans. We have had little experience with combined therapy with external-beam irradiation and radioiodine at the University of Florida, but we would generally lean toward giving the iodine-131 treatment first, on the theory that external-beam irradiation might diminish the uptake by local-regional tumor.

It is technically difficult to deliver high-dose external-beam irradiation to the thyroid, trachea, cervical esophagus, jugular lymph nodes, upper neck, and upper mediastinum without exceeding the tolerance of the spinal cord. The depth of the spinal cord from the anterior skin surface varies markedly in this anatomical region because of differences in thickness between the upper chest versus the lower neck. From a lateral approach, the contour is even more irregular, owing to the shoulders. While many authors have discounted the effect of external irradiation, the doses applied in many of their series were quite low,[65] apparently because therapists feared complications.

There is no evidence to indicate that thyroid carcinomas are any more or less curable by external irradiation than squamous cell carcinomas of equal volume. For most situations in which radiation therapy is indicated, high doses (e.g., 6000 rad to 7000 rad/6½ to 7½ weeks) are required if one expects to obtain a satisfactory rate of control. A number of techniques have been devised to deliver a high dose to this region, including high-energy electrons, oblique wedges, and a variety of arc techniques. The normal cervical lordosis and thoracic kyphosis make wedges or arcs impractical because the techniques do not allow adequate field-shaping. Simple lateral fields do not allow adequate coverage of the upper mediastinum because the shoulders get in the way. Exclusive use of high-energy electrons has the disadvantage of producing excessive subcutaneous fibrosis. An anterior cobalt-60 field directed at the neck and mediastinum plus a posterior high-energy x-ray field to the mediastinum is capable of delivering the initial 5000-rad tumor dose to the low neck and upper mediastinum.[57] Boost doses beyond the basic 5000 rad may be administered with electrons in some situations. If doses in the range of 7000 rad are required to tumors as deep as the cervical esophagus plus the upper mediastinum, a four-field box technique using compensated (with beeswax) lateral fields is recommended (see Chapter 22, Carcinoma of the Cervical Esophagus). If neck disease extends behind the plane of the spinal cord, it can be treated with electrons.

When all gross disease has been removed, but tumor was "shaved off" the larynx, trachea, or esophageal wall by sharp dissection, residual microscopic disease is presumably present. External-beam irradiation has been shown to prevent local recurrence in a high proportion of such patients and is sometimes combined with radioiodine, since the risk of distant metastases in this setting is also substantial.[92] Sheline reported results in a small series of well-differentiated thyroid cancers following external-beam irradiation (5000 rad to 6000 rad/6 to 7 weeks) after microscopically incomplete resection.[90] Follow-up was 5 to 22 years. The results were good (Table 32-2). We recommend no less than 6000 rad/6 to 6½ weeks.

External-beam irradiation is indicated if there is gross residual cancer following operation or if local disease is inoperable. Radioiodine alone is usually insufficient to control large masses in the neck, even when the tumor concentrates the substance.[92,99] Moreover, in approximately 20% of cases, the tumor does not concentrate iodine-131 at all.[40] A combination of the two treatments is advised by a number of investigators in these situations;[38,40,92,99] there are no data to show how best to time the one treatment relative to the other or to guide the doses of each modality. In some very advanced cases, only palliation is to be expected. Regression of gross disease following irradiation may continue for several months.

At the University of California, San Francisco, in 6 of 10 patients (60%) with minimum 5-year follow-up data the cancer remained locally controlled 5 to 25 years after postoperative external-beam irradiation for macroscopic residual disease; even when treatment was unsuccessful,

palliation was often substantial, since all four of the failures occurred 5 to 18 years after treatment.[90] Survival at 15 years following postoperative external-beam irradiation of gross residual cancer was 36% at the Institut Gustave-Roussy.[99,101]

The results of external-beam irradiation for inoperable tumors have not been highly satisfactory, but prolonged palliation is sometimes achieved. Frazell and Foote reported that 6 (26%) of 23 patients with advanced, inoperable primary or recurrent papillary cancer were without evidence of recurrence 5 years following x-ray therapy alone.[35] In a larger series of patients, Tubiana reported only 20% of inoperable patients alive 5 years and 10% alive 15 years after external-beam irradiation.

FOLLOW-UP

Occasionally patients with diffuse pulmonary metastases or early local-regional recurrence (especially in the mediastinum) have tumors too small or too inaccessible to be detected on routine chest roentgenogram or by clinical examination. Periodic whole-body radioiodine scans are useful in monitoring patients at high risk of developing recurrence. Tubiana recommends that scans be obtained at 6-month intervals for 2 years, then annually until the fifth year, and semiannually until 15 to 25 years.[100] Chest films are obtained at the same intervals until 5 years and annually thereafter. Technetium bone scans and bone surveys are not performed in the absence of symptoms. We have no experience with serum thyroglobulin determination in the follow-up period; the marker is said to be of value in detecting recurrent cancer in patients whose glands have been totally removed or ablated[102] and apparently provides information that is complementary to that from iodine-131 scans.[20] Since thyroid tissue is the only source of circulating thyroglobulin, patients who have no residual normal thyroid tissue should have no detectable serum thyroglobulin except that which is produced by persistent cancer. In some patients thyroglobulin is detectable only after TSH stimulation. The diagnostic accuracy of thyroglobulin determination is not satisfactory if normal residual thyroid tissue is present.[87]

TREATMENT OF DISTANT METASTASES

Five to 10% of all patients with distant metastases from well-differentiated carcinomas are believed to be permanently cured following administration of radioiodine;[15,99] in patients with lung metastases as the only site of disease, the cure rate may be as high as 30% if the tumor concentrates radioiodine.[99] In some patients who were presumed to have been cured and who died of other causes, autopsies have disclosed clinically unsuspected residual thyroid cancer.[100] If radioiodine is not taken up, long-term survival is unusual. Most of the patients in whom treatment is successful are under 40 years of age.[44] Concentration of radioiodine by invasive follicular carcinoma is frequently poor.[99] Treatment in most patients is only palliative in intent, but it is undertaken even in the absence of symptoms because all clinical evidence of disease may disappear for substantial periods of time and many who ultimately have recurrent disease will live without symptoms for years or even decades.[64] The best long-term results obtained by Sheline in the treatment of metastatic disease were in patients with diffuse miliary lung disease; since these patients also happen to be the group most likely to develop severe

TABLE 32-2.	Local Control After External-Beam Irradiation for Papillary or Follicular Carcinoma Following Microscopically Incomplete Resection

Histology	Local Control
Papillary	12/12
Follicular	3/5
Total	15/17 (88%)*

* Length of follow-up in patients with locally controlled disease was 5 to 22 years (mean 10.2 years; median 9 years). Local recurrences in two patients occured at 4 and 6 years.

Note: University of California, San Francisco, data.

(Data from Sheline GE, Galante M, Lindsay S: Radiation therapy in the control of persistent thyroid cancer. Am J Roentgenol Radium Ther Nucl Med 97:923–930, 1966)

or even fatal radiation pneumonitis or pulmonary fibrosis, large single doses of iodine-131 are to be avoided.* In the occasional patient with a large solitary pulmonary metastasis, consideration should be given to surgical resection, followed by iodine-131 scan and therapy.

As a general rule, metastases will not concentrate radioiodine as long as normal thyroid tissue is present. Following surgical or radioiodine (usually with 30 mCi to 60 mCi of iodine-131) ablation of the gland, many, but not all, metastases will concentrate radioiodine. Not all lesions in which iodine-131 concentration is demonstrated will regress, since its concentration may be poor, its distribution may be nonuniform, or the tumor may be poorly responsive.[94] In patients with multiple sites of disease, not all lesions take up iodine-131 to the same degree.[89] Concentration is enhanced by taking the patient off thyroid hormone for 5 to 6 weeks (3 to 4 weeks if the patient is on L-triiodothyronine). Patients receive a low-iodine diet for 3 to 4 weeks and a diuretic (hydrochlorothiazide, 50 mg daily, plus dietary potassium supplements) for 2 weeks prior to iodine-131 administration so as to produce an acute iodide depletion to promote iodine-131 uptake by the tumor.[39] Occasionally, elderly patients are supported with 5 μg/day of L-triiodothyronine if they are tolerating hypothyroidism poorly; this often gives marked symptomatic improvement while maintaining stimulation of thyrotropin production. Administering exogenous (bovine) thyrotropin for several days prior to radioiodine administration[19,101] does not add much to the management of most patients, provided they have been off thyroid hormone for sufficient time;† additionally, some patients develop allergic reactions following administration of bovine thyrotropin. On rare occasions, one encounters patients with tumors that are seemingly quite hormone-dependent and grow rapidly when the patient is made hypothyroid; in such patients, it is helpful to substitute L-triiodothyronine for other thyroid medications 6 weeks prior to scanning, then discontinue replacement therapy 3 (rather than 6) weeks before iodine-131 is administered, so as to minimize the duration of hypothyroidism. A shorter period of withdrawal of L-triiodothyronine along with administration of thyrotropin (10 units intramuscularly on 3 successive days) may result in less than maximal iodine uptake in metastases since peak blood levels are very transient.[7,46]

Some physicians who administer iodine-131 give 200 mCi to 300 mCi (in divided doses), then quit; we agree with Sheline that a more sensible approach to patients with demonstrable metastases is to push the dose to tissue tolerance (as indicated by marrow depression) or to the point that uptake in the tumor is low or disappears.* Successful treatment of metastases in Tubiana's hands generally required three to nine doses of 100 mCi to 150 mCi administered at 3-month intervals over one to several years, with the number of doses dependent on the results of posttherapy scintigrams.[100] Most American authors recommend a somewhat longer interval (6 to 12 months) between successive doses so as to allow more adequate marrow recovery.[7,41,61,77]

Patients with bone metastases are often over 40 years of age and have tumors that concentrate radioiodine poorly;[44,61] even if concentration is demonstrated and all evidence of cancer is made to disappear, recurrence is the rule.[6] Only occasional patients with bone metastases survive for long periods without clinical recurrence.[41,101,111] Patients with metastases to weight-bearing long bones or vertebrae and patients with bone pain should be given external-beam irradiation in addition to radioiodine.[61,68]

Medullary Carcinoma

Because of the high incidence of multicentricity and bilaterality within the gland, total thyroidectomy is recommended.[5,56] If parathyroid hyperplasia is also present, all parathyroid tissue is removed and a portion of one gland is autografted.[106]

For patients with no apparent lymph node metastases at operation, usually the central lymph nodes between the carotid sheaths from the level of the hyoid bone down into the superior mediastinum to the level of the innominate artery are dissected. If there is obvious lymphadenopathy, or if frozen section reveals positive lymph nodes, radical neck dissection(s) is performed in preference to conservation neck surgery.[5,16,56,66] For patients with positive nodes who are treated by operation alone, clinically detectable failure occurs in almost two thirds of cases and a number of others are presumed to have residual disease on the basis of persistently elevated calcitonin levels.[16] Since most of the failures occur in the mediastinum and neck, postoperative radiation therapy should be given to these patients. Medullary carcinomas do not concentrate radioiodine or suppress with thyroid hormone.

When doses of external-beam irradiation similar to those used for squamous cell carcinoma are used postoperatively, small amounts of residual tumor have been controlled.[38] At the Institut Gustave-Roussy, only the patients with the most unfavorable tumors (extensive neck disease with lymph-node involvement and/or inadequate surgical excision) were given postoperative radiation therapy; yet their survival at 20 years was approximately double that of patients with less advanced cancers treated by surgery alone.[99] There are a handful of reports of patients with gross and/or inoperable masses that were permanently controlled (8 to 17 years' follow-up) following high-dose radiation.[38,84,101] There is no documentation that medullary carcinoma requires different doses than squamous cell carcinoma of equal volume. Regression of gross disease occurs slowly.

Patients are monitored 1 or 2 weeks postoperatively, then every 6 to 12 months with provocative (pentagastrin and/or calcium infusion) testing for elevated calcitonin levels. Norton, at the National Cancer Institute, carefully studied seven asymptomatic patients who had no clinical signs of disease and negative metastatic workups but who had elevated basal or stimulated calcitonin levels 1 to 5 years after thyroidectomy.[73] By performing selective venous catheterization with pentagastrin stimulation, he was able to localize disease to the neck or superior mediastinal lymph nodes in all seven patients; in each patient, the presence of residual cancer was histologically confirmed by completion thyroidectomy and/or lymph node dissection. Since, with only 6 to 36 months of follow-up, stimulated calcitonin levels returned to normal in only one patient (suggesting residual disease in the other six), the value of such repeat surgery has been questioned by some. We would recommend the addition of external-beam irradiation in patients whose disease is apparently confined to the neck and mediastinum.

---

* Sheline GE: Personal communication, 1982.

† Sheline GE: Personal communication, September 1982.

Anaplastic Carcinomas

Most patients have advanced, incurable disease at presentation. Regardless of the type of treatment administered, only an occasional patient is cured. Anaplastic carcinoma does not concentrate radioiodine, does not suppress with exogenous thyroid hormone, and responds rather poorly to external-beam irradiation.[90] The tumors are usually locally unresectable at presentation; laryngectomy, pharyngectomy, cervical esophagectomy, and radical neck dissection(s) are rarely justifiable. The usual intent of treatment is palliation of local symptoms. Tracheostomy is often necessary to prevent death by asphyxiation and must often be carried out with the use of a bronchoscope in order to ensure an adequate airway while a search is being made for the trachea in the midst of a massive local tumor. Operative deaths have been described in this setting.[30] External-beam irradiation is administered to palliate symptoms of local or metastatic disease.

For patients with resectable lesions, total thyroidectomy is always followed by external-beam irradiation, even when resection was considered complete, since failure to do so usually results in local recurrence.[1] The best chance for cure is in the occasional patient who is incidentally found to have a small focus of anaplastic carcinoma within a predominantly well-differentiated carcinoma.[1,5] External-beam irradiation is recommended even in this setting.

At the M. D. Anderson Hospital, postoperative irradiation plus dactinomycin has been used in combination since 1965 for patients whose disease is confined to the neck.[1]

Treatment of extensive local disease is often by radiation therapy alone. In patients who are otherwise in reasonably good medical condition, efforts to obtain local control of disease are often made in an attempt to avert a miserable death secondary to local disease. There is no strong evidence at this time that combinations of chemotherapy and irradiation produce better results than irradiation alone; attempts to combine the two modalities must be made with caution to avoid excessive side-effects. Because these tumors proliferate quite rapidly, hyperfractionation and accelerated fractionation schemes that deliver two or three fractions per day may be of benefit.

RESULTS OF TREATMENT

Differentiated Carcinomas

GENERAL REMARKS

Since differentiated carcinomas often have a long natural history, 5 years is insufficient time to assess treatment results. In a review of 30 years' experience at the Lahey Clinic, Cady found that slightly over half of all cancer recurrences were manifest by 5 years and less than half of all cancer deaths had occurred by that time (Figs. 32-5 and 32-6).[15] Tumor recurrence and death due to cancer continued to occur sporadically up to 25 and 30 years, respectively, after treatment.

A number of factors correlate with decreased survival, including the following:

1. Large size of the primary lesion[111]
2. Extension of the primary lesion through the capsule of the gland or of nodal metastasis through the capsule of the lymph node into surrounding soft tissues in the neck[15,111]
3. Follicular carcinoma with moderate-marked invasiveness[24,48,112]

4. Age over 40[15,111]
5. Male sex[13–15,35,97]
6. Presence of distant metastases[15,99]

Not all of these variables are absolutely independent of each other; for example, the most aggressive histologic types tend to occur in older patients[36,48] and extension to adjacent structures tends to occur in patients with large primary lesions.[11] The presence or absence of lymph node metastasis has been shown to be of no prognostic value in a number of large series,[15,19,65,95,110] and, in fact, an inverse correlation has at times been demonstrated, with the highest rates of survival in patients with the greatest number of positive nodes.[15,48]

Radiation-induced thyroid cancer behaves no differently than that in those patients without prior irradiation.[32] For papillary carcinoma, the relative proportions of the papillary and follicular elements are of no apparent significance; multiple foci of tumor within the gland are common but have not been clearly shown to adversely affect prognosis.[22] It is difficult to assess the effect of any individual mode of treatment on prognosis since adjuvant treatments (e.g., radioiodine, external-beam irradiation, and thyroid hormone) are seldom used alone and have seldom been applied in any systematic manner for similar stage disease.

PAPILLARY CARCINOMA

At the Mayo Clinic, intraglandular papillary carcinomas less than or equal to 1.5 cm have been arbitrarily designated as "occult" lesions whether they were clinically apparent or not. In 1980, Hubert reviewed treatment results after conservative operations in 137 Mayo Clinic patients (1926–1955) with such lesions.[49] In 82 patients, the operation had been performed for a coexisting condition (e.g., multinodular goiter, Graves' disease) and cancer was clinically unsuspected. In most of the remaining 55 patients, the clinical presentation was that of lymph node metastases in the neck without any evidence of a primary lesion; in many, the enlarged nodes were massive. Surgery often consisted of unilateral or bilateral subtotal lobectomy; no total thyroidectomies were performed. For 55 patients with lymph node involvement, lymphadenectomy generally involved modified radical neck dissection or simple excision of palpably involved nodes. Only two radical and no elective lymph node dissections were performed. Ten (18%) of 55 patients with positive lymph nodes required subsequent surgery (13 total operations) for recurrent neck disease; all disease was resectable by conservative lymphadenectomy and/or completion thyroidectomy. Two (5%) of 82 patients with negative lymph nodes underwent subsequent operations for primary tumor recurrence; none required lymph node dissection. With 25 to 54 years' follow-up, only 1 of 137 patients died of thyroid cancer. Based on these data, it is concluded that such patients need not be subjected to radical operations, external-beam irradiation, or radioiodine on the basis of theoretical considerations concerning possible multicentric disease or possible residual nodal disease. Although about 10% of patients will require reoperation, the salvage rate is high. Even though many of the patients were cured by lesser procedures, the recommendation for these patients is ipsilateral total and contralateral subtotal lobectomy, judicious nodal surgery, and replacement thyroid hormone.

The survival of patients with somewhat larger lesions (>1.5 cm but still within the thyroid capsule) was almost as good as the "occult" group; with 11 to 40 years' follow-up, only 8 of 272 patients (3%) died of cancer. The 20-year survival rate of patients with extraglandular extension was half that of the other two groups (Fig. 32-7).[112]

Death from papillary carcinoma is unusual in patients diagnosed before age 40 compared with patients over 40 (Fig. 32-8).[112] A combination of extrathyroid extension and age greater than 40 carries a particularly poor prognosis (Fig. 32-9).[111]

For patients who do not undergo elective lymph node dissections, the reported failure rate in the neck is less than would be predicted from the incidence of subclinical metastases in patients who have undergone such operations.[22,24,35,49,63,72] The same is true of failure in the contralateral thyroid lobe following less than total thyroidectomy. Although failures in the retained lobe have sometimes been noted as long as 10 years or more after surgery,[82] the number of reported failures is much less than the incidence of bilaterality noted in subserially sectioned total thyroidectomy specimens.[22,24] Following conservative operations (e.g., ipsilateral total and contralateral subtotal lobectomy combined with limited neck surgery), 10% to 20% of patients have had to undergo reoperation for nodal or primary recurrent disease;[25,111] the frequency increases according to size and local extent of the primary lesion. The salvage rate is high unless the soft tissues of the neck are involved by recurrent cancer.[24,64] Occasional patients must undergo a third, fourth, or even fifth operation.[111]

Asphyxia due to locally uncontrolled cancer is the immediate cause of death in the majority of patients who die of papillary carcinoma.[30] Distant metastasis alone as a cause of death occurred in only 9 of 70 patients (13%) who died of papillary carcinoma at Memorial Sloan-Kettering Hospital.[98] Occasional patients may live 20 or more years in a relatively asymptomatic state despite pulmonary metastases.[35]

FOLLICULAR CARCINOMA

Survival of patients with follicular carcinoma correlates with the degree of histologic invasiveness (Fig. 32-10). With minimal or slight capsular invasion, only 3 of 104 patients were known to have died of cancer.[112] Patients with more invasive lesions do quite poorly, with frequent local and distant failure, and most patients eventually die of cancer; many of the deaths occur after 5 years.[24,112] Patients over 40 tend to have more invasive lesions and fare less well than those under 40.[15,24,36]

Medullary Carcinoma

Survival correlates best with nodal status. At the Mayo Clinic, the 10-year survival in 74 patients with positive nodes was approximately one half that of 65 patients with negative nodes (Fig. 32-11).[16] Following resection with curative attempt in 128 Mayo Clinic patients, clinically apparent tumor recurrences were noted in almost two thirds of the patients with positive nodes versus about 10% of those with negative nodes; the majority (36 of 44 or 82%) of recurrences were local and/or regional (i.e., neck and mediastinum), which is in general agreement with the pattern of failure observed at the M. D. Anderson Hospital.[47] In addition to the 44 patients who developed clinically obvious tumor recurrence, 12 others without clinical evidence of cancer were probably not cured because they had persistently elevated plasma calcitonin levels during follow-up. In Tubiana's series, some patients with persistently elevated calcitonin levels have remained without clinical evidence of relapse after 5 to 10 years of obser-

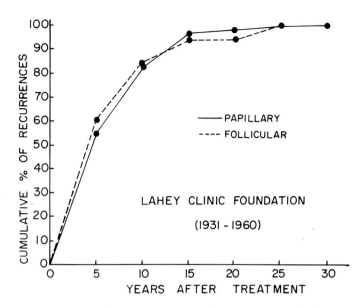

FIG. 32-5. Cumulative percentage of recurrences of differentiated thyroid carcinoma, Lahey Clinic Foundation (1931–1960). In the papillary group, first recurrences were local or regional in approximately one-half of cases, while in the follicular group, the first recurrence was most often (75%) due to distant metastasis. (Data from Cady B, Sedgwick CE, Meissner WA, Bookwalter JR, Romagosa V, Werber J: Changing clinical, pathological, therapeutic, and survival patterns in differentiated thyroid carcinoma. Ann Surg 184:541–553, 1976)

FIG. 32-6. Cumulative percentage of deaths due to differentiated thyroid carcinoma, Lahey Clinic Foundation (1931–1960). Slightly fewer than half of the patients who died of thyroid cancer did so by 5 years. (Data from Cady B, Sedgwick CE, Meissner WA, Bookwalter JR, Romagosa V, Werber J: Changing clinical, pathologic, therapeutic, and survival patterns in differentiated thyroid carcinoma. Ann Surg 184:541–553, 1976)

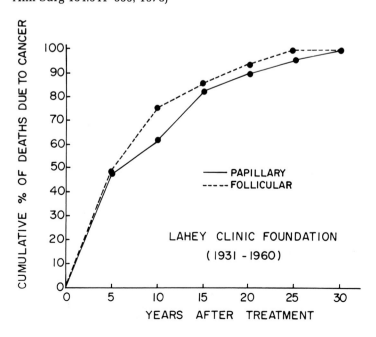

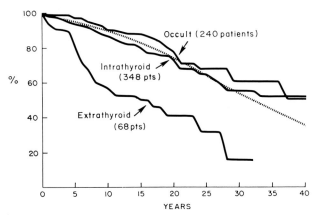

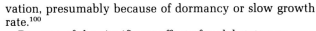

FIG. 32-7. Survival following treatment of 656 patients with papillary carcinoma of the thyroid gland (Mayo Clinic, 1926–1960). The "occult" group comprises patients whose primary lesions were less than or equal to 1.5 cm in size. The dotted line represents survival of normal people of comparable age and sex. (With permission from Woolner LB, Beahrs OH, Black BM, McConahey WM, Keating FR: Thyroid carcinoma: General considerations and followup data on 1181 cases. In Young S, Inman DR [eds]: Thyroid Neoplasia, pp 51–79. New York, Academic Press, 1968. Copyright ©: Academic Press Inc. [London] Ltd.)

FIG. 32-8. Survival following treatment of 415 traced patients with papillary carcinoma of the thyroid gland (Mayo Clinic, 1926–1960). Excluded are patients with lesions less than or equal to 1.5 cm (*i.e.*, "occult" carcinomas). The dotted lines represent survival of normal people of comparable age and sex. (With permission from Woolner LB, Beahrs OH, Black BM, McConahey WM, Keating FR: Thyroid carcinoma: General considerations and followup data on 1181 cases. In Young S, Inman DR [eds]: Thyroid Neoplasia, pp 51–79. New York, Academic Press, 1968. Copyright ©: Academic Press Inc. [London] Ltd.)

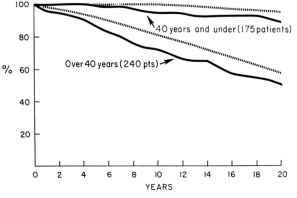

vation, presumably because of dormancy or slow growth rate.[100]

Because of the significant effect of nodal status on cure rate, early detection of familial cases with annual calcitonin screening of family members is indicated. Patients with MEN IIB syndrome are said to have very poor survival rates.[74]

Anaplastic Carcinoma

In most reported series, approximately 90% of patients are dead within 1 year after treatment. Local, regional, and distant failures are all frequent. The only patients cured with any regularity have the unusual circumstance of disease confined to the gland and regional lymph nodes, without extension into the soft tissues of the neck.[1]

There is no clear evidence that chemotherapy has improved upon the dismal results obtained with postoperative radiation therapy alone. The initial enthusiasm for combination surgery, radiation, and dactinomycin at the M. D. Anderson Hospital has waned a bit following the initial report of three of six patients cured;[79] the combined approach failed to produce a single long-term survivor in eight additional patients treated over the succeeding 6 years.[1]

COMPLICATIONS OF TREATMENT

The operative mortality rate from thyroidectomy is about 0.1%.[4]

The most serious and immediate postoperative hazard is hemorrhage. Since the blood tends to be trapped in the midline of the neck, it may lead to rapid airway collapse. In severe cases the wound must be opened immediately, wherever the patient may be. After the obstruction has been relieved, the patient is transferred back to the operating room, the bleeding is controlled, and a tracheostomy is created if necessary. Severe hemorrhage occurred after only 1 of 574 consecutive thyroidectomies at the Mayo Clinic.[4]

Mild, asymptomatic hypocalcemia occurs after thyroidectomy in about 25% of patients, is maximal 48 to 72 hours postoperatively, then disappears within 1 week.[4,106] Such transient drops in serum calcium are believed to be secondary to trauma to the glands or to their blood supply. The sooner after surgery the drop occurs and the longer it persists, the less likely is recovery, since all the parathyroid tissue may have been removed or its vascular supply so compromised that it ceases to function.

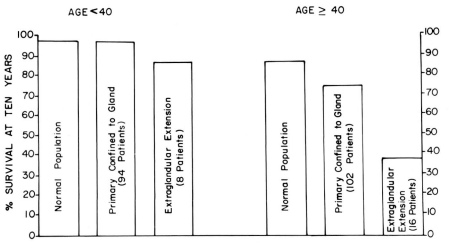

FIG. 32-9. Ten-year survival according to age and local extent of papillary carcinoma of the thyroid (Mayo Clinic, 1926–1948). The 10-year survival data for the normal population are for people of comparable age and sex. (Data from Woolner LB, Beahrs OH, Black BM, McConahey WM, Keating FR Jr: Classification and prognosis of thyroid carcinoma: A study of 885 cases observed in a thirty-year period. Am J Surg 102:354–387, 1961)

The risk of permanent hypoparathyroidism relates mainly to the extent of surgery, as dictated by the extent of disease, and to the experience and skill of the surgeon. There is little risk if only a single thyroid lobe is removed or if one leaves a small remnant of one lobe behind and then ablates the remaining gland with iodine-131. In cases in which total thyroidectomy is necessary, permanent hypoparathyroidism can be expected to occur in 15% to 20% of patients.[26,56] If parathyroid tissue is visualized at operation, it should be protected. If it appears that the parathyroid glands are going to be jeopardized, one of the glands may be identified histologically and then transplanted into the sternocleidomastoid muscle. Following an extensive operation, signs of hypoparathyroidism are sought and the serum calcium level is checked daily; replacement therapy is begun only in the presence of hypocalcemic signs.[31] Permanent hypoparathyroidism requires indefinite calcium replacement; vitamin D is also usually given.

Inadvertent section of one recurrent laryngeal nerve with resultant unilateral vocal cord paralysis has occurred in about 1% of patients whose primary treatment was by operation at the Mayo Clinic. It is advisable to control bleeding during operation with finger pressure until normal structures can be clearly identified. Indiscriminant and blind clamping in a pool of blood is liable to result in nerve injury. At no time should sharp dissection or clamping be done in the region of the nerve without its being clearly in sight.[4] The risk of nerve damage is greater in patients who must undergo reexploration of the thyroid bed following the first operation because of difficulty secondary to edema and inflammatory reaction (during the weeks immediately following surgery) and fibrosis (months to years after operation).[4,5] Bilateral recurrent laryngeal nerve injury is extremely rare and usually necessitates permanent tracheostomy or a secondary procedure such as arytenoidectomy (Woodman procedure). Transient nerve injuries, due to stretching or pinching of the nerve at operation, usually resolve within a few months.[4]

Damage to the external branch of the superior laryngeal nerve results in voice fatigue. Horner's syndrome is quite rare, but it may occur secondary to injury to the cervical sympathetic chain at the time of ligation of the inferior thyroid artery.[31]

A rare complication is pneumothorax that is secondary to injury to the lung apex.[4]

Bone marrow depression may occur following large single doses or multiple small doses of radioiodine; it is usually transient and does not require treatment.[19] The risk of developing acute leukemia or aplastic anemia is small and related to total cumulative dose.[81,92,101] The total body dose from iodine-131 is approximately 0.25 rad to 0.50 rad per millicurie administered.[82,86] Patients with multiple fine, diffuse lung metastases are at some risk of developing radiation (iodine-131)-induced pneumonitis and/or pulmonary fibrosis.[35] In two fatal cases of radiation pneumonitis reported at Memorial Sloan-Kettering Hospital, dyspnea on exertion first appeared 2 months following large single doses of iodine-131; severe respiratory distress and cyanosis were present by about 3 months, and death occurred shortly thereafter.[77] Transformation of a well-differentiated to an anaplastic carcinoma is said to contraindicate the use of radioiodine for differentiated cancers.[25] Anaplastic transformation is seen in a small percentage of patients, whether they receive radioiodine or not;[1,70] there are no data to suggest that the incidence is increased by radioiodine, but if it is, the risk is apparently

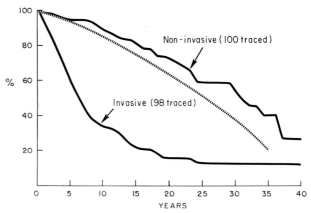

FIG. 32-10. Survival following treatment of 198 traced patients with follicular carcinoma of thyroid gland (Mayo Clinic, 1926–1960). Noninvasive cases are those with slight or equivocal capsular invasion, and invasive cases are those with moderate to marked invasion, including recurrent or inoperable tumors. The dotted line represents survival of normal people of comparable age and sex. The 5-, 10-, and 15-year survival rates are all similar to those reported by Hirabayashi and Lindsay at the University of California, San Francisco, for their localized and invasive subgroups.[48] (With permission from Woolner LB, Beahrs OH, Black BM, McConahey WM, Keating FR: Thyroid carcinoma: General considerations and followup data on 1181 cases. In Young S, Inman DR [eds]: Thyroid Neoplasia, pp 51–79. New York, Academic Press, 1968. Copyright ©: Academic Press Inc., [London] Ltd.)

FIG. 32-11. Survival following treatment of 139 patients with medullary carcinoma of the thyroid gland (Mayo Clinic, 1926–1973) according to nodal status at the time of operation. The dashed line represents survival of normal people of comparable age and sex. (Redrawn from Chong GC, Beahrs OH, Sizemore GW, Woolner LH: Medullary carcinoma of the thyroid gland. Cancer 35:695–704, 1975)

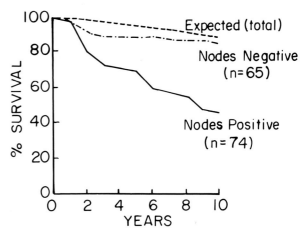

low. Long-term follow-up of patients (aged 6 to 20) treated for thyroid cancer with iodine-131 (total dose 80 mCi to 690 mCi; mean 196 mCi) has disclosed no apparent increase in occurrence of infertility or birth defects compared with the general population.[86] Of 33 married patients (13 males, 20 females) on whom follow-up was available 14 to 25 years after treatment, there were 71 live births in 29 families. Four patients (12%) were apparently infertile, and there was only one major congenital (cardiac) anomaly

(1%). The authors estimated gonadal doses to be approximately 0.1 rad per millicurie administered.

Complications of external-beam irradiation are discussed elsewhere (see Chapter 14, The Effect of Radiation on Normal Tissues of the Head and Neck). Tissues at risk include the spinal cord, larynx (edema), trachea (necrosis), subcutaneous tissues, and brachial plexus.

REFERENCES

1. Aldinger KA, Samaan NA, Ibanez M, Hill CS Jr: Anaplastic carcinoma of the thyroid. A review of 84 cases of spindle and giant-cell carcinoma of the thyroid. Cancer 41:2267–2275, 1978

2. Ashcraft MW, van Herle AJ: Management of thyroid nodules: I. History and physical examination, blood tests, x-ray tests, and ultrasonography. Head Neck Surg 3:216–230, 1981

3. Ashcraft MW, van Herle AJ: Management of thyroid nodules: II. Scanning techniques, thyroid suppressive therapy, and fine needle aspiration. Head Neck Surg 3:297–322, 1981

4. Beahrs OH: Complications in thyroid and parathyroid surgery. In Conley J: Complications of Head and Neck Surgery, pp 239–249. Philadelphia, WB Saunders, 1979

5. Beahrs OH, Kiernan PD, Hubert JP Jr: Cancer of the thyroid gland. In Suen JY, Myers EN: Cancer of the Head and Neck, pp 599–631. New York, Churchill Livingstone, 1981

6. Beierwaltes W: Discussion (pp 149–155) of Cassano C, Baschieri I, Baschieri L: Follow-up of 188 cases of thyroid carcinoma after combined surgical and radioiodine treatment. In Young S, Inman DR: Thyroid Neoplasia, pp 143–155. London, Academic Press, 1968

7. Beierwaltes WH: The treatment of thyroid carcinoma with radioactive iodine. Sem Nucl Med 8:79–94, 1978

8. Block GE: An appraisal of the hormonal control of carcinoma of the thyroid gland. Surg Gynecol Obstet 132:289–290, 1971

9. Block MA: Primary treatment of well-differentiated thyroid cancer. J Surg Oncol 16:279–288, 1981

10. Block MA, Miller JM, Horn RC Jr: Significance of mediastinal lymph node metastases in carcinoma of the thyroid. Am J Surg 123:702–705, 1972

11. Breaux EP Jr, Guillamondegui OM: Treatment of locally invasive carcinoma of the thyroid: How radical? Am J Surg 140:514–517, 1980

12. Brennan MF, Bloomer WD: Cancer of the endocrine system. In DeVita VT Jr, Hellman S, Rosenberg S (eds): Cancer: Principles and Practice of Oncology, pp 971–1035. Philadelphia, JB Lippincott, 1982

13. Buckwalter JA, Thomas CG Jr: Selection of surgical treatment for well differentiated thyroid carcinomas. Ann Surg 176:565–578, 1972

14. Byar DP, Green SB, Dor P, Wiliams ED, Colon J, van Gilse HA, Mayer M, Sylvester RJ, VanGlabbeke M: A prognostic index for thyroid carcinoma: A study of the EORTC thyroid cancer cooperative group. Eur J Cancer 15:1033–1041, 1979

15. Cady B, Sedgwick CE, Meissner WA, Bookwalter JR, Romagosa V, Werber J: Changing clinical, pathologic, therapeutic, and survival patterns in differentiated thyroid carcinoma. Ann Surg 184:541–553, 1976

16. Chong GC, Beahrs OH, Sizemore GW, Woolner LH: Medullary carcinoma of the thyroid gland. Cancer 35:695–704, 1975

17. Clark OH: TSH suppression in the management of thyroid nodules and thyroid cancer. World J Surg 5:39–47, 1981

18. Clark RL: Discussion (pp. 417–419) of Harness JK, Thompson NW, Sisson JC, Beierwaltes WH: Differentiated thyroid carcinomas. Arch Surg 108:410–419, 1974

19. Clark RL, Cole VW, Fuller LM, Healey JE Jr, Hill CS Jr, Ibanez ML, Macdonald EJ, White EC: Thyroid. In MacComb WS, Fletcher GH: Cancer of the Head and Neck, pp 293–328. Baltimore, Williams & Wilkins, 1967

20. Colacchio TA, LoGerfo P, Colacchio DA, Feind C: Radioiodine total body scan versus serum thyroglobulin levels in follow-up of patients with thyroid cancer. Surgery 91:42–45, 1982

21. Cope O, Dobyns BM, Hamlin E Jr, Hopkirk J: What thyroid nodules are to be feared? J Clin Endocrinol 9:1012–1022, 1949

22. Crile G Jr: Late results of treatment for papillary cancer of the thyroid. Ann Surg 160:178–182, 1964

23. Crile G Jr: Treatment of thyroid cysts by aspiration. Surgery 59:210–212, 1966

24. Crile G Jr: Treatment of carcinomas of the thyroid. In Young S, Inman DR: Thyroid Neoplasia, pp 39–50. London, Academic Press, 1968

25. Crile G Jr: Changing end results in patients with papillary carcinoma of the thyroid. Surg Gynecol Obstet 132:460–468, 1971

26. Crile G Jr: In Beierwaltes W, Crile G Jr, Block G, Block M, Kaplan E, Paloyan E, Seed R, Southwick H: Discussion of surgery of the irradiated gland for possible thyroid carcinoma, p 412. In DeGroot LJ, Frohman LA, Kaplan EL, Refetoff S (eds): Radiation-Associated Thyroid Carcinoma, pp 411–417. New York, Grune & Stratton, 1977

27. Crile G Jr, Hawk WA Jr: Aspiration biopsy of thyroid nodules. Surg Gynecol Obstet 136:241–245, 1973

28. Cutler SJ, Scotto J, Devesa SS, Connelly RR: Third National Cancer Survey: An overview of available information. J Natl Cancer Inst 53:1565–1575, 1974

29. DeGroot LJ: Thyroid carcinoma. Med Clin North Am 59:1233–1246, 1975

30. Djalilian M, Beahrs OH, Devine KD, Weiland LH, DeSanto LW: Intraluminal involvement of the larynx and trachea by thyroid cancer. Am J Surg 128:500–504, 1974

31. Dozois RR, Beahrs OH: Surgical anatomy and technique of thyroid and parathyroid surgery. Surg Clin North Am 57:647–661, 1977

32. Edis AJ: Natural history of occult thyroid cancer. In DeGroot LJ, Frohman LA, Kaplan EL, Refetoff S (eds): Radiation-Associated Thyroid Carcinoma, pp 155–160. New York, Grune & Stratton, 1977

33. Eycleshymer AC, Schoemaker DM: A Cross-Sectional Anatomy, p 55. New York, Appleton-Century-Crofts, 1938

34. Frable MA, Frable WJ: Thin needle aspiration biopsy of the thyroid gland. Laryngoscope 90:1619–1625, 1980

35. Frazell EL, Foote FW Jr: Papillary cancer of the thyroid. A review of 25 years of experience. Cancer 11:895–922, 1958

36. Gardet P, Parmentier C, Gerard-Marchant R, L'Heritier C, Caillou B, Cukersztein W, Tubiana M: Differentiated cancers of the thyroid: Course after treatment with special reference to frequency and chronology of the first relapse for 470 treated patients. Ann Radiol 20:831–840, 1977

37. Graze K, Spiler IJ, Tashjian AH Jr, Melvin KEW, Cervi-Skinner S, Gagel RF et al: Natural history of familial medullary thyroid carcinoma. N Engl J Med 299:980–985, 1978

38. Halnan KE: The nonsurgical treatment of thyroid cancer. Br J Surg 62:769–771, 1975

39. Hamburger JI: Diuretic augmentation of ^{131}I uptake in inoperable thyroid cancer. N Engl J Med 280:1091–1094, 1969

40. Harmer CL: External beam radiotherapy for thyroid cancer. Ann Radiol 20:791–800, 1977

41. Harness JK, Thompson NW, Sisson JC, Beierwaltes WH: Differentiated thyroid carcinomas: Treatment of distant metastases. Arch Surg 108:410–417, 1974

42. Harwick RD: Thyroid cancer: Surgical decision making. Sem Oncol 7:392–399, 1980

43. Hayles AB, Johnson LM, Beahrs OH, Woolner LB: Carcinoma of the thyroid in children. Am J Surg 106:735–743, 1963

44. Haynie TP, Nofal MM, Beierwaltes WH: Treatment of thyroid carcinoma with I-131. JAMA 183:303–306, 1963

45. Hazard JB: Nomenclature of thyroid tumors. In Young S, Inman DR: Thyroid Neoplasia, pp 3–37. London, Academic Press, 1968

46. Hershman JM, Edwards CL: Serum thyrotropin (TSH) levels after thyroid ablation compared with TSH levels after exogenous bovine TSH: Implications for ^{131}I treatment of thyroid carcinoma. J Clin Endocrinol 34:814–818, 1972

47. Hill CS Jr, Ibanez ML, Samaan NA, Ahearn MJ, Clark RL: Medullary (solid) carcinoma of the thyroid gland: An analysis of the M. D. Anderson Hospital experience with patients with the tumor, its special features, and its histogenesis. Medicine 52:141–171, 1973

48. Hirabayashi RN, Lindsay S: Carcinoma of the thyroid gland: A statistical study of 390 patients. J Clin Endocrinol 21:1596–1610, 1961

49. Hubert JP Jr, Kiernan PD, Beahrs OH, McConahey WM, Woolner LB: Occult papillary carcinoma of the thyroid. Arch Surg 115:394–398, 1980

50. Hunt PS, Poole M, Reeve TS: A reappraisal of the surgical anatomy of the thyroid and parathyroid glands. Br J Surg 55:63–66, 1968

51. Jesse RH: Discussion (pp 417–419) of Harness JK, Thompson NW, Sisson JC, Beierwaltes WH: Differentiated thyroid carcinomas. Arch Surg 108:410–419, 1974

52. Jubiz W: Endocrinology: A Logical Approach for Clinicians, pp 45–79. New York, McGraw-Hill, 1979

53. Katz AD, Zager WJ: The malignant "cold" nodule of the thyroid. Am J Surg 132:459–462, 1976

54. Klonoff DC, Greenspan FS: The thyroid nodule. Adv Intern Med 27:101–126, 1982

55. Lahey FH, Hare HF: Malignancy in adenomas of the thyroid. JAMA 145:689–695, 1951

56. Leape LL, Miller HH, Graze K, Feldman ZT, Gagel RF, Wolfe HJ, Delellis RA, Tashjian AH Jr, Reichlin S: Total thyroidectomy for occult familial medullary carcinoma of the thyroid in children. J Pediatr Surg 11:831–837, 1976

57. Lindberg RD: External beam irradiation in thyroid cancers. In Fletcher GH: Textbook of Radiotherapy, pp 384–388. Philadelphia, Lea & Febiger, 1980

58. Löwhagen T, Granberg P-O, Lundell G, Skinnari P, Sundblad R, Willems J-S: Aspiration biopsy cytology (ABC) in nodules of the thyroid gland suspected to be malignant. Surg Clin North Am 59:3–18, 1979

59. McCormack KR, Sheline GE: Retropharyngeal spread of carcinoma of the thyroid. Cancer 26:1366–1369, 1970

60. McKenzie AD: The natural history of thyroid cancer: A report of 102 cases analyzed 10 to 15 years after diagnosis. Arch Surg 102:274–277, 1971

61. Maheshwari YK, Hill CS, Haynie TP III, Hickey RC, Samaan NA: I-131 therapy in differentiated thyroid carcinoma: M. D. Anderson Hospital experience. Cancer 47:664–671, 1981

62. Mancuso AA, Hanafee WN: Computed Tomography of the Head and Neck, pp 92–111. Baltimore, Williams & Wilkins, 1982

63. Martin H: The surgery of thyroid tumors. Cancer 7:1063–1099, 1954

64. Mazzaferri EL, Young RL: Papillary thyroid carcinoma: A 10-year follow-up report of the impact of therapy in 576 patients. Am J Med 70:511–518, 1981

65. Mazzaferri EL, Young RL, Oertel JE, Kemmerer WT, Page CP: Papillary thyroid carcinoma: The impact of therapy in 576 patients. Medicine 56:171–196, 1977

66. Miller HH, Melvin KEW, Gibson JM, Tashjian AH Jr: Surgical approach to early familial medullary carcinoma of the thyroid gland. Am J Surg 123:438–443, 1972

67. Mortenson JD, Bennett WA, Woolner LB: Incidence of carcinoma in thyroid glands removed at 1000 consecutive routine necropsies. Surg Forum 5:659–662, 1954

68. Moss WT, Brand WN, Battifora H: The thyroid. In Radiation Oncology: Rationale, Technique, Results, 5th ed, pp 195–232. St. Louis, CV Mosby, 1979

69. Netter FH (ed): Anatomy of the thyroid and parathyroid glands. The CIBA Collection of Medical Illustrations, vol 4,

70. Nishiyama RH, Dunn EL, Thompson NW: Anaplastic spindle-cell and giant-cell tumors of the thyroid gland. Cancer 30:113–127, 1972

71. Nobles ER: Nonrecurrent laryngeal nerve. Arch Surg 100:741–742, 1970

72. Noguchi S, Noguchi A, Murakami N: Papillary carcinoma of the thyroid: II. Value of prophylactic lymph node excision. Cancer 26:1061–1064, 1970

73. Norton JA, Doppman JL, Brennan MF: Localization and resection of clinically inapparent medullary carcinoma of the thyroid. Surgery 87:616–622, 1980

74. Norton JA, Froome LC, Farrell RE, Wells SA Jr: Multiple endocrine neoplasia type IIb: The most aggressive form of medullary thyroid carcinoma. Surg Clin North Am 59:109–118, 1979

75. Pemberton J deJ, Beaver MG: Anomaly of right recurrent laryngeal nerve. Surg Gynecol Obstet 54:594–595, 1932

76. Psarras A, Papadopoulos SN, Livadas D, Pharmakiotis AD, Koutras DA: The single thyroid nodule. Br J Surg 59:545–548, 1972

77. Rall JE, Alpers JB, Lewallen CG, Sonenberg M, Berman M, Rawson RW: Radiation pneumonitis and fibrosis: A complication of radioiodine treatment of pulmonary metastases from cancer of the thyroid. J Clin Endocrinol 17:1263–1276, 1957

78. Robbins SL: Pathologic Basis of Disease, pp 1297–1373. Philadelphia, WB Saunders, 1974

79. Rogers JD, Lindberg RD, Hill CS Jr, Gehan E: Spindle and giant cell carcinoma of the thyroid: A different therapeutic approach. Cancer 34:1328–1332, 1974

80. Rose RG, Hartfield JE, Kelsey MP, Macdonald EJ: The association of thyroid cancer and prior irradiation in infancy and childhood. J Nucl Med 4:249–258, 1963

81. Rose RG, Kelsey MP: Radioactive iodine in the diagnosis and treatment of thyroid cancer. Cancer 16:896–913, 1963

82. Rose RG, Kelsey MP, Russell WO, Ibanez ML, White EC, Clark RL: Follow-up study of thyroid cancer treated by unilateral lobectomy. Am J Surg 106:494–500, 1963

83. Rosen IB, Walfish PG, Miskin M: The ultrasound of thyroid masses. Surg Clin North Am 59:19–33, 1979

84. Rossi RL, Cady B, Meissner WA, Wool MS, Sedgwick CE, Werber J: Nonfamilial medullary thyroid carcinoma. Am J Surg 139:554–560, 1980

85. Rouvière H: Anatomy of the Human Lymphatic System, pp 19, 63–65. Tobias MJ, trans. Ann Arbor, MI, Edwards Brothers, 1938

86. Sarkar SD, Beierwaltes WH, Gill SP, Cowley BJ: Subsequent fertility and birth histories of children and adolescents treated with ^{131}I for thyroid cancer. J Nucl Med 17:460–464, 1976

87. Schlumberger M, Fragu P, Parmentier C, Tubiana M: Thyroglobulin assay in the follow-up of patients with differentiated thyroid carcinomas: Comparison of its value in patients with or without normal residual tissue. Acta Endocrinol 98:215–221, 1981

88. Schneider AB, Favus MJ, Stachura ME, Arnold JE, Ryo UY, Pinsky S, Colman M, Arnold MJ, Frohman LA: Plasma thyroglobulin in detecting thyroid carcinoma after childhood head and neck irradiation. Ann Intern Med 86:29–34, 1977

89. Scott JS, Halnan KE, Shimmins J, Kostaki P, McKenzie H: Measurement of dose to thyroid carcinoma metastases from radioiodine therapy. Br J Radiol 43:256–262, 1970

90. Sheline GE, Galante M, Lindsay S: Radiation therapy in the control of persistent thyroid cancer. Am J Roentgenol Radium Ther Nucl Med 97:923–930, 1966

91. Silverberg E: Cancer statistics 1982. CA 32:15–31, 1982

92. Simpson WJ, Carruthers JS: The role of external radiation in the management of papillary and follicular thyroid cancer. Am J Surg 136:457–460, 1978

93. Sizemore GW, Carney JA, Heath H III: Epidemiology of med-

Endocrine System and Selected Metabolic Diseases, pp 41–42. New York, CIBA, 1965

ullary carcinoma of the thyroid gland: A 5-year experience (1971–1976). Surg Clin North Am 57:633–645, 1977

94. Smithers DW: Thyroid carcinoma treated with radioactive iodine. In Young S, Inman DR (eds): Thyroid Neoplasia. London, Academic Press, 1968

95. Staunton MD, Greening WP: Treatment of thyroid cancer in 293 patients. Br J Surg 63:253–258, 1976

96. Steinfeld CM, Moertel CG, Woolner LB: Diarrhea and medullary carcinoma of the thyroid. Cancer 31:1237–1239, 1973

97. Thomas C: Surgery of the thyroid. Med Clin North Am 59:1247–1262, 1975

98. Tollefsen HR, DeCosse JJ, Hutter RVP: Papillary carcinoma of the thyroid: A clinical and pathological study of 70 fatal cases. Cancer 17:1035–1044, 1964

99. Tubiana M: External radiotherapy and radioiodine in the treatment of thyroid cancer. World J Surg 5:75–84, 1981

100. Tubiana M: Thyroid cancer. In Beckers C (ed): Thyroid Diseases, pp 187–227. New York, Pergamon Press, 1982

101. Tubiana M, Lacour J, Monnier JP, Bergiron C, Gerard-Marchant R, Roujeau J, Bok B, Parmentier C: External radiotherapy and radioiodine in the treatment of 359 thyroid cancers. Br J Radiol 48:894–907, 1975

102. Van Herle AJ, Uller RP: Elevated serum thyroglobulin: A marker of metastases in differentiated thyroid carcinoma. J Clin Invest 56:272–277, 1975

103. Verby JE, Woolner LB, Nobrega FT, Kurland LT, McConahey WM: Thyroid cancer in Olmsted County 1935–1965. J Natl Cancer Inst 43:813–820, 1969

104. Vickery AL: Needle biopsy and the thyroid nodule. In DeGroot LJ, Frohman LA, Kaplan EL, Refetoff S (eds): Radiation-Associated Thyroid Carcinoma. New York, Grune & Stratton, 1977

105. Warwick R, Williams PL (eds): Gray's Anatomy, 35th British ed, pp 1373–1377. Philadelphia, WB Saunders, 1973

106. Wells SA Jr: The parathyroid gland. In Sabitson DC Jr (ed): David-Christopher Textbook of Surgery, The Biologic Basis of Modern Surgical Practice, 10th ed, pp 656–667. Philadelphia, WB Saunders, 1972

107. Wells SA Jr, Baylin SB, Gann DS, Farrell RE, Dilley WG, Preissig SH, Linehan WM, Cooper CW: Medullary thyroid carcinoma: Relationship of method of diagnosis to pathologic staging. Ann Surg 188:377–383, 1978

108. Wells SA Jr, Norton JA: Medullary carcinoma of the thyroid and multiple endocrine neoplasia-II syndromes. In Friesen Sr (ed): Surgical Endocrinology: Clinical Syndromes, pp 287–303. Philadelphia, JB Lippincott, 1978

109. Williams ED: The pathology of thyroid malignancy. Br J Surg 62:757–759, 1975

110. Woolner LB: Thyroid carcinoma: Pathologic classification with data on prognosis. Semin Nucl Med 1:481–502, 1971

111. Woolner LB, Beahrs OH, Black BM, McConahey WM, Keating FR Jr: Classification and prognosis of thyroid carcinoma: A study of 885 cases observed in a thirty-year period. Am J Surg 102:354–387, 1961

112. Woolner LB, Beahrs OH, Black BM, McConahey WM, Keating FR: Thyroid carcinoma: General considerations and follow-up data on 1181 cases. In Young S, Inman DR (eds): Thyroid Neoplasia, pp 51–79. London, Academic Press, 1968

Pediatric Tumors of the Head and Neck

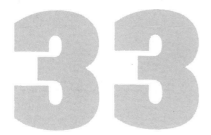

ROBERT B. MARCUS, Jr.

Excluding accidents, malignant neoplasms are the leading cause of death for all pediatric age-groups once the neonatal period is passed. Still, pediatric cancer is a rare disease, and the Third National Cancer Survey showed an incidence of only 124.5 cases per year per million white children under the age of 15 and 97.8 cases per million black children.[151] This means that over the first 15 years of life, approximately 2 of every thousand children will develop cancer. The incidence has been stable over the past 20 years, although the death rate has decreased, particularly over the years 1965 through 1975.[150]

The most common childhood cancers are shown in Table 33-1.[151] Histologic types that give rise to head and neck malignancies are rare, with neuroblastoma, soft tissue sarcomas, and bone tumors being the most common. Most histologic subtypes that occur in the head and neck also occur elsewhere in the body and are generally reported by histology rather than by anatomical site. Approximately 10% of pediatric neoplasms occur in the head and neck. The most common histologic subtypes and their estimated frequency are shown in Table 33-2.

In general, the treatment techniques applicable to cancer of the head and neck in children are similar to those used for tumors of similar histology presenting elsewhere in the body. The occurrence in the head and neck, however, does make the surgical approach more difficult for many of these lesions, particularly the sarcomas. A team approach is necessary, and many tumors that were previously fatal are now cured with an aggressive, well-planned therapeutic attack. Because of the rarity of the tumors, they are best treated in centers specializing in pediatric cancer.

Retinoblastoma is an ophthalmological problem and it will not be discussed in this text. Lymphomas, carcinomas of the thyroid, skin, nasopharynx, and major and minor salivary glands are discussed in specific chapters. A few benign lesions are also included in this chapter. Juvenile angiofibroma is discussed in a separate chapter.

MALIGNANT TUMORS

Soft Tissue Sarcomas

RHABDOMYOSARCOMA

Rhabdomyosarcomas are tumors of the skeletal muscle and comprise the overwhelming majority of soft tissue sarcomas in children. The incidence is approximately 4.5 per million children per year under the age of 15, representing approximately 3.5% of all malignant neoplasms in children. According to the First Intergroup Rhabdomyosarcoma Study (IRS), 38% of pediatric rhabdomyosarcomas occur in the head and neck (Table 33-3).[88]

TABLE 33-1. Malignant Neoplasms in US Children Under 15 Years of Age (Third National Cancer Survey)

Diagnosis	Rate (Cases/1,000,000/Year)	
	White Children	Black Children
Leukemia	42.1	24.3
Central nervous system tumor	23.9	23.9
Lymphoma	13.2	13.9
Sympathetic nervous system tumor	9.6	7.0
Soft tissue tumor	8.4	3.9
Kidney tumor	7.8	7.8
Bone tumor	5.6	4.8
Retinoblastoma	3.4	3.0
Gonadal and germ cell tumors	2.2	2.6
Liver tumor	1.9	0.4
Total	124.5	97.8

(Adapted from Young JL Jr, Miller RW: Incidence of malignant tumors in US children. J Pediatr 86:254–258, 1975)

TABLE 33-2. Incidence of Malignant Solid Tumors of the Head and Neck* in Children (Age Birth to 15 Years)

Tumor	Incidence†
Retinoblastoma	3.4
Rhabdomyosarcoma	2.1
Thyroid	1.6
Neuroblastoma	0.7
Nasopharynx	0.4
Parotid	0.3
Osteosarcoma	0.2
Fibrosarcoma	0.2
Ewing's sarcoma	0.1
Other	0.7
Total	9.7

* Excludes lymphomas and central nervous systems tumors.

† Rates per million per year. Incidence was calculated using data from Third National Cancer Survey[151] and incidences of head and neck primary lesions stated in this chapter within each histologic group.

PATHOLOGY

At the present time, rhabdomyosarcomas are divided into four histologic types. Embryonal rhabdomyosarcoma accounts for 75% of primary lesions of the head and neck.[135] The remaining 25% will be either alveolar, botryoid, or pleomorphic, with the latter primarily found in adults. Three additional small cell, mesenchymal sarcomas that behave similar to rhabdomyosarcoma have been described by the pathology committee of the IRS.[40] There is no evidence that the treatment of primary lesions of the head and neck should be modified because of the histologic type of the tumor.

PATTERNS OF SPREAD

Local Spread

About 70% of orbital rhabdomyosarcomas start in the tissues posterior to the globe. Another 20% arise in the eyelid and 5% in the conjunctiva.[67] The bony orbit, although thin, still produces a barrier for growth of tumor in all directions except anteriorly. The tumor can, however, grow posteriorly to involve the extraocular muscles and rarely may extend through the orbital foramen or supraorbital fissure into the central nervous system. In addition, if allowed to progress, these tumors will violate the medial wall of the orbit and extend into the nasal cavity or ethmoid sinuses.

Lesions starting in the nasopharynx or paranasal sinuses are usually rapidly growing tumors and quickly invade neighboring structures (Fig. 33-1). In one series, only 4 of 20 primary rhabdomyosarcomas of the nasopharynx remained confined to the nasopharynx;[14] the remainder extended to one or more nearby structures, including the orbit, nasal cavity, maxillary sinus, ethmoid sinuses, sphenoid sinuses, clivus, and base of the skull.

Middle ear lesions appear to have two different sites of origin: mastoid and petrosal.[13] Mastoid lesions are the most common. They often spread along the internal auditory canal and then to the prepontine leptomeninges. In doing so, they usually involve the facial nerve. It has been shown that the fallopian canal is a vulnerable area to tumors that "when penetrated provides a channel for direct extension into the auditory meatus and posterior fossa".[96] From there, the development of the hemibase syndrome often occurs (involvement of multiple cranial nerves on one side by an extra-axial process).

Petrosal lesions pursue a different course, probably starting in the region of the eustachian tube, tensor tympani muscle, or carotid canal. Spread occurs through the petrosal bone with early abducens nerve paralysis due to cavernous sinus involvement in the region of Dorello's canal. Further extension into the carotid canal involves the sympathetic

TABLE 33-3.	Distribution of Rhabdomyosarcoma by Primary Site (First Intergroup Rhabdomyosarcoma Study)	
Site	No. Patients	Percentage
Orbit	54	10
Other head and neck	157	28
Trunk	38	7
Extremities	98	18
Genitourinary	118	21
Intrathoracic	14	3
Gastrointestinal/hepatic	16	3
Perineum/anus	12	2
Retroperitoneum	41	7
Other	6	1
Total	554	100

(Modified from Maurer HM: The Intergroup Rhabdomyosarcoma Study: Update, November 1978. Natl Cancer Inst Monogr 56:61–68, 1981)

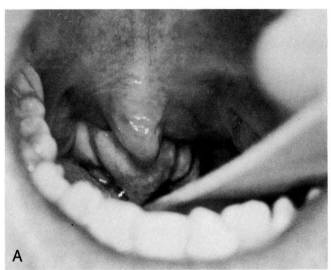

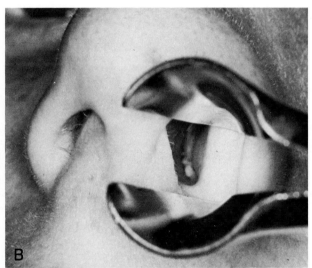

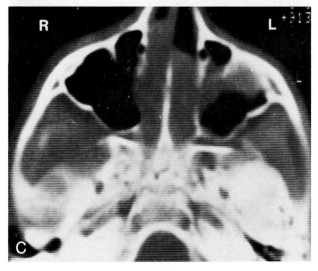

FIG. 33-1. Large polypoid rhabdomyosarcoma filling entire nasopharynx of a 14-year-old boy. (*A*) Mass is easily visible extending into the oropharynx. (*B*) Tumor is visible in left anterior nares. (*C*) CT scan section through nasal cavity shows tumor filling nasal cavity and extending into left maxillary sinus.

nerves (causing Horner's syndrome) and the trigeminal nerve as it crosses the petrous ridge. Oddly enough, even in large tumors invasion of the labyrinth is rare. Facial nerve involvement is uncommon with lesions arising in the petrosal bone. The pattern of cranial nerve involvement provides a clue as to the site of origin.

Laryngeal primary lesions appear to arise from diverse parts of the larynx, but they may have a predilection for the true cord and subglottic region.[15] A few may arise from the area of the pyriform sinus.

The other primary sites are less common but, in general, rhabdomyosarcomas arising in the oral cavity, oropharynx, scalp, and neck spread locally like primary carcinomas in these sites. However, they grow very rapidly and often reach a large size.

Meningeal Involvement by Parameningeal Primary Lesions

In addition to the routes of spread previously described, recent evidence indicates that lesions in the middle ear, nasopharynx, and paranasal sinuses (the parameningeal sites) have an increased risk of meningeal extension.

Apparently, local invasion into the base of the skull is followed by extension to the leptomeninges first, then to the brain itself by way of the Virchow-Robin spaces.[78] Ultimately, the entire subarachnoid space of the entire neural axis may be involved.

Interestingly enough, meningeal extension in orbital lesions is rare.

Lymph Node Spread

Clinically positive neck nodes at diagnosis are unusual in head and neck rhabdomyosarcoma, as is microscopic involvement found by an elective neck dissection.[76] Orbital primary lesions in particular have a very small incidence of neck node involvement.

Metastasis Beyond the Clavicles

Approximately 13% of patients with head and neck rhabdomyosarcomas present with distant metastases at the time of diagnosis, except for orbital primary lesions, which have a 4% incidence.[135]

The most common site of distant metastasis for primary lesions of the head and neck is the lung, followed by bone and liver.

CLINICAL PICTURE AND DISTRIBUTION

The location of primary head and neck rhabdomyosarcomas is shown in Table 33-4, and the age distribution is given in Figure 33-2.

The most common presenting symptom in orbital lesions is proptosis, often with rapid and alarming progression, and often accompanied by diplopia, drooping of the upper lid, and even a decrease in visual acuity or blindness. At this point, a discrete mass may be palpated in about one fourth of the patients.[67] A few patients will complain of pain or tearing early in the course of the disease, and a

FIG. 33-2. Age distribution of patients (age < 21 years) with rhabdomyosarcoma of head and neck sites. Data collected from the literature where age of patient was stated.

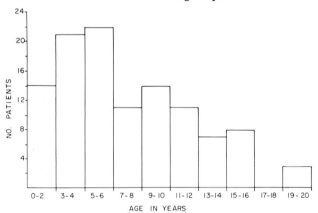

TABLE 33-4.	Location of Primary Lesion: Head and Neck Rhabdomyosarcoma (Age < 21 Years). Data Collected From Literature Where Site and Age Are Stated.	
Site	**No. Patients**	**Percentage**
Orbit	99	25
Parameningeal primaries		
Nasopharynx	76	19
Middle ear	35	9
Paranasal sinuses	53	14
Infratemporal fossa	13	3
Neck	25	6
Oropharynx	22	6
Parotid	21	5
Scalp	15	4
Oral cavity	14	4
Cheek	9	2
Larynx	4	1
Temporal muscle	5	1
Other	4	1
Total	395	100

few patients are diagnosed because of epistaxis, with the tumor having penetrated into the nasal cavity.[67]

Patients with primary rhabdomyosarcomas of the nasopharynx and sinuses usually present with ear symptoms; fullness due to eustachian tube obstruction and tinnitus are the most common. Nasal obstruction, epistaxis, dysphagia, and local pain are also common presenting symptoms. Tumor in the parapharyngeal space may cause cranial nerve deficits.

With primary lesions in the middle ear, there is almost always a painless discharge as the first symptom. A small mass may be noticed in the external auditory canal, and a diagnosis of otitis media is often made. Preliminary roentgenographic evaluation may produce a diagnosis of mastoiditis, with or without bone destruction. By the time the diagnosis is made, however, more advanced symptoms are usually present. Facial nerve palsy has been reported in as high as 88% of patients, while other cranial nerves were involved in 28%.[78] In addition, 28% of patients presented with a postauricular mass or swelling.

Primary lesions in the oral cavity or oropharynx may cause pain, but since many occur in very young children (they have even been reported at birth), symptoms such as dyspnea, dysphagia, cough, or abnormal phonation are noted. Trauma to the tumor from sucking or swallowing may cause bleeding, and blood may be found on the bed of an infant.[83]

Laryngeal lesions are extremely rare. When the patient is an infant, symptoms of croup or "noisy breathing" have been reported.[4] The onset of dyspnea may be rapid.

Rhabdomyosarcomas of the scalp, cheek, parotid, temporal region, and neck usually present as an asymptomatic, rapidly growing mass.

STAGING

The IRS staging system for rhabdomyosarcomas is shown in Table 33-5.[1,90] Most head and neck lesions are difficult to remove in their entirety, and thus group III is the largest subset.

DIAGNOSTIC EVALUATION

The workup of a patient with rhabdomyosarcoma is directed at determining both the extent of local disease as well as the possible presence of distant metastases. As a minimum, after a thorough history and physical examination, a complete blood cell count, platelet count, differential count, liver function studies, renal functional studies, and urinalysis should all be done. The lungs should be evaluated with a chest roentgenogram as well as whole-lung tomograms or computerized tomography of the thorax (CT scan). A bone scan and bone marrow aspiration and biopsy are also necessary.

To evaluate the local extent of primary tumor, conventional roentgenograms should be done, followed by a contrast-enhanced CT scan. Coaxial tomograms of the primary site and base of the skull may also be useful in primary parameningeal lesions.

In addition, for parameningeal lesions the central nervous system must be evaluated. A CT scan of the brain is probably the most accurate screening test, and the primary site can be studied simultaneously. However, since even those patients with no roentgenographic evidence of invasion of the base of the skull or overt central nervous system disease may still have involvement of the central nervous system, a spinal tap is advised for the paramen-

ingeal primary lesions, and frankly malignant cells will sometimes be found.

SELECTION OF TREATMENT MODALITIES

Surgery is the local treatment of choice for small lesions (e.g., those of the tongue, buccal mucosa, scalp, parotid gland, and neck) that can be removed with minimal cosmetic or functional deformity. Most lesions of the head and neck, however, are difficult to resect because of the anatomical location, and radiation therapy is the treatment of choice. Orbital lesions, even though operable, have a high rate of control with radiation therapy, and vision may be preserved in a few cases.

All patients with head and neck rhabdomyosarcomas should receive systemic chemotherapy. With small resectable primary lesions, good results are obtained with postoperative chemotherapy. However, with larger lesions, several cycles of chemotherapy should be given initially to decrease the amount of disease prior to local treatment (Fig. 33-3). If irradiation is given, chemotherapy should continue throughout irradiation and for 12 to 18 months after its initiation. A few patients may need combined surgery and radiation therapy at the primary site; induction chemotherapy should be given first, followed by irradiation, then excision of residual disease.

The clinically negative neck requires no treatment beyond chemotherapy and careful observation. Patients with a clinically positive neck who have resection of their primary lesion are probably best treated with a neck dissection. Even a young child whose primary lesion is irradiated may have a better end result with a neck dissection rather than irradiation of bulky adenopathy. It may be preferable to wait until after initial chemotherapy before proceeding with the neck dissection.

Surgery

The basic principle of wide resection of the primary tumor including surrounding normal tissue is a difficult concept to apply without producing considerable morbidity or deformity. For middle ear or nasopharyngeal rhabdomyosarcomas, biopsy is probably the best the surgeon can obtain, leaving most of the treatment to the radiation ther-

TABLE 33-5.	Intergroup Rhabdomyosarcoma Study Staging System	
Group	**Description**
I	Localized disease, completely resected; regional nodes not involved
IIA	Grossly resected tumor with microscopic residual disease; no evidence of regional node involvement
IIB	Regional disease (extension into adjacent organ or regional nodes), completely resected
IIC	Regional disease with involved nodes, grossly resected, but with evidence of microscopic residual
III	Gross residual disease after surgery
IV	Metastatic disease at diagnosis

(Data from Maurer HM, Moon T, Donaldson M, Fernandez C, Gehan EA, Hammond D et al: The Intergroup Rhabdomyosarcoma Study: A preliminary report. Cancer 40:2015–2026, 1977)

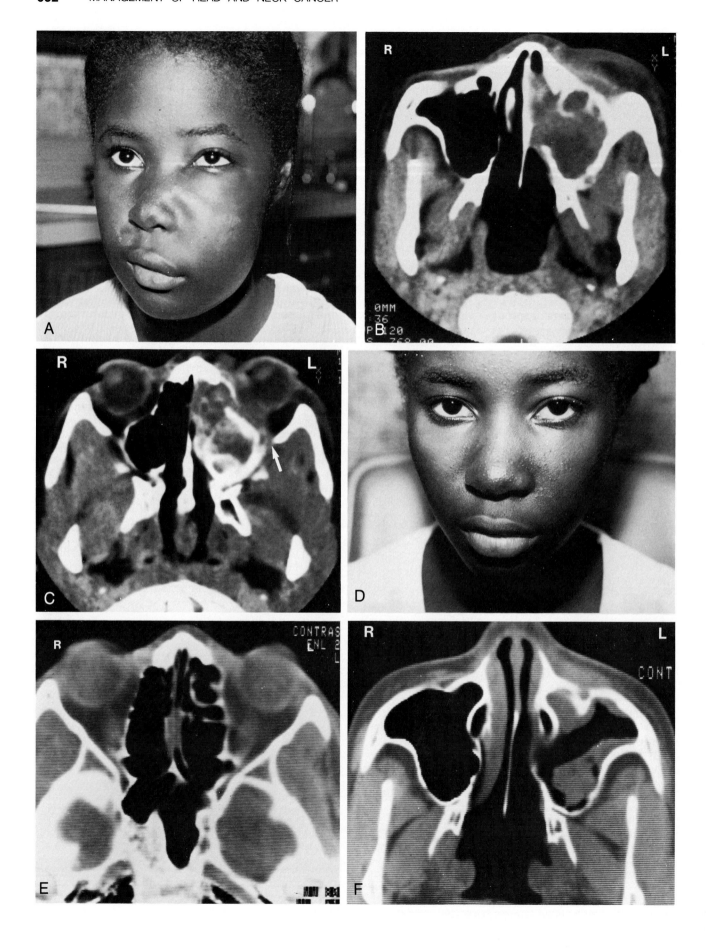

◀ **FIG. 33-3.** (A) A 14-year-old girl presented with a 3-week history of swelling in the left side of the face and a 1-week history of diplopia. Physical examination revealed a large palpable tumor mass beneath the left cheek and extending into the left alveolar ridge. (B) CT scan revealed involvement of the left maxillary sinus, the orbit, the nasal cavity, the infratemporal fossa, and the soft tissues of the premaxilla. (C) Tumor involves the left ethmoid sinus and the medial portion of the left orbit and extends through the inferior orbital fissure (arrow) to the infratemporal fossa. Biopsy revealed embryonal rhabdomyosarcoma. Chemotherapy consisting of vincristine, doxorubicin HCl (Adriamycin), cyclophosphamide, and dactinomycin was begun. (D) After 6 weeks of chemotherapy, just prior to the start of irradiation, there was no visible tumor, and physical examination also revealed no evidence of tumor. (E) Repeat CT scan showed no definite residual tumor in the left orbit. (F) There was residual tumor in the left maxillary sinus and in the premaxillary soft tissues. The fascial planes in the infratemporal fossa behind the left maxillary sinus have returned to normal.

TABLE 33-6. Local Control of Pediatric Rhabdomyosarcoma (All Sites) by Clinical Group and Dose (Intergroup Rhabdomyosarcoma Study) (No. Controlled/No. Treated)

Group	Dose (rad)		
	<4000	4001–5000	>5000
I	3/3	1/2 (50%)	14/15 (93%)
II	19/21 (95%)	20/21 (95%)	56/58 (96.5%)
III	21/25 (84%)	29/31 (93.5%)	99/115 (86%)

(Modified from Tefft M, Lindberg RD, Gehan EA: Radiation therapy combined with systemic chemotherapy of rhabdomyosarcoma in children: Local control in patients enrolled in the Intergroup Rhabdomyosarcoma Study. Natl Cancer Inst Monogr 56:75–81, 1981)

apist and chemotherapist. For operable lesions, the appropriate surgical procedures are described elsewhere in this book.

Radiation Therapy

The radiation treatment of head and neck sarcomas in children is one of the most difficult tasks in pediatric radiation therapy. The volume of tissue to be treated is usually large enough to include a number of sensitive structures, and the dose required for control is high enough to cause profound soft tissue side-effects in the growing child. Therefore, careful treatment planning is necessary to minimize long-term side-effects, particularly when concomitant chemotherapy is given. However, the natural tendency to minimize the volume of irradiation must be avoided, since it has been well shown that an insufficient volume increases the rate of local recurrence.[141]

The techniques for each site are similar to those used for primary carcinomas and are presented in other chapters of this book. It must be stressed, however, that for parameningeal lesions, the superior margin must be at least 2 cm above the base of the skull, even if no cranial nerves are involved and there is no radiologic evidence of invasion of the base of the skull.

It is not necessary to electively irradiate the neck, since the failure rate with adjuvant chemotherapy is very small.[89] If a clinically positive node is present, however, neck irradiation is recommended if a neck dissection is not done.

Until recently, it has been thought that a minimum of

TABLE 33-7. Local Control of Pediatric Rhabdomyosarcoma (All Sites) by Age and Dose (Intergroup Rhabdomyosarcoma Study) (No. Controlled/No. Treated)

Age (Years)	Dose (rad)	
	4001–5000	>5000
≤6	41/45 (91%)	69/77 (90%)
>6	15/22 (68%)	133/152 (87.5%)

(Modified from Tefft M, Lindberg RD, Gehan EA: Radiation therapy combined with systemic chemotherapy of rhabdomyosarcoma in children: Local control in patients enrolled in the Intergroup Rhabdomyosarcoma Study. Natl Cancer Inst Monogr 56:75–81, 1981)

5000 rad was necessary for the control of head and neck rhabdomyosarcomas; doses of 5500 rad to 6500 rad were recommended by some authors.[37,55] However, present data (Table 33-6) would indicate that local control is good with lower doses, particularly when only subclinical disease remains.[141] Patients over 6 years of age may need a higher dose (Table 33-7).

Therefore, patients under 6 years of age should receive

TABLE 33-8. Head and Neck Rhabdomyosarcoma: Sites of Failure by Clinical Group (Intergroup Rhabdomyosarcoma Study: 2-Year Minimum Follow-up)

Primary Site	Group	No. Patients	Site of Failure				
			P	N	CNS	DM	ID
Orbit	I	1	0	0	0	0	0
	II	10	0	1	0	0	0
	III	21	1	1	0	1	2*
Head and neck (excluding orbit)	I	5	1	0	0	0	0
	II	23	1	1	0	2	0
	III	79	12	0	13	7	8†

* One patient died of treatment toxicity, another of varicella.

† Seven patients died of treatment toxicity, one of unknown causes.

(P, primary site; N, regional nodes; CNS, central nervous system; DM, distant metastasis; ID, intercurrent disease)

(Adapted from Raney RB, Donaldson MH, Sutow WW, Lindberg RD, Maurer HM, Tefft M: Special considerations related to primary site in rhabdomyosarcoma: Experience of the Intergroup Rhabdomyosarcoma Study, 1972–1976. Natl Cancer Inst Monogr 56:69–74, 1981)

doses of 4000 rad to 4500 rad at about 180 rad/day, with larger lesions requiring the larger doses. Older children should receive 4500 rad to 5500 rad at 180 rad/day. Generous margins should be employed to start treatment, with a reduction at 3500 rad to 4000 rad. A dose of 3000 rad to 4000 rad should be adequate for subclinical disease in the neck after positive nodes have been removed. The usual doses for gross disease should be employed for clinically positive adenopathy.

Chemotherapy

Combination chemotherapy is now an integral part of the treatment of rhabdomyosarcoma in childhood. Multiple drugs have been found to be effective, including dactinomycin (actinomycin D),[137] vincristine,[133] cyclophosphamide,[49] and doxorubicin HCl (Adriamycin).[46,109]

Most regimens use a combination of drugs.[58,66,90,111,132] The VAC regimen (vincristine, dactinomycin, and cyclophosphamide) has been the most widely used in the past, but regimens containing doxorubicin HCl may be more effective.

Because of the success with chemotherapy in rhabdomyosarcoma, the chemotherapy is started first for large lesions in order to maximize the response before local treatment. The complete response rate after 6 weeks of induction chemotherapy alone is approximately 62%, with another 36% of patients showing a partial response (see Fig. 33-3).[140] There is no evidence that withholding local therapy for 6 weeks decreases survival.

RESULTS OF TREATMENT

The local control of head and neck rhabdomyosarcomas is good (Tables 33-6 through 33-8).[110,141] Orbital primary lesions in particular have an excellent prognosis and few local failures. In fact, radiation therapy alone has been shown to give good results for orbital primary lesions, although adjuvant chemotherapy may improve the survival.[119] Unfortunately, with doses of 5000 rad and above, only approximately one fourth of patients retain useful vision.[119]

The parameningeal lesions have the worst local control and the worst prognosis. In addition to the local failures that are discovered, the high incidence of central nervous system failures may mask additional local failures.

Recent survival results from the IRS-I for all sites, including the head and neck, are shown in Figure 33-4.[88] Most relapses occur within 2 years of diagnosis, but an occasional patient may relapse 5 to 10 years or more after treatment.

One of the major controversies is the treatment of parameningeal rhabdomyosarcomas. A report in 1978 from the IRS showed that 20 (35%) of 57 patients with parameningeal rhabdomyosarcomas failed in the central nervous system, even though follow-up was still short.[139] Once a patient failed in the meninges or central nervous system, the disease was universally fatal. Because of this high failure rate, treatment of these lesions in the IRS-II included 3000 rad of craniospinal axis irradiation plus intrathecal chemotherapy if there was evidence of invasion of the base of the skull, cranial nerve involvement, cytology-positive cerebrospinal fluid, or CT scan involvement of the brain.

Other data conflict with their recommendation. Chan and co-workers from M. D. Anderson Hospital reported a series of 27 patients with parameningeal rhabdomyosarcoma treated from 1961 through 1976, most of whom received the VAC chemotherapy regimen in addition to radiation therapy to the primary lesion.[19] Nineteen of the 27 were alive without evidence of disease with a 2-year minimum follow-up, and only one lesion recurred in the central nervous system. A review by Berry and Jenkin of the patients treated at Princess Margaret Hospital in Toronto revealed similar results, with only 3 documented central nervous system failures of 21 parameningeal primary lesions.[6] Two of the three patients with central nervous system failure had extensive tumors that showed substantial involvement of the central nervous system on initial workup.

Therefore, it has not been proved that patients with only cranial nerve involvement or roentgenographic evidence of invasion of the base of the skull should receive craniospinal irradiation. However, those who present with a positive cerebrospinal fluid cytology or definite intracranial extension are at high risk for dissemination throughout the central nervous system and may benefit from therapy to the central nervous system. The results of the next IRS may provide an answer.

FIBROSARCOMA

Fibroblastic tumors in children present a multitude of un-resolved conflicts. There are probably more opinions about their classification than there are affected patients, since they are extraordinarily rare. Still, they represent the most common soft tissue neoplasm in children except for rhab-domyosarcoma, and one to two cases per year will be seen at institutions treating a moderate number of pediatric neoplasms.

PATHOLOGY

Whereas the diagnosis of fibrosarcoma in adults is well established, in children it remains controversial.

There are fibroblastic proliferations that some pathol-ogists prefer to label as one of the myriad of "juvenile fibromatoses," while other pathologists lump what are probably the same lesions into a group of tumors called fibrosarcomas or "infantile fibrosarcomas." However, most pathologists experienced in the field feel that true fibro-sarcoma does occur in children and is histologically iden-tical to that occurring in adults, although clinically less aggressive.[126]

There is a distinct clinical variant of fibrosarcoma in children called congenital or infantile fibrosarcoma by most authors. These lesions are either present at birth or develop within the first year of life. Whether there is a histologic distinction is a matter yet to be resolved, but they appear to have a particularly good prognosis.[22,27,126,130]

The etiology of fibrosarcoma in childhood is speculative. A few occur in patients with prior irradiation. In addition, patients with bilateral retinoblastoma have a high inci-dence of sarcomas, particularly osteosarcomas and fibro-sarcomas, both with and without prior irradiation.[126] How-ever, most lesions occur sporadically with no history of prior irradiation or bilateral retinoblastoma.

LOCATION AND ANATOMY

The majority of lesions originate in the extremities, but about 20% of pediatric fibrosarcomas occur in the head and neck region. This is true even for those lesions pre-senting in the first year of life.[22,97,130]

The neck is the most common primary site of fibrosar-comas above the clavicles; approximately one third of pa-tients present with this as their primary site. The oral cavity, scalp, auriculoparotid region, and face are the next most common sites, in decreasing frequency. Fibrosarcomas have also been reported in the maxillary sinus, naso-pharynx, nasal cavity, and larynx.

PATTERNS OF SPREAD

Locally, fibrosarcomas of the head and neck spread by direct invasion of adjacent tissues. The skin above the lesion is usually not directly involved, but the tumor may occasionally erode underlying bone in the skull, mandible, or neck. Lymph node metastases occur in less than 10% of patients.[136]

The incidence of hematogenous metastasis to lung and bone is reported to be less than 10% for patients under 10 years of age.[22,130] For patients over 15 years of age, the metastatic rate may approach that of adults, that is, close to 50%.[130] For patients between 10 and 15 years of age, the rate of distant metastasis is less clear.

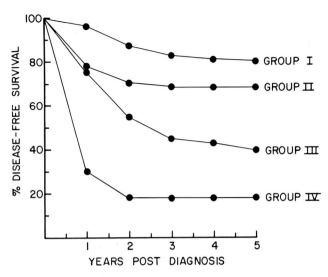

FIG. 33-4. Disease-free survival by group in 554 patients treated on the First Intergroup Rhabdomyosarcoma Study. (Modified from Maurer HM: The Intergroup Rhabdomyo-sarcoma Study: Update, November 1978. Natl Cancer Inst Mongr 56:61–68, 1981)

CLINICAL PICTURE AND WORKUP

Approximately 36% of pediatric fibrosarcomas are pres-ent at birth, while another 13% present in the first year of life. From 1 to 9 years of age, the fibrosarcomas are seen less often, with 2% to 3% of the total lesions presenting at each year of age, but the frequency rises again in the 10- to 16-year age-group. The disease has been reported slightly more often in males than females.[130]

Most patients with fibrosarcomas of the head and neck, as well as elsewhere in the body, present with a painless mass (Fig. 33-5). Some may have tense, shiny, erythematous skin over the lesion. Most patients have a history of a slowly growing mass prior to diagnosis, but they may pre-sent with a rapid growth over a period of a week to a month and require immediate attention. Other symptoms depend on the location of the disease at the time of di-agnosis. Roentgenograms of the lesion may show only a soft tissue mass or may show bone erosion or cortical thickening adjacent to the mass.

The workup should include an evaluation of the local extent of disease with the appropriate roentgenographic studies. A chest roentgenogram and a bone scan (or skeletal survey for very young children) are probably sufficient to rule out metastatic disease, although a CT scan of the lungs may be considered. The yield from these studies will be small, however, particularly in infants.

TREATMENT SELECTION AND TREATMENT RESULTS

There is general agreement that surgery alone is the preferred treatment for pediatric fibrosarcomas, especially those occurring in the first year of life. The extent of surgery depends on the age of the child and the location of the tumor. Simple excision has a high recurrence rate; reports in the literature show rates of 40% to 60%.[22,53,126,130] More radical surgery probably decreases the rate of local re-currence, but this has not been clearly established. How-ever, the rate of distant metastasis is less than 10% in

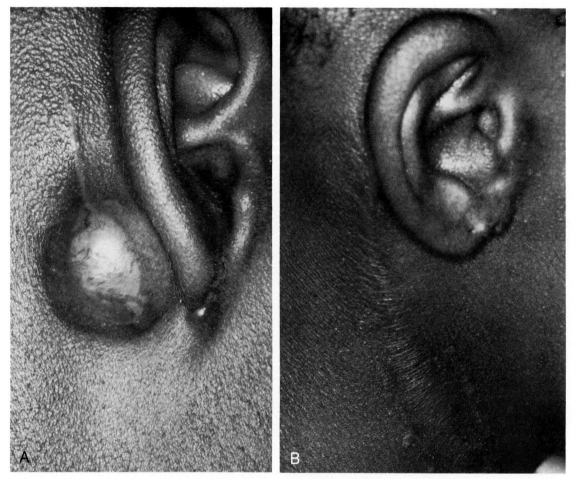

FIG. 33-5. (A) Fibrosarcoma arising in the right postauricular region in a 10-year-old girl. Two months prior to this recurrence, the patient had undergone excision of a similar-sized mass. (B) Two years after reexcision and postoperative irradiation; 6000 rad was delivered using electrons. Patient had no evidence of local recurrence or distant metastasis.

FIG. 33-6. Actuarial survival of patients with fibrosarcoma (birth to age 19 years) reported to the End Results Section of the National Cancer Institute before 1971. (Modified by permission from Neifeld JP, Berg JW, Godwin D, Salzberg AM: A retrospective epidemiologic study of pediatric fibrosarcomas. J Pediatr Surg 13:735–740, 1978)

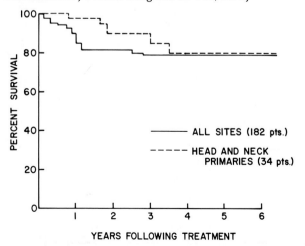

children under age 10 and the overall survival is good (Fig. 33-6).[22,53,97,126,130] Therefore, in infants, more conservative treatment may be considered to minimize morbidity, especially in the head and neck region. A wide excision with an adequate cuff of normal tissue is the preferred therapy, with more radical surgery reserved for recurrence.

Although radiation therapy has often been used postoperatively, the risks involved with treating infants to the appropriate dose should minimize its application.

The prognosis of childhood fibrosarcoma continues to be excellent, even for children up to 10 years of age. However, at some time above that age, these tumors begin to act more like the adult variety, with much higher rates of distant metastasis, although there is little, if any, difference histologically. Some authors report a survival rate of only 50% above age 10;[126] others report survival to be good up to age 19.[97] At these older ages, radiation therapy can increase the rate of local control. Postoperative doses in the range of 5000 rad to 6000 rad at 170 rad to 180 rad/day are appropriate if adequate margins cannot be obtained. Prophylactic neck irradiation is not indicated in the presence of a clinically negative neck.

There is little good information on chemotherapy. Drugs such as dactinomycin, methotrexate, cyclophosphamide, vincristine, and doxorubicin HCl have been used for metastatic tumors, but the response rates are not clear. Since the main problem initially is a local one, an improvement in survival has not yet been demonstrated by the use of adjuvant chemotherapy, but it may be a reasonable addition to treatment in an older child (age > 10) with a high-grade or unfavorable lesion.

OTHER SOFT TISSUE SARCOMAS

Except for rhabdomyosarcoma and fibrosarcoma, other soft tissue sarcomas of the head and neck region in the pediatric age-group are anecdotal. Although virtually all histologies have been reported to occur, the following three soft tissue sarcomas have some unique features in the pediatric age-group. (See Chapter 34, Adult Mesenchymal Tumors Presenting in the Head and Neck, for a discussion of histologies not included here.)

HEMANGIOPERICYTOMA

Besides the usual adult variety of hemangiopericytoma, which occurs rarely in older children, an infantile variety has been described by some authors.[31] It almost exclusively occurs in children under 1 year of age and can be congenital. The tumor starts in the subcutis and is grossly multiloculated. Histologically, there is increased mitotic activity and focal necrosis. Radiologically, calcifications are sometimes seen in the necrotic areas. Most lesions are solitary, but multiple congenital hemangiopericytomas have been reported in the head and neck.[68,122]

The treatment of infantile hemangiopericytoma is surgical excision. Local recurrence is rare, as is the development of metastatic disease. Death is a rare event, even for patients presenting with multiple lesions.[104]

The children that present with the adult variety of hemangiopericytoma are usually in their second decade of life, and there are no data indicating that treatment should be any different than that of adults.

ALVEOLAR SOFT PART SARCOMA

Alveolar soft part sarcoma is an unusual tumor of uncertain histogenesis.[21] Most commonly, these tumors present in the third decade, but presentation in the second decade is more common if the lesion is in the head or neck.[127] Seven of the 12 cases found in a review of the world's literature by Spector and co-workers presented in patients under the age of 20, with 2 children presenting in the first decade of life. The other 5 occurred in patients in their third decade. The most common primary site was the tongue (6 of 7), particularly the base of the tongue.

The natural history of these tumors is long. They are slow to grow, often recur locally, and may metastasize to regional nodes and distant sites.[127]

Most lesions were treated surgically, with an occasional patient receiving preoperative or postoperative irradiation in the range of 5000 rad to 6000 rad. Short-term survival is fair, with 59% of patients alive at 5 years and 47% at 10 years.[81] However, recurrences beyond 10 years are not uncommon, and the long-range survival may be much lower.

SYNOVIAL CELL SARCOMA

Synovial sarcoma may occur in the neck in the pediatric age-group. This is a disease of young males, with an average age of 19 years according to one series.[116]

The treatment is primarily surgical, but local control was only 7 of 17 in patients who initially had surgery alone in Roth's series. Many of these probably had inadequate surgery by today's standards, however. Postoperative irradiation for incompletely excised lesions has been reported to be effective with doses of 5500 rad to 6000 rad/ 5½ to 7 weeks.[5,16]

Approximately half of the patients with primary lesions in the neck survive 5 years.[50,116] Most deaths are caused by pulmonary metastases, but in many who die of distant metastases local failure occurs first.

Bone Sarcomas

Bone sarcomas represent approximately 4.5% of all malignant childhood tumors. Osteosarcoma is the most common, representing 63% of pediatric bone tumors. Ewing's sarcoma accounts for another 27%, while chondrosarcoma and other rare bone tumors make up the remaining 10%.[151] These figures do not include primary lymphomas of bone.

OSTEOSARCOMA

Osteosarcomas account for 2.6% of all pediatric malignant tumors and 63% of malignant bone tumors in childhood.[151] Seven to 16% of osteosarcomas occur in the head and neck, most of them in adults.[25,61]

Prior radiation therapy, Paget's disease, fibrous dysplasia, and bilateral retinoblastoma (even without radiation therapy) predispose to the development of osteosarcoma in the head and neck (Fig. 33-7).

FIG. 33-7. CT scan showing osteosarcoma of the mandible (*arrows*) developing in 32-year-old patient with fibrous dysplasia of the entire left side of his face. The patient was treated with 6000 rad preoperatively followed by a hemimandibulectomy. There is no evidence of recurrence 3 years following treatment.

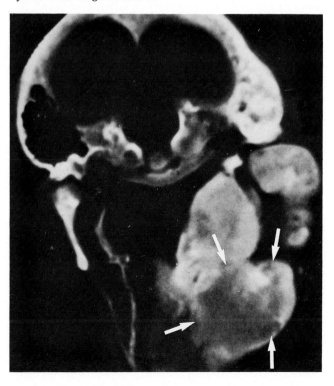

PATHOLOGY

Osteosarcoma shows considerable variation in its histologic presentation. By definition, the proliferating malignant cells must produce osteoid, or material histologically indistinguishable from it, in at least one small focus. Osteosarcoma starting in the jaws is reported to show less histologic anaplasia, according to Dahlin, but not every series confirms this.[25,42]

LOCATION

The distribution for 329 head and neck lesions is shown in Figure 33-8. The body of the mandible is most commonly involved, then, in descending frequency, the symphysis, angle, and ascending ramus. In the maxilla, the alveolar ridge and antrum are the most common sites. Involvement of the base of the skull or cervical spine is a rare occurrence.

PATTERNS OF SPREAD

By the time an osteosarcoma is diagnosed, it has generally breached the cortex and an extraosseous mass is present, which invades the surrounding soft tissues. The most common site of metastatic disease is the lung, although bone metastases are not uncommon.

CLINICAL PICTURE

Osteosarcoma of the head and neck appears to present at a later age than osteosarcoma of the extremities (Fig. 33-9). Whereas 66% of osteosarcomas of the long bones present in patients under 20 years of age, head and neck lesions have a roughly even distribution by decade from 10 years of age to 50. The male-to-female ratio is approximately 1:1, and there does not appear to be any major racial predisposition.

Most osteosarcomas present with pain in the involved bone. This is usually mild and transitory at first, but gradually develops into a more persistent, and at times very severe, pain. When the tumor breaks through the cortex of the bone into the soft tissues, a large mass may be noticed by the patient. The mass may be rock hard, but a soft or rubbery mass does not exclude osteosarcoma in the differential diagnosis.

Mandibular tumors may cause dental symptoms early in the course of the disease; a palpable mass is usually present. Maxillary primary lesions are often more insidious, with symptoms of sinusitis or nasal congestion an early complaint, and later symptoms becoming apparent when the tumor invades the orbit. Primary lesions of the cervical spine usually cause neurologic symptoms in the arms, with pain and weakness being most common. Skull lesions usually present as an asymptomatic mass, but pain and other neurologic symptoms may be present.

Roentgenographic findings vary greatly. Tumors may be either primarily sclerotic or primarily lytic, but they usually have a combination of these features. The lytic lesions are more painful in general than the sclerotic ones. The destructive process usually involves the cortex with a gradual transition from zones of marked lysis to zones of uninvolved bone, making the border indistinct. The periosteum is often elevated by penetrating tumor, and a soft tissue mass may be visible on roentgenograms, tomograms, or CT scans. There are often amorphous calcium deposits in the soft tissue mass as the growing tumor attempts to lay down an abnormal bone matrix.

Symmetrical widening of the periodontal ligament involving one or more teeth may be a clue to a developing osteosarcoma or chondrosarcoma of the mandible.[41] Root resorption of a permanent erupted tooth is unusual for an osteogenic sarcoma, being more common as a result of inflammation or a benign tumor.[26]

STAGING

A complete evaluation should be undertaken *before the biopsy is done* for suspected osteosarcoma. In addition to plain roentgenograms of the involved site, the local disease can also be evaluated with CT scan and digital vascular imaging.

The overwhelming majority of metastatic disease appears first in the lungs. A chest roentgenogram plus either a CT scan of the lung or whole-lung tomograms is an effective way of evaluating small foci of disease in the lung.

A bone scan is useful in determining the extent of local disease as well as in detecting metastatic bone lesions.

The level of serum alkaline phosphatase is usually elevated, and patients whose levels remain high after surgical resection should be strongly suspected of harboring metastatic disease. This test is also used in the follow-up, since a rise in alkaline phosphatase following treatment has been correlated with the development of metastatic disease or a local recurrence. In children, and particularly in adolescents, the serum alkaline phosphatase level is normally quite high, and caution must be used in interpreting an elevated alkaline phosphatase level in that age-group.

FIG. 33-8. Location of 329 cases of osteosarcoma of the head and neck. Data collected from the literature, 1940 to present, where location of the lesion was well specified.

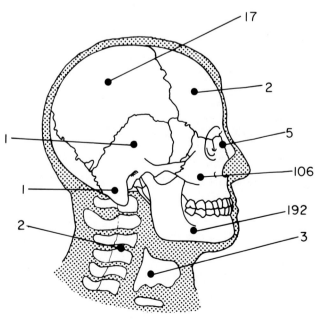

SELECTION OF TREATMENT MODALITIES

The risk of distant metastases is less for head and neck primary lesions than in other sites (Table 33-9). The emphasis of treatment is therefore local control. Surgical excision is recommended if the lesion presents in a resectable site such as the mandible, maxilla, or skull, but surgery alone is often inadequate and may be combined with preoperative or postoperative radiation therapy.

For more favorable lesions, such as those in the mandible or alveolar ridge of the maxilla, adjuvant chemotherapy is probably of minimal value; few of these patients develop distant metastases until after one or more local failures. For lesions of the maxillary antrum, skull, cervical spine, and other rare sites in the head and neck, the prognosis is so poor that it is worthwhile to consider aggressive therapy with surgery (if possible), irradiation, and chemotherapy.

Surgery

Of the lesions arising in the head and neck, mandibular osteosarcomas are most amenable to surgical resection, and resection of the involved portion of the mandible with surrounding soft tissue is recommended by some authors, while others recommend hemimandibulectomy, since local failure remains the biggest problem in controlling disease in this site (see Table 33-9). A few small lesions of the mandible can be reconstructed after initial resection, but if soft tissue extension is present, reconstruction is usually not possible. Maxillary lesions starting on the alveolar ridge usually can be resected by a limited maxillectomy, but lesions arising elsewhere in the maxilla (i.e., "antral primaries") may require a maxillectomy with or without an orbital exenteration. More extensive lesions may require a craniofacial procedure (see Chapter 23, Nasal Vestibule, Nasal Cavity, and Paranasal Sinuses). For lesions arising in the skull, surgery becomes more difficult, although still possible in most cases. However, for lesions arising in the base of the skull or cervical spine, surgery is usually not possible, and these masses must be treated with radiation therapy.

Radiation Therapy

Radiation therapy is usually recommended in combination with surgical resection because of the high rate of local failure after resection alone (see Table 33-9). The radiation therapy is usually given postoperatively in full therapeutic doses (7000 rad to 7500 rad/8 to 9 weeks). Preoperative radiation therapy (5000 rad to 6000 rad/5 to 7 weeks) is selected for lesions that are not technically resectable in the hope that sufficient regression may be followed by total resection.

For lesions that are inoperable, an occasional cure with radiation therapy alone has been reported.[39,77] The dose required for control is not clear. Usually, doses in the range of 7000 rad to 8000 rad/7 to 9 weeks are required, but the constraints of central nervous system tolerance limit the dose that can be delivered to lesions of the cervical spine

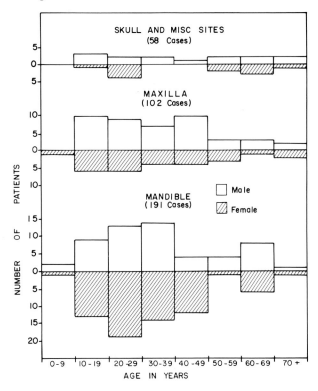

FIG. 33-9. Age and sex distribution of 351 cases of osteosarcoma of the head and neck. Data collected from the literature, 1940 to present, where the age and sex of patients were specified.

Primary Site	No. Patients	Site of Failure		
		P	P + DM	DM
Mandible	49	21 (43%)	6 (12%)	6 (12%)
Maxilla				
Antrum	11	6 (55%)	4 (36%)	0 (0%)
Alveolar ridge	19	7 (37%)	5 (26%)	2 (11%)
Skull* and miscellaneous sites	14	4 (29%)	4 (29%)	5 (36%)

TABLE 33-9. Osteosarcoma of the Head and Neck: Site of Failure (Data Collected From the Literature, 1940 to date; 5-Year Minimum Follow-up)

* Two-year minimum follow-up.
(P, primary site; DM, distant metastasis)

and base of the skull. Lower doses may sometimes be effective, at least for extending survival, particularly in conjunction with chemotherapy.[65] Special treatment programs with particles (protons) may sometimes be advised to minimize the dose to the brain stem or spinal cord.

Chemotherapy

The three drugs most effective against osteosarcoma are methotrexate, doxorubicin HCl, and cis-platinum. At present, most adjuvant regimens include two or more of these drugs.[64,87,134] Chemotherapy is probably a weak adjuvant, and therefore may not be recommended in favorable head and neck lesions.

RESULTS OF TREATMENT

Chambers and Mahoney used preoperative interstitial radium to deliver 10,000 rad to 16,000 rad to mandibular lesions followed by surgery 2 weeks later.[18] Five-year survival was obtained in 22 (73%) of 30 patients, and the rate of local control was better than 80%.

Preoperative external-beam irradiation in doses of 5000 rad to 6000 rad is also probably of value.[131] The local control rate (5-year minimum follow-up) collected from the literature (excluding Chambers and Mahoney) is better for those who received preoperative radiation therapy (8 of 13, 62%) than for surgery alone (17 of 44, 39%). Ninety percent of local failures occur within the first 2 years.

Actuarial survival by primary site for skull, maxillary, and mandibular lesions is shown in Figure 33-10. For cervical spine lesions and lesions arising around the base of the skull, for which irradiation is the primary modality of treatment, it is difficult to find a single patient who did not die of disease.

EWING'S SARCOMA

Ewing's sarcoma is a distinctive, small round-cell tumor that occurs primarily in the second and third decades of life. It is uncommon in the head and neck region. Of 58

FIG. 33-10. Actuarial survival[24] by primary site of 206 patients with osteosarcoma of the head and neck. Data were collected from literature, 1940 to present, where length of survival and primary site were clearly stated.

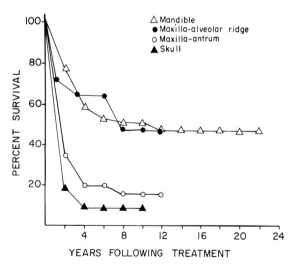

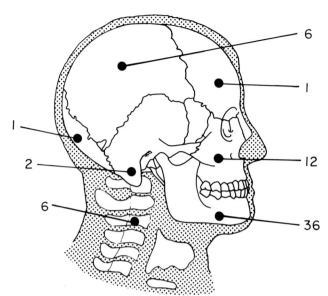

FIG. 33-11. Location of 64 cases of Ewing's sarcoma of the head and neck. Data collected from literature, 1950 to present, where location of lesion was well specified. Includes 6 patients from the University of Florida.

patients treated at the University of Florida from 1969 through 1980, only 6 had primary lesions above the clavicles. Dahlin, in reviewing 299 Ewing's sarcomas seen at the Mayo Clinic before 1975, reported only 8 occurring above the clavicles.[25]

Blacks in both the United States and Africa are rarely afflicted.[43,147]

PATHOLOGY

Ewing's sarcoma is a primitive malignant tumor of bone of uncertain origin, characterized by anaplastic small cells with round nuclei without distinct cytoplasmic borders or prominent nucleoli. They are usually glycogen positive. The differential diagnoses include metastatic neuroblastoma and primary lymphoma of bone.

LOCATION

The distribution of 64 cases of Ewing's sarcoma of the head and neck reported in the literature from 1950 to date is shown in Figure 33-11.

PATTERNS OF SPREAD

The medullary cavity appears to be the site of origin of most Ewing's sarcomas. However, even in early stages of disease, the cortex may be eroded and a large, friable, hemorrhagic, soft tissue mass can develop. In later stages of disease, almost all tumors will exhibit a soft tissue mass that encircles and envelops the involved portion of the bone. Mandibular primary lesions tend to spread laterally into the soft tissues of the masseter muscles instead of medially into the oral cavity. However, a primary lesion of the mandible that did invade the floor of the mouth is shown in Figure 33-12. Lesions of the cranium are usually slow to invade the dura and brain, preferring instead to grow outward. Cervical spine lesions tend to compress the

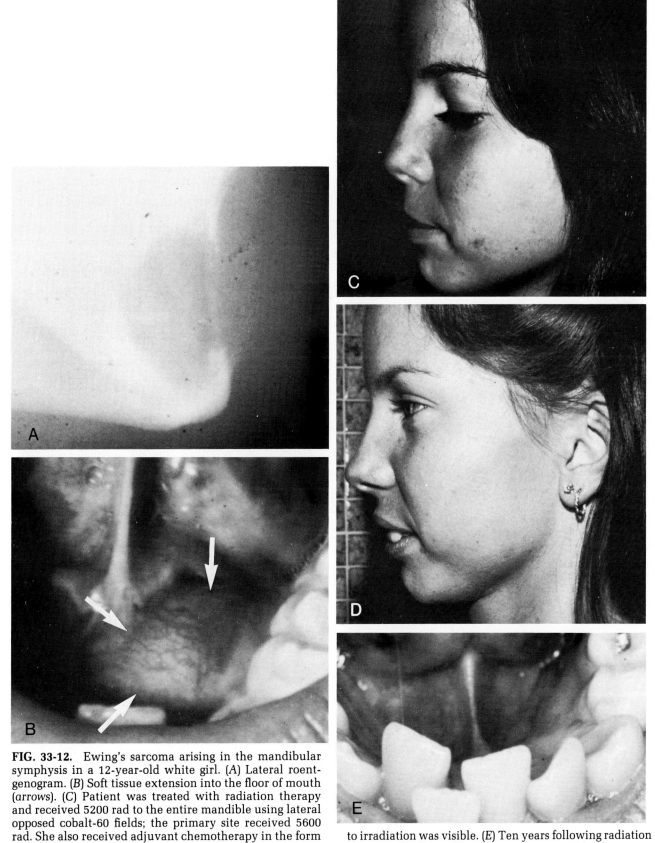

FIG. 33-12. Ewing's sarcoma arising in the mandibular symphysis in a 12-year-old white girl. (*A*) Lateral roentgenogram. (*B*) Soft tissue extension into the floor of mouth (*arrows*). (*C*) Patient was treated with radiation therapy and received 5200 rad to the entire mandible using lateral opposed cobalt-60 fields; the primary site received 5600 rad. She also received adjuvant chemotherapy in the form of cyclophosphamide and vincristine. Three years following therapy, the profile of her face was normal. (*D*) Ten years following therapy, hypoplasia of the mandible secondary to irradiation was visible. (*E*) Ten years following radiation therapy, the floor of mouth appears normal. There was crowding of the mandibular incisors secondary to hypoplasia of the mandible.

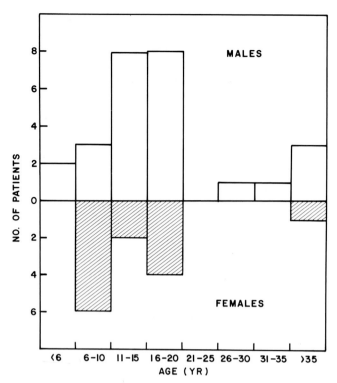

FIG. 33-13. Age and sex distribution of 39 patients with Ewing's sarcoma of the head and neck. Data are taken from the literature, 1950 to present, where age, sex, and primary site of lesion were specified.

cord early in the course of the disease. Cervical lymph node involvement is uncommon. The most common sites of distant metastasis are the lung, skeleton, and bone marrow.

CLINICAL PICTURE

Ewing's sarcoma of the head and neck most commonly presents between the ages of 6 and 20 years, with a 2:1 male to female predominance (Fig. 33-13).

Most patients present with pain or an asymptomatic mass. Often, there is a history of a rapidly increasing mass followed by a stable period lasting for a few weeks or many months. There is often local temperature elevation over the mass. In mandibular lesions, dental problems may be the first sign of the tumor, and the patient may present to the dentist. Involvement of the inferior alveolar nerve may cause paresthesias of the lips and chin.

Patients with maxillary primary lesions often present with nasal obstruction, dental problems, swelling of the zygomatic region, exophthalmos, and tearing.[36]

Systemic symptoms are often present, with a slight to moderate fever, anemia, leukocytosis, and an increased sedimentation rate. These symptoms may herald spread to bone marrow or other distant sites, but they also occur in what appears to be localized disease. They are a poor prognostic sign.

The usual roentgenographic appearance of Ewing's sarcoma in the head and neck is that of a lytic or mottled pattern of bone destruction with poorly defined margins. A few lesions are predominantly sclerotic.

STAGING

The evaluation involves roentgenograms of the primary site, including the whole bone involved, with careful analysis of the extent of disease by tomograms or CT scan. A Panorex view of the mandible is useful in evaluating lesions originating there.

A complete blood cell count, sedimentation rate, and liver function studies are necessary to evaluate systemic disease. A chest roentgenogram and either whole-lung tomograms or a CT scan of the lung are important to rule out metastatic lung disease. A bone scan as well as bone marrow aspiration and biopsy are necessary to evaluate possible spread to other bones and the bone marrow.

SELECTION OF TREATMENT MODALITIES

Radiation therapy is the principal modality used for the local treatment of Ewing's sarcoma of the head and neck. Small mandibular lesions may occasionally be selected for surgery but most other lesions are best treated with irradiation. In addition, all sites of metastatic disease at diagnosis should be irradiated. Whole-lung irradiation should be given to patients with lung metastases.

All patients should receive systemic chemotherapy. In the past, chemotherapy and radiation therapy have been started concomitantly, but good results can be obtained by inducing the patient with several cycles of chemotherapy prior to local treatment. Not only will most soft tissue masses disappear, but also areas of bone destruction will sometimes begin to heal. Chemotherapy should be continued during radiation therapy and for 6 to 12 months afterward, depending on the regimen employed.

Radiation Therapy

The dose of radiation required for local control when chemotherapy is given concomitant to radiation therapy is analyzed in Table 33-10.[112] We recommend a reducing-field technique with 3500 rad to 4000 rad to the lesion using generous margins, followed by a 1000- to 1500-rad boost to the lesion itself for a total dose of 5000 rad to 5500 rad at 180 rad to 200 rad/fraction. It is not necessary to treat the contralateral hemimandible in a patient with a small unilateral lesion.

Chemotherapy

The four drugs most commonly used in the treatment of Ewing's sarcoma are vincristine, cyclophosphamide,

TABLE 33-10.	Correlation of Local Control With Irradiation Dosage (Intergroup Ewing's Sarcoma Study— All Sites)
Tumor Dose (rad)	**No. Controlled/No. at Risk (%)**
3000–3999	6/6 (100)
4000–4999	37/43 (86)
5000–5999	80/91 (88)
≧6000	50/53 (94)

(Adapted from Razek A, Perez CA, Tefft M, Nesbit M, Vietti T, Burgert EO Jr, Kissane J, Pritchard DJ, Gehan EA: Intergroup Ewing's Sarcoma Study: Local control related to radiation dose, volume, and site of primary lesion in Ewing's sarcoma. Cancer 46:516–521, 1980)

dactinomycin, and doxorubicin HCl, although other drugs are known to be active. All have good activity against the tumor as single agents. Most regimens for the treatment of Ewing's sarcoma use a combination of these four drugs.[20,99,105-107]

Bone marrow depression is one of the major side-effects of all regimens. With lesions near the oral cavity, severe confluent mucositis secondary to the combination of radiation therapy and doxorubicin HCl or dactinomycin may render the child virtually incapable of eating and require admission to the hospital for nutritional supplementation.

RESULTS OF TREATMENT

The survival of patients with Ewing's sarcoma has improved dramatically with the advent of systemic chemotherapy. Whereas the prechemotherapy survival rate was approximately 5% at 5 years,[108] adjuvant chemotherapy has increased the rate to 50% or better at 5 years.[20,99,107,114] Survival in patients treated with radiation therapy alone is compared with survival in those treated with irradiation plus chemotherapy in Figure 33-14 and Table 33-11.[20]

There are few data on lesions of the maxilla, although the survival of those reported is good.[36,114] The Intergroup Ewing's Sarcoma Study reported six patients with skull and facial bone primary lesions and two patients with cervical spine lesions alive without evidence of disease with maximum follow-up of 5 years.[105]

A large extraosseous mass has been shown to produce a much poorer prognosis, regardless of the primary site.[93]

FIG. 33-14. Relapse-free survival of patients with Ewing's sarcoma (all sites) treated at M. D. Anderson Hospital, 1948–1975. (Chan RC, Sutow WW, Lindberg RD, Samuels ML, Murray JA, Johnston DA: Management and results of localized Ewing's sarcoma. Cancer 43:1001–1006, 1979)

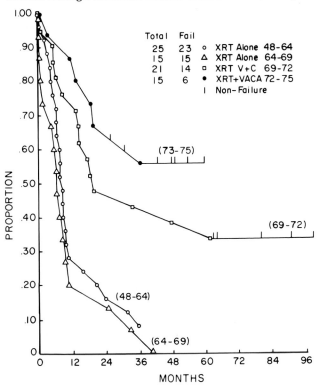

TABLE 33-11.	Survival of Patients With Ewing's Sarcoma of Mandible (Compiled from the Literature)

Treatment	No. Alive at 5 Years/ No. at Risk
Radiation therapy alone	5/17 (29%)
Radiation therapy + adjuvant chemotherapy	6/14 (43%)

A few patients who present with metastatic disease can be cured with intensive chemotherapy and radiation therapy.[106] Most successes occur in patients who have either a single bony or lung metastasis, and these patients warrant aggressive treatment with radiation therapy to all sites of gross disease as well as concomitant chemotherapy. Those with multiple bony metastases at diagnosis continue to do dismally.

CHONDROSARCOMA

In the Mayo Clinic series, of 470 patients with chondrosarcoma, only 17 presented in the second decade and only 3 were under 10 years of age.[25] In general, the treatment principles are the same for the pediatric age-group as they are for adults, and this is covered in more detail in Chapter 34, Adult Mesenchymal Tumors Presenting in the Head and Neck.

Lymphomas

Lymphomas represent the third most common malignancy in the pediatric age-group.[151] Lesions presenting in the head and neck are the most common single site of involvement. (See Chapter 35, Lymphomas and Related Diseases Presenting in the Head and Neck.)

Neuroectodermal Tumors

NEUROBLASTOMA

Neuroblastoma is the most common extracranial malignant solid tumor in infancy and childhood. It comprises approximately 7% of childhood malignancies and is slightly more common in males than females, with a ratio of 1.3: 1.0.[151] Twenty-five to 30% of neuroblastomas present in patients under 1 year of age, with another 15% to 20% at 1 to 2 years of age. Over half are older than 2 years of age at diagnosis, but only a rare patient is older than age 5.[8]

PATHOLOGY

Neuroblastoma arises from primordial neural crest cells.[121] It is one of a number of tumors that are designated by the broad term *neurocristopathy*[121] and is the most malignant variant of a spectrum of tumors that also includes the ganglioneuroblastoma and the benign ganglioneuroma. Ganglioneuromas may sometimes by derived from neuroblastomas that have matured, or they may arise *de novo*.

LOCATION

The most common site of primary neuroblastoma in the head and neck is in the cervical sympathetic chain. This represents approximately 5% of all neuroblastomas, and two thirds of those arising in the head and neck region. The only common site in the head is the olfactory bulb, but this tumor, called the esthesioneuroblastoma, primarily occurs in adults (see Chapter 23, Nasal Vestibule, Nasal Cavity, and Paranasal Sinuses).

In addition, neuroblastoma may metastasize to the head and neck area. Bilateral proptosis or supraorbital ecchymoses from bilateral orbital involvement (Fig. 33-15) are not uncommon, and the cranium is the most common site of bony metastasis.

PATTERNS OF SPREAD

Cervical neuroblastoma spreads locally by invading the surrounding tissues. It may also pass through the neural foramina into the spinal canal, thus causing neurologic sequelae. These so-called dumbbell tumors are more common with abdominal or thoracic primary lesions, but they do occur in the neck.

Neuroblastoma also has a high propensity to spread to regional nodes. The most common sites of distant metastases are the bone marrow, bony cortex, liver, and skin.

CLINICAL PICTURE

Neuroblastoma commonly presents as a painless mass. In the neck, this can be a lymph node, but more commonly it is a deeper mass that feels fixed to the underlying vertebral structure of the neck. Patients with "dumbbell" tumors may present with neurologic symptoms, although complete obstruction has occasionally been demonstrated by myelography in patients with no neurologic symptoms. Horner's syndrome is common at diagnosis.

FIG. 33-15. An 18-month-old girl with typical supraorbital ecchymoses secondary to bilateral orbital metastases from neuroblastoma.

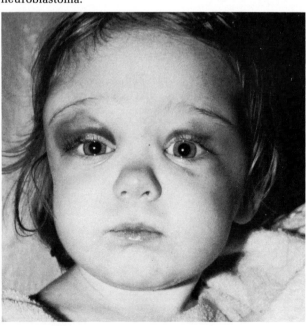

TABLE 33-12.	Evans' Staging for Neuroblastoma
Stage	**Description**
I	Tumor confined to the organ or structure of origin
II	Tumors extending in continuity beyond the organ or structure of origin but not crossing the midline; regional lymph nodes on the homolateral side may be involved
III	Tumors extending in continuity beyond the midline; regional lymph nodes may be involved bilaterally
IV	Remote disease involving skeleton, organs, soft tissues, or distant lymph node groups
IVS	Patients who would otherwise be stage I or II but who have remote disease confined only to one or more of the following sites: liver, skin, or bone marrow (without roentgenographic evidence of bone metastasis on complete skeletal survey)

(Stages from Evans AE, D'Angio GJ, Randolph J: A proposed staging for children with neuroblastoma. Cancer 27:374–378, 1971)

STAGING AND WORKUP

The most commonly used staging system is shown in Table 33-12.[34]

The routine workup should include a complete blood cell count, platelet count, differential, sedimentation rate, liver function studies, and renal function studies. A 24-hour urine collection for catecholamines and their products should be done. Most tumors will produce elevated vanillylmandelic acid and homovanillic acid levels, but more extensive testing of other metabolites will almost always reveal an elevation of at least one.[145] Radiologically, a chest roentgenogram should be done, as well as a bone scan or bone survey, since up to 70% of patients may have metastatic bone disease at diagnosis. A bone marrow aspirate and biopsy are necessary since some patients have bone marrow disease without involvement of the cortex.

The primary site in the head and neck should be evaluated with a CT scan or tomograms.

SELECTION OF TREATMENT AND TREATMENT RESULTS

In contrast to many other childhood cancers, there has been no dramatic improvement in survival due to treatment over the past 20 years. The two most important determinants in survival are the age of the patient and the stage of disease at diagnosis (Table 33-13).[8] Treatment recommendations at the present time are based on prognosis. It seems clear that for young patients with stage I or II disease, complete excision offers the best chance for cure, with 90% or more under 1 year of age surviving. Stage II patients with residual disease may benefit from postoperative irradiation, with good results reported with doses of 1000 rad to 1500 rad at 150 rad to 180 rad/day.[63]

Stage III disease, although still localized at diagnosis, has a much poorer prognosis and generally occurs in older patients. However, for those under 1 year of age, surgery alone or with postoperative irradiation yields excellent survival.[8,63]

TABLE 33-13.   Percentage Survival by Age and Stage in Neuroblastoma

Age (Years)	Stage				
	I	II	III	IV	IVS
<1	97	89	82	26	91
1–2	77	49	36	4	54
>2	67	37	26	3	42

(Breslow N, McCann B: Statistical estimation of prognosis for children with neuroblastoma. Cancer Res 31:2098–2103, 1971)

In older patients with stage III disease, adjuvant chemotherapy has been explored, but two Children's Cancer Group studies showed no changes in survival, although there may have been a longer time to relapse in one study.[32]

For stage IV disease, survival is dismal at any age, although an occasional patient under 1 year of age may survive.[8,57] Stage IVS is a special situation, with relatively good survival even with minimal or no therapy. Stage IVS occurs primarily in children under 1 year of age, and the good results probably represent activation of the immune system in some way that is not yet understood.[33]

MALIGNANT MELANOTIC NEUROECTODERMAL TUMOR OF INFANCY

This unusual tumor of early infancy is believed to arise from neural crest tissue and is now considered to be one of the neurocristopathies, although in the past it has masqueraded under a variety of names, including pigmented ameloblastoma, pigmented congenital epulis, melanotic ameloblastic odontoma, melanotic progonoma, retinal anlage tumor, congenital melanocarcinoma, and retinoblastic teratoma.[28] Pathologically, the tumor consists of melanin-containing cells and small dark cells that are similar to a conventional neuroblastoma. It occurs primarily in patients under the age of 1 year, and the most common site is the head and neck, with the maxilla accounting for the location of 71% of the cases.[101]

The only proven treatment is surgery. Excision of the tumor is accompanied by a control rate of over 80%.[101] The course is usually benign, but metastases may occasionally occur.[28]

MISCELLANEOUS BENIGN LESIONS

Histiocytosis X

Histiocytosis X is a baffling group of diseases in which the etiology, incidence, and even the cell of origin are yet to be determined. The histiocytoses are not technically thought to be cancer and, indeed, are often self-limited with little or no treatment. However, in some children the disease is lethal, even with aggressive multimodal therapy.

The mortality of the disease is primarily age-dependent (Fig. 33-16).[44] There is no obvious sex predilection, but a familial incidence has been reported.[94] At the present time, histiocytosis X is thought to be an autoimmune disorder,

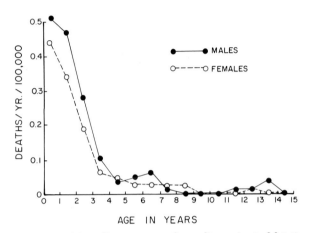

FIG. 33-16. Mortality per year from disseminated histiocytosis in white children, by age at diagnosis (United States, 1960–1964). (Glass AG, Miller RW: US mortality from Letterer-Siwe disease. Pediatrics 42:364–367, 1968. Copyright 1968, American Academy of Pediatrics)

and there is an associated immune deficiency, at least in some patients.[98]

PATHOLOGY

The common pathologic feature of histiocytosis X is a diffuse proliferation of histiocytes, with or without granuloma formation. However, the differentiation of several forms of the disease is primarily a clinical and not a histologic one.

Eosinophilic granuloma is the most benign of the entities and represents a solitary presentation of the disease. It occurs most often in the skull or long bones, although it can occur in a soft tissue site, often in the central nervous system.[69]

Disseminated forms of the disease have been classified in the past as either Hand-Schüller-Christian syndrome or Letterer-Siwe syndrome. Hand-Schüller-Christian disease encompasses the triad of exophthalmos, membranous bone defects, and diabetes insipidus, whereas the Letterer-Siwe type presents with widespread organ involvement. However, because of the overlap of the various syndromes, as well as the fact that one syndrome may evolve into another, there is now a trend to use the following groups: localized histiocytosis, chronic disseminated histiocytosis, and acute disseminated histiocytosis.

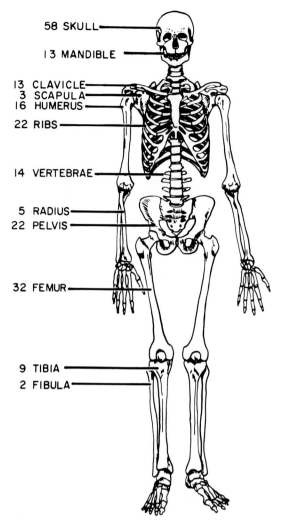

58 SKULL
13 MANDIBLE
13 CLAVICLE
3 SCAPULA
16 HUMERUS
22 RIBS
14 VERTEBRAE
5 RADIUS
22 PELVIS
32 FEMUR
9 TIBIA
2 FIBULA

FIG. 33-17. Presenting sites of 214 cases of localized histiocytosis (eosinophilic granuloma) of bone. (Bunch WH: Orthopedic and rehabilitation aspects of eosinophilic granuloma. Am J Pediatr Hematol Oncol 3:151–156, 1981. Copyright © 1981, MASSON PUBLISHING USA, INC., New York)

LOCATION

In review of the world literature, the skull is found to be the most common site for the presentation of localized histiocytosis (eosinophilic granuloma) of bone, with 27% of patients having lesions there (Fig. 33-17).[10] The mandible alone is the primary site in 6% of patients. Soft tissue primary lesions in the oral cavity, nasopharynx, and elsewhere in the head and neck have been reported.

The disseminated forms of the disease involve the same sites in approximately the same relative frequency (Fig. 33-18).

CLINICAL PICTURE

The most common presentation for localized histiocytosis (eosinophilic granuloma) is pain or swelling in the local area. However, destruction of the temporal or mastoid bones may simulate chronic otitis media. Infiltration of the maxilla and mandible may cause dental symptoms such as loose teeth or pain. Frontal or orbital masses may cause proptosis and visual dysfunction. Sphenoid bone and sella turcica involvement may cause pituitary dysfunction, particularly diabetes insipidus. Diabetes insipidus may occur secondary to focal disease in the hypothalamus or pituitary without attendant bony involvement, however. Localized histiocytosis usually occurs in older children and young adults.

The chronic disseminated form of the disease is primarily confined to bone, with multiple bones usually involved. In addition to bony involvement, however, severe seborrhea is also common, and a typical scaly, maculopapular rash, which spreads from the ear to involve both cheeks and neck, is not infrequent.

The acute disseminated form of the disease is frequently misdiagnosed because the initial signs and symptoms are quite varied and mimic other diseases. It usually occurs in infants and frequently produces fever of unknown origin, poor appetite, weight loss, failure to thrive, irritability, and lethargy. A maculopapular rash with a hemorrhagic base may be prominent, along with adenopathy and organ involvement. The liver and spleen can be massively enlarged, and the lung is also commonly involved. The acute disseminated form often pursues a malignant, rapidly fatal course, particularly in children under 2 years of age, the age at which it occurs most commonly.

STAGING

There have been several suggested staging systems for histiocytosis, but none has been commonly accepted.[47,72,75] The one proposed by Komp and co-workers is simple and of prognostic value (see Fig. 33-19).[72]

Many of the lesions of histiocytosis, particularly those in the head and neck, can be found with a careful physical examination. The skull should be palpated, searching for bony involvement, and careful attention should be given the middle ear, eyes, orbits, and oral cavity. Laboratory studies include a complete blood cell count, platelet count, sedimentation rate, liver function studies, renal function studies, and a urine specific gravity. A water deprivation test should be performed if there is suspicion of diabetes insipidus.

Roentgenographically, a chest roentgenogram and skeletal survey are essential. Histiocytosis remains one disease where conventional roentgenograms are more sensitive than a bone scan, which may be normal even with multiple bony lesions. Roentgenographically, most bony lesions are lytic, with no sclerotic border until they begin to heal. Other studies to consider are a bone marrow aspiration and biopsy, Panorex films of the mandible and maxilla, and immunologic studies.

TREATMENT SELECTION AND TREATMENT RESULTS

The usual treatment of a single bone lesion is biopsy with curettage. As many as 70% of the lesions will heal following such treatment.[82,86] For progressive lesions and those that cause symptoms at diagnosis, such as severe otitis media or exophthalmos, radiation therapy is recommended, and if radiation therapy can be instituted soon after the onset of diabetes insipidus, it may be possible to reduce this complication of the disease.[47] The dose of radiation is not clear. Treatment has been reported to be successful with as little as 300 rad, but occasional failures have been noted with doses of 3500 rad.[115,125] It certainly appears that a dose of 600 rad to 900 rad is adequate for 85% to 90% of the lesions.[125] It can be given at a rate of 150 rad to 200 rad/

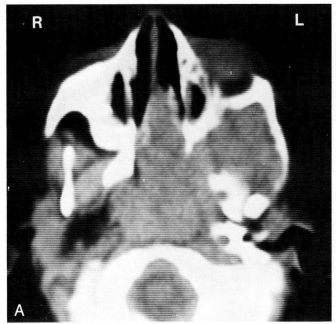

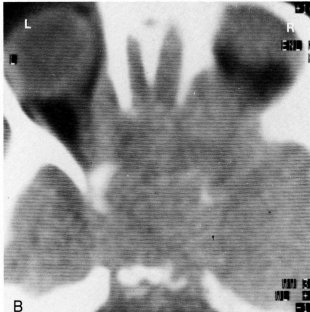

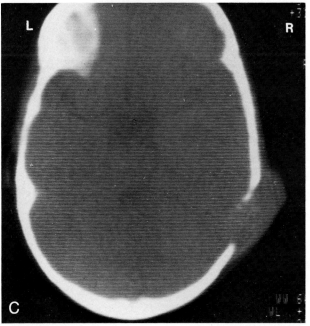

day with minimal risk of acute or late side-effects and the treatment can usually be repeated in case of persistence.

The prognosis of isolated eosinophilic granuloma is very good. It is very rare to see a patient die of this disease. In a review of 686 cases of eosinophilic granuloma by Slater and Swarm, only 9 patients died.[124] Even patients who relapse usually survive, whether the relapse is local or distant. It is not uncommon for a patient to develop several foci of bone involvement over a period of years, only to have the disease disappear eventually.

The results for the disseminated form of the disease are somewhat different. The prognosis for these patients is primarily dependent on their age, the presence or absence of organ dysfunction, and the response to therapy (Fig. 33-19).[72]

Multiple chemotherapeutic agents have been used for the disseminated form of the disease, with response rates varying from 30% to 60%, of which about one half are complete responses.[144] Vincristine, vinblastine, cyclophosphamide, chlorambucil, methotrexate, and 6-mercaptopurine are all effective, as is the combination of prednisone with any of the preceding drugs. Patients with only multifocal bone disease usually survive, even when they do not initially reach a complete remission. Patients in the "poor-risk" category are less responsive to treatment and often die rapidly, even with multiple different chemotherapeutic regimens. Low-dose total-body or hemibody irradiation has been tried in these patients, but the data are preliminary.[48]

For those patients who survive solitary bony lesions, there are virtually no long-term sequelae of treatment unless the primary lesion has affected the hypothalamic/pituitary axis, although an occasional untreated vertebral lesion may result in permanent neurologic sequelae. This is certainly not true of those patients who have more disseminated disease, since almost half have long-term sequelae (unrelated to treatment), such as permanent diabetes insipidus, chronic lung disease, orthopedic disability, neurologic defects, emotional problems, intellectual impair-

FIG. 33-18. A 6-month-old infant had several sites of involvement by histiocytosis X in the head and neck. There were no lesions elsewhere in the body. (*A*) CT scan shows massive lesion involving the nasopharynx, nasal cavity, and left infratemporal fossa. (*B*) A magnified CT image through the orbits shows involvement of both orbits and the sella. (*C*) Separate skull lesion as seen on CT scan.

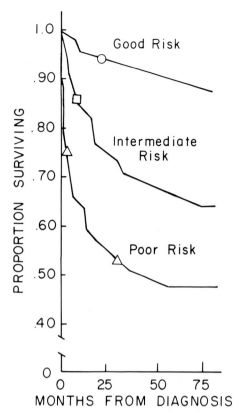

FIG. 33-19. Survival of patients with disseminated histiocytosis using the following staging system:

Good risk: Greater than 2 years of age, no organ dysfunction

Intermediate risk: Less than 2 years of age, no organ dysfunction

Poor risk: Organ dysfunction at any age

(Komp DM, Herson J, Starling KA, Vietti TJ, Hvizdala E: A staging system for histiocytosis X: A Southwest Oncology Group study. Cancer 47:798–800, 1981)

ment, and deficits in hearing.[73] Thus, even though the chances of survival are good for most patients, the disability due to the disease remains high.

Hemangiomas

It has been estimated that 10% of all children born are afflicted with a hemangioma, and since 30% occur in the head and neck, it is the most common pediatric neoplasm arising in the head and neck.[3,62] Hemangiomas are usually classified as capillary, cavernous, and juvenile, but there is a multitude of names and classification systems.[50]

Capillary hemangiomas are the most common and occur in the skin or mucous membranes and, in most cases, are congenital. They are composed of capillary vessels lined by a single layer of flattened or plump endothelial cells surrounded by a discontinuous layer of pericytes and reticular fibers.[50]

Cavernous hemangiomas are composed of dilated blood vessels and spaces lined by thin walls and may be formed by both arterial and venous vessels. They are connected with the general circulation of the body and may reach enormous sizes, resulting in large, blood-filled cul-de-sacs. They represent less than 5% of the hemangiomas in the newborn and tend to occur after infancy.[146] They may be intramuscular and located in the deep soft tissues.

Juvenile hemangiomas, called by some authors "hypertrophic hemangiomas," occur exclusively in children. They are characterized by proliferation of blood vessels, hyperplasia, and atypical endothelial cells. They do have mitotic figures and may look more ominous pathologically than their clinical course.[129]

Whereas most hemangiomas present as a single entity, there is a group of diseases that produce diffuse angiomatosis in infants. Sturge-Weber syndrome (encephalotrigeminal syndrome, encephalofacial angiomatosis) is a triad with a cutaneous hemangioma in the distribution of the trigeminal nerve, a homolateral meningeal hemangioma causing calcification and neurologic signs, and a choroidal hemangioma that sometimes causes glaucoma. Incomplete forms of the syndrome are more common than the complete triad. Lindau-von Hippel's disease consists of hemangiomatosis of the retina and cerebellum. Maffucci's syndrome (dyschondroplasia) represents hemangiomatosis of the skeletal system.

Most hemangiomas in infants pass through a phase of rapid growth for the first year of life, then begin a period of slow resolution. It is estimated by some authors that at least 80% of congenital cutaneous hemangiomas will eventually involute spontaneously.[7,84] If involution is going to occur, it will do so in most cases by 4 years of age, although a few may not begin to regress until 6 or 7 years of age.[51] Doppler monitoring of the number of arteriovenous fistulas may be of some help in predicting whether the lesion will involute.[7] If the lesion is not causing functional impairment, then simple observation is adequate, at least until school age, when treatment of the lesion may be considered if there is no regression.[51]

There are certain lesions, however, that may require immediate intervention, such as subglottic hemangiomas, eyelid hemangiomas, and those occurring in the lip or nose, where permanent functional impairment may result. Subglottic hemangiomas may be life threatening. These lesions are usually located immediately below the vocal cords in the child; they are sessile and not well demarcated from the surrounding structures, with mucosa usually covering the mass and obscuring the usual red color of a hemangioma.[12,35] Subglottic hemangiomas occur more often in girls; they usually present with stridor. With small lesions, observation (with or without tracheotomy) may be safe, but most lesions will usually require early intervention. Orbital hemangiomas, although less acute in their symptoms, may also need intervention rather than observation if they are large enough to cause proptosis and diplopia or otherwise interfere with vision; lack of the use of one eye in early childhood will prevent normal visual development. When the decision to intervene therapeutically is made, for either cosmetic or functional reasons, surgical excision is the treatment of choice for small lesions. However, surgical therapy of the more extensive lesions may result in severe hemorrhage, and perhaps even airway obstruction with oral cavity and subglottic lesions. Large resections of defects on the face may give poor cosmetic results, even with good skin grafting. In these settings, corticosteroids are recommended by many authors.[23,29,38,51] Doses of 20 mg to 40 mg of prednisone for 3 to 21 days can cause rapid cessation of growth and even involution of the lesions at times. For lesions unresponsive to corticosteroids there are several alternatives. Carbon dioxide laser has been reported to be successful in the treatment of some subglottic and intraoral hemangiomas.[54] There is minimal bleeding and a lack of postoperative edema reported with this technique, and it is usually successful in patients in whom other treatment has failed. It is not recommended for cavernous lesions, however. The argon laser has also been advocated of late for extensive capillary hemangiomas.[102] Sometimes there is extensive scarring with this technique and there is often a need for multiple treatments. Percutaneous embolization of large hemangiomas has been performed with some success.[85]

In the past, a large number of hemangiomas were treated with radiation therapy, particularly those with acute symptoms such as eyelid, orbital, or subglottic lesions. The results of radiation therapy are initially satisfactory, with a decrease in the size and cosmetic deformity of the mass in most patients, although such a change may take 2 months to a year to be complete. Doses in the range of 200 rad/1 fraction to 450 rad/3 fractions have been recommended.[138] The main problem with radiation therapy is the carcinogenic potential. However, in one review from Li and co-workers of 4746 patients treated in infancy for hemangioma of the skin at the Children's Hospital Medical Center in Boston from 1946 to 1968, only three cancer deaths were found (vs. 2.4 expected), with follow-ups of 6 to 28 years.[80] Only one tumor was in proximity to the treatment field. Therefore, external-beam irradiation may be a viable alternative for patients with lesions not easily amenable to other approaches. Electrons may be used to decrease the dose to underlying tissues.

Lymphangioma

Lymphangiomas are considered by most authors to be congenital malformations rather than neoplasms.[148] There are three types: (1) *lymphangioma simplex,* which has many thin-walled channels; (2) *cavernous lymphangioma,* which has larger cystic areas within a fibrous adventitia; and (3) *cystic hygroma,* a lesion of large, multiple cystic spaces of different sizes. The former two are more common in the oral cavity and orbit, while cystic hygroma occurs in the neck. None of the lesions is encapsulated; all send microscopic extensions into surrounding tissues. Most lesions are diagnosed early in life, often in the first year, but a few may go unnoticed for many years.

Neck lesions are usually soft, cystic masses that transilluminate and often cause respiratory compromise. Oral cavity lymphangiomas can occur submucosally, making diagnosis difficult. Orbital lesions usually have lid or conjunctival involvement with the appearance of typical dilated vascular channels into which hemorrhage may occur. Proptosis is the most common symptom.

As the affected child grows, so does the lymphangioma. Thus, there is controversy as to whether it is preferable in young children to treat the patient immediately after diagnosis or to wait until the child is older and can better withstand surgery. A few patients have been cured with needle aspiration.[120] Few lymphangiomas can be totally removed in one operation, and staged resections may be necessary. However, there is no purpose served by removing important normal structures because partial excision may cause enough scarring to prevent recurrence.

Radiation therapy has been used in lymphangiomas, and although it is considered to be of little value by most authors, it occasionally will provide a good response.[118]

Teratomas

Teratomas have been reported in most midline structures, and the head and neck is not without its representation. A teratoma will be present in the head and neck in approximately 1 of 40,000 births.[60] They are thought to be derived from pluripotential cells, and since they can grow independent of the host they are usually considered true neoplasms.

The functional classification of these tumors was proposed by Arnold in 1888 and has been accepted by many authors.[2] The two most common types are the dermoids and the true teratomas. The dermoids constitute the majority of the group and are bigerminal in origin, being composed of epidermal and mesodermal elements. They usually consist of an epithelial-lined cavity with variable numbers of skin appendages such as hair and sebaceous glands. Most arise from the midline region of the nasopharynx and are not associated with cranial abnormalities.[11,45] They also may occur in the orbit and midline and tip of the nose, as well as in the oral cavity.

The true teratomas are trigerminal in origin. Sometimes they differentiate to the degree that organs can be recognized histologically. They are associated with developmental abnormalities of the skull and are usually based in the nasopharyngeal vault, but they may also arise in the neck, orbit, or oral cavity.[59] The most highly differentiated of the trigerminal tumors have been called "epignathi," because they were initially thought to arise from the upper jaw. Actual fetal organs and limbs can be present in the epignathi, with the same axial orientation as the host.

Most of these children present with respiratory obstruction, often at birth or shortly thereafter. Immediate treatment of the infant is usually indicated to establish a satisfactory airway, using either an endotracheal tube or a tracheotomy. More careful assessment of the child can then be performed.[59] The primary treatment is surgical, and for the most common tumor, the dermoid, the prognosis is excellent. All patients who experienced surgical removal were cured. The local recurrence rate is small, even with only avulsion of the tumor.[11]

True teratomas, on the other hand, often recur locally and no more than 20% to 30% are cured.[11,59,70,103,149] Even though the prognosis is not good with a true teratoma, an aggressive surgical approach would seem indicated, since the tumor is incompatible with life if left untreated. There are no data regarding the use of radiation therapy or chemotherapy.

COMPLICATIONS OF TREATMENT

Besides the usual risks and sequelae involved in treating head and neck cancers, which are discussed elsewhere in this book, the developing child has additional risks from both radiation therapy and chemotherapy. The sequelae of radiation therapy are better known because the modality has been in use for a longer period of time, but the risks attendant with giving cytotoxic drugs are also beginning to be recognized.

Radiation Therapy

BONE AND SOFT TISSUES

There is adequate evidence that radiation doses in the range of 2000 rad or less can slow bone growth in children, and doses above this range will usually close epiphyses and completely halt bone development.[56,100,117] Obviously, the younger the age at the time of treatment, the greater the resulting deformity. In the teenage years, when the development of the skull and facial bones is virtually complete, there is little noticeable deformity, but for children in the first decade and particularly for infants, radiation in the range of 2000 rad or more can result in permanent abnormal bony development (see Fig. 33-12C, D).

The development of soft tissues such as muscles is affected by similar doses. Hypoplasia of the soft tissues within the treatment field is usual with doses above 2000 rad.

TEETH

The developing teeth are also sensitive to radiation in therapeutic doses. There is not much information regarding the dose needed to cause damage, but it is probably similar to bone doses. Sequelae in permanent teeth after radiation therapy in infancy include retarded root structures, dwarfed teeth, and occasionally failure of one or more permanent teeth to form.[71] Sometimes, permanent teeth may erupt early or may calcify prematurely.[9,128]

EYES

It is not clear whether children's eyes are more sensitive to radiation than the eyes of adults. A considerable number of children have been treated to the whole eye at various institutions for retinoblastoma with doses of 3500 rad to 5000 rad or above. Good vision is preserved in the majority of patients who received these doses if they had a small tumor at the time of treatment. There may be a slightly better chance of preserving good vision if the dose is kept below 4000 rad.[17] However, data from treating orbital rhabdomyosarcomas to 5000 rad to 6000 rad without chemotherapy show that only 5 of 14 survivors who were evaluable retained useful vision.[119] Thus, it appears that doses up to 4500 rad are probably tolerated fairly well by the eye of a child, even an infant, but doses of 5000 rad and above are poorly tolerated. The additive effect of chemotherapy may increase the risk of permanent damage at any given dose level. The most common cause of blindness is retinal or optic nerve damage, just as in adults. However, most patients with orbital tumors usually receive high doses to the lens as well as the retina, and the incidence of cataracts in children at doses of 5000 rad or above appears to be close to 100%.[119] (See Chapter 14, The Effect of Radiation on Normal Tissues of the Head and Neck, for a full discussion.)

CENTRAL NERVOUS SYSTEM

Although in most head and neck cancers (excluding brain tumors) little radiation is delivered to the brain parenchyma itself, in parameningeal rhabdomyosarcoma a considerable amount of brain tissue receives high-dose irradiation. Brain necrosis is rare, but disturbances of the hypothalamic/pituitary axis are not. Neuroendocrine abnormalities after treatment are known to be dose dependent. Less than 1800 rad probably produces no abnormality.[95] However, doses of 3000 rad or greater appear to cause growth hormone deficiencies, which is the most sensitive neuroendocrine function.[123] Not all patients with growth hormone deficiencies have decreased stature. (See section on complications of treatment in Chapter 24, Nasopharynx.)

Chemotherapy

The most common drugs used in treating cancers that occur in the head and neck in children are vincristine, doxorubicin HCl, dactinomycin, cyclophosphamide, and methotrexate. Each has its own risks and side-effects, most of which are similar in children to the side-effects in adults and are discussed in Chapter 8, General Principles for Treatment of Cancers in the Head and Neck: Chemotherapy.

Second Malignancies

One of the most serious sequelae of cancer treatment in children is the development of a second neoplasm. Although radiation has been known for a long time to produce a risk of oncogenesis, it is now becoming clear that chemotherapy has similar risks.

All ionizing radiation probably results in some risk for the development of tumors. However, because of the high dosage used in medical irradiation, as well as the relatively few patients treated, it has been hard to get exact data on the risk of tumor induction by therapeutic irradiation. According to several older reports, patients surviving 2 or more years who were treated with radiation in childhood have an incidence of 5% to 6.5% of development of a second malignancy; the most common tumors are osteosarcoma, soft tissue sarcomas, thyroid cancers, and leukemia, although a wide variety of tumors has been reported.[79,91,142] However, these studies are based on kilovoltage data, with inaccurate dosimetry and much higher doses than are presently used. In addition, the kilovoltage techniques produced a very high bone absorption dose, which may increase the risk of osteosarcoma. Present techniques with megavoltage therapy have considerably decreased the dose both to the bone and to the overlying soft tissues. One series reporting the results of just megavoltage irradiation in a pediatric population showed a very low incidence, although follow-up was not as long as in the older kilovoltage series.[52]

In adults, there are good data regarding the risks of certain chemotherapeutic drugs and the development of a second malignancy. Alkylating agents have been implicated in causing acute myelogenous leukemia.[30,113] Nitrogen mustard and procarbazine are thought to induce leukemia in patients treated for Hodgkin's disease, especially in combination with radiation.[74,143]

There is no proof that children have either an increased or decreased risk compared with adults.[92] Follow-up on childhood cancers treated with chemotherapy is still short, and more time is needed to answer this question.

Not only does the treatment of childhood cancer give rise to secondary oncogenesis, it appears that many children who develop one childhood cancer have a higher risk of developing a second at a later time, even without irradiation or chemotherapy (Table 33-14).[92] In addition, many of the tumors that arise in the field of irradiation occur in patients known to have a genetic susceptibility to devel-

TABLE 33-14. Etiology of Second Malignant Neoplasms in 200 Children*

Second Neoplasm	Radiation-Associated (in RT Field)†	Chemotherapy-Associated (Treated With Chemotherapy Alone)	Unassociated With Radiation Therapy or Chemotherapy
Bone sarcoma	34	2	7
Soft tissue sarcoma	31	0	11
Leukemia/lymphoma	21	3	9
Thyroid	15	0	3
Skin carcinoma	11	1	10
Brain tumor	5	2	14
Breast carcinoma	4	0	2
Others	12	3	7
Total	133	11	63

* There were 207 second cancers in 200 patients registered by the Late Effects Study Group.

† Some patients also had chemotherapy.

(Modified from Meadows AT, Krejmas NL, Belasco JB: The medical cost of cure: Sequelae in survivors of childhood cancer. In Van Eys J, Sullivan MP: Status of the Curability of Childhood Cancers, pp 263–275. New York, Raven Press, 1980)

TABLE 33-15. Incidence of Second Malignant Neoplasms in Children

Interval After Treatment (Years)	No. Second Malignant Neoplasms	Average Annual Rate*
0–5	26	75
5.1–10	26	302
10.1–15	27	479
15.1–20	9	307
20.1–25	5	935
25.1–30	2	1204

* Per 100,000 person-years at risk.

(Meadows AT, Krejmas NL, Belasco JB: The medical cost of cure: Sequelae in survivors of childhood cancer. In Van Eys J, Sullivan MP [eds]: Status of the Curability of Childhood Cancer, pp 263–275. New York, Raven Press, 1980)

oping second cancers, such as patients with bilateral retinoblastoma.

The incidence of second tumors begins to rise within 5 years after therapy, and the incidence continues to rise for many years after that, whether the tumor is induced by treatment or inherent in the child (Table 33-15).[92]

It has been estimated that one of each thousand adults will be a survivor of childhood cancer by the end of this decade.[92] All of the effects of therapy on the long-term quality of their lives are still unknown.

REFERENCES

1. American Joint Committee on Cancer: Manual for Staging of Cancer, 2nd ed, pp 111–116. Philadelphia, JB Lippincott, 1983
2. Arnold J: Ueber behaarte Polypen der Rachen-Mundhöhle und deren Stellung zu den Teratomen. Arch Pathol Anat 111:176–210, 1888
3. Batsakis JG: Tumors of the Head and Neck: Clinical and Pathological Considerations, 2nd ed, pp 290–293. Baltimore, Williams & Wilkins, 1979
4. Batsakis JG, Fox JE: Rhabdomyosarcoma of the larynx: Report of a case. Arch Otolaryngol 91:136–140, 1970
5. Berman HL: The role of radiation therapy in the management of synovial sarcoma. Radiology 81:997–1002, 1963
6. Berry MP, Jenkin RDT: Parameningeal rhabdomyosarcoma in the young. Cancer 48:281–288, 1981
7. Bingham HG: Predicting the course of a congenital hemangioma. Plast Reconstr Surg 63:161–166, 1979
8. Breslow N, McCann B: Statistical estimation of prognosis for children with neuroblastoma. Cancer Res 31:2098–2103, 1971
9. Bruce KW, Stafne EC: The effect of irradiation on the dental system as demonstrated by the roentgenogram. J Am Dent Assoc 41:684–689, 1950
10. Bunch WH: Orthopedic and rehabilitation aspects of eosinophilic granuloma. Am J Pediatr Hematol Oncol 3:151–156, 1981
11. Calcaterra T: Teratomas of the nasopharynx. Ann Otol Rhinol Laryngol 78:165–171, 1969
12. Campbell JS, Wiglesworth FW, Latarroca R, Wilde H: Con-

genital subglottic hemangiomas of the larynx and trachea in infants. Pediatrics 22:727–737, 1958

13. Canalis RF, Gussen R: Temporal bone findings in rhabdomyosarcoma with predominantly petrous involvement. Arch Otolaryngol 106:290–293, 1980

14. Canalis RF, Jenkins HA, Hemenway WG, Lincoln C: Nasopharyngeal rhabdomyosarcoma: A clinical perspective. Arch Otolaryngol 104:122–126, 1978

15. Canalis RF, Platz CE, Cohn AM: Laryngeal rhabdomyosarcoma. Arch Otolaryngol 102:104–107, 1976

16. Carson JH, Harwood AR, Cummings BJ, Fornasier V, Langer F, Quirt I: The place of radiotherapy in the treatment of synovial sarcoma. Int J Radiat Oncol Biol Phys 7:49–53, 1981

17. Cassady JR, Sagerman RH, Tretter P, Ellsworth RM: Radiation therapy in retinoblastoma: An analysis of 230 cases. Radiology 93:405–409, 1969

18. Chambers RG, Mahoney WD: Osteogenic sarcoma of the mandible: Current management. Am J Surg 36:463–471, 1970

19. Chan RC, Sutow WW, Lindberg RD: Parameningeal rhabdomyosarcoma. Radiology 131:211–214, 1979

20. Chan RC, Sutow WW, Lindberg RD, Samuels ML, Murray JA, Johnston DA: Management and results of localized Ewing's sarcoma. Cancer 43:1001–1006, 1979

21. Christopherson WM, Foote FW, Stewart FW: Alveolar soft-part sarcomas: Structurally characteristic tumors of uncertain histogenesis. Cancer 5:100–111, 1952

22. Chung EB, Enzinger FM: Infantile fibrosarcoma. Cancer 38:729–739, 1976

23. Cohen SR, Wang C-I: Steroid treatment of hemangioma of the head and neck in children. Ann Otol Rhinol Laryngol 81:584–590, 1972

24. Cutler SJ, Ederer F: Maximum utilization of the life table method in analyzing survival. J Chronic Dis 8:699–712, 1958

25. Dahlin DC: Bone Tumors: General Aspects and Data on 6221 Cases, 3rd ed, pp 191, 244, 275. Springfield, IL, Charles C Thomas, 1978

26. Davidoff SM: A method for early and differential diagnosis of central tumours of the jaws. Int Dent J 18:753–758, 1968

27. Dehner LP, Askin FB: Tumors of fibrous tissue origin in childhood. A clinicopathologic study of cutaneous and soft tissue neoplasms in 66 children. Cancer 38:888–900, 1976

28. Dehner LP, Sibley RK, Sauk JJ Jr, Vickers RA, Nesbit ME, Leonard AS, Waite DE, Neeley JE, Ophovan J: Malignant melanotic neuroectodermal tumor of infancy: A clinical, pathologic, ultrastructural and tissue culture study. Cancer 43:1389–1410, 1979

29. Edgerton MT: The treatment of hemangiomas: With special reference to the role of steroid therapy. Ann Surg 183:517–532, 1976

30. Einhorn N: Acute leukemia after chemotherapy (melphalan). Cancer 41:444–447, 1978

31. Enzinger FM, Smith BH: Hemangiopericytoma: An analysis of 106 cases. Hum Pathol 7:61–82, 1976

32. Evans AE, Albo V, D'Angio GJ, Finklestein JZ, Leiken S, Santulli T, Weiner J, Hammond GD: Cyclophosphamide treatment of patients with localized and regional neuroblastoma: A randomized study. Cancer 38:655–660, 1976

33. Evans AE, Catten J, D'Angio G, Gerson JM, Robinson J, Schnaufer L: A review of 17 IV-S neuroblastoma patients at the Children's Hospital of Philadelphia. Cancer 45:833–839, 1980

34. Evans AE, D'Angio GJ, Randolph J: A proposed staging for children with neuroblastoma. Cancer 27:374–378, 1971

35. Ferguson CF, Flake CG: Subglottic hemangioma as a cause of respiratory obstruction in infants. Ann Otol Rhinol Laryngol 70:1095–1112, 1961

36. Ferlito A: Primary Ewing's sarcoma of the maxilla: A clinicopathological study of four cases. J Laryngol Otol 92:1007–1024, 1978

37. Fernandez CH, Sutow WW, Merino OR, George SL: Childhood rhabdomyosarcoma: Analysis of coordinated therapy and re-

sults. Am J Roentgenol Radium Ther Nucl Med 123:588–597, 1975

38. Fost NC, Esterly NB: Successful treatment of juvenile hemangiomas with prednisone. J Pediatr 72:351–357, 1968

39. Francis KC, Phillips R, Nickson JJ, Woodard HQ, Higinbotham NL, Coley BL: Massive preoperative irradiation in the treatment of osteogenic sarcoma in children. A preliminary report. Am J Roentgenol Radium Ther Nucl Med 72:813–818, 1954

40. Gaiger AM, Soule EH, Newton WA: Pathology of rhabdomyosarcoma: Experience of the Intergroup Rhabdomyosarcoma Study, 1972–1978. Natl Cancer Inst Monogr 56:19–27, 1981

41. Gardner DG, Mills DM: The widened periodontal ligament of osteosarcoma of the jaws. Oral Surg 41:652–656, 1976

42. Garrington GE, Scofield HH, Cornyn J, Hooker SP: Osteosarcoma of the jaws: Analysis of 56 cases. Cancer 20:377–391, 1967

43. Glass AG, Fraumeni JF Jr: Epidemiology of bone cancer in children. J Natl Cancer Inst 44:187–199, 1970

44. Glass AG, Miller RW: US mortality from Letterer-Siwe disease, 1960–1964. Pediatrics 42:364–367, 1968

45. Goldman N, Hardcastle B: Nasopharyngeal teratoma. South Med J 62:1155–1156, 1969

46. Gottlieb JA, Baker LH, Burgess MA, Sinkovics JG, Moon T, Bodey GP, Rodriguez V, Rivkin SE, Saiki J, O'Bryan RM: Sarcoma chemotherapy. In M. D. Anderson Hospital: Cancer Chemotherapy: Fundamental Concepts and Recent Advances, pp 445–454. Chicago, Year Book Medical Publishers, 1975

47. Greenberger JS, Cassady JR, Jaffe N, Vawter G, Crocker AC: Radiation therapy in patients with histiocytosis: Management of diabetes insipidus and bone lesions. Int J Radiat Oncol Biol Phys 5:1749–1755, 1979

48. Griffin TW: The treatment of advanced histiocytosis-X with sequential hemibody irradiation. Cancer 39:2435–2436, 1977

49. Haddy TB, Nora AH, Sutow WW, Vietti TJ: Cyclophosphamide treatment for metastatic soft tissue sarcoma: Intermittent large doses in the treatment of children. Am J Dis Child 114:301–308, 1967

50. Hadju SI: Pathology of Soft Tissue Tumors, pp 188, 375–378. Philadelphia, Lea & Febiger, 1979

51. Handler SD, Raney RB Jr: Management of neoplasms of the head and neck in children: I. Benign tumors. Head Neck Surg 3:395–405, 1981

52. Haselow RE, Nesbit M, Dehner LP, Khan FM, McHugh R, Levitt SH: Second neoplasms following megavoltage radiation in a pediatric population. Cancer 42:1185–1191, 1978

53. Hays DM, Mirabal VQ, Karlan MS, Patel HR, Landing BH: Fibrosarcoma in infants and children. J Pediatr Surg 5:176–183, 1970

54. Healy GB, Fearon B, French R, Magil T: Treatment of subglottic hemangioma with the carbon dioxide laser. Laryngoscope 90:809–813, 1980

55. Healy GB, Jaffe N, Cassady JR: Rhabdomyosarcoma of the head and neck: Diagnosis and management. Head Neck Surg 1:334–339, 1979

56. Heaston DK, Libshitz HI, Chan RC: Skeletal effects of megavoltage irradiation in survivors of Wilms' tumor. AJR 133:389–395, 1979

57. Helson L: Management of disseminated neuroblastoma. CA 25:264–277, 1975

58. Heyn RM, Holland R, Newton WA, Tefft M, Breslow N, Hartmann JR: The role of combined chemotherapy in the treatment of rhabdomyosarcoma in children. Cancer 34:2128–2142, 1974

59. Hjertaas RJ, Morrison MD, Murray RB: Teratomas of the nasopharynx. J Otolaryngol 8:411–416, 1979

60. Holt GR, Holt JE, Weaver RG: Dermoids and teratomas of the head and neck. Ear Nose Throat J 58:520–531, 1979

61. Huvos AG: Bone Tumors: Diagnosis, Treatment and Prognosis, p 52. Philadelphia, WB Saunders, 1979

62. Jacobs AH, Walton RG: The incidence of birthmarks in the neonate. Pediatrics 58:218–222, 1976

63. Jacobson HM, Marcus RB Jr, Thar TL, Million RR, Graham-Pole JR, Talbert JL: Pediatric neuroblastoma: Postoperative radiation therapy using less than 2000 rad. Int J Radiat Oncol Biol Phys 9:501–505, 1983

64. Jaffe N, Frei E III, Watts H, Traggis D: High-dose methotrexate in osteogenic sarcoma: A 5-year experience. Cancer Treat Rep 62:259–264, 1978

65. Jenkin RDT: The treatment of osteosarcoma with radiation: Current indications. In M. D. Anderson Hospital: Management of Primary Bone and Soft Tissue Tumors, pp 151–162. Chicago, Year Book Medical Publishers, 1977

66. Jereb B, Ghavimi F, Exelby P, Zang E: Local control of embryonal rhabdomyosarcoma in children by radiation therapy when combined with chemotherapy. Int J Radiat Oncol Biol Phys 6:827–833, 1980

67. Jones IS, Reese AB, Kraut J: Orbital rhabdomyosarcoma: An analysis of 62 cases. Am J Ophthalmol 61:721–736, 1966

68. Kauffman SL, Stout AP: Hemangiopericytoma in children. Cancer 13:695–710, 1960

69. Kepes JJ, Kepes M: Predominantly cerebral forms of histiocytosis-X: A reappraisal of "Gagel's hypothalamic granuloma," "granuloma infiltrans of the hypothalamus" and "Ayala's disease" with a report of 4 cases. Acta Neuropathol (Berl) 14:77–98, 1969

70. Keswani RK, Chugh TD, Dhall JC, Mehrotra GC: Epignathus: A case report. Br J Plast Surg 21:355–359, 1968

71. Kimeldorf DJ, Jones DC, Castanera TJ: The radiobiology of teeth. Rad Research 20:518–540, 1963

72. Komp DM, Herson J, Starling KA, Vietti TJ, Hvizdala E: A staging system for histiocytosis X: A Southwest Oncology Group study. Cancer 47:798–800, 1981

73. Komp DM, El Mahdi A, Starling KA, Easley J, Vietti TJ, Berry DH, George SL: Quality of survival in histiocytosis X: A Southwest Oncology Group study. Med Pediatr Oncol 8:35–40, 1980

74. Krikorian JG, Burke JS, Rosenberg SA, Kaplan HS: Occurrence of non-Hodgkin's lymphoma after therapy for Hodgkin's disease. N Engl J Med 300:452–458, 1979

75. Lahey ME: Prognosis in reticuloendotheliosis in children. J Pediatr 60:664–671, 1962

76. Lawrence W Jr, Hays DM, Moon TE: Lymphatic metastasis with childhood rhabdomyosarcoma. Cancer 39:556–559, 1977

77. Lee ES, MacKenzie DH: Osteosarcoma: A study of the value of preoperative megavoltage radiotherapy. Br J Surg 51:252–274, 1964

78. Leviton A, Davidson R, Gilles F: Neurologic manifestations of embryonal rhabdomyosarcoma of the middle ear cleft. J Pediatr 80:596–602, 1972

79. Li FP: Second malignant tumors after cancer in childhood. Cancer 40:1899–1902, 1977

80. Li FP, Cassady JR, Barnett E: Cancer mortality following irradiation in infancy for hemangioma. Radiology 113:177–178, 1974

81. Lieberman PH, Foote FW Jr, Stewart FW, Berg JW: Alveolar soft-part sarcoma. JAMA 198:1047–1051, 1966

82. Lieberman PH, Jones CR, Dargeon HWK, Begg CF: A reappraisal of eosinophilic granuloma of bone, Hand-Schüller-Christian syndrome and Letterer-Siwe syndrome. Medicine 48:375–400, 1969

83. Liebert PS, Stool SE: Rhabdomyosarcoma of the tongue in an infant: Results of combined radiation and chemotherapy. Ann Surg 178:621–624, 1973

84. Lister WA: The natural history of strawberry naevi. Lancet 234:1429–1434, 1938

85. Longacre JJ, Benton C, Unterthiner RA: Treatment of facial hemangioma by intravascular embolization with silicone spheres: Case report. Plast Reconstr Surg 50:618–621, 1972

86. McGavran MH, Spady HA: Eosinophilic granuloma of bone: A study of 28 cases. J Bone Joint Surg 42A:979–992, 1960

87. Marcove RC: En bloc resections for osteogenic sarcoma. Cancer Treat Rep 62:225–231, 1978

88. Maurer HM: The Intergroup Rhabdomyosarcoma Study: Update, November 1978. Natl Cancer Inst Monogr 56:61–68, 1981

89. Maurer HM, Donaldson M, Gehan EA, Hammond D, Hays DM, Lawrence W Jr et al: Rhabdomyosarcoma in childhood and adolescence. Curr Probl Cancer 2:1–36, 1978

90. Maurer HM, Moon T, Donaldson M, Fernandez C, Gehan EA, Hammond D et al: The Intergroup Rhabdomyosarcoma Study: A preliminary report. Cancer 40:2015–2026, 1977

91. Meadows AT, D'Angio GJ, Evans AE, Harris CC, Miller RW, Mike V: Oncogenesis and other late effects of cancer treatment in children. Radiology 114:175–180, 1975

92. Meadows AT, Krejmas NL, Belasco JB: The medical cost of cure: Sequelae in survivors of childhood cancer. In Van Eys J, Sullivan MP (eds): Status of the Curability of Childhood Cancers, pp 263–275. New York, Raven Press, 1980

93. Mendenhall CM, Marcus RB Jr, Enneking WF, Springfield DS, Thar TL, Million RR: The prognostic significance of soft tissue extension in Ewing's sarcoma. Cancer, 51:913–917, 1983

94. Miller DR: Familial reticuloendotheliosis: Concurrence of disease in five siblings. Pediatrics 38:986–995, 1966

95. Mühlendahl KE von, Gadner H, Riehm H, Helge H, Weber B, Müller-Hess R: Endocrine function after antineoplastic therapy in 22 children with acute lymphoblastic leukaemia. Helv Paediatr Acta 31:463–471, 1976

96. Myers EN, Stool S, Weltschew A: Rhabdomyosarcoma of the middle ear. Ann Otol Rhinol Laryngol 77:949–958, 1968

97. Neifeld JP, Berg JW, Godwin D, Salzberg AM: A retrospective epidemiologic study of pediatric fibrosarcomas. J Pediatr Surg 13:735–739, 1978

98. Nesbit ME Jr, O'Leary M, Dehner LP, Ramsay NK: The immune system and the histiocytosis syndromes. Am J Pediatr Hematol Oncol 3:141–149, 1981

99. Nesbit ME Jr, Perez CA, Tefft M, Burgert EO Jr, Vietti TJ, Kissane J, Pritchard DJ, Gehan EA: Multimodal therapy for the management of primary, nonmetastatic Ewing's sarcoma of bone: An intergroup study. Natl Cancer Inst Mongr 56:255–262, 1981

100. Neuhauser EBD, Wittenborg MH, Berman CZ, Cohen J: Irradiation effects of roentgen therapy on the growing spine. Radiology 59:637–650, 1952

101. Nikai H, Ijuhin N, Yamasaki A, Niitani K, Imai K: Ultrastructural evidence for neural crest origin of the melanotic neuroectodermal tumor of infancy. J Oral Pathol 6:221–232, 1977

102. Noe JM, Barsky SH, Geer DE, Rosen S: Port wine stains and the response to argon laser therapy: Successful treatment and the predictive role of color, age, and biopsy. Plast Reconstr Surg 65:130–136, 1980

103. Ochsner A, Ayers WB: Case of epignathus: Survival of host after its excision. Surgery 30:560–564, 1951

104. Peace RJ: A congenital neoplasm of the brain of a newborn infant: Report of a case with necrospy. Am J Clin Pathol 24:1272–1275, 1954

105. Perez CA, Tefft M, Nesbit ME Jr, Burgert EO Jr, Vietti TJ, Kissane J, Pritchard DJ, Gehan EA: Radiation therapy in the multimodal management of Ewing's sarcoma of bone: Report of the Intergroup Ewing's Sarcoma Study. Natl Cancer Inst Monogr 56:263–271, 1981

106. Pilepich MV, Vietti TJ, Nesbit ME, Tefft M, Kissane J, Burgert EO, Pritchard D: Radiotherapy and combination chemotherapy in advanced Ewing's sarcoma: Intergroup study. Cancer 47:1930–1936, 1981

107. Pomeroy TC, Johnson RE: Combined modality therapy of Ewing's sarcoma. Cancer 35:36–47, 1975

108. Pritchard DJ, Dahlin DC, Dauphine RT, Dauphine RT, Taylor WF, Beabout JW: Ewing's sarcoma: A clinicopathological and

statistical analysis of patients surviving five years or longer. J Bone Joint Surg 57A:10–16, 1975

109. Ragab AH, Sutow WW, Komp DM, Starling KA, Lyon GM Jr, George S: Adriamycin in the treatment of childhood solid tumors: A Southwest Oncology Group study. Cancer 36:1567–1571, 1975

110. Raney RB Jr, Donaldson MH, Sutow WW, Lindberg RD, Maurer HM, Tefft M: Special considerations related to primary site in rhabdomyosarcoma: Experience of the Intergroup Rhabdomyosarcoma Study, 1972–1976. Natl Cancer Inst Monogr 56:69–74, 1981

111. Raney RB Jr, Gehan EA, Maurer HM, Newton WA Jr, Ragab AH, Ruymann FB, Sutow WW, Tefft M: Evaluation of intensified chemotherapy in children with advanced rhabdomyosarcoma (clinical groups III and IV). Cancer Clin Trials 2:19–28, 1979

112. Razek A, Perez CA, Tefft M, Nesbit M, Vietta T, Burgert EO Jr, Kissane J, Pritchard DJ, Gehan EA: Intergroup Ewing's Sarcoma Study: Local control related to radiation dose, volume, and site of primary lesion in Ewing's sarcoma. Cancer 46:516–521, 1980

113. Reimer RR, Hoover R, Fraumeni JF Jr, Young RC: Acute leukemia after alkylating-agent therapy of ovarian cancer. N Engl J Med 297:177–181, 1977

114. Roca AN, Smith JL Jr, MacComb WS, Jing B-S: Ewing's sarcoma of the maxilla and mandible: Study of six cases. Oral Surg 25:194–203, 1968

115. Rodrigues RJ, Lewis HH: Eosinophilic granuloma of bone: Review of literature and case presentation. Clin Orthop 77:183–192, 1971

116. Roth SA, Enzinger FM, Tannenbaum M: Synovial sarcoma of the neck: A follow-up study of 24 cases. Cancer 35:1243–1253, 1975

117. Rubin P, Casarett GW: Clinical Radiation Pathology, pp 518–554. Philadelphia, WB Saunders, 1968

118. Russo PE, Dewar JP: Congenital lymphangioma. Am J Roentgenol Radium Ther Nucl Med 85:726–728, 1971

119. Sagerman RH, Tretter P, Ellsworth RM: Orbital rhabdomyosarcoma in children. Trans Am Acad Ophthalmol Otolaryngol 780P:602–605, 1974

120. Saijo M, Munro IR, Mancer K: Lymphangioma, a long-term follow-up study. Plast Reconstr Surg 56:642–651, 1975

121. Schimke RN: The neurocristopathy concept: Fact or fiction. In Evans AE (ed): Advances in Neuroblastoma Research, pp 13–24. New York, Raven Press, 1980

122. Seibert JJ, Seibert RW, Weisenburger DS, Allsbrook W: Multiple congenital hemangiopericytomas of the head and neck. Laryngoscope 88:1006–1012, 1978

123. Shalet SM, Price DA, Beardwell CG, Morris Jones PH, Pearson D: Normal growth despite abnormalities of growth hormone secretion in children suited for acute leukemia. J Pediatr 94:719–722, 1979

124. Slater JM, Swarm OJ: Eosinophilic granuloma of bone. Med Pediatr Oncol 8:151–164, 1980

125. Smith DG, Nesbit ME Jr, D'Angio GJ, Levitt SH: Histiocytosis X: Role of radiation therapy in management with special reference to dose levels employed. Radiology 106:419–422, 1973

126. Soule EH, Pritchard DJ: Fibrosarcoma in infants and children: A review of 110 cases. Cancer 40:1711–1721, 1977

127. Spector RA, Travis LW, Smith J: Alveolar soft part sarcoma of the head and neck. Laryngoscope 89:1301–1306, 1979

128. Stafne EC, Bowing HH: The teeth and their supporting structures in patients treated by irradiation. Am J Orthod (Oral Surg Sect) 33:567–581, 1947

129. Stout AP: Hemangio-endothelioma: A tumor of blood vessels featuring vascular endothelial cells. Ann Surg 118:445–464, 1943

130. Stout AP: Fibrosarcoma in infants and children. Cancer 15:1028–1040, 1962

131. Suit HD: Radiotherapy in osteosarcoma. Clin Orthop 111:71–75, 1975

132. Sutow WW: Chemotherapeutic management of childhood rhabdomyosarcoma: In M. D. Anderson Hospital: Neoplasia in Childhood, pp 201–208. Chicago, Year Book Medical Publishers, 1969

133. Sutow WW, Berry DH, Haddy TB, Sullivan MP, Watkins WL, Windmiller J: Vincristine sulfate therapy in children with metastatic soft tissue sarcoma. Pediatrics 38:465–472, 1966

134. Sutow WW, Gehan EA, Dyment PG, Vietti T, Miale T: Multidrug adjuvant chemotherapy for osteosarcoma: Interim report of the Southwest Oncology Group studies. Cancer Treat Rep 62:265–269, 1978

135. Sutow WW, Lindberg RD, Gehan EA, Ragab AH, Raney RB Jr, Ruymann F, Soule EH: Three-year relapse-free survival rates in childhood rhabdomyosarcoma of the head and neck: Report from the Intergroup Rhabdomyosarcoma Study. Cancer 49:2217–2221, 1982

136. Swain RE, Sessions DG, Ogura JH: Fibrosarcoma of the head and neck: A clinical analysis of forty cases. Ann Otol Rhinol Laryngol 83:439–444, 1974

137. Tan CTC, Dargeon HW, Burchenal JH: The effect of actinomycin D on cancer in childhood. Pediatrics 24:544–561, 1959

138. Tefft M: The radiotherapeutic management of subglottic hemangioma in children. Radiology 86:207–214, 1966

139. Tefft M, Fernandez C, Donaldson M, Newton W, Moon TE: Incidence of meningeal involvement by rhabdomyosarcoma of the head and neck in children: A report of the Intergroup Rhabdomyosarcoma Study (IRS). Cancer 42:253–258, 1978

140. Tefft M, Fernandez CH, Moon TE: Rhabdomyosarcoma: Response with chemotherapy prior to radiation in patients with gross residual disease. Cancer 39:665–670, 1977

141. Tefft M, Lindberg RD, Gehan EA: Radiation therapy combined with systemic chemotherapy of rhabdomyosarcoma in children: Local control in patients enrolled in the Intergroup Rhabdomyosarcoma Study. Natl Cancer Inst Monogr 56:75–81, 1981

142. Tefft M, Vawter GF, Mitus A: Second primary neoplasms in children. Am J Roentgenol Radium Ther Nucl Med 103:800–822, 1968

143. Toland DM, Coltman CA, Moon TE: Second malignancies complicating Hodgkin's disease: The Southwest Oncology Group experience. Cancer Clin Trials 1:27–33, 1978

144. Vietti TJ, Strandjord SE: Histiocytosis X. In Carter SK, Glatstein E, Livingston RB: Principles of Cancer Treatment, pp 897–901. New York, McGraw-Hill, 1982

145. Voorhess ML: Neuroblastoma with normal urinary catecholamine excretion. J Pediatr 78:680–683, 1971

146. Waisman M: Common hemangiomas: To treat or not to treat. Postgrad Med 43:183–187, 1968

147. Williams AO: Tumors of childhood in Ibadan, Nigeria. Cancer 36:370–378, 1975

148. Willis RA: Pathology of Tumors, 4th ed, p 729. New York, Appleton-Century-Crofts, 1967

149. Wilson JW, Gehweiler JA: Teratoma of the face associated with a patent canal extending into the cranial cavity (Rathke's pouch) in a three-week-old child. J Pediatr Surg 5:349–359, 1970

150. World Health Organization (WHO): World Health Statistics Annuals, 1950 through 1971. Geneva, Switzerland, WHO, 1953–1974

151. Young JL Jr, Miller RW: Incidence of malignant tumors in US children. J Pediatr 86:254–258, 1975

Adult Mesenchymal Tumors
Presenting in the Head and Neck

ROBERT B. MARCUS, Jr.
WILLIAM M. MENDENHALL

In general, mesenchymal lesions in the head and neck behave as do their extremity counterparts. However, all of the tumors described in this chapter are uncommon and some are rare. It is important to diagnose them correctly and to apply the proper treatment since almost all of them are potentially curable.

BONE AND CARTILAGE TUMORS

Aneurysmal Bone Cyst

An aneurysmal bone cyst is not a true neoplasm but rather a benign lesion of bone of unknown etiology. It has been postulated that it may be caused by a local circulatory disturbance with resultant increased venous pressure and may arise either *de novo* or in conjunction with other lesions such as giant cell tumor, chondroblastoma, or fibrous dysplasia. It is half as common as giant cell tumor of bone, it occurs with a slight female preponderance, and roughly 80% of patients are under 20 years of age at the time of diagnosis. Bones of the head and neck are affected in approximately 13% of cases, usually involving either the calvarium or cervical vertebrae. The patient generally presents with a painful mass that, roentgenographically, appears as an eccentric zone of expanded, rarefied bone with a peripheral eggshell-thin rim of subperiosteal new bone.[3,6,24,25] Cervical spine lesions often present with neurologic symptoms.

Surgery has generally been accepted as the treatment of choice and may entail either curettage or *en bloc* resection. Recurrence rates after curettage vary from 21% to 44% and increase with incomplete resection, lesions that are greater than 5 cm, and age under 15 years.[31,39] The recurrence rate after *en bloc* resection is essentially zero. Radiation therapy is usually reserved for surgically inaccessible or recurrent lesions and is successful in 80% to 90% of cases.[29,31,39] Doses in the range of 2000 rad to 3000 rad in 3 to 4 weeks are adequate with megavoltage.[29]* The response to radiation therapy is generally immediate, with symptoms resolving within a few days of the initiation of treatment. Healing of the involved bone may begin by the end of treatment, but complete healing takes an average of 4 to 8 months (Fig. 34-1).[29]*

Giant Cell Tumor

Giant cell tumor of bone is of unknown etiology and involves the head and neck in about 3% of cases.[6] It occurs with a slight female preponderance,

* Marcus RB Jr: Unpublished University of Florida data, 1982.

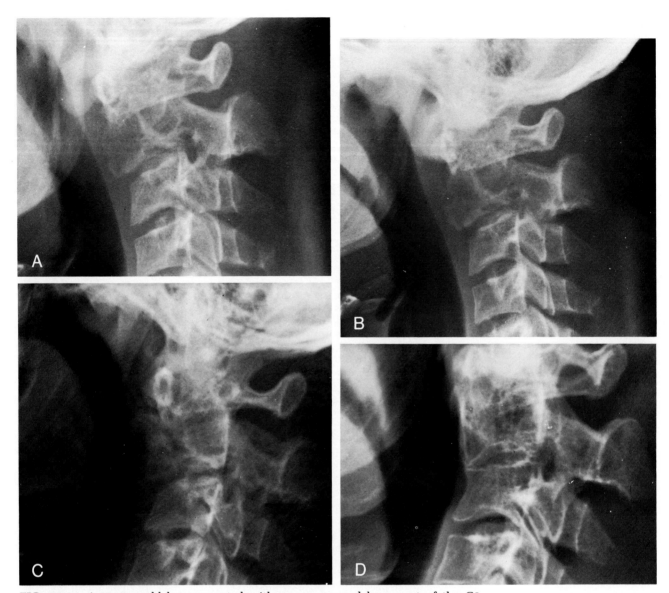

FIG. 34-1. A 15-year-old boy presented with an aneurysmal bone cyst of the C2 vertebra. (*A*) Roentgenograms of the cervical spine obtained prior to treatment (February 1964) revealed a lytic lesion of the body of C2 with ballooning of the vertebral body anteriorly. The patient received 2829 rad tumor dose in 14 fractions with 2-MV x-rays. At the time of his first follow-up visit in March 1964, he had noted complete resolution of his neck pain. (*B*) Follow-up roentgenogram in May 1964 showed little change, but over the next 4 months (September 1964), almost complete ossification occurred (*C*). (*D*) Roentgenogram of the lesion at 13 years (March 1977) shows residual abnormality but little change from appearance in *C*.

especially in younger patients; 85% of patients are over 20 years of age.[25] It usually occurs in the epiphysis and metaphysis of the long bones following closure of the growth plate; however, when the head and neck area is involved, the most common site is the sphenoid or cervical spine. If it occurs in association with Paget's disease, there is a tendency to involve the calvarium and facial bones.[25]

The patient generally presents with a painful mass that, roentgenographically, appears as an expanded zone of radiolucency with an indistinct margin; periosteal new bone formation is almost never present.[6]

There is controversy as to whether histologic grading is of prognostic value, although there is agreement that even cytologically benign giant cell tumors may develop metastasis in less than 1% of cases.[6,25] To make matters worse, it may be confused histologically with nonossifying fibroma, chondroblastoma, chondromyxoid fibroma, giant cell reparative granuloma, aneurysmal bone cyst, hyperparathyroidism, and osteosarcoma. Approximately 10% of cases may undergo malignant transformation, and when this occurs, it is associated with an 80% mortality rate.[6]

Evaluation may include an angiogram, which often

shows a hypervascular mass with an intense, nonhomogeneous capillary blush.[25] Bone and computed tomographic (CT) scans are of value.

Surgery is regarded as the treatment of choice and entails either curettage or en bloc resection. Curettage is associated with a local recurrence rate of roughly 50%.[6] Cryosurgery or cementation will decrease the rate of local recurrence to less than 10%, and local recurrence after en bloc excision is noted in less than 5% of cases.[33]

Radiation therapy is usually reserved for lesions that are incompletely excised, recurrent, or unresectable. It may achieve local control, and thus long-term cure, in over 80% of cases with doses in the range of 3500 rad to 4000 rad.[19]* Irradiation may be more successful in tumors arising from membranous bones as opposed to those arising from long bones.[10] The response of giant cell tumors to irradiation is strikingly different from that of aneurysmal bone cysts (Fig. 34-2). Some pain relief may occur toward the end of therapy, but pain may not be completely relieved for a period of months to a year or more. Little improvement is noted on roentgenograms for months. In fact, shortly after the end of treatment, absorption of the rarified rim of new bone may occur, causing great concern. However, within 6 months the mass should begin to shrink, with new bone formation around the periphery. There is rarely complete resolution of the mass, and maximum shrinkage may require 1 or 2 years.

There is little information with regard to chemotherapy for metastatic giant cell tumor. We have observed five patients who were treated with a variety of chemotherapeutic agents, including doxorubicin HCl (Adriamycin), cyclophosphamide (Cytoxan), melphalan (Alkeran), and dacarbazine (DTIC), and we have seen two complete responses and one partial response in the four patients who have been followed for at least 1 year.† However, lung metastases from giant cell tumors have a very unpredictable course, even with no chemotherapy. Some have been observed to remain stable for many years and never become a threat to the patient's life.

Chordoma

Chordoma is a tumor that arises from remnants of the primitive notochord.[6,25] It occurs almost exclusively along the axial skeleton, with 36% of cases in the base of the skull and 7% in the cervical spine.[6] There is a slight male preponderance.[21] The average age at diagnosis for head and neck lesions is 38 years, with a range of 8 to 75 years.[21] This is approximately 10 years less than the reported average age of 48 years for chordoma in general.

The tumor is slow growing, and symptoms are usually present from 6 months to 3 years prior to diagnosis.[21] Symptoms from tumor arising in the basisphenoid will depend on its route of spread, which may be intracranially or inferiorly into the nasopharynx, nasal cavity, and maxillary sinus. Patients commonly present with visual disturbances such as diplopia (secondary to involvement of the abducens nerve) or visual field deficits. In addition, they may present with headache, nasal obstruction, ear pair, or proptosis. Cervical chordoma may present as a painful mass in the lateral neck or pharyngeal wall associated with cranial nerve deficits or symptoms of spinal cord compression. Approximately 10% of patients present with or develop distant metastasis, usually to the lungs.

Roentgenographically, the lesion appears as an expansile, osteolytic lesion with areas of calcification, often associated with a soft tissue mass.[6,21] Tomograms and CT scan of the base of the skull and paranasal sinuses define the extent of the lesion.

Treatment of chordoma entails complete resection, when feasible, radiation therapy, or both of these modalities. Complete excision is rarely possible for head and neck chordoma because of the inaccessible location, although one long disease-free survival has been reported after resection alone.[47] The results of treatment with radiation alone or radiation plus surgery are dismal.[5,21,22,34,35,41,47] Treatment is followed by local recurrence in over 80% of cases within 5 years of treatment and is fatal within a time period varying from weeks to several decades.[5] Promising preliminary results have been obtained at Massachusetts General Hospital by Suit and co-workers, where a combination of photons and protons is employed in an effort to deliver a high dose (7000 rad to 7500 rad) without exceeding the tolerance of surrounding normal structures (Fig. 34-3). Six patients with chordoma of the head and neck have been treated, and all are alive and without evidence of disease at 17, 17, 20, 24, 38, and 64 months following irradiation.[45]‡

Chondrosarcoma

Approximately 5% of chondrosarcomas occur in the head and neck. Most lesions are primary, but chondrosarcomas may arise in a multitude of preexisting conditions, including enchondroma, exostosis, juxtacortical chondroma, Maffucci's syndrome, chondromyxoid fibroma, chondroblastoma, and irradiated bone. Roentgenograms show bone destruction with both calcification and ossification in the lesion.

The most common sites of head and neck chondrosarcoma are the maxillofacial areas and the jaw. Cervical spine and laryngeal lesions also occur, but primary lesions of the skull are uncommon. Chondrosarcomas often have a progressive and ultimately fatal course of disease, but many patients survive for prolonged periods with multiple recurrences. Most die of failure to control local disease, followed by extension of tumor into the cranial cavity. An occasional patient dies of metastatic disease. The mandible appears to be a worse site for chondrosarcoma than the maxilla.[2]

The primary treatment for chondrosarcoma is surgical, and if an adequate resection can be done, the local control rate is good.[11] However, lesions in the head and neck are often difficult to completely remove, particularly those in the maxillofacial region and in the cervical spine. Laryngeal lesions arise from the cricoid or thyroid cartilage.[14] Most laryngeal lesions are low grade and rarely metastasize, so that excision is usually adequate; a local recurrence can be treated with a laryngectomy.[14,16]

Chondrosarcoma is thought to be resistant to radiation therapy, but this is not necessarily the case. Harwood and co-workers reported 31 patients treated primarily with radiation therapy because the site was not suitable for excision.[20] Five of 11 patients with well-differentiated and moderately well-differentiated lesions, including two in the head and neck, remained without evidence of recurrence at 3½, 5, 5, 15, and 15 years after radiation therapy.

---

* Marcus RB Jr: Unpublished University of Florida data, 1982.
† Ellingwood KE: Unpublished University of Florida data, 1978.

‡ Suit H: Personal communication, 1982.

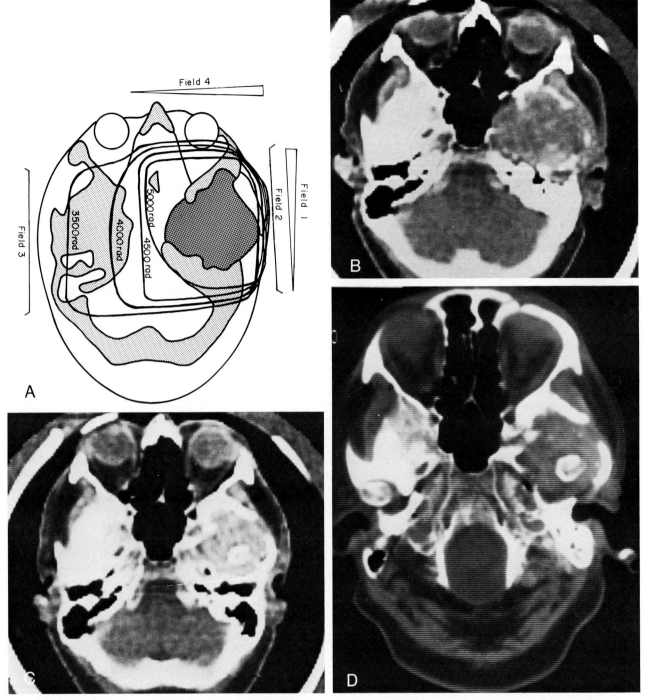

FIG. 34-2. A 75-year-old man presented with a giant cell tumor of the right temporal bone in September 1979. On physical examination, he was also noted to have a 10-cm mass overlying the right temporal bone. Initial CT scan of the head done in September 1979 (not shown) revealed a large mass of the right infratemporal and temporal fossa, extending superiorly 2 cm above the level of the optic chiasm, medially to the sphenoid sinus, and anteriorly to the posterior aspect of the orbit. (A) The patient received 5,000 rad external-beam irradiation using cobalt-60 and 17-MV x-ray with the following field arrangements:

Field 1:   Cobalt-60, SSD = 80 cm, 30° wedge, 10° posterior tilt, 750 rad given dose.
Field 2:   Cobalt-60, SSD = 80 cm, 10° posterior tilt, 2250 rad given dose.
Field 3:   17-MV x-ray, SSD = 100 cm, 3000 rad given dose.
Field 4:   17-MV x-ray, SSD = 100 cm, 15° wedge, 1500 rad given dose.

During the initial 2 weeks of treatment, the patient noted a prompt decrease in the size of the right temporal bulge. At the completion of radiation therapy he noted a modest improvement of his previously noted right facial nerve palsy. The tumor mass is represented by the dark stippled area. (B) Follow-up CT scan at 5 months (March 1980) revealed 20% to 30% decrease in size of the mass as compared with his pretreatment scan. (C) A repeat CT scan at 21 months (August 1981) revealed continued regression of the mass and reossification of the involved bones. (D) CT scan in August 1982 showed no further change.

The patients with high-grade lesions or secondary chondrosarcomas fared worse, with no controls beyond 1 year. There have been other reports of successful irradiation of head and neck chondrosarcoma.[32] Doses equivalent to those for a similar-sized squamous carcinoma should be used.

In addition, good preliminary results for inoperable lesions around the clivus have been reported by Suit and co-workers using a combination of photons and protons.[45] Doses of 6500 rad to 7500 rad were used, and the three patients treated showed no evidence of disease 16, 28, and 86 months after treatment.* McNaney and co-workers reported three patients (excluding mesenchymal chondrosarcoma) who were treated with a combination of photons and neutrons; all were alive without evidence of local recurrence at 12, 26, and 30 months, although one had developed distant metastases.[28]

However, since chondrosarcomas may recur or metastasize as late as 10 years after therapy, both of these studies need additional follow-up to confirm the early results.

MESENCHYMAL CHONDROSARCOMA

Mesenchymal chondrosarcoma is a distinctive type that occurs in both skeletal and extraskeletal forms and has a predilection for the facial bones and ribs. It is very cellular, with many undifferentiated mesenchymal cells in which islands of relatively well-differentiated cartilage exist.[2] The lesions have a high rate of distant metastasis and may recur after long periods of remission. Surgical excision is the treatment of choice. Results of radiation therapy are poor for cure, but the tumor may respond rapidly to moderate doses and provide good palliation. Our limited experience (three patients) confirms the rapid response of large primary lesions and bone metastases to radiation therapy. It has been suggested by Rosenberg and co-workers that mesenchymal chondrosarcomas be treated similar to a Ewing's sarcoma with aggressive chemotherapy and irradiation.[38]

SOFT TISSUE TUMORS

Soft tissue tumors can be divided into low-grade neoplasms that may recur after inadequate excision but rarely metastasize, and metastasizing soft tissue tumors that vary from low to high in grade.

Low-Grade, Rarely Metastasizing Lesions

INFILTRATING ANGIOLIPOMA

Angiolipoma is a distinct neoplasm characterized by a predominance of blood vessels, infiltration of skeletal muscle, and the tendency to recur locally. It presents as a slow-growing soft tissue mass, which may be fixed to underlying structures. It is most common in the extremities, but it may occur in the neck and supraclavicular regions. It is often found to have infiltrated fascia, muscle, periosteum, and even bone, with complete disregard for anatomical barriers, although it rarely infiltrates nerves.[7,15]

Angiolipomas usually have their onset in the third and fourth decades of life, but they have been reported from infancy to late adulthood.[15,26]

* Suit H: Personal communication, 1982.

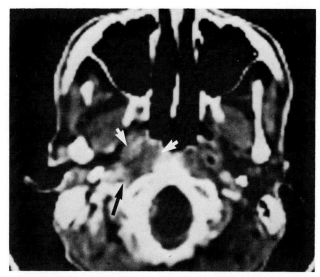

FIG. 34-3. A 63-year-old man presented with a 4-year history of diplopia and a 4-month history of retro-orbital and ocular pain associated with slurred speech and numbness of the left side of the face. Physical examination at the time of diagnosis revealed venous distention of the left fundus and paralysis of the oculomotor and trochlear nerves on the left. CT scan with contrast, angiogram, and base of skull tomograms revealed an avascular mass (arrows) arising in the left cavernous sinus and left sphenoid sinus with erosion of the posterior and lateral walls of the sphenoid sinus and extension to the left side of the clivus, parasellar region and middle cranial fossa, and the left petrous bone. Biopsy of the nasopharynx and sphenoid sinus revealed chordoma. From March 1 through May 3, 1978, the patient received 6973-rad tumor dose (initial 3900 rad delivered with x-rays and the remainder with proton beam) (administered by HD Suit, MD, Massachusetts General Hospital). The patient experienced a good response to radiation therapy and, when last seen in follow-up in November 1983, had no evidence of disease more than 5 years after treatment.

Roentgenographically, an infiltrating angiolipoma may show serpiginous densities overlying a diffuse background that is fat lucent. On CT examination, the lesion is intramuscular and the various constituents of the lesion may result in a heterogeneous appearance. The arteriographic appearance is distinctive, with hypervascularity, poor circumscription, vascular tufts, and tangled, enlarged draining veins.[4]

The lesion never metastasizes, but it has a tendency to recur locally. The treatment of choice is surgery; wide excision is necessary to prevent recurrence. Extensive resections are rarely indicated, but patients must be followed for long periods of time because late recurrence may occur. Radiation therapy has been used, but the results are inconclusive.

PLEOMORPHIC LIPOMA

A variant of lipoma has been described by Shmookler and Enzinger that can easily be confused with liposarcoma.[42]

Histologically, most of the lesion is typical lipomatous tissue but there are small atypical areas where floretlike, pleomorphic, multinucleated giant cells are common.

The lesion occurs most commonly in the neck, where half of all cases present. Most patients are male, and the tumor is rare before the fifth decade of life. Most often an asymptomatic mass that has gradually enlarged over a period of several years is reported.

Treatment is surgical excision, and there was no evidence of local recurrence in any of the patients reported by Shmookler and Enzinger.

GRANULAR CELL MYOBLASTOMA

A granular cell myoblastoma has an uncertain histogenesis and is found in nearly every tissue and organ. Approximately 50% of these lesions occur in the head and neck. It is most common in the oral cavity, especially the tongue, but it may also occur in the neck, larynx, ear, lip, eyelid, orbit, and elsewhere. The average age at onset is in the fourth to fifth decade, but it has occasionally been reported in children.[44] Multiple lesions may occur in the same person.

Granular cell myoblastoma is considered a benign lesion, but it has been reported to become malignant and to metastasize, although not all pathologists recognize the existence of a malignant type.[2,18] The lesion may be confused with a squamous cell carcinoma if the biopsy specimen is shallow. Grossly, the lesion is usually small, not larger than 2 cm in most series. It is firm, elevated, plaquelike, and not encapsulated.[18] The rare malignant lesion tends to be larger and grow more rapidly.

Local excision is the treatment of choice. Radiation therapy may be of value for lesions unsuitable for surgical resection.

AGGRESSIVE FIBROMATOSIS

Aggressive fibromatosis, first described by McFarlane in 1832, is a locally aggressive neoplasm of unknown etiology arising from musculoaponeurotic structures.[23,37] It may masquerade under many names (such as extra-abdominal desmoid or fibrosarcoma grade 1, desmoid type) but should be approached as though it is a low-grade ("grade ½") fibrosarcoma. The benign histologic appearance is misleading, since the neoplasm penetrates fascial planes, implants easily along incisions and hematomas, and may invade bone. It may occur in any anatomical location, but it has a predilection for the shoulder girdle and the thigh.[9,48] It may occur at any age, although most tend to present in young adults.[23,48] There is a female preponderance in most series.[23]

The patient often presents with a history of a firm, slowly growing mass that, late in its course, may become fixed and painful.[9,37] The duration of symptoms may vary from months to several years but is usually about 6 months.[9]

Initial treatment is usually wide resection, which is followed by local recurrence in 27% to 57% of cases.[9,23] Surgery should not be attempted unless gross total excision is possible, since radiation therapy alone has been successful even in the treatment of large unresectable lesions. Radiation therapy is used for inoperable or recurrent lesions or after resection with narrow margins and will achieve a local control rate in excess of 80% (Fig. 34-4).[17,23,48] Recommended doses are in the range of 5000 rad to 6000 rad

at 180 rad/fraction, 5 fractions/week. The regression rate is slow, and gross disease may require 6 months or longer to disappear after successful radiation therapy (Fig. 34-5). Most local recurrences after radiation therapy are marginal failures on the edge of the radiation field. Phillips reported five recurrences in 16 patients when gross lesions were treated with radiation therapy; four recurrences were outside the treatment field, which emphasizes the natural history of the disease and the need for adequate margins.*

DERMATOFIBROSARCOMA PROTUBERANS

Dermatofibrosarcoma protuberans is a low-grade malignancy arising from the dermis. It may occur at any age, but it most often occurs in the middle decades of life. It begins as a small, firm, either red or bluish subcutaneous nodule. There may be a history of a small tumor present for many years, and then a sudden growth occurs that may be painful. The lesion can occur anywhere on the body, including the head and neck area. It has the appearance of a low-grade sarcoma and often is misdiagnosed as low-grade fibrosarcoma. Metastases are uncommon but have been reported in a few cases.

The usual treatment is wide local excision. Local recurrence may develop if margins are inadequate. Initially, the lesion is usually a solitary mass, but multiple nodules may develop as it enlarges or recurs after inadequate surgery. Lindberg recommends postoperative irradiation after excision of the second local failure.†

Metastasizing Sarcomas

Most soft tissue sarcomas of the head and neck present in the parapharyngeal space or neck, but they may occur anywhere. The prognosis and response of the tumor to treatment are dependent more on the grade, size, and location of the lesion than the histologic label, but there are exceptions to this general statement. The following tumors have some unique features that require a brief discussion (see also Chapter 33, Pediatric Tumors of the Head and Neck).

Hemangiosarcoma, also called angiosarcoma, may arise from the endothelial cells of almost any organ, including the skin; the head and neck region is the most common site.

The scalp is the predominant area of involvement, with the soft tissues of the face also being a common site. The tumor is usually blue or purple with peripheral zones of erythema and satellitosis. Hemorrhage and bleeding are common. The tumor tends to infiltrate deeply into the adjacent soft tissues for long distances, often surprising the surgeon at the time of the operation. It will invade bone and cartilage, but, interestingly enough, it tends to grow around skin adnexa and leave them intact.[1]

There is a male-to-female preponderance of 4:1; the tumor is most common in the older age-groups, but it has been reported even in the pediatric age-group.[12]

According to Batsakis and Rice, there are at least two histologic grades of angiosarcoma: low grade and high grade (undifferentiated). The angiosarcomas of the scalp are most likely to be high-grade lesions and have a poor prognosis.[1]

The treatment depends on the extent of local disease, as well as on the presence of metastatic disease at the time

---

* Phillips TL: Personal communication, 1982.

† Lindberg RD: Unpublished data, 1982.

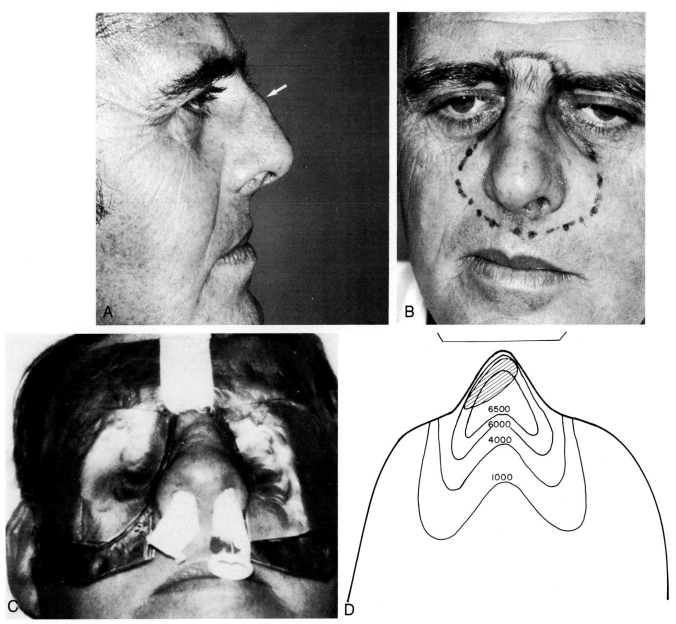

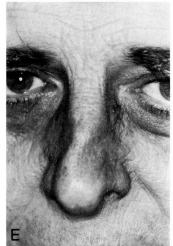

FIG. 34-4. A 47-year-old man presented with a 6-month history of a slowly growing painless subcutaneous lesion just to the left of the dorsum of the nose. (*A*) The mass (*arrow*) was fixed to the underlying cartilages, but the skin was mobile over the mass. The lesion was excised through an intranasal approach. The histologic diagnosis varied between benign fibromatosis and malignant fibrous histiocytoma. The mass quickly recurred and was reexcised, then recurred again 3 months later. Seven months after the initial excision, a transcutaneous approach was made and the diagnosis was the same. The patient then noted a slowly enlarging mass and was referred for consideration of radiation therapy. Physical examination revealed a minimal area of induration, approximately 1.5 cm in diameter, located over the junction of the nasal bone and the lateral alar cartilages. Examination of the nasal mucosa was unremarkable. Opinions regarding the histology varied from aggressive fibromatosis to a low-grade fibrosarcoma. (*B*) Outline of portal for electron-beam therapy. (*C*) A lead face mask was constructed and beeswax plugs were inserted into the nostrils to fill the air cavity. (*D*) Isodose distribution. Field 1: 14-MeV electrons, 5440-rad given dose. 10-MeV electrons, 1675-rad given dose. (*E*) At 4 years there was no evidence of recurrence. (*A*, courtesy of Maurice J. Jurkiewicz, MD, Atlanta)

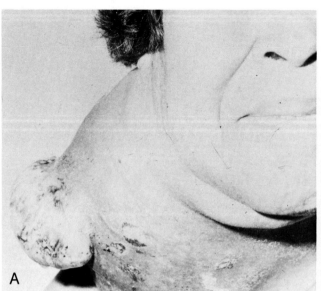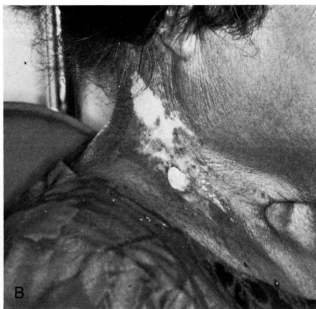

FIG. 34-5. (A) A 69-year-old Samoan woman presented with a 1-year history of a slowly enlarging mass on the right side of her neck. Roentgenogram showed erosion on the medial surface of the scapula due to pressure. Biopsy revealed aggressive fibromatosis. The lesion was considered unresectable, and 5500 rad was delivered to the mass with cobalt-60. (B) Slow resolution of the mass occurred, with complete resolution 2 years after treatment. (Hill DR, Newman H, Phillips TL: Radiation therapy of desmoid tumors. Am J Roentgenol Radium Ther Nucl Med 117:84–89, 1973)

of diagnosis. Metastases to the cervical lymph nodes and lungs are manifested in approximately one third of the patients.[1] The treatment has been primarily surgery, although local recurrences are common, and after one or more failures, patients usually develop metastases. Rosai and co-workers advise surgical excision only for lesions that are solitary and well circumscribed. They recommend that the others be treated primarily by radiation.[36] Radiation therapy has also been reported by Spittle to be effective.[43]

Since the most common mistake made in treating these patients is to underestimate the volume of tissue at risk, the entire scalp, as a minimum, should be considered at risk. Consideration should also be given to treating both sides of the neck electively as well. Doses of 5000 rad should be given the areas treated electively, and at least 6500 rad to 7000 rad should be given to the grossly involved regions at 180 rad to 200 rad/day. Multiple electron fields may be needed, at least for the boosts.

Occasionally, a very rapidly dividing tumor may be encountered for which radiation treatment with one fraction per day may not be adequate. We have treated two such patients with three fractions per day with local control of disease to date. One had a large primary tumor of the tongue and the other, a primary tumor of the scalp.

The prognosis in head and neck angiosarcomas is poor. One half of the patients die within 5 years of diagnosis, and another one fourth of the patients are still living at 5 years with persistent or recurrent tumors. Patients with scalp lesions do even worse.[30] Lesions in the nose, ear, or lip have an earlier clinical presentation and therefore a potentially better chance of cure, but these are much rarer.

Hemangiosarcoma has also been reported by Dahlin to be primary in bone, although only one of his reported cases occurred in the head and neck region (in the skull).[6] The prognosis in primary hemangiosarcoma of bone is very poor.

Malignant fibrous histiocytoma arises from tissue histiocytes and, until the 1970s, was an uncommon diagnosis. Now it is the most common histologic subtype of soft tissue sarcoma in most institutions. These tumors tend to invade along fascial planes, with well-defined margins and bulky masses that appear encapsulated but are not. They generally occur in adults over age 40. The malignant lesions primarily spread to the lung.

Liposarcoma is a tumor that most often arises in late adulthood. Occurrences in the head and neck are usually seen in the deep structures of the neck. It is possibly the most radiosensitive of the soft tissue sarcomas.

Leiomyosarcoma and rhabdomyosarcoma may at times be difficult to distinguish histologically, although rhabdomyosarcoma is more common. Most rhabdomyosarcomas in adulthood are of the pleomorphic type, although the embryonal type does occur and an occasional alveolar variant has been noted. They are usually high-grade lesions and have a high rate of metastatic disease, with perhaps the poorest prognosis of any of the adult head and neck sarcomas.

Neurosarcoma presenting in the head and neck is primarily malignant schwannoma, which often presents in early adulthood. It is essentially an orderly fibrosarcoma of nerve sheath origin that presents as a slowly expanding, encapsulated tumor. It is associated with neurofibromatosis of von Recklinghausen in a large number of patients. Most neurosarcomas occur in the parapharyngeal space and neck, but they also occur in the orbit, tongue, lip, and paranasal sinuses.

A few undifferentiated sarcomas cannot be subclassified.

The workup of patients with soft tissue sarcoma is directed at both local and metastatic disease. The primary site is evaluated with appropriate conventional roentgenograms, contrast-enhanced CT scans, tomograms, and angiograms according to the individual situation (Fig. 34-6). The most common site of metastatic disease is the lungs, so a chest roentgenogram and CT scan (or tomograms) of the lung should be performed. A bone scan will be helpful to determine not only whether bone metastases are present but also whether there is bone involvement at the primary site. This may influence the decision regarding resectability of the lesion.[8]

Although staging systems for soft tissue sarcomas have been developed, they are probably less useful in the head and neck than for primary lesions of the extremities.[40] In general, the prognosis depends on the grade, size, and resectability of the lesion.

Soft tissue sarcomas of the head and neck region are not as well suited for radical resection as the lesions of the extremities. Because of this, to obtain local control, it is often necessary to add radiation therapy. For soft tissue sarcomas of the head and neck treated with a combination of surgery and postoperative radiation therapy at M. D. Anderson Hospital, Lindberg and associates reported that 12 of 19 patients were without evidence of disease at 5 years.[27] The local control rate was 84% in these patients. They recommended postoperative radiation of 6000-rad tumor dose in 6 weeks for low-grade lesions and 6500-rad tumor dose in 6½ weeks for intermediate and high-grade lesions, with a reduction in field size at 5000 rad. The dose is higher with positive margins or gross residual disease. It is difficult to make specific recommendations regarding the volume of tissue to be treated, but it should be generous, taking into account the tissues contaminated at surgery and the extent of the hematoma. For high-grade lesions, consideration should be given to treating the regional lymphatics to 5000 rad in 5 weeks.[13]

Preoperative irradiation should be considered in situations where the lesion is borderline for resection. Our experience with very large lesions of the trunk and extremities shows major tumor regression with 5000 rad given preoperatively. A reactive fibrous rim often develops, which may aid in dissection. Good local control with preoperative radiation therapy has been reported from Massachusetts General Hospital.[38]

The role of chemotherapy in soft tissue sarcomas is still unsettled. There is no doubt that various regimens will produce a measurable response in about 50% of patients, but few of these are complete responses.[46] Trials using adjuvant chemotherapy have been even more disappointing, with only one series showing increased survival. Rosenberg and co-workers reported a 5-year disease-free survival rate of 74% using adjuvant cyclophosphamide, doxorubicin HCl (Adriamycin), and methotrexate, compared

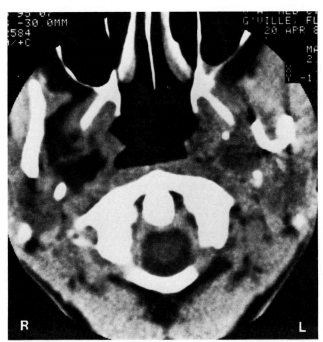

FIG. 34-6. A 30-year-old woman presented with a 2-year history of burning in the left lateral tongue and intermittent pain while eating. CT scan without contrast shows tumor present in the left parapharyngeal space and infratemporal fossa; the body of the mandible is minimally involved by tumor. Biopsy revealed hemangiopericytoma. The patient was treated with a partial resection and postoperative irradiation to 6500 rad. She was without evidence of disease at 2 years.

with 41% in historical controls.[38] However, this finding needs further confirmation in other prospective studies.

REFERENCES

1. Batsakis JG, Rice DH: The pathology of head and neck tumors: Vasoformative tumors: Part IXB. Head Neck Surg 3:326–339, 1981
2. Batsakis JG, Solomon AR, Rice DH: The pathology of head and neck tumors: Neoplasms of cartilage, bone, and the notochord: VII. Head Neck Surg 3:43–57, 1980
3. Biesecker JL, Marcove RC, Huvos AG, Miké V: Aneurysmal bone cysts: A clinicopathologic study of 66 cases. Cancer 26:615–625, 1970
4. Chew FS, Hudson TM, Hawkins IF: Radiology of infiltrating angiolipoma. AJR 135:781–787, 1980
5. Conley JJ, Clairmont AA: Some aspects of cervical chordoma. Trans Am Acad Ophthalmol Otolaryngol 84:145–147, 1977
6. Dahlin DC: Bone Tumors: General Aspects and Data on 6,221 Cases, 3rd ed, pp 99–115, 329–343, 370–375. Springfield, IL, Charles C Thomas, 1978
7. Dionne GP, Seemayer TA: Infiltrating lipomas and angiolipomas revisited. Cancer 33:732–738, 1974
8. Enneking WF, Chew FS, Springfield DS, Hudson TM, Spanier SS: The role of radionuclide bone-scanning in determining the resectability of soft-tissue sarcomas. J Bone Joint Surg 63A:249–257, 1981

9. Enzinger FM, Shiraki M: Musculo-aponeurotic fibromatosis of the shoulder girdle (extra-abdominal desmoid): Analysis of thirty cases followed up for ten or more years. Cancer 20:1131–1140, 1967

10. Friedman M, Pearlman AW: Benign giant-cell tumor of bone. Radiology 91:1151–1158, 1968

11. Fu Y-S, Perzin KH: Non-epithelial tumors of the nasal cavity, paranasal sinuses, and nasopharynx: A clinicopathologic study: III. Cartilaginous tumors (chondroma, chondrosarcoma). Cancer 34:453–463, 1974

12. Girard C, Johnson WC, Graham JH: Cutaneous angiosarcoma. Cancer 26:868–883, 1970

13. Goepfert H, Lindberg RD, Sinkovics JG, Ayala AG: Soft-tissue sarcoma of the head and neck after puberty: Treatment by surgery and postoperative radiation therapy. Arch Otolaryngol 103:365–368, 1977

14. Goethals PL, Dahlin DC, Devine KD: Cartilaginous tumors of the larynx. Surg Gynecol Obstet 117:77–82, 1963

15. Gonzalez-Crussi F, Enneking WF, Arean VM: Infiltrating angiolipoma. J Bone Joint Surg 48A:1111–1124, 1966

16. Gorenstein A, Neel HB III, Weiland LH, Devine KD: Sarcomas of the larynx. Arch Otolaryngol 106:8–12, 1980

17. Greenberg HM, Goebel R, Weichselbaum RR, Greenberger JS, Chaffey JT, Cassady JR: Radiation therapy in the treatment of aggressive fibromatoses. Int J Radiat Oncol Biol Phys 7:305–310, 1981

18. Hajdu SI: Pathology of Soft Tissue Tumors, pp 511, 516–517. Philadelphia, Lea & Febiger, 1979

19. Harwood AR, Fornaster VL, Rider WD: Supervoltage irradiation in the management of giant cell tumor of bone. Radiology 125:223–226, 1977

20. Harwood AR, Krajbich JI, Fornasier VC: Radiotherapy of chondrosarcoma of bone. Cancer 45:2769–2777, 1980

21. Heffelfinger MJ, Dahlin DC, MacCarty CS, Beabout JW: Chordomas and cartilaginous tumors at the skull base. Cancer 32:410–420, 1973

22. Higginbotham NL, Phillips RF, Farr HW, Hustu HO: Chordoma: Thirty-five-year study at Memorial Hospital. Cancer 20:1841–1850, 1967

23. Hill DR, Newman H, Phillips TL: Radiation therapy of desmoid tumors. Am J Roentgenol Radium Ther Nucl Med 117:84–89, 1973

24. Jaffe HL: Tumors and Tumorous Conditions of Bones and Joints, pp 54–62. Philadelphia, Lea & Febiger, 1958

25. Lichtenstein L: Bone Tumors, 5th ed, pp 127–157, 347–354, 419–421. St. Louis, CV Mosby, 1977

26. Lin JJ, Lin F: Two entities in angiolipoma: A study of 459 cases of lipoma with review of literature on infiltrating angiolipoma. Cancer 34:720–727, 1974

27. Lindberg RD, Martin RG, Romsdahl MM, Barkley HT Jr: Conservation surgery and postoperative radiotherapy in 300 adults with soft-tissue sarcomas. Cancer 47:2391–2397, 1981

28. McNaney D, Lindberg RD, Ayala AG, Barkley HT Jr, Hussey DH: Fifteen year radiotherapy experience with chondrosarcoma of bone. Int J Radiat Oncol Biol Phys 8:187–190, 1982

29. Marks RD Jr, Scruggs HJ, Wallace KM, Fenn JO: Megavoltage therapy in patients with aneurysmal bone cysts. Radiology 118:421–424, 1976

30. Morales PH, Lindberg RD, Barkley HT: Soft tissue angiosarcomas. Int J Radiat Oncol Biol Phys 7:1655–1659, 1981

31. Nobler MP, Higinbotham NL, Phillips RF: The cure of aneurysmal bone cyst: Irradiation superior to surgery in an analysis of 33 cases. Radiology 90:1185–1192, 1968

32. Paddison GM, Hanks GE: Chondrosarcoma of the maxilla: Report of a case responding to supervoltage irradiation and review of literature. Cancer 28:616–619, 1971

33. Parrish FF: Total resection of giant cell tumors of the extremities. In M. D. Anderson Hospital: Management of Primary Bone and Soft Tissue Tumors, pp 115–119. Chicago, Year Book Medical Publishers, 1977

34. Pearlman AW, Friedman M: Radical radiation therapy of chordoma. Am J Roentgenol Radium Ther Nucl Med 108:333–341, 1970

35. Plaut HF, Blatt ES: Chordoma of the clivus: A report of four cases. Am J Roentgenol Radium Ther Nucl Med 100:639–649, 1967

36. Rosai J, Sumner HW, Kostianovsky M, Perez-Mesa C: Angiosarcoma of the skin: A clinicopathologic and fine structural study. Hum Pathol 7:83–109, 1976

37. Rosen RS, Kimball W: Extra-abdominal desmoid tumor. Radiology 86:534–540, 1966

38. Rosenberg SA, Suit HD, Baker LM, Rosen G: Sarcomas of the soft tissue and bone. In DeVita V, Hellman S, Rosenberg S (eds): Cancer: Principles and Practice of Oncology, p 1063. Philadelphia, JB Lippincott, 1982

39. Ruiter DJ, van Rijssel TB, van der Velde EA: Aneurysmal bone cysts. Cancer 39:2231–2239, 1977

40. Russell WO, Cohen J, Enzinger F, Hadju SI, Heise H, Martin RG, Meissner W, Miller WT, Schmitz RL, Suit HD: A clinical and pathological staging system for soft tissue sarcomas. Cancer 40:1562–1570, 1977

41. Saxton JP: Chordoma. Int J Radiat Oncol Biol Phys 7:913–915, 1981

42. Shmookler BM, Enzinger FM: Pleomorphic lipoma: A benign tumor simulating liposarcoma. Cancer 47:126–133, 1981

43. Spittle MF: Radiotherapy treatment of primary angiosarcoma of the skin (abstr). Int J Radiat Oncol Biol Phys 7:1290, 1981

44. Strong EW, McDivitt RW, Brasfield RD: Granular cell myoblastoma. Cancer 25:415–422, 1970

45. Suit HD, Goitein M, Munzenrider J, Verhey L, Davis KR, Koehler A, Linggood R, Ojemann RG: Definitive radiation therapy of chordoma and chondrosarcoma of base of skull and cervical spine. J Neurosurg 56:377–385, 1982

46. Sutow WW, Maurer HM: Chemotherapy of sarcomas: A perspective. Sem Oncol 8:207–214, 1981

47. Tewfik HH, McGinnis WL, Nordstrom DG, Latourette HB: Chordoma: Evaluation of clinical behavior and treatment modalities. Int J Radiat Oncol Biol Phys 2:959–962, 1977

48. Wara WM, Phillips TL, Hill DR, Bovill E Jr, Luk KH, Lichter AS, Leibel SA: Desmoid tumors: Treatment and prognosis. Radiology 124:225–226, 1977

Lymphomas and Related Diseases Presenting in the Head and Neck

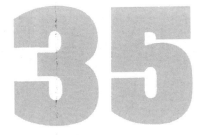

TIMOTHY L. THAR

Lymphomas are divided into two groups: Hodgkin's disease and non-Hodgkin's lymphomas. Hodgkin's disease is a single disease entity with predictable patterns of spread and well-established histologic criteria for diagnosis. On the other hand, non-Hodgkin's lymphomas are a diverse group of diseases with a common characteristic of proliferation of malignant lymphoid cells. Non-Hodgkin's lymphomas are relatively uncommon malignant diseases that range from some of the most indolent to the most aggressive malignancies. Histologic classification of non-Hodgkin's lymphoma is often difficult for the pathologist.* The modern-day treatment of lymphomas requires close cooperation among the surgeon, radiation oncologist, hematologist-oncologist, and pathologist.

ANATOMY

In the head and neck region the sites of most abundant lymphoid tissue include the lymph nodes and Waldeyer's ring (nasopharyngeal, palatine, and lingual tonsils). Smaller amounts of lymphoid tissue may be found in the salivary glands, lacrimal glands, and thyroid. Sites that are essentially without lymphoid tissue include the eyeball, middle ear, and true vocal cords.

PATHOLOGY

Hodgkin's Disease

The diagnosis of Hodgkin's disease is dependent on finding the typical Reed-Sternberg cell in an inflammatory background composed mainly of eosinophils, lymphocytes, and histiocytes. The diagnosis is usually easy to confirm for a pathologist who is familiar with lymphomas. There can be difficulties in the differential diagnosis. Occasionally, patients who have been diagnosed as having Hodgkin's disease in fact have other diseases, most commonly non-Hodgkin's lymphoma. It is important to have slides reviewed by a hematopathologist, especially for extranodal biopsies or if the clinical behavior is unusual for Hodgkin's disease.

The histologic subclassification of Hodgkin's disease most commonly used is that described by Lukes and Butler.[31] The four subtypes of Hodgkin's disease are (1) lymphocyte predominant, (2) nodular sclerosis, (3) mixed cellularity, and (4) lymphocyte depletion. The most common subtype is nodular sclerosis. Following in decreasing frequency are mixed cellularity, lymphocyte predominant, and lymphocyte depletion. The lymphocyte predominant subtype has the best prognosis and often is associated with an earlier stage and a younger median age. In the intermediate group, nodular

---

* Editor's note: The most common serious error in the management of head and neck "lymphomas" originating in extranodal sites is the incorrect interpretation of the biopsy specimen. The treating physician must be alert to this possibility and correlate the history, physical examination, and age of the patient and be properly informed on current methods of fresh tissue examination to avoid improper and sometimes fatal errors in therapy.

TABLE 35-1. Relative Distribution of NHL According to Rappaport Classification (720 patients)

Type	Nodular	Diffuse
Lymphocytic well differentiated	1%	4%
Lymphocytic poorly differentiated	18%	17%
Mixed	13%	6%
Histiocytic	6	31%
Undifferentiated		4%
Total	38%	62%

Note: Data from Bloomfield CD, Goldman A, Dick F, Brunning RU, Kennedy BJ: Multivariate analysis of prognostic factors in the non-Hodgkin's malignant lymphomas. Cancer 33:870–877, 1974; Johnson RE, Chretien PB, O'Conor GT, DeVita VT, Thomas LB: Radiotherapeutic implications of prospective staging in non-Hodgkin's lymphoma. Radiology 110:655–657, 1974; Jones SE, Fuks Z, Ball M, Kadin ME, Dorfman RF, Kaplan HS, Rosenberg SA, Kim H: Non-Hodgkin's lymphomas: IV. Clinicopathologic correlation in 405 cases. Cancer 31:806–823, 1973; and Veronesi U, Musumeci R, Pizzetti F, Gennari L, Bonadonna G: The value of staging laparotomy in non-Hodgkin's lymphoma. Cancer 33:446–459, 1974.

(Million RR: Non-Hodgkin's lymphoma. In Fletcher GH: Textbook of Radiotherapy, p 622. Philadelphia, Lea & Febiger, 1980)

sclerosis and mixed cellularity have essentially the same prognosis with proper treatment and staging. The lymphocyte depletion subtype has the worst prognosis and often is associated with advanced stage at presentation and advanced age. It is difficult to predicate any particular treatment regimen purely on the histologic subtype of Hodgkin's disease because of the inconsistencies in the histologic classification. In one review there was a 25% rate of disagreement among three expert hematopathologists over the histologic subgroups of Hodgkin's disease.[13] This situation may have improved recently, but there still remains some confusion in differentiating the mixed cellularity subtype from nodular sclerosis.

Non-Hodgkin's Lymphoma

The philosophies of one age have become the absurdities of the next, and the foolishness of yesterday has become the wisdom of tomorrow.

Sir William Osler

Non-Hodgkin's lymphomas comprise a group of neoplasms of the cells of the lymphoreticular tissue expressing varying degrees of differentiation. The classification of non-Hodgkin's lymphomas is complex and often requires the consultation of an expert hematopathologist for clarification.

Approximately 10 years ago, Rappaport proposed a histologic classification that had a major characteristic of dividing lymphomas into a nodular or diffuse pattern (Table 35-1).[4,27,28,33,45] The distinction between nodular and diffuse histologic patterns is important in terms of prognosis and therapy. The natural course of the nodular lymphomas is more indolent than the diffuse lymphomas, except diffuse

well-differentiated lymphocytic lymphoma, which may have a course similar to chronic lymphocytic leukemia.

There has been dissatisfaction with the Rappaport scheme because some of the terms used in the classification were erroneous. For example, many of the lymphomas that were termed *histiocytic* have been shown to be made up of transformed lymphocytes. True histiocytic lymphomas are thought to occur only very rarely. Newer classifications have been proposed on the basis of functional studies, such as Lukes and Collins' classification, the Kiel classification, and Dorfman's classification.[18] However, none of the newer classifications has proved to be superior to the Rappaport classification in terms of clinical utility.

A detailed discussion of the many classification systems is beyond the scope of this chapter, and only the most commonly used classification, Rappaport's, will be used. However, clinicians should be aware that the classification of non-Hodgkin's lymphoma is in a state of flux and a new international formulary of non-Hodgkin's lymphomas is being presented to provide an international system for comparing treatment methods and results.[36]

PATTERNS OF SPREAD

Hodgkin's Disease

Hodgkin's disease presents in lymph nodes in approximately 98% of cases. In approximately 90% of cases, the pattern of spread is by involvement of contiguous nodes. The general spread patterns of Hodgkin's disease are most consistent with a unifocal origin, with dissemination through lymphatic pathways.

The most common lymph node groups involved with Hodgkin's disease are the lower cervical and supraclavicular lymph nodes. Upper neck node involvement is infrequent and can be associated with preauricular node involvement in 10% to 15% of cases.[29] Patients who present with supraclavicular lymphadenopathy or bilateral neck disease have a 30% to 40% incidence of disease below the diaphragm, in the para-aortic nodes or spleen. A very favorable presentation of Hodgkin's disease is isolated involvement of the upper neck nodes, which is rarely associated with abdominal spread. Extranodal involvement such as Waldeyer's ring is very uncommon in Hodgkin's disease, and a diagnosis of Hodgkin's disease made from an extranodal site must be regarded with suspicion.

Direct extranodal extension occurs when the tumor breaks through the nodal capsule and invades an adjacent structure. This is particularly prevalent in mediastinal adenopathy, with potential invasion of the lung, pericardium, and pleura.

Non-Hodgkin's Lymphoma

Non-Hodgkin's lymphomas have an extranodal presentation in 40% to 60% of cases. In the head and neck region, the most common sites of presentation are the cervical lymph nodes and Waldeyer's ring. Of the various malignancies presenting in the Waldeyer's ring structures, lymphoma accounts for approximately 10% of nasopharynx, 5% of tonsil, and 3% of base of the tongue malignancies.[33] There is an association between involvement of Waldeyer's ring and gastrointestinal involvement in non-Hodgkin's lymphomas. Approximately 15% patients presenting with

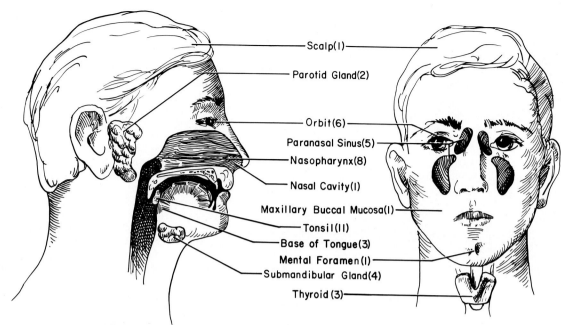

FIG. 35-1. Sites of involvement for 46 patients with primary extranodal non-Hodgkin's lymphomas of the head and neck. (University of Florida data; patients treated 5/65–3/80; analysis 4/81 by N. P. Mendenhall, MD)

non-Hodgkin's lymphomas of Waldeyer's ring will have a relapse in the gastrointestinal system and vice versa if treated with localized radiation therapy.[2,7,40] Almost all extranodal non-Hodgkin's lymphomas are of a diffuse histologic pattern, and the diffuse histiocytic lymphomas represent the single largest subgroup. The presenting sites in our series of non-Hodgkin's lymphomas are shown in Figure 35-1.

Non-Hodgkin's lymphomas tend to be generalized at the time of presentation, with a low incidence of localized disease. Histology is an important predictor, with 80% to 90% of the cases of the nodular lymphomas presenting as widely disseminated disease, whereas 30% to 40% of the cases of the diffuse lymphomas present as localized stage I and II disease. Extranodal presentations of non-Hodgkin's lymphoma have a higher incidence of localized disease than nodal presentations, and the vast majority of extranodal lymphomas have a diffuse histology.

CLINICAL PICTURE

Hodgkin's Disease

Patients presenting with Hodgkin's disease tend to be younger than those presenting with non-Hodgkin's lymphomas. The median age at onset for Hodgkin's disease is 35. There is a bimodal pattern of incidence with peaks between the ages of 15 and 25 and again at approximately 50 years of age. Hodgkin's disease is rare below the age of 5, but a patient as young as age 2 has been reported. Hodgkin's disease is slightly more common in males, and approximately 40% of patients with Hodgkin's disease will present with systemic symptoms such as fever, night sweats, or weight loss. Since the vast majority of Hodgkin's disease patients will present with positive cervical neck nodes, it is important to distinguish enlarged neck nodes

caused by infection from those caused by Hodgkin's disease. (See Chapter 16, The Unknown Primary, for differential diagnosis of a neck mass.) In general, lymph nodes involved by Hodgkin's disease tend to feel discrete, mobile, and rubbery, are nontender, and present most commonly in the anterior, lower cervical, or supraclavicular lymph nodes. Inflammatory nodes tend to be smaller, to feel softer, to be tender, and to involve both the internal jugular and spinal accessory chains. Lymph nodes involved in Hodgkin's disease may wax and wane over a period of weeks to months before slowly enlarging. The nodes may be solitary or multiple. A few patients present with numerous, bilateral, pea-sized masses. Even the most experienced oncologist cannot differentiate lymphoma, carcinoma, and inflammatory lymph nodes purely on physical examination; one must rely to a large degree on the age of the patient, the location of the nodes in the neck, and other findings in making the clinical diagnosis.

Non-Hodgkin's Lymphomas

Non-Hodgkin's lymphomas may present in either the cervical lymph nodes or extranodal sites. Involved nodes typically feel rubbery; usually numerous discrete, mobile nodes are involved. Rapidly progressive growth is more common in non-Hodgkin's lymphomas than Hodgkin's disease.

The presenting symptoms in non-Hodgkin's lymphomas depend to some degree on the primary site. In nodal presentations, the most common situation is an asymptomatic mass discovered by the patient. It is much less common to have systemic symptoms in non-Hodgkin's lymphomas than Hodgkin's disease, with 10% to 15% of patients presenting with a fever, night sweats, or weight loss.

Symptoms of non-Hodgkin's lymphomas presenting in extranodal head and neck sites are usually similar to those

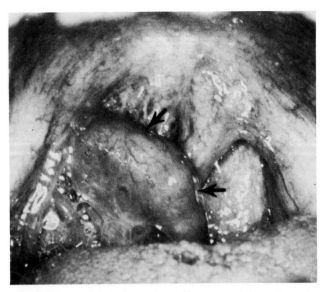

FIG. 35-2. Nodular poorly differentiated lymphocytic lymphoma (*arrows*) involving the right tonsil. Note the submucosal growth pattern that is suspicious for lymphoma.

FIG. 35-3. Diffuse histiocytic lymphoma involving the hard palate (*arrows*). This lesion could easily be confused grossly with a minor salivary gland tumor (e.g., adenoid cystic carcinoma).

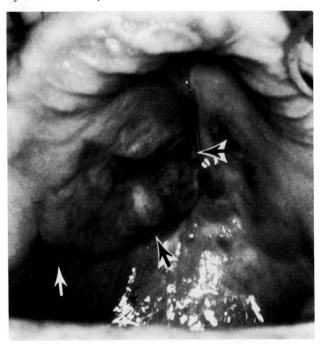

of squamous cancers of those sites. A non-Hodgkin's lymphoma of the palatine tonsil may appear as an enlarged tonsil with a reddish, smooth mucosal covering (Fig. 35-2). This can be associated with obstructive symptoms and, occasionally, pain if the lesion becomes ulcerated (Fig. 35-3). Concomitant neck adenopathy is frequent, occurring in approximately 80% of patients. These lesions may be difficult to differentiate from a hypertrophic, reactive tonsil in a young patient, and often the patient is treated with

prolonged courses of antibiotics or with incision for a tonsillar abscess. Lesions are often quite large, with the mass occluding the oropharynx.

Lesions presenting in the base of the tongue or pharyngeal walls are often submucosal and bulging in appearance. The patients may have obstructive symptoms and occasionally dysphagia or a change in voice.

Lesions presenting in the nasopharynx usually cause intermittent hearing loss secondary to unilateral or bilateral eustachian tube obstruction. Pain is rare, but patients may present with persistent nasal bleeding or nasal obstruction. Many will present with neck node adenopathy. Cranial nerve palsy is uncommon.

Patients presenting with primary orbital lymphomas usually have proptosis and diplopia as presenting symptoms (Fig. 35-4). Pain is not a prominent symptom. If there is involvement of the conjunctiva, there is usually a sensation of a mass, occasionally with local irritation and itching (Fig. 35-5).

Nasal and paranasal sinus primary lesions may produce symptoms similar to sinusitis, or the presenting symptoms may be related to invasion of adjacent structures. Initial symptoms include nasal obstruction with nasal bleeding and occasionally proptosis due to orbital invasion. Maxillary sinus lesions may produce an anterior bulging of the sinus wall.

Rarely, malignant lymphoma can present as a mass in the canine fossa.[23] Lesions in this site can frequently involve the infraorbital nerve, with resulting anesthesia of the area innervated by this nerve.

Primary lesions of the salivary gland are reported to be rare, but 6 of 46 patients (13%) with primary extranodal non-Hodgkin's lymphoma of the head and neck in the University of Florida series had parotid or submaxillary gland primary lesions. They may present as a parotitis with massive enlargement of the parotid gland. Occasionally, these cases may be confused with Sjögren's syndrome.

Non-Hodgkin's lymphomas presenting in the thyroid gland usually do not present in a manner similar to thyroid carcinoma but rather as a diffuse enlargement of one or both lobes, with or without thyroiditis.

In children, only limited numbers of non-Hodgkin's lymphomas are encountered. It is extremely rare to see a nodular lymphoma in a child below the age of 16. Most of the childhood lymphomas are high-grade malignancies, such as lymphoblastic lymphoma, Burkitt's lymphoma, or histiocytic lymphoma, and there is a high (30% to 50%) propensity for peripheral blood or leukemic involvement.

A jaw tumor is a common presentation for Burkitt's lymphoma, African type. Fifty percent of cases occurring in African children occur in the maxilla or mandible. In the United States or Europe, this presentation is quite rare, and Burkitt's lymphoma typically presents in the abdomen.

METHODS OF DIAGNOSIS AND STAGING

In both Hodgkin's and non-Hodgkin's lymphomas, the initial biopsy technique is very crucial to making the proper diagnosis. There are several general steps to follow in the diagnostic approach. The first step applies to head and neck cancers in general. In cases of cervical node presentation the clinician should first rule out the presence of a primary carcinoma or other malignancy by a thorough head and neck examination and proper biopsies. (See Chapter 16, The Unknown Primary.) Even if the patient has already had a node biopsy from the neck confirming non-Hodgkin's lymphoma, a thorough head and neck examination should be undertaken to identify any extranodal sites of disease. If the patient presents without having undergone a biopsy, the first biopsy should be performed on the extranodal tissue, if at all possible. Occasionally, lymph node tissue will also be required in order to subclassify the lymphoma, or as an aid in differentiating a lymphoma from a poorly differentiated squamous carcinoma. Whenever the size of the biopsy allows, *tissue from the initial biopsy should be subdivided and a portion placed in electron microscopy fixative.* This is often helpful in defining the cell of origin for undifferentiated or anaplastic carcinomas. If a lymphoma is suggested, fresh tissue can also be analyzed for cell surface markers, which can be a further aid in the diagnosis of lymphoma.

If there is no extranodal tissue for the primary biopsy and the patient has undergone a thorough head and neck examination and unknown primary lesion workup, then a lymph node biopsy should be done. The surgeon *should attempt to remove one of the largest nodes palpable.* Smaller nodes, while more easily removed, may not be representative, and this will necessitate repeat biopsies. The *lymph node should be removed by excisional biopsy* and, if possible, *with its capsule intact.* It is often necessary to have the entire node for determining architectural changes in a node in order to make the diagnosis and to classify the lymphoma. Even large lymph nodes can be only partially involved with lymphoma, and an incisional biopsy may miss the diagnosis. If the patient also has enlarged inguinal lymph nodes, biopsy of cervical nodes is usually preferred because of reactive or inflammatory changes frequently found in inguinal lymph nodes.

In general, the frozen section technique cannot be used to make a diagnosis of Hodgkin's disease, but it can be used as a confirmatory process to guide the surgeon as to whether the lymph node removed is likely to contain malignant tissue and, therefore, whether the surgeon needs to remove further lymph nodes or not.

Staging

The staging classification for both Hodgkin's disease and the non-Hodgkin's lymphomas is, at present, the Ann Arbor staging classification:[9]

I   Involvement of a single lymph node region or of a single extralymphatic organ or site (IE).

II   Involvement of two or more lymph node regions on the same side of the diaphragm or localized involvement of an extranodal organ or site (IIE) and one or more lymph node regions on the same side of the diaphragm.

III Involvement of lymph node regions on both sides of the diaphragm, which may also be accompanied by localized involvement of an extranodal organ or site (IIIE) or spleen (IIIS) or both (IIISE).

IV   Diffuse or disseminated involvement of one or more distant extranodal organs with or without associated lymph node involvement.

Patients with systemic symptoms are denoted by the suffix letter B. Asymptomatic patients are denoted by the suffix letter A. Systemic, or B, symptoms include unexplained fever greater than 38°C (100.4°F), night sweats, and unexplained weight loss greater than 10% of the body weight over the last 6 months.

A thorough workup is essential in deciding the best mode

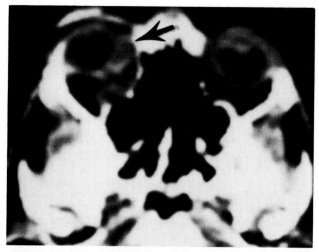

FIG. 35-4.   CT scan of diffuse histiocytic lymphoma presenting in the orbit (*arrow*). There is tumor in the medial orbit that is displacing the eye to the left.

FIG. 35-5.   Diffuse poorly differentiated lymphocytic lymphoma (*arrow*) involving the conjunctiva.

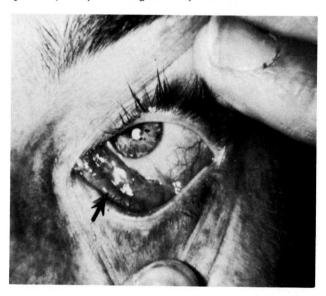

of treatment in each patient. In general, Hodgkin's disease tends to have a more consistent or predictable pattern of spread than the non-Hodgkin's lymphomas. The staging of Hodgkin's disease has been reasonably well worked out, while there remains controversy over the proper staging for non-Hodgkin's lymphomas.

Hodgkin's Disease

After a diagnosis of Hodgkin's disease has been rendered, a detailed history should be obtained with special attention on the presence of systemic symptoms. A very careful physical examination should be done with emphasis on the lymph node regions, spleen, liver, and Waldeyer's ring. The routine laboratory evaluation includes a complete blood cell count, including platelet and differential counts;

renal function evaluation; and liver function tests (serum glutamic oxaloacetic transaminase, serum glutamic pyruvic transaminase, bilirubin, alkaline phosphatase).

Routine radiologic studies should include posteroanterior and lateral chest roentgenography; lymphangiography; and computed axial tomography of the abdomen to evaluate the liver, spleen, kidneys, and upper para-aortic–celiac node region.

Supplemental tests in indicated patients include whole-chest tomography for patients with mediastinal or hilar masses, pleural effusion, or isolated parenchymal lesions (computed tomographic [CT] scanning of the chest is an alternative); intravenous pyelography if there are bulky retroperitoneal nodes or palpable abdominal masses or if abdominal radiation therapy is planned; and bone scanning in patients with suggestive symptoms.

An invasive test that should be done in Hodgkin's disease is a bone marrow biopsy, especially in patients with clinical stage III disease or greater, unexplained low blood cell counts, or B symptoms.

A decision must be made in the course of the workup in each patient with Hodgkin's disease as to whether to do a staging laparotomy. An exploratory laparotomy with splenectomy, needle and wedge biopsies of the liver, and biopsies of the para-aortic, mesenteric, portal, and splenic lymph nodes should be considered in all patients with clinical stage I, II, or III disease, if therapeutic decisions will depend on the findings at laparotomy. This decision hinges on the therapeutic policies of the physicians and varies from place to place. If the presence of splenic involvement will affect the treatment decision, then a staging laparotomy becomes more important.

Non-Hodgkin's Lymphomas

A higher percentage of patients with non-Hodgkin's lymphomas will present with advanced-stage disease; therefore, staging of these patients requires a sequential approach so unnecessary tests can be avoided. Once again, a detailed history with reference to systemic symptoms is important, although only a small percentage of non-Hodgkin's lymphomas will present with systemic symptoms. The physical examination should place a major emphasis on the nodal regions, including epitrochlear and popliteal nodes. A thorough head and neck examination should be done, with close attention to Waldeyer's ring. The routine laboratory and radiologic tests are the same as in Hodgkin's disease, except in patients with Waldeyer's ring involvement. An upper gastrointestinal series should be done in this group of patients in addition to the other radiographic studies because of frequent gastrointestinal involvement. In non-Hodgkin's lymphomas, the CT scan of the abdomen becomes more important because of the predilection for involvement of mesenteric nodes. These nodes are not seen on the lymphangiogram but can be detected by CT scan. One approach is to do the CT scan of the abdomen first, and if bulky adenopathy is present, lymphangiography may not be necessary.

All patients with non-Hodgkin's lymphomas should have a bone marrow biopsy, preferably of the bone marrow of both iliac crests. The majority of patients with nodular lymphomas will present with positive findings of bone marrow biopsies, and this will place the patient in a stage IV category.

Patients with stage I or II non-Hodgkin's lymphomas, after undergoing the above evaluation, can be considered for laparoscopy or exploratory laparotomy for purposes of staging. When a laparotomy is done in patients with non-Hodgkin's lymphomas, careful attention must be directed to the mesenteric nodes in addition to the para-aortic–celiac and pelvic nodes.

TREATMENT

Hodgkin's Disease

The curative treatment of Hodgkin's disease can consist of radiation therapy alone, chemotherapy alone, or a combination of both. In general, the early stages of Hodgkin's disease (stage I, stage II, and favorable stage IIIA) are treated with radiation therapy alone. The advanced stages (III and IV) are treated with combination chemotherapy, with MOPP (nitrogen mustard, vincristine, procarbazine, prednisone) as the most commonly used regimen. Other combination chemotherapy regimens such as ABVD (doxorubicin HCl [Adriamycin], bleomycin, vinblastine, and imidazole carboxamide) have been developed and appear to be as effective or better than MOPP, but they have not had the long follow-up experience of MOPP.[6,19] The place of combined modality therapy with radiation therapy and chemotherapy is being studied. It appears to have some advantage in patients with bulky disease, particularly large mediastinal masses, and may be of advantage in advanced-stage patients who receive chemotherapy plus low-dose irradiation to areas of bulky disease.

When Hodgkin's disease is treated with radiation therapy, a dose of 3500 rad at 150 to 170 rad/fraction appears to be sufficient for small or moderate-sized (less than 6 cm) disease. At the University of Florida, this dose resulted in an in-field recurrence rate of 7%.[43] Doses up to 3750 rad to 4000 rad may be required for disease larger than 6 cm. Doses higher than 4000 rad do not significantly improve local control rates, but they do increase the complication rate.

The actual treatment choice in each patient depends on a large number of factors, including the presence or absence of systemic symptoms, histologic subtype, number of anatomical sites involved, anatomical distribution, tumor size, the patient's overall medical condition, and any previous history of radiation therapy or chemotherapy. It is highly recommended that each patient's primary therapy be decided by collaboration between a hematologist-oncologist and a radiation oncologist. A more extensive discussion of the subtleties of treatment decisions is available in several texts.[21,29,33]

Non-Hodgkin's Lymphomas

Compared with Hodgkin's disease, non-Hodgkin's lymphomas present a much more diverse treatment challenge, and routine treatment guidelines do not exist. The treatment must be tailored to each patient. In general, the treatment of non-Hodgkin's lymphoma can be divided into treatment for the "favorable" and the "nonfavorable" histologic subtypes. The favorable lymphomas include the nodular lymphomas (except for nodular histiocytic) and diffuse well-differentiated lymphocytic lymphoma. The unfavorable histologic subtypes include diffuse poorly differentiated lymphocytic, diffuse histiocytic, diffuse undifferentiated, and nodular histiocytic lymphoma. The curative modalities for non-Hodgkin's lymphomas comprise radiation therapy, chemotherapy, occasionally surgery, or a combination of these modalities. In general, radiation therapy is considered for localized disease, stage I or II, and chemotherapy is the primary treatment for patients with stage III or IV disease.

FAVORABLE HISTOLOGIES

For patients with localized disease, stage I or II, the treatment of choice is radiation therapy. There is debate whether involved-field or extended-field irradiation gives better cure rates. If a patient's disease has been clinically staged, there may be a place for extended-field treatment with inclusion of total abdominal irradiation, since there is a very high rate of mesenteric node involvement, even if lymphangiography proves negative. This would be especially true in a patient with extensive stage II disease with numerous nodal sites involved above the diaphragm.

In patients with stage III or IV disease, chemotherapy is the usual recommended mode of treatment. There is no widely recognized curative chemotherapy program for the favorable non-Hodgkin's lymphomas. Treatment with chemotherapy can involve either a single drug or combination chemotherapy, and occasionally, in the asymptomatic patient, no therapy is recommended initially until symptoms develop. Combinations of chemotherapy and radiation therapy have not proved as yet to increase the overall survival in patients with the favorable non-Hodgkin's lymphomas.

Selected patients with stage III favorable non-Hodgkin's lymphomas can also be considered for treatment with comprehensive lymphatic irradiation, which consists of mantle radiation therapy including Waldeyer's ring, and total abdominal radiation therapy.[14,22] The dose required for local control in the favorable non-Hodgkin's lymphomas is 2500 rad to 3000 rad at 150 rad to 170 rad/fraction.

UNFAVORABLE HISTOLOGIES

Patients who have stage I or localized stage II disease should be considered for localized radiation therapy. "Localized stage II" means that the patient has only two contiguous lymph node sites involved by the disease. Patients who have stage II disease with more than two contiguous lymph node sites involved (nonlocalized) tend to have a very high relapse rate after radiation therapy alone. They can be considered for combined therapy with chemotherapy and irradiation, with improved results over irradiation alone.[34] The dose required for local control in the unfavorable histologies is 4500 rad to 5500 rad given at 180 rad/fraction. Patients with stage III or IV unfavorable non-Hodgkin's lymphomas should be treated with combination chemotherapy as a primary treatment with or without radiation therapy. The most widely used combination chemotherapy program consists of cyclophosphamide, doxorubicin HCl, vincristine, and prednisone (known as "CHOP" chemotherapy).[20] Other combinations of chemotherapy have also been shown to have a curative potential in unfavorable non-Hodgkin's lymphoma.[1,38,42]

RADIATION THERAPY TECHNIQUE

The treatment fields used in radiation therapy of extranodal non-Hodgkin's lymphoma are very similar to those used for carcinomas of the various head and neck sites. Involvement of Waldeyer's ring requires treatment of the entire Waldeyer's ring and both cervical lymph node regions. An example of the treatment portal for Waldeyer's ring disease is shown in Figure 35-6.

TREATMENT OF RECURRENCE

Treatment of patients who have recurrence is dependent on the histology of the recurrence and on the previous chemotherapy and radiation therapy given. Patients with favorable histologies in whom treatment fails can be treated with radiation therapy for local recurrences and single drug or combination chemotherapy for systemic recurrences. If the patient is asymptomatic, then he may be followed without treatment until symptoms develop. Occasionally, patients with an initially favorable non-Hodgkin's lymphoma will have a transformation into an unfavorable histologic subtype. These patients should be treated aggressively for their unfavorable lymphoma with localized radiation therapy for stage I or II disease and combination chemotherapy for more advanced disease.

Patients presenting with an unfavorable histology who have a recurrence usually require aggressive treatment. If radiation therapy was employed initially, an aggressive combination chemotherapy program should be used. Patients who fail to have their disease controlled after aggressive combination chemotherapy often respond poorly to any further treatment, but they can be considered for alternative drug combinations or radiation therapy.

RESULTS OF TREATMENT

Hodgkin's Disease

For stage I and IIA Hodgkin's disease, the 5-year continuously disease-free rates range from 80% to 90% with total nodal radiation therapy (including the mantle, para-aortic nodes, spleen, and pelvic nodes). University of Florida data on 43 patients with stage I disease indicate a 5-year survival rate of 96%. Patients with stage IIA disease had a 5-year survival rate of 84% with total or modified total nodal radiation therapy. The Joint Center in Boston has shown a 5-year survival rate of 100% in stage IA patients treated with irradiation alone, 97% continuously free of disease, and a 5-year survival rate of 93% for stage IIA patients, 80% continuously free of disease.[25] Total nodal radiation therapy for surgical stage IIB Hodgkin's disease is associated with a 5-year disease-free rate of approximately 80%.

Important prognostic indicators in early-stage disease include the total number of sites initially involved, with a recurrence rate of less than 15% when one to four sites are involved versus a recurrence rate of 50% to 60% when more than five anatomical sites are involved. The number of anatomical sites involved is probably an excellent predictor of the volume of disease and the likelihood of success with radiation therapy. Another prognostic indicator is bulky local disease, particularly mediastinal masses greater than 6 cm to 9 cm, or larger than one third of the thoracic diameter. Patients with massive mediastinal disease have a relapse rate of 20% to 40% when treated with irradiation alone. Also, the presence of systemic symptoms decreases the 5-year survival rate by approximately 20%, stage for stage.

In the more advanced stages, III and IV, chemotherapy plays a more important role. One possible exception is favorable stage IIIA (or stage III₁A), which has subdiaphragmatic disease limited to the celiac nodes or spleen. Treated with irradiation alone, these patients have a 70% to 80% relapse-free rate at 5 years. Patients with more extensive abdominal disease have a very poor relapse-free rate when treated with irradiation alone, with 10% to 20% reported to be relapse free at 5 years.[41] Patients with stage III or IV Hodgkin's disease treated primarily with MOPP have a 5-year continuously disease-free survival rate of 30% to 60%.[16] Preliminary studies of combined modality therapy of stage III and IV disease with MOPP or ABVD plus radiation therapy show continuously disease-free rates of 60% to 80% at 4 or 5 years.[5,15,37,39]

Non-Hodgkin's Lymphomas

Involved field radiation therapy is curative in 50% to 70% of patients with stage I or localized II disease. If the patients have been surgically staged, a survival rate at 5 years of 78% has been reported, versus a 5-year survival rate of 60% in patients staged I or localized stage II without laparotomy.[3,24,30] In advanced-stage, III or IV, non-Hodgkin's lymphoma, treatment is dependent on histology. In the favorable histologies, patients with stage III or IV disease can be treated with combination chemotherapy, single-agent chemotherapy, whole-body irradiation, or deferred therapy. None of these treatments appears to be curative. Some patients with stage III favorable non-Hodgkin's lymphoma can be considered for total lymphatic irradiation, which has shown a potential for being curative in 30% to 50% of patients.[14,22] Five-year survival rates for the favorable non-Hodgkin's lymphomas are 60% to 70%.

For the unfavorable histology, advanced-stage non-Hodgkin's lymphomas, the primary therapy should be aggressive, multidrug chemotherapy. At present, the commonly used regimen is CHOP, which is reported to give a 25% to 40% 5-year survival rate.[12,20] Combinations of chemotherapy and radiation therapy for advanced stage non-Hodgkin's lymphomas have not been shown to be of benefit.

FOLLOW-UP POLICY

Patients with both Hodgkin's and non-Hodgkin's lymphomas should be followed carefully, especially within the first 3 years. Relapses occur as a function of time, and approximately 80% of patients with Hodgkin's disease who are going to have a relapse will be detected in the first 3 years. In non-Hodgkin's lymphomas, the patients with unfavorable histologies tend to relapse within the first 2 years, and those with favorable histologies have a tendency to relapse later.

Patients should be seen every 6 to 8 weeks during the first 2 years, every 3 months during the third year, every 4 months during the fourth year, and every 6 months through the fifth and sixth years. After that, follow-up once a year is recommended. The follow-up examination should include a thorough physical examination, blood cell counts (including platelets), and periodic chest roent-

FIG. 35-6. (A) Treatment field to irradiate Waldeyer's ring (nasopharynx, tonsil, and base of the tongue) and upper neck nodes. The lower border is at the thyroid notch. The superior border is about 1 cm above the zygomatic arch. The posterior border coincides with the tragus and then bends posteriorly to encompass the sternocleidomastoid and occipital nodes. The anterior border extends from the orbital ridge toward the second molar region; it then bends forward along the mandible so that the submental nodes are encompassed. (B) Treatment field used to irradiate the lower neck nodes in conjunction with Waldeyer's ring and upper neck nodes. The upper border coincides with the lower border of A. Midline larynx shielding extends from the thyroid notch to the lower edge of the cricoid. The lateral margin is defined by the junction of the trapezius with the clavicle. The inferior extent is usually 2 cm below the clavicle.

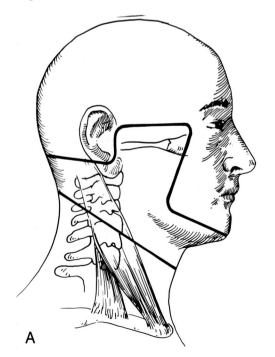

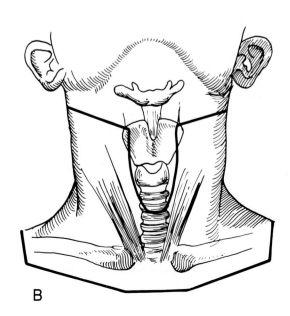

A   B

genography. A roentgenogram of the abdomen is useful in patients who have had a lymphangiogram.

COMPLICATIONS OF TREATMENT

Radiation Therapy

Radiation therapy of the head and neck region, including Waldeyer's ring, will usually result in moderate xerostomia. With a total dose of 2500 rad to 3000 rad, the patient will frequently recover good salivary function. Doses above 5000 rad usually result in persistent dryness of the mouth that is moderate to severe. All patients who are undergoing oral irradiation should have careful instruction in dental hygiene, and those receiving doses above 3000 rad should have a dental evaluation prior to or during treatment. (See Chapter 12, Dental Management for the Irradiated Patient.)

Irradiation to other sites in the head and neck, including the orbit, may include the eye as part of the treatment volume for lymphoma. With doses below 5000 rad, good vision is almost always maintained. A cataract may develop, but the cataract can be surgically removed with the same results as removal of other cataracts.

Patients irradiated in the neck region are also at risk for hypothyroidism. This is an easily managed complication if detected, and routine thyroid examination with thyroxine and thyrotropin determinations at yearly intervals is recommended to detect hypothyroidism before it is clinically manifest.

Patients irradiated to the neck may also experience Lhermitte's syndrome 4 to 6 weeks after radiation therapy. This is a transient syndrome that may last 4 to 6 weeks and consists of an electric shock–like sensation down the spinal cord on flexion of the neck. If the symptoms are disturbing, a soft cervical collar can be worn for 4 to 6 weeks.

Chemotherapy

Acute complications of chemotherapy include pancytopenia with resultant risks of infection, alopecia, and acute nausea and vomiting. A moderate to severe transient mucositis of the oral cavity can be seen with the use of some chemotherapeutic agents, such as methotrexate, 5-fluorouracil, and doxorubicin HCl.[10,11] Long-term complications include the possibility of prednisone-induced bilateral femoral head necrosis, vincristine neuropathy, cardiotoxicity due to doxorubicin HCL, cyclophosphamide-induced hemorrhagic cystitis, and sterility in young males.

Combined Modality Treatment

The complications of combined modality treatment include all of the above, plus an increased incidence of second malignancies, primarily acute leukemia. The risk of second malignancy appears to be 3% to 7% overall in patients treated with combined modalities. The risk of second malignancy may cancel the survival advantages achieved by the aggressive combined modality approach.

MYCOSIS FUNGOIDES

Mycosis fungoides is a malignant disorder of T-lymphocytes that have a special affinity for the epidermis. The disease often presents as a skin rash. This may slowly change to irregularly shaped, slightly indurated plaques. The plaques evolve into nodular skin tumors (Fig. 35-7), and eventually there is involvement of the lymph nodes and internal organs. The natural history of mycosis fungoides is exceedingly variable and the course may be prolonged irrespective of therapy.

Patients with mycosis fungoides may rarely present with oral manifestations. Sites of presentation include the tongue (most common), soft palate, hard palate, tonsils, and epiglottis. Oral lesions are most frequently seen in later stages of the disease. Clinically, the oral lesions are described most frequently as erythematous and ulcerated.

Staging

Staging of mycosis fungoides includes careful assessment of skin involvement, including size, distribution, thickness, and pigmentary changes of all lesions on the body. A careful examination of the nodal regions is also necessary, with biopsy of enlarged, suspicious nodes. All patients should have a chest roentgenogram, liver function studies, complete blood cell counts, and, in advanced-stage patients, a bone marrow biopsy. A staging system has been proposed for mycosis fungoides and is outlined in a paper by Bunn and co-workers.[8]

Treatment of mycosis fungoides is with either chemotherapy or radiation therapy. When it is confined to the skin, it can be treated with electron-beam irradiation or topical applications of chemotherapy. In the later stages, with nodal or internal organ involvement, treatment often consists of combination chemotherapy.

In the early stages, with localization to the skin, it is possible to have prolonged remissions and possible cures with electron-beam irradiation. In the Stanford experience,

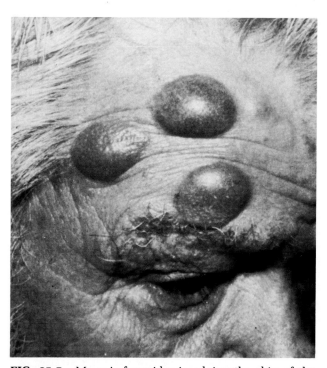

FIG. 35-7. Mycosis fungoides involving the skin of the right forehead.

approximately 40% of the patients with limited plaque disease were continuously free of disease for 8 to 10 years. When the disease has spread to extracutaneous sites, cure is rare and therapy is primarily palliative.

PEDIATRIC LYMPHOMAS

Hodgkin's Disease

Pediatric Hodgkin's disease can be likened to Hodgkin's disease occurring in the adult. The natural history and the staging are the same as outlined for adults. Pediatric patients with Hodgkin's disease tend to present more often with a favorable histology, with a higher percentage of lymphocyte-predominance cases than in adults and fewer lymphocyte-depletion histologies. Stage for stage, the relapse-free survival and cure rates in major treatment centers are as good as or better than those obtained in adult Hodgkin's disease.

Radiation therapy is often modified for the very young patient in an attempt to avoid possible late sequelae of the radiation. Bone growth retardation is a common sequela of irradiation of children under age 13 and is related to the total dose of radiation. Presently recommended is a modification of dose according to age, with 2500 rad at 150 rad to 170 rad/fraction for ages 2 through 6 and 3000 rad at 170 rad/fraction for ages 7 through 13. With these modifications, bone growth retardation and soft tissue atrophy are much less marked than with higher doses.

Chemotherapy is used as in adult Hodgkin's disease, with MOPP chemotherapy used as the standard. Usually the treatment is given for a minimum of six cycles, or for two cycles after complete response has been achieved. Combined modality treatment, with MOPP chemotherapy and low-dose radiation therapy (1500 rad to 2500 rad), is being investigated in an attempt to reduce late radiation effects, particularly growth retardation.[17,26]

Non-Hodgkin's Lymphomas

Childhood non-Hodgkin's lymphomas are different in some important aspects from adult non-Hodgkin's lymphomas. Histologically, childhood non-Hodgkin's lymphomas are usually high-grade malignancies. There is a much greater predilection for evolution to acute leukemia and a higher frequency of involvement of the central nervous system. The principles of management useful for adults with non-Hodgkin's lymphomas are not directly applicable to children.

HISTOLOGY

Rappaport's classification, with its proven relevance in adults, is less useful in the pediatric age-group. Most childhood lymphomas are diffuse; it is rare to have nodular forms in children. Generally, childhood non-Hodgkin's lymphoma can be grouped under three main headings: (1) lymphoblastic, (2) histiocytic, and (3) Burkitt's lymphoma. Burkitt's lymphoma will be discussed separately in the next section.

The childhood lymphomas are often difficult to distinguish one from another on histologic grounds, and the diagnosis must be correlated with the clinical features. Lymphoblastic lymphomas typically present as a supradiaphragmatic tumor, very often in the mediastinum. There is a marked tendency toward leukemic evolution and involvement of the central nervous system.

STAGING

The staging workup of childhood lymphomas is abbreviated due to the aggressive, rapid growth potential and the need for systemic therapy in most patients. Staging requires a history and physical examination, complete blood cell count, renal and hepatic function tests, chest roentgenogram, skeletal survey or bone scan, bone marrow aspiration and biopsies, and lumbar puncture. Additional studies such as CT scan of the abdomen, myelography, ultrasound, barium studies of the gastrointestinal tract, and lymphangiography are done in selected patients. The Ann Arbor staging system can be used, but this is an imperfect staging system for childhood non-Hodgkin's lymphomas because of their tendency for widespread dissemination and frequent bone marrow or central nervous system involvement. Other staging systems have been proposed specifically for the pediatric non-Hodgkin's lymphomas.[44]

TREATMENT

In childhood non-Hodgkin's lymphomas, the primary thrust of treatment is with combination chemotherapy. Most of the regimens use a combination of cyclophosphamide, methotrexate, doxorubicin HCl, vincristine, and prednisone. With combinations of these drugs, 80% to 90% of children are able to achieve a complete response. Patients who have localized stages of disease may benefit from adjuvant localized radiation therapy (usually 1500 rad to 2500 rad). In advanced-stage disease, irradiation is used in prophylactic treatment of the central nervous system. There is a high risk for lymphomatous involvement of the central nervous system in all patients with primary lesions of the head and neck and mediastinum and with massive abdominal disease. Without prophylactic treatment, central nervous system disease develops in approximately 30% of childhood cases at high risk and the outcome is usually fatal.

Survival in patients with localized disease (stages I and II) is quite good, approaching 70% to 90%. In patients with more advanced disease, the prognosis is much poorer, with reports of 2-year survival rates of 10% to 30%.[35]

Burkitt's Lymphoma

The classic description of Burkitt's lymphoma was made by Burkitt in his study of African patients. It is a predominantly extranodal tumor, mainly affecting the mandible and, less commonly, the abdominal viscera. This lymphoma has a unique geographic distribution in Africa and has an association with Epstein-Barr virus. Kinetic studies of Burkitt's lymphoma cells have revealed a doubling time of about 24 hours, making this one of the fastest growing human tumors. The proliferative potential of Burkitt's lymphoma is clinically apparent, with many of these tumors reaching massive sizes within days or weeks.

After its original description in Africa, a number of cases of "Burkitt-like" tumors were recognized in other parts of the world. In African patients the mean age is 7 with a range of 2 to 16 years of age; the male-to-female ratio is 2:1. In American patients the mean age is 11, with a range of 2 to 27 years of age. The majority of American patients have intra-abdominal tumors, apparently arising from

Peyer's patches or mesenteric lymph nodes. The most frequent clinical presentation is intestinal obstruction or an abdominal mass. Other areas of intra-abdominal involvement include the ovaries, kidneys, or retroperineum. A few patients present with enlarged cervical nodes.

Because of the characteristic widespread tumor distribution and urgent need for treatment due to the rapid proliferative potential, clinical staging is abbreviated. A careful history, physical examination, complete blood cell count, chest roentgenogram, renal and hepatic function tests, and bone marrow biopsy are done in all patients. CT scanning, abdominal ultrasonography, and lymphangiography have been used to identify abdominal tumor sites and in following response to therapy. The serum lactic dehydrogenase level reflects the tumor burden and is a sensitive indicator of tumor regression and relapse.

The treatment strategy in Burkitt's lymphoma is primarily systemic chemotherapy. Surgery is often used in abdominal primary lesions for diagnosis and possible bulk resection. Localized radiation therapy can be considered for slowly regressing tumor masses in combination with chemotherapy. Patients who have been treated with aggressive combination chemotherapy employing cyclophosphamide, vincristine, doxorubicin HCl, and prednisone, with intermittent high-dose, systemic and intrathecal methotrexate, have had complete response rates of 80% to 100% and 2-year survival rates of 50% to 70%.[46]

PLASMACYTOMA

Solitary plasmacytoma of the bone and soft tissue is a rare neoplasm that can involve the head and neck region. The incidence is approximately 3 per 100,000 population, with a median age of presentation of 60 years. In one series the age ranged from 28 to 74, with the majority of patients in the sixth, seventh, and eighth decades of life.[32] There is a male-to-female ratio of 4:1. Tumors can be categorized into two groups: osseous and nonosseous (extramedullary) primary lesions. Approximately 80% of the extramedullary plasmacytomas occur in the head and neck, most notably in the upper air passages. The nasopharynx, tonsil, maxillary sinus, nasal vestibule, and trachea are the more common sites of presentation. The tumors are usually submucosal masses. The regional cervical lymph nodes may be involved in 10% to 25% of cases, and an occasional patient is seen with lymph node disease and no obvious primary site. Although solitary plasmacytoma appears to be a separate disease, 10% to 40% of patients will progress to multiple myeloma on long-term follow-up. The incidence of progression to multiple myeloma is higher in patients presenting with a bone lesion as compared with an extramedullary lesion.

The recommended workup includes a bone marrow biopsy, skeletal survey and/or bone scan, urine study for Bence-Jones protein or quantitative determination of κ and λ light chains, serum protein electrophoresis and immunoelectrophoresis, serum calcium and uric acid levels, complete blood cell count, and renal function studies.

The treatment for solitary plasmacytoma is localized radiation therapy. An analysis of the dose required for local control showed that a dose of 3500 rad to 4000 rad over 4 to 5 weeks was sufficient for local control in 94% of patients.[33] There was no obvious difference in the dose required for osseous versus extramedullary lesions. The survival rate in a group of 15 patients was 87% at 5 years. Five of the 15 patients progressed to multiple myeloma

but had an indolent course. Chemotherapy is used for generalized relapse. Solitary new lesions may occur and should be treated with radiation therapy in the same manner as primary lesions.

REFERENCES

1. Anderson T, Bender RA, Fisher RI, DeVita VT, Chabner BA, Berard CW, Norton L, Young RC: Combination chemotherapy in non-Hodgkin's lymphoma: Results of long-term follow-up. Cancer Treat Rep 61:1057–1066, 1977
2. Banfi A, Bonadonna G, Ricci SB, Milani F, Molinari R, Monfardini S, Zucali R: Malignant lymphomas of Waldeyer's ring: Natural history and survival after radiotherapy. Br Med J 3:140–143, 1972
3. Bitran JD, Kinzie J, Sweet DL, Variakojis D, Griem ML, Golomb HM, Miller JB, Oetzel N, Ultmann JE: Survival of patients with localized histiocytic lymphoma. Cancer 39:342–346, 1972
4. Bloomfield CD, Goldman A, Dick F, Brunning RU, Kennedy BJ: Multivariate analysis of prognostic factors in the non-Hodgkin's malignant lymphomas. Cancer 33:870–877, 1974
5. Bonadonna G, Zucali R, De Lena M, Valagussa P: Combined chemotherapy (MOPP or ABVD)–radiotherapy approach in advanced Hodgkin's disease. Cancer Treat Rep 61:769–777, 1977
6. Bonadonna G, Zucali R, Monfardini S, De Lena M, Uslenghi C: Combination chemotherapy of Hodgkin's disease with Adriamycin, bleomycin, vinblastine, and imidazole carboxamide versus MOPP. Cancer 36:252–259, 1975
7. Brugère J, Schlienger M, Gérard-Marchant R, Tubiana M, Pouillart P, Cachin Y: Non-Hodgkin's malignant lymphomata of the upper digestive and respiratory tract: Natural history and results of radiotherapy. Br J Cancer, Suppl II, 435–440, 1975
8. Bunn PA, Lamberg SI: Report of the committee on staging and classification of cutaneous T-cell lymphomas. Cancer Treat Rep 63:725–728, 1979
9. Carbone PP, Kaplan HS, Musshoff K, Smithers DW, Tubiana M: Report of the Committee on Hodgkin's Disease Staging Classification. Cancer Res 31:1860–1861, 1971
10. Chabner BA, Myers CE, Coleman CN, Johns DG: The clinical pharmacology of antineoplastic agents (first of two parts). N Engl J Med 292:1107–1112, 1975
11. Chabner BA, Myers CE, Coleman N, Johns DG: The clinical pharmacology of antineoplastic agents (second of two parts). N Engl J Med 292:1159–1168, 1975
12. Coltman CA Jr, Luce JK, McKelvey EM, Jones SE, Moon TE: Chemotherapy of non-Hodgkin's lymphoma: 10 years' experience in the Southwest Oncology Group. Cancer Treat Rep 61:1067–1078, 1977
13. Coppelson LW, Factor RM, Strum SB, Graff PW, Rappaport H: Observer disagreement in the classification and histology in Hodgkin's disease. J Natl Cancer Inst 45:731–740, 1970
14. Cox JD: Total central lymphatic irradiation for Stage III nodular malignant lymphoreticular tumors. Int J Radiat Oncol Biol Phys 1:491–496, 1976
15. DeLena M, Monfardini S, Beretta G, Fossati-Bellani F, Bonadonna G: Clinical trials with intensive chemotherapy and radiotherapy in Hodgkin's disease. International symposium on Hodgkin's disease. Natl Cancer Inst Monogr 36:403–422, 1973
16. DeVita VT Jr, Lewis BJ, Rozencweig M, Muggia FM: The chemotherapy of Hodgkin's disease: Past experiences and future directions. Cancer 42:979–990, 1978
17. Donaldson SS, Glatstein E, Rosenberg SA, Kaplan HS: Pediatric Hodgkin's disease: II. Results of therapy. Cancer 37:2436–2447, 1976
18. Dorfman RF: Pathology of the non-Hodgkin's lymphomas: New classifications. Cancer Treat Rep 61:945–951, 1977
19. Durant JR, Gams RA, Velez-Garcia E, Bartolucci A, Wirtschafter D, Dorfman R: BCNU, Velban, cyclophosphamide,

procarbazine, and prednisone (BVCPP) in advanced Hodgkin's disease. Cancer 42:2101–2110, 1978

20. Elias L, Portlock CS, Rosenberg SA: Combination chemotherapy of diffuse histiocytic lymphoma with cyclophosphamide, Adriamycin, vincristine, and prednisone (CHOP). Cancer 42:1705–1710, 1978

21. Glatstein E: Introduction to lymphoma. In Carter SK, Glatstein E, Livingston RB: Principles of Cancer Treatment, pp 787–789. New York, McGraw-Hill, 1982

22. Glatstein E, Fuks Z, Goffinet DR, Kaplan HS: Non-Hodgkin's lymphomas of stage III extent: Is total lymphoid irradiation appropriate treatment? Cancer 37:2806–2812, 1976

23. Goldman NC: Malignant lymphoma of the canine fossa. South Med J 73:812–813, 1980

24. Hellman S, Chaffey JT, Rosenthal DS, Moloney WC, Canellos GP, Skarin AT: The place of radiation therapy in the treatment of non-Hodgkin's lymphomas. Cancer 39:843–851, 1977

25. Hellman S, Mauch P, Goodman RL, Rosenthal DS, Moloney WC: The place of radiation therapy in the treatment of Hodgkin's disease. Cancer 42:971–978, 1978

26. Jenkin D, Freedman M, McClure P, Peters V, Saunders F, Sonley M: Hodgkin's disease in children: Treatment with low dose radiation and MOPP without staging laparotomy: A preliminary report. Cancer 44:80–86, 1979

27. Johnson RE, Chretien PB, O'Conor GT, DeVita VT, Thomas LB: Radiotherapeutic implications of prospective staging in non-Hodgkin's lymphoma. Radiology 110:655–657, 1974

28. Jones SE, Fuks Z, Bull M, Kadin ME, Dorfman RF, Kaplan HS, Rosenberg SA, Kim H: Non-Hodgkin's lymphomas: IV. Clinicopathologic correlation in 405 cases. Cancer 31:806–823, 1973

29. Kaplan HS: Hodgkin's Disease, 2nd ed, pp 478–547. Cambridge, MA, Harvard University Press, 1980

30. Levitt SH, Bloomfield CD, Frizzera G, Lee KKC: Curative radiotherapy for localized diffuse histiocytic lymphoma. Cancer Treat Rep 64:175–177, 1980

31. Lukes RJ, Butler JJ: The pathology and nomenclature of Hodgkin's disease. Cancer Res 26:1063–1081, 1966

32. Mendenhall CM, Thar TL, Million RR: Solitary plasmacytoma of bone and soft tissue. Int J Radiat Oncol Biol Phys 6:1497–1501, 1980

33. Million RR: The lymphomatous diseases. In Fletcher GH: Textbook of Radiotherapy, p 584. Philadelphia, Lea & Febiger, 1980

34. Monfardini S, Banfi A, Bonadonna G, Rilke F, Milani F, Val-

agussa P, Lattuada A: Improved five year survival after combined radiotherapy-chemotherapy for stage I-II non-Hodgkin's lymphoma. Int J Radiat Oncol Biol Phys 6:125–134, 1980

35. Murphy SB: Combined modality therapy of childhood non-Hodgkin's lymphoma. Rec Results Cancer Treat 65:207–213, 1978

36. Non-Hodgkin's Lymphoma Pathologic Classification Project: National Cancer Institute sponsored study of classifications of non-Hodgkin's lymphoma: Summary and description of a working formulation for clinical usage. Cancer 49:2112–2135, 1982

37. Prosnitz LR, Farber LR, Fischer JJ, Bertino JR, Fischer DB: Longterm remission with combined modality therapy for advanced Hodgkin's disease. Cancer 37:2826–2833, 1976

38. Rodriguez V, Cabanillas F, Burgess M, McKelvey EM, Valdivieso M, Bodey GP, Freireich FJ: Combination chemotherapy ("CHOP-bleo") in advanced (non-Hodgkin) malignant lymphoma. Blood 49:325–333, 1977

39. Rosenberg SA, Kaplan HS, Glatstein EJ, Portlock CS: Combined modality therapy of Hodgkin's disease: A report on the Stanford trials. Cancer 42:991–1000, 1978

40. Rudders RA, Ross ME, DeLellis RA: Primary extranodal lymphoma: Response to treatment and factors influencing prognosis. Cancer 42:406–416, 1978

41. Stein RS, Golomb HM, Diggs CH, Mauch P, Hellman S, Wiernik PH, Ultmann JE, Rosenthal DS: Anatomic substages of stage IIIA Hodgkin's disease. Ann Intern Med 92:159–165, 1980

42. Sweet D, Golomb HM, Desser RK, Lester EP, Bitran JD, Diekamp U, Moran EM, Stein RS, Yaehnin S, Ultmann JE: Treatment of advanced histiocytic lymphoma with COMA chemotherapy (abstr). Proc AACR-ASCO 17:10, 1976

43. Thar TL, Million RR, Hausner RJ, McKetty MHB: Hodgkin's disease, stages I and II: Relationship of recurrence to size of disease, radiation dose, and number of sites involved. Cancer 43:1101–1105, 1979

44. Toledano SR, Meadows AT: Diagnosis and staging of non-Hodgkin's lymphoma in childhood. In Graham-Pole J: Non-Hodgkin's Lymphomas in Children, pp 63–80. New York, Masson Publishing, 1980

45. Veronesi U, Musumeci R, Pizzetti F, Gennari L, Bonadonna G: The value of staging laparotomy in non-Hodgkin's lymphoma. Cancer 33:446–459, 1974

46. Ziegler JL: Burkitt's lymphoma. N Engl J Med 305:735–745, 1981

Cost of Management
of Head and Neck Cancer

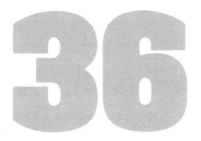

RODNEY R. MILLION
MARGUERITE C. SIGAL

In this chapter several examples are given of the costs involved in the management of head and neck cancer. The examples represent specific patients and therefore do not represent average costs based on analysis of large numbers of patients. They should be considered to be representative of uncomplicated treatment costs; if the patient develops a complication, which is all too frequent, then the cost escalates quite rapidly.

Thawley and Ogura have written one of the rare reviews on the cost of laryngeal surgery.[1] The total costs that they quote for the year 1978 are similar to the ones quoted in this chapter for operative procedures. For current surgical admissions, the semiprivate hospital room represents 25% to 30% of the cost, the surgeon's fee, 15% to 20%, the anesthetist's fee, 15% to 20%, and the use of the operating room and recovery room, 10% to 20%.

The cost of radiation therapy escalated rapidly in the past decade due to the expensive treatment equipment, more frequent use of computerized dosimetry, the use of specialized blocking techniques such as Cerrobend blocks, and the increased use of physicists, dosimetrists, and radiation therapy technologists to assist in the overall management of the patient. While these various factors have improved the sophistication and quality of delivery of radiation therapy, there has not been a corresponding increase in cures per dollar spent. Most insurance carriers reimburse the patient for outpatient radiation therapy.

The cost of multiagent chemotherapy regimens that include cisplatin and bleomycin can be quite expensive, particularly if the patient is hospitalized for part of the treatment or for complications of treatment. Unfortunately, insurance carriers still do not always reimburse for chemotherapy treatments, and the patient is often left to pay this bill out of pocket.

The costs indicated in Tables 36-1 through 36-9 (pp. 648–649) are substantial, and one could rapidly see a total bill on the order of $25,000 to $30,000 if the patient had three cycles of cisplatin and bleomycin, 5 weeks of radiation therapy, and a major operative procedure.

Residency training programs are remiss in not familiarizing young physicians with the costs their patients are incurring. The physician must constantly think in terms of the benefit-to-cost ratio.

The American Cancer Society is frequently instrumental in assisting patients with nonmedical expenses such as room, board, travel, and noncancer drugs. Many patients must leave home, particularly for radiation therapy or chemotherapy, and these added costs of day-to-day living are not paid by insurance. It is in this area that the American Cancer Society (especially in Florida) has been so generous in assisting patients.

REFERENCE

1. Thawley SE, Ogura JH: Health care costs of laryngeal surgery. Laryngoscope 89:595–600, 1979

TABLE 36-1. Radiation Therapy Costs for Carcinoma of the Vocal Cord*

Professional Fee†	$1900
Hospital Fee	1450
Travel	·300
Total	$3650

* Cobalt-60, 28 treatments.
† Includes cost of physics support.

TABLE 36-2. Radiation Therapy Costs for Carcinoma of the Floor of the Mouth*

Professional Fees	
Radiation therapy†	$2557
Radiology	100
Anesthesia	250
Pathology	90
Subtotal	$2997
Hospital Fees	
External-beam irradiation	$1300
Hospitalization/operating room	1700
Subtotal	$3000
Travel	$250
Total	$6247

* Cobalt-60, 22 treatments; radium needle implant—3 days in hospital.
† Includes cost of physics support.

TABLE 36-3. Radiation Therapy Costs for Carcinoma of the Tonsil*

Professional Fee†	$2800
Hospital Fee	2700
Travel	400
Total	$5900

* Cobalt-60, 37 treatments.
† Includes cost of physics support.

TABLE 36-4. Surgical Costs for Direct Laryngoscopy

Professional Fees	
Surgeon	$240
Anesthetist	250
Pathologist	207
Cardiologist	35
Radiologist	14
Subtotal	$746
Hospital Fees	
2-day hospitalization (including 1 hour of operating room time)	$870
Total	$1616

TABLE 36-5. Surgical Costs for Laryngectomy and Radical Neck Dissection

Professional Fees	
Surgeon*	$2330
Anesthetist	2163
Pathologist (laboratory)	375
Radiologist	95
Pathologist (surgical)	60
Subtotal	$5023
Hospital Fees	
7-day admission (including operating room time)	$4939
Total	$9962

* Laryngectomy without radical neck dissection = $1375.

TABLE 36-6. Surgical Costs for Hemimandibulectomy and Radical Neck Dissection

Professional Fees	
Surgeon	$3500
Anesthetist	1200
Pathologist (blood, laboratory, surgical pathology)	665
Radiologist	80
Cardiologist	70
Subtotal	$5515
Hospital Fees	
17-day admission (including operating room time)	$8554
Total	$14,069

TABLE 36-7. Surgical Costs for Superficial Lobe Parotidectomy

Professional Fees	
Surgeon	$920
Anesthetist	603
Pathologist	270
Radiologist	20
Cardiologist	35
Subtotal	$1848
Hospital Fees (6-Day Admission)	
Semiprivate room (6 days)	$738
Electrocardiogram × 2	48
Blood bank	85
Chest roentgenogram	24
Recovery room	140
Operating room	805
Laboratory	82
Surgical pathology	35
Pharmacy	226
Surgery supplies	77
Anesthesia supplies	195
Subtotal	$2455
Total	$4303

TABLE 36-8. Costs for Diagnostic Radiologic Procedures	
CT Scan of Larynx	
Without contrast	$360
With contrast	$465
CT Scan of Paranasal Sinuses	
Without contrast	$360
With contrast	$465
Tomograms of Larynx	$145
Tomograms of Paranasal Sinuses	$145

TABLE 36-9. Chemotherapy Costs	
Single-Agent Chemotherapy (Outpatient Treatment)	
Consultation	$110.00
Methotrexate: 8 doses × 70 mg each	248.00
Office visits × 8	216.00
Chest roentgenograms × 5	160.00
Complete blood cell counts × 12	144.00
SMA15 × 3	
To interpret	38.25
To draw	12.00
Administration of chemotherapy drugs × 8 doses	120.00
Subtotal	$1048.25
Hospitalization for leukopenia (5 days)	$1754.00
Professional fee for hospitalization	245.00
Total	$3047.25
Multiagent Chemotherapy (Outpatient Treatment)	
Cisplatin: 150 mg IV	$506.00
Bleomycin: 15 units × 5 doses	1022.00
Office visits	27.00
Complete blood cell count	12.00
Administration of chemotherapy drugs	23.00
Creatinine clearance	23.00
Total per course	$1613.00
Total for four courses	$6452.00

Index

Index

*Page numbers in **boldface** represent color plates.*